FLUID MECHANICS, FLUID MACHINES AND HYDRAULICS

3rd Edition

(With 500 Solved Problems)

By the same authors
Laboratory Manual of F...
By Dr. V.P. ...

By the same authors

Laboratory Manual of Fluid Mechanics and Machines.
By Dr. V.P. Gupta, Dr. J. Chandra and Dr. K.S. Gupta

FLUID MECHANICS, FLUID MACHINES AND HYDRAULICS

3rd Edition
(With 500 Solved Problems)

Dr. V.P. Gupta
Ex-Professor of Civil Engineering & Dean,
Faculty of Engineering, J.N.V. University, Jodhpur
Principal, JCDM College of Engineering, Sirsa (Haryana)

Professor (Dr.) Alam Singh
Ex-Professor & Head of Civil Engineering Deptt.,
Faculty of Engineering, J.N.V. University, Jodhpur

Manish Gupta
B.Tech., IIT, Kanpur; M.Tech, IIT, Mumbai

Foreword by

Professor (Dr.) Bharat Singh
Professor Emeritus (WRDTC) & Formerly Vice-Chancellor
University of Roorkee, Roorkee

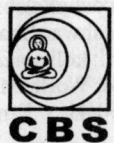

CBS
CBS Publishers & Distributors Pvt. Ltd.
New Delhi • Bengaluru • Chennai • Kochi • Kolkata • Mumbai
Hyderabad • Uttarakhand • Nagpur • Patna • Pune • Jharkhand

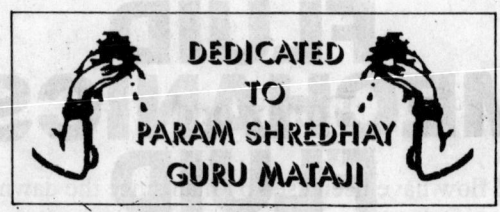

DEDICATED
TO
PARAM SHREDHAY
GURU MATAJI

ISBN: 81-239-0660-9

First Edition: 1987
Second Edition: 1992
Third Edition: 1999
Reprint: 2004, 2007, 2009, 2012, 2014, 2018, 2020

Published by **Satish Kumar Jain** and produced by **Varun Jain** for
CBS Publishers & Distributors Pvt. Ltd.,
4819/XI Prahlad Street, 24 Ansari Road, Daryaganj, New Delhi - 110002
delhi@cbspd.com, cbspubs@airtelmail.in • www.cbspd.com
Ph.: 23289259, 23266861, 23266867 • Fax: 011-23243014

Corporate Office: 204 FIE, Industrial Area, Patparganj, Delhi - 110 092
Ph: 49344934 • Fax: 011-49344935
E-mail: publishing@cbspd.com • publicity@cbspd.com

Branches:
• *Bengaluru:* 2975, 17th Cross, K.R. Road, Bansankari 2nd Stage,
  Bengaluru - 70 • Ph: +91-80-26771678/79 • Fax: +91-80-26771680
  E-mail: cbsbng@gmail.com, bangalore@cbspd.com
• *Chennai:* No. 7, Subbaraya Street, Shenoy Nagar, Chennai - 600030
  Ph: +91-44-26681266, 26680620 • Fax: +91-44-42032115
  E-mail: chennai@cbspd.com
• *Kochi:* Ashana House, 39/1904, A.M. Thomas Road, Valanjambalam,
  Ernakulum, Kochi • Ph: +91-484-4059061-65
  Fax: +91-484-4059065 • E-mail: cochin@cbspd.com
• *Kolkata:* 6-B, Ground Floor, Rameshwar Shaw Road, Kolkata - 700014
  Ph: +91-33-22891126/7/8 • E-mail: kolkata@cbspd.com
• *Mumbai:* 83-C, Dr. E. Moses Road, Worli, Mumbai - 400018
  Ph: +91-9833017933, 022-24902340/41 • E-mail: mumbai@cbspd.com

Representatives:

• Hyderabad: 0-9885175004   • Nagpur: 0-9021734563
• Patna: 0-9334159340   • Pune: 0-9623451994
• Jharkhand: 0-9811541605   • Uttarakhand: 0-9716462459

Printed at: J.S. Offset Printers, Delhi (India)

Foreword

Principles of fluid flow have been used by man since the dawn of civilization. Ancient Sumerian and Egyptian irrigation systems as well as urban drainage systems of Indus Valley sites have indicated at least qualitative knowledge of principles of flow of water. Greeks and Romans discovered certain qualitative laws as well. Hydraulics, however, remained primarily empirical till the brilliant boundary layer concept of Von Karaman and Prandtl enabled application of mathematical theory to real fluid problems. Even so fluid mechanics involves many complex problems, not all of which are amenable to purely theoretical treatment. This is particularly true for energy losses, and boundary layer separation phenomenon, where assistance from precise measurements has to be taken. Still, the phenomenal advances in this science enable design of very major hydraulic structures with reliable prediction of their behaviour in the field of civil engineering and other fields of contrivances like huge aeroplanes, water turbines and pumps.

Good textbooks are essential for good teaching. It is important that textbooks on basic engineering subjects should stress and explain fundamental principles and physical behaviour before going on to problem solving techniques.

Foreign textbooks are too expensive for Indian students and we have to aim at self-reliance in this area also. The textbooks prepared by veteran Prof. Alam Singh and his colleague Dr. V.P. Gupta meet this criterion quite well. This book gives a comprehensive coverage and explanation of the subject. I am sure it will be found very useful by the students of engineering.

Roorkee
July, 1987

Bharat Singh
Professor Emeritus (WRDTC)
Ex-Vice Chancellor,
University of Roorkee,
Roorkee

Preface to the Third Edition

The second edition of the book has received very encouraging response from the users and the present edition has been thoroughly reviewed to identify the areas requiring modifications or additions to enhance the usefulness of the book.

The significant additions in the present edition are : chapter 1 and chapter 2 have been rewritten, chapter 10–articles on surges and waves have been revised; more number of solved examinations have been included from various competitive examination papers of UPSC, ICS and Institution of Engineers (India)

The full text of the book has been set on computer and is in laser print. The figures have been redrawn on AutoCad. Objective type of questions and problems are provided at the end of each chapter to consolidate the understanding of the subject matter.

The subject matter has been dealt with the help of about 500 solved examples, 555 figures, 274 objective type of questions and 317 problems.

The present revised edition of the book will be useful to under groundnut and post graduate students of Civil, Mechanical, Electrical and Mining engineering who may be pursuing the course of Fluid Mechanics and Fluid Machines. The subject matter has been so embodied it will be quite useful to the graduate engineers appearing in various competitive examination, i.e. UPSC, ICS and PSC's.

Comments for further improvement of the book would be highly appreciated.

The authors would like to express their sincere thanks to Mr Mool Singh and his team for the preparation of computer print, to M/s CBS Publishers for publication of the text and to my wife Rama and sons Ashish and Manish for their active co-operation.

V.P. Gupta
Alam Singh

Jan. 1, 1999

Preface to the Second Edition

The popularity of the first edition of the book amongst the students and teachers of various universities prompted the authors to bring out the second edition. The main objectives of the second edition are more or less the same as those of first one's. The book has been considerably enlarged and revised. Following six new chapters have been added in the book.

14. Dynamic action of fluids

15. Fluid machines —— Turbines

16. Pumps —— Reciprocating pumps.

17. Centrifugal pumps.

18. Miscellaneous machines

19. Compressible flows.

In addition to these chapters, number of numerical examples with complete solutions have been added. The text ends with two appendices, one giving derivation of N.S. equations and the other giving ready conversion of units.

The authors are highly thankful to Professor Emeritus (Dr.) Bharat Singh, former Vice Chancellor, University of Roorkee, Roorkee, who had written the foreword. The authors also acknowledge with thanks the suggestions given by several teachers and also the students for upgrading the book. The authors also record appreciation for M/s CBS Publishers and Distributors, New Delhi, for bringing out this edition.

(*Note* : The first edition of the book was under the title "Mechanics and Engineering of Fluids").

Jodhpur

V.P. Gupta

Alam Singh

Preface to the First Edition

This is a clear comprehensive text covering all the major aspects of fluid mechanics as required for different branches of engineering, in particular for Civil and Mechanical engineering. With even emphasis on the physical basis of phenomena and the engineering practice, the principles of fluid mechanics are set out clearly and simply and the applications are illustrated by examples. The book is designed to suit students appearting for degree and diploma examinations and for professional and competitive examinations like those of AMIE, USPS(Engg.) and ICS. For this purpose, a large number of worked out examples, objective questions and unsolved problems with answers are included. Practicing engineers would find it a useful lead-in to more specialised literature. The book may also be helpful to the post- graduate students of the first course in fluid mechanics to refresh their knowledge.

The first chapter of the book deals with the physical properties of fluid and a brief exposure is given to the system of units. Chapters 2 to 5 discuss the basic principles of the fluid flow and related equations, etc. Chapter 6 on the dimensional analysis and similitude will help in analyzing the various problems and in planning requisite model testing. Chapter 7 & 8 deal with the viscous flow, whereas Chapters 9 deals with turbulent flow in pipes. The pipe network analysis is discussed in Chapter 10. Thus these four chapters represent what is known as the internal flow, whereas the external flow or flow around immersed bodies has been dealt with in Chapter 11. Chapter 12 describes the open channel flow from its basic channel characteristics to greater details of rapidly varied flow or hydraulic jump. Chapter 12 on open channel flow is written in such a manner that it can be understood independently without going into rigorous treatments of chapters 2 to 5. Chapter 13 on fluid flow measurement describes at one place various flow measuring devices with their principles of working, e.g. orifices, mouthpieces, weirs and notches, as well as modern sophisticated instruments like hot wire anemometer and transducers, etc.

In the preparation of this book, the authors had to make use of the publications of various other engineers, researchers, organisations and institutions. Care has been taken to give credit to the original workers and any omission is purely out of inadvertance. The authors record appreciation for the useful discussions they had with their colleague Professor J. Chandra and for the assistance rendered by their colleague Shri Deepak Sancheti, Assistance Professor, in solving the problems included in the book. The authors feel highly indebted to Professor Emeritus (Dr.) Bharat Singh, WRDTC & formerly Vice-Chancellor, University of Roorkee, Roorkee, who could find time to scan the book before its release and so pleasingly write the Foreword. The authors would always welcome comments and suggestions from the readers.

Illustrations 298, Examples 166, Objective questions 171 Problems 158.

Jodhpur.

Alam Singh , V.P. Gupta

Notations

$a =$ acceleration

$A, A_1, A_2 =$ area of cross section

$B =$ bottom width

$B =$ Breadth of wheel at inlet

$c =$ celerity

$C =$ Chezy's roughness coefficient

$C_c =$ coefficient of contraction

$c_f =$ coefficient of local skin friction

$C_d =$ coefficient of discharge

$C_D =$ coefficient of drag

$C_L =$ coefficient of lift

$c_p =$ specific heat at constant pressure

$c_v =$ coefficient of velocity

$c_v =$ specific heat at constat volume

$C_f =$ average drag coefficient

$C =$ a constant

$d =$ diameter of opening depth of flow

$d =$ diameter of nozzle

$D =$ diameter of pipe

$D =$ diameter of pitch circle

$= $ dia of wheel at inlet

$E =$ specific energy

$E, e =$ Specific energy, energy per unit weight

$E_L =$ energy loss

$E_v =$ modulus of elasticity

$f =$ acceleration of plunger

$= $ frequency of power supply

$f =$ Darcy's friction coefficient

$f_t =$ hoop stress

$F =$ force

$F_x =$ component of force in X- direction

$F_y =$ component of force in Y- direction

$g =$ acceleration due to gravity

$G =$ mass flow rate of compressible fluid

$G =$ shear modulus of elasticity

$h, H =$ head

$h_L =$ head loss due to blade friction

$h_s/h_d =$ static head suction/delivery

$h_{Lc} =$ head loss in the cassing

$h_{Lr} =$ head loss in the runner

$h_{Li} =$ head loss in the impeller

$H =$ enthalpy

$= $ net head

$H_d =$ delivery head

$H_m =$ manomatric head

$H_r =$ Total head across runner

$H_a =$ acceleration head/atmospheric pressure head

$H_s =$ datum head at entrance

$= $ suction head

$H_{sv} =$ total pressure head above vapour pressure

$H_{TH} =$ theoritical or ideal head

$H_v =$ Vapour pressure head

$H_l =$ gross head

$i =$ gradient of energy line

$I =$ internal energy

$J =$ joule, unit of energy

$k =$ Karman's universal constant

$k =$ coefficient of bladde friction

$k_u =$ speed ratio

$k_v =$ coefficient of velocity

$K =$ modulus of elasicity

$K =$ radius of gyration

$K_P/K_Q/K_H =$ power/discharge/head coefficient

$l =$ mixing length

$l_1 =$ length of connecting rod

$L =$ length of stroke

$l_c =$ equivalent length

$m =$ jet ratio

$M =$ total mass

$n =$ an index

$n =$ breadth ratio

$n_s =$ a dimensionless parameter, a type number

$N =$ Manning's rugosity coefficient

$N =$ speed of runner, r.p.m.

$N_c =$ Cauchy's number

$N_F =$ Froude's number

$N_M =$ Mach's number

$N_W =$ Weber's number

$p =$ pressure intensity

$P =$ total pressure

$P =$ Power

$P_i/P_c/P_M =$ power lost, impeller/casing/mechanical friction

$q =$ discharge/unit width

Q = discharge

$Q_r/Q_v/Q_i$ = volumetric flow rate through runner/leakage/impeller

r = radius of crank

R = gas constant

= hydraulic radius

= radius of a circle

R = radius of pitch circle

R_e = Reynolds number

s = slope

S = slip/suction specific speed

S = Strouhal number

t = thickness of wave

t = wall thickness

T = time interval

= top width of channel

T = torque

u or u_x = component of velocity in X–direction

u = speed of wheel at inlet

U_l = absolute vel. at outlet

U = absolube vel. at inlet

U = Velocity

U = mean velocity

U_f = velocity of flow at inlet

U_0 = free stream velocity

$V\theta$ = component of tangential velocity

U_r = component of radial velocity

U_r = relative velocity at inlet

U_w = whirl velocity at inlet

U_0 = shear or frictional velocity

v = specific volume

= component of velocity in Y-direction

V = volume

w = component of velocity in Z-direction

W = weight

x, y, z = Co-ordinates in three co-ordinate directions

z = datum head

z = number of venas

Z = section factor

ρ = specific mass or mass denisty

α = energy correction factor

α = guide blade angle in inlet

β = angle between absolute velocity and rim velocity at outlet

β = vorticity

$\xi\,\eta\,,\gamma$ = components of vorticity in the three co-ordinate directons

θ = angle

θ = inlet vane angle

ε = eddy kinematic viscosity

η_M = mechanical efficiency

η_V = volumetric efficiency

η_{man}/η_H = manometric/hydraulic efficiency

η_0 = overall efficiency

η = eddy dynamic viscosity

μ = dynamic viscosity

ν = kinematic viscosity

σ = coefficient of surface tension

ω = rotation of fluid element

Γ = circulation

τ = shear stress

Φ = potential funciton

φ = qutlet vane angle

= speed ration

ψ = flow ratio

Ψ = stream function

χ = stability parameter

δ = boundary layer thickness

δ' = thickness of laminar sublayer

δ_* = displacement thickness of boundary layer

$\theta/$ = momentoum thickness of boundary layer

δ_2 = energy thickness of boundary layer

Suffix '1' refers to outlet quantities

Suffix 'u' refers to unit quantities

Suffix 's' refers to specific quantities

CONTENTS

1

Introduction and Fluid Properties

1.1 INTRODUCTION

Fluid mechanics is that division of engineering science which is concerned with the behaviour of fluid at rest as well as in motion. Basic principles and concepts of fluid mechanics lie at the core of many engineering analysis, design and synthesis of those problems which involve the fluid as a medium. Flow of blood in arteries and breathing (through nasal system) are simple examples of fluid flow through conduits. In addition to the physical properties of fluid, the modern fluid mechanics makes use of the principles of conservation of mass, conservation of energy (i.e. first law of thermodynamics) and the conservation of momentum. Fluid mechanics has been developed from two branches of science, viz. empincal hydraulics and mathematical hydrodynamics. The laws governing the behaviour and motion of a fictitious fluid particle having neither viscosity nor compressibility are dealt within mathematical hydrodyanamics.

Fluid mechanics can be broadly classified as Fluid statics, Fluid kinematics and Fluid dynamics.

Fluid statics : it is mainly concerned with the forces exerted by fluids at rest.

Fluid kinematics : It deals with the motion of ideal and real fluid, e.g. acceleration and velocities, etc.

Fluid dyanmics : It deals mainly with the forces causing the motion of ideal and real fluid. It also deals with the accompanying energy changes being taking place during the motion.

1.2. DEFINITIONS AND FLUID PROPERTIES

All matter can be classified either as solid or fluid. Fluid state is commonly divided into liquid state and gaseous state. These three states of matter differ from each other in the spacing and latitude of motion of their molecules ; these variables (spacing and motion) being large in a gas, smaller in liquid and extremely small in a solid. Thus it follows that inter-molecular cohesive forces are large in a solid, small in a liquid and too small in a gas. A further difference between solid and fluid is that the latter has eiher no tensile strength or very little of it and only when it is kept in a container it can support compressive forces. When a fluid is subjected to a shear stress it is deformed continuosuly as long as this force is applied. This, however, does not mean that there is no shearing stress. It depndes on the magnitude of the rate

1

of deformation of the fluid element. A fluid at rest has no shearing stress. A solid can resist the tensile stress, compressive stress and even to a certain limit the shear stress also.

The two states of fluid, viz. liquid and gas, exhibit quite different characteristics. (i) Under ordinary condition liquids can be compressed slightly only when extremely high pressures are applied, and hence for all practical considerations, they are taken as incompressible fluid. Gases, on the other hand, are readily compressible whenever external pressures are exerted. (ii) Liquids have free surfaces whereas gases do not have it.

A vapour is in gaseous state whose temperature and pressure are such that it is very near the liquid phase, e.g. the steam is considered a vapour because its characteristics (state of existing) are not far from those of water.

Ideal fluid. An ideal fluid may be defind as the one which is now viscuous and incompressible. It is a fictitious fluid which is the creation of mathematician to simplify the analytical treatment of fluid flow. Such a fluid does not exist in reality. Sometimes water and air are taken as ideal fluids as they approximately exhibit the characteristics of ideal liquid and ideal gas respectively.

Real fluid. All the existing fluids have got viscosity to some extent and can be compressed slightly. Hence all the existing fluids are real fluids. In a real fluid, shearing forces always develop whenever the motion of one particle takes place past another particle (or layer).

1.3 UNIT OF MEASUREMENT

Units may be defined as those standards in terms of which physical quantities are measured. The fundamental units are mass M, length L, time T and force, F; out of which only three principal units are sufficient to describe any fiuid motion completely (M and F are connected by Newton's second law of motion). The system of units used in mechanics are based upon Newton's second law of motions which states that "the summation of all forces F acting on any body of mass M is directly proportional to the product of mass M and its acceleration 'a'.

$$F \alpha M . a \qquad ....(1.1a)$$
$$F = k . M . a \qquad ...(1.1b)$$

where k is the constant of proportionality. If the units of F, M and 'a' are so chosen that one unit of force produces a unit acceleration in one unit of mass, then k is unity. Hence

$$F = M . a \qquad ...(1.1c)$$

There are two widely used systems of measurement, namely Foot Pound Second (FPS) system used by American and British scientists and engineers and Centimetre, Gram Second (CGS) system used by continental scientists and engineers. There is another similar system of units known as MKS system in which unit of mass, length and time are kilorgram. metre and second respectively. In CGS system, corresponding units are gram centimetre and second and in FPS system these are measureed in pound, foot and second.

Geometrical properties of some plane surfaces

Shape	Area A	Vertical distance of centroid G from top of the figure $\bar{h}$	Moment of inertia about an axis passing through centroid G I_{GG}
Rectangle width b and depth d	bd	$d/2$ from top edge	$bd^3/12$
Tringle base width b and altitude h	$bh/2$	$2h/3$ from top vertex	$bd^3/36$ $[I_{\infty} = bh^3/12]$
Circel diameter d	$\pi d^2/4$	$d/2$ from top of the figure	$\pi d^4/64$
Semi circle diameter d parallel to water surface	$\pi d^2/8$	$2d/3\pi$ from the horizontal diameter	$11d^4/1600$
Quarter of a circle diameter	$\pi d^2/16$	$2d/3\pi$ from horizontal radius (parallel to water surface)	$0.0044\,d^4$
Ellipse horizontal major axis width b and vertical minor axis of height h	$\pi bh/4$	$h/2$ from top edge of plane figure	$\pi bh^3/64$
Parabola horizontal base width b and height of vertex above base h	$2bh/3$	$3h/5$ from the vertex	$8bh^3/175$

(5) They should be written without final full stop.

(6) When combined unit is formed by multiplication of two or more units, some space must be left between the units. e.g. Nm.

(7) When combined unit is formed by dividing one unit by another, this should be written as m/s or ms^{-1}.

(8) Quantities which are multiples of basic unit are formed by means of prefixes, e.g. 20 G means 20×10^9 and is read as twenty giga. Similarly, 20 M means 20×10^6 and is read as twenty mega.

1.4 PHYSICAL PROPERTIES

Some of the physical properties of fluids are (i) specific mass (ii) specifice weight (iii) viscosity (iv) compressibility and (v) surface tension, which are discussed below.

1. Specific mass

All fluids possess mass. Mass is a quantitative measure of the amount of matter in a given body and is computed by dividing specific weight by acceleration due to gravity 'g'. The basic property of the fluid mass is its inertia or its resistance to change in motion. The amount of fluid mass contained in a unit volume is defined as specific mass or mass density ρ. The unit of mass density in metric absolute system is kilogram mass per cubic metre, kg (m)/m^3 and in gravitatinal system is metric slug per cubic metre

TABLE 1.3 DERIVED UNITS OF PHYSICAL QUANTITIES

	Quantity	Symbol	Unit
1	Velocity, linear angular	metre/second radian/second	m/s rad/s
2	Acceleration, linear angular	metre/per second per second radian per second per second	m/s^2 rad/s^2
3	Force	newton	N
4	Density, mass, weight	kilogram per cubic metre Newton per culic metre	kg/m^3 N/m^3
5	Momentum, linear, angular	kilogram metre per second kilogram radian per second	kg m/s kg rad/s
6	Viscosity, dynamic, kinematic	newton second/(metre)^2 (metre)^2/second	Ns/m^2 m^2/s
7	Surface tension	newton per metre	N/m
8	Energy or work	joule	J$(=$Nm$)$
9	Power	watt	$(=$Js$^{-1})$
10	Moment of inertia	kilogram per metre squared	kg/m^2
11	Pressure intensity or stress	pascal$(=$netwon per metre$^2)$	Pa $(=$N/m$^2)$
12	Temperature interval	degree Celsius	°C

m slug/m^3. In SI system, the unit of mass remains same as in metric absolute system, i.e. kg/m^3. The mass density of water at 4°C at mean sea level is 1000 kg/m^3 (SI system) or 102 m slug/m^3 (MKS system). The mass density of fluid increases with increase in pressure and decreases with increase in temperature.

2. Specific Weight

Weight is defined as the graviational pull acting on a freely falling body and varies with its position on the earth surface, i.e. with its elevation above mean sea level and with latitude.

Specific weight is the weight of the fluid contained in unit volume and may be represented by the symbol 'w'.

$$w = \rho g \qquad ...(1.8)$$

The specifie weight of water at 4°C at mean sea level and at atmospheric pressure of 760 mm of mercury is 1000 kg (f)/m^3 (it is kilogram force/m^3) in MKS gravitational system and 9810 N/m^3 in SI system.

3. Specific volume

It is the volume 'v' occupied by either a unit weight or unit mass of fluid. It is commonly applied to gases and is usually expressed in cubic metre per newton or cubic metre per kilogram (unit of mass).

Since the two definitions will result in different numerical values, care should be taken in which sense the term is being used. In this text the latter definition is used.

4. Specific gravity

The specific gravity of a liquid is the ratio of the density of liquid to that of pure water at 4°C and at a presure of 760 mm of mercuty at mean sea level. The specific gravity of water at 4° is 1.0 and that of mercury varies from 13.5 to 13.6. Knowing specific gravity of liquid, specific weight can be calculated as

sp. weight = sp, gravity liquid× sp. wt of water   ...(1.9)

The specific gravity of a gas is the ratio of its density to that of either hydrogen or air free of carbon dioxide at some specified temperature and pressure.

5. Viscosity

Viscosity of a fluid is the property of fluid by virtue of which it offers resistance to shear or angular deformation. Viscosity is fundamentally due to cohesion and molecular momentum exchange between fluid layers. As flow occurs, these effects appear as tangential or shearing stress between moving layers.

Consider two parallel plates sufficiently large so that edge conditions may be neglected, which are placed at a distance Y apart and the space between them is filled with a fluid. The lower surface is assumed to be stationary while upper one is moving parallel to it with a velocity U by the application of a force F acting on the upper plate of surface area A. The fluid in immediate contact with the solid boundary has the same velcity as boundany, i.e., there is no slip at the boundary. The fluid in the area a b c d (Fig 1.1) flows to the new position a b'c'd with each particle moving parallel to the boundary. The velocity u varying from zero at the stationary plate to U at the upper plate,

It is evident that a shearing or frictional resistance exists between adjacent layers. Experiments show that other quantities being held constant, F is directly proportional to A and to U and inversely proportional to Y.

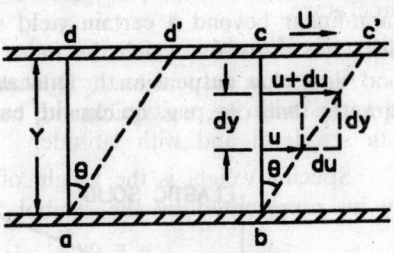

FIG. 1.1 DEFORMATION OF A FLUID ELEMENT

$$F \alpha AU/Y$$
$$F = \mu A U/Y \qquad ...(1.10a)$$

If shear stress τ (tau) is written as the ratio of force F and area of contact A, i.e. $\tau = F/A$,

Then $\qquad \tau = \mu U/Y \qquad ...(1.10b)$

The ration of U/Y is angular velocity of line 'ad'. It is also the time rate of angular deformation of the fluid. The rate of decrease of angle dad'(in contrast to solid where shear stress is proportional to magnitude of deformation) may also be written as du/dy.

Therefore

$$\tau = \mu \frac{\partial u}{\partial y} \qquad ...(1.10c)$$

The constant of proportionality μ is called the coefficient of viscosity', 'absolute viscosity', 'dynamic viscosity' or simply 'the viscosity'. Eq. 1.10 c is Newton's law of viscosity and it states that for a given rate of angular deformation of fluid the shear stress is directly proportional to its viscosity.

Fluids may be classified as Newtonian fluids or Non-Newtonian fluids. In a Newtonian fluid, there is linear variation betwen aplied shear stress τ and the resulting rate of deformation du/dy, μ is contant in Eq.1.10c. Water, air and light oils are some of the exapmples of Newtonian fluids. In a Non-Newtonian fluid, there is a nonlinear relation between the magnitude of shear stress applied and the resultant angular deformation, which is represented as

$$\tau = A (du/dy)^n + B \qquad ...(1.11)$$

where A and B are constants which depends upon the type of fluid and conditions imposed on the flow. Some examples of Non- Newtonian fluids are plastics, suspensions, paints and blood.

The ideal fluid with no viscosity is represented on the horizontal axis while the true elastic solid is represented by the vertical axis (Fig. 1.2). A true or 'Bingham plastic fluid' is the one which sustains certain amount of stress before suffering deformation. A plastic fluid can be shown by a straight line intersecting the vertical axis at the yield stress, e.g. sewage sludge and drilling mud. 'Thixotropic fluid' is that in which the angular deformation is non-linear beyond a certain yield stress, e.g.printer's ink. 'Pseudo plastic fluids', are those for which the index of Eq. 1.11 is less than one, e.g. milk, blood and clay suspension. 'Dilatant fluid' is that for which the index n is greater than one, e.g. quicksand, butter and concentrated solution of sugar.

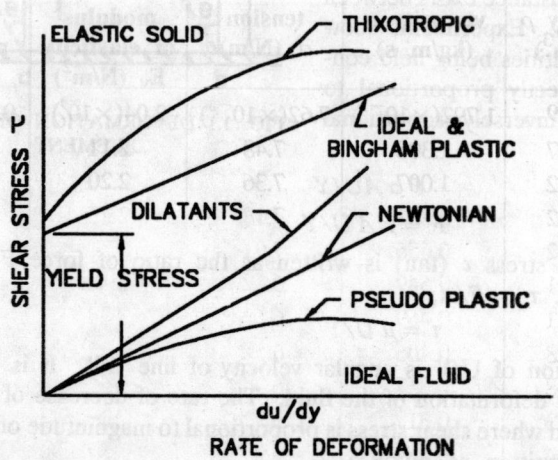

FIG. 1.2. NEWTONION AND NON-ENWTONION FLUID

(a) *Variation of viscosity with temperature and pressure.* The resistance of a fluid to shear stress depends upon its cohesion (force of attraction among its molecules) and upon its rate of transfer of molecular momentum. A liquid (in which molecules are much more closely spaced than a gas) has cohesive forces much larger than a gas and cohesion seems to be the predominant cause of viscosity in the liquid. Since the cohesion decreases with temperature, the viscosity of liquid decreases with the inccrease in temperature.

On the other hand, a gas has very small cohesive force and most of its resistance is the result of the transfer of molecular momentum when one layer moves relative to an adjacent layer. The molecular transfer of momentum sets up an apparent shear stress in the fluid which resists the relative motion. With increase in temperaturae, this inter-molecular activity increases,Hence the viscosity of gas increases with increase in temperature. The variation of some properties of water and air with temperaturte are given in Tables 1.4 and 1.5.

The absolute viscosity of fluid is practically independent of pressure for the range whoich is ordinarily encountered in enginering work. But for extremely high pressures the value of viscosity is some what higher.

Helmholtz (1821-1894) using Poisseuille's experiments found that absolute viscxosity of water and air can be given by the following equations

Air : $\mu_t = \mu_0 [1 + 0.0029\,T + 7 \times 10^{-6}\,T^2]$ poise ...(1.12b)

Water : $\mu_t = \mu_0 \dfrac{1}{1 + 0.03368\,T + 0.000221\,T^2}$ poise ...(1.12a)

where μ_t and μ_0 are the absolute viscisities in pose and T is the temperature in degree Celsius.

TABLE 1.4 VARIATION OF PROPERTIES OF WATER WITH TEMPERATURE

Tempe-rature T°C	Mass Density ρ (kg/m^3)	Dynamic viscosity μ (kg/m s)	Surface tension σ (N/m)	Bulk modulus of elasticity E_V (N/m^2)	Vapour pressure p_V (N/m^2)
0	999.9	1.792($\times 10^{-3}$)	7.62($\times 10^{-3}$)	2.04($\times 10^9$)	0.588($\times 10^3$)
10	999.7	1.308	7.48	2.11	1.117
20	998.2	1.007	7.36	2.20	2.462
30	995.2	0.801	7.18	2.23	4.316
40	995.2	0.656	7.01	2.27	7.455
50	988.1	0.549	6.82	2.30	12.36
60	983.1	0.469	6.68	2.28	19.914
70	977.8	0.406	6.50	2.25	31.392
80	971.8	0.357	6.30	2.21	70.43
90	965.3	0.317	6.12	2.16	70.436
100	958.4	0.284	5.94	2.07	101.337

(a) *Viscosity-dimensions and units.* The dimensions of absolute viscosity are derived from Eq.1.10c.

$$[\mu] = \frac{[\tau]}{[du/dy]} = \frac{[F/A]}{\left[\dfrac{L}{T} \cdot \dfrac{1}{L}\right]}$$

TABLE 1.5 VARIATION OF SOME PRPOERTIES OF AIR WITH TEMPERATURE AT ATMOSPHERIC PRESSURE

Temperature T°C	Mass density ρ (kg/m^3)	Dynamic viscosity μ (kg/ms)	Kinematic viscosity ν (m^2/s)
−40	1.52	14.94($\times 10^{-6}$)	9.83($\times 10^{-6}$)
−20	1.40	15.92	11.37
0	1.29	17.05	13.22
20	1.20	17.05	15.13
40	1.12	18.15	17.01
60	1.06	19.05	18.70
80	0.99	20.65	20.86
100	0.94	21.85	23.24
120	0.90	23.20	25.78

$$[\mu] = \left[\frac{FT}{A}\right]$$

$$[\mu] = \left[\frac{FT}{L^2}\right] \quad \text{in terms of 'FLT system'} \qquad ...(1.13)$$

The forcxe dimension may be expressed in terms of mass using Newton's second law of motion. Hence,

$$[\mu] = \left[\frac{ML}{T^2} \cdot \frac{T}{L^2}\right]$$

$$[\mu] = \left[\frac{M}{LT}\right] \quad \text{in terms of 'MLT system'} \qquad ...(1.14)$$

The CGS absolute unit of viscosity is gm/cm-sec but the more commonly used unit is poise in CGS gravitational system which is defined as

$$1 \text{ poise } = 1 \text{ dyne sec/cm}^2 \qquad ...(1.15)$$

Similarly, commonly used unit in MKS gravitational unit is kg(f) sec/m² and in SI system Ns/m²

Now, $\qquad 1\,kg\,(f) = 981 \times 10^3$ dyne

and $\qquad 1\,N = 1\,kg \times \dfrac{m}{s^2} = \dfrac{(1000\,\text{grm})\,(100\,\text{cm})}{\text{second}^2} = \dfrac{10^5\,\text{gm} \times \text{cm}}{\text{second}^2}$

$$= 10^{-5} \text{ dyne}$$

Therefore, 1 poise $= \dfrac{1}{981 \times 10^3}$ kg (f) $\times$ sec $\times \dfrac{1}{10^{-4}\,m^2}$

$$1 \text{ poise } = \dfrac{1}{98.1} \dfrac{\text{kg (f)} \times \text{sec}}{m^2} \qquad ...(1.16)$$

Similarly, 1 pois $= \dfrac{[10^{-5}\,N]\,[sec]}{[10^{-4}\,m^2]}$

$$1 \text{ poise } = 10^{-1} \dfrac{\text{NS}}{m^2} \qquad ...(1.17)$$

Most of the fluids have low viscosity, hence, a smaller unit centipoise (= 1/100 poise) is frequently used. It has a further advantage that the viscosity of water at 20° C is 1 centipoise. The value of viscosity of any fluid is an indication 'how thick a fluid is relative to water'. It is numerically equal to specific viscosity (a dimensionless ratio) of fluid relative to that of water at 20° C. Thus if viscosity of a fluid is 50 centipoise, it will be 50 times more viscous than water.

Kinematic viscosity

In many problems involving viscosity, frequently ratio of viscosity and mass density appears (μ/ρ). This is defined as kinematic viscosity ν(nue) because only dimensions of length and time are involved as in kinematics. The dimensions of ν(nue) may be dtermined as follows

$$[\nu] = [\mu/\rho]$$

$$[v] = \left[\frac{FT}{L^2} \cdot \frac{L^3}{M} \right]$$

But from Newton's law $[M] = [FT^2/L]$

$$[v] = \left[\frac{FT}{L^2} \cdot L^3 \cdot \frac{L}{FT^2} \right]$$

$$[v] = [L^2/T] \qquad \qquad ...(1.18)$$

The unit of kinematic viscosity in MKS system and SI system of units is "m^2/s". But the more commonly used unit is stokes ($=1\ cm^2/s$) named after GG Stokes. The centistokes($= 1/100$ stokes) is often a more convenient unit to be used in problems.

6. Compressibility

Fluids can be compressed by the application of pressure from outside and will expand on removal of this pressure. This property of fluid is known as compressibility of fluid. The compressibility of a fluid is inversely proportional to its volume modulus of elasticity. It is defined as

$$\beta = 1/E_v \qquad \qquad ...(1.19)$$

and

$$E_v = - dp / \frac{dv}{v} \qquad \qquad ...(1.20)$$

in which dv is the change in specific volume v of fluid produced due to application of pressure change dp. The negative sign indicates that with increase in pressure the volume of fluid decreases.

From Eq. 1.20, it is seen that the bulk modulus of elasticity is the ratio of pressure increase and volumetric strain and hence E_v can be expressed in the units of pressure, i.e. kg (f)/m^2 or N/m^2.

(a)*effect of change of pressure and temperature.*

Bulk modulus of elasticity of fluid is not constant but increases with increase in pressure. This happens because the resistance of fluid increases with pressure increase. Typical values of the bulk modulus of elasticity of some common fluids are given in Table 1.6

The mass density is the ratio of mass of fluid m and its specific volume v, therefore

$$\rho = m/v \qquad \qquad ...(1.21)$$

Since the mass in a given volume remains constant, therefore, differentiating Eq. 1.21,

$$d\rho = - \frac{m}{v^2} \cdot dv$$

$$\frac{dv}{v} = - \frac{v\, d\rho}{m} = - \frac{d\rho}{\rho}$$

From Eq. 1.20 $E_v = - dp / \frac{dv}{v}$

$$E_v = \frac{\rho\, dp}{d\rho} \qquad \qquad ...(1.22)$$

TABLE 1.6
PROPERTIES OF COMMON LIQUIDS AT 20° C

Liquid	Mass density kg/m^3	Dynamic viscosity kg/ms	Surface tension N/m	Bulk modulus N/m^2	Vapour pressure N/m^2
Water	998	$1.00(\times 10^{-3})$	$72.7(\times 10^{-3})$	$2.05(\times 10^9)$	384.0
Ethyl alcohol	789	1.197	1.32	1.32	5786.0
Benzene	879	0.647	1.10	1.10	10000.0
Carbon tetra-chloride	1632	0.972	1.12	1.12	12750.0
Mercury	13.546	1.152	26.2	26.2	0.1726
Glycerine	1262	620	1.62	1.62	0.01373
Kerosene	800	2.0	–	–	–

(b) *Incompressible fluid*. It is seen from above Eq. 1.22 that the change in mass density due to pressure is very small in liquids and therefore, the liquids are ordinarily considered incompressible. For example, water is generally considered as incompressible fluid. But in the problems involving large change in pressure, (e.g. water hammer) the effect of compressibility is to be considered. To gain some idea of incompressibility of water, consider the application of 1 kN/cm^2 pressure intensity to a cubic metre of water ($E_v = 2.1 \times 10^9$ N/m^2). Substituting in Eq.1.20 and 1.21,

$$\frac{d\rho}{\rho} = -\frac{dv}{v}$$

$$= \frac{dp}{E_v} = \left(\frac{1000\,\text{N} \times 10^4\,m^2}{2.1 \times 10^9\,\text{N/m}^2} \right) = \frac{1}{210}$$

Hence the application of 1 kN/cm^2 pressure to water under ordinary conditions causes its volume to decrease by only 1 part in 210.

(c) *Compressible fluid*. (i) For isothermal process the relationship between pressure p and specific volume v is given by

$$pv = C, \text{ (constant)}$$

$$p = C\rho$$

Differentiating this equation,

$$dp = C\,d\rho$$

This means, $dp/d\rho = C = p/\rho$

Substituting the value of $dp/d\rho$ in Eq. 1.22,

$$E_v = -\rho\frac{dp}{d\rho} = -\rho\frac{p}{\rho}$$

$$E_v = -p \qquad\qquad ...(1.23)$$

(ii) For isentropic process the relationship between pressure and specific volume is

$$p/\rho^k = C$$
$$p = C\rho^k$$

Differentiating both sides

$$dp = C \times k\rho^{k-1} d\rho$$

Therefore

$$\frac{dp}{d\rho} = Ck\rho^{k-1}$$

$$= \frac{p}{\rho^k} \times k\rho^{k-1} = kp/\rho$$

Substituting value of $dp/d\rho$ in Eq. 1.22

$$E_v = -\rho\, dp/d\rho$$
$$E_v = -\rho \times k\rho/\rho$$
$$E_v = -kp \qquad \qquad ...(1.24)$$

Pressure disturbances can not be transmitted instantaneously between two points in a fluid unless the fluid is inelastic ($E_v = \infty$) The small pressure disturbance travels through the fluid medium with celerity (velocity) c. It is given by Eq.1.25a

$$c = \sqrt{\frac{dp}{d\rho}} \qquad \qquad ...(1.25a)$$

Substituting the value of $dp/d\rho$ from Eq 1.22.

$$c = \sqrt{\frac{E_v}{\rho}} \qquad \qquad ...(1.25b)$$

where c is frequently termed as 'sonic or accoustic velocity.'

For incompressible fluid, there is no change in the volume, hence $Ev = \infty$. For a perfect gas, it has been found from experiments that there is virtually not much heat loss while the sound moves through a medium and the process is isentropic. Therefore, from Eq 1.24 and Eq.1.25 b

$$c = \sqrt{kp/\rho} \qquad \qquad ...(1.25c)$$

For a perfect gas the well known gas equation is

$$pv = RT$$
$$p/\rho = R.T \qquad \qquad ...(1.26)$$

Hence from Eq. 1.25c and Eq. 1.26

$$c = \sqrt{kRT} \qquad \qquad ...(1.25d)$$

To study the effects of compressibility, a dimensionless number, known as Mach number is used in fluid flow problems. It is the ratio of the velocity of fluid v (or the relative velocity of the body with respect to fluid) to the velocity of sound c, i.e.,

$$N_m = U/c$$

If N_m less than 1, the flow is considered as subosonic flow

N_m equal to 1, the flow is considered as sonic flow

N_m much greater than 1, the flow is considered as super sonic flow

N_m greater than 1, the flow is considered as hyper sonic flow

In general, the flow occurs at $N_m \leq 0.2$ which corresponds to a velocity of flow nearly 70 m/s and for such flows the effects of compressibility can be neglected. But for flow having large Mach number which will involve large velocity of flow and hence large change in pressure, the effect of compressibility should be considered. For example, in the problems of water hammer occurring in the power penstock or the aeroplanes moving at supersonic speed the fluid compressibility is an important parameter affecting the flow.

The bulk modulus of elasticity of liquids decreases with temperature. But in case of gases the pressure and temperature are inter-connecated and hence the bulk modulus varies both with the temperature and pressure.

7.   Surface Tention and capilliarity :

Due to molecular attraction liquids possess certain properties such as cohesion and adhesion. Cohesion is the force of attraction among the liquid molecules. Adhesion is the force of attraction between molecules of a liquid and molecules of a solid boundary surface in contact with the liquid. The force of cohesion enables a liquid surface to resist tensile stress while adhesion enables it to stick to another body. Surface tension is due to cohesion whereas capillarity is due to both cohesion and adhesion.

(a)   **Surface tension :** When the surface of liquid is in contact with another liquid or solid surface, there exists an apparant tension. The resultant of this tensile force is commonly known as "surface tension".

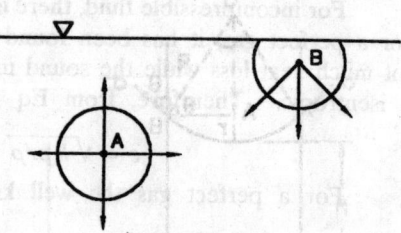

Consider fluid molecule A inside the fluid (Fig. 1.3). It is being attracted by the force of attraction by the fluid molecules surrounding it. The resultant force is, therefore, zero. Next consider a fluid molecule B on the free surface.

FIG. 1.3. DEFINITION SKETCH FOR SURFACE TENSION

It is being attracted by the fluid molecules in the fluid. There is no such force of attraction outside the free surface. Thus the unbalanced force acts on the fluid molecule 'B' in the downward direction. Such unbalanced force acts at all the points in the free surface. Thus, the free surface behaves as a stretched membrane. This unbalanced force on the surface is called

of fluid v (or the relative velocity of the body with respect to fluid) to the

"surface tension". It is designated by (σ). It is measured as the force per unit length of the liquid surface in contact of solid boundary.

$$[\sigma] = \left[\frac{Force}{Length} \right]$$

$$[\sigma] = \left[\frac{F}{L} \right]$$

$$[\sigma] = \left[\frac{N}{m} \right]$$

(b) Capilliarity : When the molecules of liquid are in contact with a solid surface. The liquid surface will stick to the solid surface. If the adhesion is more than cohesion, the liquid will rise along the solid surface. Moreover, it will wet the surface. For example, the water in contact of glass tube walls wet its surface and rises along its walls [Fig. 1.3(a)].

Similarly, when the cohesion is more than adhesion, the liquid does not wet the solid surface and liquid surface depresses along the contact surface. For example, mercury in contact of glass tube walls does not wet its surface and depresses along its wall [Fig. 1.4(b)].

This rise or drop in the liquid surface relative to the adjacent general level is known as capilliarity. This rise or drop can be calculated by the following analysis :

Consider a small fluid element ABCD on the liquid surface (Fig. 1.4 and 1.5). It is of size dx (along AB) and dy normal to it (along BC). Since the liquid surface is curved in XY plane, let the surface has radius of curvatureR_1 and R_2 in the two normal directions (Fig. 1.4). The forces acting on this curved surface are pressures pi acting downward on this curved surface and po from below it. This pressure difference is balanced by the force of surface

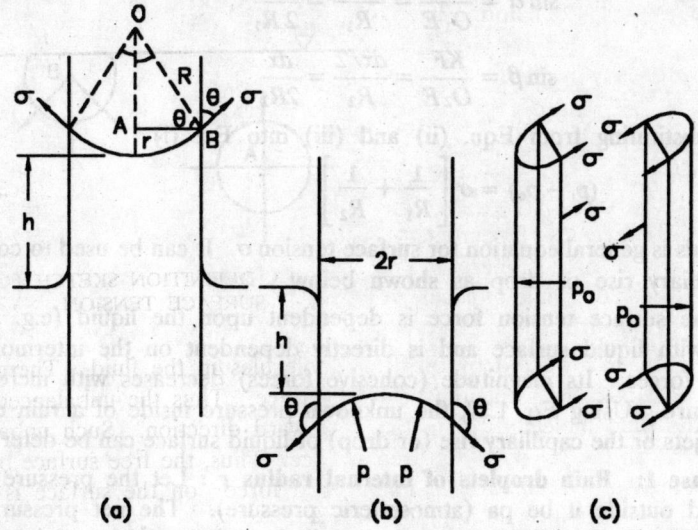

FIG. 1.4. CAPILLARY (A) RISE (B) DROP (C) CYLINDRICAL JET

tension acting tangentially along AB, BC, CD and DA for static equilibrium i.e. $\sigma \times 2\,dx + \sigma \times dy$.

Resolving the forces in normal (vertical) direction to the element.

$$\Sigma F_N = 0$$

$$(p_i - p_0)\,dx\,dy = (2\sigma\,(dx \times 1)\sin\alpha + (2\sigma\,dy \times 1)\sin\beta$$

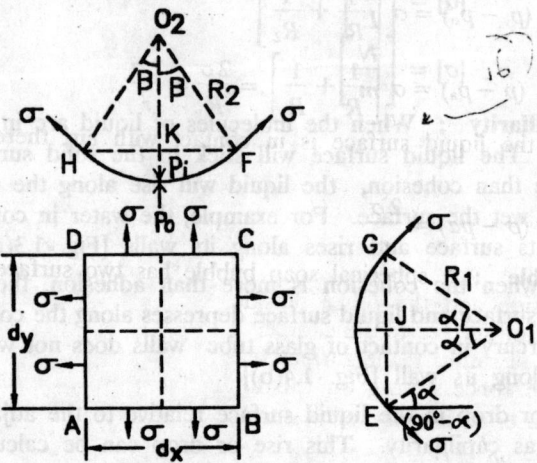

FIG. 1.5. GENERAL ANALYSIS OF CAPPILIARITY

Dividing by the area of the element dx dy on both sides

$$(p_i - p_0) = 2\sigma\left(\frac{\sin\alpha}{dy} + \frac{\sin\beta}{dx}\right) \qquad \ldots(i)$$

From Fig. 1.4, O_1 JE and O_2 KF,

$$\sin\alpha = \frac{JE}{O_1 E} = \frac{dy/2}{R_1} = \frac{dy}{2R_1} \qquad \ldots(ii)$$

$$\sin\beta = \frac{KF}{O_2 F} = \frac{dx/2}{R_2} = \frac{dx}{2R_2} \qquad \ldots(iii)$$

Substituting from Eqn. (ii) and (iii) into Eq. (i)

$$(p_i - p_0) = \sigma\left[\frac{1}{R_1} + \frac{1}{R_2}\right] \qquad \ldots(1.27)$$

This is general equation for surface tension σ. It can be used to compute the capilliary rise or drop as shown below.

The surface tension force is dependent upon the liquid (e.g. air) in contact with liquid surface and is directly dependent on the intermolecular cohesive forces. Its magnitude (cohesive forces) decreases with increase in temperature. Using Eq. 1.27, the unknown pressure inside of a rain droplet and tiny jets or the capilliary rise (or drop) of liquid surface can be determined.

Case 1: Rain droplets of internal radius r : Let the pressure inside be p and outside it be pa (atmospheric pressure). The net pressure (p - pa) will balance the surface tension acting all along the periphery of the circular section of the droplet. (Fig. 1.6 a). It is known that for spherical surfaces, the radii of curvature in the mutually perpendicular directions are equal i.e. $R_1 = R_2 = R$ (say).

If the radius of the droplet be r, then $R = r$.

Substituting in Eq. 1.27,

$$(p_i - p_o) = \sigma \left[\frac{1}{R_1} + \frac{1}{R_2} \right]$$

$$(p - p_a) = \sigma \left[\frac{1}{R} + \frac{1}{R} \right] = \frac{2\sigma}{R} = \frac{2\sigma}{r} \qquad ...(1.28a)$$

Assuming the liquid surface is in contact with air, therefore, pa = $p_{atom} = 0$.

$$\therefore \qquad (\rho - pa) = \frac{2\sigma}{r} \qquad ..(1.28b)$$

Soap Bubble : A spherical soap bubble has two surfaces in contact with air, one inside and the other outside, each one of which contributes the same amount of surface tension force. Hence, on a hemispherical section of a soap bubble of radius r, the surface tension force is $2\sigma(2\pi r)$. However, the net pressure force acting on the hemispherical section is $(pi - pa)$ πr^2 as in the case of droplet of water.

$$\therefore \qquad (pi - pa)\pi r^2 = 2\sigma(2\pi r)$$

$$(pi - pa) = \frac{4\sigma}{r} \qquad ...(1.28c)$$

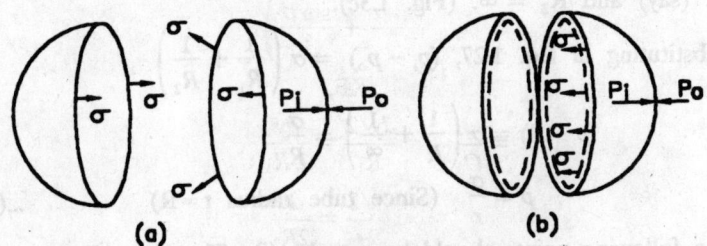

FIG. 1.6. SPHERICAL BUBBLES
(A) RAIN DROP (B) SOAP BUBBLE

Case II : Capillary rise in a cylindrical tube

Let a cylindrical tube of radius r is immersed in water (Fig. 1.4a) or mercury (Fig. 1.4b) so that liquid surface rises/drops along solid wall by h (metre).

In this case, pi = pa, po = -wh (since the pressure on liquid surface outside is atmospheric or zero and the liquid rises by a height 'h' about the liquid surface. The radii of curvature $R_1 = R_2 = R$.

Substituting in Eq. 1.27

$$(pi - po) = \sigma \left[\frac{1}{R_1} + \frac{1}{R_2} \right]$$

or $\qquad [pa - (-wh)] = \sigma \left[\dfrac{1}{R} + \dfrac{1}{R} \right]$

or $\qquad pa + wh = \dfrac{2\sigma}{2}$

or $\qquad pa + wh = \dfrac{2\sigma}{R}$

or $\qquad h = \dfrac{2\sigma}{wR}$ $\qquad\qquad (pa = patm = 0)$

Now in $\triangle O_1 AB$, (Fig 1.4 a or b) $\cos\theta = \dfrac{r}{R}$;

$$\dfrac{1}{R} = \dfrac{\cos\theta}{r}$$

Therefore,, capilliary rise or drop h in a cylindrical tube of radius r is given by

$$h = \dfrac{2\sigma\cos\theta}{wr} \qquad\qquad ...(1.29)$$

Here θ is the "angle of contact" which the liquid surface in the tube makes with the tube wall.

Case III : Cylindrical liquid jet :

Let a cylindrical jet (radius r) discharges into atmosphere (po = pa = 0). The pressure inside is p (say.). It is known that the radius of curvature, R_1 = R (say) and R_2 = ∞. (Fig. 1.3c).

Substituting in Eq. 1.27, $(p_i - p_o) = \sigma \left(\dfrac{1}{R_1} + \dfrac{1}{R_2} \right)$

or $\qquad (p - 0) = \sigma \left(\dfrac{1}{R} + \dfrac{1}{\infty} \right) = \dfrac{\sigma}{R}$

∴ $\qquad p = \dfrac{\sigma}{r}$ (Since tube radius r = R) $\qquad ...(1.30)$

The following points should be noted, (i) The above Eqs. 1.28 and 1.29 are limited to a very narrow tube (r < 2.5 mm) whereas in large diameter tubes the liquid surface will be far from spherical surface (as assumed above).

(ii) The angle θ is known as the angle of contact and it results from the phenomenon of surface tension. The magnitude of this angle is different for various liquids. For water in contact of extremely clean vertical glass surface, the angle of contact θ is 0° and for mercury in contact of extremely clean glass tube, is 130°. Evidently, in practice, such cleanliness is virtually never encountered and hence h will be smaller than found from above equations.

(iii) Gibson has found that the value of for water air interface in contact with glass is 25° 32′ and surface tension σ = 0.0075 kg/m or 0.0735

N/m. The capillary rise h (mm) in a tube of diameter 'd' (mm) is given by

$$h = \frac{27}{d} \text{ mm}$$ ...(1.30 a)

Similarly, for mercury air interface in contact with glass, was found to be $128°52'$ with $\sigma = 0.054$ kg/m or 0.53 N/m. The capillary drop h in a tube of diameter d(mm) is given by

$$h = \frac{9.6}{d} \text{ mm}$$ ...(1.30b)

(iv) To avoid the effects of capillarity in manometer a tube of 12.5 mm or larger should be used.

(v) It is found that surface tension decreases with increase in temperature but the effects is rather small on capillary rise.

In general, the surface tension forces are very small, and can be neglected. But in some engineering problems, this may be predominant such as in the mechanics of bubbles, the break up of liquid jets, the formation of liquid drops, the capillary rise in narrow spaces and model testing and interpretation of results obtained from small models. The discharge flowing over a weir at small head is also effected by surface tension.

8. Vapour Pressure

All liquids possess a tendency to vapourise, i.e. these changes from liquid to gaseous state. Such vapourisation occurs because molecules are continuously ejected through the free liquid surface. These ejected molecules exert their own partial pressure on the liquid surface and it is known as "vapour pressure p_v" of the liquid. At the same time in a confined space the molecules leaving the liquid surface rebound back and re-enter the liquid surface. This means, that partial pressure due to vapours increases until the rate of leaving equals the rate of re-entry. At this equilibrium condition, the vapour pressure is known as "saturation vapour pressure.".

Effect of temperature and · pressure :

with increase in temperature, molecular activity increases and hence saturation pressure also increases.

At any other temperature, the pressure on a liquid surface will be either equal to or greater than saturation pressure. If the pressure reduces then it will induce fast rate of evaporation known as "boiling". Hence, if the external pressure imposed on the liquid surface is reduced lower than vapour pressure (e.g. at higher elevation p_a < p_v) or temperature is increased, boiling of liquid starts. Thus boiling of liquid is dependent on the imposed external pressure as well as upon temperature. Refer Sec. 19.2.1 for Equation of state for gaseous state of fluid.

Examples 1.1 to 1.24

1.1 If the specific gravity of a liquid is 0.80, determine its mass density, specific weight (weight density) and specific volume.

Solution :

$$\text{Specific gravity} = \frac{\text{Mass density of liquid}}{\text{Mass density of water}}$$

∴ Mass density of liquid = Specific gravity × Mass density of water

$= 0.8 \times 1000$ kg/m^3 ($\because$ Mass density of water $= 1000$ kg/m^3)

$= 800$ kg/m^3

Weight density of liquid = Mass density × acceleration due to gravity

$$w = \rho g$$
$$= 800 \times 9.81 \text{ N/m}^3 = 7252 \text{ N/m}^3$$
$$= 7.252 \text{ kN/m}^3$$

$$\text{Specific volume of liquid} = \frac{1}{\text{Mass density of liquid}}$$

$$v = \frac{1}{\rho}$$

$$\frac{1}{800} = 1.25 \times 10^{-3} \text{ m}^{-3}/\text{kg}$$

1.2 : Find the kinematic viscosity of a liquid in stokes whose specific gravity is 0.95 and viscosity is 0.011 poise.

Solution :

Given $\mu = 0.011$ poise

But 1 poise $= 0.1$ Ns/m^2

Hence $\mu = 0.011 \times 0.1$ Ns/m^2

$= 0.0011$ Ns/m^2

Mass density of liquid

$= $ specific gravity × mass density of water

$= 0.95 \times 1000$ kg/m^3

$= 950$ kg/m^3

Therefore, kinematic viscosity of liquid

$$= \frac{\text{Dynamic viscosity}}{\text{Mass density}}, v = \frac{\mu}{\rho} = \frac{0.0011 \text{ Ns/m}^2}{950 \text{ kg/m}^3}$$

$$v = 1.16 \times 10^{-6} \text{ m}^2/\text{s}$$

$$v = 1.16 \times 10^{-6} \times 10^4 \text{ cm}^2/\text{s}$$

$$= 0.016 \text{ stokes}$$

$$\because \quad \frac{1 \, cm^2}{s} = 1 \text{ stokes}$$

1.3 : If a certain liquid has viscosity 5 x 10^{-4}kg$_f$ sec/m^2 and kinematic viscosity 3.503 × 10^{-2} stokes, what is its specific gravity.

Solution :

Dynamic viscosity = Mass density × kinematic viscosity

$$\text{Mass density} = \frac{\text{Dynamic viscisity}}{\text{kinematic viscosity}}$$

$$\rho = \frac{\mu}{v}$$

Dynamic viscosity $\mu = 5 \times 10^{-4}$ kgf sec / m²

From Eq. 1.16, 1 Poise = 1/98.1 kgf sec / m²

1 kg sec/m² = 98.1 Poise; $\mu = 5 \times 10^{-4} \times 98.1$ Poise.

From Eq. 1.17, 1 Poise = 0.1 Ns / m²

$\therefore \quad \mu = (5 \times 10^{-4} \times 98.1) \times 0.1 \, N s/m^2 = 490.5 \times 10^{-5} \, N s/m^2$

Also, $v = 3.503 \times 10^{-2}$ Stokes

$\because \qquad 1 \, cm^2/s = 10^{-4} \, m^2/s$

$\therefore \qquad v = 3.503 \times 10^{-2} \times 10^{-4} \, m^2/s$

Now, $\qquad \rho = \dfrac{\mu}{\rho}$

$$= \frac{490.5 \times 10^{-5} \, N s/m^2}{3.503 \times 10^{-6} \, m^2/s}$$

$$= 1400 \, kg/m^3$$

$$\text{Specific gravity} = \frac{\text{Mass density of liquid}}{\text{Mass density of water}}$$

$$= \frac{1400 \, kg/m^3}{1000 \, kg/m^3} = 1.4$$

1.4 The space between two square flat parallel plates is filled with oil. Each side of the plate is 60 cm. The thickness of oil film is 12.5 mm. The upper plate which moves at 2.5 m/s, requires a force of 100 N to maintain the speed. Determine (i) dynamic viscosity in poise, (ii) kinematic viscosity in stokes. Given that the specific gravity of oil is 0.95. (A.M.I.E. 1977 W)

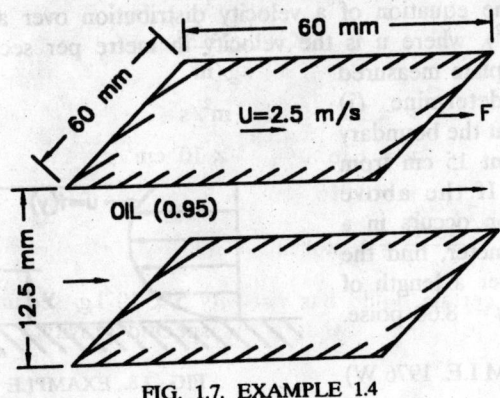

FIG. 1.7. EXAMPLE 1.4

Solution :

Shear stress acting on the top plate,

$$\tau = \mu \frac{du}{dy}$$

Let area of top plate in contact with liquid be A

Force required on the top plate to maintain given velocity = F.

$$F = \tau \times A$$

$$= \mu \frac{du}{dy} \times A$$

$$100 = \mu \times \frac{2.5 \text{ m/s}}{12.5 \times 10^{-3} \text{ m}} \times (0.6 \text{ m} \times 0.6 \text{ m})$$

$$\mu = \frac{100 \times 12.5 \times 10^{-3}}{2.5 \times 0.60 \times 0.6} \text{ N s/m}^2$$

$$= 1.388 \text{ Ns/m}^2$$

Since 1 Poise = 0.1 Ns/m²

$$\mu = 1.388 \times (1/0.1) \text{ Poise} = 13.88 \text{ Poise.}$$

The mass density of liquid ρ = specific gravity × mass density of water

$$\rho = 0.95 \times 1000 \text{ kg/m}^3 = 950 \text{ kg/m}^3$$

∴ Therefore, Kinematic viscosity $v = \dfrac{\text{Dynamic viscosity} \, \mu}{\text{Mass density} \, \rho}$

$$v = \frac{1.388 \text{ Ns/m}^2}{950 \text{ kg/m}^3}$$

$$= 1.46 \times 10^{-3} \text{ m}^2/\text{s} \quad \left(\because 1 \text{ stokes} = \frac{1 \text{ cm}^2}{\text{s}} = 10^{-4} \frac{\text{m}^2}{\rho} \right)$$

$$= 1.46 \times 10^{-3} \times 10^4 \text{ stokes}$$

$$= 14.61 \text{ stokes}$$

1.5 : If the equation of a velocity distribution over a plate is given by $u = (2y - y^2)$, where u is the velocity in metre per second at a point y metre from the plate measured perpendicularly, determine (i) The shear steress at the boundary and (ii) at a point 15 cm from the boundary. If the above velocity distribution occurs in a pipe of 3 cm diameter, find the total resistance over a length of 100 m, assuming $\mu = 8.60$ poise.

(Similar A.M.I.E. 1976 W)

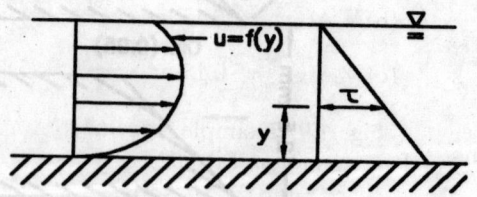

FIG. 1.8. EXAMPLE 1.5

Solution :

From Eq. 1.9c, $\tau = \dfrac{du}{dy}$

Given $\mu = 2y - y^2$

Hence $\tau = \mu \times \dfrac{d}{dy} (2y - y^2)$

$= \mu \times (2 - 2y).$

(i) Shear stress τ_0 at the boundary i.e. y = 0

$$\tau_0 = 8.6 \times 0.1 \, (2 - 2 \times 0) \, N/m^2$$

$$= 1.77 \, N/m^2$$

$\because \mu = 8.6 \text{ poise} = 8.6 \times 0.1 \dfrac{Ns}{m^2}$

$$= 1.777 \, N/m^2$$

(ii) Shear stress at a distance of 15 cm from the boundary,

i.e. $y = 0.15 \, m,$

$$\tau = 8.6 \times 0.1 \, (2 - 2 \times 0.15) = 1.462 \, N/m^2$$

(iii) Total resistance R in a pipe of 3 cm diameter and over a length of 100 m.

$= \text{wall sheaar stress} \times \text{wetted area}$

$= \tau_0 \times \pi \, DL$

$= 1.77 \times 3.14 \times 0.03 \times 100 \, N = 16.20 \, N$

1.6 : If the velocity profile over a flat plate is a parabola with vertex 15 cm from the plate, where the velocity is 1.0 m/s. Calculate the velocity gradients and shear stress at a distance 0 cm, 5 cm and 10 cm from the stationary plate. Assume $\mu = 8.5$ poise.

Solution :

Since velocity distribution is parabolic (given), assume the velocity distribution as

$$u = a + by + cy^2 \quad ..(i)$$

where a, b and c, are constants and are unknown. These are determined from boundary conditions.

(a) At y = 0 m, u = 0

(b) At y = 0.15 m, u = 1

(c) At y = 0.15 m , $\dfrac{\partial u}{\partial y} = 0$

Fig. 1.9, Example 1.6 Substituting boundary condition (a) in Eq. (i),

$$a = 0 \quad ..(iv)$$

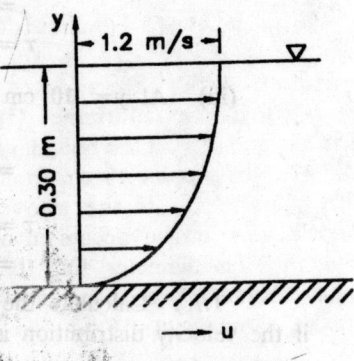

FIG. 1.9. EXAMPLE 1.6

Substituting B.C. (b) in Eq. (i)

$$1.0 = b \times 0.15 + C \times (0.15)^2 \qquad ...(v)$$

Substituting B.C. (c) in Eq. (i)

$$\frac{du}{dy} = b + 2cy$$

$$0 = b + 2c \times 0.15$$

$$0 = b + 0.3\,c \qquad ...(vi)$$

Solving Eqs. (v) and (vi), b and c can be determined

From Eq. (vi), $\quad b = -0.3\,c \qquad ...(vii)$

From Eqs. (v) and (vii)

$$0.15\,(-0.3\,c) + (0.15)^2\,c = 1.0$$

Solving $\qquad\qquad c = -4444$

and $\qquad\qquad b = 13.33$

Hence velocity distribution becomes

$$u = (13.33\,y - 44.44\,y^2) \qquad ...(i)$$

Now velocity gradient and shear stress can be computed.

(i) At $\quad y = 0 \quad$ cm. $\quad \dfrac{\partial u}{\partial y} = (13.33 - 44.44 \times 2y)$

$$= (13.33 - 88.88\,y)$$

$$= 13.33 \text{ per sec.}$$

$$\tau = \mu \frac{\partial u}{\partial y}$$

$$= (8.5 \times 0.1) \times 13.33 = 11.33 \text{ N/m}^2$$

(ii) At $y = 5$ cm $\dfrac{\partial u}{\partial y} = (13.33 - 88.88\,y)$

$$= \left(13.33 - 88.88 \times \frac{5}{100} \right)$$

$$= 8.886 \text{ per sec.}$$

$$\tau = (8.5 \times 0.1) \times 8.886 = 7.55 \text{ N/m}^2$$

(iii) At $y = 10$ cm $\dfrac{\partial u}{\partial y} = (13.33 - 88.88\,y)$

$$= \left(13.33 - 88.88 \times \frac{10}{100} \right) 4.442 \text{ per sec.}$$

$$\tau = (8.5 \times 0.1) \times 4.442$$

$$= 3.776 \text{ N/m}^2$$

1.7 : Calculate the velocity gradients for y = 0, 20, 40 and 60 cm if the velocity distribution is a quarter circle having its centre 600 mm from the boundary. Also calculate the shear stress at these points, if fluid viscosity is 78.45×10^{-2} Ns/m².

Solution :

Let the equation of circle be $(u-u_o)^2 + (y-y_o)^2 = R^2$ where (u_o, y_o) are the co-ordinates of the centre of circle of radius R. Since, the co-ordinates of the centre are given $(0, 0.6)$, the equation of circle is $(u-0)^2 + (y-0.6)^2 = R^2$

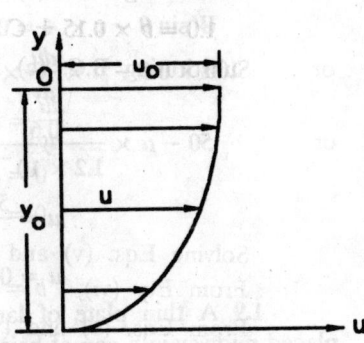

FIG. 1.10. EXAMPLE 1.7

Also at boundary,

$$u = 0, \quad y = 0.$$

$$\therefore \qquad R = 0.6 \text{ m}$$

Hence the equation of velocity profile becomes

$$u^2 + (y-0.6)^2 = (0.6)^2$$

Simplifying, $\qquad u^2 = -(y^2 - 1.2\,y)$ ...(1)

Differentiating it with respect to y,

$$\frac{du}{dy} = \frac{-(2y-1.2)}{2u} = -\frac{(y-0.6)}{u} \qquad ...(2)$$

From Eqs. (1) and (2), the velocity and velocity gradients at various points can be calculated. Thereafter the shear stress can be determined using Newton's law of viscosity $\left(\tau = \mu \dfrac{du}{dy}\right)$, Eq. 1.9 c.

y	u	du/dy	τ
m	m/s	S⁻¹	N/m²
0	0	∞	∞
0.4	0.566	0.354	0.277
0.6	0.600	0	0
0	0		

The example illustrates the variation of shear stress in a vertical section.

1.8 : A rectangular plate of size 1 m × 1 m and wweighing 100 N slides down a 30 inclined surface at a uniform velocity of 0.6 m/s. If the uniform gap of 1.2 mm between the plate and the inclined surface is filled with oil, determine its viscosity

Solution :

While the plate just starts moving, the force causing its motion should slightly exceed the frictional force on its lower surface.

In the condition of equilibrim,

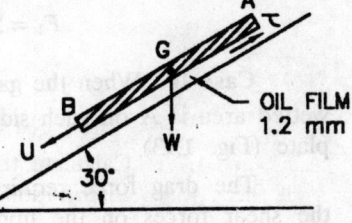

FIG. 1.11. EXAMPLE 1.8

$$\Sigma F_x = 0$$

$$W \sin \theta - \tau \times A = 0$$

or

$$100 \times 0.5 - \mu \times \frac{du}{dy} \times 1 \times 1 = 0$$

or

$$50 - \mu \times \frac{0.6}{1.2 \times 10^{-3}} \times 1 = 0 \qquad (\because \sin \theta = \sin 30° = 0.5)$$

$$\mu = \frac{50 \times 1.2 \times 10^{-3}}{0.6}$$

$$\mu = 0.1 \ \text{Ns/m}^2$$

1.9 A thin plate of large area is placed midway in a gap of height 'h' filled with oil of viscosity μ_0 and the plate is pulled at a constant velocity U. If a lighter liquid of viscosity μ_1 is then substituted in the gap and the plate is located un-symmetrically in the gap parallel to the wall, it is found that for the same velocity u the drag force will be the same as before. Find $_1$ in terms of μ_0 and the distance from the nearer wall to the plate.

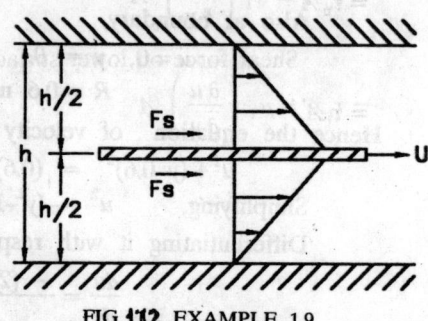

FIG. **1.12** EXAMPLE 1.9

Solution :

Case I : When the gap contains oil of viscosity μ_0, the velocity gradient is given by (Fig. 1.12).

$$\frac{du}{dy} = \frac{U}{h/2} = \frac{2U}{h}$$

Drag force $F_1 =$ (Shear stress on the upper surface + shear

stress on the lower surface) × area of contact.

As the plate is placed symmetrically the force will be same on upper surface and lower surfaces, (say) F

$\therefore$

$$F_1 = [\tau + \tau] \times A = 2\tau . A$$

$\therefore$

$$F_1 = \left[2\mu_0 \frac{\partial u}{\partial y} \right] \times A$$

Substituting the value of velocity gradient

$$F_1 = 2\mu_0 \frac{U}{h/2} . A = \frac{4\mu_0 U A}{h} \qquad ...(1)$$

Case II : When the gap contains oil of viscosity μ_1, let us assume that wetted area is A on each side and the plate is placed y distance from lower plate (Fig. 1.13)

The drag force required to pull the plate will be the summation of the shear forces on the upper and lower sides.' Hence

$$F_2 = \mu_1 \times \left(\frac{du}{dy}\right)_u \times A + \mu_1 \left(\frac{du}{dy}\right)_l \times A$$

Velocity gradient on upper

surface $= \dfrac{U}{(h-y)}$

Velocity gradient on lower

surface $= \dfrac{U}{y}$

Shear force on upper surface

$= \tau_u A = \mu_1 \left(\dfrac{\partial u}{\partial y}\right)_u A$

Shear force on lower surface

$= \tau_l A = \mu_1 \left(\dfrac{\partial u}{\partial y}\right)_l A$

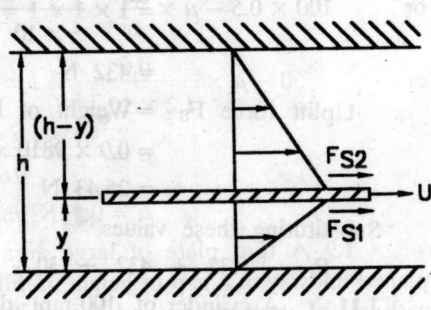

FIG. 1.13. EXAMPLE 1.9

$$\therefore \quad F_2 = \mu_1 \frac{U}{(h-y)} \times A + \mu_1 \frac{U}{y} . A$$

$$= \frac{\mu_1 U h A}{y(h-y)} \qquad \qquad ...(2)$$

Since the drag force F_1 should be equal to F_2, therefore,

$$\frac{4\mu_0 UA}{h} = \frac{\mu_1 U h A}{y(h-y)}$$

Solving, $\qquad \mu_1 = 4\mu_0 \dfrac{y}{h}\left(1 - \dfrac{y}{h}\right)$

1.10 : A vertical gap is 12 mm wide and is of infinite extent. An oil of specific gravity 0.9 is filled in the gap. A square plate 1.2 m x 1.2 m and 2 mm thick is pulled in between these two vertical walls at a velocity of 0.15 m/s. The weight of the plate is 30 N. Calculate the force required to pull the plate up. Take $\mu = 1$ Ns/m^2.

Solution :

When the vertical plate is just to be lifted, it will be in equilibrium condition, i.e.

$$\Sigma F_y = 0$$

The forces acting on it are force F required to pull it out, weight of plate W , frictional forces acting on its two sides F_1 and F_2 (= F_1) and uplift force F_B.

$$\therefore \quad F + F_B - F_1 - F_2 - W = 0$$

$$F = (F_1 + F_2 + W - F_B)$$

Viscous or frictional force $F_1 = F_2 = $ du/dy

. A

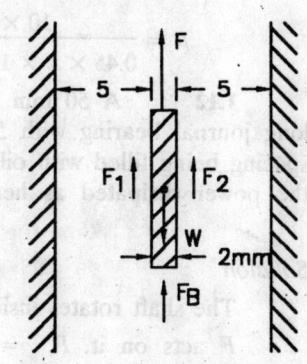

FIG. 1.14. EXAMPLE 1.10

$$= \mu \frac{U}{\Gamma} . A$$

$$= 1 \times \frac{0.15}{5 \times 10^{-3} \times 1.2 \times 1.2}$$

$$= 432 \text{ N}$$

Uplift force F_B = Weight of liquid displaced

$$= 0.9 \times 9810 \times 1.2 \times 1.2 \times 2 \times 10^3$$

$$= 25.43 \text{ N}$$

Substituting these values,

$$F = [432 + 432 + 30 - 25.43] = 868.57 \text{ N}$$

1.11 : A cylinder of 100 mm diameter, 0.15 m length and weighing 10 N slides axially in a vertical pipe of 104 mm diameter. If the space between cylinder surface and pipe wall is filled with liquid of viscosity μ and cylinder slides downwards at a velocity of 0.45 m/s, determine μ.

(A.M.I.E. 91, winter)

Solution :

While the cylinder moves down, its motion is resisted by viscous forces,

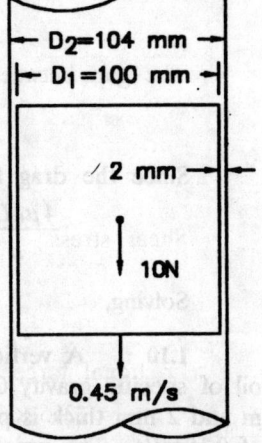

FIG. 1.15 EXAMPLE 1.11

$$\Sigma F_y = 0$$

$$W - F = 0$$

$$W - \tau . \pi D_1 L = 0$$

$$10 - \mu \times \frac{du}{dy} \times \pi \times 100 \times 10^{-3} \times 0.15 = 0$$

$$\mu = \frac{10}{(0.45/2 \times 10^{-3}) \times \pi \times 100 \times 10^{-3} \times 0.15}$$

Since $\quad \dfrac{du}{dy} = \dfrac{U}{(10 - 100)/2 \times 10^{-3}}$

$$\mu = \frac{10 \times 2 \times 10^{-3}}{0.45 \times \pi \times 100 \times 10^{-3} \times 0.15} = 0.943 \text{ Ns/m}^2$$

1.12 : A 50 mm diameter shaft rotates at 1500 rpm in a 100 mm long journal bearing with 50.5 mm internal diameter. The uniform annual spacing being filled with oil having dynamic viscosity of 0.08 Pa s. Calculate the power disipated as heat.

(A.M.I.E. 92 Winter)

Solution :

The shaft rotates inside the journal bearing and viscous (frictional force F acts on it. F = Shear stress $\times$ Area

$$= \tau \times A$$

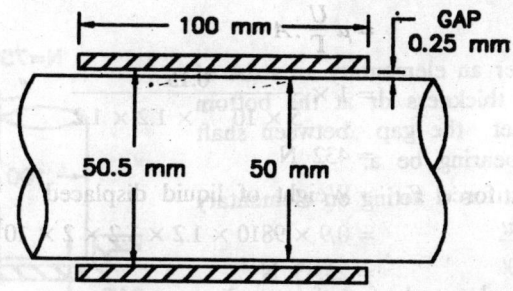

FIG. 1.16 EXAMPLE 1.12

$$= \mu \frac{du}{dy} \times A$$

The peripheral velocity of shaft $u = \frac{\pi DN}{60}$

$$= \frac{\pi \times 60 \times 10^{-3} \times 1500}{60} = 3.925 \text{ m/s}$$

The gap between shaft and bearing,

$$a = \frac{(50.5 - 50)}{2} \times 10^{-3} \text{ m}$$

$$a = 0.25 \times 10^{-3} \text{ m}$$

Shear stress $\tau = \mu \frac{du}{dy}$

$$= 0.08 \times \frac{3.925}{0.25 \times 10^{-3}} = 1256 \text{ N/m}^2$$

Frictional force $F = \tau \times \pi D L$

$$= 1256 \times 3.14 \times 50 \times 10^{-3} \times 100 \times 10^{-3} \text{ N} = 19.72 \text{ N}.$$

Torque $T = F \times D/2$

Power lost $= \text{Torque} \times \omega = F \times D/2 \times \omega.$

$$= F \times \frac{D}{2} \times \frac{2\pi N}{60}$$

$$= F \times u$$

$$= 19.72 \times 3.925 \text{ W}$$

$$= 77.4 \text{ W}$$

1.13 : The lower end of a vertical shaft rests in a foot step bearings. Assuming that the end of the shaft and the surface of bearing are both flat and are separated by an oil film of 0.5 mm thickness, find torque required to rotate the shaft at 750 r.p.m. The diameter of shaft is 100 mm and $\mu = 1.5$ poise.

(A.M.I.E. 1977, Summer)

Solution :

Consider an elementary area dA of radius r and thickness dr at the bottom of shaft. Let the gap between shaft bottom and bearing be a.

Shear stress d acting on elementary area $dA = \tau \dfrac{du}{dy}$

∴ Peripheral speed of shaft at radius r is $= \omega r$

∴ $d = d\tau = \dfrac{\mu w r}{a}$

Shear force dF acting on dA is $= d\tau \times area$

$= \dfrac{\mu w r}{a} \cdot (2\pi r\, dr)$

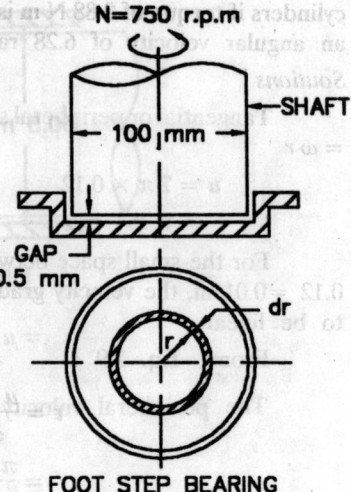

N=750 r.p.m

SHAFT

100 mm

GAP
0.5 mm

dr

r

FOOT STEP BEARING

FIG. 1.17 EXAMPLE 1.13

Torque dF acting on elementary strip $= dF \times r$

$$= \left(\mu \dfrac{\omega r}{a} \cdot 2\pi \cdot r\, dr \right) r$$

$$= \dfrac{2\pi \mu w}{a} r^3\, dr$$

∴ Torque T acting on the bottom of shaft

$$= \int_0^R dT$$

$$= \int_0^R \dfrac{2\pi \mu \omega}{a} r^3\, dr$$

$$= \dfrac{2\pi \mu \omega}{a} \cdot \dfrac{R^4}{4}$$

$$= \dfrac{\pi \mu \omega R^4}{2a}$$

The angular speed of shaft $\omega = \dfrac{2\pi N}{60} = \dfrac{2 \times 3.14 \times 750}{60}$

$= 78.5$ rad/s.

∴ $T = \dfrac{3.14 \times 1.5 \times 0.1 \times 78.5 (50 \times 10^{-3})^4}{2 \times 0.5 \times 10^{-3}}$

$= 0.231$ Nm

1.14 : A cylinder of 0.12 m radius rotates concentrically inside a fixed cylinder of 0.13 m radius. Both cylinders are 0.3 m long. Determine the viscosity of fluid which fills the space between the cylinders if torque of 0.88 N m is required to maintain an angular velocity of 6.28 rad/s.

Soutions :

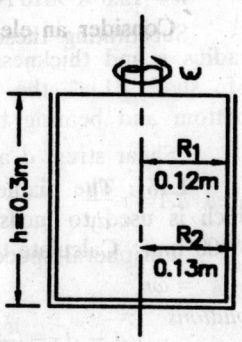

FIG. 1.18. EXAMPLE 1.14

Tangential or peripheral speed of inner cylinder

$= \omega r$

$$u = 2\pi \times 0.12$$

$$= 0.754 \text{ m/s}$$

For the small space between cylinders $= 0.13 - 0.12 = 0.01$ m. the velocity gradient may be assumed to be linear.

From Eq. 1.9 c,

$$\tau = \frac{\mu \, \partial u}{\partial y}$$

$$= \mu \times \frac{0.754}{0.13 - 0.12} = 75.4 \, \mu \text{ N/m}^2$$

Torque resisted $= \tau$ (area) (arm)

$$= 75.4 \times (2\pi R_2 h) (R_2)$$

$$= 75.4 \, \mu \, (2\pi \times 0.13 \times 0.3) (0.13)$$

Torque applied = Torque resisted

∴ $$0.88 = 75.4 \, \mu \, (2\pi \times 0.13 \times 0.3) (0.13)$$

$$\mu = \frac{0.88}{75.4 \times 2\pi \times (0.13)^2 \times 0.3}$$

$$= 0.366 \text{ Pa s (Ns/m}^2)$$

1.15 : Calculate the capillary rise in a glass tube of 3 mm diameter when immersed in (a) water (b) mercury. The temperature of both liquids is 20° C., the angle of contact for water is zero degree and for mercury, it is 130°. It is known that surface tension of water air and mercury air at this temperature are 0.0735 N/m and 0.51 N/m.

Solution :

From Eq. 1.28, $$h = \frac{2\sigma \cos\theta}{wr}$$

For water air interface, $\sigma = 0.735$ N/m $\theta = 0°$, $w = 9810$ N/m^3

and $$r = 1.5 \times 10^{-3} \text{ m}$$

Substituting these values, capillary rise is

$$h = \frac{2 \times 0.0735 \times \cos 0°}{9810 \times 1.5 \times 10^{-3}}$$

$$= 0.01 \text{ m}$$

For mercury air interface, $\sigma = 0.51$ N/m, $\theta = 130°$,

$$w = 13.6 \times 9810 \, \text{N/m}^2 \quad ; \quad \text{and} \quad r = 1.5 \times 10^{-3} \, \text{m}$$

Substituting these values capillary depression is

$$h = \frac{2 \times 0.51 \times \cos 130°}{13.6 \times 9810 \times 1.5 \times 10^{-3}}$$

$$= 0.00386 \, \text{m}$$

1.16 : The diameters of the limbs of a U-tube are 4 mm and 5 mm which is used to measure the pressure readings in the range of 10 mm to 100 mm. Calculate the percentage error at its lowest and highest readings.

Solutions :

Capillary rise in a circular tube,

$$h = \frac{2\sigma \cos\theta}{w \, r}$$

For water air contact, $\sigma = 0.00735 \, \text{N/m} \, , \theta = 0°$

In 4 mm diameter tube, $h = \dfrac{2 \times 0.0735 \times \cos 0°}{9810 \times 2 \times 10^{-3}} = 0.0075 \, \text{m}$

In 5 mm diameter tube, $h = \dfrac{2 \times 0.0735 \times \cos 0°}{9810 \times 2.5 \times 10^{-3}} = 0.0060 \, \text{m}$

Error caused due to capillarity $= (0.0075 - 0.0060) \, \text{m}$

$$= 1.5 \, \text{mm}$$

Hence, percentage error caused at lowest reading

$$= \pm \frac{\text{Error}}{\text{Gauge reading}} \times 100$$

$$= \pm \frac{1.5}{10} \times 100 = \pm 15\%$$

And, percentage error caused at highest reading

$$= \pm \frac{1.5}{10} \times 100 = \pm 15\%$$

It is to be noted that error due to capillarity will be relatively higher at lower pressure readings.

1.17 : Find the surface tension in a soap bubble of 40 mm diameter when the inside pressure is 2.4 N/m² above the atmospheric pressure.

Solution :

From Eq. 1.27 c,

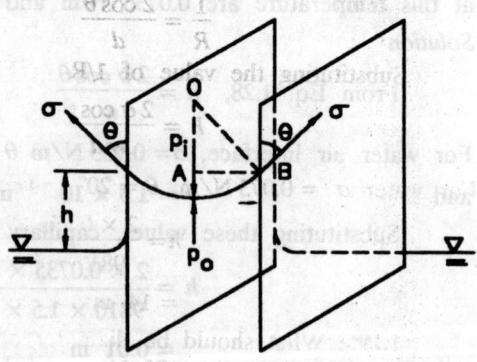

FIG. 1.19 EXAMPLE 1.17

$$(p_i - p_o) = \frac{4\sigma}{r}$$

$$2.4 = \frac{4\sigma}{\frac{40}{2} \times 10^{-3}}$$

$$\sigma = \frac{2.4}{4} \times \frac{40}{2} \times 10^{-3}$$

$$= 0.012 \text{ N/m}$$

1.18 : Two parallel wide glass plates separated by a distance of 1 mm are placed in water. How far does the water rise due to capillary action in the portion away from the ends of plate ? Assume $\sigma = 0.073$ N/m and angle of contact with glass as 20°. (A.M.I.E., 1992 Winter)

Solution :

From Eq. 1.26,

$$(p_i - p_o) = \sigma \left(\frac{1}{R_1} + \frac{1}{R_2} \right)$$

The pressure acting on the curved surface $p_i = 0$, and the pressure acting from below curved surface is $p_o = -w\,h$.

The radius of curvatures $R_1 = R$ (say) and $R_2 = \infty$.

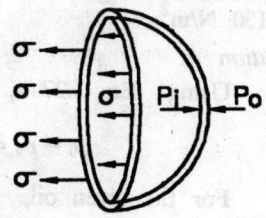

FIG. 1.20. EXAMPLE 1.18

$$\therefore \quad [\, 0 - (- w\,h)] = \sigma \left[\frac{1}{R} + \frac{1}{\infty} \right]$$

$$h = \frac{\sigma}{w} \cdot \frac{1}{R} \qquad \qquad \text{...(i)}$$

Let the spacing between plates be d (=1 mm)

From $\triangle OAB$, $\cos\theta = \dfrac{d/2}{R}$

$$\therefore \qquad \frac{1}{R} = \frac{2\cos\theta}{d} \qquad \qquad \text{...(ii)}$$

Substituting the value of 1/R in Fig. (i),

$$h = \frac{2\sigma\cos\theta}{w\,d}$$

For water $\sigma = 0.073$ N/m, $\theta = 20°$ (given) and $w = 9810$ N 4m³

$$h = \frac{2 \times 0.073 \times \cos 20°}{9810 \times 1 \times 10^{-3}} = 0.014 \text{ m}$$

$$= 14 \text{ mm}$$

1.19 : What should be diameter of a droplet of water in mm, if the pressure inside is to be 175 N/m² greater than outside ?

Solution :

From Eq. 1.27 a,

$$(p_i - p_0) = \frac{2\sigma}{r}$$

Hence

$$2r = \frac{4\sigma}{(p_i - p_0)}$$

The surface tension for water air contact is 0.0735 N/m

Hence, $2r = d = \dfrac{4 \times 0.0735}{175} = 0.00168$ m

$$= 1.68 \text{ mm}$$

1.20 In measuring the unit surface energy of a mineral oil (specific gravity = 0.85) by the bubble method, a tube having an internal diameter of 1.5 mm is immersed to a depth of 12.5 mm in the oil. Air is forced through the tube forming a bubble at the lower end. What magnitude of unit surface energy will be indicated by a maximum bubble pressure intensity of 150 N/m^2.

Solution :

Using Eq. 1.27 a,

$$p_i - p_0 = \frac{2\sigma}{r}$$

For the given oil, $w = 0.85 \times 9810 = 8338.5$ N/m^2,

$$r = 0.75 \times 10^{-3} \text{ m}$$

when the air is forced through the tube, the pressure outside the bubble p_0 = pressure due to column of 12.5 mm of oil

$$p_0 = 8338.5 \times 12.5 \times 10^{-3} = 104.23 \text{ N/m}^2$$

Pressure inside the bubble pi is given = 150 N/m^2.

Substituting these values in Eq. 1.27 a.

$$(150 - 104.23) = \frac{2\sigma}{0.75 \times 10^{-3}}$$

$$\sigma = \frac{45.77 \times 0.75 \times 10^{-3}}{2}$$

$$= 0.01716 \text{ N/m}$$

1.21 Determine the capillary rise of water in a clay soil of average diameter 0.06 mm. Assume the average size of the pores to be one fifth of the soil diameter.

Solution :

Given pore size = 1/5 soil diameter.

$$= \frac{0.06}{5} = 0.012 \text{ mm}$$

For water air contact, $\sigma = 0.0735$ N/m and $\theta = 0°$

Using Eq. 1.27 a,

$$h = \frac{2 \times 0.0735 \times \cos 0°}{9810 \times (0.012/2 \times 10^{-3}}$$;

$$= 2.5 \text{ m}$$

1.22 : Find the change in volume of 1 m^3 of water at 30°C when subjected to a pressure of 20 bar. Further, determine the bulk modulus of elasticity of water from the following test data, at 35 bar the volume of water was 1 m^3 and at 240 bar the volume reduced to 0.99 m^3.

Solution :

(a) From Table 1.4, $E = 2.23 \times 10^9$ N/m^2

Using Eq. 1.19 $dv = -\dfrac{v\,dp}{E_v}$

$$= \frac{1 \times 20 \times 10^5}{2.23 \times 10^9} \qquad (\because 1 \ bar = 10^5 \text{ N/m}^2)$$

$$= 0.00089 \text{ m}^3$$

(b) Increase in pressure $= (240 - 35) = 205$ bar

Decrease in volume $= (1 - 0.99) = 0.01$ m^3

From Eq. 1.19, $E_v = \dfrac{dp}{dv/v}$

$$= \frac{205 \times 10^5}{0.01/1}$$

$$= 2.05 \times 10^9 \text{ N/m}^2$$

1.23 : Determine the increase in pressure needed to cause 0.1 % reduction in volume of water, air aand mercury. Assume modulus of elaasticity of water and mercury as 2.075×10^9 N/m^2 and 2.431×10^{10} N/m^2 respectively.

Solution :

From Eq. 1.19, $E_v = \dfrac{p}{-(dv/v)}$

$$p = \frac{dv}{v} \times E_v$$

(i) For water : $\dfrac{dv}{v} = 0.1\% = -\dfrac{0.1}{100}$

$$E_v = 2.075 \times 10^9 \text{ N/m}^2$$

$\therefore$ Increase in pressure $p = \left[-\dfrac{0.1}{100} \times 2.075 \times 10^9 \right]$ N/m^2

$$p = 2.075 \times 10^6 \text{ N/m}^2$$

(ii) For mercury : $\dfrac{dV}{V} = 0.1\% = -\dfrac{0.1}{100}$

$$E_v = 2.431 \times 10^{10} \text{ N/m}^2$$

Increase in pressure $= \left[-\dfrac{0.1}{100} \times 2.431 \times 10^{10} \right] \dfrac{N}{m^2}$

$$= 2.431 \times 10^7 \text{ N/m}^2$$

(iii) For air subjected to isothermal process,

From Eq. 1.22, $E_v = -p$ = atmospheric pressure

$$= 10.13 \text{ N/m}^2$$

Increase in pressure $= -[-0.1/100 \times 10.13]$

$$= 0.01013 \text{ N/m}^2$$

(iv)   For air subjected to adiabatic process (k = 1.4),

From Eq. 1.23, $E_v = -kp$

$$= -1.4 \times 10.13 \text{ N/m}^2$$

$$= 14.182 \text{ N/m}^2$$

Increase in pressure $= -\left[\dfrac{0.1}{100} \times 14.182 \right]$

$$= 0.0142 \text{ N/m}^2$$

Thus, it is seen that a very high increase in pressure is required to bring 0.1 % decrease in the volume of water and mercury as compared to that of air.

1.24   : Determine the density of sea water at a depth of 1 km. if the mass density of water at the surface is 1025 kg/m^3 and the average bulk modulus of sea water is 2.35×10^9 N/m^2.

(A.M.I.E., 1992 Winter)

Solution :

The mass of sea water = mass density $\times$ volume

$$m = \rho \, v$$

Differentiating,

$$0 = \rho \, dv + v \, d\rho$$

Hence,

$$-\frac{dv}{v} = +\frac{d\rho}{\rho}$$

From Eq. 1.19, $E_v = \dfrac{p}{-dv/v}$

$$\frac{dv}{v} = -\frac{p}{E_v}$$

$$\frac{d\rho}{\rho} = \frac{\rho g d}{E_v}$$

$$= \frac{1025 \times 9.81 \times 1000}{2.35 \times 10^9}$$

$$= 4.28 \times 10^{-3}$$

∴ Change in mass density $d\rho$ at a depth of 1 km.

$$= 4.28 \times 10^{-3} \times 1025 \text{ kg/m}^3$$

$$= 4.387 \text{ kg/m}^3$$

∴ Density of sea water at a depth of 1 km.

$$= (1025 + 4.387)$$

$$= 1029.387 \text{ kg/m}^3$$

Objective Questions

1.1 A fluid is a substance that :

    (a) always expands until it fills any container

    (b) is practically incompressible

    (c) can not be subjected to shear force

    (d) can not remain at rest under action of any shear force

    (e) has the same shear stress at a point regardless of its motion.

1.2 An ideal fluid is one which:

    (a) is compressible

    (b) is incompressible

    (c) is nonviscous and incompressible

    (d) has low viscosity and incompressible

    (e) has no surface tension and compressible.

1.3 Newton's law of viscosity is a relationship between:

    (a) pressure, intensity, velocity and viscosity

    (b) shear stress and angular deformation

    (c) pressure intensity, velocity and angular deformation

    (d) pressure, temperature and velocity

    (e) none

1.4 Apparent shear forces:

    (a) can never occur when the fluid is at rest

    (b) may occur owing to cohesion when the liquid is at rest

    (c) depend upon molecular interchange of momentum

    (d) depend upon cohesive forces

    (e) can never occur in a frictionless fluid, regardless of its motion.

1.5 Viscosity of liquids

    (a) decreases with decrease in fluid temperature

    (b) increases with decrease in fluid temperature

    (c) does not change with fluid temperature

    (d) is dependent on pressure

1.6 Viscosity of gases

    (a) decreases with decrease in temperature
    (b) increases with decrease in temperature
    (c) does not change with change in temperature
    (e) none

1.8 The dimensions of dynamic viscosity are

(a) $ML^{-1}T^{-2}$ (b) $ML^{-1}T^{-1}$

(c) MLT^{-2} (d) ML^2T^{-1} (e) None

1.9 The dimensions of kinemetic viscosity are

(a) FT/L^2 (b) M/LT (c) L^2T^2

(d) L^2/T^1 (d) L^2/T^2

1.10 Viscosity expressed in poise, is converted into SI units of viscosity by multiplication by

(a) 1/98.1 (b) 1/9.81 (c) 1/10

(d) 1/1000 (e) None

1.11 The kinematic viscosity, expressed in stokes, is converted into m²/s by multiplying by

(a) 10^{-4} (b) 10^{-2} (c) 10^4 (d) none

1.12 The pressure in a dew drop is

(a) the same at the atmospheric pressure

(b) less than atmospheric pressure

(c) more than atmospheric pressure

(d) none

1.13 The dimensions of surface tension are

(a) F (b) FL^{-1} (c) FL^{-2} (d) FL^{-3} (e) none

1.14 Printer's int is a

(a) newonian fluid

(b) non newtonian fluid

(c) ideal fluid

(d) thixotropic substance

1.15 Which of the following are newtonian fluids ?

(a) water (b) air (c) blood

(d) concentrated sugar solution (e) bentonite solution

1.16 Surface tension is a phenomenon due to

(a) cohesion

(b) viscous force

(c) adhesion between liquid and solid molecules

(d) adhesion and cohesion both

(e) none

1.17 The capillary rise or drop in a small diameter tube is

    (a) directly proportional to diameter

    (b) inversely proportional to the square of the diameter

    (c) directly proportional to surface tension and diameter

    (d) directly proportional to surface tension and inversely proportional to diameter

    (e) none

1.18 The weight of liquid that rises in a tube due to capillary rise is supported by

    (a) the atmospherric pressure

    (b) by friction on the walls of the tube

    (c) vertical component of surface tension

    (d) none

1.19 In an isothermal gas

    (a) the pressure intensity varies as the tempreature

    (b) the tempreature varies directly as the elevation

    (c) the tempreature remains constant

    (d) the heat energy remains constant

    (e) none

1.20 An adiabotic flow is one in which

    (a) the fluid temperature remains constant

    (b) the heat transfer does not take place

    (c) the pressure remains constant

    (d) none

Problems

1.1 Carbon tetra chloride has mass density 1660 kg/m^3, calculate its specific weight and specific volume.

1.2 Determine the specific volume of ethyl alcohol whose mass density is 788.45 kg/m^3

1.3 Air weighs 0.0118 kN/m^3. Find the relative density and kinematic viscosity of air if the viscosity is given as 1.78×10^{-4} poise

1.4 Calculate the velocity gradient at a distance of 0,5,10 and 15 cm if the velocity profile is a parabola with a vertex 15 cm. from the surface where the velocity is 80 cm/s. Also calculate the shear stresses at these points if the fluid at these points has a viscosity of $80 \times 10^{-2} \text{ Ns/m}^3$

1.5 If the equation of velocity profile is $u = 4\,y^{2/3}$, what are the velocity gradients at the boundary and at 75 mm and 150 mm from the boundary where u is in metre/sec and y is in metre.

1.6 A very large plate is centred in the gap of width 600 mm with different oils of unknown viscosities above and below, one viscosity is twice the other. When the plate is pulled at a velocity 300 mm/s, the resulting force on one square centimeter of the plate due to viscous shear on both sides is 3 N. Assuming viscous flow and neglecting all end effects, calculate the viscosities of oil.

1.7 Through a very narrow gap of height 'h' a thin plate of very large extent is being pulled at constant velocity U. On one side of the plate is oil of viscosity μ and on other side of plate is oil of viscosity $k\mu$. Calculate the position of the plate so that the drag force on it will be a minimum.

1.8 Castor oil at 20°C fills the space between two concentric cylinders 250 mm high and with diameters of 150 mm and 155 mm. What torque is required to rotate the inner cylinder at 12 rpm, the outer cylinder remaining stationary ?

1.9 A torque of 5 Nm is required to rotate intermediate cylinder situated between two cylinder of radius 25 cm and 25.5 cm, at 30 rpm. Calculate the viscosity of oil. All cylinders are 45 cm high. Neglect end effects.

1.10 A vertical gap 2.5 cm wide of infinite extent contains oil of specific gravity 0.95, viscosity 2.5 N s/m². A metal plate 1.5 m x 0.15 m weighing 50 N is to be lifted through the gap at a constant speed of 0.1 m/s. Estimate the force requried to lift the plate.

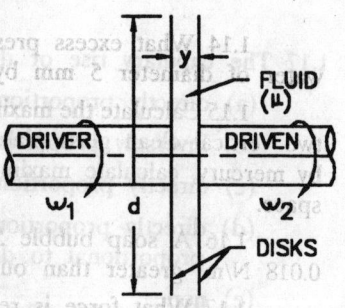

FIG. 1.21. PROBLEM 1.11

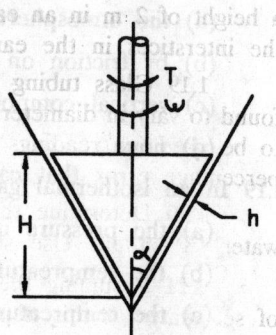

FIG. 1.22. PROBLEM 1.12

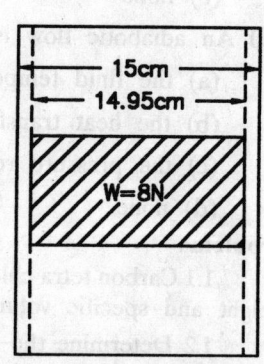

FIG. 1.23. PROBLEM 1.13

1.11 A fluid drive shown (Fig.1.26) transmits a tarque for stredy state condition (ω_1 and ω_2 constant). Derive an expression for the slip ($\omega_1 - \omega_2$) in terms of T, μ, d and h.

1.12 Oil of viscosity μ fills the gap, which is very small.Calculate the torque T required to rotate the cone at constant speed w (Fig.1.12)

1.13 Calculate the approxite viscosity of oil. The weight falls at a constant velocity of 4 cm/s (Fig.1.23) Height of piston 0.15 m.

1.14 What excess pressure may be caused within a cylindrical jet of water of diameter 5 mm by surface tension ?

1.15 Calculate the maximum capillary rise of water to be expected between two vertical clean glass plates spaced 1 mm apart. If the water is replaced by mercury, calculate maximum capillary depression of mercury in the same space.

1.16 A soap bubble 50 mm diameter contains an inside pressure of 0.018 N/m^2 greater than outside, calculate the tension in the soap film.

1.17 What force is required to lift a thin wire ring 25 mm diameter from a water surface at 20°C. ? Neglect the weight of the ring.

1.18 It is found that water at 4°C rises throught capillary action to a height of 2 m in an earth dike. To what diameter of uniform tube would the interstices in the earth correspond ?

1.19 Glass tubing to be used in a differential U tube manometer is found to vary in diameter between 6.25 mm and 7.5 mm. Assuming that gauge to be used for readings from 50 mm to 400 mm water head, estimate the percentage error that can occur.

1.20 Determine the velocity of sound at 20°C and 101.2 kPa. in (i) water (ii) in air. Use suitable values of ρ and E_vC

1.21 Assuming the depth of sea to be 11 km, find the mass density of sea water at this depth if its specific gravity at sea level is 1.026. Take a constant value of $E_v = 2.113 \times 10^9$ kPa.

2

Fluid Statics

SECTION I : PRESSURE INTENSITY AND ITS MEASUREMENT

2.1 INTRODUCTION

Fluid statics is the study of fluid problems in which there is no relative motion between fluid elements and thus velocity gradient du/dy = 0

Pressure intensity or pressure is defined as the force acting on unit area. If total force F acts uniformly on an area A, then

$$p = \frac{F}{A}$$

If the pressure intensity varies from point to point, then pressure intensity p may be defined as

$$p = \underset{\Delta A \to 0}{Lim} \frac{\Delta F}{\Delta A} \qquad ...(2.1)$$

where ΔF is the force acting on an elementary area dA. The unit of pressure intensity is N/m^2 or Pa (=Pascal).

The pressure always acts normal to the surface of the area. This statement can be proved as follows.

Let force F acts on an elementary area dA at an angle θ to the normal to the area. The force F can be resolved into two components - one tangential to the area dA and another normal to it. However, it is known that the force tangential to the area, i.e. shear force

$$F = \tau A = \frac{\mu \, du}{dy} \times A$$

is zero as there is no relative motion between two fluid elements. Therefore, only normal component of ΔF exists (Fig. 2.1a). Thus, one may conclude that pressure always acts normal to the surface. It must be remembered that since fluid is at rest, it is immaterial whether the fluid is ideal or real.

2.2 PASCAL'S LAW :

The pressure acting at a point in a fluid at rest has the same magnitude in all directions.

Consider a molecule at a point p (x,y) in fluid at rest. For mathematical analysis, let us consider the magnified shape of fluid molecule as a small wedge shaped body ABC of size dx and dy in X and Y directions respectively. Let its' length in longitudinal directions (normal to the plane of paper) be 1 metre (2-D body).

Since the fluid is at rest, the forces acting on it are (i) pressure forces px, py and ps acting normally on faces, AB, BC and AC of unit width respectively and (ii) the weight of fluid in the molecule w dx dy/2 x 1 acting vertically downward through its C.G.

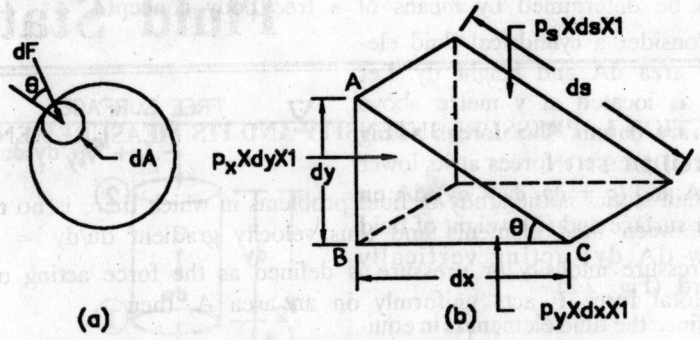

FIG. 2.1 FORCES ACTING ON A FLUID ELEMENT

For equilibrium, $\Sigma F_x = 0$, $\Sigma F_y = 0$

Resolving the forces in x-direction,

$$p_x \times dy \times 1 - ps \times ds \times 1 \times \sin \theta = 0$$

From Fig. 2.1, $\sin \theta = dy/ds$

$$p_x \, dy \times 1 - ps \times dy \times 1 = 0$$

$$p_x = ps \qquad \qquad \ldots(2.2)$$

Similarly, resolving forces in Y-direction,

$$p_y \times dx \times 1 - ps \times ds \times \cos \theta - w \frac{dx \, dy}{2} \times 1 = 0$$

From Fig. 2.1, $\cos \theta = dx/ds$

$$py \times dx \times 1 - ps \times dx \times 1 - \frac{w \, dx \, dy}{2} \times 1 = 0$$

The last term is the product of two small quantities dx and dy which will be quite small and can be neglected.

$$py = ps \qquad \qquad \ldots(2.3)$$

Therefore, from Eqs. 2.2 and 2.3,

$$px = py = ps \qquad \qquad \ldots(2.4)$$

This proves that the pressure acting at a point in the fluid at rest has the same magnitude in X, Y and S directions. The inclination of surface AC (= ds) with horizontal is chosen arbitrarily. Thus, one can conclude that pressure at a point has same magnitude in all directions and this result holds good at all points in the fluid.

Although this proof has been carried out for a two dimensional body, it may be proved for three dimensional body also by taking a tetrahydron of fluid with three faces in three co-ordinate axes and four faces inclined arbitrarily.

2.3. VARIATION OF PRESSURE WITH ELEVATION IN A FLUID :

The variation in pressure from point to point in a fluid which is at rest can be determined by means of a free body concept.

Consider a cylindrical fluid element of area dA and height dy. Let its base is ·located at y metre above an arbitrary datum. The forces acting on it are (i) pressure forces at its lower face p.dA and $(p + \partial p/\partial y \times dy)$ dA on its upper surface and (ii) weight of fluid w (= w dA dy) acting vertically downward (Fig. 2.2)

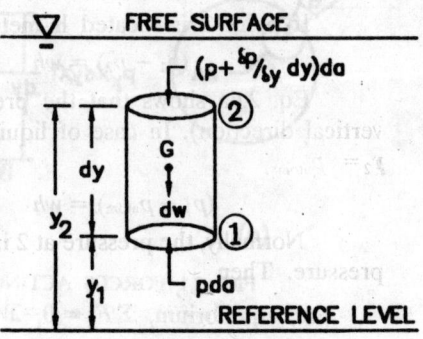

FIG. 2.2 PRESSURE VARIATION WITH ELEVATION

Since the fluid element is in equilibrium,

$$\Sigma F_x = 0, \ \Sigma F_y = 0$$

The cylindrical fluid element is symmetrical, the pressure forces acting on it in the horizontal direction will balance, i.e.

$$\Sigma F_x = 0$$

Resolving the forces in the vertical direction,

$$pdA - \left(p + \frac{\partial p}{\partial y} dy\right) dA - w \, dA \, dy = 0$$

Simplifying,

$$dp = -w \, dy \qquad \qquad ...(2.5)$$

The partial differentials are reduced to exact differentials since p can vary only in vertical direction (Y - direction). Eq. 2.5 is a general equation of fluid statics and indicates that pressure in a fluid at rest increases in downward direction at the rate of specific weight of fluid. It should be noted that p and y are of opposite nature or sign.

If dy = 0, it is a horizontal plane, then

$$dp = 0.$$

which proves that the pressure remains constant on a horizontal plane.

Eq. 2.5 can be integrated to obtain the variation of p with y if specific mass (or specific weight w) remains constant with elevation as in case of incompressible fluid. For compressible fluid, mass density varies with elevations as in meteorology, ocean, etc. Hence a relationship between mass density and pressure p is needed to integrate Eq. 2.5.

1. Pressure variation in an incompressible fluid.

For incompressible fluid, the mass density remains constant, hence Eq. 2.5 can be integrated . Let point 1 be located at a height y_1 and point 2 at y_2 above the datum. Integrating, Eq. 2.5

2.3. VARIATION OF PRESSURE WITH ELEVATION IN A FLUID :

$$\int_{p_1}^{p_2} dp = \int_{y_1}^{y_2} -\rho g \, dy$$

$$(p_2 - p_1) = -\rho g (y_2 - y_1) = -w (y_2 - y_1)$$

$$(p_1 - p_2) = w (y_2 - y_1)$$

If point 2 is located h metre above point 1, $(y_2 - y_1) = $ h(say) then,

$$(p_1 - p_2) = wh \qquad ...(2.6a)$$

Eq. 2.6a shows that the pressure varies linearly with elevation (in the vertical direction). In case of liquids, point 2 may be located at free surface, $p_2 = p_{atom}$.

$$(p_1 - p_{atom}) = wh \qquad ...(2.6 \text{ b})$$

Normally, the pressure at 2 i.e. atmospheric pressure is taken as reference pressure. Then

$$p_1 = p = wh \qquad ...(2.6c)$$

The unit for pressure intensity is N/m^2 or Pa (Pascal)

Eq. 2.6c is also written as

$$h = \frac{p}{w}$$

Hence, the pressure is also expressed in terms of liquid column or height h metre (or head) whose specific weight is w N/m^3.

2. Pressure variation in compressible fluid.

Case I : Isothermal Process :

In this process the temperature of fluid remains constant. Such a condition may be assumed to exist for a small height of atmosphere. For a perfect gas with constant temperature or isothermal process, Boyle's law is applicable and relates pressure p of a given fluid with specific volume v. If po and vo are its initial condition at some reference level (for example at earth surface, y = 0, these conditions may refer to atmospheric conditions),

$$pv = p_0 v_0 \qquad ...(2.7a)$$

$$\frac{p}{\rho} = \frac{p_0}{\rho_0} \qquad ...(2.7b)$$

$$\text{Since} \quad v = \frac{1}{\rho}$$

Substituting in Eq. 2.5

$$dp = -wdy = -\rho g \, dy$$

$$= -\frac{\rho_0 p}{p_0} \cdot g \, dy$$

$$\frac{p_0}{\rho_0} \frac{dp}{p} = -g \, dy$$

Integrating with respect to y,

$$\frac{p_0}{\rho_0} \log_e p = -gy + C$$

At reference datum (earth surface), $y = y_0 = 0$, $p = p_{atm} = p_0$

$$C = \frac{p_0}{\rho_0} \log_e p_0 \qquad \qquad ...(2.9)$$

Substituting for C,

$$\frac{p_0}{\rho_0} \log_e (p/p_0) = -gy$$

$$\log_e (p/p_0) = -\frac{gy}{p_0/\rho_0} \qquad \qquad ...(2.10)$$

For a perfect gas,

$$\frac{p_0}{\rho_0} = RT_0 \qquad \qquad ...(2.11)$$

Substituting for p_0/ρ_0,

$$\log_e (p/p_0) = -\frac{gy}{RT_0}$$

$$p = p_0 e^{-gy/RT_0} \qquad \qquad ...(2.12)$$

Eq. 2.12 gives the variation of p with elevation y measured above earth surface. For small value of gy/RT_o, the expression reduces to $p = p_o$ as for liquids of constant mass density.

Case II : Polytropic process or Isentropic process

(i) pressure variation :

For polytropic or isentropic process the relationship between pressure p and mass density is

$$\frac{p}{\rho^n} = \frac{p_0}{\rho_0^n} = C \qquad \qquad ...(2.13a)$$

In this equation C is a constant and n is an index.

For adiabatic process, n = k = cp/cv = ratio of specific heat of gases at constant pressure to specific heat at constant volume.

$$\frac{p}{\rho^n} = \frac{p_0}{\rho_0^n} = C \qquad \qquad ...(2.13b)$$

From Eq.2.13 a,

$$\rho = \rho_0 (p/p_0)^{1/n} \qquad \qquad ...(2.13b)$$

Substituting the value of in Eq. 2.5

$$dp = -\rho g \, dy$$

$$= -\rho_0 (p/p_0)^{1/n} g \, dy$$

$$dy = -\frac{1}{\rho_0 g} \frac{p_0^{1/n}}{p^{1/n}} dp$$

Integrating it from y to y_0 and assuming g to be constant,

$$\int_{y_0}^{y} dy = -\frac{p_0^{1/n}}{\rho_0 g} \int_{p}^{p_0} \frac{dp}{p^{1/n}}$$

$$(y - y_0) = -\frac{p_0^{1/n}}{\rho_0 g} \left[\frac{p^{-1/n+1}}{-1/n+1} \right]_{p}^{p_0}$$

$$(y - y_0) = \frac{p_0^{1/n}}{\rho_0 g} \frac{n}{(n-1)} \left[p_0^{(n-1)/n} - p^{(n-1/n)} \right]$$

$$= \frac{n}{n-1} \cdot \frac{p_0}{\rho_0 g} \left[1 - (p/p_0)^{n-1)/n} \right]$$

Simplifying,

$$(p/p_0)^{(n-1)/n} = \left[1 - \frac{n-1}{n} \cdot \frac{\rho_0 g}{p_0} \cdot (y - y_0) \right] \qquad ...(2.14a)$$

$$(p/p_0) = \left[1 - \frac{n-1}{n} \cdot \frac{\rho_0 g}{p_0} \cdot \Delta y \right]^{n/(n-1)} \qquad ...(2.14a)$$

For a perfect gas, from Eq. 2.11, $\dfrac{p_0}{\rho_0} = RT_0$

$$(p/p_0) = \left[1 - \frac{n-1}{n} \cdot \frac{g \Delta y}{RT_0} \right]^{n/(n-1)} \qquad ...(2.14b)$$

Here, $\Delta y = (y - y_0)$ which is the height in metre of any point y metre above earth surface (i.e. reference surface)

(ii) **Mass density variation :**

From Eq. 2.13 a,

$$\left(\frac{\rho}{\rho_0} \right) = \left(\frac{p}{p_0} \right)^{1/n}$$

Substituting the value of (p/p_0) from Eq. 2.14a,

$$\frac{\rho}{\rho_0} = \left[1 - \frac{n-1}{n} \cdot \frac{g \cdot \Delta y}{p_0/\rho_0} \right]^{1/(n-1)} \qquad ...(2.15a)$$

$$= \left[1 - \frac{n-1}{n} \cdot \frac{g \cdot \Delta y}{R T_0} \right]^{1/(n-1)} \qquad ...(2.15b)$$

(iii) **Temperature variation :** In problems of meteorology and aviation, one must know the relationship for air among pressure, specific weight, temperature and elevation. It is known that in the lower atmosphere known as troposphere, the temperature of air decreases linearly with altitude at an average rate of $0.0065°$ C per metre to $-70°$ C at an altitude of 11 km. Thereafter, for a considerable elevation (≈ 30 km), the temperature remains constant at $-70°C$. This upper region of constant temperature is known as stratosphere. From thermodynamic considerations the process is polytropic in the lower layer (troposphere) with index n = 1.235 and isothermal in the upper layer (stratosphere).

Lapse Rate : It is defined as the rate of variation of temperature and can be computed by Eq. 2.16b.

The equation of state for a gas is

$$\frac{p}{\rho} = RT \qquad \qquad ...(2.11a)$$

At the reference datum (say earth surface), the pressure is p_o, specific mass ρ_0, temperature T_o and R is the universal constant for gas.

$$\frac{p_0}{\rho_0} = RT_0 \qquad \qquad ...(2.11b)$$

Dividing Eq. 2.11a by 2.11b,

$$\frac{p}{p_0} \frac{\rho_0}{\rho} = \frac{T}{T_0}$$

Substituting for p/p_0 and ρ/ρ_0 from Eqs. 2.14b and 2.15b :

$$\frac{T}{T_0} = \left[1 - \frac{n-1}{n} \cdot \frac{g \Delta y}{R T_0} \right] = \left[1 - \frac{n-1}{n} \frac{g(y - y_0)}{RT_0} \right] \qquad ...(2.16a)$$

Differentiating w.r. to y

$$\frac{1}{T_0} \frac{dT}{dy} = - \frac{n-1}{n} \frac{g}{R T_0}$$

∴ Therefore, Temperature Lapse Rate $\dfrac{dT}{dy} = \dfrac{n-1}{n} \dfrac{g}{R}$ ...(2.16b)

(i) For n = 1, the process is isothermal and lapse rate is zero or temperature is constant.

(ii) For n > 1, the process is polytropic and lapse rate is negative or temperaature decreases with altitude.

(iii) Standard atmosphere : The value of standard atmosphere at mean sea level corresponds to $15°$ C temperature; 101.325 kN/m² (1 bar or 10^5 N/m²) pressure and 1.227 kg/m³ as mean mass density of atmospheric air.

2.4 MEASUREMENTS OF FLUID PRESSURE :

1. Absolute and Gauge Pressure

The atmospheric air exerts a normal pressure upon all surfaces with which it is in contact and is known as "atmospheric pressure". The atmospheric pressure varies with altitude and can be measured by means of a barometer. At mean sea level under normal conditions, the equivalent value of atmospheric pressure is 1 bar ($= 10^5$ N/m^2) which can be converted into 76 cm. of mercury or 10.3 m of column of water or 1.03 kgf/cm^2.

The fluid pressure at a point is to be measured with reference to some standard known pressure. The two most common reference datum are : (i) absolutely zero pressure (or complete vacuum), and (ii) local atmospheric pressure.

When the pressure is measured above absolute zero pressure, it is called "absolute pressure". (Pressure at A in Fig. 2.3). If it is measured above or below local atmospheric pressure, it is known as ."gauge pressure". If the pressure at a point is less than local atmospheric pressure, it is as known as "negative gauge pressure" or "vacuum pressure" or "suction pressure" and its gauge value is the amount by which it is below atmospheric pressure (Pressure at B, Fig. 2.3). It should be noted that there cannot be negative absolute pressure (as this will mean tension at a point which is considered impossible in any fluid). Gauge pressures are positive, if they are more than local atmospheric pressure. The relationship between local atmospheric pressure, absolute and gauge pressure can be obtained from Fig. 2.3.

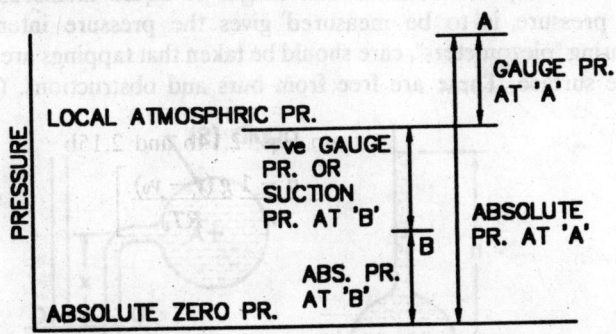

FIG. 2.3. RELATIONSHIP BETWEEN GAUGE AND ABSOLUTE PRESSURE

(i) Absolute pressure at Point A
  = [local atmospheric pressure + gauge pressure at A]

(ii) Absolute pressure at Point B
  = [local atmospheric pressure - gauge pressure at B]

2. Measurement of Pressure :

The pressure at a point can be measured by means of either (A) Manometers or (B) pressure gauges. The first one is described below whereas the pressure gauges are described later.

(A) Manometers : These are pressure measuring devices which function on the principle of balancing the fluid pressure (at the given point) to a column of same fluid or some other fluid.

Manometer may be classified as

(a) Simple manometers and (b) Differential manometers.

(a) Simple manometers are used to measure the pressure at a given point. These may be

    (i) Piezometric tube and

    (ii) U-tube manometer as shown in Fig. 2.4.

(b) Differential manometers are used to measure the differences of pressures between two points or sections. These may be :

    (i) Two tube piezometers

    (ii) U-tube differential manometer (Fig. 2.7)

    (iii) Inverted U-tube manometer (Fig. 2.7)

Most of the problems of manometers can be solved by a simple procedure given below. Besides these, micro manometers are used for accurate measurement of differential pressure (Fig. 2.8).

1. Simple manometers :

    (i) Piezometer : The simplest device for measuring fluid pressure is called "piezometer". It is a glass tube mounted vertically at the required point so that liquid rises up in the tube. The height of liquid meniscus from the point where pressure is to be measured gives the pressure intensity. (Fig. 2.4a). While using "piezometers", care should be taken that tappings are absolutely normal to the surface. These are free from burs and obstructions. (since flow

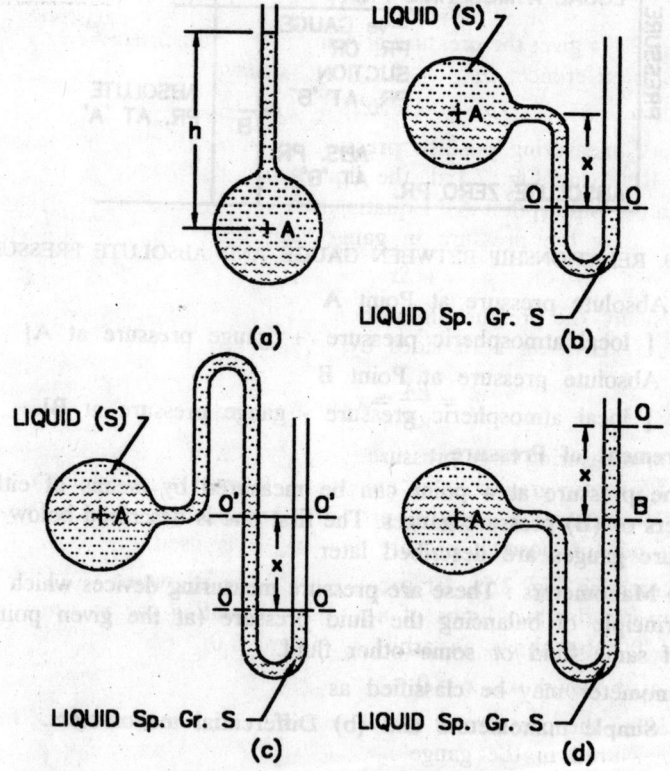

FIG. 2.4. SIMPLE MANOMETERS

around obstructions causes velocity variation and consequently pressure head reduces) and are of proper size (not more than 3 mm size for small diameter pipes and not more than 6 mm for large diameter pipes.).

The limitations of piezometer tubes are :

(i) it would not work for negative gauge pressure, and

(ii) it is impossible to measure large pressures at any point since this would need very long vertical tubes.

(ii) U-tube manometer : For measuring small gage pressures, positive or negative, various forms of U-tube manometers are used. The difference in the levels of liquid columns in the two limbs of a U-tube is the measure of the unknown pressure, Fig. 2.4b to 2.4d (if the same fluid is used). Sometimes, a different liquid of sp.gr. S_m is used in the U-tube, then one has to write down the manometer equation and solve it to determine unknown pressure.

For measuring small negative pressure, the arrangement in Fig. 2.4 b or 2.4 c is used. Referring Fig. 2.4 b and 2.4 c, the liquid of sp.gr. S is contained in the pipe. Let the pressure at A be p_A and the liquid column stands x metre below pipe centre line. Take a horizontal reference datum as 0–0. Equating the pressure in the two limbs of the U-tube above 0–0.

$$p_A + wS\,x = p_{atm}$$

$$p_A = p_{atm} - wSx \qquad ...(2.17a)$$

Eq. 2.17a gives the pressure at A in absolute units. If atmospheric pressure is taken as reference, $p_{atm} = 0$.

Then, $\qquad p_A = -w\,Sx \qquad ...(2.17b)$

For measuring positive pressure at A, the arrangement in Fig. 2.4d is used. Referring Fig. 2.4 d, the liquid column rises to C by x above the centre line of pipe (point A). Equating the pressure in the two limbs of U-tube and expressing the pressure in gauge $(p_{atm} = 0)$.

$$p_A = w\,Sx \qquad ...(2.18a)$$

Usually, the pressure intensity is expressed in terms of head h, of liquid of sp.gr. S. Dividing both sides by $w\,S$,

$$h = \frac{p_A}{wS} = x \text{ metre} \qquad ...(2.18b)$$

For measuring large pressure (gauge), both positive and negative, another liquid of specific gravity S_m is employed. It must be immiscible in the first liquid. For measuring negative pressure, arrangement in Fig. 2.5a and 2.5b is used and for positive presure Fig. 2.5 c is used.

Referring Fig. 2.5a, let pressure at A be p_A which causes a deflection of x between the two limbs of a U-tube. Equating the pressure in the two limbs of U-tube above an arbitrary datum 0-0.

$$p_A + wSy + wS_m x = 0$$

Since the pressure at the open end is atmospheric which for pressure to be measured in the gauge system, is assumed zero, i.e. $p_{atm} = 0$.

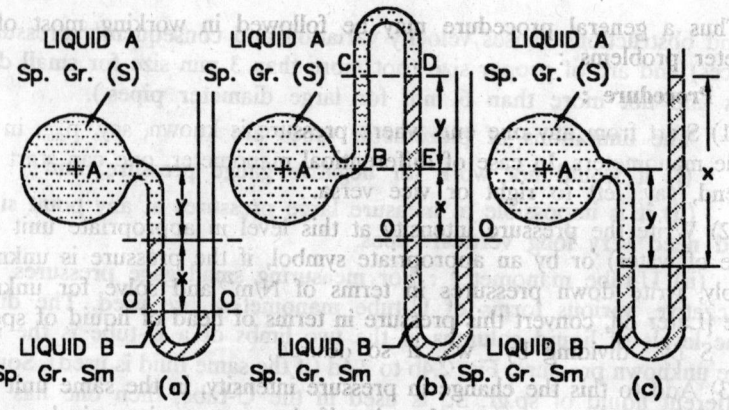

FIG. 2.5 : SIMPLE MANOMETERS FOR MEASURING LARGE PRESSURE

$$\therefore \qquad p_A = -w(Sy + S_m x) \qquad\qquad ...(2.19)$$

In Fig. 2.5b, another arrangement is shown to measure negative pressure so that liquid of sp.gr. S_m does not enter the pipe line during its operation.

Let the pressure at 'A' be p_A, then pressure at C will be lower than at A by w S y. And the pressure at D is same as at C, i.e.

$$p_c = p_A - wS\,y = p_D$$

and pressure p_E at E will be more than p_D by w S_{mx}. Here x is the deflection of liquid (sp.gr. Sm) between the two limbs of U-tube.

$$\therefore \qquad p_E = p_D + w\,Sm\,x$$
$$p_E = p_A - w\,S\,y + w\,S_m\,x$$

Equating the pressure in the two limbs above a horizontal datam 0-0,

$$p_A - w\,S\,y + w\,S_m\,x = p_{atm} = 0 \ (gauge\ system)$$
$$p_A = w\,(S_m\,x - Sy) \qquad\qquad ...(2.20a)$$

Alternatively, the pressure head h in terms of height of liquid column of sp.gr. S is,

$$h = \frac{p_A}{wS} = -\left(\frac{S_m}{S}x - y\right) \qquad\qquad ...(2.20b)$$

For positive pressure measurement, refer Fig. 2.5 c. Equating the pressure in the two limbs above horizontal datum 0-0,

$$p_A + w\,S\,y = w\,S_m\,x$$
$$p_A = w\,(S_m\,x - Sy) \qquad\qquad ...(2.21a)$$

In terms of pressure head h of liquid flowing in the pipe line (or container),

$$h = \frac{p_A}{wS} = \left(\frac{S_m}{S}x - y\right) \qquad\qquad ...(2.21b)$$

Thus a general procedure may be followed in working most of the manometer problems :

General Procedure :

(1) Start from any one end where pressure is known, say, p_{atm}, in case of simple manometers. In case of differentioal manometer, one can start from either end, say, left to right or vice versa.

(2) Write the pressure intensity at this level in appropriate unit (say,. in metre of water) or by an appropriate symbol, if the pressure is unknown. Preferably, write down pressures in terms of N/m^2 and solve for unknown pressure [Later on, convert this pressure in terms of head of liquid of specific gravity S by dividing by wS, if so desired,

(3) Add to this the change in pressure intensity, in the same unit from one meniscus to the next; use plus sign if the next meniscus is lower and minus if the next meniscus is higher.

(4) Continue until the other end of gauge is reached and equate the expression to the pressure at that point, known or unknown.

(5) Solve this equation for unknown quantity.

Refer next section and solved examples for the use of this method.

(iii) Single Tube Manometer :

The U-Tube manometers require readings of fluid levels in both the limbs, since a change in pressure will cause the rise of fluid in one limb and drop in the other limb. This demerit of U- tube manometer can be overcome by using single tube manometer which is a modified form of U-tube manometer. It consists of a reservoir of large area being connected on one of the limb of manometer (Fig. 2.6a). The area of cross section of reservoir is about 100 times larger as compared to the tube of manometer.

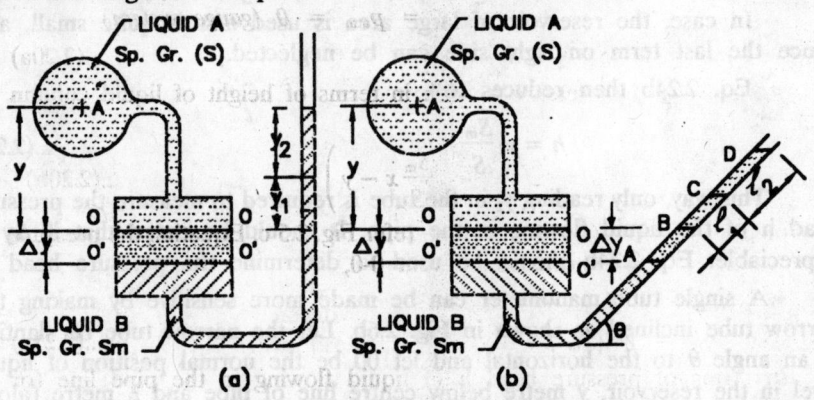

FIG. 2.6. SENSITIVE MANOMETER

The main advantage of such an arrangement is that for any change in pressure, the change in liquid level in the reservoir will be small and can be neglected. Therefore, the change in pressure is indicated by the rise of liquid column in the other limb.

When the manometer is not connected, the liquid level in the reservoir is at 0-0, i.e. y metre below the centre line of pipe and y_1 metre above 0-0 in the other limb. Fig. 2.6a. It is known as normal position of manometric liquids.,

$$Sy = S_m y_1 \qquad \ldots(2.22)$$

where S is the specific gravity of liquid in the pipe and S_m is the specific gravity of the measuring liquid. When the manometer is connected, the high pressure liquid in the pipe will enter reservoir. The liquid level in the reservoir will drop to 0'0' by Δy below 0-0 and will rise by y_2 metre above 0-0. i.e. it will stand $(y_1 + y_2)$ metre above 00 in the tube. Let the area of cross section of reservoir be A and that of tube be a. Then

$$A . \Delta y = a y_2 \qquad \ldots(2.23)$$

Use the procedure outlined above and take new reference level 0'0'. Start from open end where pressure is atmospheric (or $p_{atm} = 0$).

$$\therefore \ 0 + w \, S_m \, (y_1 + y_2 + \Delta y) - w \, S \, \Delta y - w \, S \, y = p_A$$

Substituting the values of y and Δy from Eq. 2.22 and 2.23.

$$p_A = w \, S_m \left(y_1 + y_2 + \left(\frac{a}{A} y_2 \right) \right) - wS \left(\frac{a}{A} y_2 \right) - w \left(S_m y_1 \right)$$

$$\ldots(2.24a)$$

For expressing it in terms of head of liquid h, flowing in pipe (sp.gr. S), divide by w S on both sides and solve,

$$\frac{p_A}{wS} = \left[\frac{S_m}{S} (y_2 + \frac{a}{A} y_2) - \frac{a}{A} y_2 \right]$$

$$h = y_2 \left[\frac{S_m}{S} + \left(\frac{S_m}{S} - 1 \right) \frac{a}{A} \right] \qquad \ldots(2.24b)$$

In case, the reservoir of large area is used a/A is quite small, and hence the last term on right side can be neglected.

Eq. 2.24b then reduces to

$$h = y_2 \frac{S_m}{S} \qquad \ldots(2.25)$$

This way, only reading y_2 in the tube is required to measure the pressure head h of the liquid flowing in the pipe. It should be noted that if Δy is appreciable. Eq. 2.24b should be used to determine the pressure head h.

A single tube manometer can be made more sensitive by making the narrow tube inclined as shown in Fig. 2.6b. Let the narrow tube be slanting at an angle θ to the horizontal and let 00 be the normal position of liquid level in the reservoir, y metre below centre line of pipe and l_1 metre (along the tube) in the narrow tube, such that,

$$y S = S_m l_1 \sin \theta \qquad \ldots(2.26)$$

On being connected to the pipe, liquid level in the reservoir drops by Δy to 0'0' and rises in the narrow tube by l_2 along the tube i.e. it stands at $l_1 + l_2$ metre above 00, then

$$A\,(\Delta y) = a\,(l_2) \qquad\qquad ...(2.27)$$

Write manometric equation, starting from open end D,

$$0 + w\,S_m\,l_2 \sin\theta + w\,S_m\,l_1 \sin\theta + w\,\Delta y\,S_m - wS\,\Delta y - wS\,y = p_A \qquad ...(2.28a)$$

Solving for pressure head h, using Eq.2.26 & 2.27,

$$h = \frac{p_A}{wS} = l_2\left[\frac{S_m}{S}\sin\theta + \left(\frac{S_m}{S} - 1\right)\frac{a}{A}\right] \qquad ...(2.28b)$$

Again, if reservoir of large area A is used, a/A is quite small and hence the last term on right side can be dropped, then only one reading l_2 of narrow limb is required to be read to determine the pressure head h of the fluid in the pipe. Eq. 2.28b reduces to

$$h = \frac{S_m}{S}\,l_2 \sin\theta \qquad ...(2.29)$$

Since the tube is slanted even a small pressure head will be magnified and a sufficiently large deflection l_2 will be obtained.

2. Differential Manometers :

In many cases the difference of pressure between two points on the same pipe (or container) or between two different pipes (or containers) is to be determined. When the difference is expected to be large, U-tube manometer containing higher density fluid (e.g. mercury) is used (Fig. 2.7a). For measuring smaller difference of pressure, inverted U-tube manometer containing lighter density fluid (e.g. oil or even air) may be used (Fig. 2.7b). The measuring fluid should be immiscible with the fluid whose pressure is to be determined.

(b) Inverted U-tube manometer.

U-Tube differential manometer : Consider two pipes A and B carrying a fluid of density w S and connected by a U-tube manometer containing measuring liquid of density w S_m. The centre of B is z metre above than A (Fig. 2.7a). The pressure at A and B are p_A and p_B, respectively. In order to determine the difference of pressures between two pipes, i.e. p_A - p_B write manometric equations and solve it. Let the resultant deflection in the U-tube be x.

$$p_A + wS\,(x + y) - w\,S_m\,x - wS\,(y + z) = p_B$$

or

$$p_A - p_B - w\,S\,z = w\,S_m\,x - w\,S\,x$$

Since $z = z_2 - z_1$ = difference in the elevations of A and B above a horizontal datum.,

$$(p_A + w\,S\,z_1) - (p_B + w\,S\,z_2) = w\,x\,(S_m - S) \qquad ...(2.30a)$$

The differential head h between A and B is obtained by dividing wS on both sides.

$$\left(\frac{p_A}{wS} + z_1\right) - \left(\frac{p_B}{wS} + z_2\right) = h = x\left(\frac{S_m}{S} - 1\right) \qquad ...(2.30b)$$

Inverted U-tube manometer : Fig. 2.7b shows an inverted differential U-tube manometer connected between two points A and B on a pipe line. The pipe is carrying a fluid of density w S and inverted U-tube contains a lighter liquid of density w S_m. Usually the lighter density fluid is used as measuring fluid ($S_m < S$).

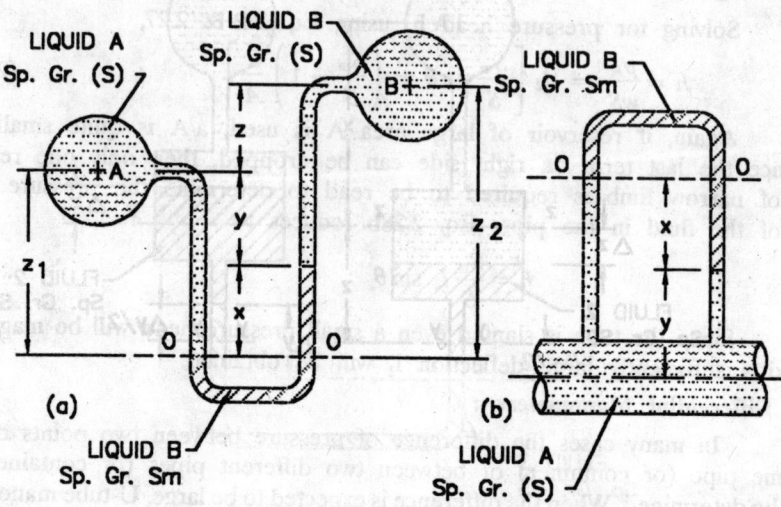

(a)

(b)

FIG. 2.7 (A) DIFFERENTIAL U–TUBE MANOMETER
(B) INVERTED U–TUBE MANOMETER

Writing manometric equation following above mentioned procedure.

$$p_A - w S (x + y) + w S_m x + w S y = p_B$$

or

$$p_A - p_B = w x (S - S_m) \qquad \ldots(2.31a)$$

Alternatively, the differential pressure head h is,

$$\left(\frac{p_A}{wS} - \frac{p_B}{wS}\right) = x \left(1 - \frac{S_m}{S}\right) \qquad \ldots(2.31b)$$

If the differential pressure ($p_A - p_B$) is expected to be small, lighter density fluid (i.e. S_m) is used. As the density of measuring fluid S_m approaches to that of the density of fluid S in the pipe, ($1 - S_m/S$) approaches zero. This means a larger deflection x is obtained (Eq. 2.31b) for small value of ($p_A - p_B$), thus increasing the sensitivity of the gauge. It is often satisfactory to use air as lighter fluid in an inverted U-tube manometer in Fig. 2.7b. As the density S_m of air is much smaller[1] ($S_m \approx 0$) than any other liquid, the pressure exerted by it can be considered to be nearly zero and can be neglected. In that case, the deflection x between two limbs of inverted U-tube directly gives the pressure difference between two sections A and B.

3. Micromanometers :

These are used for measuring very small differences in pressure intensities between two points or precise determination of large pressure differences.

---

1. If the air at very high pressure is used to measure the high pressure in A and B, S_m can not be neglected.

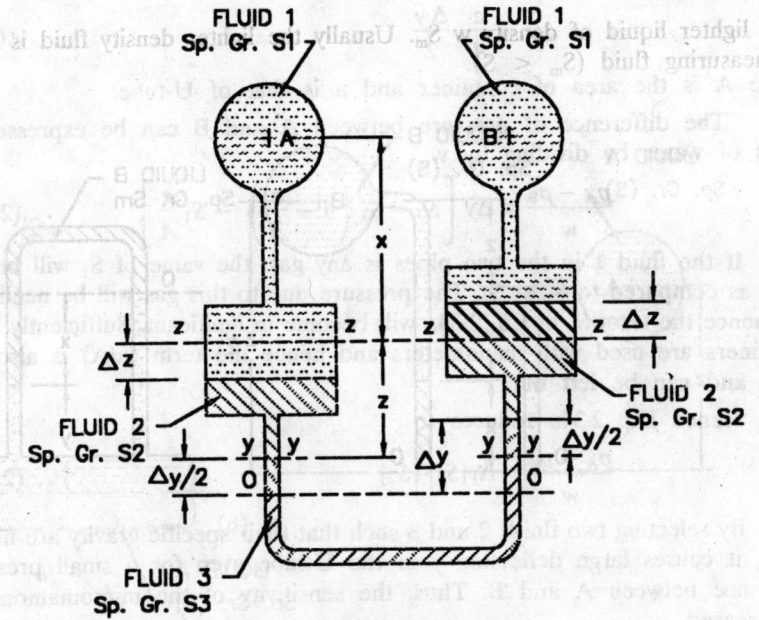

FIG. 2.8 MICRO–MANOMETER

They essentially consists of a U-tube with two large size containers connected between two points A and B. One of the many arrangements is shown in Fig. 2.8.

Two pipes A and B carry a fluid of specific gravity S_1 and a U-tube is connected to them. The U-tube contains fluid of specific gravity S_2 on the upper side and S_3 below it. In the normal condition, the fluid 2 stands at horizontal level z z in the large containers and fluid 3 at y y in the U-tube. On application of pressure at one of its end, say A, the fluid is depressed by Δz in the left container and rises by same amount in right side container. At the same time, the level of fluid 3 in the U-tube dropped by $\Delta y/2$ in the left leg of U-tube and rises by $\Delta y/2$ in the right leg. That is to say, the fluid 3 in the U-tube is deflected by Δy.

Write manometric equation starting from left side. Take 0-0 as horizontal datum.

$$p_A + wS_1(x + \Delta z) + w S_2\left(z - \Delta z + \frac{\Delta y}{2}\right)$$
$$- wS_3(\Delta y) - w S_2(z + \Delta z - \Delta y/2) - w S_1(x - \Delta z) = p_B$$

Solving, it reduces to

$$(p_A - p_B) = w[S_3 \cdot \Delta y + S_2(2\Delta z - \Delta y) - S_1(2\Delta z)] \qquad ...(2.32)$$

Under equilibrium condition, one can write the relationship

$$A \cdot \Delta z = a \cdot \Delta y/2$$

or
$$\Delta z = \frac{a}{A} \cdot \frac{\Delta y}{2} \qquad \qquad ...(2.33)$$

where A is the area of container and a is that of U-tube.

The difference of pressure between A and B can be expressed in terms of water by dividing by w.

$$\frac{p_A - p_B}{w} = \Delta y \left[S_3 - S_2 \left(1 - \frac{a}{A} \right) - S_1 \frac{a}{A} \right] \qquad ...(2.34a)$$

If the fluid 1 in the two pipes is any gas, the value of S_1 will be too small as compared to S_2 or S_3. The pressure due to this gas will be negligible and hence the term S_1 in Eq. 2.34a will become insignificant. Sufficiently large containers are used with manometers and hence the term (a/A) is also too small and can be left out.

Hence Eq. 2.34a reduces to

$$\frac{p_A - p_B}{w} = \Delta y [S_3 - S_2] \qquad \qquad ...(2.34b)$$

By selecting two fluids 2 and 3 such that their specific gravity are nearly equal, it causes large deflection y in the U-tube even for a small pressure difference between A and B. Thus, the sensitivity of the micromamometer is increased.

In another type of micromanometer, initially the meniscus is maintained at predetermined location and indicated by a mark or hairline. On application of pressures, the meniscus tends to move and is then brought to original level by the movement of one of the limb of manometere by a rotation of a screw gauge. This rotation of screw gauge is pre-calibrated and thus difference in pressure is measured.

2.5 MECHANICAL GAUGES :

These are mechanical devices used to measure high pressures. It consists of an elastic element which is deflected on the application of pressure. This deflection is then measured on a pre-calibrated scale by means of a lever system.

Mainly there are two types of pressure gauges frequently used. These are :

(i) Bourden gauge

(ii) Diaphragm gauge or aneroid barometer.

Besides these two types, another pressure gauge called "dead weight pressure gauge" is used mainly to calibrate pressure gauges.

(i) Bourden Gauge :

It consists of a mettalic bent tube of elliptical cross-section, Fig. 2.9a. The open end of this tube A is connected to the fluid for which the pressure is to be measured and end B is attached rigidly to the frame. The free end C is connected by a linkage D to a pointer E. A circular dial with graduaated scale in kN/m^2 (or Pascal) as well as in centimeters of mercury is mounted on the top of gauge.

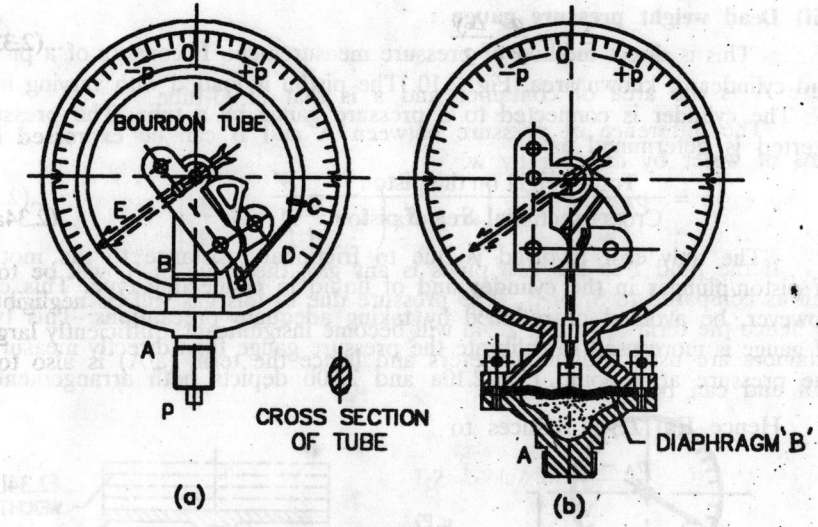

FIG. 2.9. (A) BOURDON TUBE PRESSURE GAUGE
(B) DIAPHRAGM PRESSURE GAUGE

In the properly adjusted position while the gauge is not connected to any point, the printer reads zero on the dial. When the gauge is connected to a high pressure fluid, the mettalic tube expands and its cross section tends to be circular. This deflection makes the linkage to move the needle on the scale. If the pressure measured happens to be more than local atmospheric pressure, the pointer moves to the right and pressure is generally measured in kN/m^2 or pascal on the scale. If the pressure is less than local atmospheric pressure, the pointer moves to the left and the pressure is measured in centimeter of mercury. It is to be noted that since the local atmospheric pressure acts outside the tube, the gauge measures the difference of pressure inside and outside the tube. Thus, the local atmospheric pressure and not the standard atmospheric pressure is used as reference pressure in the gauge system of measurement.

(ii) Diaphragm pressure gauge :

It essentially consists of a short cylinder A which is covered with a corrugated diaphragm B, instead of the Bourden tube (Fig. 2.9b). Elastic deformation of the diaphragm under pressure is transmitted by a similar arrangement to the pointer needle. This type of gauge is used to measure relatively low pressures. The instrument should be calibrated before its use.

The Aneroid barometer operates on this principle. It consists of cylinder A covered with diaphragm. All the air from this cylinder is evacuated and so the pressure remains zero. The pressure imposed over the diaphragm B outside is higher which is to be measured.

This pressure deflects the diaphragm and, in turn, moves the pointer needle on the graduated scale. Thus, the pressure in absolute system is found.

(iii) Dead weight pressure gauge :

This is direct method of pressure measurement. It consists of a piston and cylinder of known area. Fig. 2.10. The piston is loaded with varying load W. The cylinder is connected to a pressure gauge by a tube. The pressure exerted is determined as

$$p = \frac{\text{Total weight on the piston}}{\text{Cross-sectional area of piston}} = \frac{W}{A} \qquad ...(2.35)$$

The only eror involved is due to frictional resistance to the motion of piston/plunger in the cylinder and of liquid in connecting type. This can, however, be avoided or reduced by taking adequate precautions. This type of gauge is more used to calibrate the pressure gauge than directly measuring the pressure at a point. Fig. 2.10a and 2.10b depicts both arrangements.

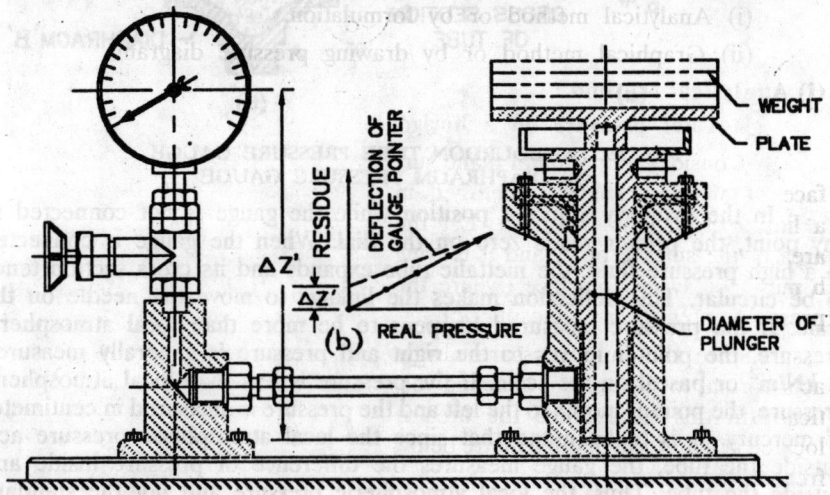

FIG. 2.10. DEAD WEIGHT PRESSURE GAUGE AND CALIBRATION INSTRUMENT

(iv) Barometer :

The absolute pressure of atmosphere at any place (local atmospheric pressure) is measured by mercury manometer (invented by Torricelli in 1643). It consists of a glass tube filled with mercury with its one end closed. It is inverted with its open end beneath the mercury surface in the receptacle, Fig. 2.11. The mercury columns in the tube will stand to a height h above mercury surface in the receptacle which is indicative of the local atmospheric pressure; the space above AB contains the vapour of the fluid.

The pressure exerted by these vapour should be as small as possible so as to correspond to absolute zero (above level AB).

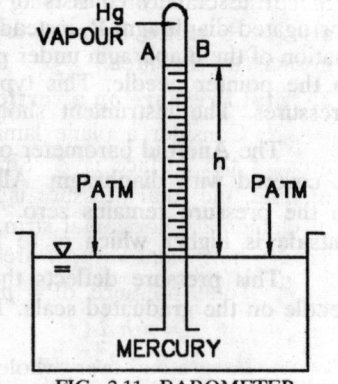

FIG. 2.11. BAROMETER

Mercury is generally preferred as manometric fluid. It additionally offers another advantage - being of higher density, a reasonably short tube is needed. Barometric reading varies with the location of the place as well as with temperature. The standard atmospheric pressure at 50° latitude and at mean sea level is taken as 760 mm of mercury column or 1 bar which is equal to 100 kPa.

SECTION II·; TOTAL PRESSURE AND ITS LOCATION

2.6 HYDROSTATIC FORCE ON PLANE SURFACES :

In the preceding sections the variation of pressure intensity throughout a fluid at rest has been considered. In this section the calculation of the magnitude, direction and location of the total pressure due to fluid pressure on submerged plane surface will be made.

There are two methods to compute the total pressure and its location.

(i) Analytical method or by formulation.

(ii) Graphical method or by drawing pressure diagram.

(i) Analytical Method :

1. Total pressure on a horizontal plane surface :

Consider a horizontal plane surface of arbitrary shape submerged in a liquid of specific weight w. Let the area of the surface be A and it is lying h metre below free surface (where the pressure intensity is atmospheric).

Since the fluid pressure always acts normal to the area; it is acting vertically in this case. Since the area is located at a uniform depth h metre below free surface, 0–0.

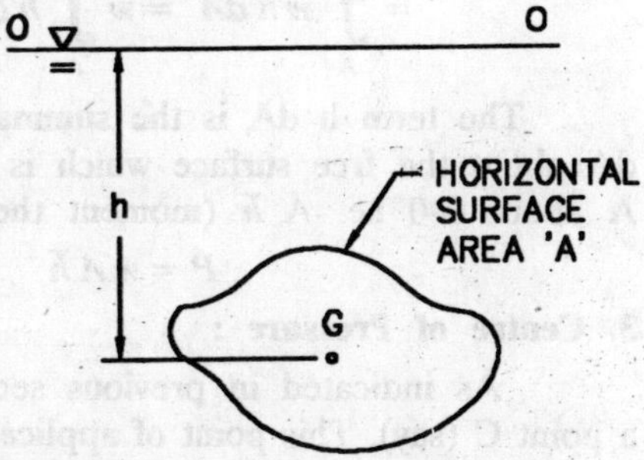

$$P = pA$$

$$P = whA$$

FIG. 2.12. A HORIZONTAL PLANE SUR-
FACE IMMERSED IN FLUID
...(2.36)

The total pressure P acts through a point C called "centre of pressure". Since the plane area is lying at a uniform depth, the centre of pressure will also be h metre below 0–0. The direction of this force is downward and normal to the area.

2. Total Pressure on a vertical plane surface :

Consider a plane lamina of any shape lying vertically in a fluid. The area of the surface is A. Since the pressure intensity varies with the depth of fluid, the total pressure is computed as the sum of total pressure on each of elementary horizontal strip of the area dA.

Take a horizontal strip of area dA at a depth h below free surface O-O.

Total pressure $dP = p \times dA$

$$= w h \, dA$$

Integrating over whole area,

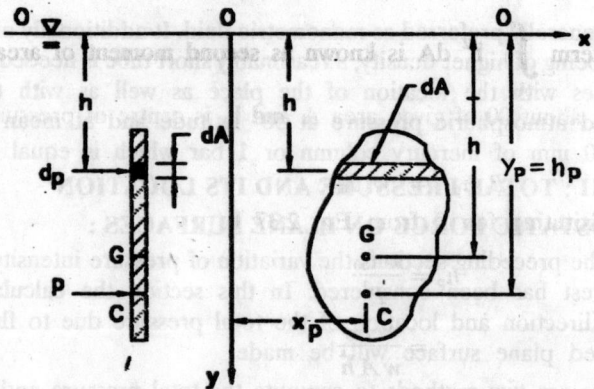

FIG. 2.13. A VERTICAL PLANE SURFACE IMMERSED IN FLUID

Total pressure $P = \int_A dP$

$$= \int_A w h \, dA = w \int_A h \, dA \qquad \text{...(2.37a)}$$

The term h dA is the summation of the moment of elementary area dA about the free surface which is equal to the moment of the total area A about 0–0 i.e. A $\bar{h}$ (moment theorem).

$$P = w A \bar{h} \qquad \text{...(2.37b)}$$

3. Centre of Pressure :

As indicated in previous section, the total pressure P acts through a point C (say). This point of application of resultant total pressure is defined as "centre of pressure". Let the co-ordinates of C are (x_p, y_p) as shown in Fig. 2.13. x_p is the horizontal distance from an arbitrarily chosen vertical surface and y_p is the vertical distance from the free surface 0–0.

Consider an elementary area dA at a depth h from free surface 00. The total pressure dP acting on it is given by Eq. 2.37a.

$$dP = w h \, dA$$

Take the moment of both sides about 0–0.

$$dP \times h = w h^2 \, dA$$

Summing up for all the similar strips of the given area A,

$$dP \times h = \int_A w h^2 \, dA$$

or $\qquad\qquad P h_p = w \int_A h^2 \, dA \qquad \text{...(2.38a)}$

The term $\displaystyle\int_A h^2\, dA$ is known as **second moment** of area or moment of inertia I_{00} about 00 of given area A and h_p is centre of pressure as defined above.

$$P\, h_p = w\, I_{00}$$

Substituting for P from Eq. 2.37 b.

$$h_p = \frac{w\, I_{00}}{P}$$

$$= \frac{w\, I_{00}}{w\, A\, \overline{h}}$$

$$= \frac{I_{00}}{A\, \overline{h}} \qquad\qquad ...(2.38b)$$

From the theorem of **parallel axis**, the moment of inertia I_{00} about 00 can be expressed as the sum of moment of inertia I_{GG} about an axis passing through the centroid G of the area and the product of area with the square of the distance of centroid from 00,

i.e. $$I_{00} = I_G + A\, \overline{h}^2$$

Hence $$h_p = \frac{I_G + A\, \overline{h}^2}{A\, \overline{h}}$$

$$h_p = \overline{h} + \frac{I_G}{A\, \overline{h}} \qquad\qquad ...(2.39a)$$

It can be further simplified as

$$(h_p - \overline{h}) = \frac{I_G}{A\, \overline{h}} \qquad\qquad ...(2.39b)$$

Since the term on right side is always positive, it means that $h_p - \overline{h} \geq 0$ i.e. the centre of pressure always lies below centre of gravity or at the most both these points may coincide (as in case of horizontally placed surfaces).

4. Total pressure on Inclined plane surfaces :

Consider a plane surface MN of area A immersed in liquid of specific weight w and inclined at an angle θ with the free surface. (The free surface is the reference plane surface on which the pressure is assumed zero). The trace of the area MN intersects the free surface along 0–0, Fig. 2.14.

Take an elementary area dA located at a distance y from the line of intersection of the area A with free surface, i.e. 00. Total pressure acting on elementary area dA is given by dP

$$dP = p.\, dA$$

$$= w\, y \sin\theta\, dA \qquad\qquad ...(2.40a)$$

Summing it up over the whole surface area A,

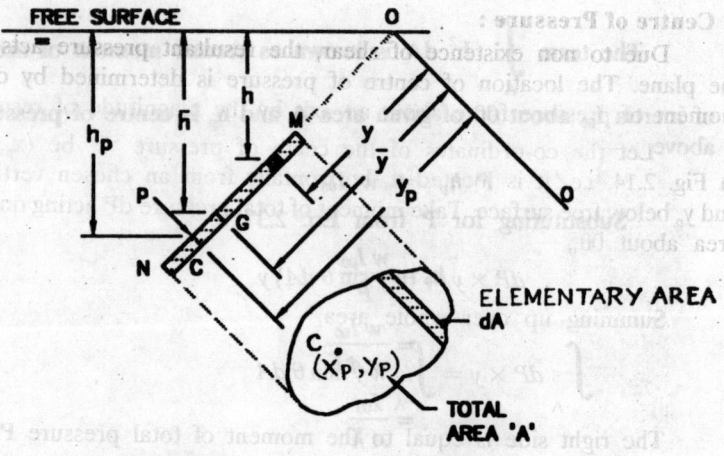

FIG. 2.14. TOTAL PRESSURE ON AN INCLINED PLANE SURFACE.

$$P = \int_A dP$$

$$= \int_A w\, y \sin\theta\, dA$$

$$= \int_A w \sin\theta\, y\, dA$$

The term $\int_A y\, dA$ is the summation of the moment of elementary area dA about 0–0 and is equal to the moment of whole area A about the same axis (moment principle) or in other words the product of A and the perpendicular distance of centroid of the area, i.e. $A\bar{y}$

$$P = w \sin\theta\, A\, \bar{y}$$

where $\bar{y}$ is the distance of the centroid of the area from 0–0 along the trace MN.

$$P = w A \bar{y} \sin\theta \qquad \qquad ...(2.40b)$$

If $\bar{h}$ is the vertical distance of the centroid from free surface, i.e. $\bar{h} = y\sin\theta$

Then $\qquad \qquad P = w A \bar{h} \qquad \qquad ...(2.40c)$

The above expression gives the magnitude of the resultant or total force acting on an inclined plane surface. It is seen that Eq. 2.40c does not contain angle θ, hence it is general expression and can be used to determine total pressure on horizontal, vertical or inclined plane surfaces. Acutally, the effect of θ is included in the value of $\bar{h}$.

5. Centre of Pressure :

Due to non existence of shear, the resultant pressure acts normal to the plane. The location of centre of pressure is determined by dividing the moment of pressure force about an axis by the magnitude of resultant force.

Let the co-ordinates of the cente of pressure 'C' be (x_p, y_p) shown in Fig. 2.14, i.e. it is located x_p horizontally from an chosen vertical surface and y_p below free surface. Take moment of total pressure dP acting on elementary area about 00.,

$$dP \times y = (w y \sin \theta \, dA) y$$

Summing up over whole area,

$$\int_A dP \times y = \int_A w y^2 \sin \theta \, dA$$

The right side is equal to the moment of total pressure P about 0–0, then

$$P \times y_p = w \sin \theta \int_A y^2 \, dA$$

where y_p is the distance of centroid of area from 0–0 measured along MN.

The term $\int y^2 \, dA$ is moment of inertia I_{00} of area A about the axis of rotation 0–0.

$$\therefore \qquad P \times y_p = w \sin \theta \, I_{00}$$

Substituting the value of P from Eq. 2.40b,

$$y_p = \frac{w \sin \theta \, I_{00}}{w A \bar{y} \sin \theta}$$

$$y_p = \frac{I_{00}}{A \bar{y}} \qquad \qquad ...(2.41a)$$

It is known from the theorem of parallel axis for moment of inertia that the moment of inertia about 00, is equal to the sum of moment of inertia about an parallel axis passing through G and the product of area A and square of the distance between two axis, ie.

$$I_{00} = I_G + A \bar{y}^2 \qquad \qquad ...(2.42)$$

Substituting the value of I_{00} in Eq, 2,41a

$$y_p = \frac{I_G + A \bar{y}^2}{A \bar{y}}$$

$$y_p = \left(\bar{y} + \frac{I_G}{A \bar{y}} \right) \qquad \qquad ...(2.41b)$$

Fig. 2.41b gives the location oof centre of pressure along inclined surface.

From Fig. 2.14, $h_p = y_p \sin\theta$

$$h = y \sin \theta$$

$$\bar{h} = \bar{y} \sin \theta$$

Hence, Eq. 2.41b becomes

$$\frac{h_p}{\sin \theta} = \frac{\bar{h}}{\sin \theta} + \frac{I_G}{A \bar{h}/\sin \theta}$$

$$h_p = \left(\bar{h} + \frac{I_G \sin^2 \theta}{A \bar{h}} \right) \qquad ...(2.41c)$$

Eq. 2.41c gives the location of centre of pressure in the vertical direction.

To determine the lateral location of centre of pressure, i.e. x_p, similar procedure is used.

Take moment of total pressure acting on elementary area, dP about OY and equate it with the moment of resultant pressure P about the same axis.

Moment of dP about OY,

$$dP \times x = w y \sin \theta \, dA . x \qquad ...(i)$$

Intergrate it over whole area, A,

$$\int_A dP \, x = w \sin \theta \, y \, dA . x$$

Moment of resultant pressure P about OY

$$= P \times x_p$$
$$= w A \bar{y} \sin \theta \, x_p \qquad ...(ii)$$

Equating Eqs. (i) and (ii)

$$w A \bar{y} \sin \theta . \dot{x}_p = w \sin \theta \int_A x y \, dA$$

or
$$x_p = \int \frac{x y \, dA}{A \bar{y}}$$

The term $\int x y \, dA = I_{xy}$ represents moment of inertia or second moment of area about OY

$$x_p = \frac{I_{xy}}{A \bar{y}} \qquad ...(2.42a)$$

From the theorem of parallel axis,

$$I_{xy} = I_{xy}' + A \times \bar{x} \bar{y}$$

where I_{xy}' represents moment of inertia of area about an axis parallel to OY and passing through centroid of area G.

$$x_p = \left[\bar{x} + \frac{I_{xy}'}{A \bar{y}} \right] \qquad ...(2.42b)$$

Thus C is suitably located by its co-ordinates (x_p, y_p).

Corollary : From Eq. 2.41c,

$$(h_p - \overline{h}) = \frac{I_G \sin^2 \theta}{A\overline{h}} \qquad ...(2.42c)$$

The right hand side of this Eq. 2.42c is always positive, that means $(h_p - \overline{h})$ should be either positive or at the most it can be zero. This shows that centre of pressure either lies below the centre of gravity of the area or at the most these two points can coincide (as in the case of horizontal planes). Furthermore, as the depth of immersion of the area increases (h becomes larger) the right hand side tends to be smaller, which reduces the difference between h_p and h (i.e. $h_p - \overline{h}$).

It should be noted that the above formula have been derived with zero pressure at free liquid surface. If the pressure on the surface is different than zero, a new surface of zero pressure should be first determined by converting the pressure acting on the surface into equivalent head and the calculations are then made with reference to this new surface.

B. Graphical Method (Method of Pressure Diagraams) :

Another method of determining total pressure P acting on a surface immersed in a fluid and its location is by means of drawing pressure diagrams for the surface. This method is quite useful when the surface is immersed in or supports more than one fluid. For example, a tank contains more than one liquid and thus its vertical walls supports more than one fluid on one of its side.

It is known that (i) when the fluid is at rest, the fluid pressure p always acts normal to the surface and (ii) from Eq. 2.6c, it is seen that the pressure intensity p varies linearly with the depth, i.e.

$$p = wh \qquad ...(2.6c)$$

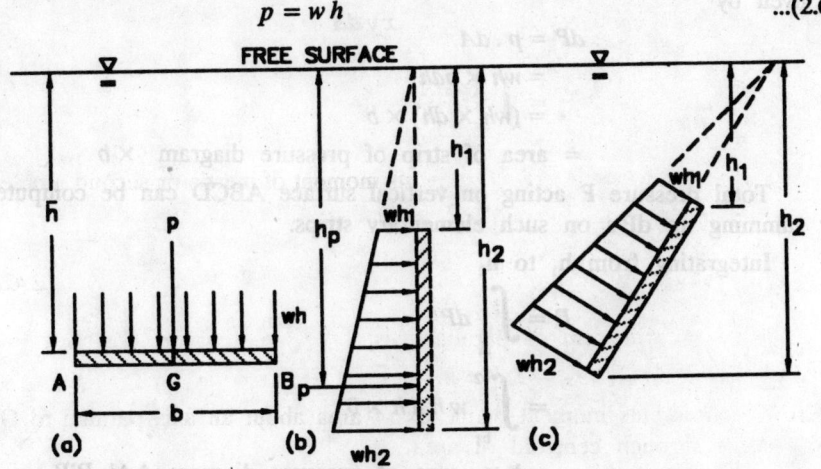

FIG. 2.15. PRESSURE DIAGRAMS ON (A) HORIZONTAL (B) VERTICAL AND (C) INCLINED SURFACE

Thus, pressure diagrams can be drawn over immersed surface and magnitude and location of total pressure can be computed. Three typical pressure diagrams on horizontal, vertical and inclined plane surfaces are shown in Fig.

2.15. The shaded area apearing as rectangle /trapezoidals are really volumes (for unit thickness normal to the plane of paper) and are known as pressure prisms.

A vertical surface A B C D of width B and height H is immersed in a fluid of specific weight w, Fig. 2.16. Consider an elementary strip of height dh (and width b) and at a depth h from free surface. The pressure acting at this depth

$$p = wh$$

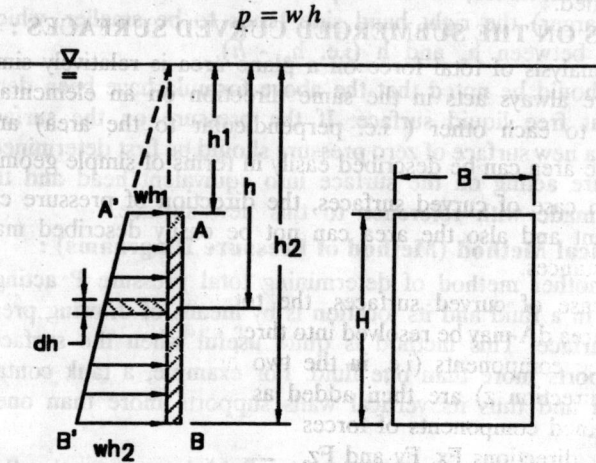

FIG. 2.16. COMPUTATION OF TOTAL PRESSURE

The total pressure dP acting on an elementary area dA (= b dh) is given by

$$dP = p \cdot dA$$

$$= wh \times bdh$$

$$= (wh \times dh) \times b$$

$$= \text{area of strip of pressure diagram} \times b$$

Total pressure P acting on vertical surface ABCD can be computed by summing up dP's on such elementary strips.

Integrating from h_1 to h_2

$$P = \int_A dP$$

$$= \int_{h_1}^{h_2} whdh \times b$$

$$= b \times \text{ area of pressure diagram AA' B'B.}$$

$$= w \times \text{ volume of pressure prism} \qquad ...(2.43)$$

Eq. 2.43 gives the magnitude of total pressure P acting on one side of the surface. The total pressure P passes through the centroid of the pressure prism which can be computed by Eq. 2.44.

$$h_p = \left[h_1 + \frac{h_2 - h_1}{3} \left(\frac{w h_1 + 2 w h_2}{w h_1 + w h_2} \right) \right]$$

$$h_p = \left[h_1 + \frac{h_2 - h_1}{3} \left(\frac{h_1 + 2 h_2}{h_1 + h_2} \right) \right] \quad ....(2.44)$$

The total pressure P and its location h_p as found from Eq. 2.43 and 2.44 can also be obtained from Eq. 2.40c and 2.41c and hence the results can be verified.

2.7 FORCES ON THE SUBMERGED CURVED SURFACES :

The analysis of total force on a plane area is relatively simple because : (i) pressure always acts in the same direction on an elementary area and are parallel to each other (i.e. perpendicular to the area) and

(ii) the area can be described easily in terms of simple geometric shapes.

But in case of curved surfaces, the direction of pressure changes from point to point and also the area can not be easily described mathematically in many instances.

In case of curved surfaces, the total force dP (= p dA) on an elementary area dA may be resolved into three mutually perpendicular directions and the three components (i.e. in the two horizontal directions x and y and in vertical direction z) are then added as scaler in the respective dirctions.

These combined components of forces in x, y and z directions Fx, Fy and Fz, are then added algebraically to determine the resultant pressure force F and its directions.

A curved surface AB submerged in a fluid as shown in Fig. 2.17. Consider an elementary are dA which is inclined at an angle α with the horizontal. The pressure p will act normal to it (according to Pascal's law).

The pressure force dP acting on dA = p × dA

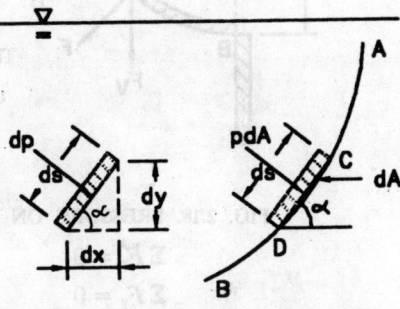

FIG. 2.17 PRESSURE ACTING ON A CURVED SURFACE

Horiozntal component of $dP = p\, dA \sin \alpha$

$$= p \times (dA \sin \alpha)$$

$$= p \times \text{vertical projection of dA}$$

Similarly, vertical compoennt of $dP = p\, dA \cos \alpha$

$$= p\, (dA \cos \alpha)$$

$$= p \times \text{horizontal projection of dA}$$

This means, total pressure acting on an area in any direction

= pressure intensity at that point

× [projection of area in the normal direction] ..(2.45)

If the curved surface is regular and symmetrical, the line of action of these forces will be in the same plane.

Suppose it is required to determine the total pressure force in the curved surface AB shown in Fig. 2.18. On each element of surface AB, the pressure force dP is marked in magnitude and direction and the location of total pressure force may be determined by forgoing principles.

Draw the free body diagram of fluid ABC, (Fig. 2.18). Let F_H and F_v are the fluid pressure components in horizontal and vertical direction. The surface AB exerts reactions F_H' and F_v' equal in magnitude and in opposite respective dirctions. W is the weight of the fluid supported by the surface AB. Then by statics, one can write

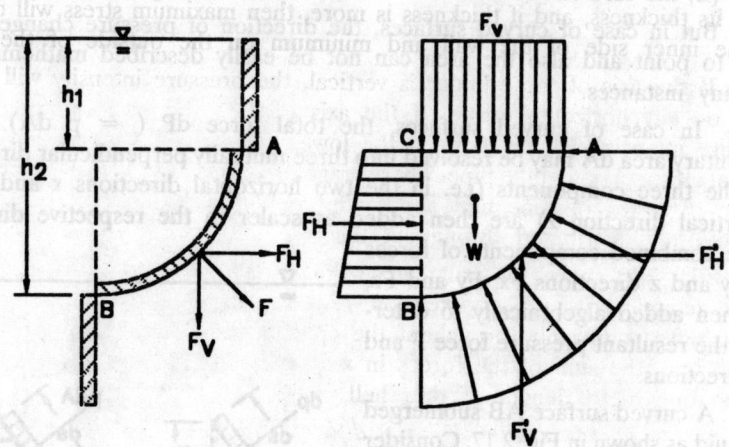

FIG. 2.18. PRESSURE ON A QUADRANT OF A CIRCLE

$$\Sigma F_x = 0$$
$$\Sigma F_y = 0$$

Hence, $\quad F_H' - F_H = 0$ ...(2.46a)

and $\quad F_v' - W_{AB} - F_v = 0$ ...(2.46b)

Simplifying, $\quad F_H' = F_H$ ...(2.46c)

and $\quad F_v' = W_{AB} + F_v$ ...(2.46d)

in which F_H and F_v easily determined from Eq. 2.37b. This means that "total horizontal force is equivalent to a force on vertical projection CB of submerged area below liquid surface by h and total vertical force is equal to the weight of liquid suported by AB over it."

In some cases, the lower side of surface is subjected to a hydrostatic pressure while upper side is not. In such problems, an imaginary volume is supposed to occupy the upperside of the surface. The magnitude of F_H and F_v is calculated by above method and then the direction of these forces are reversed.

2.8 SIMPLE APPLICATIONS :

There are numerous engineering problems where the principles of fluid statics are used. In many hydraulic machines fluid pressures are used for their operation, e.g. hydraulic press, jack, crane, rivetter, etc. Many of the structures are subjected to hydraulic pressures such as (i) different type of gates used in the irrigation structures, (ii) masonry dams, (iii) overhead tanks, (iv) lock gates, and even (v) water power mains. Some of these problems are analysed hereinunder.

1. Pipes and cylindrical shells under internal pressures :

Tanks, pipes, boiler, shells and many other structures are cylindrical in shape. When they are filled with fluid under pressure the shell walls are subjected by tensile stresses - known as hoop stress. If shell wall thickness is small as compared to its diameter, the hoop stress can be taken as uniform along its thickness, and if thickness is more, then maximum stress will develop on the inner side of the wall and minimum on the outside of the wall.

If the axis of the cylinder is vertical, the pressure intensity will be the same on any horizontal plane. If the axis of the cylinder is horizontal, the pressure intensity will be more at the lower side then the upperside on any vertical cross section of the pipe. The average pressures are too high as compared to the diameter of pipe and hence the pressures at the centre are taken as uniformly distributed throughout the pipe diameter.

Fig. 2.19 shows the half cut section of a shell lying horizontally. The forces acting on it are hoop tension T across its thickness t and pressure p distributed uniformly throughout the cross section. Since the forces are in equilibrium, the sum of the forces in x-direction should be equated to zero. Taking one metre length of the shell,

$$2T = F = p \times d \times 1$$

or
$$T = \frac{pd}{2} \qquad \qquad ...(2.47a)$$

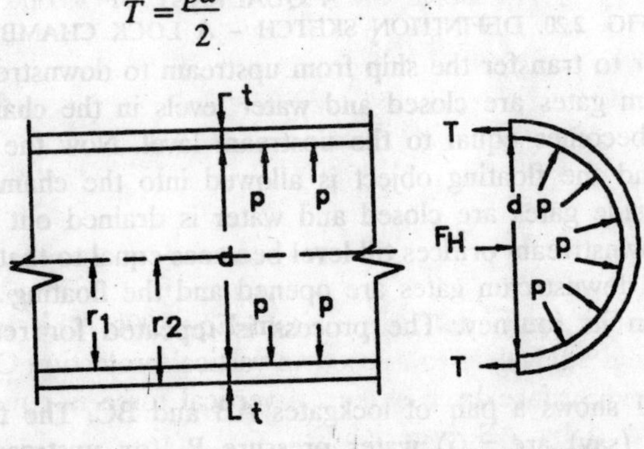

FIG. 2.19. FORCES ACTING ON A THIN SHELL

If the thickness of wall is t and f_t is the permissible hoop stress in the shell material, one can write

$$2T = 2f_t \times t \times 1$$

$$f_t \times t = \frac{pd}{2}$$

or

$$f_t = \frac{pd}{2t} \qquad ...(2.47b)$$

For thick wall cylinders, Gibson has shown by his stress distribution analysis that maximum stress f_{tmax} is given by

$$f_{tmax} = p \left[\frac{r_1^2 + r_2^2}{r_1^2 - r_2^2} \right] \qquad ...(2.48)$$

r_1 and r_2 are outer and inner radii of the shell respectively.

2. Static pressure on lock gates :

Many a times during the course of travel floating objects like boats, ships, etc. come across a sharp drop in water level in the canal/river. To facilitate their movement from one side to other, lock chambers (Fig. 2.20) are constructed in the canal/river. These chambers are provided with a pair of gates on upstream as well as on downstream side. On the lower side of these chambers are provided a set of orifices to fill or empty the lock chamber.

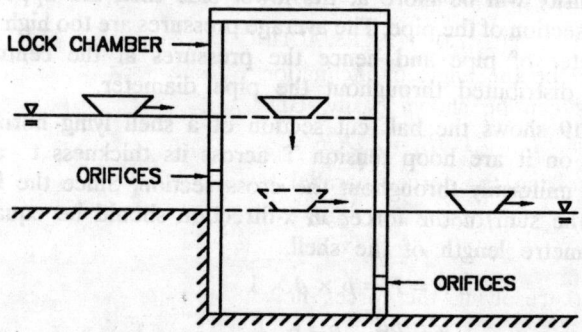

FIG. 2.20. DEFINITION SKETCH – A LOCK CHAMBER

In order to transfer the ship from upstream to downstream side initially the downstream gates are closed and water levels in the chamber is allowed to rise till it becomes equal to the upstream level. Now the upstream gates are opened and the floating object is allowed into the chamber. Thereafter, the upstream side gates are closed and water is drained out of the chamber through the downstrteam orifices till level becomes equal to that on downstream side. Now the downstream gates are opened and the floating object proceeds downstream on its journey. The process is repeated for return journey of water vehicle.

Fig. 2.21 shows a pair of lockgates AB and BC. The forces acting on each gate BC (say) are : (i) water pressure P_1 (on upstream side) and P_2 (downstream side), acting at $2H_1/3$ and $2H_2/3$ from water surface. (ii) reaction of gate AB on BC, i.e. T acting normally to the surface of contact between two gates and (iii) reaction of hinges R_T (top hinge) and R_B (bottom hinge) on which gate BC is hanging. The net reaction is R ($= R_1 + R_2$). The magnitude and direction of R is not known. Thus gate BC (and also AB) is in equilibrium while all these forces are acting on it. These forces P (net water pressure), T (reaction of AB on BC) and R (reaction of hinges) must be colinear and intersect at one point for the gate to remain in equilibrium. Thus, the force diagram can be drawn as shown in Fig. 2.21.

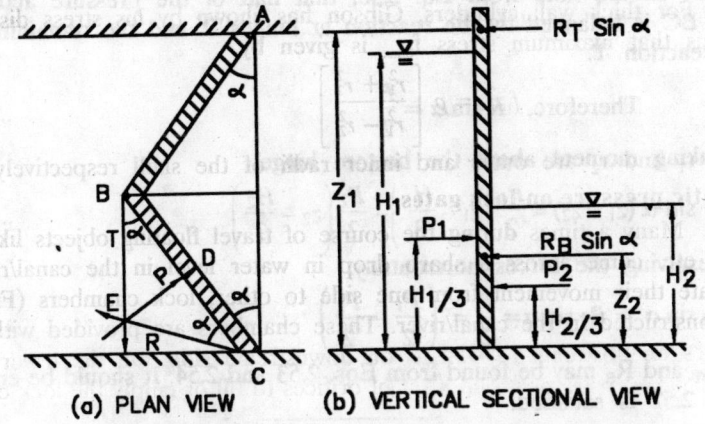

(a) PLAN VIEW   (b) VERTICAL SECTIONAL VIEW

FIG. 2.21. FORCES ACTING ON A LOCK GATE

Let α be the angle of inclination of gate with the normal to the side of lock. As can be shown easily, BDE and CDE are similar triangles.

$$\angle DBE = \angle DCE = \alpha$$

Resolving the forces parallel to the gate,

$$T \cos \alpha = R \cos \alpha$$

$$T = R \qquad ..(2.49)$$

Also, resolving the forces normal to the gate,

$$R \sin \alpha + T \sin \alpha - P = 0$$

or

$$R = \frac{P}{2 \sin \alpha} \qquad ...(2.50)$$

The water pressure P_1 and P_2 can be calculated as follows. From Eq. 2.37b

$$P_1 = \frac{w H_1}{2} \times \text{ wetted area of the gate on u/s}$$

$$P_2 = \frac{w H_2}{2} \times \text{ wetted area of the gate on d/s}$$

Then

$$P = P_1 - P_2 \qquad ...(2.51)$$

The resultant reaction of hinges R can be computed from Eqs. 2.50 and 2.51 and also T from Eqs. 2.49 and 2.51. Thus T is known in magnitude and direction. The reaction R is known in magnitude and its direction will be inclined at an angle α to the surface of the gate BC. Let the reaction of top hinge is R_T at an elevation Z_1 and that of bottom hinge is R_B at Z_2 metre above floor. Then,

$$R = R_B + R_T \qquad ...(2.52)$$

Since the reaction R is inclined at an angle α to the surface BC, the components of it acting in the plane of water pressures will be $R_B \sin \alpha$ and $R_T \sin \alpha$.

One should note from Eq. 2.50, that half of the pressure acting on the gate BC is balanced by the reaction at hinges R and the remaining half by the reaction T.

Therefore, $\quad R \sin \alpha = \dfrac{P}{2} \qquad ...(2.50)$

Taking moment about the bottom hinge,

$$R_T \sin \alpha \,(z_1 - z_2) = \frac{P_1}{2}\left(z_1 - \frac{H_1}{3} \right) - \frac{P_2}{2}\left(z_2 - \frac{H_2}{3} \right) \qquad ...(2.53)$$

Resolving the forces horizontally,

$$R_B \sin \alpha + R_T \sin \alpha = \frac{P}{2} = \left(\frac{P_1}{2} - \frac{P_2}{2} \right) \qquad ...(2.54)$$

R_T and R_B may be found from Eqs. 2.53 and 2.54. It should be ensured that Eq. 2.52 is satisfied.

3. Water pressure on masonary dam :

Fig. 2.22 shows the section of a gravity dam. The forces acting on the dam are (a) its self weight W acting on its centre of gravity, (b) the net hydrostatic pressure P acting at centre of pressure and, (c) uplift pressure U acting at the base of dam.

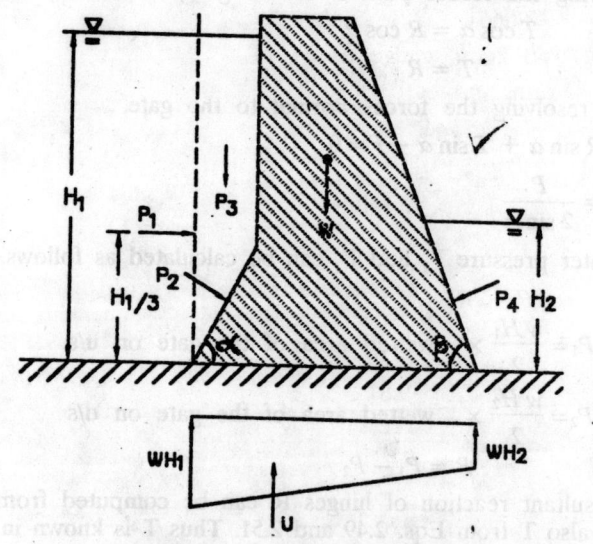

FIG. 2.22. FORCES ACTING ON A GRAVITY DAM.

Resolving these forces in horizontal and vertical directions,

$$F_H = P_1 + P_2 \sin \alpha - P_4 \sin \beta \qquad ...(2.55)$$

$$F_V = W + P_2 \cos \alpha + P_3 + P_4 \cos \beta - U \qquad ...(2.56)$$

where, P_1, P_2, P_3 and P_4 are water pressure components and U is uplift pressure at the base. These can be calculated from Eq. 2.37b.

The magnitude and direction of the resultant of horizontal forces F_H and vertical forces F_V can be found from force polygon. For the stability of dam section, the resultant R of these forces should pass through the middle third of the base. i.e. the resultant R should cut the base within b/3 and 2b/3 from the upstream end. Details of the analysis of stability of dam section can be obtained elsewhere (Refer books on water resources engineering).

4. Static pressure on tank :

The static pressure acting on the walls of water tanks can be obtained either. by analytical method of Eq. 2.37b (Sec. 2.6.2 and 2.6.3) or if it contains more than one fluid, then by graphical method (Sec. 2.6, Part B) by drawing pressure diagrams. The base of the tank supports the weight of water contained in it and hence the pressure force at the base is equal to the weight of water.

EXAMPLES 2.1 TO 2.46

SECTION A : FLUID PRESSURE AND ITS MEASUREMENT

2.1 A vacuum gauge reads a negative pressure of 27.95 k Pa. Express this pressure in the following units (i) kg/sq.cm. gauge, (ii) kg./sq.m. absolute, (iii) metre of water gauge, (iv) metre of an oil (sp.gr. = 0.82) absolute, (v) cm. of mercury (sp.gr. = 13.6) gauge.

Solution :

(i) $p = \dfrac{27.95 \times 1000}{9.8066}$ (1 kg_f = 9.8066 N $\approx$ 9.81 N)

     = 2850 kg/m² gauge or vacuum.

(ii) p = (atm. pressure + gauge pressure)

     = $p_a + p$ gauge

     = 10300 – 2850

     = 7450 kg/m² absolute = 73.059 kN/m² also.

(iii) $p = wh$

     h (water) = $\dfrac{\text{Pressure in kN/m}^2\ \text{(gauge)}}{\text{specific weight of water}}$

     = $\dfrac{27.95}{9.81}$ = 2.85 m gauge

(iv) h (oil) abs = $\dfrac{\text{Pressure in kN/m}^2\ \text{(abs.)}}{\text{sp. weight of oil}}$

     = $\dfrac{73.059}{0.82 \times 9.81}$ = 9.08 m abs

(v) h (mercury) gauge = $\dfrac{\text{Pressure in kN/m}^2\ \text{(gauge)}}{\text{sp. weight of mercury}}$

     = $\dfrac{27.95}{13.6 \times 9.81}$ = 0.2095 m

= 20.95 cm (gauge)

2.2 The barometric pressure at sea level is 760 mm of mercury while on top of mountain is 720 mm. If specific weight of air is assumed constant as 0.01185 N/m³, calculate the elevation of mountain top.

Solution :

The elevation of mountain = the change in the reading of barometer.

The difference in air pressure (i.e. change in reading of barometer) at mean sea level and the mountain top

$$= 13.6 \times 9.81 \times \frac{(760 - 720)}{1000} \, kPa$$

$$= 5.336 \ kPa$$

$$\text{Height of mountain} = \frac{5.336}{\text{sp. wt. of air}}$$

$$= \frac{5.336}{0.01185}$$

$$= 450.33 \ m.$$

2.3 A tank contains various fluids as shown in Fig. 2.23. A vacuum gauge at the top reads -21.0 kPa. Find the elevation of liquids in the piezometric tubes F and H and the deflection of mercury in the U-tube. The oil fills the U-tube in the right hand tube upto a level of EL 10.2.

Solution :

Since the pressure at the top is negative, actual free surface will be below B.

Pressure at the top

$$= - 21.0 \ kPa = \frac{- 21.0}{0.7 \times 9.81}$$

= 3.06 m of oil (sp. gr. 0.7).

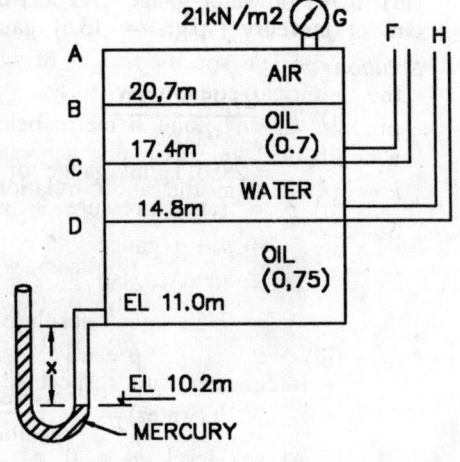

FIG. 2.23. EXAMPLE 2.3

Therefore, the free surface of the oil will be at EL (20.7 − 3.06) = EL 17.64 m

(a) The tube F indicates the pressure at the level of surface 'C'

Since $p_c = 0.7 \times 9.81 \times (17.64 - 17.4)$

$$= 1.648 \ kPa$$

∴ $$h = \frac{1.648}{0.7 \times 9.81} = 0.24 \ m \ of \ oil$$

Therefore, the level in the tube F = (17.4 + 0.24)

$$= \text{EL } 17.64 \text{ m.}$$

(b) The tube H will indicate the pressure at surface D.

Since
$$p_D = p_c + 9.81 \times (17.4 - 14.8)$$
$$= 1.648 + 25.506$$
$$= 27.154 \text{ kPa}$$

$$\therefore \quad h = \frac{27.154}{9.81}$$
$$= 2.768 \text{ m of water.}$$

The level in the tube H = 14.8 + 2.768 = EL 17.768 m

(c) Pressure at the bottom of tank
$$= p_D + 9.81 \times 0.75 \times (14.8 - 11.0)$$
$$= 27.154 + 9.81 \times 0.75 \times 3.8$$
$$= 55.11 \text{ kPa.}$$

(d) Apply manometric equation to the U-tube
$$0 + 13.6 \times 9.81 \times x - 0.75 \times 9.81(11.0 - 10.2) = 55.11$$
$$13.6 \times 9.81x = 55.11 + 0.75 \times 9.81 \times 0.8$$

$$x = \frac{60.996}{13.6 \times 9.81} = 0.457 \text{ m.}$$

2.4 The specific weight of water in the ocean may be calculated from the empirical equation $w = w_0 + 10 \, k \sqrt{h}$. Derive an expression for the pressure at any point h metre below free surface and calculate pressure at a depth of 2 km., assuming $w_0 = 10.3$ kN/m^3. The height h is in metre and $k = 9 \times 10^{-5}$ in the above relation.

Solution :

From Eq. 2.5 dp/dh = w
$$dp/dh = (w_0 + 10 \, k \, h)$$
$$dp = (w_0 + 10 \, k \, \sqrt{h}) \, dh$$

Integrating with respect to h,
$$p = w_0 h + 20/3 \, k \, h^{3/2} + C$$

At sea level, $h = 0$, $p = 0$.

Therefore, $C = 0$

Hence required expression is
$$p = w_0 h + 20/3 \, k \, h^{3/2}$$

At sea surface, $w_0 = 10.3$ kN/m^3, $k = 9 \times 10^{-5}$
$$p = 10.3 h + 20/3 \times 9 \times 10^{-5} h^{3/2}$$
$$= 10.3 \, h + 60 \times 10^{-5} \, h^{3/2}$$

At h = 2 km below free surface,
$$p = 10.3 \times 2 \times 1000 + 60 \times 10^{-5} \times (2 \times 1000)^{3/2}$$

$$= 20.6 \times 1000 + 53.666 = 20653 \text{ kPa.}$$

2.5 Fig. 2.24 shows a conical vessel having the outlet in the bottom at A to which a U-tube manometer is connected.
The reading of U-tube is given in the figure
when the water surface is at A. Find out the
reading of the manometer when the vessel is
completely filled with water. Specific weight
of water is 9.81 kN/m³.

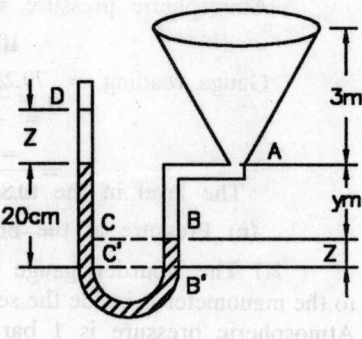

FIG. 2.24. EXAMPLE 2.5

Solution,

Initially let the water level be y metre
above B in the right limb. Using manometric
equation, start from open end.

$$0 - 13.6 \times 9.81 \times 0.2 - 9.81y = 0$$

$$y = 2.72 \text{ m.}$$

When the water is filled in conical vessel, the mercury level is lowered to B' by z (say) in the right limb and mercury level at D will be pushed up by the same amount to D' in the left limb. Now take B'C' as reference level and write manometric equation

$$0 + 13.6 \times 9.81 \times (0.2 + z + z) - 9.81(z + y + 3) = 0$$

$$13.6 \times 9.81 \times (0.2 + 2z) - 9.81(z + 5.72) = 0$$

$$z = 0.1145 \text{ m}$$

New reading of manometer $= (0.2 + 2z)$

$$= (0.2 + 2 \times 0.1145) \text{ m}$$

$$= 429.0 \text{ mm}$$

2.6 Calculate the gauge reading in the Fig. 2.25. Specific gravity of oil is 0.85. Barometric pressure is 750 mm of mercury.

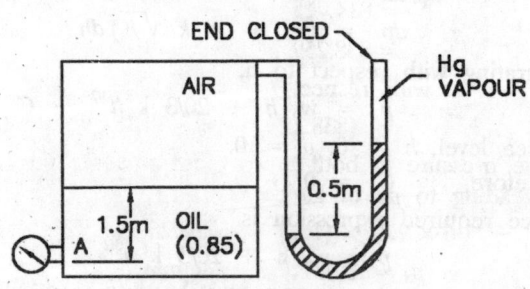

FIG. 2.25. EXAMPLE 2.6

Solution :

As the right limb of U-tube is closed and contains mercury vapour only, the pressue due to these vapour will be negligible.

The pressure of air (inside tank) $= 13.6 \times 9.81 \times 0.5$

$$= 66.708 \text{ k Pa abs.}$$

Pressure at the level of gauge $= 66.708 + 0.85 \times 9.81 \times 1.5$

$$= 79.215 \text{ kPa abs.}$$

Atmospheric pressure $= 13.6 \times 9.81 \times 0.75$

$$= 10.062 \text{ k Pa}$$

Gauge reading $= 79.215 - 100.062$

$$= -20.847 \text{ k Pa gauge}$$

$$= \frac{-20.847}{0.85 \times 9.81}$$

$$= -2.50 \text{ m oil gauge.}$$

2.7 The Bourden gauge connected to the manometer is inside the sealed tank. Atmospheric pressure is 1 bar absolute. Calculate the gauge reading p_x.

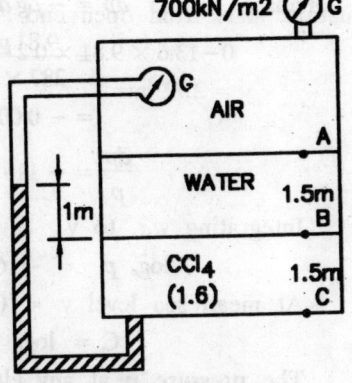

FIG. 2.26. EXAMPLE 2.7

Solution :

Since atmospheric pressure $= 1$ bar $= 100$ kPa

Therefore, pressure at A $=$ atm.pressure $+ 700$ k Pa gauge

$$= 800 \text{ k Pa absolute.}$$

Pressure at B $=$ Pressure at A $+$ Pressure due to water column.

$$= 800 + 9.81 \times 1.5 = 814.715 \text{ kPa abs.}$$

Pressure at C $=$ Pressure at B $+$ Pressure due to Carbon tetra chloride

$$= 814.715 + 9.81 \times 1.6 \times 1.5$$

$$= 838.259 \text{ kPa.}$$

Pressure at C with respect to local pressure of air at A

$$= (838.259 - 800) = 38.259 \text{ kPa gauge}$$

Now the pressure in both limbs of U-tube are equated to compute the unknown reading to px of gauge G.

$$p_x + 1.6 \times 9.81 \times (1.0 + 1.5) = 38.259$$

$$p_x = 0.981 \text{ k Pa vacuum}$$

2.8 Compute the berometric pressure in bar at an altitude of 1200 m if the pressure at sea level is 1.013 bar. Assume isothermal condition at 21°C.

Solution :

From Eq. 2.5, $dp = -\rho g \, dy$

In this Eq. 2.5, δ is unit weight of air at 21° C

The unit weight at 21°C $\rho g = \dfrac{1}{v} \cdot g$

From Eq. of state $\rho v = RT$

or

$$\frac{1}{v} = \frac{p}{RT}$$

Thus, $\rho g = g \cdot \dfrac{p}{RT}$

Assuming $R = 287$ J/kg K, and $T = 273 + 21 = 294°K$

$$\rho g = g \cdot \frac{p}{287\,(294)}$$

Thus, $dp = -\rho g\, dy$

$$= -\frac{9.81\, p\, dy}{287 \times 294}$$

$$= -0.000116\, p\, dy$$

$$\frac{dp}{p} = -116 \times 10^{-6}\, dy$$

Integrating w.r. to y

$$\log_e p = -116 \times 10^{-6}\, y + C$$

At mean sea level $y = 0$, $p = 1.013 \times 10^5$ Pa absolute,

$$C = \log_e (1.013 \times 10^5).$$

The pressure p at any elevation y is given by

$$\log_e p = -116 \times 10^{-6}\, y + \log_e (1.013 \times 10^5)$$

$$\log_e (1.013 \times 10^5)/p = 116 \times 10^{-6}\, y$$

The pressure at an altitude of $y = 1200$ m,

$$2.3 \log_{10} \frac{(1.013 \times 10^5)}{p} = 116 \times 10^{-6} \times 1200$$

Solving, $p = 88122.7\ Pa = 0.881$ bar

2.9 Determine the drop in temperature for an altitude of 2000 m above earth's surface. Assume adiabatic conditions to prevail and take temperature at earth surface as 15°C and gas constant $R = 287$ J/kgK. Also determine the temperature lapse rate. If the pressure at earth surface is 1.013 bar, what is the pressure at that altitude for polytropic atmosphere. n can be taken as 1.24.

Solution :

(i) From Eq. 2.16 a, viz.

$$\frac{T}{T_0} = \left[1 - \frac{n-1}{n} \cdot \frac{g \cdot \Delta y}{R\, T_0}\right]$$

The temperature drop is given by $= \dfrac{T_0 - T}{T_0}$

$$\frac{T_0 - T}{T_0} = \frac{n-1}{n} \cdot \frac{g \cdot \Delta y}{R \, T_0}$$

Absolute temperature $T° = (273 + 15) = 288°\text{K}$

Substituting the given values,

$$\left[\frac{T_0 - T}{T_0}\right] = \frac{1.24 - 1.0}{1.24} \times \frac{9.81 \times 2000}{2.87 \times 288}$$

$$T = 274.77° \text{ K or abs.}$$

Therefore, Temperature drop $= (288 - 274.77) = 13.13°\text{C}$

(ii) From Eq. 2.16b, Lapse rate $\dfrac{dT}{dy} = \dfrac{n-1}{n} \cdot \dfrac{g}{R}$

$$\frac{dT}{dy} = \frac{1.24 - 1}{1.24} \times \frac{9.81}{2.87}$$

$$\frac{dT}{dy} = 6.6157° \text{ K/m}$$

(iii) From Eq. 2.14 b,

$$\left(\frac{p}{p_0}\right) = \left[1 - \frac{n-1}{n} \cdot \frac{g \, \Delta y}{R \, T_0}\right]^{n/(n-1)}$$

$$T_0 = (273 + 15°) = 288°\text{K}$$

$$\left(\frac{p}{p_0}\right) = \left[1 - \frac{0.24 \times 9.81 \times 2000}{1.24 \times 287 \times 288}\right]^{(1.24/1.24 - 1)}$$

$$p = 0.7944 \text{ bar.}$$

2.10 Taking the lapse rate in the international standard atmosphere as 0.0065 °K/m, determine the pressure at an altitude of 5 km.

Solution :

From Eq. 2.5, $dp = -\rho \, g \, dy$

It is known from Eq.2.11 a

$$\frac{p}{\rho} = RT$$

or

$$\rho = \frac{p}{RT}$$

Substituting the value of ρ in Eq. 2.5,

$$dp = -\frac{pg}{RT} dy$$

$$\frac{dp}{p} = -\frac{g}{RT} dy$$

$$= -\frac{g}{RT} \cdot \frac{dy}{dT} \cdot dT$$

Writing lapse rate as $L = -\dfrac{dT}{dy}$

$$\frac{dp}{p} = \frac{g}{LR} \cdot \frac{dT}{T}$$

Integrating with respect to T,

$$\log_e p = \frac{g}{LR} \log_e T + C$$

At mean sea level, $p = p_0$, $T = T_0$

$$C = \left(\log p_0 - \frac{g}{LR} \log T_0 \right)$$

Substituting the value of C

$$\log_e (p/p_0) = \frac{g}{LR} \log_e (T/T_0)$$

$$\left(\frac{p}{p_0} \right) = \left(\frac{T}{T_0} \right)^{g/LR}$$

Temperature at 5 km altitude $= T_0 - y \times \dfrac{dT}{dy}$

$$= 288 - 5000 \times 0.0065$$

$$= 255.5°K$$

Substituting in the above relationship

$$p = p_0 (T/T_0)^{g/LR}$$

$$= 10^5 \left(\frac{255.5}{288} \right)^{\frac{9.81}{0.0065 \times 288}}$$

$$= 10^5 (0.887)^{5.24} \ N/m^2$$

$$= 0.5339 \ bar.$$

2.11 What will be the mass density of atmospheric air at the top of a mountain 8000 m above sea level ? Take $p_0 = 101.325 \ kN/m^2$, $= 1.208 \ kg/m^3$ and $n = 1.20$.

Solution :

From Eq. 2.15a,

$$\frac{\rho}{\delta_0} = \left[1 - \frac{n-1}{n} \cdot \frac{g \cdot \Delta y}{p_0/\rho_0} \right]^{1/n - 1}$$

$$= \left[1 - \frac{1.2 - 1}{1.2} \cdot \frac{9.81 \times 8000}{101.325 \times 1000/1.208} \right]^{1/(1.2 - 1)}$$

$$= [1 - 0.1559]^{1/0.2}$$

$$\rho = 1.208 \, (0.844)^{1/0.2}$$

$$= 0.5173 \ kg/m^3$$

2.12 Calculate the pressure in the pipe M by means of an open manometer shown in Fig. 2.27.

Solution :

Pressure at C = 25 cm of mercury

$= 1.36 \times 9.81 \times 0.25 = 33.354$ N/m^2

Pressure at B = Pressure at C

= Pressure at A = 33.354 N/m^2

Pressure at M = Pressure at A + Pressure due to 0.75 m of Fluid column AA'

$= 33.354 + 0.8 \times 9.81 \times 0.75$

$= 39.24$ N/m^2 gauge

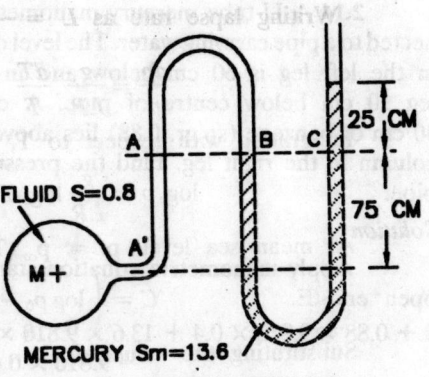

FIG. 2.27 EXAMPLE 2.12

2.13 Find the pressure (gauge) at A in mm of water and in kN/m^2. Also determine the absolute pressure at A in kN/m^2 in Fig. 2.28. Fluid P is air and fluid Q is oil of specific gravity 0.8. Take barometric reading as 740 mm of mercury.

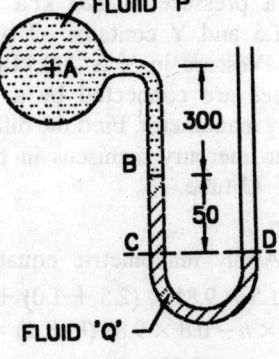

Solution :

Pressure at open end D is atmosphere or zero

Pressure at C = Pressure at D

$= pa = 0$

Pressure at B = Pressure at C– Pressure due to 0.05 m of column of Fluid Q

FIG. 2.28. EXAMPLE 2.13

$= 0 - 9810 \times 0.8 \times 0.05$

$= -392.4$ N/m^2

Pressure at A = Pressure at B–Pressure due to column of fluid P.

Since specific weight of air is too small as compared to liquid, the pressure due to A'B can be neglected.

Therefore, Pressure at A = - 392.4 N/m^2 (gauge)

Pressure head at A $= -\dfrac{392.4}{9810}$ m of water

$= -40$ mm of water (gauge)

Absolute pressure at A = [Atmospheric pressure

+ Gauge pressure at A]

$= 13.6 \times 9810 \times 0.740 - 392.4$

$= 98335$ N/m^2 = 98.335 kN/m^2

2.14 A U-tube mercury manometer is connected to a pipe carrying water. The level of mercury in the left leg is 60 cm below and in the right leg 10 cm below centre of pipe. A column of 40 cm of benzene (sp.gr. 0.88) lies above mercury column in the right leg. Find the pressure in the pipe.

Solution :

Apply manometric equation starting from open end E.

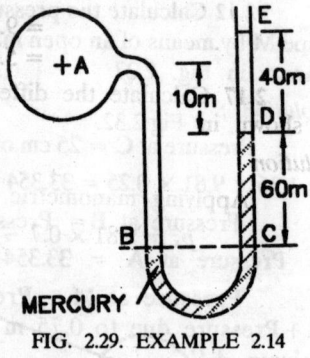

FIG. 2.29. EXAMPLE 2.14

$$0 + 0.88 \times 9.810 \times 0.4 + 13.6 \times 9.810 \times 0.50 - 9.810 \times 0.60 = p_A$$

$$p_A = 3.453 + 66.708 - 5.886$$

$$p_A = 64.275 \text{ kN/m}^2 \text{ (gauge)}$$

2.15 Pipe X contains a liquid under a pressure of 120 kPa and of sp.gr. 1.5 and Y contains oil of sp.gr. of 0.8. Pressure in Y is 200 kPa. Both the pipes are connected by a U-tube mercury manometer. Find the difference h in the mercury meniscus in the two legs of U-tube.

Solution :

Apply manometric equation :

$$120 + 1.5 \times 9.81 \times (2.5 + 1.0) + 13.6 \times 9.81 \times h - 0.8 \times 9.81 (h + 1) = 200$$

Solving, $h = 0.289$ m.

FIG. 2.30. EXAMPLE 2.15

2.16 Pipe A carries a liquid (sp.gr. 0.8) under pressure and pipe B carries water under pressure. Both the pipes are connected by a U-tube manometer as shown in Fig. The liquid B in right limb stands at a height of 2.5 m above the level of liquid A in the left limb. Find the difference in pressures between pipe A and B. The manometric liquid is of sp.gr. 1.25.

Solution :

Apply manometric equation,

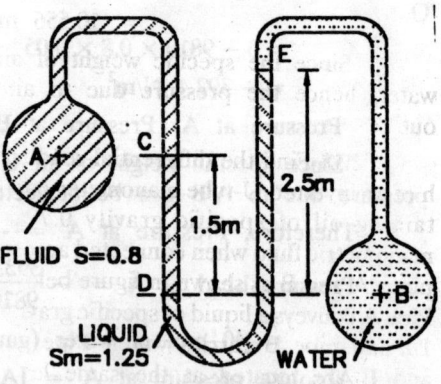

FIG. 2.31. EXAMPLE 2.16

$$p_A + 0.8 \times 9.81 \times 1.5 - 1.25 \times 9.81 \times 2.5 + 9.81 \times 2.5 = p_B$$

$$p_B - p_A = 9.81(0.8 \times 1.5 - 1.25 \times 2.5 + 2.5)$$

$$= 9.81 \times (0.575)$$
$$= 5.64 \text{ N/m}^2$$

2.17 Calculate the difference of pressure in the two pipes X and Y as shown in Fig.2.32.

Solution

Applying manometric equation, starting from X,

$$p_x + 9.81 \times 0.7 - 13.6 \times 9.81 \times 0.45 + \rho g \times 0.3$$
$$-13.6 \times 9.81 \times 0.36 - 9.81 \times 0.24 = p_y$$

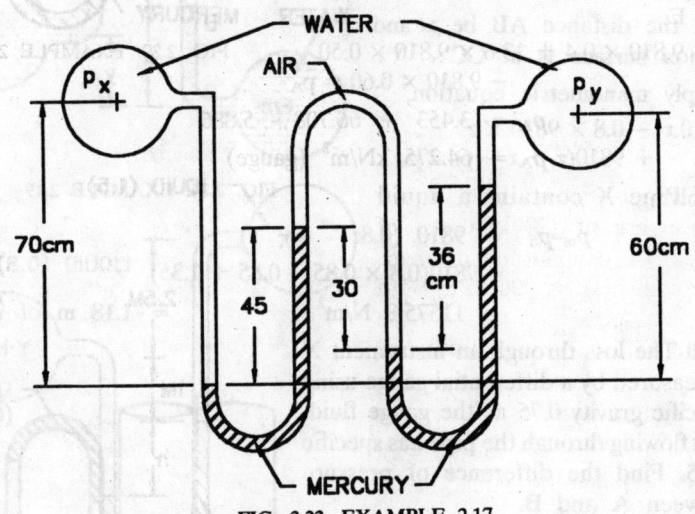

FIG. 2.32. EXAMPLE 2.17

Solving it,

$$(p_x - p_y) = 103.554 \text{ kPa}$$
$$= 10.556 \text{ m of water.}$$

Since the specific weight of air is too small as compared to that of water, hence the pressure due to air column will be negligible and is left out.

2.18 Find the differential reading h of an inverted U-tube manometer containing oil of specific gravity 0.7 as manometric fluid when connected across pipes A and B as shown in figure below, Pipe A conveys a liquid of specific gravity 1.2 and pipe B carries water. Pipes A and B are located at the same level and the pressure in the two pipes are equal.

Solution,

Apply manometric equation,

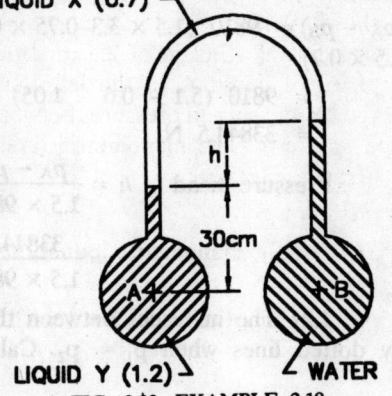

FIG. 2.33. EXAMPLE 2.18

$$p_A - 1.2 \times 9810 \times 0.3 - 0.7 \times 9810 \times h + 9810(h + 0.3) = p_B$$

Since $p_A = p_B,$

$$0.3\ h = 0.06$$

$$h = 0.2 \text{ m or } 20 \text{ cm.}$$

2.19 Compute the difference of pressure between two pipes m and n with the given data in the figure; y = 135 cm and z = 85 cm.

Solution,

Let the distance AB be x and the common surface is at CC'.

Apply manometric equation,

$$p_m - 9810x - 0.8 \times 9810 \times z$$
$$+ 9810(z + x - y) = p_n$$

Solving,

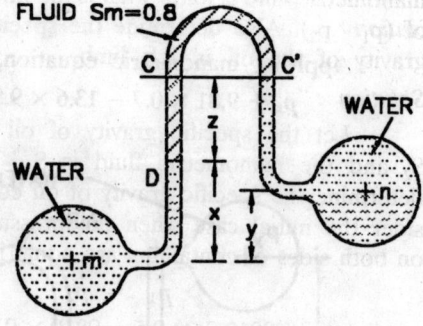

FIG. 2.34. EXAMPLE 2.19

$$p_m\text{–}p_n = 9810\ (0.8z - z + y)$$
$$= 9810(0.8 \times 0.85 - 0.85 + 1.35)$$
$$= 11575.8 \text{ N/m}^2 \qquad = 1.18 \text{ m of water.}$$

2.20 The loss through an instrument X is to be measured by a differential gauge using oil of specific gravity 0.75 as the gauge fluid. The liquid flowing through the pipe has specific gravity 1.5. Find the difference of pressure head between A and B.

Solution :

Let the pressure at A and B be p_A and p_B respectively.

Using manometric equation,

$$p_A - 1.5 \times 9810 \times (4.5 - 1.2) - 0.75 \times 9810$$
$$(4.5 - 3.7) - 1.5 \times 9810 \times (3.7 - 3.0) = p_B$$

$$(p_A - p_B) = 9810\ (1.5 \times 3.3 - 0.75 \times 0.8 - 1.5 \times 0.7)$$

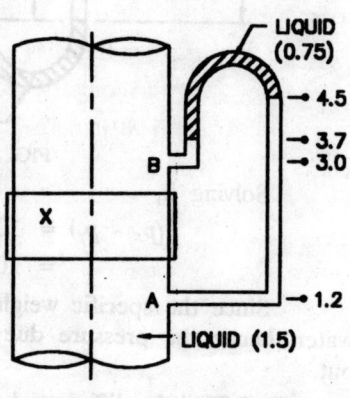

FIG. 2.35. EXAMPLE 2.20

$$= 9810\ (5.1 - 0.6 - 1.05)$$
$$= 33844.5 \text{ N}$$

Pressure head $\quad h = \dfrac{p_A - p_B}{1.5 \times 9810}$

$$= \dfrac{33844.5}{1.5 \times 9810} = 2.3 \text{ m}$$

2.21 The meniscus between the oil and water is in the position shown by dotted lines when $p_1 = p_2$. Calculate the pressure difference $(p_1 - p_2)$

in terms of specific gravity of manometric fluid S_1 which will cause the meniscus to rise 5 cm in the U- tube. If the manometric fluid is water what is the value of $(p_1 - p_2)$. Also determine the specific gravity of the oil in left limb.

Solution :

Let the specific gravity of oil is S_2 and the manometric fluid is S_1. To determine the specific gravity of oil consider the initial case when the pressure on both sides of containers are equal i.e.

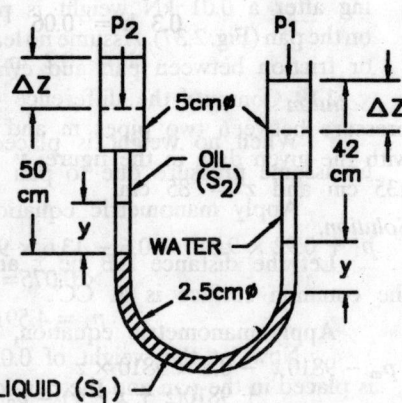

FIG. 2.36. EXAMPLE 2.21

$$p_1 = p_2$$
$$9810\, S_2 \times 0.5 = 9810 \times 0.42$$
$$S_2 = \frac{0.42}{0.50} = 0.84$$

When the pressure difference (p_1-p_2) is increased, the meniscus in the right side container will drop by Δz (say) and simultaneous the meniscus in the right leg of U-tube will be lowered by y. This will cause corresponding rise y in the left leg of U-tube and Δz in the left side container.

The new condition is shown by dark line in the Fig.2.36

Applying manometric equation,

$$p_1 + 9810\,(0.42 + y - \Delta z) - 9810\, S_1 \times 2y$$
$$- 9810 \times 0.84\,(0.5 + \Delta z - y) = p_2$$

Solving it,

$$(p_1 - p_2) = 9810\,[1.84 \times \Delta z - y\,(1.84 - 2S_1)]$$

But

$$\Delta z \times A = 2y \times a$$

$$\Delta z = 2y \times \frac{a}{A}$$

$$= 2y \left(\frac{0.0025}{0.0050}\right)^2 = \frac{y}{2}$$

Substituting the value of Δz

$$(p_1 - p_2) = 9810\,[1.84 \times y/2 - y\,(1.84 - 2S_1)]$$
$$= 9810\,[2S_1 - 0.92]\,y$$

If manometric fluid is water, $S_1 = 1.0$

$$(p_1 - p_2) = 9810\,(2 - 0.92)\,y \ \text{N/m}^2$$

For a rise of 5 cm of meniscus,

$$(p_1 - p_2) = \frac{9810 \times 1.08 \times 0.05}{1000} \ \text{kN/m}^2$$
$$(p_1 - p_2) = 0.5297 \ \text{kPa}$$

2.22 Predict the manometer reading after a 0.01 kN weight is placed on the pan (Fig. 2.37). Assume no leakage or friction between pan and cylinder.

Solution :

When no weight is placed, let us assume pressure due to pan is p_1.

Apply manometric equation

$$p_1 + 0.92 \times 9.810 \times 0.6 - 13.6 \times 9.810 \times 0.075 = 0$$

$$p_1 = 4.591 \text{ kPa}$$

Now let the weight of 0.01 kN is placed in the pan and the pan lowers by Δz. This will cause the lowering of meniscus in the left leg by z and corresponding rise z in the right leg.

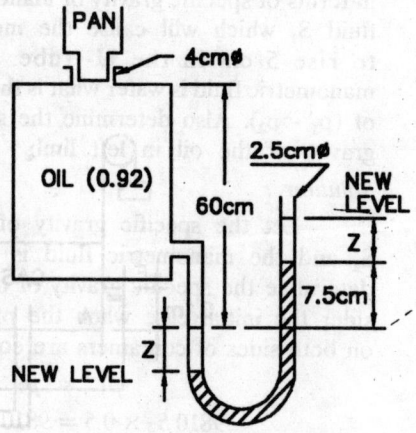

FIG. 2.37. EXAMPLE 2.22

Let the new pressure due to pan and weight be p_2.

$$p_2 + 9.81 \times 0.92 \ (0.6 + z - \Delta z) - 9.81 \times 13.6 \ (0.075 + 2z) = 0$$

But
$$\Delta z \times A = 2z \times a$$

or
$$\Delta z = 2z \ (a/A)$$

$$= 2z \times \left(\frac{0.025}{0.040} \right)^2 = 0.78125z$$

Substituting the value of Δz

$$p_2 + 9.810 \times 0.92 \ (0.6 + z - 0.78125 z) - 9.810 \times 13.6 \ (0.075 + 2z) = 0$$

$$p_2 - 264.857 z = 4.951$$

The area of pan base $= \dfrac{\pi}{4} \times (0.04)^2 = 0.00125 \text{ m}^2$

Therefore $\qquad p_2 = \dfrac{0.01}{0.00125} = 7.955 \text{ kPa}$

Substituting for p_2 in the above equation ,

$$z = 0.0127 \text{m} \quad \text{or} \quad 1.27 \text{cm}.$$

New reading of manometer $= (1.27 + 7.5 + 1.27)$

$$= 10.04 \text{ cm}$$

2.23 The pressure head at level AA is 0.9 m of water and the specific gravity of gas and air are 5.5 N/m³ and 12.4 N/m³ respectively. Determine the reading of the water column in the U- tube gauge which measures the gauge pressure at level B in the figure.

Solution :

(1) The specific weight of gas and air are assumed to remain constant for 100 m difference in elevation.

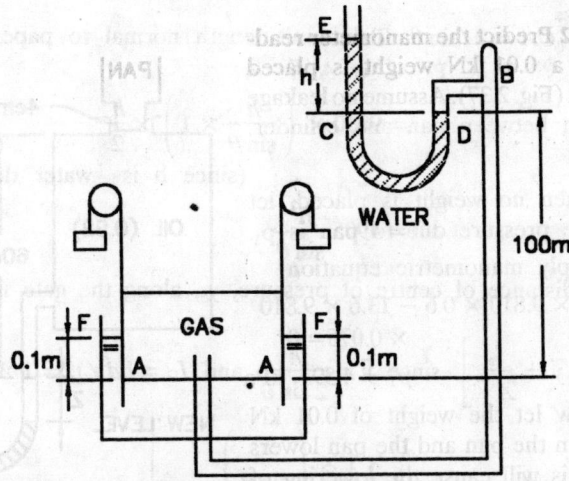

FIG. 2.38. EXAMPLE 2.14

(2) Since the specific weight of gas and air are of the same magnitude, the change of atmospheric pressure with altitude must be taken into account.

(3) Write down the equation in absolute units.

Since the end E is open, the pressure p_E is atmospheric, then pressure at F will be

$$p_F = \text{atmospheric pressure at } E + 12.4 \ (h + 100{-}0.1) \qquad ...(i)$$

The pressure at A is then computed, as

$$p_A = (p_F + 9810 \times 0.1) \qquad ...(ii)$$

Substituting from Eq. (i) into Eq. (ii)

$$p_A = p_E + 12.4 \ (h + 100{-}01) + 9810 \times 0.1 \qquad ...(iii)$$

Now pressure at C = pressure at D

$$p_c = P_E + 9810 \times h = \text{pressure at } A{-}5.5 \times 100 \qquad ...(iv)$$

From Eqs. (iii) and (iv)

$$p_E + 9810 \times h = p_E + 12.4 \ (h + 100{-}0.1) + 9810 \times 0.1{-}5.5 \times 100$$

Solving and neglecting small qauntities,

$$h = 0.17 \text{ m or } 17 \text{ mm of water.}$$

SECTION B - TOTAL PRESSURE AND ITS LOCATION

2.24 The plane gate weighs 2000 N/m normal to the plane of figure with its c.g. 2m from the hinge 0. Find h as a function of θ for equilibrium of gate.(AMIE, 93 Summer)

Solution :

Let the total pressure P acts at the centre of pressure C which is y_p distance away from water surface (measured along the gate).

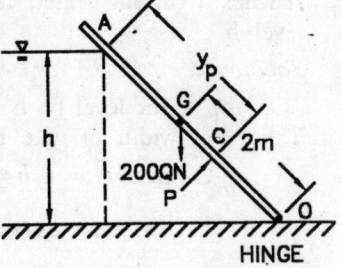

FIG. 2.39. EXAMPLE 2.24

Then, $OA = h/\sin \theta$. Take unit length normal to paper

$\therefore \qquad P = w\, A\, \bar{h}$

$$= 9810 \times \left(\frac{h}{\sin \theta} \times 1 \right) \times \frac{h}{2}$$

(since h is water depth, $\bar{h} = h/2$)

$$= 4905 \frac{h^2}{\sin \theta}$$

The distance of centre of pressure, y_p, along the gate is given by Eq. 2.41b.

$$y_p = \left[\bar{y} + \frac{I_a}{A\bar{y}} \right] \quad \text{since } \bar{y} = \frac{\bar{h}}{2\sin \theta} \text{ and } I_G = bd^3/12 = 1 \times (h/\sin \theta)^3/12$$

$$y_p = \left[\frac{h}{2\sin \theta} + \frac{\frac{1}{12} \times 1 \times \left(\frac{h}{\sin \theta} \right)^3}{\left(1 \times \frac{h}{\sin \theta} \right) \times \left(\frac{h}{2\sin \theta} \right)} \right]$$

$$= \frac{h}{\sin \theta} \left[\frac{1}{2} + \frac{1}{6} \right]$$

$$= \frac{2}{3} \frac{h}{\sin \theta}$$

Now $\qquad OC = OA - AC$

$$= \frac{h}{\sin \theta} - \frac{2}{3} \frac{h}{\sin \theta} = \frac{1}{3} \frac{h}{\sin \theta}$$

The gate will be in equilibrium, if moment of W (= 2000N) and P about hinge 0 is zero.

Hence, $\quad 2000 \times 2 \cos \theta - \left(4905 \frac{h^2}{\sin \theta} \right) \times \frac{h}{3\sin \theta} = 0$

$$4000 \cos \theta - \frac{4905\, h^3}{3 \sin^2 \theta} = 0$$

Solving, $\qquad h = 1.348\, (\sin^2 \theta \cos \theta)^{1/3}$

2.25 The automatic tipper shown in Fig. 2.40 operates when water level reaches a certain height, calculate the water level h.

Solution :

Let the water level be h metre above bed. Take unit width of gate normal to paper.

Given $DE = h, \bar{h} = h/2$

$$AD = \frac{h}{\sin \theta} = 1.155\ h$$

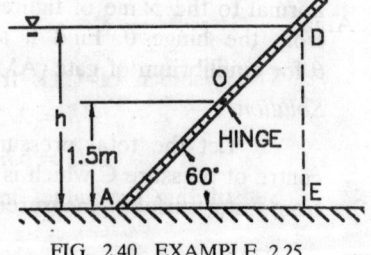

FIG. 2.40. EXAMPLE 2.25

$$A = AD \times 1$$
$$= 1.155\,h \times 1 = 1.155h$$
$$I_G = bd^3/12$$
$$= \frac{1}{12} \times 1 \times (1.155\,h)^3 = 0.1283\,h^3$$

From Eq. 2.41 c,

$$h_p = \left[\bar{h} + \frac{I_G \sin^2\theta}{A\,\bar{h}} \right]$$

$$= \left[0.5\,h + \frac{0.1283\,h^3 \times \sin^2 60°}{1.155\,h \times 0.5\,h} \right]$$

$$= [0.5\,h + 0.167\,h] = 0.667\ \text{h}$$

The gate will tip automatically, as soon as, centre of pressure rises above hinge 0 i.e. it becomes equal to (h - 1.5) as seen from figure.

$$(h-1.5) = 0.667\ h$$

$$h = \frac{1.5}{0.337} = 4.5\ \text{m}$$

Hence, the depth of water required for tipping of gate is 4.5 m.

2.26 Determine the centre of pressure of submerged plane lamina in the following cases.

(a) an equilateral triangle with its edge of length 'b' submerged such that one of its vertices is in the water surface and edge in front of it is horizontal. The lamina is held in vertical plane.

(b) A circular ring radius '2a' held vertical with its centre '3a' below water surface.

Solution :

(a) The triangular surface ABC is immersed in water with its vertex A in the water surface.

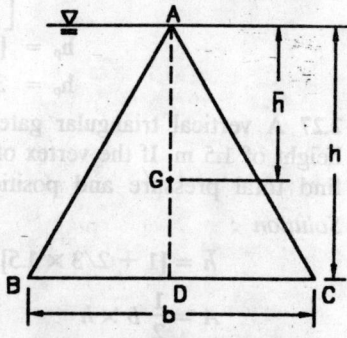

FIG. 2.41. EXAMPLE 2.26

$$h = b \sin 60$$
$$= \sqrt{3/2}\,.b = 0.866\ \text{b} \quad ...(i)$$

Area $\qquad A = \dfrac{b \times h}{2}$

The distance of C.G. from A $= \bar{h}$

$$\bar{h} = 2/3\ h$$

$$I_G = b\,h^3/36$$

Substituting the values in Eq. 2.39 a,

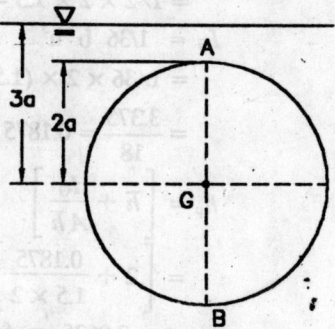

FIG. 2.42. EXAMPLE 2.26

$$I_p = \left[\overline{h} + \frac{I_G}{A\overline{h}} \right]$$

$$= \left[\frac{2}{3}h + \frac{1/36\, b\, h^3}{bh/2 \times 2/3\, h} \right]$$

$$= [2h/3 + h/12] = 3h/4$$

Substitute the value of h in terms of b from Eq.(i) derived above.

$$h_p = 3/4 \times 0.866\; b$$
$$= 0.65\; b$$

(b) Circularning: h = 3 a

$$A = \frac{\pi D^2}{4}$$

$$= \frac{1}{4} \pi (2 \times 2a)^2$$

$$= 4\pi a^2$$

From Eq. 2.39 a,

$$h_p = \left[\overline{h} + \frac{I_G}{A\overline{h}} \right]$$

$$= \left[30a + \frac{\pi/64 \,.\, (4a)^4}{4\pi a^2 \times 3a} \right]$$

$$h_p = [\; 3a + 1/3\, a\;]$$

$$h_p = 3.33a \text{ or } 0.33a \text{ below C.G.}$$

2.27 A vertical triangular gate with vertex·up has a base width of 2m and height of 1.5 m. If the vertex of the gate is one metre below the water surface, find total pressure and position of centre of pressure. [AMIE 1988 W]

Solution :

$$\overline{h} = [1 + 2/3 \times 1.5] = 2\; m$$

$$A = \frac{1}{2} b \times h$$

$$= 1/2 \times 2 \times 1.5 = 1.5\; m^2$$

$$I_G = 1/36\, b\, h^3$$

$$= 1/36 \times 2 \times (1.5)^3$$

$$= \frac{3.375}{18} = 0.1875\; m^4$$

$$h_p = \left[\overline{h} + \frac{I_G}{A\overline{h}} \right]$$

$$= \left[2 + \frac{0.1875}{1.5 \times 2} \right]$$

$$= 2.0625\; m \text{ from w.s.}$$

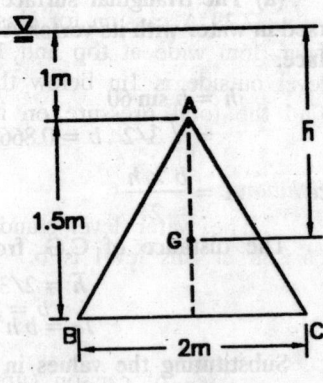

FIG. 2.43. EXAMPLE 2.27

2.28 A square lamina, length 3a, with a hole of radius 'a' cut centrally, held with its surface inclined at 30° to the horizontal and one of its surface at water surface is immersed in water. Calculate total pressure and location of centre of pressure.

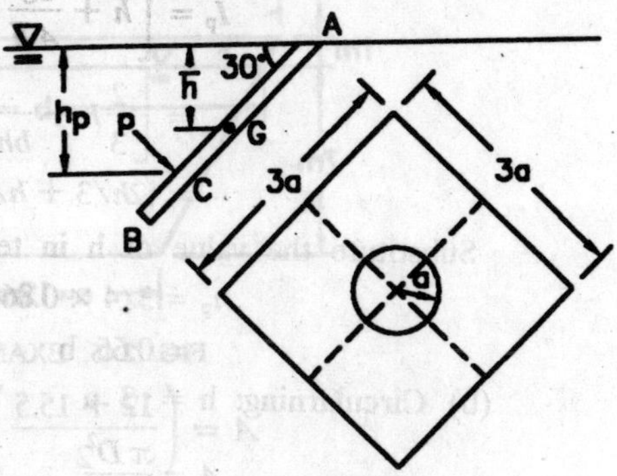

Solution :

$$P = w A \bar{h}$$

where,

$$\bar{h} = 1/2 \, (3a \sin 30°)$$

$$= 3/4 \, a$$

$$A = [(3a)^2 - \pi a^2]$$

$$= 5.86 \, a^2$$

FIG. 2.44. EXAMPLE 2.28

$$I_G = \left[\frac{1}{12} \times 3a \times (3a)^3 - \frac{\pi}{64} (2a)^4 \right]$$

$$= \left[\frac{1}{12} \times 3a \times (3a)^3 - \frac{\pi}{64} (2a)^4 \right]$$

$$= (6.74 \, a^4 - 0.7857 \, a^4)$$

$$= 5.964 \, a^4$$

From Eqs. 2.40c, and 2,41c

$$P = 9810 \times 5.86 \, a^2 \times 0.75a \, \text{N}$$

$$= 43.115 \, a^3 \, \text{kN}$$

$$h_p = \left[h + \frac{I_G \sin^2 \theta}{A \bar{h}} \right]$$

$$= \left[0.75 \, a + \frac{5.964 \, a^4 \times (\sin 30°)^2}{5.86 \, a^2 \times 0.75 \, a} \right]$$

$$= 0.75 \, a + 0.3393 \, a$$

$$= 1.089 \, a.$$

2.29 A cassion for closing the entrance to a dry dock is of trapezoidal form 16m wide at top and 12m wide at bottom and 8m deep. If the water level outside is 1m below the top level of caisson and the dock is empty, find the total pressure on it and the depth of centre of pressure.

[AMIE 1980 Nov.]

Solution :

The water level stand 1 m below the top level, therefore, width of caisson at this level is b.

$$b = 12 + \left(\frac{16 - 12}{8} \right) \times 7 = 15.5 \, \text{m}$$

Area of caisson (upto 7m depth) $= \dfrac{a + b}{2} \times h$

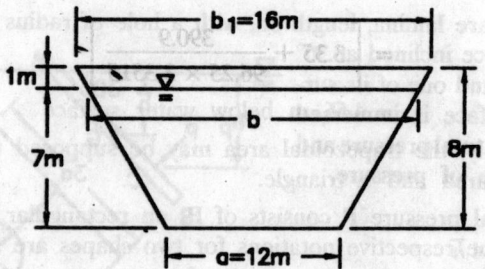

FIG. 2.45. EXAMPLE 2.29

$$A = \left(\frac{12 + 15.5}{2} \right) \times 7 = 96.25 \text{ m}^2$$

The centre of gravity lies $\bar{h}$ below free water surface.

$$\bar{h} = \left(\frac{2a + b}{a + b} \right) \frac{h}{3}$$

$$= \left(\frac{2 \times 12 + 15.5}{12 + 15.5} \right) \frac{7}{3} = 3.3515 \text{ below w.s}$$

From Eq. 2.37 b,

$$P = wA\bar{h}$$
$$= 9810 \times 96.25 \times 3.3515 \text{ N}$$
$$= 3164.54 \text{ kN}$$

Moment of inertia about an axis passing through C.G is given by

$$I_G = \left(\frac{a^2 + 4ab + b^2}{36(a + b)} \right) h^3$$

$$= \left[\frac{(12)^2 + 4 \times 12 \times 15.5 + (15.5)^2}{36(12 + 15.5)} \right] (7)^3$$

$$= 390.9 \text{ m}^4$$

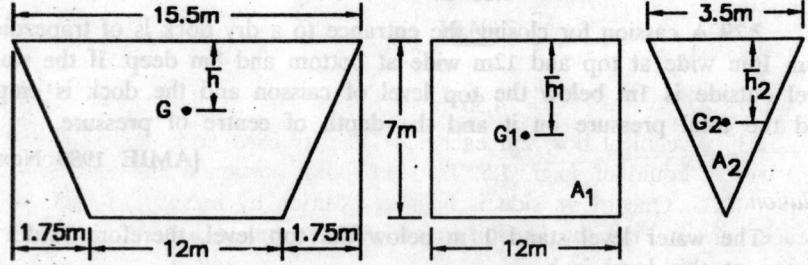

FIG. 2.46 EXAMPLE 2.29

From Eq. 2.39 a,

$$h_p = \left[\bar{h} + \frac{I_G}{A\bar{h}} \right]$$

$$= \left[3.35 + \frac{390.9}{96.25 \times 3.3515} \right]$$

$$= 4.56 \text{ m below water surface}$$

Alternatively, the trapezoidal area may be supposed to be composed of a rectangular area and a triangle.

Let the total pressure P consists of P_1 on rectangular area and P_2 on triangular area. The respective notations for two shapes are shown in figure.

$$\overline{h_1} = \frac{7}{2} = 3.5 \text{ m}, \ \overline{h_2} = \frac{1}{3} \times 7 = 2.33 \text{ m}$$

$$A_1 = 12 \times 7 = 84 \text{ m}^2, \ A_2 = 1/2 \times 3.5 \times 7 = 12.25 \text{ m}^2$$

$$P_1 = 9.81 \times 84 \times 3.5 = 2884.14 \text{ kN}$$

$$P_2 = 9.81 \times 12.25 \times 7/3 = 280.40 \text{ kN}$$

$$P = P_1 + P_2 = 3164.54 \text{ kN}$$

Centre of pressure of total pressure P_1

$$h_{p1} = \left[\overline{h_1} + \frac{I_G}{A_1 \overline{h_1}} \right]$$

$$= \left[3.5 + \frac{1/12 \times 12 \times 7^3}{84 \times 3.5} \right] = 4.667 \text{ m}.$$

Centre of pressure of total pressure P_2

$$h_{p2} = \left[\overline{h_2} + \frac{I_G}{A_2 \overline{h_2}} \right]$$

$$= \left[2.33 + \frac{1}{36} \times \frac{3.5 \times 7^3}{3.5 \times 7/2 \times 7/3} \right] = 2.4967 \text{ m}.$$

Centre of pressure of total pressure P

$$h_p = \frac{P_1 h_{p1} + P_2 h_{p2}}{P_1 + P_2}$$

$$= \frac{2884.14 \times 4.667 + 280 \times 2.4967}{3164.54}$$

$$= 4.56 \text{ m}.$$

2.30 A cubical box, 2m each side has its base horizontal and is half filled with a liquid of sp.gr. 1.5. The remaining portion is filled with an oil of sp.gr. 0.95. One of its side is held in position by means of four screws, at each corner. Find the tension in each screw due to hydrostatic pressure.

(Similar in 1987 Nov.)

Solution :

This problem is solved by graphical method.

The hydrostatic pressure on the vertical gate A B C D consists of total pressure P_1 on A B F E (shown by pressure diagram L M N) and

$P_2 + P_3$ on E F C D (shown by pressure diaagram M N T Q). To compute P_1, P_2 and P_3 and their locations, use Eq. 2.43.

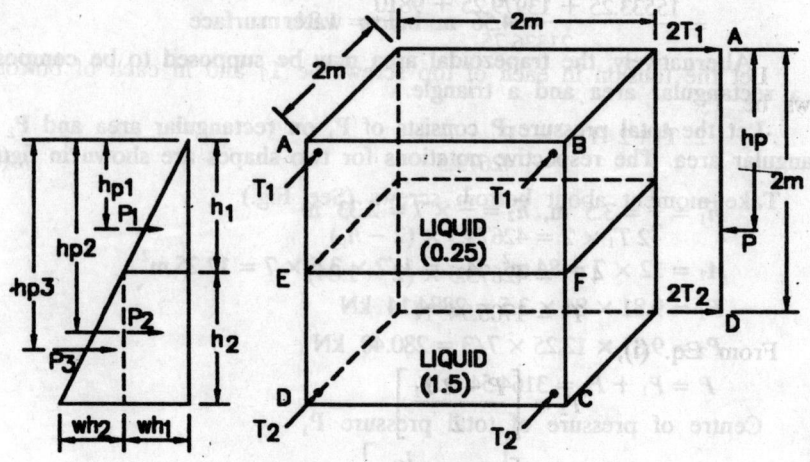

FIG. 2.47. EXAMPLE 2.30

Given $w_1 = 0.95 \times 9810 \text{ N/m}^3$, $h_1 = 1\text{m}$

$w_2 = 0.5 \times 9810 \text{ N/m}^3$, $h_2 = 1\text{m}$

Total poressure $P = P_1$ on ABFE + $(P_2 + P_3)$ on EFCD.

$= b$ [area of pressure diagram LNTQM]

$= b$ [area of (LNM + MNTS + MSQ)]

$$= 2 \left[\frac{(0.95 \times 9810 \times 1)\,(1)}{2} + (0.95 \times 9810 \times 1)\,(1) + \frac{(1.5 \times 9810 \times 1)\,(1)}{2} \right]$$

$= 2$ [4659.75 + 9319.5 + 7357.5]

$= 42673.5$ N or 42.673 kN

Centre of pressure wil be at h_p below free surface.

$$h_p = \frac{P_1 h_{p1} + P_2 h_{p2} + P_3 h_{p3}}{P}$$

where. $P_1 = 2 \times 4659.75$ N; $h_{p1} =$ centroid of L M N

$= \dfrac{h_1}{3} = 1/3$ m

$P_2 = 2 \times 9319.5$ N; $h_{p2} =$ centroid of MNTS

$= (1 + 1/2) = 1.5$ m

$P_3 = 2 \times 7357.5$ N; $h_{p3} =$ centroid of M S Q

$= (1 + 1/3\ h_2)$

$= (1 + 1/3 \times 1) = 1.33$ m

$$\therefore \quad h_p = \left[\frac{2 \times 4659.75 + 2 \times 9319.5 \times 1.5 + 2 \times 7357.5 \times 1.33}{42673.5}\right]$$

$$= \frac{15533.25 + 13979.25 + 9810}{21336.75} = 1.84 \text{ m}$$

Let the tension in each of top screws be T_1 and in each of bottom screws be T_2.

$$\therefore \quad 2\,T_1 + 2\,T_2 = P$$
$$= 42673.5 \qquad \qquad \qquad ...(i)$$

Take moment about bottom screws (See Fig.)

$$2\,T_1 \times 2 = 42673.5 \times (2 - h_p)$$
$$4\,T_1 = 42673.5 \times (2 - 1.84)$$
$$T_1 = 1706.94 \text{ N}$$

From Eq. (i),

$$T_2 = \left[\frac{P - 2\,T_1}{2}\right]$$
$$= \left[\frac{42673.5 - 2 \times 1706.94}{2}\right]$$
$$= 19629.81 \text{ N}$$

Tension in each of top screws = 1706.94 N

Tension in each of bottom screws = 19629.81 N

2.31 : A pipe line which is 4m diameter contains a circular disc valve, the pressure at the centre of valve is 196 kPa. If the pipe contains oil of sp.gr. 0.87, find the force exerted by the oil upon the gate and the position of centre of pressure. The valve can rotate about a horizontal diameter, find the torque required to maintain it in the vertical positon.

(Similar AMIE 90 S)

Solution,

The pipe runs under pressure and the pressure at the centre of valve is 196 kPa. Therefore, the free surface should be h metre above cntre line of pipe.

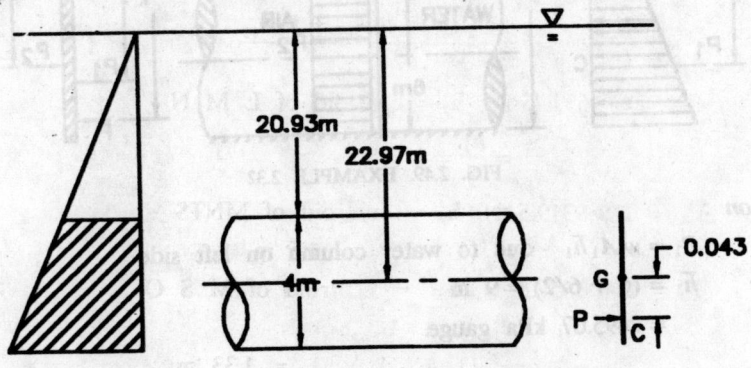

FIG. 2.48. EXAMPLE 2.31

$$h = \frac{p}{w}$$

$$= \frac{196}{9.81 \times 0.87} = 22.97 \text{ m}$$

$\bar{h} = h$ = distance of C.G. from free surface.

Now

$$P = wA\bar{h}$$

$$= 0.87 \times 9.81 \times (\pi/4 \times 4^2) \times 22.97$$

$$= 2463.537 \text{ kN}$$

$$h_p = \left[\bar{h} + \frac{I_G}{A\bar{h}} \right]$$

$$= \left[22.97 + \frac{\pi/64 \times (4)^4}{\pi/4\,(4)^2 \times 22.97} \right]$$

$$h_p = 2.97 + 0.043 = 23.013\text{m} \quad \text{below free surface}$$

$$= 0.043 \text{ m below centre line.}$$

Torque required to maintain the gate in vertical position

$$= \text{moment of } P \text{ about axis of rotation}$$

$$= P \times (h_p - \bar{h})$$

$$= 2463.537 \times 0.043$$

$$= 105.93 \text{ kN-m}$$

2.32 : A vertical circular gate of 6m diameter is fitted in a cylindrical tunnel. There is water on one side of the gate with water surface at 12 m above the invert of the tunnel and air on the other side having pressure of 122.5 kPa absolute. Determine the magnitude and location of the resultant force acting on the gate. (AMIE 92 winter)

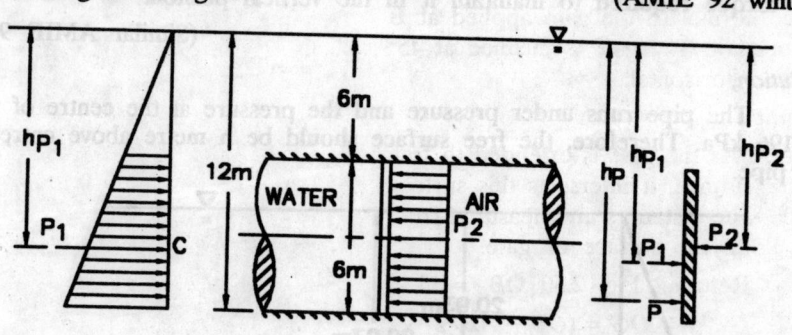

FIG. 2.49. EXAMPLE 2.32

Solution :

$$P_1 = wA_1\bar{h}_1 \quad \text{due to water column on left side}$$

where $\bar{h}_1 = (6 + 6/2) = 9$ m

$$= 2495.07 \text{ kPa gauge}$$

$$h_{p1} = \left(\bar{h} + \frac{I_G}{Ah_1} \right)$$

$$= \left[9 + \frac{\pi/64 \times (6)^4}{\pi/4\,(6)^2 \times 9} \right]$$

$= [9 + 1/16 \times 36/9] = 9.25$ m below free surface

$P_2 = 122.5$ kPa absolute.

Assuming atmospheric pressure as 1 bar $= 10^5$ N/m²

$\qquad = 100$ kPa

$P_2 = 122.5 - 100$

$\qquad = 22.5$ kPa gauge

Therefore, net pressure on the gate $P = P_1 - P_2$

$P = 2495.07 - 22.5$

$\qquad = 2472.57$ k Pa gauge

Let the net total pressure P acts h_p metre below free surface.

$$h_p = \frac{P_1 h_{p1} - P_2 h_{p2}}{P}$$

$$= \frac{2495.07 \times 9.25 - 22.5 \times 9}{2472.57}$$

$= 9.2522$ m below free surface.

2.33 : An inclined sluice gate AB (1.2m x 5m size) as shown in Fig. 2.50 is installed to control the discharge of water. End A is hinged. Determine the force normal to the gate applied at B to open it. The gate is inclined at 45° to the horizontal.

Solution :

As the gate is extended to free water surface, it intersects this surface at 00. The distances are measured from 00 along the surface of gate.

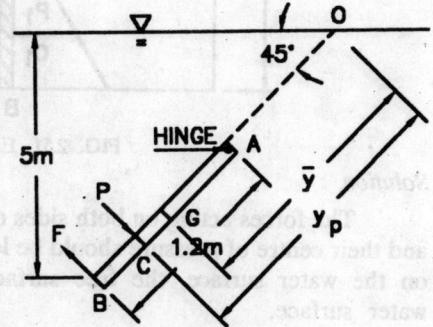

FIG. 2.50. EXAMPLE 2.33

Refering Fig. 2.50 OB $= 5 \cos 45 = 5\sqrt{2}$ m

$\bar{y} = OG = (OB - AB/2)$

$\qquad = (5\sqrt{2} - 1.2/2) = 6.471$ m

$$y_p = \left[\bar{y} + \frac{I_G}{A\bar{y}} \right]$$

$$= \left[6.471 + 1/12 \times \frac{5 \times (1.2)^3}{5 \times 1.2 \times 6.471} \right]$$

$= 6.4895$ m

$$P = wA\overline{h}$$
$$= 9.81 \times (1.2 \times 5) \times (6.471 \sin 45°)$$
$$= 269.325 \text{ kN}$$

To find F, take moment about hinge at A

$$F \times AB = P \times AC$$
$$F \times 1.2 = P[OC - OA] = P[OC - (AG - AB/2)]$$
$$F = \frac{269.325 \times [6.4895 - (6.471 - 0.6)]}{1.2}$$
$$= 138.81 \text{ kN.}$$

2.34 Gate AB shown in Figure below is 1.2 m wide and is hinged at A. Gauge G reads -0.147 bar and oil of sp.gr. 0.75 is filled in the right side tank. What horizontal force must be applied at B for equilibrium of gate AB.

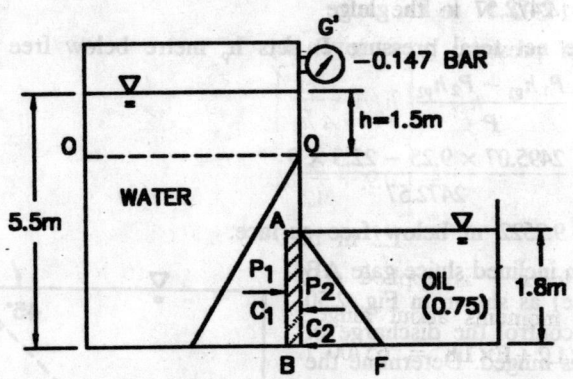

FIG. 2.51. EXAMPLE 2.34

Solution :

The forces acting on both sides of AB due to liquids should be evaluated and their centre of pressure should be located. Since there is a negative pressure on the water surface, the free surface will be h metre (say) below actual water surface.

$$h = \frac{-0.147 \times 10^5}{9810} = -1.5 \text{ m}$$

This means the free water surface lies 1.5 m below actual water surface and depth of water should be taken as (5.5 - 1.5) = 4 m for computation.

$$\overline{h_1} = (OA + AB/2) \quad \because \quad OA = OB - 1.8$$
$$= 4 - 1.8 = 2.2\text{m}$$
$$= \left(2.2 + \frac{1.8}{2}\right) = 3.1 \text{ m}$$

The total pressure acting on AB from left side,
$$P_1 = wA\overline{h_1}$$

$$= 9810 \times 1.2 \times 1.8 \times 3.1$$
$$= 65700 \text{ N to the right}$$

The centre of pressure h_{p1} measured from 00 is

$$h_{p1} = \left[\bar{h}_1 + \frac{I_G}{A\bar{h}_1} \right]$$

$$= \left[3.1 + \frac{1}{12} \times \frac{1.2 \times (1.8)^3}{1.2 \times 1.8 \times 3.1} \right]$$

$$= 3.2 \text{ m below 00}$$

The total pressure acting on AB from right side is

$$P_2 = wA_2\bar{h}_2$$

$$= 0.75 \times 9810 \times 1.8 \times 1.2 \times \left(\frac{1.8}{2} \right) \left(\because h_2 = \frac{1.8}{2} = 0.9 \text{ m} \right)$$

$$= 14302 \text{ N to the left.}$$

Centre of pressure h_{p2} is given by

$$h_{p2} = \left[\bar{h}_2 + \frac{I_G}{A\bar{h}_2} \right]$$

$$= \left[0.9 + \frac{1}{12} \times \frac{1.2 \times (1.8)^3}{1.2 \times 1.8 \times 0.9} \right]$$

$$= 1.2 \text{ m below liquid surface at A.}$$

Let a force F is applied at B from right to left side.
Taking moments about hinge at A

$$14302 \times 1.2 + F \times 1.8 = 65700 \text{ (A } C_1)$$

where $\quad A C_1 = (h_{p1} - OA) = (3.2 - 2.2) = 1 \text{ m}$

$$\therefore F \times 1.8 = 65700 \times 1 - 14302 \times 1.2$$

Solving, $\qquad F = 2700 \text{ N to the left.}$

2.35 : A vertical gate AB of size 3.8m x 1.4m wide is held vertical to close the opening of a sluice in the body of a dam. It is hinged at 15 cm below the C.G. of the gate. The total depth of water from B on u/s side is 6m. What force must be applied at the bottom of gate to keep it closed.

(Similar, A.M.I.E., 86 W)

Solution,

Since height of gate AB is 3.8m

$$OA = (6 - 3.8) = 2.2 \text{ m}$$

$$\therefore \quad \bar{h} = (2.2 + 1/2 \times 3.8) = 4.1 \text{ m}$$

$$P = wA\bar{h}$$

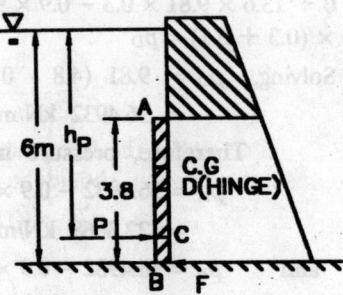

FIG. 2.52. EXAMPLE 2.35

$$= 9.81 \times (3.8 \times 1.4) \times 4.1$$
$$= 213.957 \text{ kN}$$

$$h_p = \left[\bar{h} + \frac{I_G}{A\bar{h}} \right]$$

$$= \left[4.1 + \frac{1}{12} \times \frac{1.4 \times (3.8)^3}{1.4 \times 3.8 \times 4.1} \right]$$

$$h_p = [4.1 + 0.293] = 4.393 \text{ m}$$

To find force F applied at B, take moment about hinge at D.

$$F \times (BD) = P \times (CD)$$

where,

$$CD = (h_p - OD)$$
$$= [h_p - (\bar{h} + GD)]$$
$$= [4.393 - (4.1 + 0.15)]$$
$$= 0.143 \text{ m}$$

$$F \times \frac{3.8}{2} = 213.957 \times 0.143$$

Solving, $F = 16.103 \text{ kN}$

2.36 : Calculate the minimum force F required to keep the cover of the box closed, shown in figure below. The cover is 1.5 m wide perpendicular to the plane of paper. The U-tube mercury manometer reads 0.30 m which is fitted at the bottom. The box contains an oil of sp.g. 0.9.

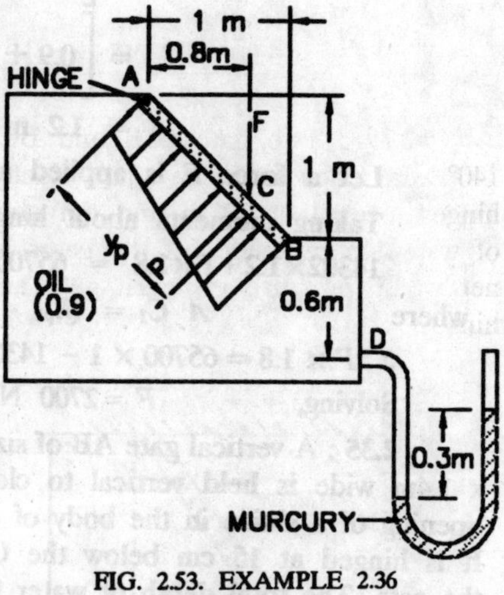

Solution :

Apply manometric equation to determine pressure at D. Start from open end,

$$0 + 13.6 \times 9.81 \times 0.3 - 0.9 \times 9.81$$
$$\times (0.3 + 0.1) = p_D$$

Solving, $p_D = 9.81 (4.8 - 0.36)$
$$= 36.4932 \text{ kN/m}^2$$

FIG. 2.53. EXAMPLE 2.36

Therefore, pressure intensity at A and B will be

$$p_A = 36.4932 - 0.9 \times 9.81 \times (0.6 + 1.0)$$
$$= 22.3668 \text{ kN/m}^2$$

and $p_B = 36.4932 - 0.9 \times 9.81 \times 0.6$
$$= 31.1958 \text{ kN/m}^2$$

These pressures will act normal to the inclined cover AB. The pressure diagram on AB is shown in figure.

The total pressure P acting on cover AB can now be determined by graphical method.

$$P = b \times \text{ area of pressure diagram}$$

$$= 1.5 \times \left[\frac{p_A + p_B}{2} \times AB \right]$$

where $AB = \sqrt{(1)^2 + (1)^2} = \sqrt{2} = 1.414$ m

$$P = 1.5 \left[\frac{22.3668 + 31.1958}{2} \times 1.414 \right]$$

$$= 1.5 \times 26.7813 \times 1.414 = 56.803 \text{ kN}$$

The centre of pressure will be at the centroid of pressure prism.

$$y_p = AC = \frac{[2 \times p_B + p_A]}{(p_B + p_A)} \times \frac{AB}{3}$$

$$= \frac{2 \times 31.1958 + 22.3668}{(31.1958 + 22.3668)} \times \frac{1.414}{3}$$

$$= 0.7458 \text{ m}$$

To find F_1, take moment about hinge at A,

$$F \times 0.8 = P \times y_p$$

$$F = \frac{56.803 \times 0.7458}{0.8} = 52.958 \text{ kN}$$

2.37 : Two gates AB and BC of a lock chamber make an angle of 140° with each other in plan. Each gate is supported at one end by two hinges located at 12 m and 6m above the bottom of the lock. The depth of water on two sides of the gates are 9m and 4.5 m respectively. Find the net water pressure on each gate and the reaction at the top and bottom hinges.

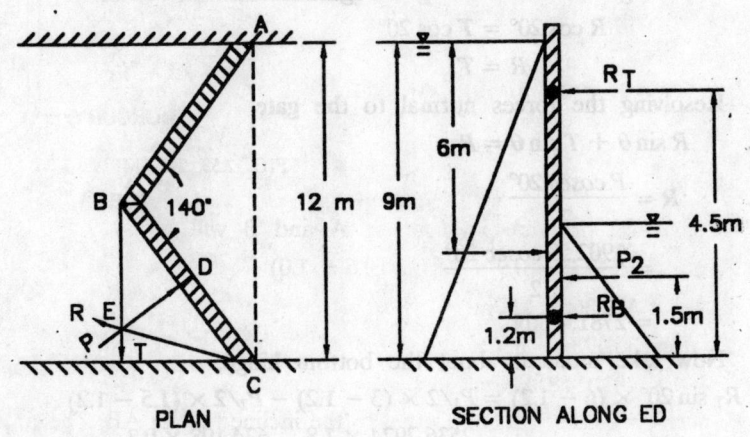

PLAN   SECTION ALONG ED

FIG. 2.54. EXAMPLE 2.37

Solution :

Width of each gate (AB = BC) = 6 Cosec 70°

= 6.385 m normal to plane of paper.

$P_1 = w A_1 \overline{h_1}$

= 9.81 × (6.385 × 9) × 9/2

= 2536.7924 kN towards right

$P_2 = w A_2 \overline{h_2}$

= 9.81 × (6.385 × 4.5) × 4.5/2

= 634.198 kN towardss left.

Therefore, the net water pressure P acting on gate ,

$P = P_1 - P_2$

= 2536.7924 - 634.198

= 1902.59 kN towards right.

Since the pressure distribution on both sides is triangular,

$h_{p1} = 2/3 × 9 = 6$ m from water surface or 3 m from bottom

and $h_{p2} = \dfrac{2}{3} × 4.5 = 3$ m from water surface or 1.5 from bottom

Hence, net pressure will act h'$_p$ distance from bottom

$$h'_p = \frac{P_1 × 3 - P_2 × 1.5}{P}$$

$$= \frac{2536.7924 - 634.198 × 1.5}{1902.59}$$

= 3.5 m from bottom.

Let the reactions at bottom and top hinges are R_B and R_T.

Resolving the forces along the gate

$R \cos 20° = T \cos 20°$

$R = T$

Resolving the forces normal to the gate

$R \sin \theta + T \sin \theta = P$

or $R = \dfrac{P \, cosec \, 20°}{2}$

$$= \frac{1902.59 \, cosec \, 20°}{2}$$

= 2781.4 kN

Now take moment about the bottom hinge,

$R_T \sin 20° × (6 - 1.2) = P_1/2 × (3 - 1.2) - P_2/2 × (1.5 - 1.2)$

$$R_T × 4.8 \sin 20° = \frac{2536.7924 × 1.8}{2} - \frac{634.198 × 0.3}{2}$$

$$R_T = 1332.76 \text{ kN}$$

Since, $\quad R_B + R_T = R$

$$R_B = (2781.4 - 1332.76)$$
$$= 1448.64 \text{ kN}.$$

2.38 : Determine the magnitude and direction of the resultant force acting on the radial gate of radius 4m shown below. The length of gate is 5m.

Solution :

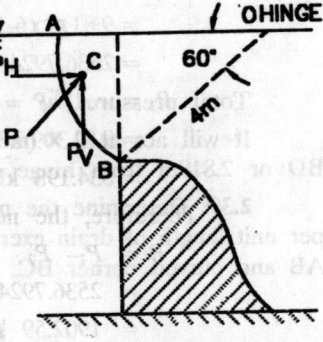

P_H = Pressure intensity × Projection of area in the normal direction.

= Total pressure acting on projection of AB in the vertical plane i.e. BD.

From Eq. 2.55, BD = 4 Sin 60° = 3.464 m

FIG. 2.55. EXAMPLE 2.38

$$OD = 4 \cos 60° = 2.0 \text{ m}$$
$$P_H = w A \bar{h}$$
$$9.81 \times (3.464 \times 5) \times \frac{3.464}{2}$$
$$= 294.283 \text{ kN}$$

It will act at 2h/3 from water surface

$$h_p = 2/3 \times 3.464 = 2.309 \text{ m}$$

The vertical component P_v of total pressure is equal to the weight of liquid displaced, i.e. weight of water in volume A B D.

$$P_v = 9.81 \times 5 \times (Area\ A\ O\ B - Area\ B\ O\ D)$$
$$= 9.81 \times 5 \times \left[\pi (4)^2 \times \frac{60°}{360°} - \frac{1}{2} \times 3.464 \times 2 \right]$$
$$= 9.81 \times 5 [8.381 - 3.464]$$
$$= 9.81 \times 5 \times 4.917$$
$$= 241.179 \text{ kN acting upward}$$

Thus the resultant pressure P must pass through 0.

$$P = \sqrt{(P_H)^2 + (P_v)^2}$$
$$= \sqrt{(294.283)^2 + (241.179)^2}$$
$$= 380.486 \text{ kN}$$

It will act at an angle θ with horizontal

$$\tan \theta = \frac{P_v}{P_H}$$
$$= \frac{241.179}{294.283} = 0.8195$$

$$\theta = 39.33°$$

Since P_H acts at C at 2.309m below water surface

$$OE = E\,C \cot \theta$$
$$= 2.309 \cot 39.33° = 2.818\text{m}$$
$$ED = (OE - OD)$$
$$= (2.818 - 4 \cos 60°) = 0.818 \text{ m}$$

Total pressure $\quad P = 380.486$ kN

It will act at 2.309m below water surface and 0.818m to the left of BD or 2.818m from hinge at 0.

2.39: Determine the magnitude direction and line of action of forces per unit length of drain exerted upon its horizontal bottom CD, vertical side AB and curved corner BC. The normal depth of water in the drain is 2m.

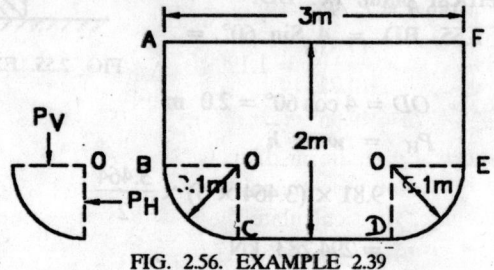

FIG. 2.56. EXAMPLE 2.39

Solution :

Total pressure on vertical surface AB.

$$P_H = w\,A\,\bar{h}$$
$$= 9.81 \times (1 \times 1) \times 1/2 = 4.905 \text{ kN/m}$$
$$h_p = \left[\bar{h} + \frac{I_G}{A\,\bar{h}} \right]$$
$$= \left[0.5 + \frac{1}{12} \times \frac{1 \times (1)^3}{1 \times 1 \times 0.5} \right] = 0.667 \text{ m}$$

Total pressure on horizontal surface CD

$$P_v = w\,A\,\bar{h}$$
$$= 9.81 \times (1 \times 1)\,(2)$$
$$= 19.62 \text{ kN}$$

It will act vertically downward at the centre of CD.

Curved surface BC : From Eq. 2.45

$$P_H = (w \times \text{ vertical projection of BC} \times \text{ depth of centre of mass of vertical projection})$$
$$= 9.81 \times (1 \times 1) \times (1 + 1/2)$$

Similarly, P_v = [weight of water in BC + total pressure on horizontal projection of BC]

$$= [9.81 \times \pi/4 \,(1)^2 \times 1 + 9.81 \times (1 \times 1) \times 1]$$
$$= 17.514 \text{ kN}$$

It will act through centre of mass at $\dfrac{4r}{3\pi}$ from OC

$$= \frac{4 \times 1}{3\pi} = 0.425, \text{ from vertical OC.}$$

Resultant pressure on BC is given by P and it will act at an angle θ with the horizontal

$$P = \sqrt{P_H{}^2 + P_v^2}$$
$$= \sqrt{(14.715)^2 + (17.514)^2}$$
$$= 22.875 \text{ kN.}$$
$$\tan\theta = P_v/P_H$$
$$= \frac{17.514}{14.715} = 1.1902$$
$$\theta = 49.96°$$

2.40 : A cylindrical gate 2m in diameter and 3m long is held in position as shown in figure. Calculate the magnitude and location of resultant water force exerted on the gate. Also calculate the least weight of the gate to ensure that it will not float away from bottom. [A.M.I.E., 81 Summer]

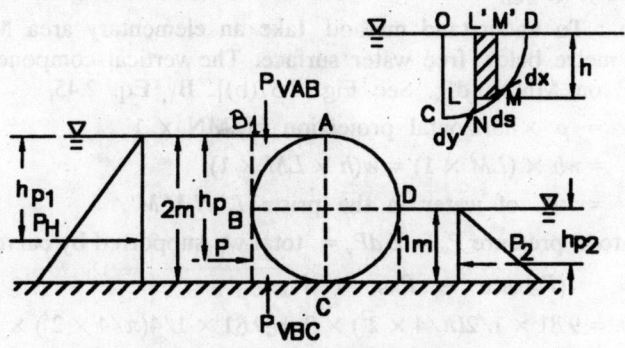

FIG. 2.57. EXAMPLE 2.40

Solution :

Horizontal component : Let the horizontal component P_{H1} acts on ABC and P_{H2} on CD. The length of gate is 3m.

From Eq. 2.45,

$$P_{H1} = \int w \times \text{vertical projection of } ABC \times h.$$
$$= 9.81 \times (3 \times 2) \times 2/2$$
$$= 58.86 \text{ kN towards right}$$

It will act at 2/3 h from water surface or 1/3 h from bottom,

$$h_{p1} = 2/3 \times 2 = 4/3 \text{ m}$$

Similarly,
$$P_{H2} = 9.81 \times (3 \times 1) \times 1/2$$
$$= 14.715 \text{ kN towards left.}$$
$$h_{p2} = 2/3 \times (1) = 1/3 \text{ from water surface}$$

Net horizontal force $P_H = P_{H1} - P_{H2}$
$$P_H = 58.86 - 14.715$$
$$= 44.145 \text{ kN towards right}$$

To locate centre of pressure of P_H, take moment about C.

$$P_{H1} \times (2 - 4/3) - P_{H2} \times (1 - 1/3) = P_H \times h' P$$

$$h' P = \frac{58.86 \times 2/3 - 14.15 \times 1/3}{44.145}$$

$$= 0.77 \text{ m above bottom}$$

Vertical components : The vertical component of total pressure will act downward on segment AB whereas on BC and CD these will act upwards.

$(P_v)_{AB}$ = weight of water in AB_1 B acting downwards

$(P_v)_{BC}$ = weight of water in AB_1 BCA acting upwards

$(P_v)_{ABC}$ = weight of water in (AB_1 BCA-AB_1 B)acting upward

= weight of water in ABC upwards

Similarly, $(P_v)_{CD}$ = weight of water in OCD acting upwards

[Note : To understand method, take an elementary area MN of unit length at h metre below free water surface. The vertical component of total pressure dP on MN is dP_v. See Fig. 2.57(b)]. By Eq. 2.45,

$$d P_v = p \times \text{horizontal projection of MN x 1.}$$
$$= wh \times (LM \times 1) = w(h \times LM \times 1)$$
$$= \text{wt. of water in the prism } L' N M M'.$$

The total pressure $P_v = \Sigma dP_v =$ total wt. supported by curved surface.]

$$(P_v)_{ABCD} = P_{ABC} + P_{CD}$$
$$= 9.81 \times 1/2(\pi/4 \times 2^2) \times 3 + 9.81 \times 1/4(\pi/4 \times 2^2) \times 3$$
$$= 46.247 + 23.124$$
$$= 69.37 \text{ kN acting upward.}$$

The resultant water pressure will be vectorial sum of P_H and P_v

$$P = \sqrt{P_H{}^2 + P_v{}^2}$$
$$= \sqrt{(44.145)^2 + (69.37)^2}$$
$$= 82.225 \text{ kN}$$

$$\tan \theta = \frac{P_v}{P_H}$$

$$= \frac{69.37}{44.145} = 1.5714$$

$$\theta = 57.53°$$

Least weight required to keep the cylinder down

W acting downward = Pv acting upward

$$= 69.37 \text{ kN}$$

2.41: The profile of the water face of a dam is given by the equation $324y = 5x^{5/2}$, where y is the height in metre above the floor level and x is the set back of the free surface from the vertical line of reference. Determine the resultant force per metre of the length of the dam, its inclination to the vertical and the location of the point of intersection of the resultant force with horizontal floor.

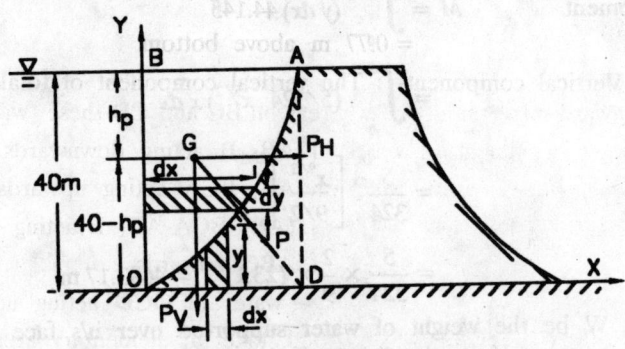

FIG. 2.58 EXAMPLE 2.41

Solution :

Horizontal force P_H :

$$P_H = \int w \times \text{vertical projection of A x h}$$

$$= 9.81 \times (40 \times 1) \times 40/2$$

$$= 7848 \text{ kN to the right.}$$

$$h_p = 1/3 \times h$$

$$= 1/3 \times 40 = 40/3 \text{ below water surface}$$

Vertical force Pv : It is equal to the weight of volume of water OAB supported by dam

$$P_v = w \times \text{ area OAB} \times 1$$

$$P_v = w \times \text{ area (OBAD-OAD)} \times 1$$

To find area OAD :The equation of curve OA is

$$y = \frac{5}{324}x^{5/2}$$

when $y = 40, x \left[\frac{324 \times 40}{5}\right]^{2/5} = 23.1 \text{ m}$

Now, area $OAD = \int_{0}^{23.1} y \, dx$

$$= \int_{0}^{23.1} 5/324 \times x^{5/2} \, dx = 256 \text{ m}^2$$

Also, area $OBAD = 40 \times 23.1 = 924 \text{ m}^2$

Therefore, $Pv = 9.81 \times (924 - 256) \times 1$

$$= 6553.1 \text{ kN}$$

To find location of G : Take moment of OAD about vertical line OB and integrate,

Moment $M = \int_{0}^{23.1} (y \, dx) \, x$

$$= \int_{0}^{23.1} (5/324 \cdot x^{5/2}) \, x \, dx$$

$$= \frac{5}{324} \cdot \left[\frac{x^{9/2}}{9/2} \right]_{0}^{23.1}$$

$$= \frac{5}{324} \times \frac{2}{9} \times (23.1)^{9/2} = 4693.17 \text{ m}^3$$

Let W be the weight of water supported over u/s face of the dam and let its center of gravity lies at $\bar{x}$ from OB.

Take moment of W about OB,

$$W \times \bar{x} = \text{summation of moment of OAB}$$

$$\bar{x} = \frac{9.81 \, [40 \times 23.1 \times 23.1/2 - 4693.17] \times 1}{6553.1}$$

$$= \frac{9.81 \, (10672.2 - 4693.17)}{6553.1} = 8.95 \text{ m}$$

Resultant pressure $P = \sqrt{P_H^2 + Pv^2}$

$$= \sqrt{(7848)^2 + (6553.1)^2}$$

$$= 10224 \text{ kN}$$

Inclination with horizontal, $P_H \tan \theta = \dfrac{Pv}{P_H}$

$$\tan \theta = \frac{6553.1}{7848.0} = 0.835$$

$$\theta = 39.86°$$

To locate the point of intersection of P with horizontal base at D, i.e. OD

$$OD = OE + ED$$

$$= 8.95 + (40 - h_p) \cot \theta$$
$$= 8.95 + (40 - 2/3 \times 40) \cot \theta$$
$$= \left(8.95 + \frac{40}{3} \times \frac{1}{0.835}\right)$$
$$= 24.91 \text{ m from vertical OB.}$$

2.42 : Figure below shows a tank full of water under pressure. The length of tank is 2m. An empty cylinder lies along length of the tank on one of its corner. Find the horizontal and vertical force acting on curved surface ABC.

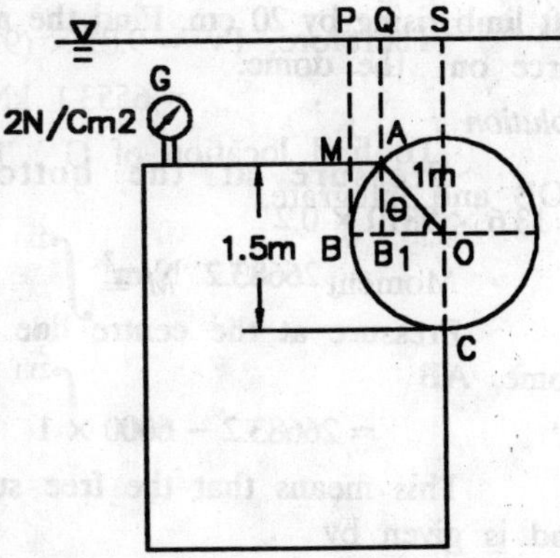

Solution :

Pressure at the top of tank $= 2 \text{ N/cm}^2$
$= 20 \text{ k Pa}$
$= \dfrac{20 \times 1000}{9810} = 2.038 \text{ m of water}$

Hence, the free surface exists at 2.038 m above the top of tank.

FIG. 2.59. EXAMPLE 2.42

Horizontal component of pressure P_H on ABC :

$$P_H = w A \bar{h}$$
$$= 9.81 \times (2 \times 1.5) \times (2.038 + 1.5/2)$$
$$= 82.05 \text{ kN towards right}$$

Vertical component of pressure P_v :- It will be the sum of $(P_v)_{AB}$ acting in the downwards direction and $(P_v)_{BC}$ acting in upward direction.

In $\triangle OAB_1$, since radius $= 1$m, $AB_1 = 0.5$, $OA = 1$ m $\sin \theta = 0.5, \theta = 30°$

$\therefore OB_1 = 1 \cos 30° = 0.866$ m and $BB_1 = (1 - 0.866) = 0.134$ m

$$(P_v)_{AB} = w \times 2 \times area \; ((OAB_1 + AMBB_1 - OAB) + AQPM)$$
$$= 2 \times 9.81 \left[\frac{1}{2} \times 0.866 \times 0.5 + 0.134 \times 0.5 \right.$$
$$\left. - \pi (1)^2 \times \frac{30°}{360°} + 0.134 \times 2.038 \right]$$
$$= 5.784 \text{ kN acting downward.}$$

$(P_v)_{BC} =$ weight of volume BCSP
$$= w \times 2 \times area \; (BOC + OSPB)$$
$$= 9.81 \times 2 \times [1/ \times 4 \pi (1)^2 + 1 \times (2.038 + 1.5)]$$
$$= 65.205 \text{ kN acting upward.}$$

Net $\quad\quad (P_v) = [65.205 - 5.784]$
$$= 59.421 \text{ kN acting upward.}$$

2.43 : Figure below shows a pressure vessel with a hemi spherical dome. The dome is filled with oil of sp.wt. 6 kN/m³ at such a pressure that a manometer connected at the bottom of the vessel has mercury column in the left limb rising by 20 cm. Find the net force on the dome.

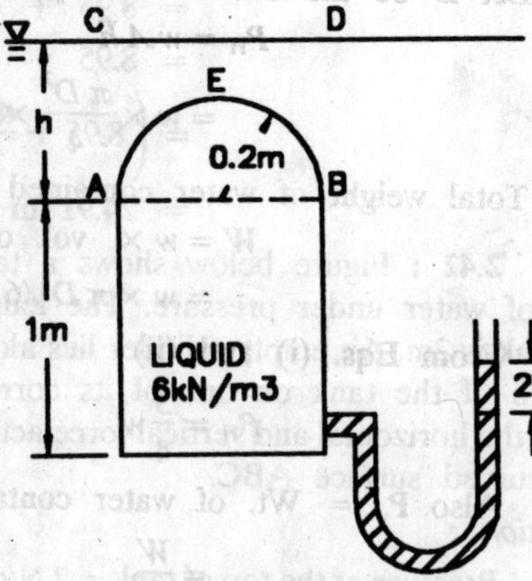

Solution :

Pressure at the bottom

= 13.6 × 9810 × 0.2

= 26683.2 N/m²

Pressure at the centre line of dome, AB

FIG. 2.60. EXAMPLE 2.43

= 26683.2 − 6000 × 1 = 20683.2 N/m² .

This means that the free surface must lie at a height h above AB and is given by

$$h = p/w$$

$$= \frac{20683.2}{6000} = 3.4472 \text{ m of liquid above AB}$$

Net force on the dome = w [vol. of cylinder ACDB− vol. of hemi sphere AEB]

$$= 6000 \left[\pi (0.2)^2 \times 3.447 - \frac{1}{2} \times 4/3 \pi \times (0.2)^3 \right]$$

= 2497.2 N or 2.497 kN acting upward.

2.44 : A spherical vessel is filled completely with water of weight W. Show that the resultant pressure on each halves into which it is divided by a vertically diametric plane is W √13/4. If the diametric plane is horizontal, show that the resultant fluid pressure on one halve is five times the other.

[AMIE, 1977 Summer]

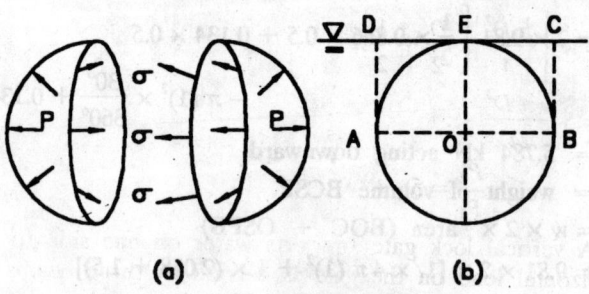

FIG. 2.61. EXAMPLE 2.44

Solution :

Case I : Sphere devided by vertical plane :

Let D be the diameter of sphere,

$$P_H = wA\bar{h}$$

$$= w \times \frac{\pi D^2}{4} \times \frac{D}{2} = \frac{w\pi D^3}{8} \quad ...(i)$$

Total weight of water contained in sphere = W

∴ $\qquad W = w \times$ vol. of sphere

$$= w \times \pi D^3/6 \quad ...(ii)$$

From Eqs. (i) and (ii)

$$P_H = \frac{3}{4} w \quad ...(iii)$$

Also P_v = Wt. of water contained in hemi sphere

$$= \frac{W}{2}$$

Resultant pressure $P = \sqrt{P_H^2 + P_v^2}$ $\qquad ...(iv)$

$$P = \sqrt{(3/4\,W)^2 + (W/2)^2} = W\sqrt{13}/4$$

Case II : Sphere cut by horizontal diameter

Since ADE and ECB are symmetrical there will be no horizontal force P_H

Therefore, net resultant fluid pressure on ADCB is $P_{v1} = P_1$

P_1 = Wt. of fluid in (ADE + ECB)

$\qquad = w \times$ (vol. of cylinder ADCB-vol.of hemi sphere AEB)

$$= w \times \left(\frac{\pi D^2}{4} \times \frac{D}{2} - \frac{1}{2} \times \frac{\pi D^3}{6} \right)$$

$$= \frac{w\pi D^3}{24}$$

Similarly, net resultant pressure on bottom half portion

AFB = P_{v2} = P_2

P_2 = wt. of fluid in (cylinder ADCB+hemi sphere AFB)

$$= w \left[\frac{\pi D^2}{4} \times \frac{D}{2} + \frac{1}{2} \cdot \frac{\pi D^3}{6} \right]$$

$$= 5 \frac{w\pi D^3}{24}$$

Hence $\qquad \dfrac{P_2}{P_1} = 5$

2.45 : A vertical lock gate supports water on one side to a depth of 8 m. The horizontal load on the gate is carried by three beams parallel to the surface. Find the depths of the beams below the surface if each is to carry one third of the load.

Solution :

For three equally loaded beams, three portions of the pressure distribution diagram i.e. ACD, CDHE and EHJB must have equal areas and beams must be at depths corresponding to the centres of pressure of these areas. Moreover, the total pressure will pass through the centroid of the areas. Assuming the gate to be 1 m wide,

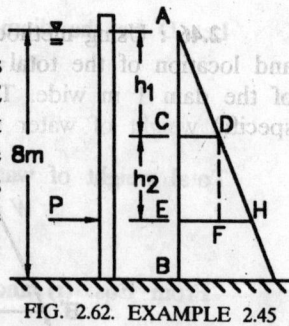

FIG. 2.62. EXAMPLE 2.45

$$P = w A \bar{h}$$
$$= w \times 8 \times 1 \times 8/2 = 32 \ w \ kN \qquad ...(i)$$

Therefore, load per beam $= 32/3 \ w \ kN$ ...(ii)

For top beam, $P_1 = \dfrac{32 \ w}{3} = \dfrac{w \ h_1^2}{2}$

$$h_1 = 4.619 \ m. \qquad ...(iii)$$

Therefore, depth of top beam $= \dfrac{2}{3} h_1$

$$= \dfrac{2}{3} \times 4.619 = 3.08 \ m. \qquad ...(iv)$$

Now let the middle beam is located h_2 m below first beam

Then $\qquad CD = w \ h_1 = 4.619 \ w$ ...(v)

$$EH = w \ (h_1 + h_2) \qquad ...(vi)$$

Therefore, area CDHFE $= wh_1 \times h_2^2 + wh^2 \times h_2/2$ ...(vii)

From Eqs. (vi) and (vii)

$$\dfrac{32}{3} w = w \left(4.619 \times h_2 + \dfrac{h_2^2}{2} \right)$$

Solving, $\qquad h_2 = 1.913 \ m$

Let P_2 acts at y_2 metre below CD, therefore take moment about CD.

$$\dfrac{32}{3} w y_2 = w \times 4.619 \times \dfrac{1.913}{2} + w \times \dfrac{1.913}{2} \times \dfrac{2}{3} \times 1.913$$

$$y_2 = 1.01 \ m$$

Therefore, second beam will be at a depth from water surface

$$= (4.619 + 1.01) = 5.629 \ m$$

Let bottom beam be at a depth h_3 from water surface.

Take moment about water surface.

$$\dfrac{32}{3} w \ (3.08 + 5.629 + h_3) = 32 \ w \times \dfrac{2}{3} (8)$$

$$h_3 = 7.291 \ m$$

Thus, top beam will be at a depth of 3.08, middle beam at 5.629 m and bottom beam will be at a depth of 7.291 m from water surface.

2.46 : Using method of components, calculate the magnitude, direction and location of the total force acting on the upstream face of the section of the dam 1 m wide. Take specific weight of masonry as 20 kN/m² and specific weight of water as 9.81 kN/m³.

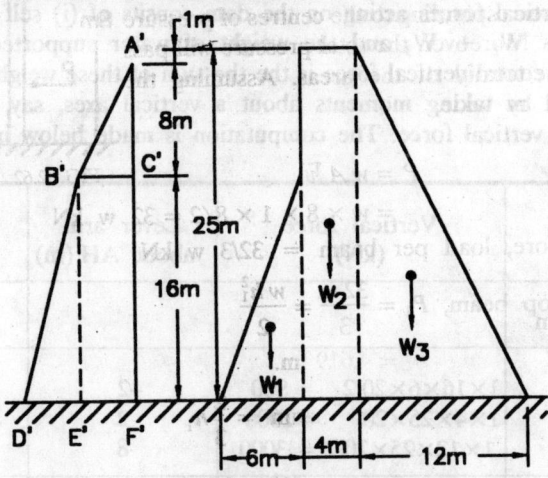

FIG. 2.63. EXAMPLE 2.46

Solution :

The upstream face ACE consists of vertical face AC and inclined face CE. Only horizontal force acts on AC whereas horizontal and vertical forces will act on CE.

Pressure intensity on $AC = wh = 9.81 \times 8$ kPa

Pressure force on face $AC = P_1$ = area of prism $A'B'C''$

$$= 1/2(9.81 \times 8) \times 8 = 313.892 \text{ kN}$$

Pressure intensity at bottom = $E'F' + E'D' = B'C' + E'D'$

$$= (9.81 \times 8 + 9.81 \times 16)$$

$$= 9.81 \times 24 \text{ kPa}$$

Horizontal pressure force on CE = area of prism B'C'F'E'D'

$$= area (B'C'E' + B'F'E'D')$$

$$= (w \times 8 \times 16 + w \times 16 \times 16/2)$$

$$= 256 \times 9.81$$

$$= 2511.3 \text{ kN}$$

Total force acting horizontally $= 313.892 + 2511.36$

$$= 2825.25 \text{ kN}$$

Alternatively, the vertical projection of the upstream face is a plane surface 24 m high and 1 m wide.

Therefore, $P_H = wA\bar{h}$

$$= 9.81 \times 24 \times 1 \times 24/2$$

$$= 2825.28 kN$$

$$h_p = 2/3 \times \text{ depth of water}$$

$$= 2/3 \times 24 = 16 \text{ m from water surface}$$

The vertical forces acting on the dam consits of (i) self weight of dam section $W_1 + W_2 + W_3$ and the weight of water supported by upstream face ACE. The total vertical force is the the sum of these weights. Its location is determined by taking moments about a vertical axes, say, AH and then diving by net vertical force. The computation is made below in tabular form.

Item	Vertical force (kN)	Lever arm about AH (m)	Moment kN–m
Weight of dam			
W_1	$1 \times 16 \times 6 \times 20/2 \quad = 960$	-2	-1920
W_2	$1 \times 4 \times 25 \times 20 \quad = 2000$	2	4000
W_3	$1 \times 12 \times 25 \times 20/2 = 3000$	8	24000
Weight of water behind AC Over CE	$9.81 \times 1 \times 6 \times 8 = 470.88$ $9.81 \times 1 \times 6 \times 16/2 = 470.88$	-3 -4	-1412.64 -1883.52
Sum	$= 6901.76 kN$		$= 22783.84$ kN-m

Total vertical force $P_v = 6901.76$ kN

Total moment about AH $= 22783.84$ kN-m clockwise

Therefore, the vertical force will act at a distance $\bar{x}$ from AH

$$\bar{x} = \frac{22783.84}{6901.76} = 3.301 \text{ m}$$

The resultant pressure $P = \sqrt{P_H^2 + P_v^2}$

$$= \sqrt{(2825.28)^2 + (6901.76)^2}$$

$$= 7457.64 \text{ kN}$$

The resultant will act at an angle θ with horizontal,

$$\tan \theta = \frac{P_v}{P_H}$$

$$= \frac{6901.76}{2825.28} = 2.4428$$

$$\theta = 67.73°$$

Objective Questions :

2.1 The pressure intensity in the air space above an oil (sp. gr. 0.75) surface in a tank is 1.6 k Pa. The pressure 2 m below the surface of the oil, in metre of water, is

(a) 3.6   (b) 4.5   (c) 16.3

(d) 20.0   (e) none of these.

2.2 Select the correct statement

(a) Local atmospheric pressure is always below standard atmospheric pressure.

(b) Local atmospheric pressure depends upon elevation of locality only.

(c) Standard atmospheric pressure is the mean local atmospheric pressure at sea level.

(d) A barometer reads the difference between local and standard atmospheric pressure.

2.3 With the barometer reading 70 cm mercury, 50 kPa is equivalent to

(a) 0.51 atm.   (b) 0.55 atm.   (c) 43.4 kPa suction

(d) 65 cm. of mercury abs.   (e) none

2.4 A mercury water manometer has a gauge difference of 0.5 m (difference in the elevation of meniscus). The difference in pressure intensity in metre of water is

(a) 0.5   (b) 6.3   (c) 6.8

(d) 5.8   (e) none of these

2.5 Absolute pressure is measured by

(a) Bourden gauge   (b) Aneroid barometer

(c) differential gauge   (d) vacum gauge

2.6 Gauge pressures of flowing fluid are measured by

(a) manometers   (b) Aneroid barometer

(c) Bourden gauge   (d) vacuum gauge

2.7 Mercury is generally used in manometers because

(a) it is heavy fluid   (b) it has low vapour pressure

(c) it has low surface tension (d) it measures acurately

2.8 For precise measurement of low pressure by a U-tube manometer which fluid is suitable ?

(a) water   (b) mercury

(c) carbon tetra chloride   (d) air

2.9 Location of centre of pressure is such that it is always

(a) at the centroid of the submersed area

(b) always above the centroid of the plane

(c) at the centroid of the pressure prism

(d) independent of the orientation of area

2.10 The hydrostatic pressure at a point is given by

(a) $p = z/w$ (b) $p = wz$

(c) $p = wz + constant$ (d) $p = constant$

(e) $p = z \times constant$

2.11 The piezometric head is expressed by

(a) $p + wz$ (b) $p - wz$ (c) $z + p/w$

(d) $p/\rho + gz$ (e) $\rho z + p/g$

2.12 The vertical distance of the centre of pressure below the centroid of the plane area is

(a) $I_G/A\bar{h}$ (b) $I_G \sin^2\theta/A\bar{h}$ (c) $I_0 \sin^2\theta/A\bar{h}$

(d) $I_G \sin\theta/A h^2$ (e) none of these

2.13 The pressure acting at the bottom of hemispherical vessel 4 m diameter full of water is

(a) 5.14 kN   (b) 2.57 kN

(c) 9.81 kN   (d) none of these

2.14 A free surface used in Eq. 2.37c is

(a) a surface of zero pressure

(b) a surface of atmospheric pressure

(c) a given surface

(d) none of these

2.15 The vertical component of pressure force on a submerged curved surface is equal to

(a) its horizontal component

(b) the force on a vertical projection on the curved surface

(c) the weight of liquid vertically above the curved surface

(d) the product of pressure at the centroid and surface area

(e) none

Problem

2.1 Prove that pressure always acts normal to the surface.

2.2 State Pascal's law. Give some of the examples where this principle is used.

2.3 Derive fundamental equation of hydrostatic and show that pressure varies linearly with elevation for an incompressible fluid.

2.4 Derive an equation for pressure variation with elevation for compressible fluid subjected (a) to isothermal process, (b) to adiabatic process with $c_p/c_v = k$

2.5 Explain gauge, absolute and vacuum pressure. How will you determine absolute pressure from gauge and vacuum pressure.

2.6 Describe Bourden tube pressure gauge.

2.7 Prove that centre of pressure always lies below centre of gravity of the plane lamina immersed in fluid.

2.8 What are sensitive manometers. Describe one of them.

2.9 An closed vessel contains 1 m of carbontetrachloride, 0.5 m of water, 0.30 m of of crude oil (sq. gr. = 0.8) and air above it. If the bourden gauge at the bottom reads 150 kPa what is the reading of Bourden gauge at the top of the tank ?

2.10 Barometric pressure is 100 kPa. Calculate the vapour pressure of the liquid and the gauge reading (Fig. 2.64)

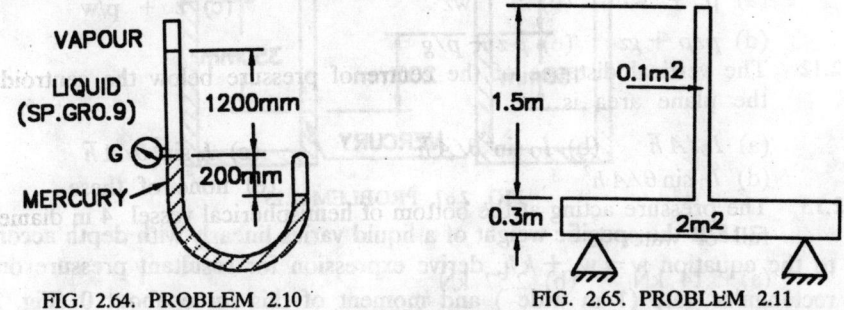

FIG. 2.64. PROBLEM 2.10   FIG. 2.65. PROBLEM 2.11

2.11 In Fig. 2.65, the cross sectional areas of the tank and the tube are respectively 2 and 0.1 m². (a) compute the total force on the bottom of the tank due to the water pressure, (b) compute the total weight of water. Why is there a difference between the two answers.

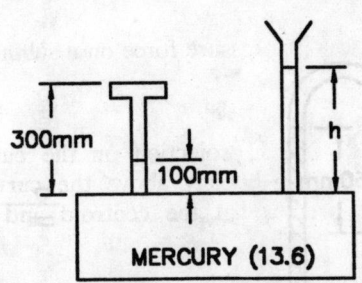

FIG. 2.66. PROBLEM 2.11

2.12 The vessel shown in Fig. 2.66 is initially filled with mercury. The left tube is then closed and mercury is added to the right tube until it is 10 cm. high in the left tube. Compute the height h of mercury column in the right tube. Assume the system to remain isothermal. The barometric reading is 72 cm of mercury.

2.13 Figure 2.67 shows a differential manometer which is connected to two sections of two parallel oil pipes. Calculate the pressure difference $(p_A - p_B)$.

2.14 The differential head for a flow meter in a converging pipe carrying water is measured by means of the inverted U-tube manometer. What is the difference in piezometric head between A and B (a) if the space above the water column is filled with a liquid with air and (b) if the space is filled with a liquid having a specific gravity of 0.8 (Fig. 2.68)

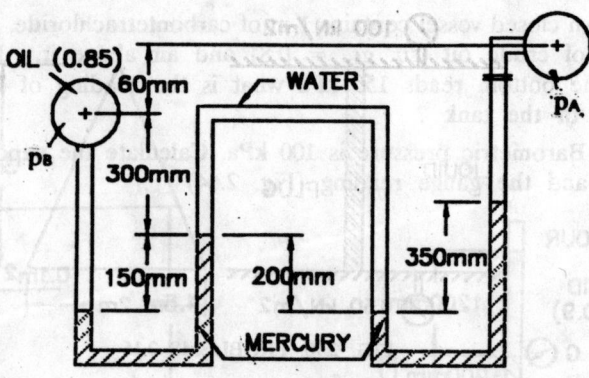

FIG. 2.67. PROBLEM 2.13

2.15 If the specific weight of a liquid varies linearly with depth according to the equation $w = w_0 + k h$, derive expression for resultant pressure on the rectangular gate (1 m wide) and moment of this force about 0 (Fig. 2.69)

2.16 A triangular area of 2 m base and 1.5 m altitude has its base horizontal and lies in a 45° plane with its apex below the base and 3 m below a water surface. Calculate the magnitude, direction and location of the resultant force on the area.

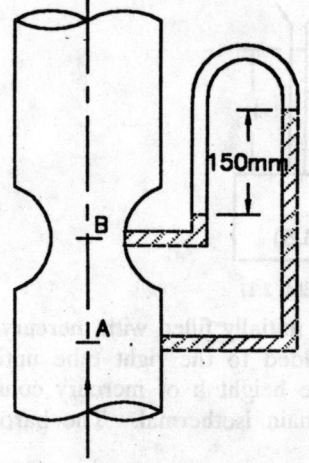

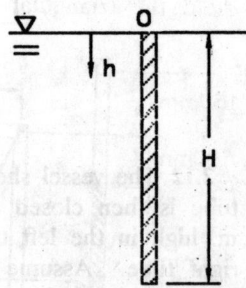

FIG. 2.68. PROBLEMS 2.16   FIG. 2.69. PROBLEM 2.15

2.17 Calculate the magnitude and location of the resultant force of the liquid on the tunnel plug shown in Fig.2.70

2.18 Calculate the intensity of pressure required to keep the rectangular gate in equilibrium position. The gate is hinged at the top A. Assume the system to be frictionless Fig. 2.71

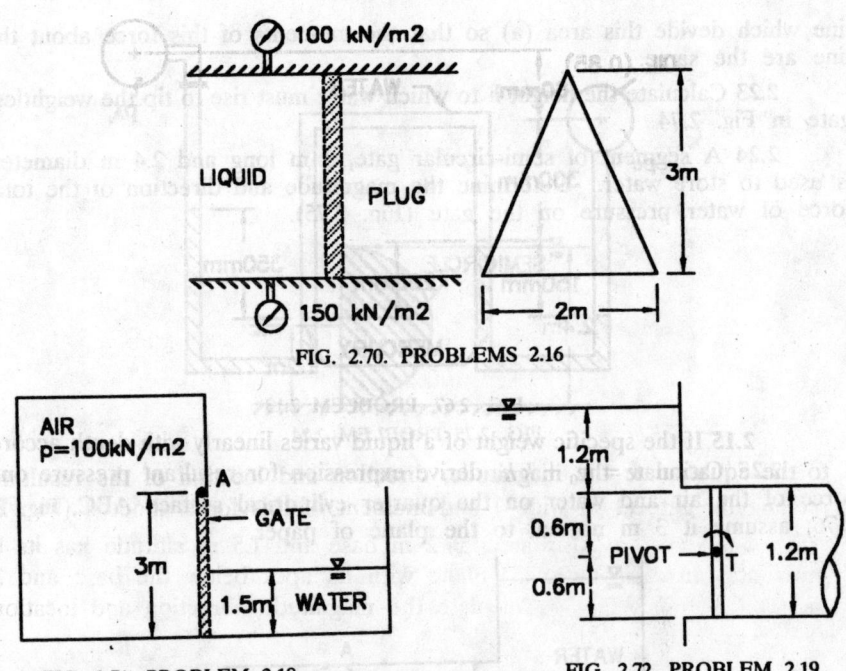

FIG. 2.70. PROBLEMS 2.16

FIG. 2.71. PROBLEM 2.18

FIG. 2.72. PROBLEM 2.19

2.19 A circular butterfly gate, 1.2 m diameter, is pivoted about a horizontal axis passing through its diameter. Compute the torque T required to keep the gate in the closed position (Fig 2.72).

2.20 Calculate L if W = 0.05 kN and exact position of the pointer to hold the triangular gate in equilibrium in Fig. 2.73

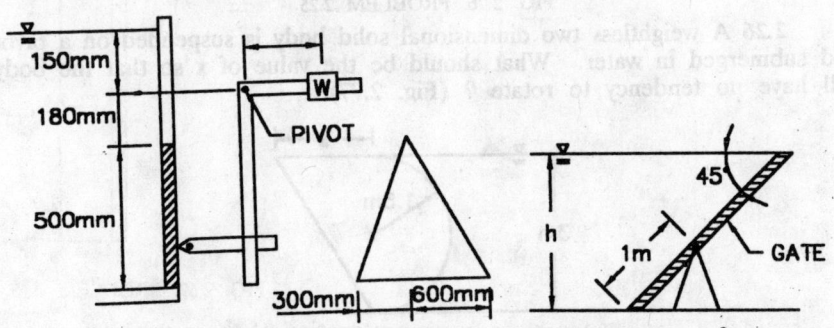

FIG. 2.73 PROBLEM 2.20

FIG. 2.74. PROBLEM 2.23

2.21 A submerged rectangular gate located in a vertical plane has its base 7 m below, and its centre of pressure 5 m below a water surface. Calculate the height of the rectangle.

2.22 A vertical rectangular gate, 4 m high and 2.5 m wide, has a depth of water on its upper edge of 5 m. What is the location of a horizontal line which devide this area (a) so that the moments of this force about the line are the same.

2.23 Calculate the height h to which water must rise to tip the weightless gate in Fig. 2.74

2.24 A segment of semi-circular gate, 3 m long and 2.4 m diameter, is used to store water. Determine the magnitude and direction of the total force of water pressure on the gate (Fig. 2.75).

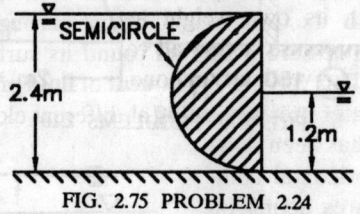

FIG. 2.75 PROBLEM 2.24

2.25 Calculate the magnitude, direction and location of the resultant force of the air and water on the quarter cylindrical surface ABC, in Fig 2.76; assume it 3 m normal to the plane of paper.

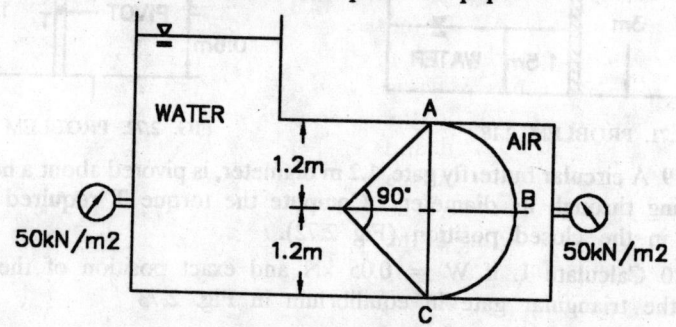

FIG. 2.76. PROBLEM 2.25

2.26 A weightless two dimensional solid body is suspended on a pivot and submerged in water. What should be the value of x so that the body will have no tendency to rotate ? (Fig. 2.77)

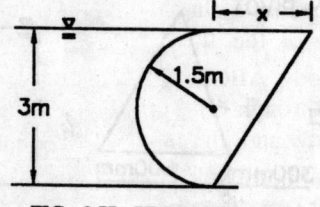

FIG. 2.77. PROBLEM 2.26

Buoyancy of Fluid

3.1 INTRODUCTION

If a body is floating in a fluid and is at rest, it will be in equilibrium in a vertical plane with its own weight acting through its centre of gravity and the resultant fluid pressure acting all round its surface. This upward force is known as 'Buoyancy'. This vertical component of fluid pressure can be calculated easily by summing the water pressure acting at different elements of the submerged portion of the body (as has been done in Section 2.6). The horizontal components of fluid pressures acting on two sides of a symmetrical vertical axis will be equal in magnitude and opposite in direction.

Consider a body ABCD immersed in fluid in Fig. 3.1. The vertical component of pressure forces acting on its two ends are p dA on the top surface acting downward and (p + w H) dA on the bottom surface acting in the upward direction. The resultant pressure force acting in the upward direction is F_B.

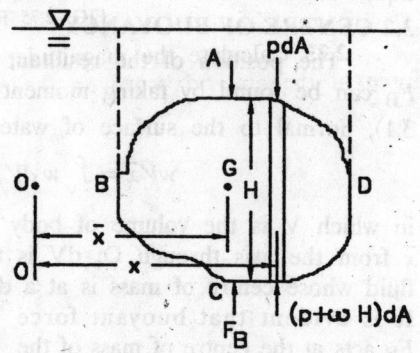

FIG. 3.1 FORCES ON SUBMERGED BODY

1. Principle of buoyancy

If the whole body is imagined to be made up of similar vertical prisms, the total resultant upward pressure force is equal to the weight of fluid displaced by the body. (Archimedes principle). This is the familiar law of buoyancy.

2. Principle of floatation

If a body is floating in a fluid either partially or fully submerged, it displaces its own weight of the fluid in which it floats.

In Fig. 3.1, the body ABCD submerged in a fluid is in equilibrium and its weight W (acting through G) and buoyant force are equal which means that the densities of body and fluid are also equal.

When $W > F_B$, the body will sink. If the body happens to be more compressible than the fluid, its density will increase more rapidly with depth than that of fluid and it will sink to the bottom. If the body is less compressible than the fluid, it will sink to the depth at which the two densities are equal. If such a body has a density which is initially only slightly greater than that of fluid, the depth to which it will sink will be small. But if the density of the body is quite large the depth required is also large and hence the body will sink.

When $W < F_B$, the body will rise until its density and that of the fluid are equal as is the case of balloon ascending in air.

If the body happens to the more compressible than the fluid it will rise indefinitely, provided the fluid has no definite limit of height, as in the case of earth's atmosphere. If the body is less compressible, it will rise to a certain height where the densities of body and fluid equalise and will remain in equilibrium at this level.

If a body is immersed in a liquid with free surface and its weight is less than that of the same volume of liquid, it will rise and float on the liquid surface.

3.2 CENTRE OF BUOYANCY

The position of the resultant upward pressure or force of buoyancy F_B can be found by taking moment about an axis passing through O (Fig. 3.1), normal to the surface of water. Therefore,

$$w V \overline{x} = \int_v w \, dV \times x$$

in which V is the volume of body whose centre of mass is at a distance $\overline{x}$ from the axis through O; dV is the volume of the elementary prism of fluid whose centre of mass is at a distance x from the same axis (Fig. 3.1). It is evident that buoyant force F_B acts at the centre of mass of the displaced liquid. It is known as the 'centre of buoyancy'.

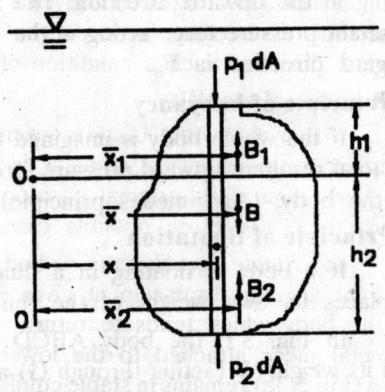

When the body floats at the interface of two fluids (Fig.3.2) of specific weights w_1 and w_2, the buoyant force on a vertical prism of cross section dA is

$$\delta F_2 = (p_2 - p_1) \, dA$$

$$= (w_2 h_2 + w_1 h_1) \, dA$$

Integrating over the whole area of the body,

$$F_2 = \int w_2 h_2 \, dA + \int w_1 h_1 \, dA$$

FIG. 3.2. A BODY FLOATING AT THE INTERFACE OF TWO FLUIDS

and the location of its line of action can be determined by taking moment about an axis OO

$$\overline{x} = \frac{\int^1 w_1 \, dV_1 \times x + \int w_2 \, dV_2 \times x}{w_1 V_1 + w_2 V_2} = \frac{w_1 V_1 \overline{x}_1 + w_2 V_2 \overline{x}_2}{w_1 V_1 + w_2 V_2}$$

in which V_1 and V_2 are the volumes of the two fluids displaced and their corresponding centres of mass acting at $\bar{x}_1$ and $\bar{x}_2$ respectively from the axis OO, i.e. at their centroids.

For a body floating at the free surface of liquid the specific weight of air, w_a, is negligible as compared to specific weight of the liquid. Consequently, the buoyant force is equal to the weight of the liquid displaced. Since the floating body is in static equilibrium,

$$\sum F_y = 0$$

Upward buoyant force F_B = weight of liquid displaced, W.

3.3. STABILITY OF FLOATING BODIES

A body floating in a fluid may have following types of stability.

(1) Vertical stability

(2) Linear stability

(3) Rotational stability

1. Vertical stability

When a body floating in a static liquid is given a slight upward displacement, the volume of fluid displaced reduces resulting in an unbalanced downward force which tends to bring back the body to its original position. Similarly , a downward displacement causes an unbalanced upward force which brings back the body to its original stability.

2. Linear stability

When a floating body is given a slight linear displacement in any direction, it sets up a restoring force on the body tending to return the body to its original position. Such a condition of the body is known as 'Linear stability'.

3. Rotational stability

When a floating body is given a slight angular displacement, either a restoring or overturning moment is set up on the body. In the first case, the body regains its original position whereas in the latter case it overturns. Thus, there are three possible cases of rotational stability.

(a) Stable equilibrium. A body is said to be in stable equilibrium if a slight angular displacement given to the body sets up a rotational couple in the body which tends to return it in the original position. For example, a metal piece attached to the lower end of a wooden piece4 floating in a fluid (Fig. 3.3a) remains in stable equilibrium. When a slight angular displacement is given to it, a restoring couple is set up on it which brings it in the original position. Such a condition of the body is said to be 'stable equilibrium.'

(b) Unstable equilibrium. A body is said to be in unstable equilibrium if the angular displacement given to the body sets up an additional overturning moment on the body and finally the body overturns, e.g. the metal piece attached to the top of the wood floating in the liquid (Fig. 3.3b) will overturn on giving a slight angular displacement. Such a condition of the body is said to be 'unstable equilibrium.'

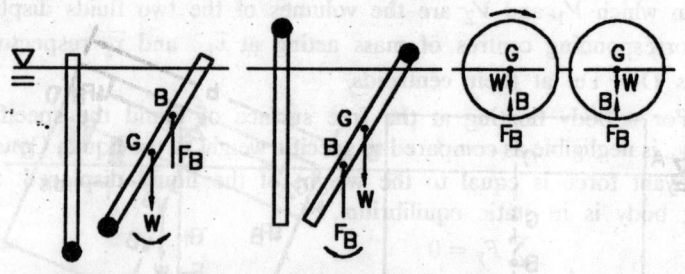

RESTORING MOMENT OVERTURNING MOMENT
(a) STABLE   (b) UNSTABLE   (c) NEUTRAL

FIG. 3.3 CONDITIONS OF EQUILIBRRIUM OF A FLOATING BODY

(c) Neutral equilibrium. A body is said to be in neutral equilibrium if the angular displacement given to the body sets up no couple on the body and the body remains floating in its displaced position, e.g. a sphere or a right circular cylinder floats in neutral equilibrium. Such a condition of the body is said to be in 'neutral equilibrium'.

Normally, it is found that if the centre of buoyancy lies above centre of gravity, the body is said to be in stable equilibrium. A slight displacement of the body sets up a rightening couple on the body to return the body to its original position. But in case of marine ships, the centre of buoyancy should be lower than centre of gravity for it to be stable (see Fig. 3.4).

In practice, the actual test whether the body is in a stable equilibrium or not depends on the couple which develops on the body.

3.4 METACENTRE AND METACENTRIC HEIGHT

Consider a ship of length L floating in water (Fig. 3.4). The weight of the ship W acts through its centre of gravity G whereas the buoyant force F_B acts at centre of buoyancy B. These two forces act in a vertical line and the ship is in equilibrium. Due to slight angular displacement, the centre of buoyancy shifts from B to new location B_1 which is the centroid of the submerged volume after it is tilted.

Now if the vertical line through B_1 is extended up, it cuts the line joining B and G at M, Fig. 3.4c. This point of intersection M, of the vertical line through B_1 and extended line BG is known as metacentre.

The distance MG is known as the 'metacentric height', when θ is infinitely small.

It is obvious from Fig 3.4c that if M lies above G then F_B and W form a rightening couple which tries to restore the ship to its original position. But if M lies below G, then F_B and W form a couple which would overturn the ship. Thus the location of M is a measure of the stability of the floating ship and hence accurate estimates of metacentric height are made under various

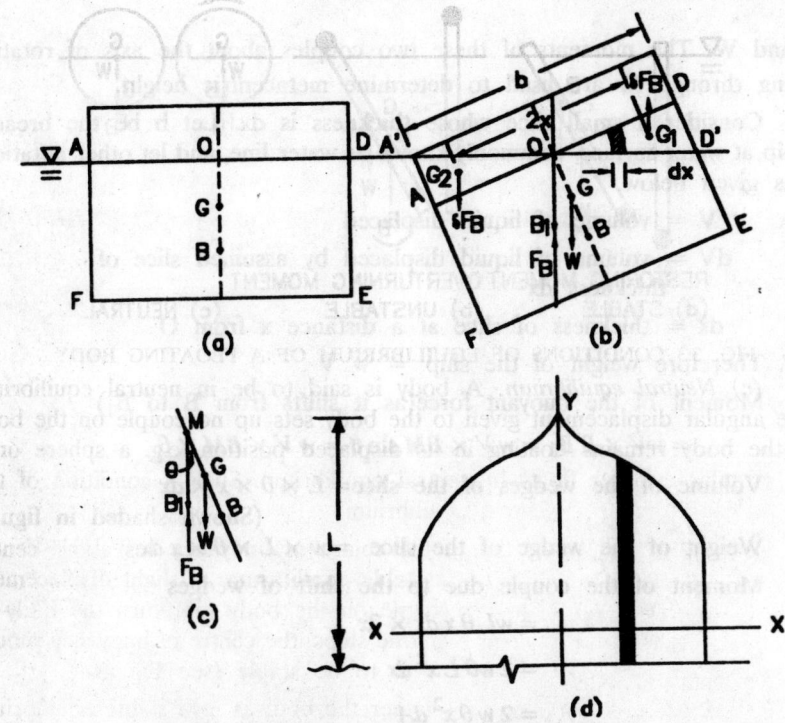

FIG. 3.4. STABILITY OF A FLOATING SHIP

conditions of loading to ensure the stability of the ship. It varies from 0.5 m to 2 m.

3.5 DETERMINATION OF METACENTRIC HEIGHT

The metacentric height can be determined either by (1) Analytical method or by (2) Experimental method.

1. Analytical method

Consider a tranverse section of a floating ship (or a floating body) whose length is L (Fig. 3.4). Let the ship heel in an anticlockwise direction through a small angle due to which the immersed portion of the ship changes from ADEF to A' D' E F. Actually, the ship rotates about 'O' on the water line. But for very small angle θ, it may be assumed to rotate about M as it lies very near to the water line. Since the volume of displaced liquid remains the same, the new water line cuts the old water line at the mid point 'O' and the immersed volume of ship ODD' comes out of water and an equivalent volume of ship OAA' on the other side is immersed in water. The emerged portion ODD' causes a reduction in F_B by δF_B but at the same time it is brought to its original value of F_B by an additional δF_B on the left hand side due to the immersion of equivalent portion of the ship. This shift of force sets up a couple on the ship. The apparent movement of the wedges causes the shift of B to B_1. This, in turn, sets up another couple due to

F_B and W. The moments of these two couples about the axis of rotation passing through M are used to determine metacentric height.

Consider a small slice whose thickness is dx. Let b be the breadth of ship at water surface, commonly known as water line, and let other notations be as given below.

V = volume of liquid displaced

dV = volume of liquid displaced by assumed slice of thickness dx

dx = thickness of slice at a distance x from O

Therefore weight of the ship = w V

Moment of the buoyant force (as it shifts from B to B_1)

$$= wV \times BB_1 = wV \times BM \sin\theta = wV \times BM \times \theta \qquad ...(i)$$

Volume of the wedges of the slice = $L \times \theta \times x \times dx$

(Shown shaded in figure)

Weight of the wedge of the slice = $w \times L \times \theta \times x\, dx$

Moment of the couple due to the shift of wedges

$$= wL\,\theta\,x\,dx \times 2x$$

$$= 2w\theta L x^2 dx$$

$$= 2w\theta x^2 dA$$

Summing up for the whole width of the wedge

$$= 2w\theta \int x^2 dA \qquad ...(ii)$$

Here $dA\ (=L\,dx)$ is the area of slice in the plane of the water surface.

Equating Eqs. (i) and (ii)

$$w \times V \times BM \times \theta = 2w\theta \int x^2 dA$$

$$BM = \left(2 \int x^2 dA\right)/V$$

But $\left(2\int x^2 dA\right) = 2\int dI = I$, is second moment of the area at water line about the axis of rotation YY. Therefore,

$$BM = I/V \qquad ...(3.5)$$

Hence, metacentric height $\overline{MG} = \overline{BM} - \overline{BG}$ $\qquad ...(3.6)$

Then rightening couple $C = F_B \times MG \sin\theta$

$$C = w \times V \times (I/V - \overline{BG})\,\theta \qquad ...(3.7)$$

(for small angle θ)

Since BG is the distance between the centre of buoyancy and centre of gravity of the ship which is known and BM is determined from Eq. 3.5, MG and C can be calculated from Eqs. 3.6 and 3.7.

Thus the condition for stability of a floating body is that

$$BM \geq BG \qquad (3.8)$$

Note that the ship will be unstable if
$$BM - BG < O$$
$$BG > BM; BG > I/V \qquad (3.9)$$

In the above Eq. 3.5, the second moment of area of the ship at the water surface (generally known as the deck) can be easily determined for regular shape of the deck. If the shape of the deck is other than a rectangle, I for it can be determined by dividing the deck into simple figures. Alternatively, the moment of inertia is given as a function of the second moment of area of the circumscribing rectangle.

I of a deck $= k$ (I of circumscribing rectangle)

For the pitching of ship (rotation of ship about axis XX; see Fig. 3.4) second moment of area should be found about XX. For overall stability of the ship, smaller of I_{xx} and I_{yy} should be used in Eq. 3.5.

2. Experimental method

With the position of the centre of buoyancy of a floating body (or a ship) known (by computation of the centroid of the fluid displaced), the metacentric height and centre of gravity of the body can be determined experimentally (see Fig. 3.5).

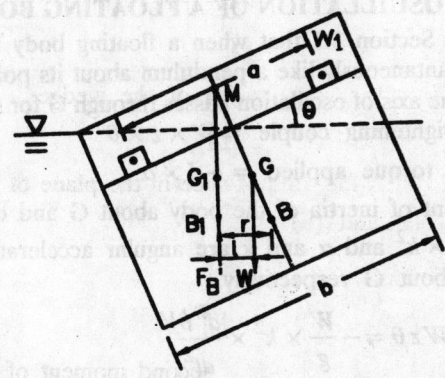

FIG. 3.5. EXPERIMENTAL DETERMINATION OF THE METACENTRIC HEIGHT

Initially the body is so adjusted that it is vertical with weight W_1 on the right hand side. Now the weight W_1 is shifted from right side to the left side by a distance 'a' which causes the body to tip by angle θ. The angle of tip is measured on a scale by means of a plumb bob suspended on the deck. Since the body remains in equilibrium, the shifted location of centre of gravity and centre of buoyancy, i.e. G_1 and B_1 respectively will be in the same vertical line.

Moment due to shifting of weight $W_1 = W_1 \times a$

Moment due to shifting of G to $G_1 = W \times l$

where W is the weight of the floating body and $l = MG \times \sin\theta$
Equating two moments,

$$MG = \frac{W_1 \times a}{W \sin\theta} \qquad \qquad ...(3.10)$$

3. Determination of c.g.

Referring of Fig. 3.5, if the sides of the ship are vertical at the water line, the moment due to shift of B to B_1 is equal to the moment of the couple of the two wedges. Therefore,

$$w V r = w \times \frac{1}{2} \times \frac{b}{2} \times \frac{b}{2} \tan\theta \times 2b/3 \qquad (\angle\, G M G_1 = \theta)$$

$$r = \frac{b^3}{12} \frac{\tan\theta}{V}$$

From Fig. 3.5 $r = BM \sin\theta$

$$BM = \frac{b^3}{12 V} \sec\theta \qquad \qquad ...(3.11)$$

Knowing MG from Eq. 3.10 and BM from Eq. 3.11, the location of G, i.e. BG, can be determined.

$$BG = BM - MG \qquad \qquad ...(3.12)$$

3.6 TRANSVERSE OSCILLATION OF A FLOATING BODY

It is shown in Section 3.3 that when a floating body is given a lateral heel, it oscillates instantaneously like a pendulum about its point of suspension. If it is assumed that the axis of oscillation passes through G for small metacentric height z, then the rightening couple $= W \times z \times \theta$

Inertia of the torque applied $= - I \times \alpha$

where I is the moment of inertia of the body about G and can be computed by formula, $I = W/g \times k^2$ and α and k are angular acceleration $d^2\theta/dt^2$ and radius of gyration about G respectively.

Therefore, $\quad Wz\theta = -\dfrac{W}{g} \times k^2 \times \dfrac{d^2\theta}{dt^2}$

$$d^2\theta/dt^2 + z g\theta/k^2 = 0$$

The solution of this differential equation is

$$\theta = A \sin\left(\sqrt{\frac{zg}{k^2}} \times t\right) + B \cos\left(\sqrt{\frac{zg}{k^2}} \times t\right)$$

where A and B are the constants of integration. The boundary condition are (i) when $t = 0$, $\theta = 0$ and hence $B = 0$ and (ii) when $T = I/2$, $\theta = 0$, hence

$$\theta = A \sin\left(\sqrt{\frac{zg}{k^2}} \times \frac{T}{2}\right) = 0 \qquad \qquad ...(3.13)$$

A cannot be zero, therefore

$$\sin\left(\sqrt{\frac{zg}{k^2}} \times \frac{T}{2}\right) = 0$$

Solving, $\qquad T = 2\pi \sqrt{\dfrac{k^2}{zg}}$ \qquad ...(3.14)

From this Eq. 3.14, the time of oscillation of the floating body can be calculated for known values of z and k. It will be noticed that if z is increased, the time of oscillation is shorter and vice versa. This is noticeable with a ship travelling in ballast, as the effect of the ballast is to lower the centre of gravity G and thus increase z.

Example 3.1 - 3.16

3.1 Determine the maximum ratio of a to b for the stability of a rectangular block of mass density ρ_b for a small angle of tilt when it floats in a liquid of mass density ρ_1. The dimension a is greater the b.

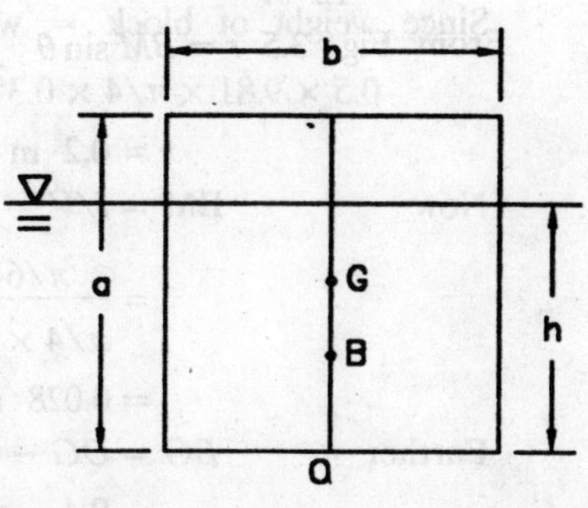

Solution

Consider 1 m length of block normal to the plane of paper.

Let the depth of immersion be h

Now weight of the block = weight of liquid displaced

FIG. 3.6. EXAMPLE 3.1

$$\rho_b g \times ab \times 1 = \rho_1 g \times bh \times 1$$

Solving, $\qquad h = \dfrac{\rho_b}{\rho_1} \times a$ \qquad ...(i)

The centre of buoyancy will lie at $\dfrac{h}{2}$ from the bottom. Hence,

$$OB = \frac{h}{2} = \frac{1}{2}\frac{\rho_b}{\rho_1} \times a \qquad ...(ii)$$

Then, $\qquad BG = OG - OB$

$$= \frac{a}{2} - (\rho_b a)/2\rho_1 = \frac{a}{2}(1 - \rho_b/\rho_1)$$

Now $BM = \dfrac{\text{Moment of inertia of surface area at the waterline}}{\text{volume of body immersed in liquid}}$

$$= (1/12 \times 1 \times b^3)/(b \times h \times 1) = b^2/12h$$

Substitute the value of h from Eq. (i)

$$BM = (\rho_1 b^2)/(12a\,\rho_b)$$

For stability.

$$BM \geq BG$$

$$\frac{b^2}{12\,a} \times \frac{\rho_1}{\rho_b} \geq \frac{a}{2} - (1 - \rho_b/\rho_1)$$

$$\frac{a}{b} \leq \frac{\rho_1}{\sqrt{6\rho_b\,(\rho_1 - \rho_b)}}$$

3.2 Determine the position in which a solid cylindrical block of wood of diameter 0.3 m and length 0.4 m will float in water. Take specific gravity of wood as 0.5.

Solution

Case I. Consider first the possibility of its floating with its axis vertical so that it cuts the base at O.

Let x be the submerged depth.

Since weight of block = weight of liquid displaced

$$0.5 \times 9.81 \times \pi/4 \times 0.3^2 \times 0.4 = 9.81 \times \pi/4 \times 0.3^2 \times x$$

$$x = 0.2 \text{ m}$$

Now $\qquad BM = I/V$

$$= \frac{\pi/64 \times (0.3)^4}{\pi/4 \times (0.3)^2 \times 0.2}$$

$$= 0.028 \text{ m}$$

Further $\qquad BG = OG - OB$

$$= \frac{0.4}{2} - \frac{x}{2}$$

$$= 0.1 \text{ m}$$

$$MG = BM - BG$$

$$= 0.028 - 0.1 = -0.072 \text{ m}$$

That means M lies below G and hence the cylinder will not be stable in this position.

Case II. Now consider it to float with its axis horizontal and its sumbmerged depth as x.

Again, weight of cylinder = weight of liquid displaced

$$0.5 \times 9.81 \times \pi/4 \times 0.3^2 \times 0.4$$

$$= 9.81 \times 0.4 \ (\text{area } OA'C'B - \text{ area } OA'B')$$

$$0.0353 = (\pi r^2/2\,\pi \times 2\theta \times \pi/180 - 2 \times 1/2 \times 0.15 \sin\theta \times 0.15 \cos\theta)$$

Solving it, $\theta = 90°$ and $x = r = 0.15$ m

Now $\qquad I = 1/12 \times 0.4 \times (0.3)^3 = 0.0009 \text{ m}^4$

$$V = \frac{1}{2} \times \pi/4 \times (0.3)^2 \times 0.4 = 0.0045\,\pi \text{ m}^3$$

$$BM = I/V$$

$$= 0.0009/(0.0045\,\pi)$$

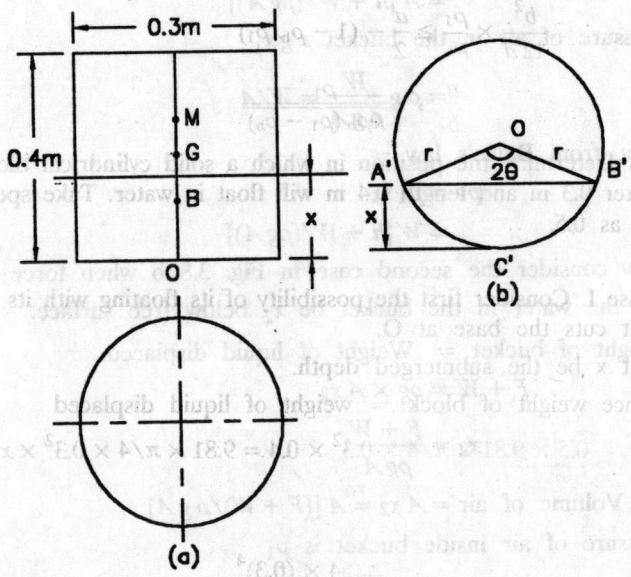

FIG. 3.7. (A) & (B) EXAMPLE 3.2

$$= \frac{0.2}{\pi} \text{ m}$$

Further, the centre of buoyancy will lie at the centroid of the liquid displaced which is a hemisphere, i.e. at $4r/3\pi$ below the centre.

Therefore, $OB = \dfrac{4}{3\pi} \times \dfrac{0.3}{2} = \dfrac{0.2}{\pi}$ metre

Since, the C.G. of cylinder will be at the centre O, hence

$$BG = OB = (0.2/\pi) \text{ metre}$$

Also $MG = BM - BG$

$$= 0.2/\pi - 0.2/\pi = 0$$

Hence, the cylinder will float half immersed in the liquid.

3.3 A cylindrical bucket with one end open, 2R in diameter and H metre high, is submerged in a liquid of mass density ρ. The bucket weights W kN and it floats in the liquid with height h above the liquid surface. Determine the force required just to submerge the bucket. Neglect thickness of the bucket wall and assume that the air follows the isothermal law.

Solution

Let the water level be x_1 inside the bucket.

Weight of bucket = Weight of liquid displaced

$$W = \rho g A x_1$$

$$x_1 = W/\rho g A$$

Volume of air = $A (h + x_1)$

$$= A\left[h + W/(\rho g A)\right]$$

Pressure of air in the bucket $\rho g x_1$

$$= \rho g \frac{W}{\rho g A} = W/A$$

Now, from Boyle's law.

$$pv = p_1 v_1$$
$$= W\left[h + W/(\rho g A)\right] \qquad \text{...(i)}$$

Now consider the second case in Fig. 3.8 b when force is applied. Let the water in the bucket be x_2 below free surface.

Weight of bucket = Weight of liquid displaced.

$$F + W = \rho g \times A\, x_2$$
$$x_2 = \frac{F + W}{\rho g A}$$

Volume of air $= A\, x_2 = A\left[(F + W)/\rho g A\right]$

Pressure of air inside bucket is p_1

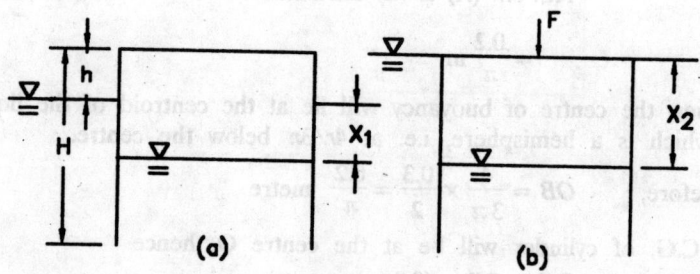

FIG. 3.8 (A) & (B) EXAMPLE 3.3

$$p_1 = \rho g x_2$$
$$= \rho g \times \frac{F + W}{\rho g A}$$
$$= \frac{F + W}{A}$$

Then, $\qquad p_1 v_1 = \dfrac{F + W}{A} \times \dfrac{F + W}{\rho g} \qquad \text{...(ii)}$

Equating Eqs. (i) and (ii)

$$W\left(h + \frac{W}{\rho g A}\right) = \frac{(F + W)^2}{\rho g A}$$

Solving, $\qquad F = \sqrt{W^2 + \rho g A h} - W$

3.4 A pontoon whose all transverse and longitudinal cross sections are rectangle has a length of 7m and a width of 3m. The weight of pontoon is 30 tonnes (1 tonne = 9.81 kN). Determine the position of centre of gravity above the base of the pontoon such that it does not overturn in still water. Sea water weighs 10.006 kN/m³

Solution

Let the pontoon be immersed in water by h metre.

Weight of body = Weight of liquid displaced

$$30 \times 9.81 = 10.006 \ (3 \times 7 \times h)$$

$$h = \frac{30 \times 9.81}{10.006 \times 21} = 1.4 \text{ m}$$

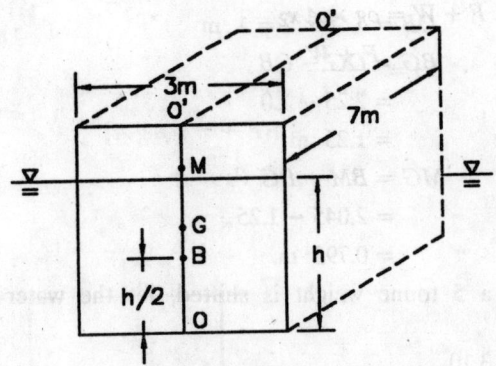

FIG. 3.9. EXAMPLE 3.4

Hence, $OB = h/2 = 0.7$ m

$$BM = I/V$$

$$BM = \frac{1/12 \times 7 \times (3)^3}{3 \times 7 \times 1.4} = 0.535 \text{ m}$$

$$BM \geq BG$$

In the extreme case G may lie at M.

Therefore, G will lie at $OB + BM$ metre from the bottom.

$$OG = 0.535 + 0.7$$

$$= 1.235 \text{ m above bottom.}$$

3.5 A barge 20 m long × 7 m wide has a draft of 2 m when floating in upright position. Its C.G. is 2.25 m above the bottom, (a) what is it's initial metacentric height ? (b) If a 5 tonne weight is shifted 4 m across the barge, to what distance does the water line rise on the side ? Find the rightening moment for this lift.

Solution

(a) $$BM = I/V$$

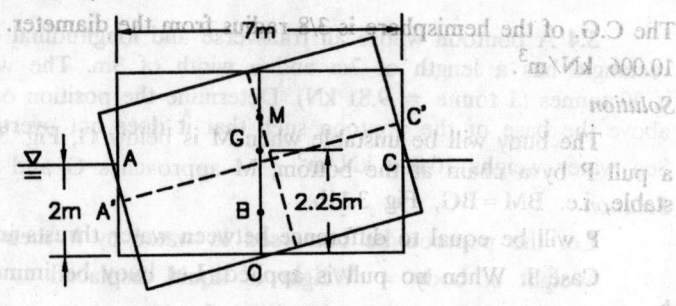

FIG. 3.10. EXAMPLE 3.5

$$= [1/12 \times 20 \times 7^3/(20 \times 7 \times 2)]$$
$$= 2.045 \text{ m}$$
$$OB = 1/2 \times 2 = 1 \text{ m}$$
$$BG = OG - OB$$
$$= 2.25 - 1.0$$
$$= 1.25 \text{ m}$$
$$MG = BM - BG$$
$$= 2.045 - 1.25$$
$$= 0.795 \text{ m.}$$

(b) When a 5 tonne weight is shifted, let the water line be shifted to $A'\,C'$.

From Eq. 3.10,

Rightening moment = moment caused due to shifting of weight
$$W \times MG \sin \theta = W_1 \times a$$
$$\sin \theta = (5 \times 9.81 \times 4)/(9.81 \times 20 \times 7 \times 2 \times 0.795)$$
$$= 0.0904$$
$$\theta = 5° 12'$$

Rise of water line on one side $= 3.5 \tan \theta$
$$= 3.5 \tan (5°12')$$
$$= 0.318 \text{ m}$$

Rightening moment $= W \times MG \tan \theta$
$$= 9.81 \times 20 \times 7 \times 2 \times 0.79 \tan (5°12')$$
$$= 197.1 \text{ kN m}$$

3.6 A solid buoy (specific gravity 0.6 times of sea water) floats in sea water. The buoy consists of an upright cylinder, 1 m diameter and 2.0 m long, with a hemi-sphere 1 m diameter at the lower end. A chain is attached to the lowest point of the hemisphere. Find the required pull in the chain so that the buoy just floats with the axis of the cylindrical portion vertical.

The C.G. of the hemisphere is 3/8 radius from the diameter. Sea water weighs 10.006 kN/m³.

Solution

The buoy will be unstable when M is below G, Fig. 3.11a. By applying a pull P by a chain at the bottom, M approaches G and buoy will be just stable, i.e. BM = BG, Fig 3.11b.

P will be equal to difference between water thrusts in these two cases.

Case I. When no pull is applied. Let buoy be immersed by a depth h_1.

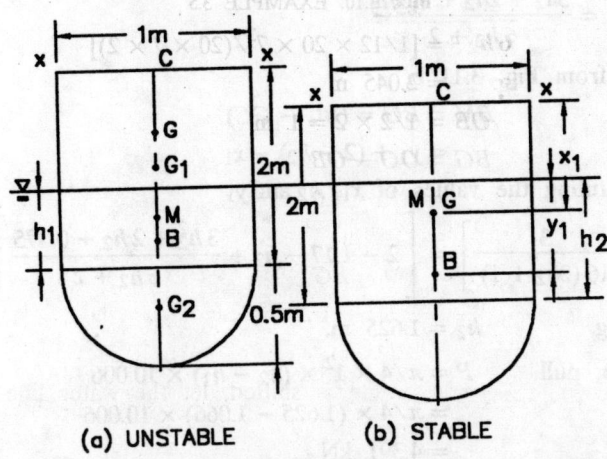

(a) UNSTABLE   (b) STABLE

FIG. 3.11. EXAMPLE 3.6

Weight of buoy = weight of liquid displaced.

$$[\pi \times 0.5^2 \times 2 + \tfrac{2}{3} \times \pi \times 0.5^3] \, 0.6 \times 10.006$$

$$= [\pi \times 0.5^2 \times h_1 + \tfrac{2}{3}\pi \, 0.5^3] \, 10.006$$

$$h_1 = 1.066 \text{ m}$$

Case II. When the pull P is applied by the chain, let the buoy be immersed by depth h_2.

$$BM = BG = I/V$$

$$= [\pi/64 \times (1)^4/[\pi/4] \times 1^2 \times h_2 + \tfrac{1}{2}\pi \times 0.5^3]$$

$$= \frac{3}{16\,(3\,h_2 + 1)} \qquad \qquad ...(i)$$

Location of combined centre of gravity. Take moment about top surface XX.

$$[\pi/4 \times 1^2 \times 2 \times 1 + \tfrac{2}{3} \times \pi \times 0.5^3 \times (2 + \tfrac{3}{8} \times 0.5)]$$

$$= [\pi/4 \times 1^2 \times 2 + \frac{2}{3} \times \pi \times 0.5^3] \times x_1$$

$$x_1 = 1.17 \text{ m}$$

Location of centre of buoyancy. It will be the centroid of the liquid displaced. Let it be located at depth y_1 from water surface.

$$[\pi/4 \times 1^2 \times h_2 \times (h_2/2) + \frac{2}{3}\pi \times 0.5^3 \times (h_2 + \frac{3}{8} \times 0.5)]$$

$$= y_1 [\pi/4 \times 1^2 \times h_2 + \frac{2}{3}\pi \times 0.5^3]$$

$$y_1 = \frac{3h_2^2 + 2h_2 + 0.375}{6h_2 + 2} \qquad \text{...(iii)}$$

Now from Fig. 3.11 b,

$$BM = BG = (BC - GC)$$

$$= y_1 + (2 - h_2) - x_1 \qquad \text{...(iv)}$$

Substituting the values of x_1, h_2 and y_1

$$\left[\frac{3}{16(3h_2 + 1)}\right] = \left[2 - 1.17 - h_2 + \frac{3h_2^2 + 2h_2 + 0.375}{6h_2 + 2}\right]$$

Solving, $\qquad h_2 = 1.625 \text{ m.}$

Hence, pull $\qquad P = \pi/4 \times 1^2 \times (h_2 - h_1) \times 10.006$

$$= \pi/4 \times (1.625 - 1.066) \times 10.006$$

$$= 4.391 \text{ kN}$$

3.7 A right solid cone with apex angle equal to 60° is of density C relative to that of fluid in which it floats with apex downward. Determine what range of C is compatible with stable equilibrium.

Solution

Let $\qquad w = $ specific weight of fluid

$\qquad w_1 = $ specific weight of cone

Then, $\qquad C = w_1/w \qquad \text{...(i)}$

Weight of cone $= w_1 \times \pi \dfrac{R_1^2}{3} \times \sqrt{3} R_1 \qquad \text{...(ii)}$

Weight of fluid displaced $= w \times \pi \dfrac{R^2}{3} \times \sqrt{3} R \qquad \text{...(iii)}$

From Eqs. (ii) and (iii) $w_1/w = R^3/R_1^3$

From (i) $\qquad C = R^3/R_1^3$

Now $\qquad BM = \dfrac{I}{V} = \dfrac{\pi/4 \times R^4}{\pi R^2/3 \times \sqrt{3} \cdot R} = \dfrac{\sqrt{3}}{4} R \qquad \text{...(v)}$

$$BG = OB - OG$$

$$= OB - (AG - AO)$$
$$= h/4 - [h_1/4 - (h_1 - h)]$$
$$= \tfrac{3}{4}(h_1 - h) = \tfrac{3}{4}\sqrt{3}\,(R_1 - R)$$
...(iv)

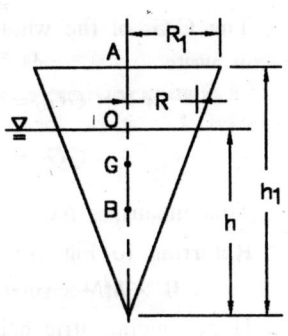

For stability, $BM \geq BG$

$$\frac{\sqrt{3}}{4} R \geq \frac{3\sqrt{3}}{4}(R_1 - R)$$

$$R/R_1 \geq \frac{3}{4}$$

From (iv) and (vii) $C^{1/3} \geq \frac{3}{4}$ and

FIG. 3.12. EXAMPLE 3.7

$$C > 27/64$$
...(vii)

Therefore, the range of C should be 27/64 and 1.0

3.8 A rectangular pontoon 6 m wide, 16 m long and 2 m deep, weighs 80 tonnes when loaded but without ballast water. A vertical diaphragm divides the pontoon longitudinally into two compartments each 3 m wide and 16 m long. 20 tonnes of water ballast are admitted to the bottom of each compartment, the water surface being free to move. The C.G. of pontoon without ballast water is 1.5 m above the bottom and on the geometric centre of the plan. (a) Calculate the metacentric height for rolling, (b) If 2 tonne of deck load is shifted 3 m laterally, find the approximate angle of heel.

Solution

When the loaded vessel heels through a small angle θ, B moves to B_O (Fig.3.13b) which is given by

$$BB_O = BM \times \theta = I/V \times \theta$$

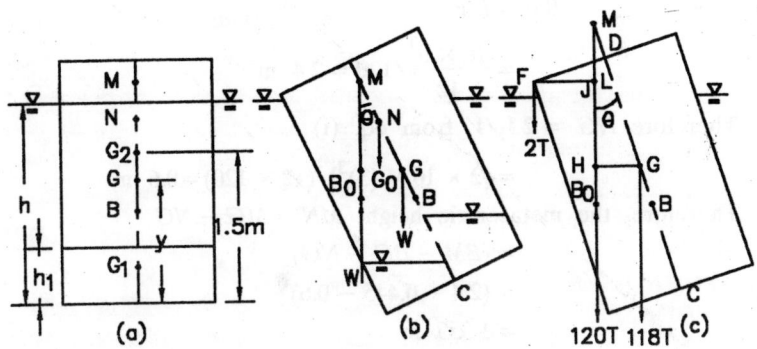

FIG. 3.13. EXAMPLE 3.8

At the same time, C.G. of each tank is also displaced and the shift is given by $I_1/V_1 \times \theta$. The subscript 1 refers to the tank.

The C.G. of the whole pontoon moves from G to G_o and therefore, one can write

$$w V \times GG_o = 2 w V_1 \times I_1/V_1 \times \theta$$

$$GG_0 = \frac{2 I_1}{V} \times \theta$$

This means, $\quad NG = 2I_1/V \qquad \qquad \qquad ...(i)$

Referring to Fig. 3.13b, the rightening couple is equal to
$$W \times MN \times \sin \theta.$$

Hence metacentric height in this case is MN. Let G_1 be the C.G. of tank volume, G_2 be the C.G. of unloaded pontoon, and G be the resultant C.G. of loaded ship.

Now $\qquad \qquad V_1 = 16 \times 3 \times h_1 = \dfrac{20 \times 9.81}{9.81}$

$$h_1 = 0.416 \text{ m}$$

Also $\qquad \qquad V = (80 + 40) \times 9.81/9.81 = 120 \ m^3$

$$h = \frac{120}{16 \times 6} = 1.25 \text{ m}$$

The centre of buoyancy will lie at B, i.e. $BC = 0.625$ m above the base of the pontoon.

To determine the combined C.G., take moments about the base,

$$80 \times 9.81 \times 1.5 + 40 \times 9.81 \times \frac{0.416}{2} = 120 \times 9.81 \times y$$

$$y = 1.07 \text{ m}$$

$$BG = (CG - CB) = (1.07 - 0.625) = 0.445 \text{ m}.$$

Now $\qquad \qquad BM = I/V$

$$= \frac{16 \times 6^3}{12}/120 = 2.4 \text{ m}$$

Therefore $NG = 2 I_1/V$ from eq. (i)

$$= [2 \times 16 \times (3)^3]/(12 \times 120) = 0.6 \text{ m}$$

Therefore, the metacentric height $MN = MG - NG$

$$= (BM - BG - NG)$$

$$= (2.4 - 0.445 - 0.6)$$

$$= 1.355 \text{ m}$$

(b) When the 2 tonne load moves to F, the C.G. of the loaded pontoon will shift from G and M will also be displaced. For small load and small angle of pitch, these two points are assumed fixed relative to pontoon. Taking moment about M,

$$2 \times FJ = 118 \times HG \qquad \qquad ...(ii)$$

Now
$$MD = BM - BD$$
$$= BM - (CD - CB)$$
$$= (2.4 - 2 + 0.625)$$
$$= 1.025 \text{ m}$$
$$MG = (BM - BG)$$
$$= (2.4 - 0.445) = 1.955 \text{ m}$$
$$HG = MG \sin \theta \text{ and } FJ = (3 - MD \tan \theta) \cos \theta$$

Substituting in Eq. (ii)
$$2 \cos \theta (3 - 1.025 \tan \theta) = 118 \times 1.955 \sin \theta$$
$$\tan \theta = 0.02578$$
$$\theta = 1.477°$$

3.9 A ship has a displacement of 6000 tonnes (1 tonne = 9.81 kN) and water plane area is 1200m². The C.G. and centre of area of water plane are respectively 50 m and 60 m from the stern. The metacentric height for pitching is 120 m. Obtain the alteration of the draught at the stern when the ship passes from sea water into a fresh canal water. Assume metacentric height and water plane area remain unaltered by the change of draught.

Solution

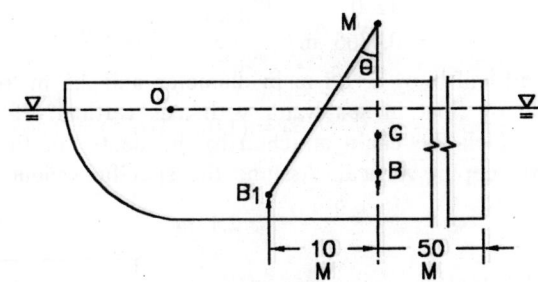

FIG. 3.14. EXAMPLE 3.9

Let the subscripts 1 and 2 refer to the sea water and fresh water respectively. Since the specific weight of sea water is more than fresh water $V_2 > V_1$

The weight of the ship = Weight of sea water displaced
$$= w_1 v_1$$

When the ship is in fresh water, only an upthrust of $w_2 V_1$ will act at B and the remaining upthrust $(V_2 - V_1) w_2$ will act at the C.G. of the extra volume $(V_2 - V_1)$ i.e. on the vertical through O.

Therefore centre of buoyancy will be displaced forward from B by $B B_1 = x$ (say)

Taking moments about B_1

$$V_1 w_2 x = (V_2 - V_1) w_2 (10 - x)$$

$$x = 10 (V_2 - V_1)/V_2$$

But

$$V_2 = \frac{6000 \times 9.81}{9.81} = 6000 \text{ m}^3$$

and

$$V_1 = \frac{6000 \times 9.81}{10.3} = 5724 \text{ m}^3$$

(Specific weight of sea water $= 10.3 \text{ kN/m}^3$)

From Eq. (i) $x = 10 (6000 - 5714)/6000 = 0.476$ m

This ship will not be in equilibrium unless B_1 is below G.

Therefore, the ship will lower its stern until above condition is satisfied. This means the ship will rotate through an angle θ, which is given by.

$$\theta = \frac{B B_1}{BM} = \frac{B B_1}{MG} \text{ as MG is too large.}$$

Therefore, extra draught at stern

= increase due to change of water
+ increase due to rotation through θ about G.

$$\text{Extra draught} = \frac{V_2 - V_1}{area} + \frac{x}{MG} \times 50$$

$$= \frac{286}{1200} + \frac{0.476 \times 50}{120}$$

$$= 0.4366 \text{ m}$$

3.10 A cylindrical buoy is 1.5 m in diameter and 2.5 m long. It weighs 15 kN. Will the buoy float in sea water with axis vertical? If not, find the vertical pull with which the chain attached to the centre of the base of the buoy be pulled to keep it vertical. Assume the specific weight of sea water as 10.25 kN/m^3

Solution

Displaced volume$= \dfrac{15.0}{10.25} = 1.463 \text{ m}^3$

The depth of immersion

$$= \frac{1.463}{\dfrac{\pi}{4} (1.5)^2} = 0.828 \text{ m}$$

Therefore, the centre of buoyancy B will lie at $0.828/2 = 0.414$ m below the water line and C.G. of buoy lies at $(1.25 - 0.828) = 0.422$ m above the water line.

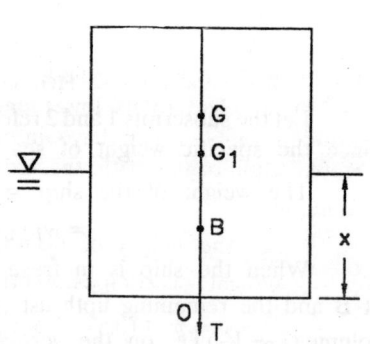

FIG. 3.15. EXAMPLE 3.10

$$BG = 0.414 + 0.422 = 0.836 \text{ m}$$

$$BM = \frac{I}{V} = \frac{\pi/64 \times (1.5)^4}{\pi (1.5)^2 \times 0.828} = 0.17 \text{ m}$$

$BM < BG$, the buoy will not float with its axis vertical. Hence, a chain is attached at its bottom in which the tension is T, the depth of immersion is now x (say).

$$\text{Depth of immersion } x = \frac{\dfrac{(15.0 + T)}{10.25}}{\dfrac{\pi}{4}(1.5)^2}$$

$$x = \frac{(15.0 + T)}{18.1} \text{ m}$$

Now

$$(BM)_1 = I/V_1 = \pi/64 \times (1.5)^4/[\pi/4 \, (1.5)^2 \times x]$$

$$= \frac{2.25 \times 18.1}{16 \times (15.0 + T)} = \frac{2.546}{(15.0 + T)}$$

Let the combined C.G. of the weight of buoy W and T be at G_1 It can be determined by taking moments about O. Thus

$$(15.0 + T) \times OG_1 = 15.0 \times 1.25$$

$$OG_1 = 18.75/(15.0 + T)$$

Therefore, $\quad (BG)_1 = (OG_1 - x/2)$

$$= \frac{18.75}{(15.0 + T)} - \frac{15.0 + T}{36.2}$$

For stability of ship, $(BM)_1 > (BG)_1$

$$\frac{2.546}{15.0 + T} > \frac{18.75}{15.0 + T} - \frac{15.0 + T}{36.2}$$

Solving it, $T > 9.22$ kN

Thus pull in the chain should be greater than 9.22 kN

3.11 A wooden cylinder 500 mm in diameter (specific gravity equal to 0.5) has a concrete cylinder 1 m long of the same diameter (specific gravity = 2.5) attached to its lower end. Determine the minimum length which the wooden cylinder can have in order that the system may float in water in stable equilibrium with the axis horizontal.

Solution

Let the height of cylinder be h m

Weight of composite cylinder

$$= \pi/4 \, (0.5)^2 \, [h \times 0.5 \times 9.81 + 1.0 \times 2.5 \times 9.81]$$

$$= 9.81 \times \pi/4 \times (0.5)^2 \, [0.5 \, h + 2.5) \qquad \text{...(i)}$$

Let depth of immersion be $(y + 1) \, m$

Then weight of liquid displaced

$$= \pi/4 \, (0.5)^2 \times (y + 1) \times 9.81 \quad ...(ii)$$

Therefore, equating (i) and (ii)

$$9.81 \times \pi/4 \times (0.5)^2 \, (0.5 \, h + 2.5)$$

$$= 9.81 \times \frac{\pi}{4} \, (0.5)^2 \, (y + 1)$$

$$y = (0.5 \, h + 1.5) \quad ...(iii)$$

Let the combined C.G. of the wooden and concrete cylinders lie at G at distance x below the top of the cylinder. Taking moments about the point O,

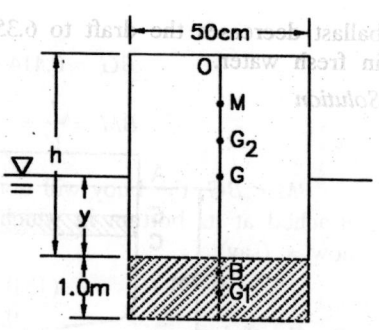

FIG. 3.16. EXAMPLE 3.11

$$\pi/4 \times (0.5)^2 \times h \times 9.81 \times 0.5 \times h/2 + (\pi/4) \, (0.5)^2$$
$$\times 1.0 \times 2.5 \times 9.81 \times (h + 0.5)$$
$$= 9.81 \times \pi/4 \, (0.5)^2 \times (0.5 \, h + 2.5) \times x$$

$$x = OG = \frac{[0.25 \, h^2 + 2.5 \, (h + 0.5)]}{(0.5 \, h + 2.5)} \quad ...(iv)$$

The centre of buoyancy B will lie at a distance z metre below the top of the cylinder. Therefore

$$OB = z = (h + 1) - (1 + y)/2$$

Substituting the value of y from (iii)

$$OB = z = 0.75 \, h - 0.25 \quad ...(v)$$

Hence, $BG = OB - OG$ ...(vi)

$$= (0.75 \, h - 0.25) - \frac{(0.25 \, h^2 + 2.5 \, h + 1.25)}{(0.5 \, h + 2.5)}$$

Now $BM = I/V$

$$= \frac{\left\{ \dfrac{\pi}{64} \, (0.5)^4 \right\}}{\left\{ \dfrac{\pi}{4} \, (0.5)^2 \times (y + 1) \right\}}$$

$$= \frac{1}{64 \, (y + 1)}$$

For stable equilibrium $BM \geq BG$

$$\frac{1}{64 \, (y + 1)} \geq (0.75 \, h - 0.25 - \frac{(0.25 \, h^2 + 2.5 \, h + 1.25)}{(0.5 \, h + 2.5)}$$

Solving it for h, minimum height of wooden cylinder = 7.9 m

3.12 A ship with vertical sides near the water line, of mass 4000 tonne draws 6.7 m in salt water ($\rho = 1025 \, kg/m^3$). Discharge of 200 tonne of water ballast decreases the draft to 6.35 m. What would be the draft of the ship in fresh water.

Solution

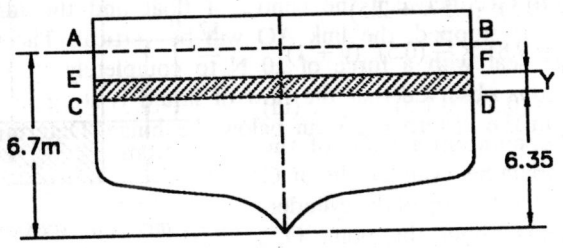

FIG. 3.17. EXAMPLE 3.12

Let the ship is immersed in salt water by 6.7 m so that the area at water line be AB. As the ballast of 200 tonne is reduced, the new water line is CD. The area at this water lines is also A.

A decrease in draft of 0.35 m is caused by the decrease in ballast of 200 tonne. Therefore.

Decrease in Wt. of ballast = decrease in the weight of the liquid displaced.

$$(200 \times 9.81 \times 1000) = (1025 \times 9.81) (A \times 0.35)$$

Solving $A = 557.5 \text{ m}^2$ ...(i)

Since the buoyant force $F_B = w \times$ volume of liquid displaced

Volume of liquid displaced $= F_B/w$.

The difference in the volume displaced in salt water and fresh water can be expressed as

$$= \left[\frac{(4000 - 200)}{1000} - \frac{(4000 - 200)}{1025} \right] \times 1000 \text{ m}^3 \qquad ...(ii)$$

Let the draft in fresh water be $(6.35 + y) \, m$.

Then change in the volume of fresh water displaced can also written as $(A \times y)$ (shown hatched in the figure).

$$= (557.5 \times y) \qquad ...(iii)$$

From Eqs. (ii) and (iii)

$$= \left(\frac{3800}{1000} - \frac{3800}{1025} \right) \times 1000 = 557.5 \, y$$

Solving, $y = 0.166 \, m$.

The draft in fresh water $= (6.35 + 0.166)$

$$= 6.516 \text{ m}$$

3.13 A float valve regulates the flow of liquid of sp. gr. 0.8 into a cistern. The spherical float is 15 cm in diameter. AOB is a weight-less link carrying the float at one end and a valve at the other end which closes the pipe through which the oil flows into the cistern. The link in mounted on a frictionless hinge at O and the angle AOB is 135°. The length OA is 20 cm and the distance between the centre of float and the hinge is 50 cm. When the flow is stopped, the link AO will be vertical. The valve is to be pressed on the seat with a force of 10 N to completely stop the flow into the cistern. It was observed that the flow of liquid is stopped when the free surface of oil in the cistern is 35 cm below the hinge. Determine the weight of the float.

Solution

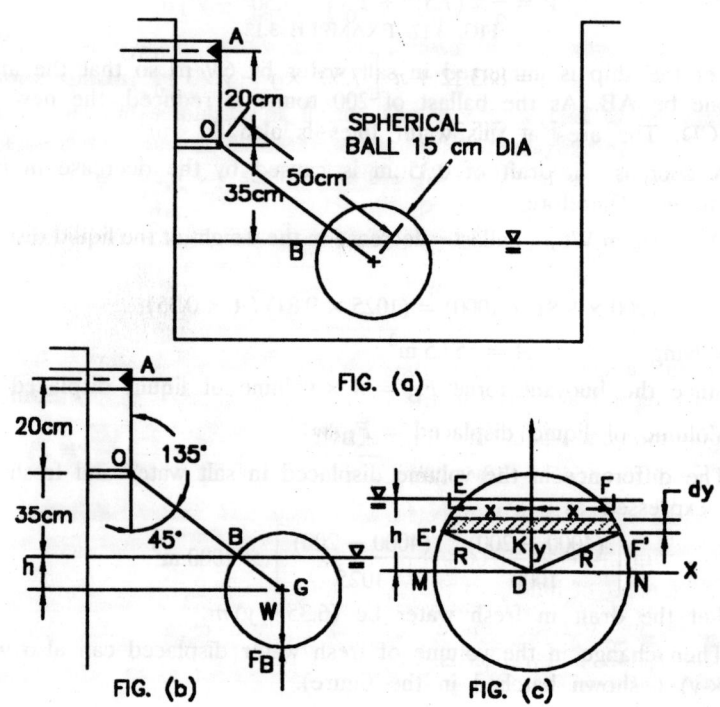

FIG. 3.18. EXAMPLE 3.13

Let the weight of the float be W and the buoyant force F_B act on it in the upward direction. Let the centre of graving of the float lie at h meter below liquid level.

Then $h = (50 \cos 45° - 35) = 0.355$ cm

According to the principle of floatation.

F_B = weight of liquid displaced.

= $0.8 \times w \times$ volume of liquid displaced ...(i)

To find the volume of liquid displaced : Consider an elementary disc of radius x at a distance y from horizontal diameter MN.

V = volume of liquid displaced.

$$= \frac{2}{3} \pi R^3 + \int_0^{0.355} \pi (x)^2 \, dy$$

From $\Delta KDF, x^2 = R^2 - y^2$

$$V = \frac{2}{3} \pi R^3 + \int_0^{0.336} \pi [R^2 - y^2] \, dy$$

$$V = \frac{2}{3} \pi (7.5)^3 + \int_0^{0.355} [7.50^2 - y^2] \, dy$$

$$= 883.12 + \pi \left[7.50^2 \times y - y^3/3 \right]_0^{0.355}$$

Solving, $V = 945.36 \, cm^3$ or $945.36 \times 10^{-6} \, m^3$

Therefore, $F_B = 0.8 \times 9810 \times 945.36 \times 10^{-6}$ N

$$= 7.419 \text{ N}$$

The net vertical force acting on the float

$$= F_B - W$$

$$= (7.419 - W)$$

Since the hinge is frictions, the moment about O of the net vertical force on the float is transferred to the valve A without any loss of magnitude,

Taking moment about the hinge O

$(7.419 - W) \times 50 \cos 45° = 10 \times 20$

$$W = 1.76 \text{ N}$$

3.14 A ship displaces 50.00 kN of sea water of mass density 1025 kg/m^3. The second moment of inertia of the water line section about an axis through centre is 12000 m^4 and the centre of buoyancy is 2 m below the centre of gravity. It the radius of gyration is 3.7 m, calculate the period of oscillation.
Solution

From Eq. 3.14.

$$T = 2\pi \sqrt{k^2/zg}$$

where z is meta centric height.

$$MG = \frac{I}{V} - BG$$

Volume of sea water displaced $= \dfrac{50,000 \times 10^3}{1025 \times 9.81}$

$$= 4972.5 \text{ m}^3$$

$$\therefore \qquad MG = \left[\frac{12000}{4972.5} - 2.0 \right]$$
$$= (2.413 - 2)\, m$$
$$MG = 0.413 \text{ m}$$

Hence, $\qquad T = 2\pi \sqrt{\dfrac{3.7^2}{0.413 \times 9.81}}$

$$= 11.54 \text{ s}$$

It is seen that although large metacentric height yields greater stability, it reduces the time period of oscillation. This means frequent oscillation of the ship causes discomfort.

3.15. A cylindvical buoy (Fig. 3.20) 1.8 m diameter, 1.2 m high weighing 10 kN floats in salt water of density 1025 kgm^{-3}. It's centre of gravity is 0.45 m from bottom. If a load of 2 kN is placed on the top, find the maximum height of centre of gravity of this load above the bottom if the buoy is to remetin is stable equilibrium.

Solution :

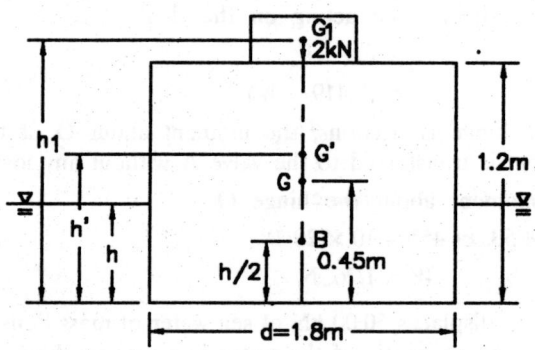

FIG. 3.19. EXAMPLE 3.15

Let G be C.G. of buoy 0.45 m above bottom, G_1 be C.G. of load at h_1 m above bottom and G' be the C.G. of combined buoy and load at a height of h' bottom.

Let V be the volume of liquid displaced by the bouoy when the load W_1 is in position and buoy is immersed h meter in salt water. W be the weight of buog

Then buoyancy force = weight of salt water displaced.

$$= \rho g V$$
$$= \rho g \left(\frac{\pi}{4} . d^2 \times h \right) \qquad \qquad \text{...(i)}$$

Also buoyarrcy force = Weight of buoy + W_1 \qquad ...(ii)

From Eqs. (i) and (ii)

$$\rho g \times \frac{\pi}{4} d^2 \times h = W + W_1$$

$$\therefore \qquad h = \frac{4 (W + W_1)}{\rho g \pi d^2}$$

$$= \frac{4 [10 + 2] \times 10^3}{1025 \times 9.81 \times \pi \times (1.8)^2} = 0.47 \text{ mm}$$

The centre of buoyancy B will be at $\frac{h}{2} = 0.235$ m above bottom.

It the buoy and the load are in guest equilibrium, then meta centre and combined centre of gravity G' must coincide, i.e. $BG' = B'M$.

$$BM = BG' = \frac{I}{V}$$

$$= \frac{\frac{\pi}{64} d^4}{\frac{\pi}{4} d^2 \times h} = \frac{d^2}{16 h}$$

$$= \frac{(1.8)^2}{16 \times 0.47} = 0.431 \text{ m}$$

The combined centre of gravity G' will lie at $\left(\dfrac{h}{2} + BG'\right)$ above bottom

$$\therefore \qquad OG' = \left(\frac{0.47}{2} + 0.431\right) = 0.66 \text{ m above bottom}$$

To locate G_1, take moment of weights about bottom

$$W_1 \times h_1 + W \times 0.45 = (W + W_1) OG'$$

$$h_1 = \frac{(10 + 21) \times 10^3 \times 0.666 - 10 \times 10^3 \times 0.45}{2 \times 10^3}$$

$$h_1 = 1.746 \text{ m above bottom.}$$

3.16 A vessel carries a tank of oil weighing 'S' kN/m³ amid ships. Prove that the effect of fluidity of the oil on the rolling stability of the vessel is equivalent to a decrease in the value of metacentric height by an amount $A k^2 \cdot S / w V_1$ kN/m³ where w kN/m³ is the sp. wt of water in which the vessel floats ; V_1 is the displacement of the ship and $A k^2$ is the second moment of area of the oil surface in the tank about the longitudinal axis. To what extent will this alteration in the metacentric height be decreased by fitting of a central longitudinal partition in the tank.

Solution

When the ship heels by an angle θ, B shifts to B_1 and this shift is given by

$$BB_1 = BM \times \theta = \frac{I}{V_1} \times \theta$$

If 'o' refers to oil conditions, the shift of C.G. of oil is given by

$$\frac{I_o}{V_o} \times \theta \text{ parallel to } BB_1.$$

This means G shifts to G_1 parallel to BB_1 and may be determined to by

$$W_1 \times GG_1 = W_o \times \frac{I_o}{V_o} \times \theta \text{ (see Fig. 3.15)}$$

$$\text{...(i)}$$

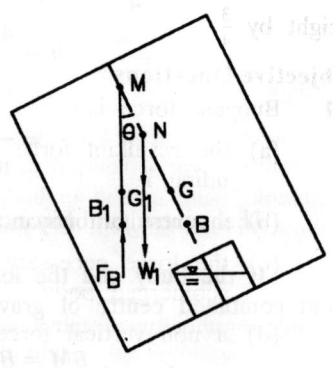

FIG. 3.20. EXAMPLE 3.16

$$GG_1 = \frac{W_o}{W_1} \times \frac{I_o}{V_o} \times \theta = \frac{V_o S I_o \theta}{w V_1 V_o} = \frac{I_o S \theta}{V_1 w}$$

$$= \frac{A k^2 S \theta}{V_1 w}$$

Hence, $GN = \dfrac{A k^2 S}{V_1 w}$

The rightening couple $= W_1 \times MN \times \sin \theta$, i.e. MN is the metacentric height when G shifts due to fluidity of oil.

If G has not shifted, the metacentric height would have been M.G. Therefore the reduction in metacentric height.

$$= MG - MN$$

$$= GN$$

$$= A k^2 S/V_1 w$$

For two tanks let subscript 2 refer to oil conditions in each tank. Then from Eq. (i)

$$W_1 \times GG_1 = 2 (W_2 \times I_2/V_2) \theta$$

or
$$GG_1 = (2 W_2 I_2 \theta)/(W_1 V_2)$$

and
$$GN_1 = (GN) \theta$$

$$= \frac{2W_2}{W_1} \times \frac{I_2}{V_2} = \frac{2 I_2 S}{V_2 w}$$

But
$$I_o = (1/12) bd^3$$

$$I_2 = (1/12) b (d/2)^3$$

Hence
$$I_2 = \frac{1}{8} I_o = \frac{1}{8} A k^2$$

Therefore, $GN = \frac{1}{4} (A k^2 S/V_1 w)$

This means that the partition reduces the above change in metacentric height by $\frac{3}{4}$

Objective Questions

3.1 Buoyant force is

    (a) the resultant force on a body due to the fluid surrounding it

    (b) the resultant force acting on a floating body

    (c) the force necessary to maintain equilibrium of a submerged body

    (d) a non vertical force for nonsymmertical bodies

    (e) equal to the volume of liquid displaced

3.2 The line of action of the buoyant force acts through the

    (a) centre of gravity of any submerged body

    (b) centroid of the volume of any floating body

    (c) centroid of the displaced volume of fluid

    (d) centroid of the volume of fluid vertically above the body

    (e) centroid of the horizontal projection of the body

3.3. A body floats in a stable equilibrium

    (a) when centre of gravity is below centre of buoyancy

    (b) when centre of buoyancy is below centre of gravity

    (c) when centre of gravity is at the centre of buoyancy

    (d) none of the above

3.4 The criterion for stability of a floating body depends on

    (a) the relative position of centre of buoyancy and the centre of gravity

    (b) the relative position of centre of buoyancy and metacentre

    (c) the relative position of centre of gravity and metacentre

    (d) none of the above

3.5 The metacentric height of a floating body depends

    (a) directly on the shape of its water line area

    (b) on the volume of liquid displaced by the body

    (c) second moment of area at water line

    (d) the distance between metacentre and the centre-of gravity

(e) none of the above

3.6 Differentiate between centre of pressure, centre of buoyancy and metacentre.

3.7 A floating body displaces a volume of liquid equal to

(a) its submerged weight   (b) its own volume

(c) its own weight   (d) none of these answers

3.8 A slab of wood is $1m \times 1m \times 0.5$ m (its specific gravity 0.5) floats in water with a 1.5 kN load on it. The volume of slab submerged in m^3, is

(a) 3.952   (b) 0.403   (c) 1.75

(d) 0.178   (e) none of these answers

3.9 A closed cubical metal box 1 m on an edge is made of uniform sheet and weighs 6 kN. It's metacentric height, in meter, when placed on oil of specific gravity 0.9, with sides vertical is

(a) 0.122   (b) 0.680   (c) –0.181

(d) 0.302   (e) none of these answers

Problems

3.1 A 2.7 m high wooden rod free to rotate at the bottom (in the vertical plane) has cross section 10 mm × 10 mm in Fig 3.21. The specific weight of wood is 7.5 kN/m^3, find the angle α to keep the rod floating.

3.2 The plug valve in Fig 3.22 weights 1 kN/m^3. Calculate the diameter D of the floating sphere for the valve to open when the water is 1.5 m deep. Consider the cable and sphere to be weightless.

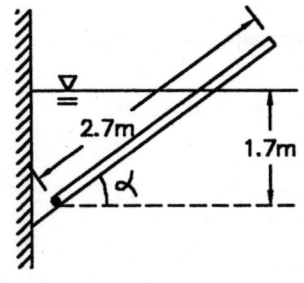

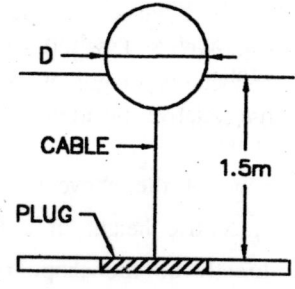

FIG. 3.21. PROBLEM 3.1   ,   FIG. 3.212 PROBLEM 3.2

3.3 A balloon having a total weight of 0.4 kN contains 600 m^3 of hydrogen. How many kilo newton of ballast is necessary to hold the balloon on the ground ? Barometric pressure is 1.03 bar ; temperature of air and hydrogen is 15.5° C.

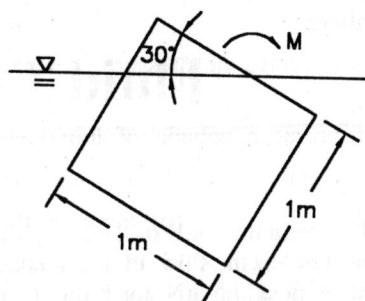

FIG. 3.23. PROBLEM 3.3

3.4 A cubical piece of wood (specific gravity = 0.9) with an edge of length 1 m floats in water. What couple M is required to hold the cube in position, shown in Fig. 3.23

3.5 A rectangular barge is 20 m long, 10 m wide and 3 m deep its draft is 1 m and is increased to 2.5 m when fully loaded. Assuming in each case that the centre of gravity of the barge and its load coincide with the geometric centre of the entire cross section, compute the position of the metacentre of both drafts.

3.6 A 15 m cube of aluminium weighs 0.05 kN when immersed in water. What will its apparent weight be when immersed in oil of sp. gr. 0.75.

3.7 A stone weighs 0.6 kN. When it was lowered into a square tank 0.60 m on a side, the weight of stone in water was 0.35 kN. How much did the water rise in the tank.

3.8 A rectangular barge with outside dimensions of 6 m width, 20 m length and 3 m height, weighs 1.750 kN. It floats in salt water ($w=10.3$ kN/m^3) and the centre of gravity of the loaded barge is 1.5 m from the top. Locate (a) the centre of buoyancy when floating on an even keel and (b) when the barge tilts at 10°, (c) locate the metacentre for 10° tilt.

3.9 An empty balloon and its equipment weighs 0.5 kN. When inflated with gas (weighing 0.3 N/m^3) the balloon is spherical and 7 m in diameter. What is the maximum weight of cargo that the balloon can lift assuming air to weigh 0.06 N/m^3

Fluid Kinematics

4.1 INTRODUCTION

Fluid kinematic deals with the study of the space-time relationship without considering the force involved in the flow. Fluids, unlike soilds, are composed of particles whose relative position are not fixed from time to time Each fluid particle has its own velocity and acceleration at any instant of time. They change both with respect to time as well as space. For describing the motion of fluid, the motion of these particles should be observed at various locations in space and at successive instant of time.

There are two methods which are used to describe the fluid motion (a) Lagrangian method and (b) Eulerian method.

In the *Lagrangian method*, the motion of individual particle is observed at various instants of time. Consider that the co-ordinates of some fixed point (reference co-ordinates) in space are, $x = x_0\, y = y_0\, , z = z_0$ at some time interval $t = t_0$, then the co-ordinates of individual particle (x,y,z) can be described as

$$x = f_1 (x_0 y_0 , z_0 , t_0) \qquad ...(4.1a)$$

$$y = f_2 (x_0 , y_0 , z_0 , t_0) \qquad ...(4.1b)$$

$$z = f_3 (x_0 , y_0 z_0 , t_0) \qquad ...(4.1c)$$

These are known as parametric equations of the path of fluid particles at any time t. The velocity and acceleration components at any instant of time can be described as

$$x - \text{ component } u = dx/dt , a_x = du/dt \qquad ...(4.2a)$$

$$y - \text{ component, } v = dy/dt , a_y = dv/dt \qquad ...(4.2b)$$

$$z - \text{ component, } w = dz/dt , a_z = dw/dt \qquad ...(4.2c)$$

In a deformable system such as fluid, it will be unmanageable to observe the motion of each fluid particle. Instead, the motion of various fluid particles is observed at some fixed point in space. The velocity of fluid particle is then expressed as

$$\overline{U} = U(x,y,z,t) \qquad ...(4.3)$$

where x,y,z and t are independent variables at which the motion (or the velocity) is observed. This method of describing the flow characteristics is known as the *Eulerian method.* Moreover, in most of the fluid mechanics problems, the velocities and accelarations are required at various points in the flow field and the behaviour of individual fluid particle is not needed. The Eulerian method is simple and is mostly used. The **Lagrangian** method involves a lot of mathematical difflculties in solving the flow equations, Eq. 4.1a to Eq. 4.1c.

The components of velocity in x, y and z direction are expressed as.

$$u = F_1(x, y, z, t) \qquad ...(4.4a)$$
$$v = F_2(x, y, z, t) \qquad ....(4.4b)$$
$$w = F_3(x, y, z, t) \qquad ....(4.4c)$$

The equations for velocity of the first method are related to the velocity of the second method by the following relationships with the help of Eqs. 4.1 and 4.4.

$$u = dx/dt \qquad ...(4.5a)$$
$$v = dy/dt \qquad ...(4.5b)$$
$$w = dz/dt \qquad ...(4.5c)$$

It is interesting to know that these velocity components measured by means of an electronic instrument (hot wire set, laser amplifier, etc.) are spectrum of fluctuations and hence these fluctuations are averaged for some fixed interval of time, i.e.

$$\bar{u} = \frac{1}{T} \int_0^T u \, dt \qquad ...(4.6)$$

$\bar{u}$ represent the average of velocity in X direction over a period T (bar over u represents the time average) and u is the instantaneous velocity at any time instant t.

4.2. TYPES OF FLOW

Any general pattern of fluid motion, as visible by clouds, of smoke in the atmosphere will have different configuration at different points and which changes continuosly in form with time. Such a variation of velocity with time constitutes unsteadiness. The velocity variation with respect to location of particle is termed as non-uniformity and is caused by the manner in which particles of a fluid layer move with respect to adjacent layers.

1. Steady and unsteady flow

If none of the variables, such as velcoity, acceleration and density, in a flow problem varies with time, the flow is said to be 'steady', e.g. flow in a uniform diameter pipe line. If any one of the variables changes with time, the flow is said to be unsteady, e.g. motion of tidal wave. Mathematically,

Steady flow : $\partial/\partial t = 0$ \qquad ...(4.7a)

Unsteady flow : $\partial/\partial t \neq 0$ \qquad ...(4.7b)

2. Uniform and non-uniform flow

If at any given instant of time the velocity, and acceleration, etc. remain the same at all sections of flow, the flow is termed as 'uniform flow', e.g. flow in a laboratony channel. If the velocity of flow (or depth of flow, etc.) changes from section to section, the flow is termed as 'non-uniform flow', e.g., flow in a converging channel. Mathematically.

Uniform flow : $\partial/\partial s = 0$ \qquad ...(4.8a)

Non-uniform flow : $\partial/\partial s \neq 0$ ...(4.8b)

3. Laminar flow and turbulent flow

If fluid particles move in smooth paths in layers or laminas with one layer sliding over an adjacent layer, the paths of individual particle do not cross or interesect. Such a flow is said to be 'laminar' e.g. flow through sandy soils. If the path of various particles irregular and random with no systematic pattern of flow (which is not discernible), the flow is termed as 'turbulent flow'. Majority of flows which are met in practice are of turbulent type.

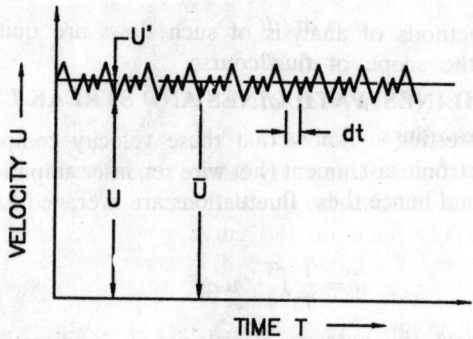

FIG. 4.1. VARIATION OF VELOCITY WITH TIME

In turbulent flow, the velocity fluctuates with time and this specturm of velocity variation can be recorded by electronic instruments (like hot wire anemometer or laser amplifier). The time average velocity $\bar{u}$ can be found as

$$\bar{u} = \frac{1}{T} \int_0^T u\, dt \qquad \text{...(4.9a)}$$

and $$u = \bar{u} + u' \qquad \text{...(4.9b)}$$

u is known as the instantaneous veloccity and u' is the flucturation from the mean value. T is the time period over which the time averaging is made. For accuracy, sampling time T should be large enough so that

$$\bar{u'} = 0 \qquad \text{...(4.10)}$$

(bar over u' indicates the time averaging quantity)

4.3 ONE, TWO AND THREE DIMENSIONAL FLOW

In a one dimensional flow, the variations of fluid property or flow parameters transverse to the main flow are absent. This means that fluid and flow characteristics remain constant at any cross-section normal to the main flow. However, the variation in velocity at any cross section in case of real fluid flow is assumed to be small and the average values of velocity, density, etc, are constant. For examples, the flow along a streamline is one dimensional flow. Many engineering problems are solved on the assumption of one dimensional flow. Mathematically.

$$\bar{u} = u(x, t) \qquad \text{...(4.11a)}$$

In a two dimensional flow, the variation in the flow and fluid parameters takes place in X and Y direction only. This means that all the particles move in parallel planes along identical paths in each plane. There is no variation in these parameters in the direction normal to this plane XY.

$$\bar{u} = u\,(x,y,t) \qquad\qquad ...(4.11b)$$

The flow around a cylinder or flow in a conduit is treated as two dimensional flow.

In case of three dimensional flow, the flow parameters may have variation in all the three directions X,Y and Z. Mathematically,

$$\bar{u} = u\,(x,y,z,t) \qquad\qquad ...(4.11c)$$

The methods of analysis of such flows are quite complex and hence are beyond the scope of this course.

4.4 STREAMLINES, PATH LINES AND STREAK LINES

1. Streamlines

Streamlines are imaginary curves drawn through a fluid flow to indicate the direction of motion in various sections of the flow of the fluid system. A tangent at any point on the curve represents the instantaneous direction of velocity of the fluid particles at that point. Thus, a streamline is defined as an imaginary line or curve drawn in the fluid flow such that the tangent drawn at any point of it indicates the direction of velocity at that point.

Since the velocity vector has a zero component normal to streamline, there can be no flow across a streamline at any point.

2. Equation of Streamline

Consider a point P in a fluid and moving a small distance ds along a streamline in time, Fig.4.2. The velocity at point P is U and has velocity components u, v and w in X, Y, and z directions respectively. Then one can write

$$\frac{dx}{u} = \frac{dy}{v} = \frac{dz}{w} \qquad ...(4.12a)$$

For a two dimensional flow,

$$u\,dy - v\,dx = 0 \qquad ...(4.12b)$$

Eq. 4.12 b is the equation of streamline. It relates the velocity along the streamline to the displacement along streamline.

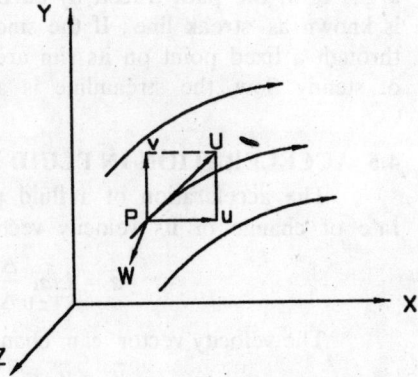

FIG. 4.2. A SET OF STREAMLINE

3. Streamtube

A streamtube represents the elementary portion of a flowing fluid bounded by a group of streamlines which confines the flow. If the cross sectional area of the streamtube is sufficiently small, the velocity at the mid point of any cross section may be taken as the average velocity for the section as a whole. The concept of streamtube has practical significance because it behaves as if it were a solid tube. There can be no flow across the wall of a streamtube.

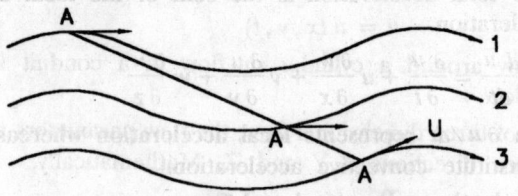

FIG. 4.3. DEFINITION SKETCH – PATH LINE

4. Path lines

A pathline is the locus or path of a single fluid particle during its motion in a given time. Consider a point A being situated at time t_1 on stream line 1. At time t_2, it may be found on streamline 2 and still later on streamline 3.

If the path of this particle is joined by a smooth curve then this curve is known as the path line.

In case of steady flow, the streamline has a fixed inclination at any point and each particle always moves tangential to the streamline, hence the path line of a particle is a streamline.

5. Streak lines

When a dye is injected into a fluid or the smoke is introduced in a gas flow, the path traced by all the particles passing through a fixed point is known as 'streak line'. If the smoke coming out of a chimney and passing through a fixed point on its rim are joined, it will trace a streakline. In case of steady flow, the streamline is also streakline.

4.5 ACCELERATION IN FLUID MOTION

The acceleration of a fluid particle in motion is defined as the time rate of change of its velocity vector.

$$\bar{a} = \underset{\Delta T \pm 0}{Lim} \frac{\Delta u}{\Delta T} \qquad \ldots(4.14a)$$

The velocity vector can change both in magnitude and direction

$$\bar{u} = \bar{u}\,(x,y,z,t)$$

Similarly, $\qquad \bar{a} = a\,(x,y,z,t)$ $\qquad\qquad \ldots(4.13)$

In case of steady flow, the velocity of all the fluid particles passing any given section remains same at all times. However, the velocity may change from section to section at the given instant of time, e.g. converging or diverging flow in a pipe or channel. Thus the acceleration of stream line will be due to displacement. It is termed as 'convective acceleration.'

In case of unsteady flow, the velcoity changes from instant to instant and the corresponding acceleration is known as 'local acceleration'.

Thus, the total acceleration is the sum of the local acceleration and convective acceleration.

$$\bar{a} = \frac{d\,\bar{u}}{dt} = \frac{\partial u}{\partial t} + u\frac{\partial u}{\partial x} + v\frac{\partial u}{\partial y} + w\frac{\partial u}{\partial z} \qquad ...(4.14\ b)$$

The term $\partial u/dt$ represents local acceleration whereas the remaining three terms constitute convective acceleration.

1. Acceleration in three dimcunsional flows

Consider a fluid particle $P(x,y,z)$ in a flow field. The velocity at this point is $\bar{u}(x,y,z)$ and the acceleration in any direction, say, X direction is given by

$$a_X = \frac{du}{dt}$$

Here du/dt is the total derivative of u with repsect to time t. The various components of velocity in X, Y and Z directions may be written as

$$\bar{u} = u(x,y,z,t) \qquad ...(4.15\ a)$$
$$\bar{v} = v(x,y,z,t) \qquad ...(4.15\ b)$$
$$\bar{w} = w(x,y,z,t) \qquad ...(4.15\ c)$$

The toal change in velocity du may now be written as

$$du = \frac{\partial u}{\partial t}dt + \frac{\partial u}{\partial x}dx + \frac{\partial u}{\partial y}dy + \frac{\partial u}{\partial z}dz$$

Then the acceleration in X direction $a_X\ (= du/dt)$ becomes

$$a_x = \frac{du}{dt} = \frac{\partial u}{\partial t} + \frac{\partial u}{\partial x}\times\frac{dx}{dt} + \frac{\partial u}{\delta y}\times\frac{dy}{dt} + \frac{\partial u}{\partial \theta}\times\frac{dz}{dt}$$

$$a_x = \frac{\partial u}{\partial t} + u\frac{\partial v}{\partial x} + v\frac{\partial u}{\partial y} + w\frac{\partial v}{\partial z} \qquad ...(4.16\ a)$$

Similarly,

$$a_y = \frac{\partial v}{\partial t} + u\frac{\partial v}{\partial x} + v\frac{\partial v}{\partial y} + w\frac{\partial v}{\partial z} \qquad ...(4.16b)$$

and $$a_z = \frac{\partial w}{\partial t} + u\frac{\partial w}{\partial x} + v\frac{\partial w}{\partial y} + w\frac{\partial w}{\partial z} \qquad ...(4.16c)$$

and $$a = i\,a_x + j\,a_y + k\,a_z \qquad ...(4.16d)$$

For two dimensional flow, Z-conponent of velocity w vanishes and hence the fourth term on right hand side of Eqs. 4.16a to 4.16c drops out.

In case of steady flow, the local acceleration is zero and only convective acceleration is present, whereas, in case of uniform flow, only local acceleration is present and convective acceleration is absent.

A similar analysis for cylindrical polar co-ordinates, in which radial and tangential velocities (u_r and u_θ) are both functions of r and θ in a plane corresponding to X-Y plane, leads to

$$u_r = \frac{dr}{dr}, \quad u_\theta = r\frac{d\theta}{dt} \qquad ...(4.17)$$

The acceleration in radial and tangential direction is given by

$$a_r = u_r\frac{\partial u_r}{\partial r} + u_\theta \times \frac{\partial u_r}{r\,\partial\theta} - \frac{u_\theta^2}{r} + \frac{\partial u_r}{\partial t} \qquad ...(4.18a)$$

$$a_\theta = u_r\frac{\partial u_\theta}{\partial r} + \frac{u_\theta\,\partial u_\theta}{r\,\partial\theta} - \frac{u_r u_\theta}{r} + \frac{\partial u_\theta}{\partial t} \qquad ...(4.18b)$$

2. Tangential and normal acceleration

Consider a fluid particle A in Fig. 4.4, which moves a distance ds in infinitesimal time interval dt. The velocity of fluid particle U and A changes to $U + dU$ as the particle reaches B in this time dt, thus the net change in velocity is dU. The change in velocity dU can be resolved in to two components, viz. ∂U_t in the direction tangent to the point A and ∂U_n in the direction normal to it, Fig. 4.4. The rate of change of velocity in tangential direction gives rise to tangential acceleration and rate of change of velocity in normal direction causes normal acceleration. Each of these two accelerations consists of local acceleration due to unsteadiness of flow and convective acceleration due to non-uniformity of flow.

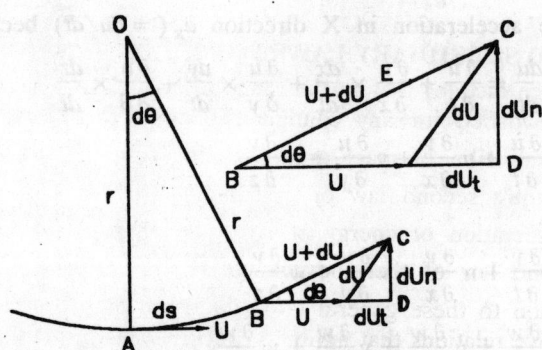

FIG. 4.4. TANGENTIAL AND NORMAL ACCELERATION

For small angle $d\theta$ in Fig. 4.4, $\sin d\theta \approx d\theta, \cos\theta \approx 1$

Hence from $\triangle BCD$, $U + \partial Ut = (U + dU)\cos d\theta \approx (U + dU)$

$$\partial Ut \approx dU$$

Similarly from $\triangle BCD$, $\partial U_n = (U + dU)\sin d\theta = (U + dU)d\theta$

$\partial U_n \approx U\,d\theta$; neglecting $d\,U\,d\theta$ being the product of two small quantities.

Therefore, tangential acceleration a_t = local acceleration + convective acceleration

$$a_t = \frac{\partial u}{\partial t} + \frac{\partial u}{\partial t} \times \frac{\partial s}{\partial s}$$

$$= \frac{\partial u}{\partial t} + \frac{\partial u}{\partial s} \times \frac{\partial s}{\partial t}$$

$$= \frac{\partial u}{\partial t} + u \frac{\partial u}{\partial s}$$

$$= \frac{\partial u}{\partial t} + \frac{1}{2} \frac{\partial u^2}{\partial s} \qquad ...(4.19a)$$

Similarly, normal acceleration a_n = local acceleration + convective acceleration

$$a_n = \frac{\partial u_n}{\partial t} + \frac{\partial u_n}{\partial s} \times \frac{\partial s}{\partial t}$$

$$= \frac{\partial u_n}{\partial t} + u \times \frac{\partial u_n}{\partial s} \qquad ...(4.19b)$$

From similar triangles, ΔOAB and ΔBCD ,

$$\frac{ds}{r} = \frac{\partial u_n}{u}$$

$$\frac{\partial u_n}{ds} = \frac{u}{r}$$

Introducing this vlaue of $\partial u_n/\partial s$ in Eq. 4.19b,

$$a_n = \frac{\partial u_n}{\partial t} + \frac{u^2}{r} \qquad ...(4.19c)$$

4.6 BASIC AND SUBSIDIARY LAWS FOR CONTINUOUS MEDIA

Experience dictates that in the range of engineering interest four basic laws must be satisfied for any continuous media. These are

(1) Conservation of mass or continuity equation.

(2) Newton's second law or momentum equation.

(3) Conservation of energy or first law of thermodynamics, and

(4) Second law of thermodynamics.

In addition to these general laws, there are numerous subsidiary laws called constitutive relations that apply to specific types of media, e.g. equation of state for the perfect gas, Newton's law of viscosity for liquids and Hook's law for elastic solids.

1. Continuity Equation - Three Dimensional Flow

The general continuity equation for unsteady three dimensional flow is derived by equating the rate of net mass flow into the parallelepiped to the time rate of increase of mass within the volume and then the limit is taken as the volume is shrunk to a point.

Consider a fluid volume (parallelopiped) having lengh δx, δy. and δz parallel to the co-ordinate axes X, Y and Z respectively, Fig. 4.5, Let the velocity components at the centroid $P(x, y, z)$ be u, v and w. The rate at which the fluid is entering the vertical surface $JKLM$ passing through P is $\rho u\, \delta y\, \delta z$. The mass inflow at the left hand face $ABCD$ is

$$\rho u\, \delta y\, \delta z - \frac{\partial}{\delta x}(\rho u\, \delta y\, \delta z)\frac{\delta x}{2}$$

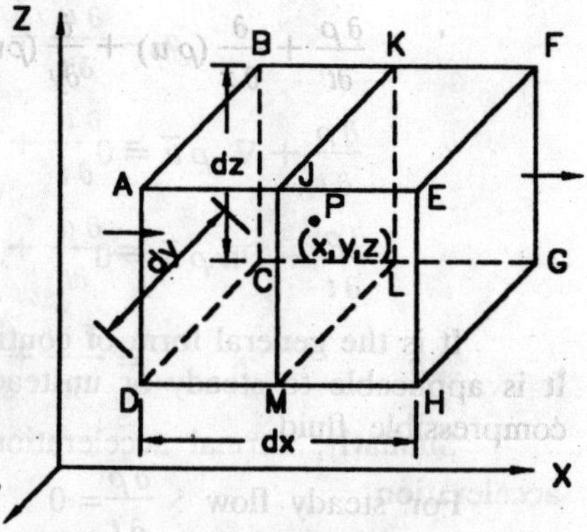

and the mass of fluid going out of the face $EFGH$ is

FIG. 4.5. CONTIUNITY EQUATION FOR THREE DIMENSIONAL FLOW

$$\rho u\, \delta y\, \delta z + \frac{\partial}{\partial x}(\rho u\, \partial y\, \delta z)\frac{\delta x}{2}$$

Therefore, the mass of the fluid retained in the parallelopiped through these two faces is

$$= Q_{ABCD} - Q_{EFGH}$$

$$= -\frac{\partial}{\partial x}(\rho\, u\, \delta y\, \delta z)\, \delta x \qquad \text{...(i)}$$

Similarly, the rate at which the fluid is stored in the parallelopiped between the pair of faces $AEHD$ and $BFGC$ in the Y-direction is

$$= -\frac{\partial}{\partial y}(\rho v\, \delta x\, \delta z)\, \delta y \qquad \text{...(ii)}$$

and between the face $DCGH$ and $ABFE$ is in the Z- direction is

$$= -\frac{\partial}{\partial z}(\rho w\, \delta x\, \delta y)\, \delta z \qquad \text{...(iii)}$$

Thus, the net amount of fluid which is stored in the parallelopiped is the sum of these three gains, that is,

$$-\left[\frac{\partial}{\partial x}(\rho\, u) + \frac{\partial}{\partial y}(\rho\, v) + \frac{\partial}{\partial z}(\rho w)\right]\delta x\, \delta y\, \delta z \qquad \text{...(iv)}$$

The amount of fluid contained in the parallelopiped is

$$= \rho\, \delta x\, \delta y\, \delta z$$

The time rate of increase of mass within the volume

$$= \frac{\partial}{\delta t}(\rho\, \delta x\, \delta y\, \delta z) \qquad \text{...(v)}$$

Equating Eqs. (iv) and (v)

$$-\left[\frac{\partial}{\partial x}(\rho\, u) + \frac{\partial}{\partial y}(\rho\, v) + \frac{\partial}{\partial z}(\delta\, w)\right]\delta x\, \delta y\, \delta z = \frac{\delta}{\delta t}(\rho\, \delta x\, \delta y\, \delta z)$$

$$\frac{\partial \rho}{\partial t} + \frac{\partial}{\partial x}(\rho u) + \frac{\partial}{\partial y}(\rho v) + \frac{\partial}{\partial z}(\rho w) = 0 \qquad \ldots(4.20a)$$

$$\frac{\partial \rho}{\partial t} + \nabla . \rho \,\overline{u} = 0 \qquad \ldots(4.20b)$$

$$\frac{\partial \rho}{\partial t} + Div . \rho \,\overline{u} = 0 \qquad \ldots(4.20c)$$

It is the general form of continuity equation for three dimensional flow. It is applicable to steady or unsteady flow as well as to compressible or incompressible fluid.

For steady flow : $\dfrac{\partial \rho}{\partial t} = 0$

Then Eq. 4.20a, b, and c, modifies to

$$\frac{\partial}{\partial x}(\rho u) + \frac{\partial}{\partial y}(\rho v) + \frac{\partial}{\partial z}(\rho w) = 0 \qquad \ldots(4.21a)$$

$$\nabla . \rho \,\overline{u} = 0 \qquad \ldots(4.21b)$$

$$\text{Div} \qquad \rho \,\overline{u} = 0 \qquad \ldots(4.21c)$$

Here $\dfrac{D}{Dt}$ is known as the 'total derivative' or 'substantive derivative, or 'Eulerian'.

For incompressible fluid, ρ remains constant so that Eq. 4.21a reduces to

$$\frac{\partial u}{\rho x} + \frac{\partial v}{\partial y} + \frac{\partial w}{\partial z} = 0 \qquad \ldots(4.22a)$$

$$\nabla . U = 0 \qquad \ldots(4.22b)$$

For two dimensional flow, there will be no component of velocity in Z-direction so that the continuity equation will become

$$\frac{\partial u}{\partial x} + \frac{\partial v}{\partial y} = 0 \qquad \ldots(4.23)$$

It states that the net rate of volume increase per unit time at any point in an incompressible fluid is zero.

2. Continuity Equation - Cylindrical Polar Co-ordinates

Consider a fluid element (parallelopiped) as shown in Fig. 4.6, situated at a radius r. Let the sides of the fluid element $A'D'$ be dr and the angle enclosed between two horizontal sides $A'D'$ and $B'C'$ be $d\theta$. The thickness of the fluid element is assumed to be dz, which is located at a distance z above the horizontal plane XY. The velocity components in the r, θ and z directions may be assumed to be U_r , U_θ and U_z respectively.

Let us first consider the mass flow in the radial direction.

The mass of the fluid entering through face $ABB'A'$

$$= \rho \, U_r \,(r \, d\theta \, dz)$$

The mass of the fluid going out through face $CDD'C'$

$$= \rho \, U_r \, (r \, d\theta \, dz) + \frac{\partial}{\partial r} (\rho \, U_r r \, d\theta \, dz) \, dr$$

The net mass of fluid remained in the parallelopiped per second

$$= - \frac{\partial}{\partial r} (\rho \, U_r \times r \, d\theta \, dz \, dr) \qquad ...(i)$$

Similarly, the net mass of fluid retained per second between $AA'D'D$ and $CBB'C'$

$$= - \frac{\partial}{\partial \theta} (\rho \, U_\theta \, dz \, dr) \, d\theta \qquad ...(ii)$$

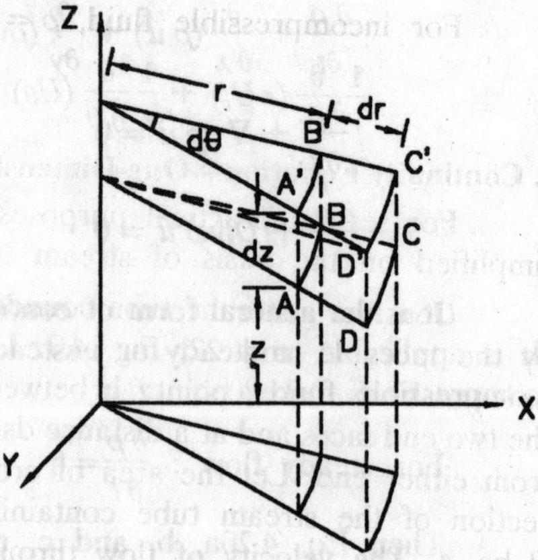

Similarly, the net mass of fluid retained per second across ABCD and $A'B'C'D'$

FIG. 4.6. CONTIUNITY EQUATION CYLINDRICAL POLAR CO–ORDINATES

$$= - \frac{\partial}{\partial \theta} (\rho \, U_z r \, d\theta \, dr \, dz) \qquad ...(iii)$$

Add all the three expressions, Eqns. (i), (ii) and (iii). The total mass of the fluid retained per second in the parallelopiped

$$- \left[\frac{1}{r} \frac{\partial}{\partial r} (\rho \, r \, U_r) + \frac{1}{r} \frac{\partial}{\partial \theta} (\rho \, U_\theta) + \frac{\partial}{\partial z} (\rho \, U_z) \right] r \, d\theta \, dz \, dr \qquad ...(iv)$$

The mass of the fluid in the paralleloped

$$= (\rho \, dr \cdot r \, d\theta \cdot dz)$$

The rate of change of mass with respect to time

$$= \frac{\partial}{\partial t} (\rho \, dr \, r \, d\theta \, dz) \qquad (v)$$

Equating the two expressions, Eqns. (iv) and (v)

$$- \left[\frac{\partial}{\partial r} \rho r \, U_r + \frac{1}{r} \frac{\partial}{\partial \theta} (\rho \, U_\theta) + \frac{\partial}{\partial z} (\rho \, U_z) \right] r \, d\theta \, dz \, dr = \frac{\partial}{\partial t} (\rho \, dr \cdot r \, d\theta , dz)$$

Dividing by the volume of parallelopiped $r \, d\theta \, dr \, dz$

$$\left[\frac{\partial \rho}{\partial t} + \frac{1}{r} \frac{\partial}{\partial r} (\rho \, r \, U_r) + \frac{1}{r} \frac{\partial}{\partial \theta} (\rho \, U_\theta) + \frac{\partial}{\partial z} (\rho \, U_z) \right] = 0 \qquad ...(4.24a)$$

It is the general form of continuity equation which is applicable in cylindrical polar co-ordinates, irrespective of the flow is steady or unsteady and uniform or non-uniform.

For steady flow, $\dfrac{\partial}{\partial t} = 0$

$$\frac{1}{r} \frac{\partial}{\partial r} (\rho r \, U_r) + \frac{1}{r} \frac{\partial}{\partial \theta} (\rho \, U_\theta) + \frac{\partial}{\partial z} (\rho \, U_z) = 0 \qquad ...(4.25)$$

For incompressible fluid, $\rho = $ constant

$$\frac{1}{r}\frac{\partial}{\partial r}(r\,U_r) + \frac{1}{r}\frac{\partial}{\partial\theta}(U_\theta) + \frac{\partial}{\partial z}(U_z) = 0 \qquad \ldots(4.26)$$

3. Continuity Equation—One-Dimensional Flow

For several practical purposes, the continuity equation can be greatly simplified on the basis of stream tube concept.

Consider a stream tube bounded by the faces 11 and 22, Fig. 4.7. Let its length be ds. Take a point P in between the two end faces and at a distance ds/2. from either end. Let the area of cross section of the stream tube containing P be A. The velocity of flow through this section (containing P) is assumed to be U_s and the mass density of the fluid is assumed as ρ . Since the flow is always in the tangential direction and there is no component of velocity in nor-

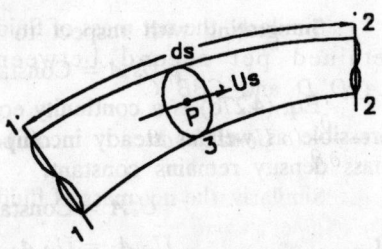

FIG. 4.7. CONTIUNITY EQUATION STREAM–TUBE CONCEPT

mal direction, both the velocity of flow U_s and cross sectional area 'A' will vary in the s- direction, i.e. along the axis of the stream tube.

The mass of the fluid going through cross section 3

$$= \rho\,U_s A$$

The mass of the fluid entering thorugh face 1

$$= \rho\,U_s A - \frac{\partial}{\partial s}(\rho\,U_s A)\frac{ds}{2}$$

The mass of the fluid going out through face 2

$$= \rho\,U_s A + \frac{\partial}{\partial s}(\partial\,U_s A)\frac{ds}{2}$$

The net mass of the fluid remained in the stream tube per second

$$= -\frac{\partial}{\partial s}(\rho\,U_s\,.A)\,ds \qquad \ldots(i)$$

The mass of fluid contained in the stream tube

$$= \rho A\,ds$$

The rate of increase of mass in the stream tube

$$= \frac{\partial}{\partial t}(\rho A\,ds)$$

Since ds is not a function of time, it can be written as

$$= \frac{\partial}{\partial t}(\rho A\,ds) \qquad \ldots(ii)$$

Equating Eqns. (i) and (ii) .

$$\frac{\partial}{\partial t}(\rho A)\,ds = -\frac{\partial}{\partial s}(\partial U_s A)\,ds$$

$$\frac{\partial}{\partial t}(\rho A)\,ds + \frac{\partial}{\partial s}(\rho U_s A)\,ds = 0 \qquad ...(4.27a)$$

For steady flow, $\dfrac{\partial}{\partial t} = 0$

$\therefore \quad \dfrac{\partial}{\partial s}(\rho U_s A)\,ds = 0$

Integrating with respect to s,

$$\rho\, Us\, A = \text{Constant} \qquad ...(4.27b)$$

Eq. (4.27b) is a continuity equation which is applicable for steady compressible as well as steady incompessible fluid. For incompressible fluid the mass density remains constant.

$$U_s A = \text{Constant}$$

or $\qquad U_{s1} A_1 = U_{s2} A_2 \qquad ...(4.27c)$

4. Equation of continuity

The application of the principle of conservation of mass (mass can neither be created nor destroyed) to asteady flow in a streamtube results in the equation of continuity. In other words, for steady flow the rate of fluid mass flowing across any cross section in the stream tube remains constant.

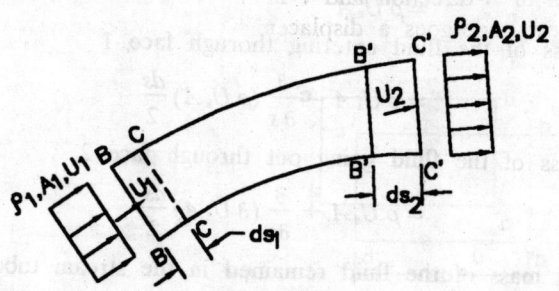

FIG. 4.8. CONTIUNITY EQUATION ONE DIMENSIONAL FLOW

Consider a streamtube through which a compressible fluid is flowing, as shown in Fig. 4.8. The cross sectional area and mass density at section B are A_1 and ρ_1 respectively. The corresponding values at B' are A_2 and ρ_2. If the fluid mass occupying position BBB'B' moves to CCC'C' in time dt, the conservation of mass principle yields,

$$\rho_1 \times A_1\, ds_1 = \rho_2 \times A_2\, d s_2$$

Dividing boty sides by dt,

$$\rho_1 \times A_1\, ds_1/dt = \rho_2 \times A_2\, ds_2/dt$$

The mean velocity at section B is $U1 = ds1/dt$

and at section B' is $U_2 = d s_2/dt$

Therefore, $\rho_1 A_1 U_1 = \rho_2 A_2 U_2$ ...(4.27d)

which is the continuity equation for one dimensional compressible fluid flows.

For incompressible fluids, ρ remains constant, hence,

$$A_1 U_1 = A_2 U_2 = Q$$ ...(4.27e)

The product of area and velocity is known as the (volume flow rate and has the dimensions of cubic metre per second, or m³/sec . Eq (4.27 e) gives accurate results if the areas A_1 and A_2 are small and the velocity distribution is uniform over the area. Otherwise the total area A should be subdivided into small areas and the discharge, i.e. flow rate passing through each of the elementary areas is then summed up to obtain total discharge. The average velocity distribution over the whole cross sectional area A

$$U = (1/A) \int u \, dA$$ ...(4.28)

Here u is the point velocity in the flow.

4.7 MOTION OF A FLUID ELEMENT

During motion a fluid element may undergo any of the four types of displacement. These are (i) pure translation, (ii) rotation, (iii) angular deformation and (iv) linear or volumetric distortion. The deformation of a fluid element may be expressed in terms of velocity and its gradients. Consider a two dimentional fluid element a b c d in X-Y plane whose sides ab and ad measure dx and dy respectively in Fig. 4.9. The velocity of fluid at lowermost left corner is u in X-direction and v in Y- direction. In a time interval dt, the fluid particle undergoes a displacement and occupies the new position

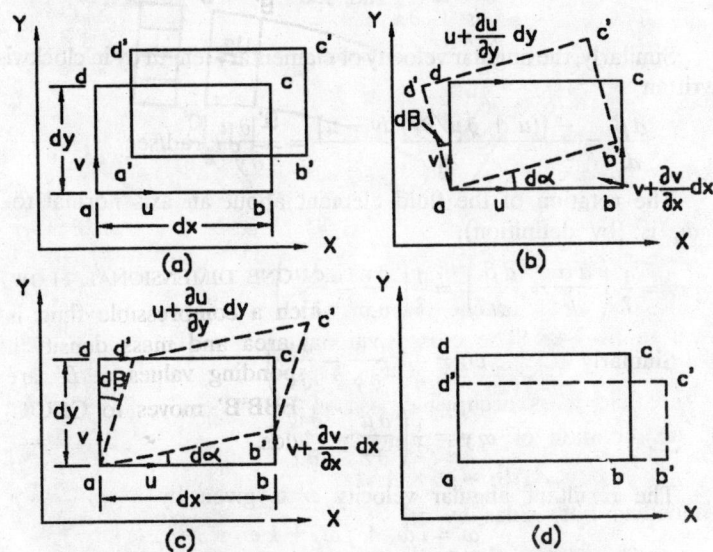

FIG. 4.9. DEFORMATION OF A FLUID ELEMENT
(A) PURE TRANSLATION (B) ROTATION
(C) ANGULAR DEFORMATION (D) VOLUMETRIC DISTORTION

a'b'c'd'. For smaller values of dx, dy and dt, Taylor series expansion may be used to obtain the velocity of corner point b and d as shown in Fig. 4.9.

In Fig. 4.9a, the fluid element shifts bodily from original location to another. Such a motion of the fluid element is known as 'pure translation'. During motion, the fluid element a b c d moves by u dt in X-direction and v dt in Y-direction in time, dt, and thus occupies the position a' b' c' d' The fluid flow with straight parallel stream lines is an example of pure translation in which fluid elements are shifted bodily from one location to another.

Fig. 4.9b shows the case of a pure rotation of a fluid element. In general, the rotation of an element of solid is measured by noting the angular displacement of a line in the plane of rotation from a reference line. Since the fluid element is deformable, the rotation of a fluid element is defined as the average angular velocity of any two infinitesimal lines perpendicular to each other and lying in the plane of rotation. Let such two lines ab and ad be taken parallel to X and Y axes. The corner b displaces to b' in time dt with a velocity $v + (\partial v/\partial x) dx$. Similarly, the corner d moves to d' with velocity $\bar{u}(\partial u/\partial y) dy$ in the counter clockwise direction. The angular displacement of ab is the determined by dividing the bb' by the side a b. Therefore,

$$d\alpha = \frac{[v + (\partial v/\partial x) dx - v] dt}{dx} = \frac{\partial v}{\partial x} dt$$

The angular velocity of the elementary length dx in anticlockwise direction (assumed to be positive) is given by

$$\frac{d\alpha}{dt} = \frac{\partial v}{\partial x} \text{ rad/sec} \qquad \qquad ...(4.29a)$$

Similarly, the angular velocity of elementary length dy in clockwise direction is written

$$\frac{d\beta}{dt} = \frac{-[(u + \partial u/\partial y) dy - u]}{dy} = \frac{-\partial u}{\partial y} \text{ rad/sec} \qquad ...(4.29b)$$

The rotation of the fluid element about an axis normal to XY plane, i.e., ω_z is (by definition),

$$\omega_z = \frac{1}{2}\left(\frac{d\alpha}{dt} + \frac{d\beta}{dt}\right) = \frac{1}{2}\left(\frac{\partial v}{\partial x} - \frac{\partial u}{\partial y}\right) \qquad ...(4.30a)$$

Similarly $\qquad \omega_x = \frac{1}{2}\left(\frac{\partial w}{\partial y} - \frac{\partial v}{\partial z}\right) \qquad ...(4.30b)$

and $\qquad \omega y = \frac{1}{2}\left(\frac{\partial u}{\partial z} - \frac{\partial w}{\partial x}\right) \qquad ...(4.30\ c)$

The resultant angular velocity ω is given by

$$\omega = i\,\omega_x + j\,\omega_y + k\,\omega_z \qquad ...(4.31a)$$

$$\omega = \frac{1}{2}\nabla \times U \qquad ...(4.31b)$$

$$2\omega = \nabla \times U \qquad ...(4.31c)$$

The term 2ω is known as 'vorticity' and is obtained from Eqs. 4.30 a, b and c. The fluid flow in a curved path in such a way that velocity increases away from the centre is an example of this type of fluid element deformation i.e. (forced vortex motion).

In Fig. 4.9c is shown the case of angular deformation of a fluid element. Let sides a b and a d be displaced in opposite directions so that $d\alpha$ is positive and $d\beta$ negative. Therefore, the angular deformation of the fluid element about Z-axis is given by the average of the angular deformation of two mutually perpendicular sides and is given by

$$e_z = \frac{1}{2}\left(\frac{d\alpha}{dt} - \frac{d\beta}{dt}\right)$$

$$= \frac{1}{2}\left[\frac{\partial v}{\partial x} - \left(\frac{-\partial u}{\partial y}\right)\right]$$

$$= \frac{1}{2}\left(\frac{\partial v}{\partial x} + \frac{\partial u}{\partial y}\right) \qquad ...(4.32a)$$

Similarly
$$e_x = \frac{1}{2}\left(\frac{\partial w}{\partial y} + \frac{\partial v}{\partial z}\right) \qquad ...(4.32b)$$

and
$$e_y = \frac{1}{2}\left(\frac{\partial u}{\partial z} + \frac{\partial w}{\partial x}\right) \qquad ...(4.32c)$$

These rates of angular deformation cause tangential stress (or shear strain) in the fluid elements. The above relations Eqs. 4.32a, b and c are used in obtaining the Navier-Stokes' equations of motion of real fluid. The flow in curved path with velocity decreasing away from the centre (of rotation) is an example of this class, i.e., (free vortex motion).

In Fig. 4.9d is shown the volumetic distortion of a fluid element. Let the fluid element abcd be deformed linearly such that ab is elongated to ab' and ad to ad'. Obviously, the length normal to the plane of paper is reduced. The rate of linear deformation of elemetary length dx is $(\partial u/\partial x)\,dx$. Similarly, for other two sides the rates of deformation in Y and Z directions are $(\partial v/\partial y)\,dy$ and $(\partial w/\partial z)\,dz$ respectively. Hence the increments in volume of the fluid element by each of these deformations are

$$\left(\frac{\partial u}{\partial x}dx\right)dy\,dz, \quad \left(\frac{\partial v}{\partial y}dy\right)dx\,dz \quad \text{and} \quad \left(\frac{\partial w}{\partial z}dz\right)dx\,dy$$

Therefore, rate of increment of the entire volume/unit volume

$$\left(\frac{\partial u}{\partial x} + \frac{\partial v}{\partial y} + \frac{\partial w}{\partial z}\right) \qquad ...(4.33)$$

This volume increment is known as 'dilation'. For incompressible fluid, above Eq. 4.33 is modified to

$$\nabla . U = 0 \qquad ...(4.22)$$

which is known as the 'equation of continuity'. The fluid flow in a converging channel causes the fluid element to be elongated in the direction of flow and reduce in dimension normal to the direction of flow. It is an example of volumetric distortion.

4.8. ROTATIONAL AND IRROTATIONAL FLOW

A flow is said to be irrotational if the fluid elements do not rotate about their mass axes which are perpendicular to the plane of motion. This means that the angular velocity ω_z given by Eq. 4.30a, should be zero everywhere in the fluid

$$\omega_z = \frac{1}{2}\left(\frac{\partial v}{\partial x} - \frac{\partial u}{\partial y}\right) = 0 \qquad \text{...(4.34a)}$$

Thus the condition of 2-D irrotational flow is

$$\frac{\partial v}{\partial x} = \frac{\partial u}{\partial y} \qquad \text{...(4.34b)}$$

In the same way, the rotation of the fluid element about X,Y and Z axes, i.e. ω_x, ω_y and ω_z should be equated to zero for 3-D irrotational flow. This means

$$\omega_x = \frac{1}{2}\left(\frac{\partial w}{\partial y} - \frac{\partial v}{\partial z}\right) = 0 \qquad \text{...(4.34c)}$$

$$\omega_y = \frac{1}{2}\left(\frac{\partial u}{\partial z} - \frac{\partial w}{\partial x}\right) = 0 \qquad \text{...(4.34d)}$$

$$\omega_z = \frac{1}{2}\left(\frac{\partial v}{\partial x} - \frac{\partial u}{\partial y}\right) = 0 \qquad \text{...(4.34a)}$$

Thus the condition of 3-D irrotational flow becomes

$$\frac{\partial w}{\partial y} = \frac{\partial v}{\partial z}, \frac{\partial u}{\partial z} = \frac{\partial w}{\partial x} \text{ and } \frac{\partial v}{\partial x} = \frac{\partial u}{\partial y} \qquad \text{...(4.35)}$$

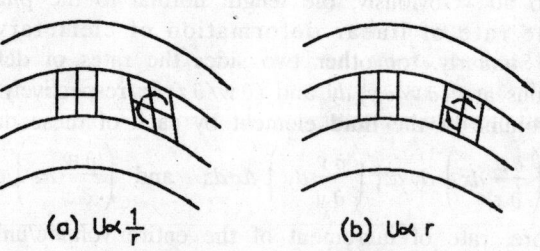

(a) $U \propto \frac{1}{r}$ (b) $U \propto r$

FIG. 4.10. (A) IRROTATIONAL FLOW (B) ROTATIONAL FLOW

If at every point in the flow this condition is not satisfied, the flow is known as 'rotational flow'. Examples of both these types of flows are shown in Fig. 4.10. In Fig. 4.10a, the fluid element deforms in such a way that the clockwise rotation of the horizontal median line is equal to the anticlockwise rotation of the vertical median line. In this way the net rotation of the fluid element in the plane of paper is zero and hence this flow is known as irrotational flow.

Flow of an ideal fluid is an irrotational flow. Similarly for the flow of fluids of small viscosity, the effect (of viscosity) is limited within a narrow region near the boundary and the flow outside is assumed to be irrotational. Flow through wash basin is another example of irrotational flow. In Fig. 4.10b, both median lines rotate in the clockwise direction and hence the fluid element rotates about its mass axis. Examples of rotational flow can be seen in the mechanical mixer or in the boundary layer region. In such cases, the fluid elements rotate about their mass axes besides moving alongwith stream lines.

4.9 CIRCULATION AND VORTICITY

The circulation Γ of the fluid around the closed path S is defined as the summation or line integral of the tangential component of the velocity about any closed contour path S in a flow field. Consider a closed path S, (Fig. 4.11) in a typical two dimensional flow field which is represented by the pattern of streamlines. The circulation is defined as

$$\Gamma = \int_{s} U_s \times d_s \qquad \qquad ...(4.36)$$

The symbol $\displaystyle\int_{s}$ denotes the line in-
tegral and is to be done once around the closed curve and U_s is the velocity at the given point and tangential to the path. As a convention, the counter clockwise direction is assumed as positive. To illustrate the application of the concept of circulation, let us consider the square element of fluid in Fig. 4.9b as a closed curve. Proceed from the left lowermost corner 'a' in the counter clockwise direction around the boundary of the element and set down the product

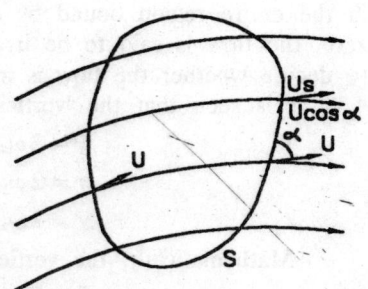

FIG. 4.11. CIRCULATION IN A 2D FLOW FIELD

of velocity component and distance in order. Then one gets the circulation around this infinitesimal fluid element as.

$$d\Gamma = \left[udx + \left(v + \frac{\partial v}{\partial x} dx \right) dy - \left(u + \frac{\partial u}{\partial y} dy \right) dx \right.$$

$$\left. - vdy \right] = \left(\frac{\partial v}{\partial x} - \frac{\partial u}{\partial y} \right) dx\, dy$$

The product dx dy is the area of the fluid element, therefore,

$$\frac{d\Gamma}{dx\, dy} = \left(\frac{\partial v}{\partial x} - \frac{\partial u}{\partial y} \right) \qquad \qquad ...(4.37)$$

The right hand side of this expresssion is termed as the vorticity of the fluid. Thus the limiting value of circulation per unit area of the fluid element is equal to the vorticity around an axis normal to the plane of the curve. In other words,

$$\gamma = \lim_{\substack{dx \to 0 \\ dy \to 0}} \frac{d\Gamma}{dx\,dy} = \left(\frac{\partial v}{\partial x} - \frac{\partial u}{\partial y}\right) \qquad ...(4.38a)$$

Similarly

$$\xi = \frac{d\Gamma}{dy\,dz} = \left(\frac{\partial w}{\partial y} - \frac{\partial v}{\partial z}\right) \qquad ...(4.38b)$$

$$\eta = \frac{d\Gamma}{dz\,dx} = \left(\frac{\partial u}{\partial z} - \frac{\partial w}{\partial x}\right) \qquad ...(4.38c)$$

Therefore

$$\beta = i\,\xi + j\,\eta + k\,\gamma \qquad ...(4.39)$$

Thus it is seen that the circulation around a closed contour is equal to the sum of the vorticities within the area of the contour. This is known as 'Stokes theorem' and may be stated for a general case of any contour S (Fig. 4.11).

$$\Gamma = \int_s U\cos\alpha \times ds = \int_s \beta\,dA \qquad ...(4.40)$$

For irrotational flow, the vorticity about three co-ordinate directions X, Y and Z, i.e. ξ, η and γ should be zero. Alternatively, if the circulation in the entire region bound by closed path S (i.e. about closed path S) is zero, the flow is said to be irrotational. Eqs. 4.38a, b and c may be used to decide whether the flow is irrotational or not. Comparing Eqs. 4.34 and 4.38, it is seen that the 'vorticity is twice the angular velocity'.

$$\xi = 2\,\omega_x \qquad ...(4.41a)$$

$$\eta = 2\,\omega_y \qquad ...(4.41b)$$

$$\gamma = 2\,\omega_z \qquad ...(4.41c)$$

Mathematically, the vorticity β is defined as curl of U, i.e.

$$\beta = \nabla \times U = curl\,U \qquad ...(4.42)$$

where

$$\beta = i\,\xi + j\,\eta + k\,\gamma$$

The circulation Γ may also be obtained by integrating Eq. 4.42.

$$\Gamma = \int\!\!\int (\nabla \times U)\,dA \qquad ...(4.43)$$

The vorticity ξ about X axis is expressed in cylindrical coordinates as

$$\xi = \frac{\partial U_z}{\partial r} + \frac{U_z}{r} - \frac{1}{r}\frac{\partial U_r}{\partial \theta} = 2\,w_z \qquad ...(4.44)$$

where U_r and U_z are velocities in the radial and normal directions respectively. The other components may also be similarly expressed in cylindrical co-ordinates.

The concept of circulation is very important in the theory of lifting surfaces such as airfoils and blades of rotodynamic machines.

4.10 VELOCITY POTENTIAL AND STREAM FUNCTION

One of the mathematical methods of describing the 2-D flow field is by means of a set of functions known as potential function and stream function and hence their study is very useful for understanding the flow phenomenon of ideal fluid (or where the viscosity of fluid is too small).

1. Potential Function

It is defined as a scaler function of space and time such that its negative derivative with respect to any direction is the velocity in that direction. Mathematically, it is defined by the Eq. 4.45 for 3-D flows as

$$u = -\frac{\partial \varphi}{\partial x} \qquad \text{...(4.45a)}$$

$$v = -\frac{\partial \varphi}{\partial y} \qquad \text{...(4.45b)}$$

$$w = -\frac{\partial \varphi}{\partial z} \qquad \text{...(4.45c)}$$

in which u, v and w are the components of velocities in X, Y and Z directions. The negative sign is used as a convention to indicate that φ decreases in the direction of flow, e.g. in case of electric flow field, the electrical potential decreases in the direction of flow.

(a) Differentiation of Eq. 4.45a with respect to y and of Eq. 4.45b with respect to x shows that

$$\frac{\partial u}{\partial y} = -\frac{\partial^2 \varphi}{\partial y \partial x}$$

$$\frac{\partial v}{\partial x} = -\frac{\partial^2 \varphi}{\partial x \partial y}$$

For φ to be a continuous function, the order of differentiation can be interchanged. Then

$$\frac{\partial u}{\partial y} = \frac{\partial v}{\partial x}$$

or

$$\frac{\partial u}{\partial y} - \frac{\partial v}{\partial x} = 0$$

which is the condition of irrotationality of flow, Eq. 4.34a.

Thus it is seen that the existence of the velocity potential for a flow implies it to be 'irrotational flow'. Flow of ideal fluid is thus frequently referred to as 'irrotational flow or potential flow'.

(b) The continuity equation in 3-D flow is

$$\frac{\partial u}{\partial x} + \frac{\partial v}{\partial y} + \frac{\partial w}{\partial z} = 0$$

Substituting the values of u, v and w from Eq. 4.45,

$$\frac{\partial^2 \varphi}{\partial x^2} + \frac{\partial^2 \varphi}{\partial y^2} + \frac{\partial^2 \varphi}{\partial z^2} = 0$$

$$\nabla^2 \varphi = 0 \qquad \qquad ...(4.46)$$

In which $\nabla^2 = \dfrac{\partial^2}{\partial x^2} + \dfrac{\partial^2}{\partial y^2} + \dfrac{\partial^2}{\partial z^2}$

is an operator. Eq. 4.46 is known as 3-dimensional form of Laplace equation. Any function of φ that satisfies Eq. 4.46 alongwith continuity equation is a possible case of irrotational flow with the given boundary conditions. There may be number of solutions of Eq. 4.46 with different boundary conditions. Thus main difficulty is the proper selection of φ for the particular problem in hand to solve it fully. Lines drawn in the flow field along which φ is constant are known as 'equipotential lines'.

The Eq. 4.45 can also be written as

$$U = grad\ \Phi = \nabla \varphi \qquad \qquad ...(4.47)$$

where ∇ is a vector notation and is written as

$$\nabla = i\frac{\partial}{\partial x} + j\frac{\partial}{\partial y} + k\frac{\partial}{\partial z} \qquad \qquad ...(4.48)$$

In case of curved flows, it is more convenient to express φ in polar co-ordinates as

$$\varphi = f(r,\theta,z) \qquad \qquad ...(4.49a)$$

Then $\qquad U_r = -\dfrac{\partial \varphi}{\partial r}$

and $\qquad U_\theta = \dfrac{-\partial \varphi}{r\,\partial \theta} \qquad \qquad ...(4.49b)$

$$U_z = \frac{-\partial \Phi}{\partial z}$$

where U_r, U_θ, U_z are the velocities in the r, θ and z direction respectively.

In cylindrical polar co-ordinates, Laplace equation is

$$\frac{1}{r}\frac{\partial \varphi}{\partial r} + \frac{\partial^2 \varphi}{\partial r^2} + \frac{1}{r^2}\frac{\partial^2 \varphi}{\partial \theta^2} + \frac{\partial^2 \varphi}{\partial z^2} = 0$$

2. Stream function

The concept of stream function is based on the principle of continuity and the properties of the stream line. It provides a mathematical means of plotting and interpreting flow fields.

A stream function is defined as the scaler function of space and time such that the partial derivative of it with respect to any direction gives the velocity component in the normal direction (to be measured in the counter clockwise direction). It exists for two dimensional flow and for certain special cases of three dimensional flows.

Consider any two stream lines A and B and a point C lying in the same XY plane. The flow rate across any of the lines joining C and a point on the streamline A such as CE or CG is ψ. By definition, there can be no flow across the streamline. Accordingly, ψ is a constant of the streamline A and is a function of the location of point $C(x,y)$ only. Similarly, the flow rate between C and adjacent streamline B is $\psi + d\psi$. Therefore, the flow rate in the streamtube bounded by streamlines A and B is $d\psi$. The flow rate entering into any triangular element DEF should be the same as going out from it (continuity principle).

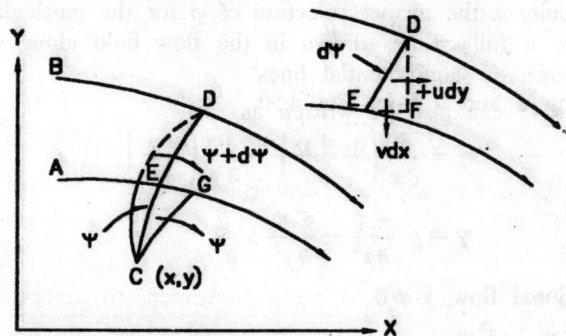

FIG. 4.12. DEFINITION SKETCH – STREAM FUNCTION

(a) Flow rate entering through face $DE = d\psi$

Flow rate coming out through both faces DF and EF $= u\,dy - v\,dx$ Since inflow should be equal to outflow, therefore,

$$d\psi = u\,dy - v\,dx \qquad \qquad ...(i)$$

The stream function ψ is a function of x and y. Hence the total derivative $d\psi$ can be written as

$$d\psi = \frac{\partial \psi}{\partial x}dx + \frac{\partial \psi}{\partial y}dy \qquad \qquad ...(ii)$$

Comparing Eqs. (i) and (ii)

$$u = \frac{\partial \psi}{\partial y} \qquad \qquad ...(4.50a)$$

$$v = -\frac{\partial \psi}{\partial x} \qquad \qquad ...(4.50b)$$

Thus, if $\psi = F(x,y)$ is known, u and v can be determined from Eq. (4.50) Conversely, if u and v are known, ψ can be derived as

$$\psi = \int \frac{\partial \psi}{\partial x}dx + \int \frac{\partial \psi}{\partial y}dy + C \qquad \qquad ...(4.51)$$

(b) Substituting u and v from Eq. 4.50 into 2-D continuity equation, Eq. 4.23

$$\frac{\partial u}{\partial x} + \frac{\partial v}{\partial y} = 0$$

$$\frac{\partial}{\partial x}\left(\frac{\partial \psi}{\partial y}\right) + \frac{\partial}{\partial y}\left(-\frac{\partial \psi}{\partial x}\right) = 0$$

or
$$\frac{\partial^2 \psi}{\partial x \partial y} = \frac{\partial^2 \psi}{\partial y \partial x}$$

It shows that ψ is a continuous function of x and y (then only the order of differentiation can be interchanged).

(c) The equation of vorticity, Eq. 4.38a is

$$\gamma = \frac{\partial v}{\partial x} - \frac{\partial u}{\partial y}$$

Substituting u and v from Eq. 4.50,

$$\gamma = \frac{\partial}{\partial x}\left(-\frac{\partial \psi}{\partial x}\right) - \frac{\partial}{\partial y}\left(\frac{\partial \psi}{\partial y}\right)$$

$$\gamma = -\frac{\partial^2 \psi}{\partial x^2} - \frac{\partial^2 \psi}{\partial y^2}$$

For rotational flow, $\gamma \neq 0$

$$\frac{\partial^2 \psi}{\partial x^2} + \frac{\partial^2 \psi}{\partial y^2} = 0 \qquad \qquad ...(4.52)$$

which is Laplace equation of flow
For rotational flow, $\gamma = 0$

$$\frac{\partial^2 \psi}{\partial x^2} + \frac{\partial^2 \psi}{\partial y^2} = -2\omega_z \qquad \qquad ...(4.53)$$

which gives the vorticity of the given rotational flow.

(d) In curved flows, the stream function ψ is convenient to use in cylindrical co-ordinates.

$$U_r = \frac{1}{r}\frac{\partial \psi}{\partial \theta} \qquad \qquad ...(4.54a)$$

and
$$U_\theta = -\frac{\partial \psi}{\partial r} \qquad \qquad ...(4.54b)$$

3. Relation between stream function and potential function

(a) A streamline can be described by Eq. 4.12b

$$u \, dy - v \, dx = 0$$

Substituting u and v from Eq. 4.50

$$\frac{\partial \psi}{\partial x} dx + \frac{\partial \psi}{\partial y} dy = 0 \qquad \qquad ...(4.54)$$

By definition left hand side is equal to the total derivation $d\psi$, hence,

$$d\psi = 0$$

which means ψ is a constant along a streamline.

Various values of this constant give a set of streamlines or flow lines. Eq. 4.54 yields the slope of streamline

$$\left(\frac{dy}{dx}\right)_{\psi \, constant} = -\frac{\partial \psi/\partial x}{\partial \psi/\partial y} = \frac{v}{u} \qquad \qquad ...(i)$$

Similarly, the total derivative of φ can be written as

$$d\varphi = \frac{\partial \varphi}{\partial x}dx + \frac{\partial \varphi}{\partial y}dy \qquad \qquad ...(4.55)$$

Along a equipotential line, φ is a constant. Therefore.

$$d\varphi = 0$$

Hence $$\left(\frac{dy}{dx}\right)_{\varphi \, constant} = -\frac{\partial \varphi/\partial x}{\partial \varphi/\partial y} = -\frac{u}{v} \qquad \qquad ...(ii)$$

From Eqs. (i) and(ii)

$$\left(\frac{dy}{dx}\right)_{\varphi \, constant} \times \left(\frac{dy}{dx}\right)_{\psi \, constant} = -1 \qquad \qquad ...(4.56)$$

This shows that the streamlines intersect equipotential lines orthogonally.

(b) It may also be seen that

$$u = -\frac{\partial \varphi}{\partial x} = \frac{\partial \psi}{\partial y}$$

$$= -\frac{\partial \varphi}{\partial y} = -\frac{\partial \psi}{\partial x}$$

These equations are known as "Cauchy-Rieman equations" and enable the stream functions to be calculated if the potential function is known and vice versa in a potential flow.

In cylindrical polar co-ordinates

$$u_r = -\frac{\partial \Phi}{\partial r} = \frac{1}{r}\frac{\partial \psi}{\partial \theta}$$

$$u_\theta = -\frac{1}{r}\frac{\partial \varphi}{\partial \theta} = -\frac{\partial \psi}{\partial r}$$

(c) The potential function exists only for irrotational flows whereas stream function may exist for both rotational and irrotational flows.

(d) Potential function exists for 2D and 3D flows whereas stream function exists for 2-D flows and some special cases of 3-D flows.

(e) Potential function satisfies Laplace equation whereas stream function for 'irrotational flow' only satisfies the Laplace equation.

4.11 FLOW NET

The mathematical solution of Laplace equation is required for obtaining the flow pattern for steady two dimensional flow with the given boundary conditions. These methods are too much involved and complicated. A simple approach to solve two dimensional irrotational flow is to use graphical method known as 'a flow net'.

A flow net is a network of mutually perpendicular streamlines and equipotential lines. The streamlines show the direction of flow at any point and are so spaced that equal rate of flow $\Delta q \, passes$ through each stream tube. The discharge Δq passing between two consecutive streamlines of a flow net equals $\Delta \psi$ (*i.e.*, the change in value of ψ from one streamline to next). Similarly, equipotential lines are also so spaced that the change in velocity potential is constant from one line to the next. Furthermore, the changes in both sets of lines are made equal, *i.e.* $\Delta \psi = \Delta \varphi$ Hence, these lines form approximate squares. It should be noted that there can be only one flow net possible for a given flow, though spacing between streamlines and equipotential lines can be varied at will. The following points should be noted about flow net.

(1) Flow net can be used for irrotational flows and for ideal fluid only. Some fluids like water and air have rather small viscosity and hence the condition of irrotationality can be approximately attained.

(2) Flow net can be constructed for both the flows within solid boundaries and flow around a solid body. In either flow, the solid boundary surfaces represent streamlines.

(3) It is observed that local velocity depends on the configuration of the boundary surface.

(4) In case of real fluid, even when the viscosity of the fluid is small, the flow does not remain irrotational immediate near the boundary and hence assumption of ideal fluid breaks down.

(5) Experiments show that in the region of converging streamlines, the flow net yields rather correct results. But in the region of divergence of streamlines, many times the flow separates from the boundary. In this region, the space between stream lines will increase and consequently the velocity will decrease in the direction of flow. The velocity of flow of real fluid is zero at the boundary. It is not possible to reduce further the zero velocity at the boundary in divergent region. The stream lines, therefore, separate from the boundary and in some cases even backward flow may take place. Thus the flow net in the separated region where streamlines are drawn up to the boundary does not yield correct result.

(6) Flow nets are useful for the confined flows only where fluid weight does not govern the flow phenomenon. This condition is fulfilled by light weight fluids.

(7) Flow net construction is purely a graphical exercise by trial and error, i.e. drawing orthogonal sets of lines within given boundaries so that they form approximate squares.

(8) Another practical method of obtaining a flow net for particular set of boundaries is 'electric analogy'. The boundaries of the model are made up of strips of non-conducting material mounted on a flat non conducting surface and the end equipotential lines are formed out of a conducting strip, e.g., brass or copper plate. A electrolyte of uniform depth is placed in the flow space and a voltage potential is applied to the two end conducting strips. By means of a probe and other electrical instruments, lines with constant voltage drop are located and drawn on a graph paper. The stream lines are then drawn normal to the equipotential lines forming approximate squares.

Use of flow net

After a flow net has been obtained for the given boundary configuration it can be used to solve the problem of irrotationl flows. If the velocity at a certain point A in the flow net is known the velocity at any other point can be determined as $U_2 = (\Delta n_2/\Delta n_1) U_1$ where Δn_1 and Δn_2 is the spacing between adjacent stream lines at two different locations in the flow. If the pressure at a point is known, the pressure at any other point in the flow field can be determined using Bernoulli's equation (Eq. 5.23).

Examples 4.1-4.21

4.1. The velocity distribution around the front part of a sphere held in the wind is given by

$$U = 1.5\, U_0 \sin \beta$$

in which U_0 is the velocity of approach and β is the angle which the radius to the required point makes with the direction of wind. Find the velocity and acceleration at a point 60° (from the front radius) on a sphere of 1 m diameter for a wind velocity of 15 m/s. Assume the flow to be irrotational.

Solution

The velocity at any point P at angle β with horizontal radius is given by

$$U = 1.5\, U_0 \sin \beta$$
$$= 1.5 \times 15 \times \sin 60° = 1.95 \text{ m/s}$$

Acceleration at point P in the tangential and normal directions is determined using Eq. 4.19a and c.

$$a_s = \frac{\partial U_s}{\partial t} + \frac{1}{2}\frac{\partial}{\partial s} U_s^2$$

and

$$a_n = \frac{\partial U_n}{\partial t} + \frac{U_s^2}{r}$$

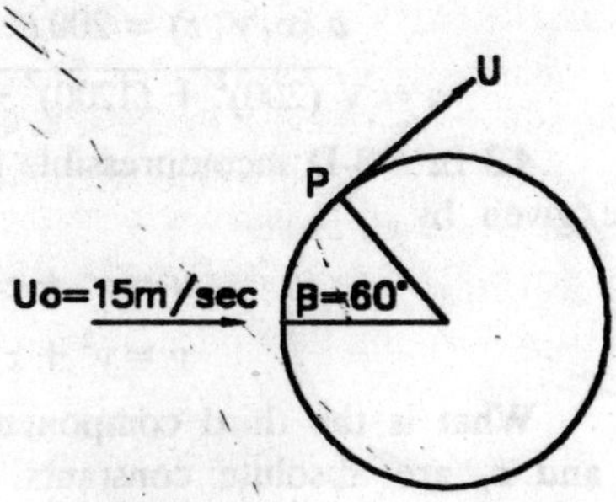

For steady flow $\dfrac{\partial U_s}{\partial t} = 0$ and

$$\frac{\partial U_n}{\partial t} = 0$$

$$a_s = \frac{1}{2}\left[\frac{\partial}{\partial s}(1.5\, U_0 \sin \beta)^2\right]$$

FIG. 4.13. EXAMPLE 4.1

$$= \frac{1}{2} \times \frac{9}{4} \times U_0^2 \frac{\partial}{\partial s} (\sin^2 \beta)$$

$$= \frac{9}{8} \times 15^2 \times 2 \sin \beta \cos \beta \frac{\partial \beta}{\partial s}$$

$$= 506.25 \sin \beta \cos \beta \frac{\partial \beta}{\partial s}$$

Now since $\partial s = r \partial \beta$, hence $\partial \beta / \partial s = 1/r$

$$a_s = 506.25 \times \frac{\sin 60° \cos 60°}{0.5} = 438.71 \text{ m/s/s}$$

and $a_n = \frac{U^2}{r} = \frac{(1.5 \times 15 \times \sin 60)^2}{0.5} = 759.4 \text{ m/s/s}$

4.2 Determine the velocity and acceleration of a particle at position $x = 1$, $y = 2$, $z = 5$ and $t = 0.1$ for the velocity field given by

$$U(x, y, z, t) = 10 x^2 i + 20 xyj + 100 tk$$

-Solution

i, j and k are unit vectors in X, Y and Z directions. The velocity of particle at (1, 2, 5) position is given by

$$U = 10 (1)^2 i + 20 \times 1 \times 2 \times j + 100 \times 0.1 \times k$$

$$= 10 i + 40 j + 10 k$$

$$U = \sqrt{(10)^2 + (40)^2 + (10)^2} = 42.43 \text{ units}$$

The acceleration at the given point is now calculated by Eq. 4.16d.

$$a_x = \left(u \frac{\partial u}{\partial x} + v \frac{\partial u}{\partial y} + w \frac{\partial u}{\partial z} \right)$$

$$= [(10 x^2) (20 x) i + (20 xy) (0) + 0 + 0] = 200 x^3$$

Similarly $a_y = 600 x^2 y$ and $a_z = 100$

Substituting the values of x, y and t,

$$a (x, y, z) = 200 x^3 i + 600 x^2 yj + 100 k$$

$$a (x, y, z) = 200 i + 1200 j + 100 k$$

$$a = \sqrt{(200)^2 + (1200)^2 + (100)^2} = 1220.6 \text{ units}$$

4.3 In a 3-D incompressible fluid flow, the two components of velocities are given by

$$u = x^2 + z^2 + c_1$$

$$v = y^2 + z^2 + c_2$$

What is the third component of velocity w ? Is this flow irrotational? c_1 and c_2 are absolute constants.

Solution

The equation of continuity (Eq. 4.22) is

$$\frac{\partial u}{\partial x} + \frac{\partial v}{\partial y} + \frac{\partial w}{\partial z} = 0$$

From given data, $\dfrac{\partial u}{\partial x} = 2x$

$$\frac{\partial v}{\partial y} = 2y.$$

Hence
$$\frac{\partial w}{\partial z} = -\frac{\partial u}{\partial x} - \frac{\partial v}{\partial y}$$

Integrating above equation,
$$w = -2xz - 2yz + c_3$$

Here c_3 is a constant which should be independent of z but may be a funciton of x and/or y.

The conditions of irrotationality (Eq. 4.34) are

$$\frac{\partial u}{\partial y} - \frac{\partial v}{\partial x} = \omega_z = 0$$

$$\frac{\partial v}{\partial z} - \frac{\partial w}{\partial y} = \omega_x = 0$$

$$\frac{\partial w}{\partial x} - \frac{\partial u}{\partial z} = \omega_y = 0$$

Alternatively, curl of U should be zero.

Curl $\quad U = \nabla \times U = \begin{vmatrix} i & j & k \\ \dfrac{\partial}{\partial x} & \dfrac{\partial}{\partial y} & \dfrac{\partial}{\partial z} \\ u & v & w \end{vmatrix}$

Substituting the values

$$i\left[\frac{\partial}{\partial y}(-2xz - 2yz + c_3) - \frac{\partial}{\partial z}(y^2 + z^2 + c_2)\right]$$

$$+ j\left[\frac{\partial}{\partial z}(x^2 + z^2 + c_1) - \frac{\partial}{\partial x}(-2xz - 2yz + c_3)\right]$$

$$+ k\left[\frac{\partial}{\partial x}(y^2 + z^2 + c_2) - \frac{\partial}{\partial y}(x^2 + z^2 + c_1)\right] = \nabla \times U$$

or $\quad i(-2z - 2z) + j(2z + 2z) + k(0 - 0) = \nabla \times U$

or $\quad i(-4z) + j(4z) = \nabla \times U$

Since curl U is not zero the flow is not irrotational.

4.4 Determine the equations of a stream line passing through the point $(n, 0)$ if the 2D flow is described by

$$u = -y/m^2 \quad \text{and} \quad v = x/n^2$$

Solution

The equation of a stream line is given by

$$\frac{dx}{u} = \frac{dy}{v}$$

$$\frac{dx}{-y/m^2} = \frac{dy}{x/n^2}$$

$$\frac{x\,dx}{n^2} + \frac{y\,dy}{m^2} = 0$$

Integrating,

$$\frac{x^2}{n^2} + \frac{y^2}{m^2} = 2A$$

where A is the constant of integration.

The above equation is the general expression for stream lines representing above 2-D flow field.

For the stream line passing through $(n, 0)$,

$$\frac{n^2}{n^2} + 0 = 2A$$

$$A = \frac{1}{2}$$

Hence, $\dfrac{x^2}{n^2} + \dfrac{y^2}{m^2} = 1$ is the requisite equation of streamline.

4.5 The following velocity components for steady, incompressible flow are:

(i) $u = 2x - 3y, v = x - 2y$ and $w = 0$

(ii) $u = 2x^2 - xy + z^2$, $v = x^2 - 4xy + y^2$, $w = 2xy - yz + y^2$

(iii) $u = 2x^2 + y^2$, $v = -4xy$

Is the equation of continuity satisfied.

Solution

The equation of continuity for 3-D steady flow of an incompressible fluid is given by

$$\frac{\partial u}{\partial x} + \frac{\partial v}{\partial y} + \frac{\partial w}{\partial z} = 0$$

(i) Substituting the values

$$L.H.S. = \frac{\partial}{\partial x}(2x - 3y) + \frac{\partial}{\partial y}(x - 2y) + \frac{\partial}{\partial z}(0)$$

$$(2 - 0) + (0 - 2) + 0 = 0$$

Hence, the flow satisfies the continuity equation.

(ii) L.H.S. $= \dfrac{\partial}{\partial x} (2x^2 - xy + z^2) + \dfrac{\partial}{\partial y} (x^2 - 4xy + y^2)$

$\qquad\qquad + \dfrac{\partial}{\partial z} (2xy - yz + y^2)$

$\qquad = (4x - y + 0) + (0 - 4x + 2y) + (0 - y + 0)$

$\qquad = 0$

The flow satisfies the continuity equation.

(iii) It is two dimensional flow, so that

$\qquad$ L.H.S. $= \dfrac{\partial}{\partial x} (2x^2 + y^2) + \dfrac{\partial}{\partial y} (-4xy)$

$\qquad = (4x + 0) + (-4x)$

$\qquad = 0$

The given flow satisfies the continuity equation.

4.6 Check whether the following function represents the possible flow phenomenon of irrotational flow

$$\varphi = \frac{4x}{(x^2 + y^2)}$$

Solution

For the flow to be irrotational flow, it should satisfy Laplace's equation

$$\frac{\partial \varphi}{\partial x} = \frac{(x^2 + y^2)(4) - 4x(2x)}{(x^2 + y^2)^2} = \frac{4(-x^2 + y^2)}{(x^2 + y^2)^2}$$

$$\frac{\partial^2 \varphi}{\partial x^2} = \frac{(x^2 + y^2)^2 \, 4(-2x) - 4(-x^2 + y^2)(2)(x^2 + y^2)(2x)}{(x^2 + y^2)^4}$$

$$= \frac{(x^2 + y^2)[-8x(x^2 + y^2) - 16x(-x^2 + y^2)]}{(x^2 + y^2)^4}$$

$$= \frac{8x^3 - 24xy^3}{(x^2 + y^2)^3}$$

Similarly, $\qquad \dfrac{\partial \varphi}{\partial y} = \dfrac{(x^2 + y^2)(0) - 4x(2y)}{(x^2 + y^2)^2} = \dfrac{-8xy}{(x^2 + y^2)^2}$

$$\frac{\partial^2 \varphi}{\partial y^2} = \left[\frac{(x^2 + y^2)^2 (8x) - (8xy)(2)(x^2 + y^2)(2y)}{(x^2 + y^2)^4} \right]$$

$$= - \frac{(x^2 + y^2)[8x(x^2 + y^2) - 32xy^2]}{(x^2 + y^2)^4}$$

$$= \left[\frac{-8x^3 + 24xy^2}{(x^2 + y^2)^3} \right]$$

The Laplace equation is

$$\frac{\partial^2 \varphi}{\partial x^2} + \frac{\partial^2 \varphi}{\partial y^2} = 0$$

L.H.S. $= \dfrac{(8x^3 - 24xy^3)}{(x^2 + y^2)^3} + \dfrac{(-8x^3 + 24xy^2)}{(x^2 + y^2)^3}$

$= 0$

Since the given function satisfies the Laplace equation, it is possible phenomenon of irrotational flow.

4.7 The x and y components in a 2-D flow field for an incompressible fluid are expressed as

$$u = 2xy \text{ and } v = a^2 + x^2 - y^2$$

(a) Show that the motion is possible.

(b) Check whether the flow is irrotational or not ?

(c) Calculate φ

Solution

(a) The continuity equatin for 2-D flow is

$$\frac{\partial u}{\partial x} + \frac{\partial v}{\partial y} = 0$$

Substituting the values of u and v.

L.H.S. $= \dfrac{\partial}{\partial x}(2xy) + \dfrac{\partial}{\partial y}(a^2 + x^2 - y^2)$

$= (2y) + (0 + 0 - 2y) = 0$

Thus, the given flow satisfies the continuity equation.

(b) Further, $\dfrac{\partial u}{\partial y} = 2x$ and $\dfrac{\partial v}{\partial x} = 2x$

The necessary condition for irrotational flow is

$$\frac{\partial v}{\partial x} - \frac{\partial u}{\partial y} = 0$$

$$2x - 2x = 0$$

Thus, the given flow is irrotational.

(c) $\qquad u = -\dfrac{\partial \varphi}{\partial x} = 2xy \text{ (given)} \qquad \qquad \text{...(i)}$

$\qquad v = -\dfrac{\partial \varphi}{\partial y} = a^2 + x^2 - y^2 \text{ (given)} \qquad \text{...(ii)}$

Integrating Eq. (i) with respect to x,

$$\varphi = -2y\frac{x^2}{2} + f(y)$$

$$= -x^2 y + f(y) \qquad \qquad \text{...(iii)}$$

Differentiating Eq. (iii) with respect to y.

$$\frac{\partial \varphi}{\partial y} = -x^2 + f'(y) \qquad \qquad \text{...(iv)}$$

From Eqns. (ii) and (iv),

$$-(a^2 + x^2 - y^2) = -x^2 + f'(y)$$

$$f'(y) = -(a^2 - y^2) \qquad \qquad \text{...(v)}$$

Integrating with respect to y,

$$f(y) = -(a^2 y - y^3/3) + c \qquad \qquad \text{...(vi)}$$

Substituting the vlaue of $f(y)$ into Eq. (iii)

$$\varphi = -x^2 y - a^2 y + \frac{y^3}{3} + c$$

$$\varphi = -x^2 y + y\left(\frac{y^2}{3} - a^2\right) + c$$

4.8 Velocity components in a 2-D flow for an incompressible fluid are as follows,

$$u = (3x + 2y) \ , \ v = (2x - 3y)$$

Determine the expressions for ψ

Solution

$$u = \frac{\partial \psi}{\partial y} = (3x + 2y) \qquad \qquad \text{(i)}$$

$$v = -\frac{\partial \psi}{\partial x} = (2x - 3y) \qquad \qquad \text{(ii)}$$

So that

$$\frac{\partial \psi}{\partial x} = (-2x + 3y)$$

Integrating Eq. (i) with respect to y,

$$\psi = 3xy + y^2 + f(x) \qquad \qquad \text{...(iii)}$$

Differentiating Eq. (iii) with respect to x,

$$\frac{\partial \psi}{\partial x} = 3y + f'(x) \qquad \qquad \text{...(iv)}$$

From Eq. (ii) and (iv)

$$-2x + 3y = 3y + f'(x)$$

$$f'(x) = -2x \qquad \qquad \text{...(v)}$$

Integrating, $\quad f(x) = -x^2 + c \qquad \qquad \text{...(vi)}$

Substituting the vlaue of $f(x)$ into Eq. (iii)

$$\psi = 3xy + y^2 - x^2 + c$$

$$= (y^2 - x^2) + 3xy + c$$

Where c is a numerical constant.

4.9 Velocity potential for a $2-D$ flow is given by $\Phi = c\,(x^2 - y^2)$. Determine the corresponding stream function, what will be the velocity of flow at the point (2,1) in the flow field ?

Solution

(a) $$\varphi = c\,(x^2 - y^2)$$

Differentiating w.r. to x,

$$\frac{\partial \varphi}{\partial x} = 2\,cx$$

$\therefore$ $$u = -\frac{\partial \varphi}{\partial x} = -2\,cx \qquad \text{...(i)}$$

Similarly $$v = -\frac{\partial \varphi}{\partial y} = 2\,cy \qquad \text{...(ii)}$$

Also $$u = \frac{\partial \psi}{\partial y} = -2\,cx \qquad \text{...(iii)}$$

and $$v = -\frac{\partial \psi}{\partial x} = 2\,cy$$

or $$\frac{\partial \psi}{\partial x} = -2\,cy \qquad \text{...(iv)}$$

Integrate Eq. (iii) w.r. to y,

$$\psi = -2\,cxy + f(x) \qquad \text{...(v)}$$

Differentiate Eq. (v) w.r. to x,

$$\frac{\partial \psi}{\partial x} = -2\,cy + f'(x) \qquad \text{...(vi)}$$

From Eqn. (iv) and (vi)

$$-2\,cy = -2\,cy + f'(x)$$

or $$f'(x) = 0$$

On integration, $f(x) = c_1$ $\qquad$ ...(vii)

From Eqns. (v) and (vii)

$$\psi = -2\,cxy + c_1$$

where c_1 is a constant of integration.

(b) At point (2,1),

$$u = 2c\,(2 \times 1) = -4\,c$$

$$v = 2c\,(1) = 2\,c$$

$\therefore$ $$U = \sqrt{u^2 + v^2}$$

$$= \sqrt{(-4c)^2 + (2\,c)^2}$$

$$= \sqrt{20}\ \text{c m/s}$$

4.10 A two dimensional fluid flow is described by the velocity components $u = 5x^3$, $v = -15x^2 y$. Evaluate the stream function. Also determine velocity and acceleration at point $P(x = 1$ m, $y = 2$ m).

Solution

The velocity components in terms of stream function are given by Eq. 4.50

$$\frac{\partial \psi}{\partial y} = u = 5x^3 \qquad ...(i)$$

$$\frac{\partial \psi}{\partial x} = -v = 15x^2 y \qquad ...(ii)$$

Integrating Eq. (i) with respect to y,

$$\psi = 5x^3 y + c_1$$

where c_1 is independent of y but may be a function of x.

Differentiating Eq. (iii) w.r. to x and equating it with eq.(ii),

$$\frac{\partial \psi}{\partial x} = 15x^2 y + \frac{\partial c_1}{\partial x} \qquad ...(iv)$$

$$\frac{\partial \psi}{\partial x} = 15x^2 y \qquad ...(ii)$$

Hence, $\qquad \dfrac{\partial c_1}{\partial x} = 0$

Integrating with respect to x,

$$c_1 = c$$

where c should be independent of x and at the same time should be independent of y as mentioned earlier, *i.e.* c may be a numerical constant. Hence,

$$\psi = 5x^3 y + c$$

The velocity at any point

$$U = iu + jv$$

$$= i(5x^3) + j(-15x^2 y)$$

$$= i(5 \times 1^3) + j(-15 \times 1^2 \times 2)$$

$$= i(5) + j(-30)$$

$$U = \sqrt{u^2 + v^2} = \sqrt{(5)^2 + (-30)^2}$$

$$= 30.41 \text{ m/s}$$

The acceleration at any point is given by Eq. 4.16 a and b. For 2-D flow w is zero.

$$ax = \frac{\partial u}{\partial t} + u \frac{\partial u}{\partial x} + v \frac{\partial u}{\partial y}$$

$$= 0 + 5x^3 \times \frac{\partial}{\partial x}(5x^3) + (-15x^2 y)\frac{\partial}{\partial y}(5x^3)$$

$$= 5x^3 \times 15x^2 + 0$$

$$= 75x^5$$

$$= 75 \times 1^5$$

$$= 75 \text{ m/s}$$

Similarly, $\qquad a_y = \dfrac{\partial v}{\partial t} + u \dfrac{\partial v}{\partial x} + v \dfrac{\partial v}{\partial y}$

$$= 0 + 5x^3 \dfrac{\partial}{\partial x}(-15x^2 y) + (-15x^2 y)\dfrac{\partial}{\partial y}(-15x^2 y)$$

$$= 5x^3(-30xy) + 15^2 y (15x^2) \; = 75x^4 y$$

$$= 75 \times 1^4 \times 2$$

$$= 150 \text{ m/s/s}$$

$$\bar{a} = \sqrt{a_x^2 + a_y^2}$$

$$= \sqrt{(75)^2 + (150)^2}$$

$$= 167.7 \text{ m/s/s}$$

4.11 Sketch the streamlines represented by

(i) $\qquad\qquad\qquad \psi = x^2 + y^2$ and $\qquad$ (ii) $\psi = 2xy$

Also find the velocity and its direction at point (1,1). Also verify the conditions of continuity and irrotational flow are satisfied.

Solution

Case I: The velocity components are given by

$$u = \dfrac{\partial \psi}{\partial y} = 2y \qquad\qquad\qquad\qquad\text{...(i)}$$

$$v = -\dfrac{\partial \psi}{\partial x} = -2x \qquad\qquad\qquad\text{...(ii)}$$

Hence, the velocity at point (1,1)

$$U = \sqrt{u^2 + v^2}$$

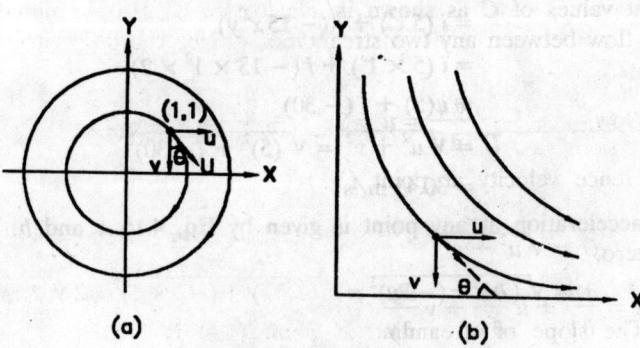

(a) (b)

FIG. 4.14. EXAMPLE 4.5

$$= 4y^2 + 4x^2 = \sqrt{4(1)^2 + 4(1)^2}$$
$$= 2\sqrt{2} \text{ m/s}$$

The slope of velocity vector at ‾point (1,1) is

$$\tan \theta = \frac{dy}{dx} = \frac{v}{u} = -1$$

The equation of stream line (Eq. 4.12b) is

$$u \, dy - v \, dx = 0$$
$$2y \, dy - (-2x) \, dx = 0$$

Integrating, $y^2 + x^2 = C$ Constant.

This is the equation of circle, hence the streamlines are concentric circles of radius equal to $\sqrt{C}$. In the above case, the velocity components in the first quadrant are $u = 2 \text{ m/s}$, and $v = -2 \, m/s$. Therefore, the direction of stream lines is clockwise as seen from Fig. 4.14a From Eqs. (i) and (ii),

$$\frac{\partial u}{\partial x} = 0 \; , \; \frac{\partial u}{\partial y} = +2 \; , \; \frac{\partial v}{\partial x} = -2 \; , \; \frac{\partial u}{\partial y} = 0$$

The continuity equation is

$$\frac{\partial u}{\partial x} + \frac{\partial v}{\partial y} = 0$$

Substituting the values, it is seen that continuity equation is satisfied. Furthermore, condition of irrotationality is

$$\frac{\partial v}{\partial x} - \frac{\partial u}{\partial y} = 0$$

Substituting the values it is seen that this condition is not satisfied, Hence the flow is rotational.

Case II : $\psi = 2xy$

It can be written as $2xy = C$ constant along a streamline.

The given equation represents a family of rectangular hyperbolas for different values of C as shown in Fig. 4.14b. It is to be noted that volume rate of flow between any two streamlines will be the difference between their constants.

Now, $\qquad \dfrac{\partial \psi}{\partial y} = u = 2x \; ; \; -\dfrac{\partial \psi}{\partial x} = v = -2y$

Hence velocity at point (1,1)

$$U = \sqrt{u^2 + v^2}$$
$$= \sqrt{(2x)^2 + (-2y)^2} = \sqrt{(2 \times 1)^2 + (-2 \times 1)^2} = 2\sqrt{2} \text{ m/s/s}$$

The slope of streamline at point (1,1) is

$$\tan \theta = \frac{dy}{dx} = \frac{v}{u} = -1$$

i.e., $\theta = 45°$

Furthermore, at point (1,1)

$$\frac{\partial u}{\partial x} = 2 \, , \, \frac{\partial u}{\partial y} = 0$$

$$\frac{\partial v}{\partial x} = 0 \, , \, \frac{\partial v}{\partial y} = -2$$

continuity equation is

$$\frac{\partial u}{\partial x} + \frac{\partial v}{\partial y} = 0$$

Substituting the values, it is seen that this equation is satisfied. Condition of irrotational flow is

$$\frac{\partial v}{\partial x} - \frac{\partial u}{\partial y} = 0$$

It is also satisfied. Therefore, this flow is irrotational.

4.12. The velocity components in a 2-D incompressible flow field are expressed as

$$u = y^3/3 + 2x - x^2y$$
$$v = xy^2 - 2y - x^3/3$$

(a) Show that these equations represent a possible case of irrotational flow. (b) Obtain an expression for φ and also for ψ .

Solution

(a) The condition of irrotationality of flow is

$$\frac{\partial v}{\partial x} - \frac{\partial u}{\partial y} = 0$$

Here,

$$\frac{\partial u}{\partial y} = \frac{\partial}{\partial y}(y^3/3 + 2x - x^2y)$$

$$= y^2 - x^2$$

$$\frac{\partial v}{\partial x} = \frac{\partial}{\partial x}(xy^2 - 2y - x^3/3)$$

$$= y^2 - x^2$$

Substituting these values in the above equation it is seen that flow is irrotational.

(b) Now,

$$u = -\frac{\partial \varphi}{\partial x} = \left(\frac{y^3}{3} + 2x - x^2y\right) \qquad \text{...(i)}$$

$$v = -\frac{\partial \varphi}{\partial y} = (xy^2 - 2y - x^3/3) \qquad \text{...(ii)}$$

Integrate Eq. (i) with respect to x

$$\varphi = -\left(\frac{xy^3}{3} + x^2 - \frac{x^3 y}{3}\right) + c_1$$

where $\qquad c_1 = f(y)$ ...(iii)

Differentiate Eq. (iii) with respect to y.

$$\frac{\partial \varphi}{\partial y} = -(xy^2 - x^3/3) + \frac{\partial c_1}{\partial y} \qquad ...(iv)$$

Equating Eq. (ii) and (iv)

$$\frac{\partial \varphi}{\partial y} = -\left(xy^2 - 2y - \frac{x^3}{3}\right) = -\left(xy^2 - x^3/3\right) + \frac{\partial c_1}{\partial y}$$

$$\frac{\partial c_1}{\partial y} = 2y$$

Integrating

$$c_1 = y^2 + c$$

Therefore $\qquad \varphi = -\left(\dfrac{xy^3}{3} - \dfrac{x^3 y}{3} + x^2 - y^2\right) + c$

$$= -(x^2 - y^2)(1 - xy/3) + c$$

(ii) $\qquad u = \dfrac{\partial \psi}{\partial y} = (y^3/3 + 2x - x^2 y)$ ...(v)

$$v = -\frac{\partial \psi}{\partial x} = (xy^2 - 2y - x^3/3) \qquad ...(vi)$$

Integrate Eq. (v) with respect to y

$$\psi = \frac{y^4}{12} + 2xy - x^2 y^2/2 + c_2 \qquad ...(vii)$$

Differentiate Eq. (vii) with respect to x,

$$\frac{\partial \psi}{\partial x} = 2y - xy^2 + \frac{\partial c_2}{\partial x} \qquad ...(viii)$$

Equating two values of $\dfrac{\partial \psi}{\partial x}$ in Eqs. (vi) and (viii)

$$-xy^2 + 2y + x^3/3 = 2y - xy^2 + \frac{\partial c_2}{\partial x}$$

Therefore, $\qquad \dfrac{\partial c_2}{\partial x} = \dfrac{x^3}{3}$

Integrate it with respect to x,

$$c_2 = \frac{x^4}{12} + c \qquad ...(ix)$$

Substituting the value of c_2 in Eq. (vii)

$$\psi = \frac{x^4 + y^4}{12} - \frac{x^2 y^2}{2} + 2xy + c$$

4.13 : A conical pipe 2m long has inlet of 100 mm diameter and outlet of 200 mm diameter. It is laid horizontally. The velocity over any cross section is considered uniform. It carries a constant discharge of 0.2 m³/s. Determine (a) total acceleration at a section 1.5 m away from its inlet. (b) If the discharge increases from 0.2 m³/s to 0.4 m³/s in 2 section, determine total acceleration at this section at t = 1 sec. from the initial condition.

Solution :

The diameter D_x at section XX is given by

$$D_x = \left(D_1 + \frac{D_2 - D_1}{L} . x \right)$$

$$= \left(0.1 + \frac{0.2 - 0.1}{2} x \right) = 0.1 \left(1 + \frac{x}{2} \right)$$

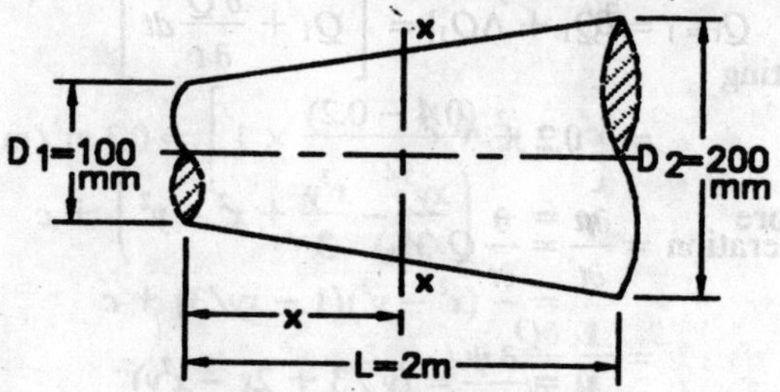

FIG. 4.15. EXAMPLE 4.13

Area of flow $A_x = \pi/4 . D_x^2$

Velocity of flow $u = \dfrac{Q}{A_x}$

$$= \frac{Q}{\pi/4 \, [0.1 \, (1 + x/2]^2}$$

$$= \frac{127.39 \, Q}{(1 + x/2)^2}$$

Case I : Constant discharge

Total acceleration = local acc. + convective acc.

For steady flow,

local acceleration = 0

$$u = 127.39 \, Q \, (1 + x/2)^{-2}$$

$$\frac{\partial u}{\partial x} = 127.39 \, Q \times (-2) \, (1 + x/2)^{-3} \, (0 + 1/2)$$

$$= -127.39 \, Q \, (1 + x/2)^{-3}$$

Convective acceleration $= u \dfrac{\partial u}{\partial x}$

Since flow is unidirectional, $u = u_x \, v = 0, w = 0,$

$$u\frac{\partial u}{\partial x} = (-127.39 \ Q)(1 + x/2)^{-2} \times (-127.39 \ Q)(1 + x/2)^{-3}$$

At $x = 1.5$ m from inlet, and $Q = 0.2$ m^3/s

Total acceleration, as $= \left[\frac{\partial u}{\partial t} + u\frac{\partial u}{\partial x}\right]$

$$= 0. - (127.39 \times 0.2)^2 \left(1 + \frac{1.5}{2}\right)^{-5}$$

$$= -39.55 \ \text{m/s/s}$$

Case II : Varying discharge :

Discharge across XX is to be computed for this case at t = 1 sec.

$$Q_{t=1} = [Q_1 + \Delta Q_1] = \left[Q_1 + \frac{\partial Q}{\partial t} dt\right]$$

$$= \left[0.2 + \frac{(0.4 - 0.2)}{2} \times 1\right] = 0.3 \ \text{m}^3/\text{m}$$

Local acceleration $= \dfrac{\partial u}{\partial t} = \dfrac{\partial}{\partial t} Q/A_x)$

$$= \frac{1}{A_x}\frac{\partial Q}{\partial t}$$

$$= \frac{1}{\pi/4 \ (0.1)^2 \ (1 + x/2)^2} \times \frac{(0.4 - 0.2)}{2}$$

Since the discharge varies from 0.2 m^3/s to 0.4 m^3/s in 2 seconds

$$\frac{\partial u}{\partial t} = 12.739\left(1 + \frac{x}{2}\right)^{-2}$$

For $x = 1.5$ m, $\dfrac{\partial u}{\partial t} = 12.739\left(1 + \dfrac{1.5}{2}\right)^{-2}$

$$= 4.16 \ \text{m/s/s}$$

Convective acceleration $= u\dfrac{\partial u}{\partial x}$

$$u = \frac{Q_t}{A_x} = \frac{Q_t}{\pi/4 \ (0.1)^2 \ (1 + x/2)^2}$$

$$= 127.39 \ Q_t \ (1 + x/2)^{-2}$$

$$\frac{\partial u}{\partial x} = 127.39 \ Q_t \ (-2) \ (1 + x/2)^{-3} \ (1/2)$$

$$= -127.39 \ Q_t \ (1 + x/2)^{-3}$$

$$u\frac{\partial u}{\partial x} = [127.39 \ Q_t \ (1 + x/2)^{-2}]$$

$$\times [-127.39 \ Q_t \ (1 + x/2)^{-3}]$$

$$= - (127.39 \, Q_t)^2 \, (1 + x/2)^{-5}$$

For $\quad x = 1.5$ m and $Q_t = 0.3$ m³/s

$$u \frac{\partial u}{\partial x} = - (127.39 \times 0.3)^2 \left(1 + \frac{1.5}{2} \right)^{-5}$$

$$= - 88.986 \text{ m/s/s}$$

Total acc. a_s = local acc. + convective acc.

$$= 4.16 - 88.986$$

$$= - 84.826 \text{ m/s/s}$$

4.14 : In a 3-D flow of incompressible fluid, two components of velocities are given by

(a) $u = 2 \, x^3$, $v = 2$ xyz

(b) $u = 2 \, x^2 + 2$ xy, $w = z^3 - 4$ xz

(c) $w = 2 \, y^2$, $w = 2$ xyz.

Find the third component.

Solution :

(a) It should satisfy continuity equation (Eq. 4.22)

$$\frac{\partial u}{\partial x} + \frac{\partial v}{\partial y} + \frac{\partial w}{\partial z} = 0$$

From given data, $u = 2x^2, \dfrac{\partial u}{\partial x} = 6x^2$

$$v = 2xyz, \frac{\partial v}{\partial y} = 2xz$$

Therefore, $\quad \dfrac{\partial w}{\partial z} = - \dfrac{\partial u}{\partial x} - \dfrac{\partial v}{\partial y}$

$$= - 6x^2 - 2xz$$

Integrating w.r. to z,

$$w = 6x^2 z - 2x . \frac{z^2}{2} + f(x, y, t)$$

$$w = 6x^2 z - x z^2 + c$$

where c is a constant of integration which should be independent of z but may be function of x and/or y.

(b) From given data, $u = (2x^2 + 2xy), \dfrac{\partial u}{\partial x} = 2x + 2y$

$$w = z^3 - 4xz, \frac{\partial w}{\partial z} = z^2 - 4x$$

From Eq.4.22, $\quad \dfrac{\partial v}{\partial y} = - \dfrac{\partial u}{\partial x} - \dfrac{\partial w}{\partial z}$

$$= -(2x + 2y) - (3z^2 - 4x)$$

$$= (2x - 2y - 3z^2)$$

Integrating w.r. to y,

$$v = 2xy - 2y^2/2 - 3z^2 . y + f(x,z,t)$$

$$v = 2xy - y^2 - 3yz^2 + c$$

There $f(x, y, t)$ or c is a constant of integration which is indepe- ndent of y.

(c) From given data, $v = 2y^2, \dfrac{\partial v}{\partial y} = 4y$

$$w = 2xyz, \dfrac{\partial w}{\partial z} = 2xy$$

From Eq. 4.22, $\dfrac{\partial u}{\partial x} = -\dfrac{\partial v}{\partial y} - \dfrac{\partial w}{\partial z}$

$$= -(4y) - (2xy)$$

Integrating w.r. to x,

$$u = -4xy - 2.\dfrac{x^2}{2}.y + f(y,z,t)$$

$$= -4xy - x^2 y + c$$

where $f(y, z, t)$ or c is a constant of integration and is independent of x.

4.15 : Plot the flow field defined by $\varphi = x^2 - y^2$

Solution :

For the given φ to be a possible case of flow field or to exit, the flow must be irrotational. This can be checked either by finding Laplacian or should satisfy continuity equation.

$$\varphi = x^2 - y^2$$

$$\dfrac{\partial \varphi}{\partial x} = 2x, \dfrac{\partial^2 \varphi}{\partial x^2} = 2$$

$$\dfrac{\partial \varphi}{\partial y} = -2y, \dfrac{\partial^2 \varphi}{\partial y^2} = -2$$

Therefore, Laplace equation is $\dfrac{\partial^2 \varphi}{\partial x^2} + \dfrac{\partial^2 \varphi}{\partial y^2} = 0$

L.H.S., $2-2 = 0 = $ R.H.S.

Hence given φ represents an irrotational flow field.

To sketch flow field determine φ.

$$u = -\dfrac{\partial \varphi}{\partial x} = -2 \qquad \qquad ...(i)$$

$$v = -\frac{\partial \varphi}{\partial y} = -(-2y) = 2y \qquad \text{...(ii)}$$

Also
$$u = \frac{\partial \psi}{\partial y} = -2x \qquad \text{...(iii)}$$

and
$$v = -\frac{\partial \psi}{\partial x} = 2y$$

$$\frac{\partial \psi}{\partial x} = -2y \qquad \text{...(iv)}$$

Integrate Eq. (iii) w.r. to y
$$\psi = -2x \cdot y + f(x) \qquad \text{..(v)}$$

Differentiate Eq. (v) w.r. to x
$$\frac{\partial \psi}{\partial x} = -2y + f'(x) \qquad \text{...(vi)}$$

Equating Eq. (iv) and Eq. (vi)
$$-2y = -2y + f'(x)$$
$$f'(x) = 0 \qquad \text{...(vii)}$$

Integrating Eq. (vii) w.r. to x
$$f(x) = c \qquad \text{...(viii)}$$

Substitute the value of f(x) in Eq.(v)
$$= -2xy + c$$

Here c is a numerical constant and its value is to be determined from given boundary condition. For the given case,

ψ = constant along a streamline or flow line, hence c is meaningless.

Hence
$$\psi = -2xy$$

This is the equation of flow lines. Now the flow field can be sketched for different values of .

$$y = -\psi/2x$$

$\psi = 10$	$x = 1$	2	3	4	5
$\psi = 10$	$y = -5$	–2.5	–5/3	–5/4	–1
$\psi = 20$	$y = -10$	–5	–10/3	–5/2	–2

4.16 : A 2-D flow field as given by
$$U = 2 x^3 i - 6 x^2 y j$$

Check whether the flow is rotational. If so compute (a) angular velocity, (b) vorticity, (c) shear strain and (d) dilatancy. Also compute circulation about the circle $x^2 + y^2 = c^2$.

Solution :

For the possible flow field, given equation should satisfy continuity equation.

$$\frac{\partial u}{\partial x} + \frac{\partial v}{\partial y} = 0$$

Given
$$u = 2\,x^3, \quad v = -6\,x^2\,y.$$

Substituting the values of u and v,

$$\text{L.H.S.} = \frac{\partial\,(2x^3)}{\partial x} + \frac{\partial\,(-6x^2y)}{\partial y}$$

$$= 6x^2 - 6x^2 = 0 = \text{R.H.S.}$$

Thus the flow is physically possible.

Rotational flow :

For rotational flow, $w_z = \dfrac{1}{2}\left(\dfrac{\partial v}{\partial x} - \dfrac{\partial u}{\partial y}\right) \neq 0$

$$\frac{\partial u}{\partial y} = 0 \ , \ \frac{\partial v}{\partial x} = -12xy$$

Since, $\dfrac{\partial v}{\partial x} - \dfrac{\partial u}{\partial y} \neq 0$, the flow is rotational.

(a) Angular velocity

$$\omega_z = 1/2\left(\frac{\partial v}{\partial x} - \frac{\partial u}{\partial y}\right)$$

$$= 1/2\,(-12xy - 0) = -6xy$$

(b) Vorticity $\quad = 2\,\omega_z$

$$= 2\,(-6\ xy) = -12\ xy$$

(c) Shear strain $e_z = 1/2\left(\dfrac{\partial v}{\partial x} + \dfrac{\partial u}{\partial y}\right)$

$$= 1/2\,(-12xy + 0)$$

$$= -6xy$$

(d) Dilatancy in x direction $= \dfrac{\partial u}{\partial x}$

$$= \frac{\partial}{\partial x}\,(2x^3) = 6x^2$$

and in Y- direction $= \dfrac{\partial v}{\partial y}$

$$= \frac{\partial\,(-6x^2y)}{\partial y} = -6x^2$$

(e) Circulation = Vorticity × area

$$= -12xy \times \pi c^2$$

Since $\qquad c = $ radius of circle

$$= -12\pi xy\,c^2$$

4.17 : For the following flows, determine the components of rotation about various axis.

(a) $u = xy$, $v = 1/2 (x^2 - y^2)$

(b) $u = xy^3z$, $v = -y^2z^2$, $w = y z^2 - y^3 z^2/2$

Solution :

(a) $u = xy$, $v = 1/2 (x^2 - y^2)$

It is 2-D flow and hence the fluid molecules will have rotation about z-axis only and $\omega_x = \omega_y = 0$.

$$\omega_z = 1/2 \left(\frac{\partial v}{\partial x} - \frac{\partial u}{\partial y} \right)$$

$$= 1/2 \left[\frac{\partial}{\partial x} \left(\frac{x^2}{2} - \frac{y^2}{2} \right) - \frac{\partial (xy)}{\partial y} \right]$$

$$= 1/2 [(1/2 . 2x - 1/0) - (x)]$$

$$= 1/2 [x - x) = 0$$

Since $\omega_x = \omega_y = \omega_z = 0$, hence given flow field is irrotation.

(b) $u = x y^3 z$, $u = -y^2 z^2$, $w = y z^2 - y^3 z^2/2$

Here

$$\omega_x = 1/2 \left(\frac{\partial w}{\partial y} - \frac{\partial v}{\partial z} \right)$$

$$= 1/2 \left[\frac{\partial}{\partial y} (yz^2 - y^3 z^2/2) - \frac{\partial}{\partial z} (-y^2 z^2) \right]$$

$$= 1/2 \left[\left(z^2 - \frac{3 y^2 z^2}{2} \right) - (-2y^2 z) \right]$$

$$= 1/2 (z^2 - 3/2 y^2 z^2 + 2y^2 z)$$

$$\omega_y = 1/2 \left(\frac{\partial u}{\partial z} - \frac{\partial w}{\partial x} \right)$$

$$= 1/2 \left[\frac{\partial}{\partial z} (x y^3 z) - \frac{\partial}{\partial x} \left(y z^2 - \frac{y^3 z^2}{2} \right) \right]$$

$$= 1/2 [xy^3 - (0 - 0)]$$

$$= 1/2 xy^3$$

$$\omega_z = 1/2 \left(\frac{\partial v}{\partial x} - \frac{\partial u}{\partial y} \right)$$

$$= 1/2 \left[\frac{\partial}{\partial x} (-y^2 z^2) - \frac{\partial}{\partial y} (x y^3 z) \right]$$

$$= 1/2 [0 - 3 x y^2 z]$$

$$= -3/2 x y^2 z$$

Hence, $\omega_x = 1/2 (z^2 - 3/2 y^2 z^2 + 2y^2 z)$,

$\omega_y = 1/2 x y^3$

$$\omega_z = -3/2xy^2z.$$

4.18 : A two dimensional flow field is given by $\varphi = 2$ xy. Determine (a) corresponding stream function, (b) velocities at A (1,3) and B (3,2) and (c) difference of pressure between A and B. Also determine discharge passing through stream tube located between these points.

Solution :

(a) Given $\varphi = 2xy$

$$u = -\frac{\partial \varphi}{\partial x} = -2y$$

$$v = -\frac{\partial \varphi}{\partial y} = -2x$$

Also

$$u = \frac{\partial \psi}{\partial y} = -2y \qquad \qquad ...(i)$$

$$v = -\frac{\partial \psi}{\partial x} = -2x$$

$$\frac{\partial \psi}{\partial x} = 2x \qquad \qquad ...(ii)$$

Integrating Eq. (i) w.r. to y,

$$\psi = -2y^2/2 + f(x)$$

or

$$\psi = -y^2 + f(x) \qquad \qquad ...(iii)$$

Differentiating Eq.(iii) w.r. to x,

$$\frac{\partial \psi}{\partial x} = 0 + f'(x) \qquad \qquad ...(iv)$$

Equating Eq. (ii) and (iv),

$$2x = f'(x) \qquad \qquad ...(v)$$

Integrating Eq. (v) w.r. to x,

$$f(x) = 2.x^2/2 + c$$

$$= x^2 + c$$

Substituting the value of f (x) in Eq. (iii)

$$\psi = -y^2 + x^2 + c$$

$$\psi = (x^2 - y^2) + c$$

Here c is a numerical constant which is determined from given boundary conditions.

For $\psi = 0$, at the origin, i.e., (0,0); $c = 0$

$$\psi = (x^2 - y^2)$$

(b) At A (1,3),

$$u_A = -2y$$

$$u_A = -2 \times 3 = -6$$

and

$$v_A = 2 \times$$

$$v_A = 2 \times 1 = 2$$

Therefore, $U_A = \sqrt{u_A^2 + v_A^2}$

$$= \sqrt{(-6)^2 + (2)^2} = \sqrt{40} \text{ units.}$$

At B (3, 2)

$$u_B = -2y$$

$$u_B = -2 \times 2 = -4$$

and

$$v_B = 2x$$

$$v_B = 2 \times 3 = 6$$

Therefore, $U_B = \sqrt{u_A^2 + v_B^2}$

$$= \sqrt{(-4)^2 + (6)^2} = \sqrt{52} \text{ units.}$$

(c) For 2-D flow,

$$\frac{p_A}{w} + \frac{U_A^2}{2g} = \frac{PB}{w} + \frac{U_B^2}{2g}$$

$$\left(\frac{p_A}{w} - \frac{p_B}{w}\right) = \left(\frac{U_B^2}{2g} - \frac{U_A^2}{2g}\right)$$

$$\left(\frac{p_A - p_B}{w}\right) = \left[\frac{(\sqrt{52})^2}{2g} - \frac{(\sqrt{40})^2}{2g}\right]$$

$$\left(\frac{p_A - p_B}{2}\right) = \frac{12}{2 \times 9.81} = 0.611 \text{ units.}$$

(d) Discharge between these two stream lines passing through A and B = Q_{AB}

$$\psi_B (3, 2) = (x^2 - y^2)$$

$$= [(3)^2 - (2)^2] = 5 \text{ units}$$

$$\psi_A (1, 3) = (x^2 - y^2)$$

$$= [(1)^2 - (3)^2] = -8 \text{ units.}$$

$$Q_{AB} = [5 - (-8)]$$

$$= 13 \text{ units.}$$

4.19 : In a 2-D flow, the velocity component in y-direction is given by v = A y e^x. Calculate X - component of velocity that would satisfy continuity equation. (A.M.I.E. 92 S)

Solution :

Continuity equation for 2-D flow is

$$\frac{\partial u}{\partial x} + \frac{\partial v}{\partial y} = 0$$

Given $\qquad v = A\,y\,e^x,\ \dfrac{\partial u}{\partial y} = A\,e^x$

$$\frac{\partial u}{\partial x} = -\frac{\partial v}{\partial y} = -A\,e^x$$

Integrating w.r. to x,

$$u = -\int A\ e^x\ dx$$

$$u = -A\ e^x + f\ (y)$$

where f (y) is independent of x, its value can be computed from given flow conditions, if any.

4.20 : Verify whether the following function represents a possible irrotational flow,

(a) $\psi = 6x - 4y + 7\,xy + 9$

(b) $\psi = A\,(x^2 + y^2)$

(c) $\varphi = \sin\,(x + y + z)$

(d) $\varphi = (r - 2/r)\,\theta$

Solution :

(a) For irrotation flow,

$$\omega_z = 1/2\left(\frac{\partial v}{\partial x} - \frac{\partial u}{\partial y}\right) = 0$$

Given $\psi = 6x - 4y + 7xy + 9$

$$u = \frac{\partial \psi}{\partial y} = -4 + 7x$$

$$v = -\frac{\partial \psi}{\partial x} = 6 + 7y$$

Therefore, $\qquad \omega_z = 1/2\left[\dfrac{\partial}{\partial x}(6 + 7y) - \dfrac{\partial}{\partial y}(-4 + 7x)\right]$

$$= 1/2\,[0 - 0] = 0$$

Given function represents irrotational flow

(b) Given $\qquad \psi = A(x^2 + y^2)$

$$u = \frac{\partial \psi}{\partial y} = 2Ax$$

$$v = \frac{\partial \psi}{\partial x} = -2Ay$$

Therefore, $\qquad \omega_z = 1/2\left(\dfrac{\partial v}{\partial x} - \dfrac{\partial u}{\partial y}\right)$

$$= 1/2\left[\frac{\partial}{\partial x}(-2Ay) - \frac{\partial}{\partial y}(2Ax)\right]$$

$$= 1/2 \, (0 - 0) = 0$$

Given function represents irrotational flow

(c) Given $\qquad \varphi = \sin (x + y + z)$

$$u = -\frac{\partial \varphi}{\partial x} = - \cos (x + y + z)$$

$$v = -\frac{\partial \varphi}{\partial y} = - \cos (x + y + z)$$

$$w = -\frac{\partial \varphi}{\partial z} = - \cos (x + y + z)$$

For irrotational flow to exist,

$$\omega_x = \omega_y = \omega_z = 0$$

Since, these are not zero, the given flow is not irrotational flow. Alternatively, given φ function should satisfy Laplace equation.

$$\frac{\partial^2 \varphi}{\partial x^2} + \frac{\partial^2 \varphi}{\partial y^2} + \frac{\partial^2 \varphi}{\partial z^2} = 0$$

Here $\qquad \dfrac{\partial \varphi}{\partial x} = \cos (x + y + z),$

$$\frac{\partial^2 \varphi}{\partial x^2} = - \sin (x + y + z),$$

$$\frac{\partial \varphi}{\partial y} = \cos (x + y + z),$$

$$\frac{\partial^2 \varphi}{\partial y^2} = - \sin (x + y + z),$$

$$\frac{\partial \varphi}{\partial z} = \cos (x + y + z),$$

$$\frac{\partial^2 \varphi}{\partial z^2} = - \sin (x + y + z),$$

$$\text{L.H.S.} = \frac{\partial^2 \varphi}{\partial x^2} + \frac{\partial^2 \varphi}{\partial y^2} + \frac{\partial^2 \varphi}{\partial z^2}$$

$$= - [3 \sin (x + y + z)] \neq 0$$

The given function does not represent irrotational flow.

(d) Given $\varphi = (r - 2/r) \sin \theta$

$$\frac{\partial \varphi}{\partial r} = \left(1 + \frac{2}{r^2} \right) \sin \theta$$

$$\frac{\partial^2 \varphi}{\partial r^2} = - \frac{4}{r^3} \sin \theta$$

$$\frac{\partial \varphi}{\partial \theta} = (r - 2/r) \cos \theta$$

$$\frac{\partial^2 \varphi}{\partial \theta^2} = \left(r - \frac{2}{r}\right)(- \sin \theta)$$

For irrotational flow, Laplace Eq. (in cylindrical polar coordinates) be satisfied.

$$\frac{\partial^2 \varphi}{\partial r^2} + \frac{1}{r}\frac{\partial \varphi}{\partial r} + \frac{1}{r^2}\frac{\partial^2 \varphi}{\partial \theta^2} = 0$$

Substituting the values on L.H.S.

$$-\frac{4}{r^3}\sin \theta + \frac{1}{r}\left(1 + \frac{2}{r^2}\right)\sin \theta + \frac{1}{r^2}\left\{-\left(r - \frac{2}{r}\right)\sin \theta\right\} = 0$$

$$= \sin \theta \left[-\frac{4}{r^3} + \frac{1}{r} + \frac{2}{r^3} - \frac{1}{r} + \frac{2}{r^3}\right]$$

$$= 0 = \text{R.H.S.}$$

Since Laplace equation is satisfied by given φ function, therefore, it represents irrotational flow.

4.21 : For the following functions in 2-D irrotational flow, determine the conjugate functions :

(a) $\psi = a. \ln . r$ (b) $\varphi = \dfrac{a \sin \theta}{r}$

Solution :

In cylindrical polar coordinates

$$u_r = -\frac{\partial \varphi}{\partial r} = \frac{1}{r}\frac{\partial \psi}{\partial \theta}$$

$$u_\theta = -\frac{1}{r}\frac{\partial \varphi}{\partial \theta} = -\frac{\partial \psi}{\partial r}$$

(a) Given = a. ln. r

$$u_r = \frac{1}{r}\frac{\partial \psi}{\partial \theta} = \frac{1}{r}\frac{\partial}{\partial \theta}(a \, l_n r) = 0 \qquad \qquad ...(i)$$

$$u_\theta = -\frac{\partial \psi}{\partial r} = -\frac{\partial}{\partial r}(a \, l_n r) = -\frac{a}{r} \qquad \qquad ...(ii)$$

Also

$$u_r = -\frac{\partial \varphi}{\partial r} = 0 \qquad \qquad ...(iii)$$

$$u_\theta = -\frac{1}{r}\frac{\partial \varphi}{\partial \theta} = -\frac{a}{r}$$

or

$$\frac{\partial \varphi}{\partial \theta} = a \qquad \qquad ...(iv)$$

Integrate Eq. (iii) w.r. to r

$$\varphi = f(\theta) \qquad \qquad \text{...(v)}$$

Differential Eq. (v) w.r.t.,

$$\frac{\partial \varphi}{\partial \theta} = f'(\theta) \qquad \qquad \text{...(vi)}$$

Equating Eqs. (iv) and (vi)

$$f'(\theta) = a \qquad \qquad \text{...(vii)}$$

Integrating w.r. to θ

$$f(\theta) = a\theta + c \qquad \qquad \text{...(viii)}$$

Substitute $f(\theta)$ in Eq. (v)

$$\varphi = a\theta + c$$

(b) Given $\qquad \varphi = \dfrac{a \sin \theta}{r}$

$$u_r = \frac{\partial \varphi}{\partial r} = \frac{\partial (a \sin \theta / r)}{\partial r} = -\frac{a}{r^2} \sin \theta \qquad \qquad \text{...(i)}$$

$$u_\theta = -\frac{1}{r} \frac{\partial \varphi}{\partial \theta} = -\frac{1}{r} \frac{\partial}{\partial \theta} \frac{(a \sin \theta)}{r}$$

$$= \frac{1}{r^2} a \cos \theta \qquad \qquad \text{...(ii)}$$

Also $\qquad u_r = \dfrac{1}{r} \dfrac{\partial \psi}{\partial \theta} = -\dfrac{a}{r^2} \sin \theta$

$$\frac{\partial \psi}{\partial \theta} = -\frac{a \sin \theta}{r} \qquad \qquad \text{...(iii)}$$

$$u_\theta = -\frac{\partial \psi}{\partial r} = -\frac{a}{r^2} \cos \theta$$

$$\frac{\partial \psi}{\partial r} = \frac{a \cos \theta}{r^2} \qquad \qquad \text{...(iv)}$$

Integrate Eq. (iii) w.r.t. θ

$$\psi = -\frac{a}{r} \cos \theta + f(r) \qquad \qquad \text{...(v)}$$

Differentiating Eq. (iv) w.r.t. r

$$\frac{\partial \psi}{\partial r} = -\frac{a \cos \theta}{r^2} + f'(r)$$

Equating Eqs. (v) and (vi)

$$\frac{a \cos \theta}{r^2} = \frac{-a \cos \theta}{r^2} + f'(r)$$

$$f'(r) = \frac{2a \cos \theta}{r^2}$$

Integrate w.r.t. r

$$f(r) = \frac{2 a \cos \theta}{r} + c \qquad \qquad ...(vii)$$

Substitute the value of f (r) in Eq. (v)

$$\psi = \frac{-a}{r} \cos \theta + \frac{2 a \cos \theta}{r} + c$$

$$\psi = \frac{a \cos \theta}{r} + c$$

Objective Questions

4.1 Normal acceleration exists when

(a) stream lines are curved

(b) stream lines are straight and parallel

(c) the flow is non-uniform

(d) none of the above answers

4.2 Fluid flow is taking place in a straight converging pipe then the acceleration is

(a) tangential local   (b) tangential convective

(c) normal local   (d) normal convective

(e) none

4.3 Stream lines in fluid flow are

(a) lines along which the velocity is constant

(b) lines along which φ is constant

(c) lines which exist in irrotational flow only

(d) lines along with ψ is constant

(e) none

4.4 In steady irrotatinal flow of a light fluid, points of equal streamline spacing also represents the points of equal

(a) tangential acceleration   (b) pressure gradient

(c) pressure intensity   (d) none of these answers

4.5 The existence of velocity potential indicates that

(a) the flow is irrotational   (b) the flow is rotational

(c) vorticity is zero   (d) none

4.6 The stream function exists for

(a) two dimensional flow only

(b) three dimensional flow

(c) irrotational flow only

(d) rotational flow only

(e) all types of flow

4.7 The continuity equation

(a) requires that Newton's second law of motion be satisfied at every point

(b) relates mass rate of flow along a stream tube

(c) states that velocity at the boundary should be zero

(d) none

4.8 A equipotential line

(a) has no velocity component tangent to it

(b) is composed of stream lines

(c) is stream line

(d) is none of these

4.9 Select the relation that must hold if the flow is irrotaional

(a) $\dfrac{\partial u}{\partial x} + \dfrac{\partial v}{\partial y} = 0$

(b) $\dfrac{\partial u}{\partial x} = \dfrac{\partial v}{\partial y}$

(c) $\dfrac{\partial^2 u}{\partial x^2} + \dfrac{\partial^2 v}{\partial y^2} = 0$

(d) $\dfrac{\partial u}{\partial y} = \dfrac{\partial v}{\partial x}$

(e) none

4.10 Select which relation is true for irrotational flow

(a) $\dfrac{\partial \varphi}{\partial x} = \dfrac{\partial \psi}{\partial y}$

(b) $\dfrac{\partial \varphi}{\partial x} = - \dfrac{\partial \psi}{\partial y}$

(c) $\dfrac{\partial \varphi}{\partial y} = \dfrac{\partial \psi}{\partial x}$

(d) $\dfrac{\partial \varphi}{\partial x} = \dfrac{\partial \psi}{\partial y}$

(e) none

4.11 In a 2-D flow, uniform flow in X direction is given by

(a) $\varphi = x$ (b) $\varphi = -y$ (c) $\psi = x$

(d) $\varphi = y$ (e) $\psi = -y$

Problems

4.1 Prove that the 2-D continuity equation in cylindrical co-ordinates for the steady plane flow of an incompressible fluid is

$$\frac{\partial U_r}{\partial r} + \frac{U_r}{r} + \frac{1}{r}\frac{\partial U\theta}{\partial \theta} = 0$$

in which U_r is the radial component and $U\theta$ is the tangential component of velocity.

Hint: The flow is assumed to take place through an elementary area of sides $r\,d\theta$ and dr

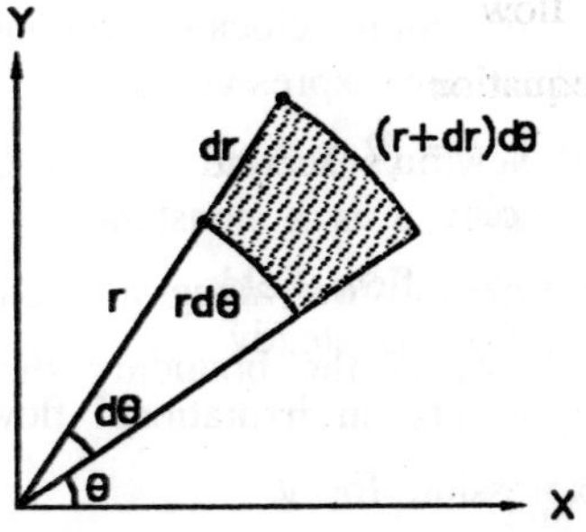

Y

FIG. 4.16. PROBLEM 4.1

4.2 In a two dimensional flow of an incompressible fluid the tangential component of velocity is given by

$$U_\theta = - C \sin\theta/r^2$$

where C is a constant. Determine U_r and the magnitude of resultant velocity.

4.3 Determine whether the flow represented by velocity components indicate irrotational flow or not ?

(a) $u = x^2 - y^2 + z^2$; $v = x^2 - 2xy - 3yz^2$; $w = x^3 + y^3 + z^3$

(b) $u = cx$; $v = cy$; $w = - 2cz$

(c) $u = Ayz/x$; $v = Azx/y$; $w = Axy/z$

(d) Two dimensional flow, $u = 2xy$; $v = x^2 - y^2$

4.4 $u = 3x^2$ and $v = 4xyz$ represent two available velocity components of a three dimensional steady flow. Find the missing component of velocity of flow.

4.5 The velocity components of the 2-D plane motion of a fluid are

$$u = (y^2 - x^2)/(x^2 + y^2)^2$$
$$v = - 2xy/(x^2 + y^2)^2$$

(a) show that the fluid is incompressible and the flow is irrotational

(b) show that the points (2,2) and $(1,2 - \sqrt{3})$ are located on the same streamline

(c) determine the discharge across a line joining the points (1,1) and (2,2); given that the thickness of the fluid stream normal to the $X - Y$ plane is 't'.

4.6 What is the irrotational velocity field associated with the velocity potential

$$\varphi = 3x^2 - 3x - 3y^2 + 16\,t^2 + 12\,tz$$

Does the flow field satisfy the incompressible continuity equation?

4.7 Determine whether the velocity field, as given below, of 2−D flow satisfies the condition of irrotationality.

(a) $u = (x + y)$; $v = (x^2 - y)$

(b) $u = f(x); v = f(y)$;   (c) $u = 0$, $v = f(x,y)$

4.8 The X and Y direction velocity components in a 2-D flow field for an incompressible fluid are expressed as

(a) $u = (x^2 + x - y^2)$, $v = (2xy + y)$

(b) $u = ax$, $v = -ay$; a is a constant

For each of the above flow fields

(a) show that the flow is steady

(b) flow field represents an irrotational flow

(c) obtain an expression for ψ

(d) also obtain an expression for φ

4.9 A two dimensional flow field is given by velocity potential function $\varphi = x^2 y - xy^2 + 1$. Derive an expression for stream function and show that each of these functions satisfies Laplace equation.

4.10 A flow field is characterised by stream function $\psi = 2xy$. Show that

(a) it represents steady flow

(b) the flow field is irrotational

(c) derive an expression for velocity components in X and Y directions. Determine the magnitude and direction of velocity vector at points $(0, -2)$ and $(2,4)$

(d) plot the streamlines $\psi = 0$, 8, 16 and try to find analogy of flow field with some practical flow case

(e) obtain an expression for velocity potential.

4.11 Show that the velocity potential $\varphi = Ax$, where A is constant, represents a possible fluid flow case. Hence, determine stream function and draw a set of streamlines and equipotential lines.

4.12 Calculate the unknown velocity components so that they satisfy the following conditions:

(a) $u = 2x^3$, $v = 2xyz$, $w = ?$

(b) $u = 2x^2 + 2xy$, $v = ?$ $w = z^3 - 4xz + 2yz$

(c) $u = ?$, $v = ax^3 - by^2cz^2$, $w = bx^3 - cy^2 + az^2x$

4.13 Check whether the following functions represent possible flow phenomenon of irrotational flow :

(a) $\varphi = x^2 - y^2 + y$ (b) $\varphi = \sin(x + y + z)$

(c) $\varphi = U \cos \theta / r$

4.14 The velocity potential $\varphi = a \cos xy$. Find the velocity components.

4.15 Given $u = (x^2 y + z^2 + 2t)$, $v = (x\dot{y} + z^2 x^2 + 2t^2)$ and $w = (4xyz - 3t)$. Find the acceleration in x- direction, at $(1,1,1)$ and $t = 1$sec. Is the flow steady. Give reasons.

Fluid Dynamics

5.1 INTRODUCTION

In the previous chapter on fluid kinematics the variation of velocity of flow with time and space co-ordinantes were studied. The change in velocity of fluid mass is produced by a set of forces. In fluid dynamics, one studies about these forces and thus it involves the principles of mass and acceleration. Two basic laws involved in it are obtained from Newton's laws of motion which will be studied here. These basic laws are

(i) conservation of energy or first law of thermodynamics and

(ii) impulse momentum equation.

The first law of motion given by Newton describes the characteristic of matter, *i.e.* inertia and the second law along with third law states that the accelerative action of a force is countered by an inertial reaction of the matter on which the force acts.

Newton's second law of motion states that the summation of all the external forces acting on a fluid mass is proportional to the product of mass and acceleration produced in the direction of forces by them. The constant of proportionality is considered to be absorbed both numerically and dimensionally by one or another quantity involved, *i.e.*

$$\Sigma F_x = M a_x \qquad \qquad ...(5.1)$$

In the solutions of problems of solid mechanics, the basic laws are applied to a fixed quantity of matter, called a system. This system may change its shape or position but contains same mass of the matter and hence, it is known as a 'closed system'. In fluid mechanics, it is convenient to focus attention on a fixed region. The fixed region is called 'control volume' and the boundary of this control volume is known as 'control surface'. The amount of matter and its position may change with time but this volume remains the same. Since the fluid is allowed to move through its boundaries, it is known as an 'open system'.

The force term in Eq. 5.1 per unit volume is referred as f. Therefore,

$$\Sigma f_x = \rho \, a_x \qquad \qquad ...(5.2)$$

The dynamical behaviour of the fluid motion is governed by a set of equations, known as equation of motion. The forces which may be involved in the fluid flow problems may be numerous. Some of these are (i) gravity force F_g (ii) pressure force F_p (iii) force due to viscosity F_v (iv) compressibility force F_e (v) Force due to turbulence F_t and (vi) surface tension force F_s. From Eq. 5.1

$$(F_g + F_p + F_v + F_c + F_s + F_t)_x = m \times a_x \qquad ...(5.3)$$

When volume chagnes are small, F_c is negligible. Usually the velocity of flow is sufficiently high and in that case F_s can also be neglected. Hence Eq. 5.3 reduces to

$$(F_g + F_p + F_v + F_t)_x = m. a_x \qquad ...(5.4)$$

Similar equations can also be written in Y and Z directions. These equations are known as 'Reynolds equations of motion'. For the flow at low values of Reynolds number, the turbulence forces are of no significance and can be neglected. Hence

$$(F_g + F_p + F_v)_x = m. a_x \qquad ...(5.5)$$

The set of equations X, Y and Z directions as in Eq. 5.5 are known as 'Navier-Stokes' equations'.

For ideal fluid flow, the fluid possesses no viscosity and hence forces due to viscosity are not present. Then Eq. 5.5 becomes

$$F_g + F_p = m. a_x \qquad ...(5.6 \text{ a})$$

Expressing the forces in terms of unit volume,

$$f_g + f_p = \rho . a_x \qquad ...(5.6 \text{ b})$$

Eq. 5.6 along with similar equations in Y and Z directions are known as 'Euler's equations of motion'. Euler's equation of motion (section 5.2) and Bernoulli's equations of motion (section 5.4) are governed by the basic law of conservation of energy.

5.2 EULER'S EQUATIONS OF MOTION

Consider a parallelopiped fluid element as shown in Fig. 5.1 having sides dx, dy and dz in the three co-ordinate directions X, Y and Z respectively. The forces acting on a fluid element are basically of two types, namely (i) body forces and (ii) surface forces.

Body forces. The body forces are external forces acting through the centriod of fluid mass, e.g. gravitational force, electromagnetic force or coriolis force due to motion of earth. Let the body force per unit mass be B. It has three components X, Y and Z in three co-ordinate directions, *i.e.*

$$B = iX + jY + kZ$$

Surface forces. The normal and the tanngential forces exerted upon a fluid element on its surface by the fluid which is in contact with it are known as surface forces.

These may be normal pressure forces acting in three co-ordinate directions and shear stresses acting on its six faces.

Referring to Fig. 5.1 the normal forces σ_x, acting in the X-directions are pressure forces p_x and $p_x + (\partial px/\partial x) \times dx$ on the two opposite faces of the fluid element $ABFE$ and $CDHG$. The shear forces acting on these faces are also shown in the figure. Here the first suffix x indicates the direction of normal on the face under consideration and second suffix y or z indicates the direction of tangential stress. Similarly, the forces acting in Y & Z direction may be marked on the other faces of fluid element.

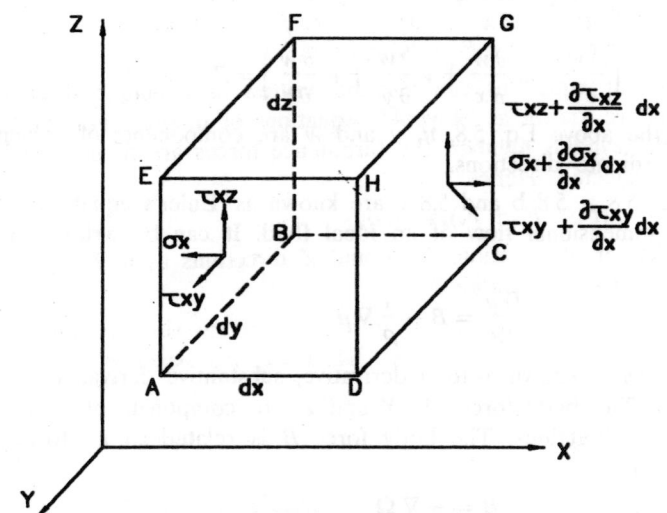

FIG. 5.1 NORMAL AND TANGENTIAL FORCES ACTING ON THE FLUID ELEMENT

The pressrue force F_p acting in X-direction

$$= p\, dy\, dz - \left(p + \frac{\partial p}{\partial x} \times dx \right) dy\, dz$$

$$= -\frac{\partial p}{\partial x} dx\, dy\, dz$$

Therefore, pressure force/unit volume acting in X- direction,

$$f_{px} = \frac{-F_{px}}{dx\, dy\, dz}$$

$$f_{px} = \frac{-\partial p}{\partial x} \qquad \qquad ...(5.7a)$$

Similarly, the pressure force/unit volume acting in Y-direction

$$f_{py} = \frac{-\partial p}{\partial y} \qquad \qquad ...(5.7b)$$

and the pressure force/unit volume acting in Z-direction

$$f_{px} = \frac{-\partial p}{\partial z} \qquad \qquad ...(5.7c)$$

In case of an ideal fluid, no viscous force acts on the fluid element; therefore, the shear forces acting in X, Y and Z directions τ_{xy} , τ_{yz} and τ_{zx}.

respectively are zero. Substituting the values of acceleration and pressure forces from Eq. 4.16 and Eq. 5.7 in Eq. 5.6, one obtains,

$$\left(\frac{\partial u}{dt} + u \frac{\partial u}{\partial x} + v \frac{\partial u}{\partial y} + w \frac{\partial u}{\partial z} \right) = X - \frac{1}{\rho} \frac{\partial p}{\partial x} \qquad ...(5.8a)$$

$$\left(\frac{\partial v}{dt} + u \frac{\partial u}{\partial x} + v \frac{\partial v}{\partial y} + w \frac{\partial v}{\partial z} \right) = Y - \frac{1}{p} \frac{\partial p}{\partial y} \qquad ...(5.8b)$$

$$\left(\frac{\partial w}{\partial t} + u \frac{\partial w}{\partial x} + v \frac{\partial w}{\partial y} + w \frac{\partial w}{\partial z} \right) = Z - \frac{1}{\rho} \frac{\partial p}{\partial z} \qquad ...(5.8c)$$

In the above Eq. 5.8, u, v and w are components of velocity in the three co-ordinate directions.

Eqs. 5.8 a, 5.8 b and 5.8 c are known as 'Euler's equations of motion' for three dimensional flow of an ideal fluid. It can be written in a vector form as

$$\frac{Du}{Dt} = B - \frac{1}{\rho} \nabla p \qquad ...(5.9)$$

DU/Dt is known as 'total derivative, substantive derivative' or Eulerian of velocity. The body forces X, Y and Z are componets of B in the three co-ordiantne directions. The body force B is related to a force potential Ω such that

$$B = -\nabla\Omega \qquad ...(5.10\ a)$$

or $\qquad (i\,X + j\,Y + k\,Z)$

$$= -\left[i \frac{\partial\Omega}{\partial x} + j \frac{\partial\Omega}{\partial y} + k \frac{\partial\Omega}{\partial z} \right] \qquad ...(5.10\ b)$$

Potential Ω is the potential energy per unit mass. Since only gravity is the body force, the potential Ω may be considered identical with gh; the work done against gravity to raise a unit mass through height h (height h is measured in Z-derection). Therefore,

$$X = 0,\ Y = 0 \qquad \text{and} \qquad Z = \partial\Omega/\partial z = -g \qquad ...(5.11)$$

The negative sign is indicative that acceleration g is acting against the direction of Z. Substituting these values in Eq. 5.8,

$$\frac{Du}{Dt} = -\frac{1}{\rho} \frac{\partial p}{\partial x} \qquad ...(5.12\ a)$$

$$\frac{Dv}{Dt} = -\frac{1}{\rho} \frac{\partial p}{\partial y} \qquad ...(5.12\ b)$$

$$\frac{Dw}{Dt} = -g - \frac{1}{\rho} \frac{\partial p}{\partial z} \qquad ...(5.12\ c)$$

As a corollary, for static fluid the velocities in three directions u, v and w are zero. Hence, Eqs. 5.12 a, b and c yield.

$$p = -wh \qquad ...(5.13)$$

5.3 EULER'S EQUATION ALONG A STREAM TUBE

Let us consider a streamtube of crosssectional area da and length ds (Fig. 5.2). The streamtube is inclined at an angle θ to the vertical. The velocity of fluid in the direction of flow is U_s and normal to it is U_n (say). The various forces acting on the fluid element are shown in Fig. 5.2.

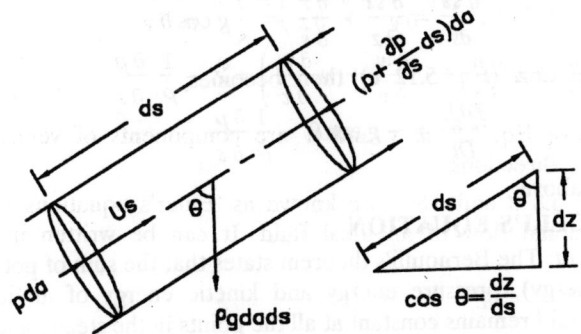

FIG. 5.2 FLOW THROUGH A STREAM TUBE

(1) *Surface force.* The pressure forces acting on its two ends are pda and $\left(p + \partial p/\partial s \, ds\right) da$. Therefore, the net pressure force acting in the direction of flow

$$= pda - \left(p + \frac{\partial p}{\partial s} ds \right) da$$

$$= - \frac{\partial p}{\partial s} ds \, da$$

The net pressure force/unit volume $= - \partial p/\partial s$ \qquad ...(5.14)

(2) *Body force.* The body force acting on the fluid element is only its self weight. Therefore, the body force acting in the direction of flow

$$F_B = - \rho g \, da \, ds \cos \theta$$

The body force/unit volume $= - \rho g \cos \theta$

But from Fig. 5.2, $\cos \theta = dz/ds$

Hence, body force/unit volume $= - \rho g \, dz/ds$ \qquad ...(5.15)

Substituting the values from Eqs. 5.14 and 5.15 into Eq. 5.6b,

$$\rho \, a_s = - \frac{\partial p}{\partial s} - \rho g \frac{dz}{ds}$$

$$a_s = - \frac{\partial}{\partial_s} (p/\rho + gz)$$ \qquad ...(5.16 a)

Similarly, the equation of motion can be written in the normal direction to the flow.

$$a_n = - \frac{\partial}{\partial_n} (p/\rho + gz)$$ \qquad ...(5.16 b)

Eqs. 5.16a and 5.16b are known as Euler's equations of motion along and normal to the streamline.

Alernatively, the same results could be obtained by usign Eq. 5.12c. The direction of flow is now S instead of Z and hence replace velocity w by U_s. The compnent of body force along the streamline is

$$\frac{\partial \Omega}{\partial s} = \frac{\partial \Omega}{\partial z} \times \frac{\partial z}{\partial s} = - \dot{g} \cos \theta$$

The relation (Eq. 5.12 c) then becomes,

$$\frac{DU_s}{Dt} = - g \cos \theta - \frac{1}{\rho} \frac{\partial p}{\partial s} \qquad \qquad ...(5.17)$$

as derived above.

5.4. BERNOULLI'S EQUATION

Statement: The Bernoulli's theorem states that the sum of potential energy (or datum energy), pressure energy and kinetic energy of an ideal and incompressible fluid remains constant at all the points in the steady and irrotational fluid flow. The Bernoulli's equation is obtained by integration of Euler's equations, Eqs. 5.16a and 5.16b.

$$\rho \, a_s = - \frac{\partial p}{\partial s} - \rho \, g \frac{dz}{ds} \qquad \qquad ...(5.16a)$$

The acceleration along streamline is given by Eqs. 4.19a

$$a_s = \frac{\partial U_s}{\partial t} + U_s \frac{\partial U_s}{\partial s}$$

For steady flow, $\partial U_s / \partial t = 0$

$$a_s = U_s \frac{\partial U_s}{\partial s} = \frac{\partial (U_s^2/2)}{\partial s} \qquad \qquad ....(4.19a)$$

Hence, $$\rho \frac{\partial (U_s^2/2)}{\partial s} = - \frac{\partial p}{\partial s} - \rho g \frac{\partial z}{\partial s} \qquad \qquad ...(5.16c)$$

Divide by ρ on both sides and multiply by ds on both sides and integrate

$$\int \frac{\partial}{\partial s}(U_s^2/2)ds = - \int \frac{\partial}{\partial s} (p/\rho) \, ds - \int g \frac{\partial z}{\partial s} ds + c$$

or $$\frac{U_s^2}{2} + \int \frac{dp}{\rho} + gz = c \qquad \qquad ...(5.18)$$

The equation is valid for steady flow of compressible fluid. For incompressible fluid, mass density ρ is constant. Eqs. 5.18 then becomes,

$$\frac{U_s^2}{2} + \frac{p}{\rho} + gz = c \qquad \qquad ...(5.19)$$

Eq. 5.19 is valid along streamlines. The values of constant c is different for various streamlines. Now, consider Eq. 5.16b

Divide by ρ on both sides and multiply by ds on both sides and integrate

$$\rho a_n = -\frac{\partial p}{\partial n} - \rho g \frac{\partial z}{\partial n} \qquad \qquad ...(5.16b)$$

The acceleration, a_n is given by Eq. 4.19 b.

$$a_n = \frac{\partial U_n}{\partial t} + U_s \frac{\partial U_n}{\partial s} \qquad \qquad ...(4.19b)$$

For steady flow, $\qquad a_n = U_s \, \partial U_n / \partial s$

Eq. 5.16b then becomes

$$\rho U_s \frac{\partial U_n}{\partial s} = -\frac{\partial p}{\partial n} - \rho g \frac{\partial z}{\partial n} \qquad \qquad ...(5.16d)$$

This equation cannot be integrated directly. Therefore, subtract $\rho U_s \dfrac{\partial U_s}{\partial n}$ from both sides and simplify

$$\rho U_s \left(\frac{\partial U_n}{\partial s} - \frac{\partial U_s}{\partial n} \right)$$

$$= -\frac{\partial p}{\partial n} - \rho g \frac{\partial z}{\partial n} - \rho U_s \frac{\partial U_s}{\partial n} \qquad ...(5.20)$$

The term on left side is the vorticity of flow. For irrotational flow the vorticity should be zero. Therefore, Eq. 5.20 simplifies to

$$\frac{\partial}{\partial n} \frac{(U_s^2)}{2} + \frac{\partial (p/\rho)}{\partial n} + g \frac{\partial z}{\partial s} = 0 \qquad ...(5.21)$$

Integrating Eq. 5.21 in the normal direction

$$\frac{U_s^2}{2} + \int \frac{dp}{\rho} + gz = c_1 \qquad \qquad ...(5.22)$$

For incompressible fluid, ρ is constant and hence,

$$\frac{U_s^2}{2} + \frac{p}{\rho} + gz = c_1 \qquad \qquad ...(5.23a)$$

Eq. 5.23 is valid along all lines normal to the stream lines. The constant c_1 may vary from one line to another. From Eqs. 5.19 and 5.22, it is observed that both relations are similar whereas one is valid along a streamline and another along a normal line. This means that either Eq. 5.19 or Eq. 5.23 is applicable to the points in the flow with following limitations.

Limitations of Bernoulli's equation.

(1) The fluid is ideal and nonviscous.

(2) The fluid is incompressible.

(3) The fluid flow is steady.

(4) The fluid flow is irrotational.

Eq. 5.19 may be written in different forms.

$$\frac{p}{\rho} + gz + \frac{U^2}{2} = c_1 \qquad \qquad ...(5.23a)$$

$$\frac{p}{w} + z + \frac{U^2}{2g} = c_2 \qquad \text{...(5.23b)}$$

$$p + wz + \frac{\rho U^2}{2} = c_3 \qquad \text{...(5.23c)}$$

Each term of Eq. 5.23a expresses the energy of unit mass of fluid, *i.e.*, in terms of N m/kg or J/kg whereas Eq. 5.23b expresses the energies as per unit weight or N m/N or simply metre. Eq. 5.23b is widely used for liquids with free surface. The last equation Eq. 5.23c represents the energy per unit volume or N m/m³ and is convenient to use for compressible gases. Since the specific weight of gases are small, the term wz in Eq. 5.23 c may be dropped. Then, the eqn. 5.23c reduces to

$$p + \frac{\rho U^2}{2} = c_3 \qquad \text{...(5.24)}$$

1. Significance of various terms

Each of the terms of the Bernoulli's equation represents a form of energy. The term z is known as potential energy (P.E.) of the unit weight of the fluid. If a weight W is placed at a height z above an arbitrary datum (or a reference line), it has a capacity to do work which is equal to Wz. Therefore, the potential energy per unit weight is equal to $Wz/W = z$ N m/N or z metre of fluid. Since this form of energy is due to the displacement of force, it is termed as 'potential energy'. It is also termed as 'datum head'.

The second term of Bernoulli's equation is p/w which represents pressure energy. It is also known as 'flow work'. It is defined as the work that a fluid is capable of doing by virtue of sustained pressure. Consider a fluid element of cross sectional area dA over which a sustained pressure p acts in the direction of flow. While the fluid element moves a distance ds, the work done by pressure is $pdAds$. The work done per unit weight of the fluid is

$$\frac{PdA\,ds}{w\,dA\,ds}$$

or   p/w $N m/N$ or metre of fluid.

The third term $U^2/2g$ is the kinetic energy (K.E.) of the unit weight of fluid. Consider a fluid element of weight W (or mass m) moving with a velocity U in the direction of flow. The kinetic energy of this fluid element is m $U^2/2 = W/g\,U^2/2$. This means that kinetic energy per unit weight is $\frac{W U^2}{2g}/W = U^2/2g$ Nm/N or metre of fluid.

The sum of potential, pressure and kinetic energies is called the 'total energy'. Thus, the Eq. 5.23 states that the total energy at all points in a steady flow field of an ideal incompressible fluid remains constant. It is the well known Bernoulli's theorem. It can be written between two sections as

$$\frac{p_1}{w_1} + z_1 + \frac{U_1^2}{2g} = \frac{p_2}{w_2} + z_2 + \frac{U_2^2}{2g} \qquad \qquad ...(5.25)$$

2. Kinetic energy correction factor

For an ideal fluid, the velocity of flow remains same throughout the cross section and its kinetic energy is determined easily. In case of a real fluid, the velocity varies from one point to another, hence, one should know the velocity distribution in the given cross section to determine the kinetic energy.

Consider a pipe of cross sectional area A in Fig. 5.3 which carries discharge Q. Let us take one of the streamtube of area dA of this pipe flow. The velocity of flow through the stream tube is u.

Kinetic energy of fluid flow in the stream tube $= \rho u . dA$

$$\frac{u^2}{2} = \rho u^3 dA/2.$$

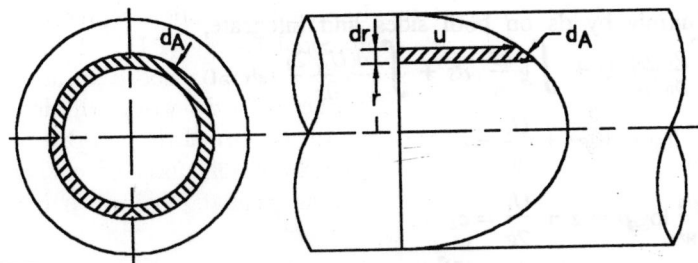

FIG. 5.3. VELOCITY DISTRIBUTION IN A PIPE

Integrate it over the whole area of the pipe. Total kinetic energy of fluid passing per unit time

$$= \int_A \frac{\rho u^3 dA}{2} \qquad \qquad ...(5.26a)$$

However, in most of the engineering problems, it is easy to deal with mean velocity of flow U. Therefore, the kinetic energy of the fluid passing per unit time $= \alpha \rho U^3 A/2$ \qquad ...(5.26b)

These two expressions may be related as

$$\alpha \rho U^3 A/2 = \int_A \frac{\rho u^3 dA}{2}$$

$$\alpha = \int_A \frac{u^3 dA}{U^3 A} \qquad \qquad ...(5.27)$$

The multiplying factor α is known as coefficient of 'kinetic energy or coriolis coefficient'. Its value is always found greater then 1.0 and depends on the velocity distribution of the flow. The value of α varies from 1.0 to

2.0; being higher for laminar flow than for turbulent flow. Since the velocity distribution for turbulent flow is logarithmic the value of α tends to be unity.

5.5 BERNOULLI'S EQUATION FOR COMPRESSIBLE FLUIDS

Two flow cases for compressible fluid are discussed below. These are (1) Isothermal flow and (2) Isentropic flow.

(1) *Isothermal flow*. For this case, Boyle's law for gases is applicable, i.e.,

$$\frac{p}{\rho} = \frac{p_0}{\rho_0}$$

$$\frac{1}{\rho} = \frac{p_0}{\rho_0} \frac{1}{p} \qquad \qquad ...(5.28)$$

Substitute the value of $1/\rho$ into Eq. 5.16a

$$\frac{p_0}{\rho_0} \frac{1}{p} \frac{\partial p}{\partial s} + g \frac{\partial z}{\partial s} + \frac{\partial (U_s^2/2)}{\partial s} = 0$$

Multiply by ds on both sides and integrate,

$$\int \frac{p_0}{\rho_0} \frac{dp}{p} ds + \int g \frac{\partial z}{\partial s} \cdot ds + \int \frac{\partial (U_s^2/2)}{\partial s} \cdot ds = 0$$

$$\frac{p_0}{\rho_0} \log_e p + gz + \frac{U_s^2}{2g} = c_1$$

$$\frac{p_0}{w} \log_e p + z + \frac{U_s^2}{2g} = c_2$$

$$\frac{p_0}{\rho_0} \log_e p + gz + \frac{U_s^2}{2} = c_1$$

$$= \frac{p_0}{w_0} \log_e p_2 + z_2 + \frac{U_2^2}{2} \qquad \qquad ...(5.29)$$

(2) *Isentropic flow*: In this case, the relationship between p and ρ is given by

$$p/\rho^k = p_0/\rho_0^k = c$$

Again substitute the value of $1/\rho$ in Eq. 5.16a

$$\frac{1}{\rho_0} \left(\frac{p_0}{p} \right)^{1/n} \frac{dp}{ds} + g \frac{dz}{ds} + \frac{d (U_s^2/2)}{ds} = 0$$

Multiply by ds on both sides and integrate

$$\frac{p_0^{1/n}}{\rho_0} \frac{n}{n-1} p^{\frac{n-1}{n}} + gz + \frac{U_s^2}{2} = c \qquad \qquad ...(5.3a)$$

Simplying between any two points 1 and 2

$$\frac{n}{n-1} \frac{p_1}{\rho_1} + gz_1 + \frac{U_{s1}^2}{2g}$$

$$= \frac{n}{n-1} \frac{p_2}{\rho_2} + gz_2 + \frac{U_{s2}^2}{2g} \qquad \qquad ...(5.30b)$$

For relatively small difference in elevations $(z_2 - z_1)$, the variation in potential energy for gases is insignificant. Therefore, Eq. 5.30b reduces to.

$$\frac{n}{n-1}\frac{p_1}{\rho_1} + U_1^2/2g$$

$$= \frac{n}{n-1}\frac{p_0}{\rho_0} + U_{s2}^2/2g$$

5.6 GENERAL FORM OF BERNOULLI'S EQUATION

The general form of Bernoulli's equation for the fluid flow is essentially a complete account of work done on the fluid, heat flow into or out of fluid system and resulting change in energies of the fluid.

The energy contained by the fluid particles may be recognised as (a) stored energy and (b) energy in transit or flow energy.

1. Stored energy

Among the various forms of stored energy, (a) the kinetic energy (b) the potential energy and (c) the internal energy of the fluid are important and hence these are only included in the general energy equation. The various forms of energy per unit weight are considered in the following treatment,.

(a) Kinetic energy (K.E.) of unit weight of fluid

$$= \frac{1}{2}\alpha m \, U^2/mg.$$

$$= \alpha \, U^2/2g \qquad \qquad ...(5.31a)$$

(b) Potential energy (P.E) of unit weight of fluid z metre above arbitrary reference datum $= (1/mg) Wz = z$ \qquad ...(5.14b)

(c) Internal Energy (I.E.) of fluid is partly in the form of K.E. produced by the random motion of the individual fluid particles and partly in the form of potential energy of fluid molecules due to relative positions of individual molecules and is written as I.

Internal energy/unit weight $= I$ \qquad ...(5.31c)

2. Energy in transit

The other class of energies is the energy in transit.

(a) The heat energy and the work done by pressure and shear are the energies in transit. The heat energy flows from higher temperature to lower temperature and is expressed in Joule.

Heat energy/unit weight $= e_H$ \qquad ....(5.31d)

(b) When the fluid flows, it either does work on the control surface through its pressure and shear stress or the control surface does work on the fluid. The mechanical work is transferred to the fluid or from the fluid by means of shaft (which is the main moving element of a pump or a turbine unit). The work done by shear forces on a control surface of properly chosen control volume reduces to zero and hence net work done by the pressure forces per unit weight of fluid on the control surface in moving a small distance δL

$$-\Delta p\, \delta A\, \delta L/w\, \delta A\, \delta L = \Delta p/w^{\bullet} \quad ...(5.31e)$$

(c) Also mechanical work done/unit weight $= e_M$ ....(5.31f)

Let us consider the fluid volume bounded by a streamtube (Fig. 5.4). The average velocities of flow at section 1 and 2 are U_1 and U_2 and the pressure of fluid at the respective sections are p_1 and p_2. In an infinitesimal time interval dt, the fluid in the control volume 1 1 2 2 moves to $1'\, 1'\, 2'\, 2'$. Therefore,

Energy of fluid at $1'\, 1'\, 2'\, 2'$ at time t_2 − Energy of fluid at 1 1 2 2 at time t_1

= work done on the fluid in time interval dt

± heat energy transferred ...(5.32)

For steady flow, the velocity and pressure of the fluid in the region $1'\, 1'\, 2\, 2$ remains invariant.

The energy of $2\, 2\, 2'\, 2'$ at t_2 - energy of $1\, 1\, 1'\, 1'$ at time t_1 = work done on fluid in time dt ± heat transfer in transit.

Substituting for various terms from Eq. 5.32

$$d\,(P.E) + d\,(K.E.) + d\,(I.E)$$

$$= d\,(\text{flow work}) \pm d\,(\text{Mech.work}) \pm d\,(\text{Head energy})$$

or $$(z_2 - z_1) + \alpha\,\frac{(U_2^2 - U_1^2)}{2g} + (I_2 - I_1)$$

$$= \frac{p_1 - p_2}{w} \pm e_M \pm e_H \quad ...(5.33)$$

In the above equation, e_M and e_H are mechanical and heat energies of fluid.

The above Eq. 5.33 is known as 'general energy equation' and is applicable to compressible and incompressible fluids. If no heat is supplied to the fluid from outside the boundary or from the fluid, e_H is zero. Also if no machine has been interposed between sections 1 and 2, the mechanical work e_M is also zero. For incompressible fluid, p_1 is equal to p_2 and for ideal fluid, the internal energy remains invariant. Thus Eq. 5.33 reduces to

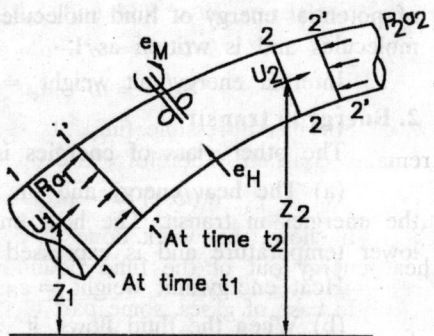

FIG. 5.4 CHANGE OF ENERGY OF FLOWING FLUID

$$p_2/w + z_2 + \alpha\, U_2^2/2g = p_1/w_1 + z_1 + \alpha\, U_1^2/2g$$

which is Bernoulli's equation, Eq. 5.25. also known as equation of motion for the flowing fluid. Thus Bernoulli's equation is a special form of energy equation which is applicable to ideal fluid and assume no transfer of heat energy from this fluid, Further, no mechanical work is added or substracted from it.

5.7 BERNOULLI'S EQUATION FOR A REAL FLUID

The real fluid possesses the viscosity and hence, the Bernoulli's equation need to be modified to include the effect of viscosity. The fluid viscosity causes the resistance to flow and produces eddies and turbulence. All these forms of energy are eventually transferred in to thermal energy. Part of this thermal energy is transformed out of flow system and part of it increases the internal energy of the fluid (it is insulated) and thereby the temperature of fluid is increased. For non- insulated flow system, the internal energy remains same and whole of the thermal energy produced due to the effect of viscosity flow out of the fluid boundaries and it is non-recoverable as useful energy, This non- recoverable energy is termed as 'loss of useful energy.

Eq. 5.25 and Eq. 5.33 are written in the differential form and compared. Eq. 5.25 for ideal fluid is

$$\frac{dp}{w} + dz + d\,(U^2/2g) = 0$$

When the effect of visocity or friction is also included,

$$\frac{dp}{w} + dz + \frac{UdU}{g} + d\,(loss) = 0 \qquad \qquad ...(5.34)$$

The energy equation Eq. 5.33 is

$$d\,(p/w) + dz + (UdU/g) + dI = de_1 + de_H \qquad ...(5.35)$$

If no mechanical energy is added or subsracted, the Eq. 5.35 is written as

$$pd\,(1/w) + dp/w + dz + UdU/g + dI = d_{eH} \qquad ...(5.36)$$

Comparing Eqs. 5.34 and 5.36,

$$d\,(loss) = dI - d_{eH} + pd\,(1/w)$$
$$= dI - d_{eH} + pdv/\rho$$

For incompressible fluid, its specific weight w and its internal energy remains constant. Therefore, the energy loss becomes

$$d\,(loss) = -d_{eH}$$

It shows that work done to overcome the friction causes the flow of heat energy out of the fluid boundaries, i.e. $-d_{eH}$.

In case of gases, some part of the work done is utilised in the increase of specific volume of the fluid and is equal to $(p/\rho)\,dv$

Thus Bernoulli's equation for real fluid between two point is written as

$$H = p_1/w + z_1 + U_1^2/2g \pm e_M = p_2/w + z_2 + U_2^2/2g + h_L$$
$$= constant \qquad \qquad ...(5.37)$$

It states that the sum of potential energy, z, pressure energy p/w and velocity energy or kinetic energy, $U^2/2g$, all expressed in terms of Nm/N of fluid or metre of flowing fluid at any section remains constant, provided adjustment for loss or addition of energies between these section is made. Most of the flow in the nature are turbulent flow and hence α is assumed as unity.

It is to be remembered that the potential energy has been measured with reference to an arbitary datum and hence, will change with the change of datum line. Moreover, in a flowing fluid from one section to another, the loss of energy also expressed in terms of Nm/N of fluid or metre of fluid written as h_L is subtracted from energy at section 1 Similarly if some machine is placed between section 1 and 2, which supplies the energy e_M to the flowing fluid, than e_M is added to the energy at section 1, e.g. a pump. If it draws the energy from the fluid, e.g. a turbine. e_M is subtracted from it. If there is no machine between section 1 and 2 e_M zero.

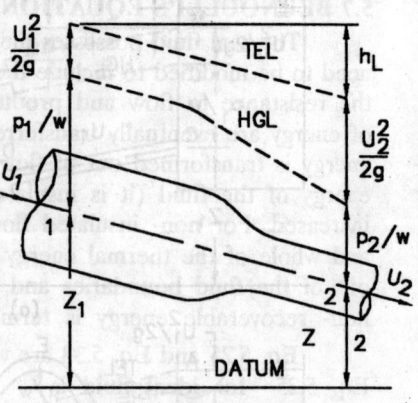

FIG. 5.5 GRAPHICAL REEPRESENTA-TION OF MODIFIED BERNOULLI'S EQUATION

The sum of $p/w + z$ is known as the 'piezometric head' and the line joining piezometric head between consecutive section is known as hydraulic gradient line, H.G.L. (Fig. 5.5).

The line drawn by joining the points representing total energy at successive sections is known as total energy line T.E.L. The slope of energy line is equal to the rate of energy loss and is given by

Energy gradient $= h_L/L$

$$i = \frac{H_1 - H_2}{L}$$

5.8 GRAPHICAL REPRESENTATION OF PRESSURE ENERGY AND TOTAL ENERGY

Let us consider the liquid flowing from reservoir A to reservoir B which are connected by pipe CDE in Fig. 5.6a. If a piezometric tube be erected at C, the liquid will rise to a height CC' equal to the pressure head at that point. If the end of the pipe were closed so that no flow takes place, the height of this column would be then CM. The drop from M to C' is due to two factors; namely (i) parital conversion of pressure head into velocity head and (ii) loss on energy at the entrance to pipe and friction loss from A to C. If a number of piezometric tubes are erected along the pipe, the liquid would rise into them to various levels, The line joining the top level of water columns in the piezometric tubes is known as a 'hydraulic energy line' or HGL. It represents the variation of pressure energy along the pipe (or flow channel). If Fig. 5.6a, the diameter of pipe increases at D and hence the pressure is higher in the pipe segment DE and therefore, the HGL rises in this segment. In Fig 5.6b, a siphon pipe has been shown connecting these

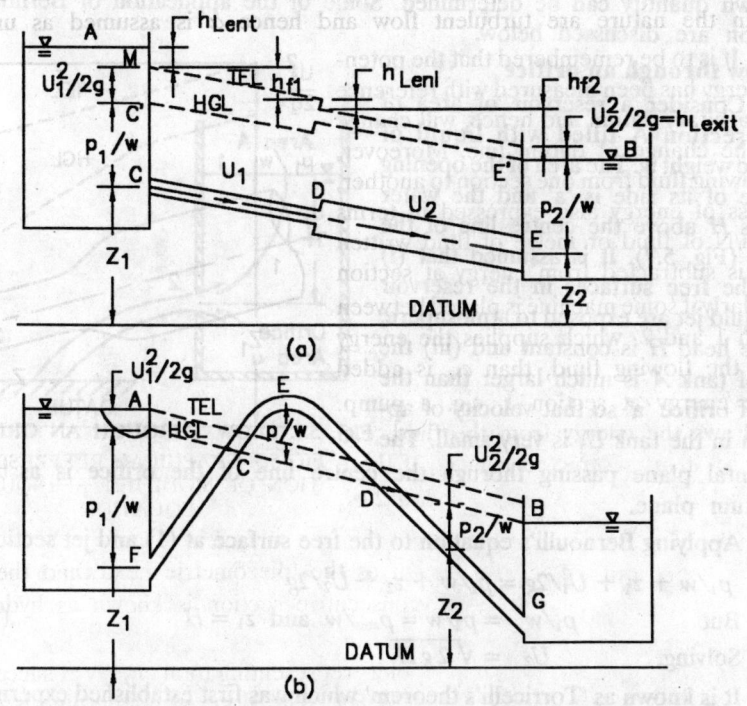

FIG. 6. HYDRAULIC GRADIENT LINE AND TOTAL ENERGY LINE.

two reservoirs A and B. The hydraulic gradient line is drawn in the same way. It is to be noted that the pressure head (or the intercept between pipe centreline and HGL) in the segment FC is reducing in the direction of flow. The pressure is zero at C and D where the pipe centreline intersects the HGL. Between C and D, the pipe rises above HGL and hence, the pressure becomes lower than atmospheric or it is negative. Thus, wherever a pipe lies above HGL, the pressure can be taken as negative

In Fig. 5.6a, the velocities of water through CD and DE are U_1 and U_2 respectively. The addition of ordinate $U_1^2/2g$ to HGL at any section represents the total energy at that section of pipe segment CD. The line joining all such points is known as the 'total energy line' or TEL. Similarly TEL can be drawn for pipe segment DE. Alternatively, if values of head loss h_L are laid off below the horizontal line through point A, the resulting line represents values of total energy H measured above any arbitrary datum plane. Indeed, the slope of TEL is the rate of loss of energy in the direction of flow which will always drop in the direction of flow (unlike HGL which may rise intermediately) unless some energy supplying device is interposed at any section of pipeline.

5.9 APPLICATIONS OF BERNOULLI'S EQUATION

For irrotational flow of an incompressible fluid, the Bernoulli's equation may be applied over the flow field alongwith the continuity equation and hence unknown quantity can be determined. Some of the application of Bernoulli's equation are discussed below.

1. Flow through an orifice

Consider a reservoir of area of cross section A filled with liquid of specific weight w. The area of the opening on one of its side is 'a' and the water level is H above the centre line of the orifice (Fig. 5.7). It is assumed that (i) both the free surfaces in the reservoir and liquid jet are exposed to atmoshpere, (ii) the head H is constant and (iii) the area of tank A is much larger than the area of orifice 'a' so that velocity of approach in the tank U_1 is very small. The horizontal plane passing thorugh the centre line of the orifice is assumed as datum plane.

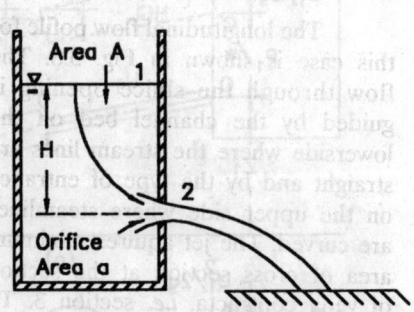

FIG. 5.7. FLOW THROUGH AN ORIFICE

Applying Bernoulli's equation to the free surface at (1) and jet section(2)

$$p_1/w + z_1 + U_1^2/2g = p_2/w + z_2 + U_2^2/2g$$

But $\qquad p_1/w = p_2/w = p_{stm}/w$ and $z_1 = H$ $\qquad$ ...(5.39)

Solving, $\qquad U_2 = \sqrt{2gH}$

It is known as 'Torricelli's theorem' which was first established experimentally in 1643.

The following points should be noted.

(1) The streamlines approaching the orifice are first curved. Then they become parallel and later become curved again in the opposite direction while falling freely.

(2) The velocity of flow through all the points of section 2 remains invariant due to parallel streamlines.

(3) The pressure, therefore, remains invariant at all points of section2.

(4) The pressure is atmoshperic on the outer boundary of the section2.

(5) Hence the pressure remains atmoshperic at all points of this section, including at its centre (as used in Eq. 5.39). This section is known as 'the section of vena contracta', the area of jet at this cross section is minimum. It lies approximately at a distance of half the diameter of the opening (from u/s face).

Further details of orifices and mouthpieces are discussed in chapter 13.

2. Flow under a sluice gate

Consider a wide open channel in which a sharp edged sluice gate is fixed. The width of opening is 'b' at section 2. The liquid with a depth y_1

approaches the section 2 with a velocity U_1 and attains a nearly zero velocity at the liquid surface. The depth in turn will increase to y_2

The longitudinal flow pofile for this case is shown in Fig. 5.8. The flow through the sluice opening is guided by the channel bed on the lowerside where the stream lines are straight and by the type of entrance on the upper side where steamlines are curved. The jet aquires minimum area of cross section at the section

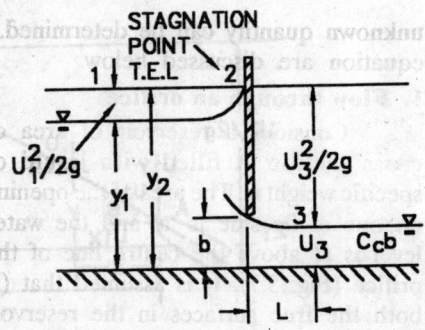

FIG. 5.8. FLOW UNDER A SLUICE GATE

of vena contracta, *i.e.* section 3. The ratio of the area of section 3 and the area of the opening is defined as the coefficient of contraction C_c. The upstream depth y_1 should be three times the width of opening for the flow to be free of vortices and eddies.

Applying Bernoulli's equations between sections 1 and 3,

$$y_1 + \frac{U_1^2}{2g} = C_c \times b + \frac{U_3^2}{2g} \qquad ...(5.40)$$

neglecting the loss of energy between section 1 and 3.

Using continuity equation

$$q = U_1 y_1 = C_c \times b \times U_3 \qquad ...(5.41)$$

where q is the discharge per unit width of the channel.

Solving Eqs. 5.40 and 5.41, the unknown quantity can be determined.

Appling Bernoulli's equation to section 1 and 2,

$$y_1 + \frac{U_1^2}{2g} = y_2$$

$$(y_2 - y_1) = U_1^2 / 2g \qquad ...(5.42)$$

The water level will rise by $(y_2 - y_1)$ behind the gate.

3. Geometry of liquid jet

Consider the jet of liquid issuing from a nozzle as shown in Fig. 5.9 with a veloicity U_1. The jet follows a curvilinear path under the influence of gravity and the pressure intensity at every poinnt of the jet is atmoshperic (or zero gauge). The vertical distance are measured above a reference horizontal plane passing through point D. The velocity of jet at any point, U, can be resolved into horizontal and vertical componens,

$$U_x = U \cos\theta \qquad ...(5.43a)$$

$$U_y = U \sin\theta \qquad ...(5.43b)$$

The horizontal accedleration at any point is given by Eq. 4.16

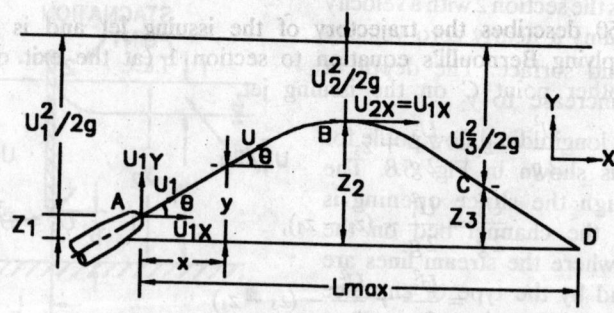

FIG. 5.9. GEOMETRY OF A LIQUID JET

$$a_x = \frac{dU_x}{dt} = 0 \qquad ...(5.44a)$$

Since, there is no horizontal acceleration a_x acting on the jet $(a_x = 0)$.

$$a_y = \frac{dU_y}{dt} = -g \qquad ...(5.44b)$$

Integrating Eqs. 5.44a and 5.44b,

U_x = constant

$$U_y = -g.t + \text{constant} \qquad ...(5.45b)$$

At $\qquad t = 0$, $U_x = U_{lx}$ and $U_y = U_{ly}$ $\qquad ...(5.45b)$

Substituting these values,

$$U_x = U_{lx} \qquad ...(5.46a)$$
$$U_y = U_{ly} - gt \qquad ...(5.46b)$$

The velocity vector can now be expressed as

$$U_x = dx/dt \qquad ...(5.47a)$$
$$U_y = dy/dt \qquad ...(5.47b)$$

Integration of Eqs. 5.47a and 5.47b results in Eqs. 5.48a and 5.48b,

$$x = U_{lx}.t + \text{constant} \qquad ...(5.48a)$$

$$y = U_{ly} \times t - \frac{1}{2}gt^2 + \text{constant} \qquad ...(5.48b)$$

At $t = 0$, $\qquad x = 0$, $\quad y = z_1$. Therefore,

$$x = U_1.t \qquad ...(5.49a)$$

$$y = U_1y.t - \frac{1}{2}gt^2 + z_1 \qquad ...(5.49b)$$

Eliminating t from Eqs. 5.49a and 5.49b,

$$(y - z_1) = \left[\frac{U_1y}{U_1x}x - \frac{gx^2}{2U_{lx}^2} \right] \qquad ...(5.50)$$

Eq. 5.50 describes the trajectory of the issuing jet and is parabolic in shape. Applying Bernoulli's equation to section 1 (at the exit of nozzle) and at any other point C on the issuing jet,

$$\frac{U_1^2}{2g} + z_1 = \frac{U_3^2}{2g} + z_3$$

$$\frac{U_3^2}{2g} = \frac{U_1^2}{2g} - (z_3 - z_1), \qquad \left(\because U_1^2 = U_{1x}^2 + U_{1y}^2 \right)$$

$$= \frac{U_{1x}^2}{2g} + \frac{U_{1y}^2}{2g} - (z_3 - z_1) \qquad \ldots(5.51a)$$

At point 2, Eq. 5.51a becomes

$$\frac{U_2^2}{2g} = \frac{U_{1x}^2}{2g} + \frac{U_{1y}^2}{2g} - (z_2 - z_1) \qquad \ldots(5.51b)$$

The vertical component of velocity at point 2 (or B) is zero. Therefore $U_2 = U_{2x} = U_{1x}$. Hence

$$(z_2 - z_1) = h_{max} = \frac{U_{1y}^2}{2g} \qquad \ldots(5.52)$$

This point of maximum height B lies $U_{1x}^2/2g$ below the total energy line (see Fig. 5.9).

The time required by a fluid particle to reach this maximum height is t (say). Then, from Eq. 5.46b

$$0 = U_1 y - gt$$

$$t = \frac{U_1 y}{g} \qquad \ldots(5.53)$$

Further, the maximum distance travelled by a fluid element in the horizontal direction is given by

$$L_{max} = \frac{U_1^2 \sin 2\theta}{g} \qquad \ldots(5.54)$$

5.10 IMPULSE MOMENTUM EQUATION

1. Dynamic force

Whenever the velocity of a stream is changed either in direction or in magnitude, a force is required to bring this change. By the Newton's third law of motion, an equal and opposite force is exerted by the fluid upon the body producing this velocity change. This is called a dynamic force to distinguish it from the forces due to hydrostatic pressures.

2. Impulse momentum equation

This is also called conservation of momentum equation. Newton's second law expresses the relation between the force F and the acceleration 'a' brought by it into a mass m.

$$F = ma = m \frac{dU}{dt}$$

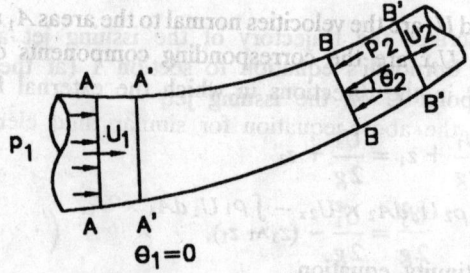

FIG. 5.10. CHANGES IN MOMENTUM OF FLUID MASS

$$Fdt = mdU \qquad \qquad ...(5.55)$$

The term on left hand side is the impulse and the term on the right hand side represents the change in momentum. Hence momentum equation states that the impulse of a force F acting over a short time interval dt is equal to the resulting change in momentum of the body in the direction of force.

The force exerted on a pipe bend, the reaction of a jet, the analysis of flow in a hydraulic jump and the force exerted on turbine blade are some of the well known applications of momentum equation.

Although energy equation and momentum equation are derived from the Newton's second law of motion, they are independent and can be applied to fluid flow separately. The application of energy equation requires prior knowledge of various losses (of frictional or otherwise) occurring between the two sections. The momentum equation just needs the knowledge of bulk characteristics of flow at the boundary of the flow. The only requirement is that the Newton's second law of motion should be applicable to the flow. The internal forces between any two mass particles remain in equilibrium as per the third law of motion. Hence the summation of unbalanced forces acting on the control surface are to be accounted for in Eq. 5.55.

Consider the free body of the fluid bounded by AABB at any instant of time t. After an interval of time dt, (say at time t_1), it occupies the position of $A'A'B'B'$. The velocities and pressure at these sections are shown in the Fig. 5.10.

The change in momentum in time dt of the mass of fluid AABB

= Momentum of fluid $A'A'B'B'$ at time t_1 − momentum of fluid $AABB$

at time t.   ...(5.56)

For steady flow, the velocity and mass density of the fluid do not change with time and hence the momentum of the mass bounded by $A'A'BB$ which is common to both the terms on right hand side of the Eq. 5.56, does not change with time. Hence the rate of change of momentum is given by

$$\frac{d M_x}{dt} = \rho_2 U_2 dA_2 \times U_{2x} - \rho_1 U_1 d A_1 \times U_{1x}$$

Here U_1 and U_2 are the velocities normal to the areas A_1 and A_2 respectively, whereas U_1x and U_2x are the corresponding components of the velocities at sections A and B in the directions in which the external forces are applied.

Integrating the above equation for similar fluid elements in the given fluid mass,

$$\frac{\Sigma\, d\, M_x}{dt} = \int_{A_2} \rho_2\, U_2\, dA_2 \times U_{2x} - \int_{A_1} \rho_1\, U_1\, dA_1 \times U_{1x}$$

From continuity equation,

$$\int_{A_2} \rho_2\, U_2\, dA_2 = \int_{A_1} \rho_1\, U_1\, dA_1 = Q$$

The mass density remains invariant for incompressible fluid. Therefore,

$$\frac{\Sigma\, d\, M_x}{dt} = \rho\, Q\, (U_{2x} - U_{1x}) \qquad \ldots(5.57)$$

Basically, the summation of all the external forces acting on the control volume in any direction is equal to the rate of change of momentum in the same direction (Eq. 5.55), hence

$$\Sigma\, F_1 x = \rho\, Q\, (U_{2x} - U_{1x}) \qquad \ldots(5.58a)$$

It is the force exerted by the body on the fluid element. By Newton's third law of motion, the fluid will exert a force on the body equal in magnitude and opposite in direction. Thus,

$$\Sigma\, Fx = -\Sigma\, F_{1x} = \rho\, Q\, (U_{1x} - U_{2x})$$
$$= \rho\, Q\, (U_1 \cos\theta_1 - U_2 \cos\theta_2) \qquad \ldots(5.58b)$$

Similarly, the expression in Y and Z directions may be written as

$$\Sigma\, F_y = \rho\, Q\, (U_{1y} - U_{2y}) \qquad .(5.58c)$$

and
$$\Sigma\, F_z = \rho\, Q\, (U_{1z} - U_{2z}) \qquad \ldots(5.58d)$$

In these expressions, the term $\rho\, QU$ is known as 'momentum flux' and may be considered to be a fictitious force which has magnitude, direction and position. The magnitude of the fictitious force at any section is expressed as $\rho\, Q\, U$, its direction is the same as that of velocity U and it acts through the centre of the flow cross section.

The external forces acting on the control volume are (i) the fluid pressure acting at the end sections, (ii) the body force acting on the control volume or its own self weight and (iii) the reactions acting at periphery of the control volume. The fluid pressure acting at the inlet and outlet sections of the control volume (e.g. a pipe bend, a channel section, etc.) and the body force, *i.e.* self weight of the fluid in the control volume may be determined from the flow configuration. Hence the reactions, which are generally unknown, may be determined from Eq. 5.58.

3. Momentum correction factor

If the velocity across a section is not uniform, the actual momentum transferred through this section is found to be greater than that computed by using mean velocity of flow. Consider a stream tube of area dA. let the velocity of flow through it be u.

The momentum transferred across it $= \rho u \, dA \times u$

$$= \rho u^2 \, dA$$

Therefore, the momentum transferred across the whole cross section A

$$= \int_A \rho u^2 \, dA$$

The momentum transferred across the section using mean velocity is $= \rho U^2 A$

Hence, momentum correction factor β is given by

$$\beta = \frac{\int_A \rho u^2 \, dA}{\rho U^2 A}$$

$$\beta = \frac{\int_A u^2 \, dA}{U^2 A} \qquad \qquad ...(5.59)$$

For incompressible flow, β is also known as 'Boussinesq coefficient'. Its value for laminar flow occurring in a circular pipe is 1.334 whereas for turbulent flow it varies from 1.005 to 1.05. Its value is found greater for the channel flows than for pipe flows. Unless otherwise given, β is taken unity.

5.11 APPLICATION OF MOMENTUM EQUATION

The momentum equation, alongwith energy equation, continuity equation and equation of state are basic fluid mechanics relations which can be used to solve various flow problems. Primarily, the two approaches (using energy equation and/or momentum equation) differ in the following aspects.

(1) Each term of the energy equation is a scaler whereas the momentum equation represents vector quantities.

(2) Energy equation describes the conservation of energy and average changes in the energy along the passage of flow whereas momentum equation relates overall external forces acting on the control surface and weight of the fluid in the control volume.

(3) Momentum equation does not require the prior knowledge of the energy loss occurring between the bounding surfaces; only the average velocity of flow and the external forces acting on the boundaries are required to be known.

Some of the flow problems using momentum equation are discussed below.

1. Thrust on a pipe bend

Consider a control volume of fluid of mass density ρ between section 1 and 2 of a pipe bend in Fig. 5.11. The forces acting on it are (i) fluid pressures p_1 and p_2 acting at the centre of sections, (ii) its self weight W acting vertically downward through the centre of gravity of the fluid in the control volume and (iii) the reaction R exerted by the bend in the opposite direction to that of resultant external forces acting on the control volume.

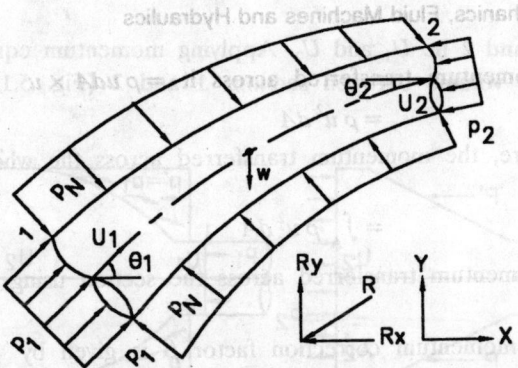

FIG. 5.11. FORCES ACTING ON A PIPE BEND

R is, indeed, the resultant of the force (exerted by the bend on the fluid) distributed nonuniformly over the curved surfaces. Applying momentum equation, Eq. 5.58d, to the fluid mass between sections 1 and 2.

X component :

$$p_1 A_1 \cos \theta_1 - p_2 A_2 \cos \theta_2 - R_x$$
$$= \rho Q (U_2 \cos \theta_2 - U_1 \cos \theta_1) \qquad ...(5.60a)$$

Y component:

$$p_1 A_1 \sin \theta_1 - p_2 A_2 \sin \theta_2 - R_y - W$$
$$= \rho Q (U_2 \sin \theta_2 - U_1 \sin \theta_1) \qquad ...(5.60b)$$

These equations, Eqs. 5.60a and 5.60b are solved to compute unknown reactions R_x and R_y exerted by the fluid on the bend.

In the same manner the forces acting on a nozzle, discharginng freely in the atmosphere may be determined. Since the nozzle is a converging pipe segment, the velocity changes take place only in its magnitude. The forces acting on the fluid in the nozzle are the pressure at its inlet end p_1 and the reaction R_x : p_2 being zero. Therefore, the X-component of mometum equation becomes,

$$p_1 A_1 + R_x = \rho Q (U_2 - U_1) \qquad ...(5.61)$$

while the nozzle is placed in the horizontal direction, no force acts in the normal direction and hence reaction R_y will be zero.

2. Mechanical energy loss due to sudden enlargement

The energy loss between two sections due to sudden enlargement can be calculated using momentum equation Eq. 5.58. alongwith energy equation Let the incompressible steady fluid flow be occurring in a pipe of area A_1 which expands suddenly to area A_2, Fig. 5.12(a). While the fluid is flowing from the smaller pipe to the bigger, it expands and some of the fluid is enclosed in the corners of bigger pipe. The pressure of the enclosed fluid still remains p_1 as has been established experimentally. Let the mean velocities at sections 1 and 2 be U_1 and U_2. Applying momentum equation Eq. 5.58a, to the control volume between sections 1 and 2 (Fig. 5.12b),

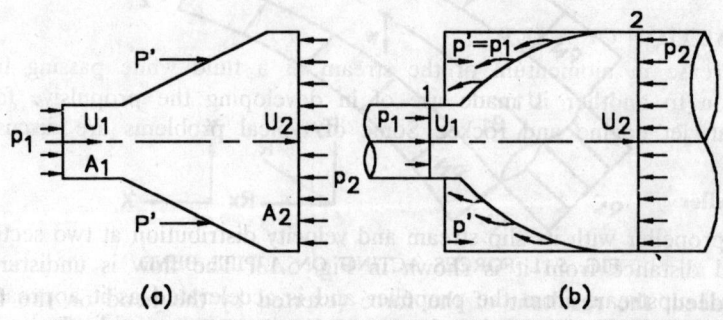

(a)   **(b)**

FIG. 5.12. (A) FREE BODY DIAGRAM (B) SUDDEN EXPANSION

$$p_1 A_1 + p_1 (A_2 - A_1) - p_2 A_2 = w \, Q/g \, (U_2 - U_1)$$

or

$$p_1 A_2 - p_2 A_2 = \frac{w \, Q}{g} (U_2 - U_1)$$

or

$$(p_1 - p_2) = \frac{w \, U_2}{g} (U_2 - U_1) \qquad \qquad ...(i)$$

Applying energy equation between sections 1 and 2,

$$\frac{p_1}{w} + \frac{U_1^2}{2g} = \frac{p_2}{w} + \frac{U_2^2}{2g} + h_L$$

where h_L is the energy loss due to sudden enlorgerment between section 1 and 2.

$$h_L = \frac{p_1 - p_2}{w} + \frac{U_1^2 - U_2^2}{2g} \qquad \qquad ...(ii)$$

From Eqs. (i) and (ii),

$$h_L = \frac{U_2}{g} (U_2 - U_1) + \frac{U_1^2 - U_2^2}{2g} \qquad \qquad ...(iii)$$

From continuity equation,

$$A_1 U_1 = A_2 U_2 \qquad \qquad ...(iv)$$

From Eqs. (iii) and (iv),

$$h_L = \frac{(U_1 - U_2)^2}{2g} \qquad \qquad ...(5.62)$$

The head loss is sometimes expressed as

$$h_L = k \, U_1^2 / 2g \qquad \qquad ...(5.63)$$

Eq. 5.63 is known as the 'Borda-Carnot' equation. It shows that mechanical energy loss in a turbulent flow varies as the square of the incoming velocity of flow.

Momentum equation can be used to solve many more fluid problems, e.g. determination of propelling thrust for boats, jets and rockets, loss of energy in a hydraulic jump (chapter 12), force exerted by a jet on the vanes (chapter 14), etc.

5.12 REACTION OF A JET

Increase in momentum of the stream of a fluid while passing from one section to another is made use of in developing the propulsive force for a boat, jet engine and rocket. Some of typical problems are discussed below.

1. Propeller

A propeller with its slip stream and velocity distribution at two sections at a fixed distance from it is shown in Fig. 5.13. The flow is undisturbed at section 1 upstream from the propeller and is accelerated as it approaches the propeller owing to the reduced pressure on its upstream side. In passing through the propeller, the fluid pressure is increased, and the fluid is accelerated

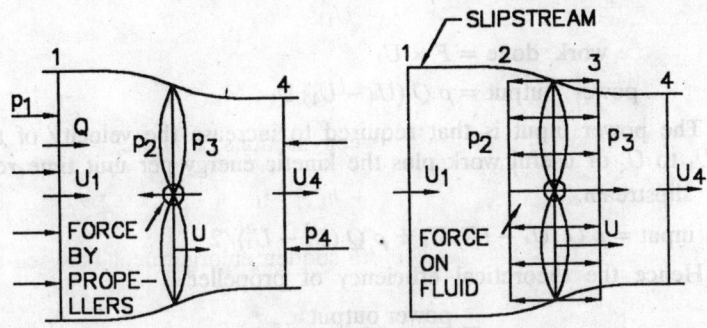

FIG. 5.13. PROPELLER

as it reaches section 4. The cross section at 4 is reduced to accommodate the higher velocity. The velocity of flow at the propeller disc is U which does not change from 2 to 3. The pressure intensity at 1 and 4 are those of undisturbed fluid and same as that existing along the slip boundaries. Consider the control volume of the fluid bounded by sections 1 and 4 and the slip boundaries. The only force acting on it in the flow direction is that due to propeller F_p, since pressure on the outer boundary of control volume is same. If A is the cross section at the propeller disc, then,

$$F = \rho\, Q\, (U_4 - U_1) = (p_3 - p_2)A \qquad ...(5.64)$$

The force on the propeller must be equal and opposite to the force on the fluid. Using continuity equation,

$$Q = A U$$

and simplifying,

$$\rho\, U\, (U_4 - U_1) = p_3 - p_2 \qquad ...(5.65)$$

Applying Bernoulli's equations between 1 and 2, and also between 3 and 4,

$$p_1 + \frac{\rho U_1^2}{2} = p_2 + \frac{\rho U_2^2}{2} \qquad \text{...(5.66a)}$$

$$p_3 + \frac{\rho U_3^2}{2} = p_4 + \frac{\rho U_4^2}{2} \qquad \text{...(5.66b)}$$

From these Eqs. 5.66a and b and using $p_1 = p_4$,

$$p_3 - p_2 = \frac{\rho}{2}(U_4^2 - U_1^2) \qquad \text{...(5.66c)}$$

From Eq. 5.65 and 5.66c

$$U = \frac{U_1 + U_4}{2} \qquad \text{...(5.67)}$$

which shows that the velocity through the propeller area is the average of velocities at upstream and downstream sections from it.

The work done by a propeller moving through still air with velocity U_1 is

$$\text{work done} = F \times U_1 \qquad \text{...(5.68)}$$

$$\text{power output} = \rho Q (U_4 - U_1) U_1 \qquad \text{...(5.69)}$$

The power input is that required to increase the velocity of the fluid from U_1 to U_4 or useful work plus the kinetic energy per unit time remaining in the slipstream.

$$\text{Power input} = \rho Q (U_4 - U_1) U_1 + \rho Q (U_4^2 - U_1^2)/2 \qquad \text{...(5.70)}$$

Hence the theoretical efficiency of propeller

$$= \frac{\text{power output}}{\text{power input}}$$

$$\eta_p = \frac{2 U_1}{U_1 + U_4} = \frac{U_1}{U} \qquad \text{...(5.71a)}$$

If $\Delta U = U_4 - U_1$ is the increase in the slipstream velocity,

$$\eta_p = \frac{U_1}{U_1 + \Delta U/2} \qquad \text{...(5.71b)}$$

which shows that the maximum efficiency is obtained for those propellers which increase the velocity as little as possible. Owing to the effect of compressibility the maximum efficiency of propellers of an aeroplane, which is nearly 85%, drops rapidly with speed (above 6500 km/hr). The maximum efficiency obtained for the propeller of the ship is nearly 65%.

2. Jet propulsion

Jet propulsion principle can also be applied to boat. Water is taken in through an opening either in the bows of the vessel, Fig. 5.14, or on either side and pumped out of a jet pipe at the stern at high velocity. In both cases, the control volume taken for analysis is fixed relative to the vessel.

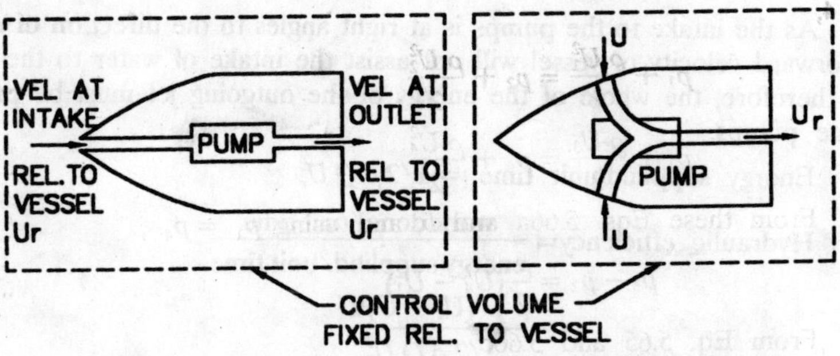

(a) INTAKE AT BOW (b) INTAKE AT SIDE

FIG. 5.14. JET PROPULSION

The two cases differ in that the water entering at the bows has a velocity relative to the vessel in the direction of the jet equal to the absolute velocity of the vessel U, while in Fig. 5.14b, for side intake, water entering into boat has no component velocity in the direction of the jet.

(a) *Intake at the bows* Let a mass of water ρQ enter the pipe intake in unit time with a velocity U and leave it with velocity U_r. Assuming the pressure of water at inlet and outlet to be same, the propelling force is computed from Eq. 5.58a,

$$F_p = \rho Q (U_r - U) \qquad ...(5.72)$$

Work done/unit time= propelling force × speed of boat

$$= \rho Q (U_r - U) U \qquad ...(5.73)$$

Kinetic energy of water/unit time at inlet $= \frac{1}{2} \rho Q U^2$

Kinetic energy of water/unit time at outlet $= \frac{1}{2} \rho Q U_r^2$

K.E. supplied by pump/unit time $= \frac{1}{2} \rho Q (U_r^2 - U^2)$ $\qquad ...(5.74)$

Hence, hydraulic efficeincy $\eta_p = \dfrac{\text{work done/unit time}}{\text{K.E./unit time}}$

$$\eta_p = \frac{\rho Q (U_r - U) U}{\rho Q (U_r^2 - U^2)/2}$$

$$= \frac{2 U}{(U_r + U)} \qquad ...(5.75)$$

(b) *Intake on either side.* For intake at right angles to the direction of motion, the control volume will be the same as in (a), and so also the rate of change of momentum through the control volume. Therefore, the propelling force will be the same as found in (a).

Work done/unit time $= \rho Q (U_r - U) U$

As the intake to the pumps is at right angles to the direction of motion, the forward velocity of vessel will not assist the intake of water to the pumps and, therefore, the whole of the energy of the outgoing jet must be provided by the pumps.

Energy supplied/unit time $= 1/2 \rho \, Q \, U_r^2$

$$\text{Hydraulic efficiency} = \frac{\text{work done/unit time}}{\text{energy supplied/unit time}}$$

$$= \frac{\rho \, U \, (U_r - U) \, U}{1/2 \rho \, Q \, U_r^2}$$

$$= \frac{2 \, (U_r - U) \, U}{U_r^2} \qquad \ldots(5.76)$$

3. Jet engine of missiles

A jet engine of missile or aircraft is shown in Fig. 5.15. Consider a stationary control volume with respect to the engine around it. the jet engine carries the fuel only and sucks in the atmoshpheric air through the jet propulsive unit at the front with a velocity U_1 (relative to the jet unit). This air then

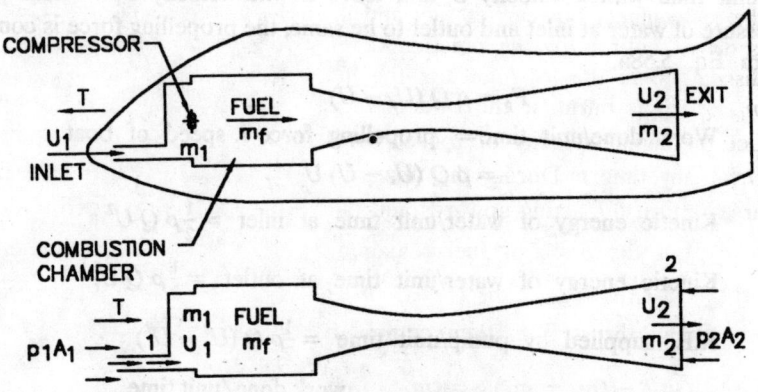

FIG. 5.15. JET ENGINE OF MISSILE

passes through a compresser before being heated by the combustion of fuel in the combustion chamber. The higher heated air containing combustion gases is then discharged into the atmosphere through the exhaust nozzle at the rear with a velocity U_2 relative to the propulsive unit. Let the air enter the jet engine with a pressure p_1 through an inlet of area A_1 and come out with a pressure p_2 . The area of the outlet is A_2 (say).

The total force exerted on the fluid in the control volume in the direction of jet = increase in momentum in the direction of jet

$$F = m_2 U_2 - m_1 U_1 \qquad \ldots(5.77)$$

where m_1 is the initial mass of air taken in by the unit which gets mixed with m_f mass of fuel to produce m_2 mass of hot gases. Therefore,

$$m_2 = m_1 + m_f \qquad ...(5.78)$$

From Eqs. 5.77 and 5.78, using $r = m_f/m_1$

$$F = (m_1 + m_f) U_2 - m_1 U_1$$

$$F = m_1 [U_2 (1 + r) - U_1] \qquad ...(5.79)$$

It T is the thrust exerted on the engine by the fluid (taken $+$ ve in the direction of motion of jet engine) and F_1 is the reaction exerted on the fluid by the engine, then $F_1 = -T$. Moreover, the fluid surrounding the control volume will also exert a force $(p_1 A_1 - p_2 A_2)$ on the fluid in the control volume. Therefore, the forces exerted on the fluid are

$$F = -T + (p_1 A_1 - p_2 A_2) \qquad \cdot$$

Substituting the value of F from Eq. 5.79,

$$T = p_1 A_1 - p_2 A_2 - m_1 [U_2 (1 + r) - U_1] \qquad ...(5.80)$$

The force exerted on the engine in the forward direction,

$$= m_1 [U_2 (1 + r) - U_1] - p_1 A_1 + p_2 A_2 \qquad ...(5.81)$$

4. Rocket engine

It does not require atmospheric air for combustion (as required by the jet engines) but carries fuel and oxidising agent along with it. The rocket is driven entirely by the reaction developed from the momentum per second discharged in the jet rear. Let the initial mass of fuel carried by rocket be m_{fo} which is burnt at the rate of m per unit time during its upward flight. Let the initial velocity of rocket be U_r which goes on varying and become U_t at any time t. During the upward flight, the forces acting on the rocket are the thrust T acting upwards and the weight $(m_r + m_{ft}) g$ acting downwards.

Let the mass of fuel remaining at any time t be m_{ft}, then

$$m_{ft} = m_{fo} - mt \qquad ...(5.82)$$

The thrust T is then computed using Eq. 5.58,

$$T - (m_r + m_{ft}) g = (m_r + m_{ft}) \cdot \frac{dU_t}{dt}$$

$$\frac{dU_t}{dt} = \frac{[T - (m_r + m_{ft}) g]}{(m_r + m_{ft}) g} \qquad ...(5.83a)$$

The initial thrust is given by

$$T = m U_r \qquad ...(5.84)$$

Therefore,

$$\frac{dU_t}{dt} = \frac{m U_r - (m_r + m_{ft}) g}{(m_r + m_{ft}) g} \qquad ...(5.83\ b)$$

This Eq. 5.83b can be integrated to determine the speed of the rocket at any time t. The height z, attained by the rocket at any time t is then computed as

$$z = \int U_t \times dt \qquad ...(5.85)$$

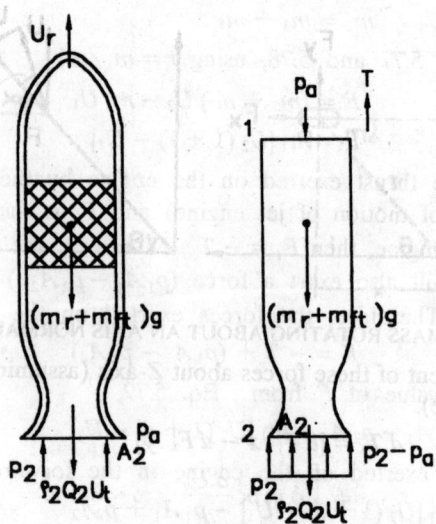

FIG. 5.16. ROCKET ENGINE

When the whole fuel is exhausted it has ascended a height z_1 and has acquired a kinetic energy $m_r U_t^2 / 2g$. The rocket moves further z_2 in the upward direction until this K.E. is converted in to P.E. Thus the maximum height attained is the summation of z_1 and z_2.

$$z_{max} = z_1 + z_2 \qquad \qquad ...(5.86)$$

5.13. ANGULAR MOMENTUM THEOREM

This theorem is useful in the design and study of the performance of turbines (axial flow type), pumps, fans, and sprinklers where torques are more important than forces.

Statement: The sum of all the externally applied torque on a given control volume of fluid is equal to the time rate of change in angular momentum of the control volume about an axis of rotation normal to the plane of rotation. The torque is the moment of the force and angular momentum is the moment of momentum about the axis of rotation.

Consider a small element of mass δm contained in a given control volume which is located at point P at a radial distance r from the origin (Fig. 5.17). The radius r makes an angle θ with X axis. The summation of forces acting on the elementary mass δm in X and Y directions are respectively F_x and F_y. These forces are caused due to the time rate of change of velocities U_x and U_y in X and Y directions, *i.e.*, due to acceleration a_x and a_y of fluid element in the two respective directions, Therefore,

$$\delta F_x = \delta_m \times a_x = \delta m \, \frac{d U_x}{dt} \qquad \qquad ...(i)$$

$$\delta F_y = \delta m \times a_y = \delta m \, \frac{d U_y}{dt} \qquad \qquad ...(ii)$$

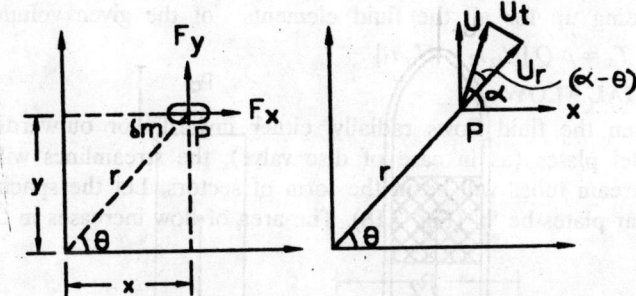

FIG. 5.17. FLUID MASS ROTATING ABOUT AN AXIS NORMAL TO ITS PATH.

Taking moment of these forces about Z-axis (assuming counter clockwise rotation as positive).

$$d\,T_x = [d\,F_y\cdot x - d\,F_x\cdot y]$$

$$= \left[\delta m \times \frac{d\,U_y}{dt} \times x - \delta m \times \frac{d\,U_x}{dt} \times y\right]$$

$$= \delta m \left[x\,\frac{d\,U_y}{dt} - y\,\frac{d\,U_x}{dt}\right] \qquad \qquad \text{...(iii)}$$

Add and subtract $\delta m\,U_x\,U_y$ hence

$$d\,T_x = \delta m \left[\left(x\,\frac{d\,U_y}{dt} + U_x\,U_y\right) - \left(y\,\frac{d\,U_x}{dt} + U_x\,U_y\right)\right]$$

$$= \delta m \left[\left(x\,\frac{d\,U_y}{dt} + U_y\,\frac{dx}{dt}\right) - \left(y\,\frac{d\,U_x}{dt} + U_x\,\frac{dy}{dt}\right)\right]$$

$$= \delta m \left[\frac{d}{dt}\left(x\,U_y - y\,U_x\right)\right]$$

Since δm is not a function of t, hence

$$d\,T_x = \frac{d}{dt}\left(\delta m\,x\,U_y - \delta\,m\,y\,U_x\right) \qquad \qquad \text{....(5.87)}$$

The velocity vector makes an angle α with X axis. Moreover, the velocity can be resolved in two components, i.e., in the direction tangential to the path of rotation called U_t and the other normal to it say, U_n. Therefore, the following substitution can be made in Eq. 5.87.

$$x = r\cos\theta \;\; ; U_x = U\cos\alpha \;\; ; \;\; U_t = U\sin(\alpha - \theta)$$

$$y = r\sin\theta \;\; ; U_y = U\sin\alpha \;\; ; \;\; U_n = U\cos(\alpha - \theta)$$

$$d\,T_z = \frac{d}{dt}[\delta m \times r\cos\theta \times U\sin\alpha - \delta m \times r\sin\theta \times U\cos\alpha]$$

$$= \frac{d}{dt}[\delta m \times r\,U\sin(\alpha - \theta)]$$

$$= \frac{d}{dt}[\delta m\,U_t]$$

Adding up for all the fluid elements of the given volume of fluid,

$$T_z = \rho Q [U_{t2} r_2 - U_{t1} r_1] \qquad ...(5.88)$$

5.14 RADIAL FLOW

When the fluid flows radially, either inwardly or outwardly, between two parallel plates (as in case of disc valve), the streamlines will be radial and the stream tubes will be in the form of sectors. Let the spacing between two circular plates be 'b' (Fig. 5.18). The area of flow increases in the outward

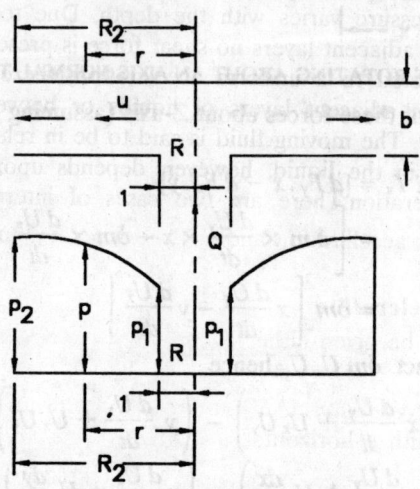

FIG. 5.18. RADIAL FLOW

direction, causing the velocity to decrease. Let the velocity of flow at any point at a radius r be u and the corresponding pressure be p. Since the flow is symmetrical, the total energy per unit weight of fluid H of all the streamlines at all the points remains invariant. Therefore, one can write

$$H = p/w + u^2/2g = \text{ constant} \qquad ...(5.89)$$

Applying continuity equation,

$$Q = 2\pi r b \times u$$

$$u = Q/2\pi br \qquad ...(5.90a)$$

$$u \propto 1/r \qquad ...(5.90b)$$

From Eqs. 5.89 and 5.90a,

$$H = \frac{p}{w} + \frac{Q^2}{8\pi^2 b^2 g r^2}$$

$$p = w \left[H - \frac{Q^2}{8\pi^2 b^2 g r^2} \right] \qquad ...(5.91)$$

It shows that the pressure increases in the radially outward direction. The variation of pressure with radius r is plotted as a parabolic curve, sometime known as 'Barlow's curve. If the pressure is atmospheric at the outer discharging end as in case of disc valve, the pressure at any intermediate point will be lower than atmospheric pressure (From Eq. 5.91). This difference of pressure opposes the flow between parallel plates. But at the same time the static pressure forces out the fluid. Thus the flow will be intermittent.

5.15. RELATIVE EQUILIBRIUM

When a liquid is at rest, the pressure always acts normally to the surface and the intensity of pressure varies with the depth. Due to the absence of relative motion between adjacent layers no shear force is present. If a confined body of liquid is subjected to a uniform acceleration, there still will be no relative motion between adjacent layers of liquids or between the layer of liquid and the boundary. The moving fluid is said to be in relative equilibrium. The pressure variation in the liquid, however, depends upon the magnitude and direction of acceleration. There are two cases of interest,

(i) uniform linear acceleration and (ii) uniform rotation about a vertical axis.

1. Uniform linear acceleration

A container can be given either a horizontal acceleration or a vertical acceleration.

(a) *Horizontal acceleration*. An open container of area A containing a fluid is accelerated with a horizontal acceleration a_x . The horizontal liquid

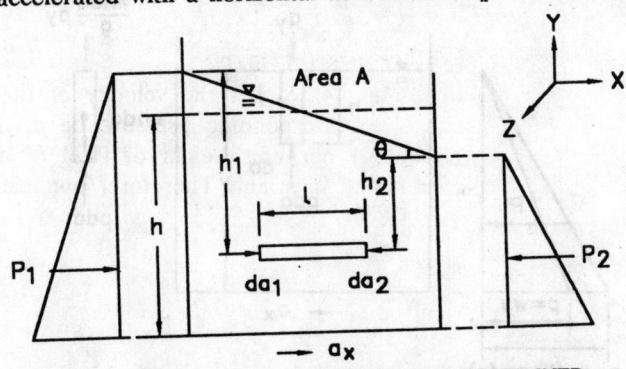

FIG. 5.19. HORIZONTALLY ACCELERATED CONTAINER.

level at rest drops at the front and rises at the rear. The water surface thus makes an angle θ with the horizontal, Fig. 5.19. Consider a fluid element of length l the water depths at its two ends are h_1 and h_2' respectively.

The forces acting on the fluid element are the fluid pressures at its two ends and inertia pressure due to horizontal acceleration a_x . Since there is no vertical acceleration, the pressure will vary in vertical direction according to the law of hydrostatics.

$$\Sigma F_x = \text{mass} \times \text{acceleration in } x\text{-direction}$$

$$(p_1 - p_2) \, da = \frac{w \, da \cdot l}{g} \times a_x$$

Solving it for the whole fluid in the tank,

$$(p_1 - p_2) = \frac{wl}{g} ax \qquad \qquad ...(5.92a)$$

$$\frac{h_1 - h_2}{l} = \frac{a_x}{g} \qquad \qquad ...(5.29b)$$

$$\tan \theta = (a_x/g) = \text{ slope of water surface} \qquad ...(5.29c)$$

Then it is seen from Eq. 5.92b that the slope of the free surface depends on the horizontal acceleration imparted to the liquid mass. The liquid pressure on any plane parallel to the water surface will be constant and is still given by Eq. 5.92a. However, if the container is moving with a constant velocity, there will be no acceleration imparted to the container and hence the liquid surface will remain horizontal.

(b) *Vertical acceleration :* Consider that the liquid contained in vessel, Fig. 5.20, is imparted an acceleration a_y in the vertically upward direction. Consider a fluid element of height h and cross-sectional area da. The forces acting on it are the pressure acting upwards and the self-weight (W) acting downwards along with inertia forces. Applying Newton's second law of motion to the fluid mass in the container,

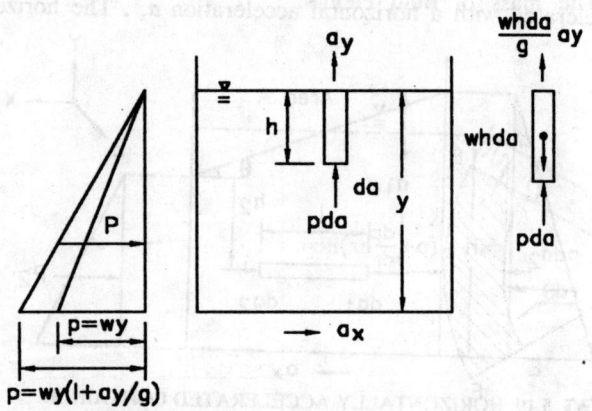

FIG. 5.20. VERTICALLY ACCELERATED FLUID MASS.

$$\Sigma F_y = m \, a_y$$

$$p \, da - wh \, da = \frac{w \, h \, da}{g} a_y$$

$$p = wh \left(1 + \frac{a_y}{g} \right) \qquad \qquad ...(5.93)$$

Eq. 5.93 shows that the pressure variation in the vertical direction is linear. It is to be noted that the magnitude of this pressure at any elevation will be greater by $(w h a_y/g)$ as compared to hydrostatic pressure if the container is accelerated upwards and will be lower if the container is accelerated downwards. In case the container falls freely under gravity $a_y = -g$ then p is equal to zero. This means that the pressure intensity is the same throughout the liquid mass and will be equal to the pressrue existing at the liquid surface.

If the vessel containing liquid is closed at the top and is imparted acceleration in vertical direction, the planes of constant pressure intensity are still given by Eq. 5.93. If the pressure at any point in the fluid is known, the pressure at all other points can be easily computed by Eq. 5.93.

2. Uniform rotation about a vertical axis

When a container filled with liquid is rotated about its central vertical axis at constant angular velocity ω , the liquid rotates as a solid body after some time interval. In this situation, no shear stress exists in the liquid and only radial acceleration acts on the fluid in the inward direction. This radial acceleration gives rise to a centripetal force acting on the fluid.

To study the variation in pressure, consider a fluid element (parallelopiped) in a stream tube and moving in a curved path, Fig.5.21. The fluid element is bounded by side AE at radius r and BF at radius $r + dr$. The angle enclosed between two sides OB and OF is $d\theta$. Let the thickness of fluid element AD be dz in the Z-direction. Thus, the area of fluid element in XY plane be da_1 and equal to $r\,d\theta\,dr$ whereas its area in XZ plane be $d\,a_2$ and is equal to $r\,d\theta\,dz$. The mass of fluid element is $\delta\,da_1\,dz$.

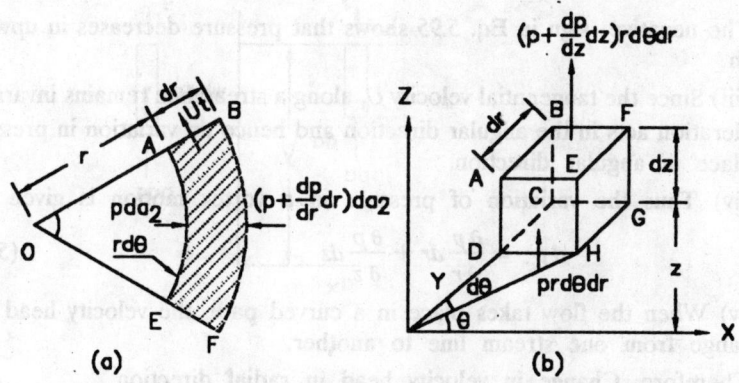

FIG. 5.21. VORTEX MOTION (A) PLAN (B) ELEVATION

The pressure forces acting in the radial direction, i.e., on two vertical faces $AEHD$ and $BFGC$ may be assumed to be pda_2 and $\left(p + \dfrac{\partial p}{\partial r}\,dr\right) da_2$. The area da_2 is equal to $rd\theta\,dz$.

The tangential velocity along streamline EA is U_t and along FB is $(U_t + \delta\,U_t)$. The corresponding radius of curvature for EA and FB are r and $r + dr$.

Besides pressure, other forces acting an fluid element are centrigugal forces acting outwardly in the radial direction and the weight of the fluid element acting vertically downward.

(i) Equating the forces in the radial direction

$$\left(p + \frac{\partial p}{\partial r} dr \right) da_2 - p \, da_2 = (\rho \, da_2 \, dr) \times U_t^2 / r$$

$$\frac{\partial p}{\partial r} = \rho \, U_t^2 / r \qquad \qquad ...(5.94a)$$

For incompressible fluid ρ is consntant; therefore, the variation of pressure head in the radial direction is

$$\frac{\partial h}{\partial r} = \frac{U_t^2}{gr} \qquad \qquad ...(5.94b)$$

(ii) Since there is no motion in the vertical direction, the pressure variation will be hydrostatic. Let the pressure force acting on DCGH be $p \, da_1$ acting upward and on ABFE be $(p + \frac{\partial p}{\partial z} dz) \, da_1$ acting downward.

Therefore,

$$p \, da_1 - (p + \frac{\partial p}{\partial z} dz) \, da_1 = \rho \, g \, da_1 \, dz$$

$$\frac{\partial p}{\partial z} = - \rho \, g \qquad \qquad ...(5.95)$$

The negative sign in Eq. 5.95 shows that pressure decreases in upward direction.

(iii) Since the tangenntial velocity U_t along a streamline remains invariant, no acceleration acts in the angular direction and hence no variation in pressure takes place in angular direction.

(iv) Thus the variation of pressure in a vortex motion is given as

$$dp = \frac{\partial p}{\partial r} dr + \frac{\partial p}{\partial z} dz \qquad \qquad ...(5.96)$$

(v) When the flow takes place in a curved path, the velocity head will also change from one stream line to another.

Therefore, Change in velocity head in radial direction

$$= \frac{(U_t + d \, U_t)^2}{2g} - \frac{U_t^2}{2g}$$

Rate of change of velocity head

$$= \left[\frac{(U_t + d \, U_t)^2}{2g} - \frac{U_t^2}{2g} \right] \times \frac{1}{dr}$$

Neglecting the product of small quantities and simplifying,
Rate of change of velocity head

$$= \frac{U_t}{g} \frac{d U_t}{dr} \qquad ...(5.97)$$

The rate of change of total head H may now be determined, as the rate of change of pressure and velocity head.

$$= \frac{d H}{dr} = \frac{dh}{dr} + \frac{d}{dr} \frac{U_t^2}{2g} \qquad ...(5.98a)$$

Substituting the values from Eqs. 5.94 b and 5.97.

$$\frac{d H}{dr} = \frac{U_t^2}{gr} + \frac{U_t}{g} \frac{d U_t}{dr}$$

$$= \frac{U_t}{g} \left[\frac{U_t}{r} + \frac{d U_t}{dr} \right] \qquad ...(5.98b)$$

The left hand side represents the 'vorticity of the fluid'.

There are two possible cases of vortex motion, namely,

(a) forced vortex motion and (b) free vortex motion which are discussed henceafter.

(a) *Forced vortex motion* : When a constant torque is applied to a body of fluid, it rotates around its central axis and forced vortex motion is obtained. (Fig. 5.22). The rotating fluid in the impeller of a centrifugal pump, rotatinng runner of a' turbine and the central core of a mixer are few examples of this class. The pressure variation is given by Eq. 5.96.

$$dp = \frac{\partial p}{\partial r} dr + \frac{\partial p}{\partial z} dz \qquad ...(5.99)$$

Substituting the values from Eqs. 5.94 and 5.95 and integrating between any two points 1 and 2 in the fluid,

$$\int_{p1}^{p2} dp = \int_{r1}^{r2} (\rho U_t^2 / r) \, dr + \int_{z1}^{z2} (\rho g) \, dz$$

In the forced vortex motion, streamlines are concentric and the velocity of any fluid element located at a radius r from the axis of rotation has a constant magnitude $(U_t \alpha r)$,

i.e. $$U_t = \omega r \qquad ...(5.85)$$

Substituting the value of U_t and solving

$$\int_{p1}^{p2} dp = \int_{r1}^{r2} \rho \omega^2 r \, dr - \int_{z1}^{z2} \rho g \, dz$$

$$\frac{p_2 - p_1}{\rho} = \frac{\omega^2}{2} (r_2^2 - r_1^2) - g (z_2 - z_1)$$

Rearranging the terms,

$$\frac{p_2 - p_1}{w} = \frac{\omega^2}{2g} (r_2^2 - r_1^2) + (z_1 - z_2) \qquad ...(5.99b)$$

Other characteristics of forced vortex motion are given below.

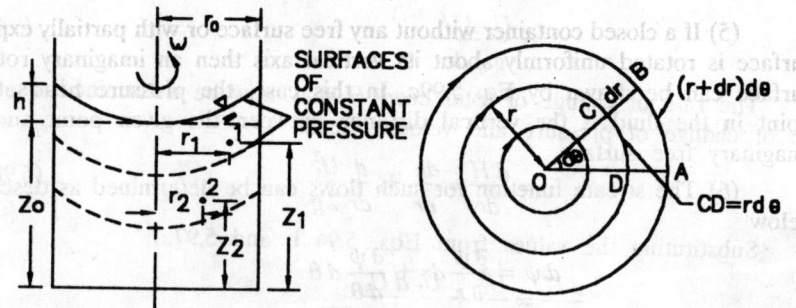

FIG. 5.22. FORCED VORTEX MOTION

(1) On any horigental surface $z_1 = z_2$, therefore, the pressure distribution is given by $\dfrac{(p_2 - p_1)}{w} = \dfrac{\omega^2}{2g} \cdot (r_2^2 - r_1^1)$

It shows that the pressure increases in the radial direction and the variation in pressure is expressed as the square of the radius.

(2) On the free surface the pressure remains atmospheric every where, i.e. $p_a = 0$ (gauge), hence p_1 and $p_2 = 0$

$$(z_1 - z_2) = \frac{\omega^2 (r_1^2 - r_2^2)}{2g} \qquad ...(5.99c)$$

If the point 2 lies at the centre of the vortex motion $r_2 = 0$. Then,

$$(z_1 - z_2) = \frac{\omega^2 r_1^2}{2g} = \frac{U_{t1}^2}{2g} \qquad ...(5.99d)$$

It shows that the point 1 rises above point 2 or the centre by the velocity head. If the point 1 lies at the rim or the container of radius r_o, the liquid will rise along the rim by a height h above the centre and is given by

$$h = \frac{\omega^2 r_o^2}{2g} \qquad ...(5.99e)$$

Eq. 5.99e defines the free surface as the paraboloid of revolution.

(3) On any other surface of constant pressure, $p_1 = p_2$ and hence above relation, Eq. 5.99d still holds good. This shows that the surfaces of constant pressures are paraboloids of revolution.

(4) It is known that the volume of paraboloid is one half of the volume of circumscribing cylinder. The volume of liquid within a container remains constant, therefore, the liquid surface will rise along the rim from its original level equal to the drop at the centre. This means the liquid level will rise by $h/2$ from its original level which can be computed from Eq. 5.99e.

(5) If a closed container without any free surface or with partially exposed surface is rotated uniformly about its vertical axis then an imaginary rotating surface can be drawn by Eq. 5.99c. In this case, the pressure head at any point in the fluid is the vertical distance between the given point and the imaginary free surface.

(6) The stream function for such flows can be determined as described below

$$d\psi = \frac{\partial \psi}{\partial r} dr + \frac{\partial \psi}{d\theta} d\theta \qquad \text{...(i)}$$

Integrating Eq. (i)

$$\psi = \int \frac{\partial \psi}{\partial r} d\psi + \int \frac{\partial \psi}{d\theta} d\theta$$

But $\qquad U_t = -\frac{\partial \psi}{\partial r}$ and $U_r = \frac{1}{r} \cdot \frac{\partial \psi}{\partial \theta}$

Then $\qquad \psi = -\int U_t \, dr + \int U_r \, r \, d\theta$

As the motion takes place in concentric circles and the velocity varies with radius, therefore, $U_t = -\omega r$ for clockwise vortex. Moreover, the radial velocity U_r is zero. Substituting $U_t = -\omega r$ in the above equation

$$\psi = \int \omega r \, dr$$

$$\psi = \frac{\omega r^2}{2} + C$$

As the centre, $\psi = 0$ and therefore $C = 0$

Hence $\qquad \psi = \frac{\omega r^2}{2}$ \qquad ...(5.100)

(7) Circulation around any differential element of fluid $ABCD$ is given by $d\Gamma$ (See Fig. 5.22)

$$d\Gamma = d\Gamma_{AB} + d\Gamma_{BC} + d\Gamma_{CD} + d\Gamma_{DA}$$

$$= [-\omega (r + dr)(r + dr) \, d\theta] + 0 + \omega r (r \, d\theta) + 0]$$

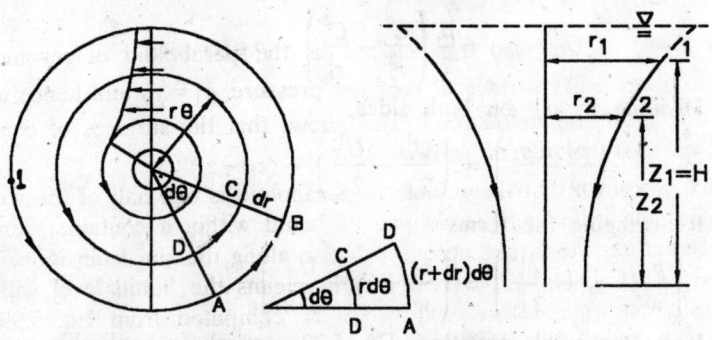

(a) VELOCITY DISTRIBUTION   (b) SHAPE OF WATER SURFACE

FIG. 5.23. FREE VORTEX MOTION

$$= - 2\omega r \, dr \, d\theta$$

The surface area of differential element is $r \, d\theta \, dr$. Therefore,

$$\frac{d\Gamma}{r \, dr \, d\theta} = - 2\omega = - \text{(vorticity } \gamma \text{ around vertical axis)}$$

It shows that either the fluid element moves around its own axis or the flow is rotational.

(b) *Free Vortex Motion* When the fluid mass moves naturally (by virtue of internal forces) in a curved path, the free vortex motion occurs. In this case no external torque acts on the fluid. Flow through an outlet at the bottom of tank, flow around the bend in a pipe system, flow in the volute chamber outside the impeller of a centrifugal pump and flow in cyclones are some of the examples of this class.

Since no external torque acts on the fluid, the time rate of change of angular momentum should be equal to zero.

Torque $\qquad T = \dfrac{\partial}{\partial t}(m \, U_t \times r) = 0 \qquad$ ...(5.101)

Integrating,

$$U_t \times r = C \qquad \qquad \text{...(5.102)}$$

where C is constant and is known as strength of the vortex formed at radius r. Thus, the tangential velocity varies inversely with the radius. Substituting the values from Eqs. 5.94a and 5.95 into Eq. 5.96.

$$\int dp = \int \frac{\partial p}{\partial r} dr + \int \frac{\partial p}{\partial z} dz$$

$$\int dp = \int \frac{\rho \, U_t^2}{r} dr - \int \rho g \, dz$$

Substituting the value of U_t from Eq. 5.102

$$\int dp = \int \frac{\rho \, C^2}{r^3} dr - \int \rho g \, dz \qquad \qquad \text{...(i)}$$

Integrate Eq. (i) between any two points 1 and 2 in the fluid

$$(p_1 - p_2) = \frac{\rho}{2}\left(\frac{C^2}{r_2^2} - \frac{C^2}{r_1^2}\right) - \rho g (z_1 - z_2)$$

Dividing by ρg on both sides,

$$\left(\frac{p_1}{w} - \frac{p_2}{w}\right) = \left(\frac{U_{t2}^2}{2g} - \frac{U_{t1}^2}{2g}\right) - (z_1 - z_2)$$

Rearranging the terms

$$\left(\frac{p_1}{w} + z_1 + \frac{U_{t1}^2}{2g}\right) = \left(\frac{p_2}{w} + z_2 + \frac{U_{t2}^2}{2g}\right) = H \qquad \text{...(5.103)}$$

It is Bernoulli's equation, Eq. 5.23b, which is applicable everywhere in the irrotational flow. Hence, Eq. 5.103 shows that the free vortex motion is an irrotational flow. It can also be verified experimentally by putting a match stick on the rotating water surface in a wash basin (freely draining). It is found that match stick does not rotate (on its own accord) about its mass axis although it moves along with the streamlines.

In case of free vortex flows, the streamlines are concentric and the velocity varies with radius in such a way that the total energy per unit weight of the fluid remains same from streamline to streamline, i.e. $(dH/dr) = 0$. From Eq. 5.98b,

$$\frac{dH}{dr} = \frac{U_t}{g}\left[\frac{U_t}{r} + \frac{dU_t}{dr}\right] = 0$$

or
$$\frac{dU_t}{U_t} + \frac{dr}{r} = 0 \qquad \ldots(5.104)$$

The left hand side is the vorticity of fluid which is zero. It further proves that free vortex motion is an irrotational motion.

Integrating Eq. 5.104 and simplifying,

$$\log U_t + \log r = \text{constant}$$

or
$$U_t \times r = C \qquad \ldots(5.102)$$

where C is a constant and is known as the strength of the vortex.

The other characteristics of free vortex motion are discussed below :

(1) On the free surface, $p_1 = p_2 = p_{atm} = 0$ (gauge), so that Eq. 5.103 becomes

$$(z_1 - z_2) = \frac{C^2}{2g}\left(\frac{1}{r_2^2} - \frac{1}{r_1^2}\right)$$

or
$$z_2 = z_1 - \frac{C^2}{2g}\left(\frac{1}{r_2^2} - \frac{1}{r_1^2}\right) \qquad \ldots(5.105)$$

It shows that the free surface of a free vortex is hyperbola asymptotic to the axis of rotation and to the horizontal plane through $z_1 = H$, as shown in Fig. 5.23.

(2) From Eqs. 5.102 and 5.103 it is found that the velocity increases and pressure decreases as one moves towards the centre of the vortex.

$$\frac{p_1}{w} = \left[H - z_1 - \frac{U_{t1}^2}{2g}\right] = \left[H - z_1' - \frac{C^2}{2gr^2}\right] \qquad \ldots(5.106)$$

(3) At the centre of a free vortex, the velocity approaches infinity $(r \to 0)$ that is not physically possible. The centre is a singular point. Indeed, the assumption of total head remaining constant ceases to be true in the vicinity of the centre, i.e. in the core. This type of motion is a combination of free vortex motion $r_0(U_1 = C/r)$ upto certain radius outside the core and forced vortex motion $(U_1 = \omega r)$ in the core. The rotational motion in the core region is due to the viscous effect of fluid. Most frequent example of this type

of motion is the flow of air in a tornado. This compound type of motion is known as 'Rankine compound vortex".

(4) If the radius of core is r_o, the tangential velocity should be the same at the periphery of the core for the two types of vortex motion. Therefore,

Free vortex motion outside the core, $U_1 = C/r_o$

Forced vortex motion inside the core, $U_t = \omega r_o$.

Hence $\qquad C = \omega r_o^2 \qquad$ ...(5.107a)

or $\qquad r_o = \sqrt{C/\omega} \qquad$ ...(5.107b)

Eq. 5.107a gives the value of constant of strength of free vortex motion whereas Eq. 5.107b yields the radius of the core.

(5) Circulation: Consider a small element of the fluid, *i.e.* ABCD and write down the expression for circulation around it in the anti-clock-wise (positive) direction.

$$d\Gamma = d\Gamma_{AB} + d\Gamma_{BC} + d\Gamma_{CD} + d\Gamma_{DA}$$
$$= (U_t + dU_t)(r + dr)\,d\theta + 0 - U_1 t r\,d\theta + 0$$
$$= U_t\,dr + r\,dU_t$$
$$= d(U_t \cdot r) \qquad ...(5.10a)$$

Since the circulation around a curve should be zero for irrotational flow

$$d\Gamma = d(U_t r) = 0$$

Integrating, $\quad U_t \times r = $ constant,

which is same as Eq. 5.102,

(6) The circulation around any closed curve which coincide with any stream line is given by

$$\Gamma = 2\pi r U_t = 2\pi C \qquad ...(5.109a)$$

or $\qquad C = \dfrac{\Gamma}{2\pi} \qquad$ ...(5.109b)

Thus the circulation around any stream line of a free vortex motion is a constant

(7) Stream function. The stream function ψ for the flow may be obtained by integration of $d\psi$. Since

$$d\psi = \frac{\partial \psi}{\partial r}\,dr + \frac{I}{r}\frac{\partial \psi}{\partial \theta}\,d\theta$$

Integrating,

$$\int d\psi = \int \frac{\partial \psi}{\partial r}\,dr + \int \frac{1}{r}\frac{\partial \psi}{\partial \theta}\,d\theta = -\int U_t\,dr + \int U_r\,d\theta$$

From Eq. 5.109a, $U_t = -\dfrac{\partial \psi}{\partial r} = \dfrac{\Gamma}{2\pi r}$

and
$$U_r = \frac{1}{r}\frac{\partial \psi}{\partial \theta} = 0$$

Since there is no motion in the radial direction. therefore,

$$\psi = -\int \frac{\Gamma}{2\pi r}\, dr + \int (0)\, d\theta$$

$$= -\frac{\Gamma}{2\pi}\log_e^{\,r} + A \qquad\qquad ...(5.110)$$

where A is a constant of integration. Let at $r = r_1$, the stream function be zero, Hence

$$A = \frac{\Gamma}{2\pi}\log_e (r_1/r_1) \qquad\qquad ...(5.111)$$

And finally the stream funtion is given by

$$\psi = \frac{\Gamma}{2\pi}\log_e (r_1/r) \qquad\qquad ...(5.112)$$

Example 5.1 - 5.31

5.1 A pipeline carrying oil of specific gravity 0.87 changes in size from 200 mm diameter at a position A to 500 mm at a position B which is 4 m at higher level (Fig. 5.24). If the pressure at A and B are 100 kPa and 60 kPa and the discharge is 200 lit/sec, determine the head loss and direction of flow.

Solution

The velocity at section A

$$U_A = \frac{0.2}{\pi/4\,(0.2)^2} = 6.37\ \text{m/s}$$

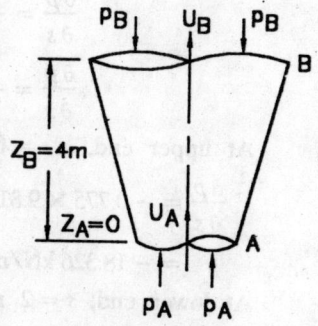

FIG. 5.24. EXAMPLE 5.1

$$U_s = 6.37\frac{(0.2)^2}{(0.5)^2} = 1.0186\ \text{m/s}$$

Total energy at $A = H_A = p_A/ws + z_A + U_A^2/2g$

$$= \frac{100}{0.87 \times 9.81} + 0 + \frac{(6.37)^2}{2 \times 9.81} = 13.785\ \text{m}$$

Total energy at $B = H_B = p_B/ws + Z_B + U_B^2/2g$

$$= \frac{60}{0.87 \times 9.81} + 4 + \frac{(1.0186)^2}{2 \times 9.81}$$

$$= 11.083\ \text{m}$$

Since $H_A > H_B$, the flow will take place from A to B in the upward direction. Applying Bernoulli's theorem between A and B,

$$H_A = H_B + h_L$$

$$h_L = H_A - H_B$$

$$= 13.785 - 11.083 = 2.702 \text{ m}$$

5.2 A section of convergent pipe is so shaped that the velocity of flow along the centre line varies linearly from 2 to 20 m/s in a distance of 2.0 m. The pipe is installed with its centre line inclined at 45° below the horizontal. Determine the magnitude of the pressure gradients at the beginning and end of the 2 m distance when the fluid has a specific gravity of 0.775.

Solution

The velocity of flow along the centre line of the convergent pipe section may be written as

$$u = 2 + \frac{(20 - 2)}{2} \times s = 2 + \partial s$$

and $\qquad \partial u / \partial s = 9.0$

Here s is measured along the centre line of convergent pipe line from the upper section.

From Eq. 5.16a,

$$\frac{\partial p}{\partial s} = -w \frac{\partial z}{\partial s} - \rho u \frac{\partial u}{\partial s}$$

$$\frac{\partial p}{\partial s} = -w \frac{\partial z}{\partial s} - \rho (2 + 9s)(9)$$

At upper end, $s = 0$

$$\frac{\partial p}{\partial s} = -0.775 \times 9.81 \times \cos 45° - \frac{9.81 \times 0.775}{9.81} \times (2) \times 9$$

$$= -18.326 \text{ kN/m}^2 \text{ per metre length}$$

At lower end, $s = 2$ m

$$\frac{\partial p}{\partial s} = -0.775 \times 9.81 \times \cos 45° - \frac{0.775 \times 9.81}{9.81} \times (2 + 9 \times 2) 9$$

$$= -144.876 \text{ kN/m}^2 \text{ per metre length}$$

5.3 A pipeline as shown in Fig. 5.25 discharges water from a reservoir. A 10 cm pipeline leads water from the reservoir. At the discharge end the pipe diameter is reduced to 5.0 cm. If the losses in the pipeline between $1-2$ is 1 m and between $2-4$ is 1.5 m, find the (a) the discharge through the pipeline and (b) the pressure at point 2. What can be the maximum elevation of point 2 above 1 if the vapour pressure is 27.5 *kPa* and the loss of head increases to 1.5 m in each segment. Assume atmoshperic pressure as 1 bar (100 *kPa*).

Solution

(a) Applying Bernoulli's equation between 1 and 4

$$\frac{p_1}{w} + z_1 + U_1^2 / 2g = \frac{p_4}{w} + z_4 + \frac{U_4^2}{2g} + h_{L12} + h_{L24} \qquad \dots(i)$$

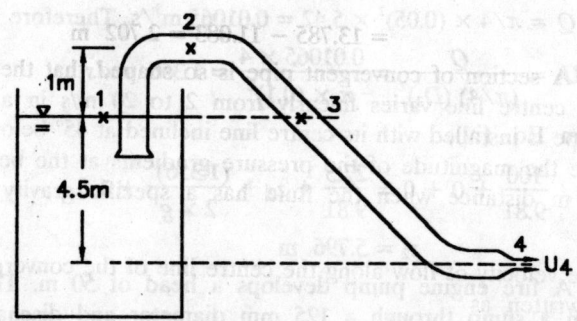

FIG. 5.25. EXAMPLE 5.3

Since the pressure at the water surface in the reservoir is atmospheric and jet discharges in the atmosphere, $p_1 = p_4 = p_a$

$$\frac{p_a}{w} + 4.5 + 0 = \frac{p_a}{w} + 0 + U_4^2/2g + 1 + 1.5$$

$$U_4 = 6.264 \text{ m/s} \qquad \ldots\text{(ii)}$$

Hence, $Q = \pi/4 \times (0.05)^2 \times 6.264 = 0.01488 \text{ m}^3/\text{s}$

(b) From continuity equation, $a_2 U_2 = a_4 U_4$

$$U_2 = (a_4/a_2) \times U_4 = (0.05/0.01)^2 \times U_4 = 1.56 \text{ m/s}$$

Applying Bernoulli's equation between 1 and 2,

$$p_1/w + z_1 + U_1^2/2g = p_2/w + z_2 + U_2^2/2g + h_{L12} \qquad \ldots\text{(iii)}$$

Substituting the values,

$$p_a/w + 0 + 0 = p_2/w + 1 + \frac{(1.56)^2}{2g} + 1$$

$$p_2/w = \frac{p_a}{w} - 2.124$$

$$p_2 = 100 - 2.124 \times 9.81 = 79.163 \text{ kPa abs}$$

$$= 20.836 \text{ kPa gauge}$$

This shows that the pressure at 2 is below atmoshperic pressure by 20.836 *kPa*.

(c) Now let us assume that point 2 can be raised to a height z_2 to maintain the limiting pressure (27.5 kN/m^2) at 2. Again applying Bernoulli's equation between 1 and 2,

$$\frac{p_1}{w} + z_1 + U_1^2/2g = p_2/w + z_2 + U_2^2/2g + h_{L12} \qquad \ldots\text{(iv)}$$

The discharge will also change as the losses are increased. Hence, again applying Bernoulli's theorem between 1 and 4,

$$0 + 4.5 + 0 = 0 + 0 + U_4^2/2g + (1.5 + 1.5) \qquad \ldots\text{(v)}$$

$$U_4 = 5.42 \text{ m/s}$$

$$Q = \pi/4 \times (0.05)^2 \times 5.42 = 0.01065 \ \text{m}^3/\text{s} \quad \text{Therefore}$$

$$U_2 = \frac{Q}{(\pi/4)\,(D_2)^2} = \frac{0.01065 \times 4}{\pi \times (0.1)^2} = 1.356 \ m/s$$

From Eq. (iv),

$$\frac{100}{9.81} + 0 + 0 = \frac{27.5}{9.81} + z_2 + \frac{(1.356)^2}{2 \times g} + 1.5$$

$$z_2 = 5.796 \ \text{m}$$

5.4 A fire engine pump develops a head of 50 m. The pump draws water from a sump through a 125 mm diameter and discharges it through a nozzle 50 mm diameter fitted at the end of a delivery pipe 100 mm diameter. The outlet of nozzle is located 30 m above the pump. The loss of head in the suction pipe is given as $5\,U_1^2/2g$ whereas in the delivery pipe the loss of energy is expressed as $10\,U_2^2/2g$. Calculate (a) the velocity of the jet issuing from the nozzle (b) the pressure in the suction pipe at the inlet to the pump located at B. Fig. 5.26.

Solution

Applying Bernoulli's theorem between A and C

Total energy at C = [Total energy at A]

+ [Energy supplied by pump]

− [Energy losses in suction pipe and delivery pipe]   ...(i)

The pressure is atmospheric at A and C and is taken as reference pressure. The velocity of flow at A in the reservoir is too small and is assumed as zero. Therefore,

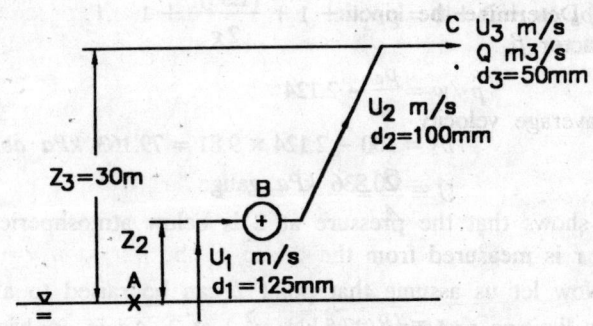

FIG. 5.26. EXAMPLE 5.4

$$\frac{p_c}{w} + z_e + \frac{U_3^2}{2g} = \frac{p_A}{w} + z_A + \frac{U_A^2}{2g} + e_M - \frac{5\,U_1^2}{2g} - \frac{10\,U_2^2}{2g}$$

Substituting the values,

$$0 + 30 + \frac{U_3^2}{2g} = 0 + 0 + 0 + 50 - 5\frac{U_1^2}{2g} - 10\,U_2^2/2g$$

$$U_3^2/2g = 20 - 5\,U_1^{\,2}/2g - 10\,U_2^2/2g \qquad ...(1)$$

From continuity equation

$$a_1 U_1 = a_2 U_2 = a_3 U_3$$

$$\frac{\pi}{4}(0.125)^2 \times U_1 = \frac{\pi}{4}(0.100)^2 \times U_2 = \frac{\pi}{4}(0.05)^2 \times U_3$$

$$U_1 = 0.16\,U_3\,;\ U_2 = 0.25\,U_3 \qquad ...(2)$$

Substituting in (1),

$$U_3^2/2g = 20 - \frac{5}{2g}(0.16\,U_3)^2 - \frac{10}{2g}(0.25\,U_3)^2$$

Solving it, $U_3 = 14.96$ m/s; $U_1 = 0.16\,U_3 = 2.3936$ m/s

(b) If ps is the pressure in suction pipe at B, then again applying Bernoulli's theorem between A and B.

$$\frac{p_A}{w} + z_A + U_A^2/2g = ps/w + z_s + U_s^2/2g + 5\,U_1^2/2g$$

$$0 + 0 + 0 = ps/w + 2 + \frac{U_1^2}{2g}(1+5)$$

Solving, $\dfrac{ps}{w} = -\,3.752$ m gauge, or ps $= 63.192$ kPa abs.

5.5 The velocity distribution in turbulent flow in a smooth round pipe is expressed by one seventh power law (Prandtl's formula)

$$u = U_{max}\,(y/R)^{1/7}$$

in which u is the point velocity at any distance y from the pipe wall, U_{max} is the maximum point velocity at the centre of pipe and R is the radius of the pipe. Determine the kinetic energy correction factor and momentum correction factor β.

Solution

The average velocity

$$U = \frac{Q}{A} = \frac{\int_A u\,dA}{\pi R^2} = \frac{\int u \times 2\pi r\,dr}{\pi R^2}$$

Since r is measured from the centre of the pipe and y from the wall of the pipe,

$$r = (R - y)$$

and $\qquad dr = -\,dy$

Therefore, $\qquad U = 2\int_0^R \frac{u\,r\,dr}{R^2}$

Substituting the value of u from one seventh power law,

$$U = \frac{2}{R^2} \int_0^R U_{max} (R - y) \, (-dy) \, (r/R)^{1/7}$$

$$= \frac{98}{120} U_{max}$$

From Eq. 5.27,

$$\alpha = \int_A \frac{u^3 \, dA}{A \, U^3}$$

$$\alpha = \int_0^R \frac{U_{max}^2 (y/R)^{3/7} (2\pi r) \, dr}{\pi R^2 \times (98/120 \times U_{max})^3}$$

Solving, $\qquad \alpha = 1.06$

Similarly from Eq. 5.59,

$$\beta = \int_A \frac{u^2 \, dA}{A \, U^2}$$

$$= \int_0^R \frac{U_{max}^2 (y/R)^{2/7} (2\pi r) \, dr}{\pi R^2 (98/120 \times U_{max})^2}$$

$$= \frac{2 \int_0^R \dfrac{(R-r)^{2/7}}{R^{2/7}} \times r \, dr}{R^2 (98/120)^2}$$

$$= 1.02$$

5.6. A fluid flows in a rectangular duct in such a manner as to have uniform velocity in the lower two third of the duct and there is no flow in the upper ove third. Calculate enengy correction factor α and momentum correction factor β. If the velocity distrilution is instead triangular with velocity U at the bottom and zero at the top of duct, calculate α and β.

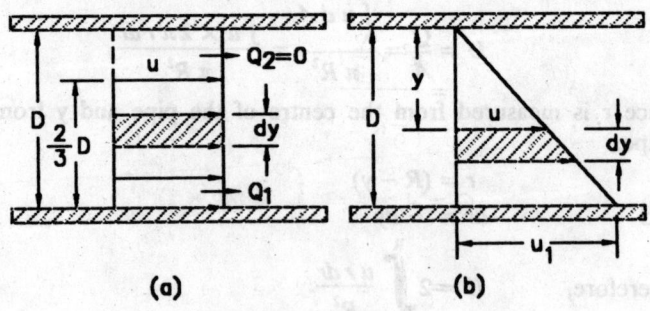

FIG. 5.27. EXAMPLE 5.6

Solution :

(a) Let the uniform velocity in lower two theird β be u. consisder unit width normal to the plane of paper.

Discharge $Q = Area \times velocity = A_1 U_1 + A_2 U_2$

$$= \left[1 \times \frac{2}{3} D \times u + 0 \right]$$

$$= \frac{2}{3} D \times u$$

Average velocity $U = \dfrac{Q}{Area \ of \ flow}$

$$\frac{\frac{2}{3} D \times u}{1 \times D} = \frac{2}{3} u$$

Then

$$\alpha = \frac{\left[\displaystyle\int_D^{2/3D} u^3 \, dy + \int_{2/3D}^D u^3 \, dy \right]}{D \times U^3}$$

$$= \frac{u^3 \times [y]_0^{2/3D} + 0}{D \left(\dfrac{2}{3} u \right)^3}$$

$$= \frac{u^3 \left(\dfrac{2}{3} D \right)}{D \times 8/27 \, u^3}$$

$$\alpha = \frac{9}{4} = 2.25$$

and

$$\beta = \frac{\displaystyle\int_0^{2/3D} u^2 \, dy + \int_{2/3D}^D u^2 \, dy}{U^2 D}$$

$$= \frac{u^2 [y]_0^{2/3D} + 0}{[\frac{2}{3} u]^2 D}$$

$$= \frac{u^2 \times \dfrac{2}{3} D}{\dfrac{4}{9} u^2 D} = 1.5$$

(v) $\qquad Q = A \times U = \displaystyle\int_0^D u \, (dy \times 1)$

$$= \int_0^D u \times dy \times 1$$

From Fig. 5.27, $\dfrac{u_u}{u_1} = \dfrac{y}{D}$ $\qquad\qquad$ ...(i)

$$Q = \int_0^D u_1 \frac{y}{D} \, dy \qquad \text{...(ii)}$$

Also, $\qquad Q = \text{Area} \times \text{av. velocity}$

$$= (1 \times D) \times U \qquad \text{...(iii)}$$

From Eqs. (ii) and (iii)

$$\therefore \qquad U \times D = u_1 \frac{D}{2}$$

$$\therefore \qquad U = \frac{u_1}{2} \qquad \text{...(iv)}$$

Alternatively, for triangular vel. distribution, one can write. $U = u_1/2$

$$\alpha = \frac{\int_0^D u^3 \, dy}{U^3 D}$$

Substituting values of u and U from Eq. (i) and Eq. (iv)

$$\alpha = \frac{\int_0^D u_1^3 (y/D)^3 \, dy}{\left(\dfrac{u_1}{2}\right)^3 D}$$

$$\alpha = \frac{u_1^3 \left(\dfrac{y^4}{4}\right)_0^D}{u_1^3 D/8} = 2.0$$

Also $\qquad \beta = \dfrac{\int_0^D u^2 \, dy}{U^2 D}$

$$= \frac{\int_0^D u_1^2 (y/D)^2 \, dy}{(u_1/2)^2 D}$$

$$= \frac{u_1^2 \cdot \left[\dfrac{y^3}{3}\right]_0^D}{\left(\dfrac{u_1^2}{4}\right) D}$$

$$= 1.33$$

5.7 Find the force exerted on a fireman holding a water hose ending in a nozzle issuing a 20 mm diameter jet of water. Pressure of water in the 60 mm diameter fire hose is 700 kPa, (FIg. 5.27).

Solution

The discharge is determined by the use of Bernoulli's theorem applied at the end of hose pipe and end of nozzle,

$$\frac{p_1}{w} + z_1 + \frac{U_1^2}{2g} = \frac{p_2}{w} + z_2 + \frac{U_2^2}{2g} + \text{Losses}$$

In this problem $z_1 = z_2$, pressure at section 2 is atmospheric which is taken as zero and the losses in the nozzle are too small, hence can be neglected. Therefore,

$$\frac{700}{9.81} + \frac{U_1^2}{2g} = 0 + 0 + \left(\frac{U_1 a_1}{a_2}\right)^2 \times \frac{1}{2g} + 0$$

$$a_1 = \frac{\pi}{4}(0.06)^2 = 0.00282 \text{ m}^2$$

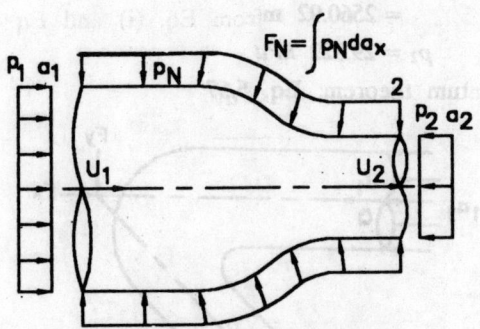

FIG. 5.28 EXAMPLE 5.7

$$a_2 = \frac{\pi}{4}(0.02)^2 = 0.000314 \text{ m}^2$$

$$U_2 = Q/a_2 = \frac{U_1 a_1}{a_2}$$

Solving, $U_1 = 4.183 \text{ m/s}$

$$U_2 = 9 U_1 = 37.65 \text{ m/s}$$

$$Q = a_1 U_1 = 0.0118 \text{ m}^3/\text{s}$$

Now the momentum theorem is applied to the free body diagram between section 1 and 2.

$$p_1 a_1 - p_2 a_2 - F_N = \frac{w Q}{g}(U_2 - U_1)$$

Here F_N is the force exerted by the nozzle on the jet in the direction of flow

$$70 \times 0.00282 - 0 - F_N = \frac{9.81}{9.81} \times 0.0118 (37.65 - 4.183)$$

Solving, $F_N = 1.579 \text{ kN}$

5.8 In a $135°$ bend (Fig. 5.28) a rectangular duct of $1 \, m^2$ cross sectional area is gradually reduced to $0.5 \, m^2$. Find the magnitude and direction of the force required to hold the duct in position if the velocity of flow at larger section is $10 \, m/s$ and the pressure is $30 \, kPa$. Take specific weight of air as $0.0116 \, kN/m^3$

Solution

From continuity equation,

$$U_2 = U_1 a_1/a_2 = \frac{10 \times 1}{0.5} = 20 \, m/s$$

$$Q = a_1 U_1 = 1 \times 10 = 10 \, m^3/s$$

Applying Bernoulli's theorem between sections 1 and 2,

$$p_1/w + z_1 + U_1^2/2g = p_2/w + z_2 + U_2^2/2g$$

Since the duct is in a horizontal plane, $z_1 = z_2 = 0$. Therefore,

$$\frac{p_2}{w} = \frac{30}{0.0116} + \frac{(10)^2}{2 \times 9.81} - \frac{(20)^2}{2 \times 9.81}$$

$$= 2560.92 \, m$$

$$p_2 = 29.822 \, kPa$$

Using momentum theorem, Eq. 5.57

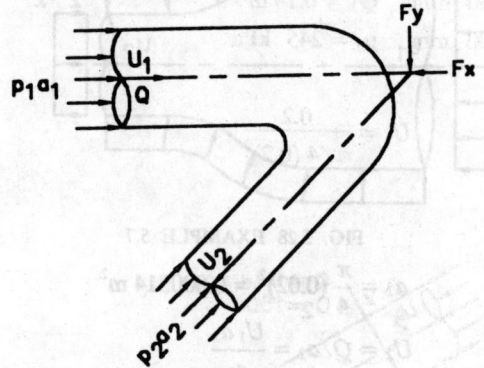

FIG. 5.29. EXAMPLE 5.8

$$p_1 a_1 - p_2 a_2 \cos 45° - F_X = (w \, Q/g) [U_2 \cos 135° - U_1]$$

Note that the horizontal component of U_2 is in the opposite direction to that of initial velocity U_1 while the jet of fluid turns by an angle of $135°$. The components of pressure at both sections will be acting in the same direction.

$$30 \times 1 + 29.822 \times 0.5 \times \frac{1}{\sqrt{2}} - F_x$$

$$= \frac{0.0116}{9.81} \times 10 \left[20 \left(\frac{-1}{\sqrt{2}} \right) - 10 \right]$$

$$F_X = 40.829 \text{ kN}$$

Similarly, F_y acting in Y-direction is computed,

$$p_2 a_2 \sin 45° - F_y = \frac{wQ}{g} [U_2 \sin 135° - 0]$$

$$29.822 \times 0.5 \times \frac{1}{\sqrt{2}} - F_Y$$

$$= \frac{11.6 \times 10}{9.81} [-20 \times \frac{1}{\sqrt{2}} - 0]$$

$$F_Y = 10.711 \text{ kN}$$

Hence, resultant force $F = \sqrt{F_X^2 + F_Y^2} = 42.21$ kN.

The direction of F with X-axis is given as

$$\tan \theta = F_Y/F_X = \frac{10.711}{40.829}$$

$$\theta = 14.70°$$

5.9 Find the resultant force acting on the horizontal pipe section shown in Fig. 5.30. The data are given below.

$$D_1 = 200 \text{ mm} \quad Q_1 = 0.20 \text{ m}^3/\text{s} \quad \theta_1 = 60°$$
$$D_2 = 150 \text{ mm}, \quad Q_2 = 0.14 \text{ m}^3/\text{s} \quad \theta_2 = 30°$$
$$D_3 = 300 \text{ mm}, \quad p_3 = 245 \text{ kPa}$$

Solution

$$U_1 = \frac{0.2}{\pi/4 \, (0.2)^2} = 6.37 \text{ m/s}$$

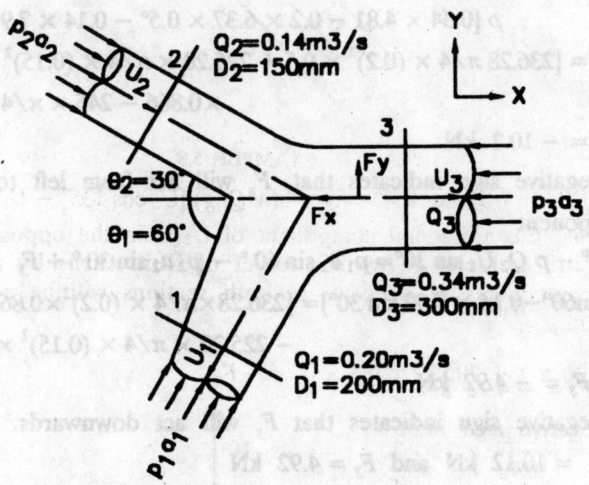

FIG. 5.30. EXAMPLE 5.9

$$U_2 = \frac{0.14}{\frac{\pi}{4} \times (0.15)^2} = 7.92 \text{ m/s}$$

and

$$U_3 = \frac{0.34}{\pi/4 (0.30)^2} = 4.81 \text{ m/s}$$

Applying Bernoulli's theorem between sections 2 and 3 along a stream line

$$\frac{p_2}{w} + \frac{U_2^2}{2g} = \frac{p_3}{w} + \frac{U_3^2}{2g}$$

$$p_2/w = p_3/w + U_3^2/2g - U_2^2/2g$$

$$= \frac{245}{9.81} + \frac{(4.81)^2}{2g} - \frac{(7.92)^2}{2g}$$

$$= 22.9566$$

$$p_2 = 225.20 \text{ kPa}$$

Similarly applying Bernoulli's equation between 1 and 3

$$p_1/w = \frac{245}{9.81} + \frac{(4.81)^2 - (6.37)^2}{2g}$$

$$= 24.085 \text{ m}$$

$$p_2 = 236.28 \text{ kPa}$$

Applying momentum theorem to the control volume bounded by the control surface. Assume the direction of F_x & F_y as shown in Fig. 5.30.

X-component

$$\rho Q_3 U_3 - \rho Q_1 U_1 \cos 60° - \rho Q_2 \times U_2 \times \cos 30$$

$$= p_1 a_1 \cos 60° + p_2 a_2 \cos 30° - p_3 a_3 - F_x$$

$$\rho [0.34 \times 4.81 - 0.2 \times 6.37 \times 0.5° - 0.14 \times 7.92 \times 0.866°]$$

$$= [236.28 \pi/4 \times (0.2)^2 \times 0.5 + 225.20 \times \pi/4 \times (0.15)^2$$

$$\times 0.866 - 245 \times \pi/4 (0.3)^2 \times F_x]$$

$$F_x = -10.2 \text{ kN}$$

The negative sign indicates that, F_x will act from left to right.

Y-component

$$\rho Q_1 U_1 \sin 60° - \rho Q_2 U_2 \sin 30° = p_1 a_1 \sin 60° - p_2 a_2 \sin 30° + F_y$$

$$\rho [0.2 \times 6.37 \sin 60° - 0.14 \times 7.92 \sin 30°] = [236.28 \times \pi/4 \times (0.2)^2 \times 0.866$$

$$- 225.20 \times \pi/4 \times (0.15)^2 \times (0.5) + F_y]$$

$$F_y = -4.92 \text{ kN}$$

The negative sign indicates that F_y will act downwards.

Therefore $F_x = 10.12 \text{ kN}$ and $F_y = 4.92 \text{ kN}$

5.10 Water flows at a velocity of 2 m/s through a 90 cm diameter pipe at the end of which there is a reducer connecting it to a 60 cm diameter pipe. If the gauge pressure at the entrance to the reducer is 400 kN/m², determine the thrust on the reducer assuming the loss of head in the reducer is 1.5 m of water.

Solution

From continuity equation

$$\frac{\pi}{4} \times (0.9)^2 \times 2 = \frac{\pi}{4} \times (0.6)^2 \times U_2$$

$$U_2 = 4.5 \text{ m/s}$$

Applying Bernoulli's equation between two sections,

$$\frac{p_1}{w} + \frac{U_1^2}{2g} = \frac{p_2}{w} + \frac{U_2^2}{2g} + h_L$$

$$\frac{400 \times 1000}{9810} + \frac{(2)^2}{2 \times 9.81} = \frac{p_2}{w} + \frac{(4.5)^2}{2 \times 9.81} + 1.5$$

$$p_2 = 377.16 \text{ kN/m}^2$$

Let F_x be the force exerted by the reducer on the fluid, in the direction opposite to the flow. The liquid will exert equal and opposite force on the reducer.

Applying momentum equation,

$$p_1 A_1 - p_2 A_2 - F_x = \frac{wQ}{g}(U_{2x} - U_{1x})$$

$$400 \times 10^3 \times \pi/4 \times (0.9)^2 - 377.16 \times 10^3 \times \pi/4 \times (0.6)^2 - F_x$$

$$= \frac{9810 \times \pi/4 \times (0.9)^2 \times 2}{9.81}(4.5 - 2.0)$$

$$F_x = 144.575 \text{ kN}$$

Force exerted on the reducer in the direction of flow

$$= 144.575 \text{ kN}$$

5.11 A closed tank 1 m × 1 m × 4 m high and weighing 1.2 kN has an orifice in the side with effective area 6.5 cm² and situated 150 mm above the tank bottom (Fig. 5.31). The tank is filled with water to a depth of 3 m. If the coefficient of friction between ground and the wheels, on which the tank is mounted, is 0.01, determine the air pressure which should be maintained in the tank in the space above the water level so that it begins to move.

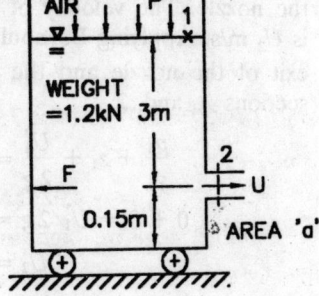

FIG. 5.31. EXAMPLE 5.11

Solution

Let the pressure of air be p kp_a. Therefore, total weight acting on the wheels

$$W = 1.2 + 1 \times 1 \times 3 \times 9.81$$
$$= 30.63 \text{ kN}$$

Applying the momentum theorem to the free body diagram of the control volume, the horizontal force F is given by

$$\Sigma F = \rho \, Q \, (U_2 - U_1) = \rho \times a \times U^2$$
$$\Sigma F = 1000 \times 6.5 \times 10^{-4} \times U^2 \qquad \text{...(ii)}$$

From Eqs. (i) and (ii)

$$\mu = \frac{F}{W}$$

$$0.01 = \frac{0.65 \, U^2}{30.63 \times 1000}$$

Solving, $\qquad U = 21.70$ m/s

Applying Bernoulli's equation to 1 and 2,

$$\frac{p}{w} + 3 + 0 = p + 0 + \frac{U^2}{2g}$$

Solving, $\qquad p = 206.015 \text{kN/m}^2$

5.12 A large disc weighing 0.05 kN is so mounted that it may move freely along a vertical axis, the plane of the plate remaining horizontal. A jet of water, 5 cm diameter, strikes the plate on the underside of the plate with a velocity of 8 m/s. Assuming that the disc deflects the jet horizontally, how high above the nozzle will the disc be held in equilibrium by the force of the jet ?

Solution

Let the jet keep the plate h metre above the nozzle. The velocity of jet at this elevatin is U_2 m/s. Applying Bernoulli's equation at the exit of the nozzle and the plate, *i.e.* between sections 1 and 2,

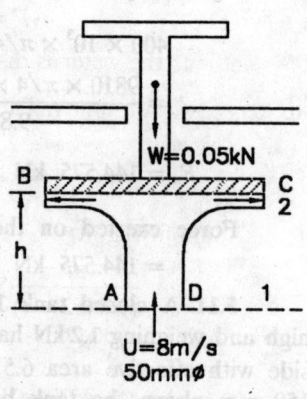

FIG. 5.32. EXAMPLE 5.12

$$\frac{p_1}{w} + z_1 + \frac{U_1^2}{2g} = \frac{p_2}{w} + z_2 + \frac{U_2^2}{2g}$$

$$0 + 0 + U_1^2/2g = 0 + h + U_2^2/2g$$

$$U_2 = \sqrt{U_1^2 - 2gh} \qquad \text{...(i)}$$

Applying momentum equation to the fluid in the control volume *ABCD*,

$$F_y = (w\,Q/g)\,(U_2 - U_1)$$
$$= \frac{9.81 \times \pi/4 \times (0.05)^2 \times 8}{9.81}\,[\sqrt{(8)^2 - 2gh} - 8] \qquad ...(ii)$$

Since the weight of the plate is 0.05 kN which is to be supported by the jet, hence,

$$0.05 = 0.0157\,[\sqrt{64 - 2gh} - 8]$$

Solving, $\qquad h = 3.114$ m

5.13 A pump and water storage tank are mounted on a flat car that runs on a horizontal and frictionless track. When 0.1 m³/s water is discharged through a 50 mm diameter nozzle parallel to the track, determine the speed of the car after 30 sec. if the original weight of the car was 75 kN. Neglect all types of resistances.

Solution

The velocity of jet relative to the car is

$$U_r = \frac{0.1}{\dfrac{\pi}{4}(0.05)^2} = 50.93 \text{ m/s}$$

The change in velocity of liquid is U_r and therefore,

$$F = \rho\,Q\,U_r$$
$$= 1000 \times 0.1 \times 50.93 \text{ N} = 5.093 \text{ kN}$$

The acceleration of the car is given by Newton's second law of motion.

$$F = \text{mass} \times \text{acceleration} = \text{mass} \times (dU/dt)$$

Since the water is discharged at the rate of 0.1 m³/s , the mass continues to decrease with time t. The speed of car is U and hence $\dfrac{dU}{dt}$ is its acceleration.

$$5.093 = \left(\frac{75}{9.81} - \frac{1000 \times 0.1 \times t}{1000} \right) \frac{dU}{dt}$$

Simplifying it,

$$\frac{dt}{(76.452 - t)} = \frac{dU}{50.93}$$

Integrating it,

$$- \log (76.452 - t) = \frac{1}{50.93} \times U + c$$

When $\quad t = 0$, $U = 0$, $\quad$ hence $c = - \log (76.452)$

Substituting the value of c in the above equation,

$$U = 50.93 \log_e \left(\frac{76.452}{76.452 - t} \right)$$

The speed of car after $t = 30$ sec,

$$U = 50.93 \log_e \left(\frac{76.452}{76.452 - 30} \right)$$

$$= 25.375 \, m/s$$

5.14 A water sprinkler consists of 15 mm jets at either end of a rotating arm as shown in Fig. 5.33. What torque must be applied to the arm to hold it stationary when the velocity of jet is 7m/s? If mechanical friction is neglected, what constant angular velocity should the arm attain ?

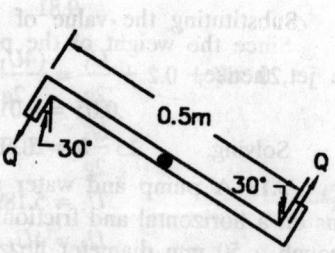

FIG. 5.33. EXAMPLE 5.14

Solution

The torque produced by the two jets is T. Therefore,

$$T = F \times r$$

$$= \rho \, Q \, (U \cos \theta - 0) \, r$$

$$= \rho \, a \, U^2 \cos \theta \times r$$

$$= \frac{9.81}{9.81} \times \frac{\pi}{4} (0.015)^2 \times (7)^2 \cos 30° \times 0.25$$

$$= 0.001875 \quad kN \quad m$$

The maximum angular velocity will be attained when the absolute velocity of water is radial.

Hence, $7 \cos 30° = \omega \, r = 0.25 \, \omega$

$$\omega = 24.25 \quad rad/sec$$

5.15 A jet of water coming out from a 50 mm diameter round nozzle attached to a 100 mm diameter pipe is directed vertically downwards. If pressure in the 100 mm diameter pipe 0.2 m above nozzle is 200 kN/m² gauge, determine the diameter of jet 5 m below nozzle level.

Solution :

Apply continuity eq. to (1) and (2)

$$A_1 \, U_1 = A_2 \, U_2$$

$$\frac{\pi}{4} \times (0.1)^2 \times U_1 = \frac{\pi}{4} (0.05)^2 \, U_2$$

$$U_2 = 4 \, U_1 \qquad \ldots(i)$$

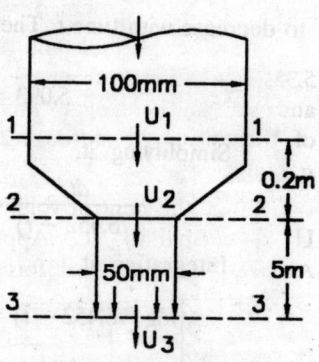

FIG. 5.34. EXAMPLE 5.15

Apply Bernoulli's equation between (1) and (2).

$$\frac{p_1}{w} + z_1 + \frac{U_1^2}{2g} = \frac{p_2}{w} + z_2 + \frac{U_2^2}{2g} + \text{losses neglect.}$$

$$\frac{200 \times 1000}{9810} + 0.2 + \frac{U_1^2}{2g} = 0 + 0 + \frac{U_2^2}{2g}$$

Substituting the value of U_2

$$20.387 + 0.2 + \frac{U_1^2}{2g} = \frac{(4U_1)^2}{2g}$$

$$15 \frac{U_1^2}{2g} = 20.587$$

$$U_1 = 5.189 \text{ m/s}$$

$$U_2 = 4U_1 = 20.75 \text{ m/s}$$

Now apply Bernoulli's equation between 2 and 3,

$$0 + 5 + \frac{U_2^2}{2g} = 0 + 0 + \frac{U_3^2}{2g}$$

$$5 + \frac{(20.75)^2}{2 \times 9.81} = \frac{U_3^2}{2 \times 9.81}$$

Solving, $\qquad U_3 = 23 \text{ m/s}$

Apply continuity equation between 2 and 3,

$$\frac{\pi}{4}(d_3)^2 \times U_3 = \frac{\pi}{4}(0.05)^2 \times U_2$$

$$d_3^2 = (0.05)^2 \frac{U_2}{U_3}$$

$$= (0.05)^2 \times \frac{20.75}{23.0} = 2.2544$$

$$d_3 = 0.0475 \text{ m} = 47.5 \text{ mm.}$$

5.16 : A tank and a trough are placed on a trolley as shown in Fig. 5.35. Water issues from the tank through a 50 mm diameter nozzle at 5 m/s and strikes the trough which turns it at 45°. Determine the compression of the spring of stiffness 2 kN/m.

Solution :

Let the control volume be ABCD and BC is so chosen that velocity U is normal to it. Apply momentum equation to this control volume ABCD. The external force acting on it is spring reaction R_x.

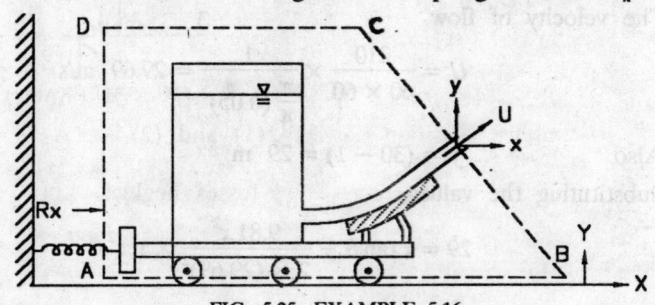

FIG. 5.35, EXAMPLE 5.16

Mass flow rate $= 1000 \times \dfrac{\pi}{4} \times (0.05)^2 \times 5$

$= 9.8125$ kg/s.

Apply momentum equation, Eq. 5.57

$$\Sigma F_x = \rho\, Q\, (U_{2x} - U_{1x})$$

$$R_x = 9.8125\, [5 \cos 45° - 0]$$

$$= 9.8125 \times 5 \cos 45°$$

$$= 34.69 \text{ N}$$

Hence force acting on the spring $= -R_x$

$$= -34.69 \text{ N} \quad \text{which tends to compress it.}$$

Compression in spring $= \dfrac{34.69}{2 \times 1000} = 0.0175$ m

$$= 17.35 \text{ mm}$$

5.17 A window in a vertical wall is located at 30m above the ground level (Fig. 5.36). A jet of water 50 mm diameter (and located 1m above the ground) strikes the window and supplies 210 m³/hr . Find the greatest distance from the wall at which fire nozzle be located so that the jet of water strikes the window.

Solution

Let the nozzle be situated x distance from the wall making an angle θ to the horizontal. Therefore,

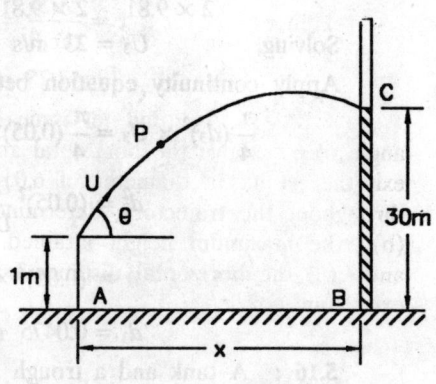

FIG. 5.36, EXAMPLE 5.17

$$x = U \cos\theta \times t \qquad \text{...(i)}$$

$$y = U \sin\theta \times t - (1/2)\, g t^2 \qquad \text{...(ii)}$$

From Eq. (i) $\quad t = x/U \cos\theta$

From Eq. (ii) $\quad y = U \sin\theta \times (x/U \cos\theta) - g/2 \times (x/U \cos\theta)^2$

$$= x \tan\theta - (g x^2/2 U^2)\, sec^2\theta$$

The velocity of flow

$$U = \dfrac{210}{60 \times 60} \times \dfrac{1}{\dfrac{\pi}{4}(0.05)^2} = 29.69 \text{ m/s}$$

Also $\quad y = (30 - 1) = 29$ m

Substituting the values,

$$29 = x \tan\theta - \dfrac{9.81\, x^2}{2 \times (29.69)^2} \times sec^2\theta$$

$$x \tan \theta - \frac{0.0055\, x^2}{\cos^2 \theta} - 29 = 0 \qquad ...(iii)$$

For maximum value of x, $dx/d\theta$, should be zero.

$$x \sec^2 \theta + \tan \theta \times \frac{dx}{d\theta} - 0.0055 \times \left[x^2 \frac{(-2)}{\cos^3 \theta} \times (-\sin \theta) \right.$$

$$\left. + \frac{1}{\cos^2 \theta} \times 2x \frac{dx}{d\theta} \right] = 0$$

Solving it, $\qquad x = \dfrac{90.9}{\tan \theta}$

Substituting this value of x in the above Eq. (iii)

$$\frac{90.9}{\tan \theta} \times \tan \theta - \frac{0.0055}{\cos^2 \theta} \times \left(\frac{90.9}{\tan \theta} \right)^2 - 29 = 0$$

Solving it, $\qquad \theta = 58° \, 58'$

Hence $\qquad x = \dfrac{90.9}{\tan \theta} = \dfrac{90.9}{\tan 58° \, 58'}$

$$= 54.75 \text{ m}$$

5.18 : A liquid jet issues out of a nozzle into atmosphere at an angle of 60° above the horizontal and with a velocity 7.0 m/s. At the nozzle exit the jet has a diameter of 6.0 cm. Assuming the jet to be unbroken throughout the trajectory, determine : (a) the equation of the trajectory, (b) the maximum height attained by the jet and its size at that location and (c) the horizontal distance travelled by the jet at the elevation of its exit from nozzle.

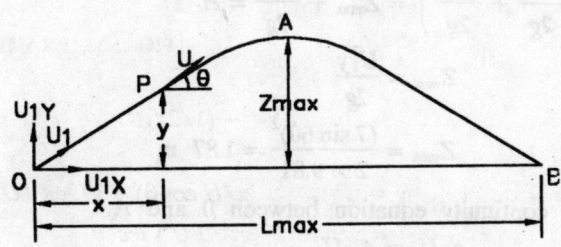

FIG. 5.37, EXAMPLE 5.18

Solution :

Let the nozzle is located at 0 and issues a jet. Let OAB is the trajectory traversed by the jet. Consider a point P (x,y) on the trajectory.

At point 0, the jet issues out with a velocity U_1 at angle θ with horizontal, then

$$U_1 x = U_1 \cos \theta = \text{ constant}$$

$$- l \cos 60°$$

$$U_1 y = U_1 \sin \theta = 7 \sin 60°$$

In time t_1 the fluid molecule travels horizontal distance x and vertical distance y.

$$x = U_1 x \cdot t \qquad \qquad ...(i)$$

$$y = U_1 y \times t - \frac{1}{2} g t^2 \qquad \qquad ...(ii)$$

From Eq. (i) $\quad t = \dfrac{x}{U_1 x}$

From Eq. (ii) $\quad y = U_1 y \times \dfrac{x}{U_1 x} - \dfrac{1}{2} g \cdot \left(\dfrac{x}{U_1 x} \right)^2$

$$y = U_1 \sin \theta \frac{x}{U_1 \cos \theta} - \frac{1}{2} g \left(\frac{x}{U_1 \cos \theta} \right)^2$$

$$y = x \tan \theta - \frac{g \cdot x^2}{2 U_1^2 \cos^2 \theta} \qquad \qquad ...(iii)$$

It is the equation of the trajectory of jet (Eq. 5.49 a)

(i) Given $U_1 = 7$ m/s, $\theta = 60°$

$$y = x \tan 60° - \frac{9.81 x}{2 (7)^2 \cos^2 60°}$$

$$y = \sqrt{3} \, x - 0.4 x^2 \qquad \qquad ...(iv)$$

(ii) At the highest point A, $U_{1y} = 0$ so that $U_A = U_{1x}$

Apply Bernoulli's theorem between 0 and A

$$0 + \left(\frac{U_1^2 x}{2g} + \frac{U_1^2 y}{2g} \right) = Z_{max} + \frac{U_1^2 x}{2g} = H$$

$$Z_{max} = \frac{U_1^2 y}{2g}$$

$$Z_{max} = \frac{(7 \sin 60)^2}{2 \times 9.81} = 1.87 \text{ m}$$

Apply continuity equation between 0 and A.

$$a_1 U_1 = A_A U_A$$

$$\frac{\pi}{4} (0.06)^2 \times 7 = \frac{\pi}{4} (d)^2 \times 3.5$$

Since $\qquad U_A = U_1 x$

$\therefore \qquad\qquad d = \sqrt{2} \times 0.06$ m

$$= 8.48 \text{ cm}$$

(iii) Horizontal distance at the elevation of jet exit,

$$OB = L_{max}$$

At B, $\qquad\qquad y = 0$,

From Eq. (iv), equation of trajectory,

$$y = \sqrt{3}\,x - 0.4x^2$$

$$0 = x\,(\sqrt{3} - 0.4x)$$

or $$x = L_{max} = \frac{\sqrt{3}}{0.4}$$

∴ $$L_{max} = 4.33 \text{ m}$$

5.19 A rectangular tank 2.5 m wide, 5 m long and 3 m deep contains oil of specific gravity 1.8 to a depth of 2.0 m (Fig. 5.38). When it is accelerated at 3.5 m/s in the direction of its length, calculate the pressure on each end of the tank. If the tank is accelerated at double the rate, how much volume of water is spilled out of the tank ?

Solution

Case I. From Eq. 5.92b

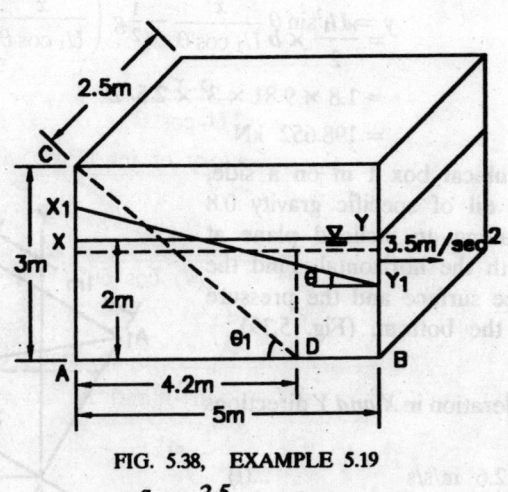

FIG. 5.38, EXAMPLE 5.19

$$\tan \theta = \frac{a_x}{g} = \frac{3.5}{9.81} = 0.3571$$

$$\theta = 19.65°$$

The water level will rise by $xx_1 = 5/2 \tan 19.65° = 0.9$ m

The pressure at A is due to 2.0 m + 0.9 m = 2.9 metres and the pressure at B is due to 2.0 m − 0.9 m = 1.1 metres

$$P_A = b \times \text{ area of pressure triangle}$$

$$= wh \times (h/2) \times b$$

$$= 1.8 \times 9.81 \times 2.9 \times (2.9/2) \times 2.5$$

$$= 185.63 \text{ kN}$$

$$P_B = 1.8 \times 9.81 \times \left(\frac{1.1 \times 1.1}{2} \right) \times 2.5$$

$$= 26.707 \text{ kN}$$

Case II. Here

$$\tan \theta_1 = \frac{a_x}{g} = \frac{7.0}{9.81} = 0.7142$$

$$\theta_1 = 35.53°$$

The water level at A will touch the top edge and some volume of water will spill over. The new water level will meet the base of the tank at $3 \cot 35.53° \, m = 4.2 \, m$

Volume of water retained $= 2.5 \times (3.0 \times 4.2)/2 = 15.75 \, m^3$

Hence volume of water spilled out

$$= (2.5 \times 3.0 \times 5) - 15.75 = 21.75 \, m^3$$

Now the pressure at A

$$= \frac{w h^2}{2} \times b$$

$$= 1.8 \times 9.81 \times 3^2 \times 2.5/2$$

$$= 198.652 \, kN$$

5.20 A cubical box 1 m on a side, half filled with oil of specific gravity 0.8 is accelerated along an inclined plane at angle of 30° with the horizontal. Find the slope of the free surface and the pressure intensity along the bottom. (Fig. 5.39).

Solution

The acceleration in X and Y directions are a_x and a_y

$a_x = 3 \cos 30° = 2.6 \, m/s/s$ ...(i)

$a_y = 3 \sin 30° = 1.5 \, m/s/s$ ...(ii)

The pressure at a distance x from A is given by Eq. 5.92a,

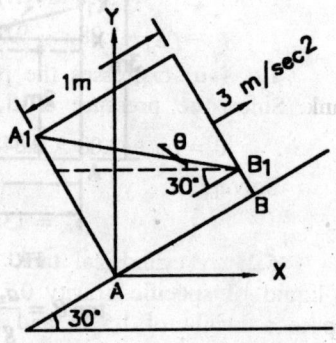

FIG. 5.39, EXAMPLE 5.20

$$p = p_A - \frac{wx}{g} a_x$$

where p_A is the pressure at A

$$p = p_A - \frac{0.8 \times 9.81 \times x \times 2.6}{9.81}$$

$$= p_A - 2.08 x$$ ...(iii)

Similarly, the pressure at an elevation y from A is given by Eq. 5.93.

$$p = p_A - wy (1 + a_y/g)$$

$$= p_A - 0.8 \times 9.81 \times y (1 + 1.5/9.81)$$

$$= p_A - 9.048 y$$ ...(iv)

Equating Eqs. (iii) and (iv), the slope of free surface is obtained.

$$p_A - 2.09 x = p_A - 9.048 y$$

But $\tan \theta = y/x$

Hence, $\tan \theta = 0.23$

$$\theta = 12.95°$$

The water surface thus makes an angle of $(30° + 12° = 42.95°$ with the sloping plane.

Let the water depth at B be z. Then the water depth at A will be $1 \times \tan (30 + 12.95°) = 0.93$ metre above B_1. To determine z, equate the volume of the fluid in the newly occupied space by the original volume of the liquid.

$$1 \times 1 \times \left(\frac{0.93 + 2z}{2} \right) = 0.5 \times 1 \times 1 \times 1$$

$$z = 0.035 \text{ metre} \qquad \text{...(v)}$$

Hence, the location of point B_1 is given by

$$x = 1 \times \cos 30° - z \times \sin 30° = 0.8485 \text{ m}$$

$$y = 1 \times \sin 30° + z \times \cos 30° = 1.3054 \text{ m} \qquad \text{...(vii)}$$

From Eqs. (iii) and (iv),

$$p = p_A - 2.08 x - 9.048 y \qquad \text{...(vi)}$$

Eq. (vii) expresses the pressure at any point along the bottom of the tank. Since the pressure at B_1 is zero, therefore,

$$0 = p_A - 2.08 \times 0.8485 - 9.048 \times 1.3054$$

Solving it,

$$p_A = 13.576 \ kPa$$

5.21 A cylindrical tank 2 m in diameter and closed at top contains a liquid of specific gravity 0.75. The tank is 2 m high and contains liquid up to a height of 1.5 m and air above it under a pressure of $- 2.25 \ kPa$. Calculate the force acting on the bottom of the tank, when it accelerated

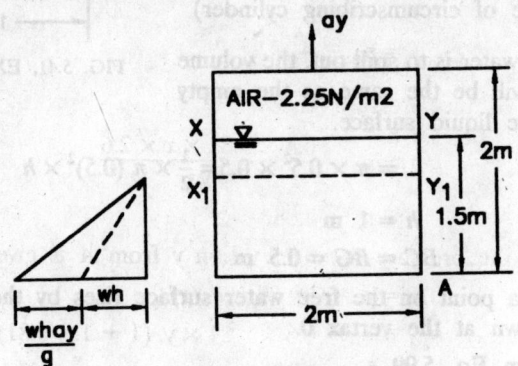

FIG. 5.40,   EXAMPLE 5.21

vertically upward at 4.9 m/s² . What is the acceleration required to have zero absolute pressure at the bottom ? (Fig. 5.40).

Solution

The free surface will shift below *xy* level by= $2.25/(0.75 \times 9.81)$

$$= 0.306 \text{ m}$$

Hence, the free surface will be at $x_1 y_1$, *i.e.* $(1.5 - 0.306)$

$$= 1.294 \text{ m above bottom.}$$

(a) $$p_A = w h (1 + a_y/g)$$

$$= 0.75 \times 9.81 \times 1.294 \left(1 + \frac{4.9}{9.81}\right)$$

$$= 14.276 \text{ kN/m}^2 \text{ gauge}$$

(b) When the pressure at the bottom is zero.

$$p_A \text{ (absolute)} = p_{atm} + p_A(\text{gauge})$$

Assume atmospheric pressure as $100 \, kPa(= 1 \text{ bar})$

$$p_A \text{ (absolute)} = 100 + 0.75 \times 9.81 \times 1.294 \left(1 + \frac{a_y}{9.81}\right)$$

$$0 = 100 + 9.52 \left(1 + \frac{a_y}{9.81}\right)$$

Solving it, $a_y = - 112.85 \text{ m/s}^2$

5.22 An open cylindricak tank, 2 m high and 1 m in diameter, contains 1.5 m of water (Fig. 5.41). If the cylinder rotates about its central axis, (a) what angular velocity can be obtained without spilling any water ? (b) what is the pressure at the bottom of the tank at E and F when angular velocity is equal to 6 radians/sec?

Solution

Volume of paraboloid of revolution

$$= \tfrac{1}{2} \text{ (volume of circumscribing cylinder)}$$

Since no water is to spill out, the volume of paraboloid will be the same as the empty space above the liquid surface.

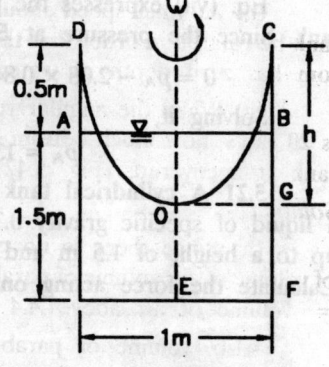

FIG. 5.41, EXAMPLE 5.22

$$= \pi \times 0.5^2 \times 0.5 = \tfrac{1}{2} \times \pi (0.5)^2 \times h$$

∴ $$h = 1 \text{ m}$$

Hence $$BC = BG = 0.5 \text{ m}$$

That is, a point on the free water surface rises by the same amount as it drops down at the vertax 0.

Now from Eq. 5.99 e.

$$h = \frac{\omega^2 r^2}{2g}$$

$$1 = \frac{\omega^2}{2g} \times (0.5)^2$$

$$\omega = 8.86 \text{ rad/sec}$$

(b) When $\omega = 6$ radians/sec, the highest point on the water surface will lie between B and C, *i.e.* $r = 0.5$ m

$$h = \frac{\omega^2 r^2}{2g}$$

$$h = \frac{(6)^2 \times (0.5)^2}{2 \times 9.81} = 0.468 \text{ m}$$

The vertex O will drop by $(0.468/2)$ m and hence head at E will be $1.5 - 0.234 = 1.266$ m above bottom and $1.5 + 0.234 = 1.734$ m above F.

Pressure intensity *at* $E = 9.81 \times 1.266 = 12.419$ kPa

Pressure intensity at $F = 9.81 \times 1.734 = 17.01$ *kPa*

5.23 The tank in Example 5.22, is closed at the top and contains air under a pressure of 150 kPa.

(a) What will be the pressure at D and E when $\omega = 10$ rad/s?

(b) At what speed should the tank be rotated in order that the bottom has zero depth of water ?

(c) When the angular velocity is 20 rad/s, how much bottom of the tank is uncovered, (Fig. 5.42) ?

Solution

(a) Since there is no change of volume of air, volume of paraboloid = volume of air above AA

Also, volume of paraboloid

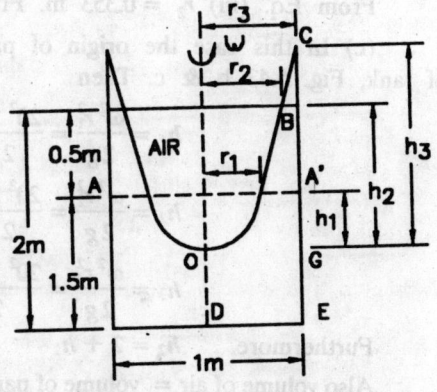

FIG. 5.42. (a) EXAMPLE 5.23

$= 0.5 \times$ volume of circumscribing cylinder

When the tank is rotated at 10 rad/sec, the water surface touches the top cover at radius of r_2 *i.e.* at B in Fig. 5.42a

Hence $\frac{1}{2} \pi r_2^2 \times h_2 = \pi \times 0.5^2 \times 0.5$

$$r_2^2 h_2 = 0.25 \qquad \text{...(i)}$$

Also, $h_2 = (\omega^2 r_2^2 / 2g)$

$$h_2 = \frac{10^2 \times r_2^2}{2g} \qquad \text{...(ii)}$$

Solving Eqs. (i) and (ii)

$$r_2 = 0.47 \text{ m}$$

$$h_2 = 1.13 \text{ m}$$

Also $\qquad h_3 = \omega^2 r_3^2/2g = 10^2 \times (0.5)^2/2g = 1.274 \text{ m}$

The depth of water at $D = 2 - h_2 = 0.87 \text{ m}$

Pressure at $\qquad D = 150 + 9.81 \times 0.87 = 158.534 \text{ } kPa$

Pressure at $\qquad E = 150 + 9.81 (1.274 + 0.87) = 171.032 \text{ } kPa$

(b) Let the speed of cylinder be ω rad/sec for obtaining zero depth at D, Fig. 5.43a.

Again, volume of paraboloid = volume of space above AA'

$$\frac{\pi}{2} r_2^2 \times 2 = \pi \times 0.5^2 \times 0.5 \qquad \qquad \text{...(iii)}$$

Further, $\qquad h_2 = \dfrac{\omega^2 r_2^2}{2g}$

$$2 = \frac{\omega^2 r_2^2}{2 \times 9.81} \qquad \qquad \text{...(iv)}$$

From Eq. (iii) $r_2 = 0.353$ m. From Eq. (iv) $\omega = 17.72$ rad/sec

(c) In this case the origin of paraboloid may lie below the bottom of tank, Fig. 5.43 b & c. Then

$$h_1 = \frac{\omega^2 r_1^2}{2g} = \frac{20^2 \times r_1^2}{2g} \qquad \qquad \text{...(v)}$$

$$h_2 = \frac{\omega^2 r_2^2}{2g} = \frac{20^2 \times r_2^2}{2g} \qquad \qquad \text{...(vi)}$$

$$h_3 = \frac{\omega^2 r_3^2}{2g} = \frac{20^2 \times 0.5^2}{2g} \qquad \qquad \text{...(vii)}$$

Furthermore, $\qquad h_2 = 2 + h_1 \qquad \qquad \text{...(viii)}$

Also volume of air = volume of paraboloid OBB' − volume of paraboloid OFF'

$$\pi \times 0.5^2 \times 0.5 = \frac{1}{2} \times \pi \times (r_2^2 h_2 - r_1^2 h_1) \qquad \qquad \text{(ix)}$$

From Eq. (vii) $h_3 = 3.097$ m

From Eq. (v) and (viii), $h_2 = 2 + 20^2 \times r_1^2/2g \qquad \text{...(x)}$

From Eq. (vi) $h_2 = 20^2 \times r_2^2/2g \qquad \qquad \text{...(xi)}$

Equating Eq. (x) and (xi)

$$2 + \frac{20^2 \times r_1^2}{2g} = \frac{20^2 \times r_2^2}{2g}$$

$$r_2^2 = 0.0981 + r_1^2 \qquad \qquad \text{...(xii)}$$

Substituting the values in Eq. (ix)

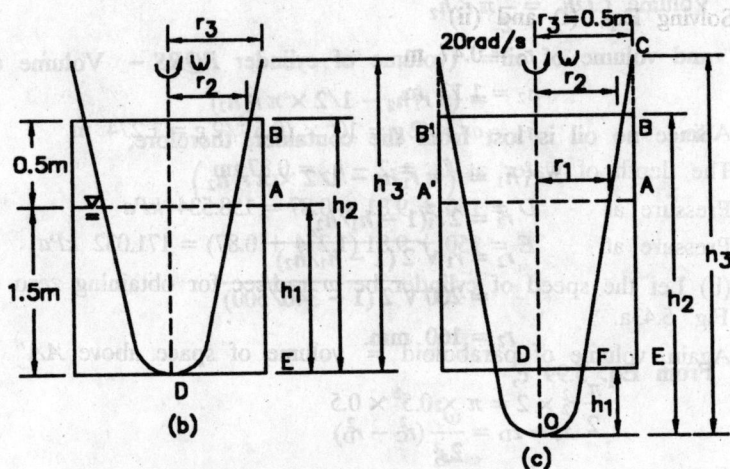

FIG. 5.43. (b) & (c) EXAMPLE 5.23

$$r_2^2 \left(\frac{400 \times r_2^2}{2g} \right) - r_1^2 \left(\frac{4000 \times r_1^2}{2g} \right) = 0.25$$

$$(0.0981 + r_1^2)^2 - r_1^4 = 0.25 \times 2g/400$$

Solving, $\qquad r_1 = 0.116$ m ; $r_2 = 0.334$ m

Hence, area of the bottom uncovered $= \pi r_1^2 = 0.0422 \, \text{m}^2$

$$h_2 = 2.275 \text{ m}$$

$$h_1 = 0.275 \text{ m}$$

5.24 A closed vertical cylinder 400 mm diameter and 500 mm high is filled with oil of specific gravity 0.9 to a depth of 340 mm, the remaining volume containing air at atmosphere air. The cylinder revolves about vertical axis at such a speed that the oil just begins to uncover the base. Calculate (a) the speed of rotation for this condition and (b) the upward force on the cover.

Solution

(a) When stationary, the surface will be at AB, a height h_1 above the base (Fig. 5.44)

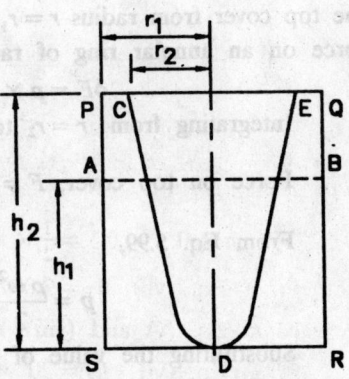

FIG. 5.44. EXAMPLE 5.24

Volume of oil $= \pi r_1^2 h_1$

When rotating at the required speed ω , a forced vertex is formed and the free surface will be the paraboloid, CDE.

Since volume of a paraboloid is equal to the half the volume of the circumscribing cylinder,

Volume $CDE = \dfrac{1}{2}\pi\, r_2^2\, h_2$

and volume of oil= (volume of cylinder $PQRS$ – Volume CDE)

$$= (\pi\, r_1^2 h_2 - 1/2 \times \pi\, r_2^2 h_2)$$

Since no oil is lost from the container, therefore,

$$\pi\, r_1^2 h_1 = \left(\pi\, r_1^2 h_2 - 1/2 \times \pi\, r_2^2 h_2\right)$$

$$r_2^2 = 2\, r_1^2(1 - h_1/h_2)$$

$$r_2 = r_1\sqrt{2\,(1 - h_1/h_2)}$$

$$= 200\sqrt{2\,(1 - 340/500)}$$

$$r_2 = 160 \text{ mm.}$$

From Eq. 5.99 c,

$$z_C - z_D = \frac{\omega^2}{2g}(r_C^2 - r_D^2)$$

For point C and D, $z_D = 0$, $Z_c = h_2$, $r_D = 0$ and $r_C = r_2$

$$h_2 = \frac{\omega^2 r_2^2}{2g}$$

$$\omega = \sqrt{\frac{2g h_2}{r_2^2}}$$

Solving,

$$= \sqrt{\frac{2 \times 9.81 \times 0.500}{(0.16)^2}}$$

$$= 19.6 \text{ rad/s.}$$

(b) While the cylinder is revolved, the oil will be in contact with the top cover from radius $r = r_1$. If p is the pressure at any radius r, the force on an annular ring of radius r and width dr is given by

$$\delta F = p \times 2\pi r\, dr$$

Integrating from $r = r_2$ to $r = r_1$

Force on top cover, $F = 2\pi \displaystyle\int_{r_2}^{r_1} pr\, dr$ ...(1)

From Eq. 5.99,

$$p = \frac{\rho\,\omega^2}{2}(r^2 - r_2^2)$$

Substituting the value of p into Eq. (1)

$$F = 2\pi \int_{r_2}^{r_1} \frac{\rho\,\omega^2}{2}(r^2 - r_2^2)\, r\, dr$$

$$= \rho\,\omega^2 \pi \int_{r_2}^{r_1} (r^3 - r\, r_2^2)\, dr$$

$$= \rho \, \omega^2 \, \pi \left[\frac{r^4}{4} - \frac{r^2}{2} . r_2^2 \right]_{r_2}^{r_1}$$

$$= \rho \, \omega^2 \, \pi \left[\left(\frac{r_1^4}{4} - \frac{r_1^2 r_2^2}{2} \right) - \left(\frac{r_2^4}{4} - \frac{r_2^4}{2} \right) \right]$$

$$= \frac{\pi \, \omega^2 \, \pi}{4} \left[r_1^4 + r_2^4 - 2 r_1^2 r_2^2 \right]$$

$$= \frac{0.9 \times 1000 \times (19.60)^2}{4} \times \pi \left(0.2^2 - 0.16^2 \right)^2$$

$$= 56.3 \ \text{N}$$

5.25 A U-tube with two arms 150 mm apart and filled to a depth of 200 mm is rotated about its central axis to cause water to vaporise at the lowest point of the tube. What should be the speed of rotation ? (Fig. 5.45)

Solution

From Eq. 5.99a, the difference of pressure between two points is given by

$$\frac{p_2 - p_1}{w} = \frac{\omega^2}{2g} (r_2^2 - r_1^2) + (z_1 - z_2)$$

Assume atmospheric pressure $p_1 = 10.0$ metre of water and vapour pressure, $p_2 = 2.5$ metre of water

$$r_2 \ (\text{at centre}) = 0 \, , z_2 = 0$$

$$r_1 = 150/2 = 75 \ \text{mm}; \ z_1 = 200 \ \text{mm}$$

Substituting these values,

$$2.5 - 10 = \omega^2 / 2g \ (0 - 0.075^2) + (0.2 - 0)$$

Solving, $\omega = 44.88$ rad/sec

Hence, $N = 60 \, \omega / 2 \pi$

$$= 60 \times 44.88 / (2 \times \pi)$$

$$= 428 \ \text{r.p.m.}$$

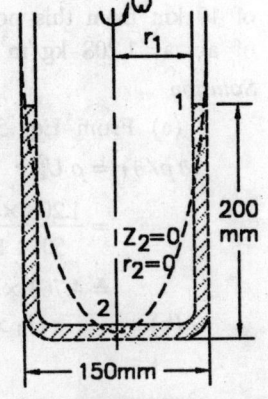

FIG. 5.45. EXAMPLE 5.25

5.26 A straight tube 1.2 m long, closed at bottom and filled with a liquid (specific weight 9.6 kN/m^3), is inclined at 45° with vertical and rotated about a vertical axis through its midpoint at 8 rad/sec. Determine the pressure at midpoint and at the bottom of the tube. (Fig. 5.46).

Solution

As it is a case of forced vortex motion,

$$h = \frac{\omega^2 r^2}{2g}$$

$$= \frac{(8)^2 \times (0.6 \sin 45°)^2}{2g}$$

$= 0.578$ m

i.e., the vortex O will be 0.578 m below A

Pressure at $G = w \times OG$

$\quad = 9.6 \times (0.6 \cos 45° - 0.578)$

$\quad = -1.476 \, kPa$

Pressure at the bottom of tube at C

$\quad = w \times$ vertical height BC

$\quad = 9.6 \times 1.2 \cos 45°$

$\quad = 8.146 \, kPa$

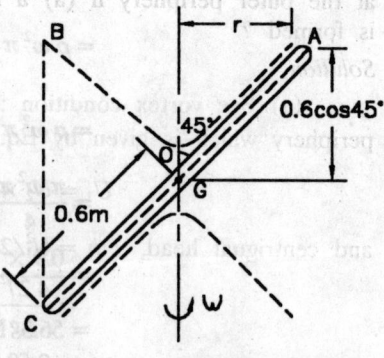

FIG. 5.46. EXAMPLE 5.26

5.27 The wind velocity in a cyclone is assumed to be according to free vortex motion law. If the velocity is 16 km/hr at 50 km from the centre of the cyclone, what pressure gradient should be obtained at this point ? What reduction in barometric pressure should occur over a radial distance of 10 km from this point towards the centre of storm ? Take mass density of air as 1.208 kg/m³.

Solution

(a) From Eq. 5.94a,

$\partial p / \partial r = \rho \, U_t^2 / r$

$\quad = \dfrac{1.208 \times 4.44^2}{50 \times 1000}$ Since 16 km/hr $= \dfrac{16 \times 1000}{3.600} = 4.44$ m/s

$\quad = 4.763 \times 10^{-4} \, \text{N/m}^2/\text{m}$

(b) $\qquad U_{t1} \times r_1 = U_{t2} \times r_2$

$\qquad U_{t2} = \dfrac{4.44 \times 50 \times 1000}{40 \times 1000} = 5.55$ m/s

(c) From Eq. 5.103 ,

$\dfrac{p_1 - p_2}{w} = \dfrac{U_2^2 - U_1^2}{2g} + z_2 - z_1$

$\qquad = \dfrac{5.55^2 - 4.44^2}{19.62}$

assuming both points at same level

$\qquad p_1 - p_2 = 1.208 \times 9.81 \times 0.565 = 6.697 \, \text{N/m}^2$

If the pressure is atmospheric at 50 km radius, the pressure at 40 km from centre will reduce by 6.697 N/m²

5.28 The water contained in an annular space of centrifugal pump of outer radius 480 mm and inner radius 250 mm is rotated so as to form a vortex. At the inner periphery, the velocity of whirl (*i.e.* at the outer tip of the blade) is 8.2 m/s and pressure is 244 *kPa*. What will be the pressure at the outer periphery if (a) a free vortex is formed, (b) a forced vortex is formed ?

Solution

(a) Fee vortex condition : Let U_1 be the velocity of whirl at outer periphery which is given by Eq. 5.102.

$$U_1 = U_2 \times r_2/r_1 = 8.2 \times \frac{0.25}{0.48} = 4.27 \text{ m/s}$$

and centrigual head, $h = U_1^2/2g \ (r_1^2/r_2^2 - 1)$

$$= \frac{4.27^2}{2g} \times \left(\frac{0.48^2}{0.25^2} - 1 \right)$$

$$= 2.50 \text{ m}$$

Hence, corresponding pressure rise $= w h$

$$= 9.81 \times 2.5 = 24.52 \, kPa$$

Pressure at out periphery $= 244 + 24.52$

$$= 268.52 \, kPa$$

(b) Forced vortex condition : $U_1 = U_2 \times r_1/r_2$

$$= 8.2 \times \frac{0.48}{0.25} = 15.74 \text{ m/s}$$

Centrifugal head $h = \frac{U_1^2}{2g} - \frac{U_2^2}{2g}$

$$= \frac{15.74^2}{2g} - \frac{8.2^2}{2g} = 9.2 \text{ metre}$$

pressure $= 9.81 \times 9.2 = 90.25 \, kPa$

Pressure at outer periphery $= 244 + 90.25$

$$= 334.25 \, kPa$$

5.29 : A two dimensional flow occurs through a rectangular duct and a bend of same width (0.5m) with a mean velocity 2 m/s. Assuming the flow to be irrotational and of free-vortex type, find the velocities at the inner ($R_1 = 0.5$ m) and outer walls ($R_2 = 1.0$ m) of the wall of duct. Also compute the difference between outer and inner walls of the duct.

Solution :

Given $B = 0.5$ m, $R_1 = 0.5$, $R_2 = 1.0$, $U_0 = 2$ m/s, $u = \frac{C}{r}$.

Consider unit depth of duct and take a small fluid element at a radius r and thickness dr.

Discharge/unit depth $q = \int_{R_1}^{R_2} u \ (dr \times 1)$

Since the flow is free vortex type, $u = C/r$

$$q = \int_{R_1}^{R_2} \frac{c}{r}\,dr$$

$$q = [C \log_e r]_{R_1}^{R_2}$$

$$q = C \log_e \frac{R_2}{R_1} \qquad \qquad ...(i)$$

Also

$$q = \text{area} \times \text{velocity}$$

$$= (0.5 \times 1) \times (2) = 1 \text{ m}^3/\text{s/m} \qquad ...(ii)$$

From Eqs. (i) and (ii),

$$\therefore \qquad 1 = C \log_e \left(\frac{1}{0.5} \right)$$

$$C = \frac{1}{\log_e 2} = 1.443$$

Hence

$$U_1 = \frac{C}{R_1}$$

$$= \frac{1.443}{0.5} = 2.886 \text{ m/s}$$

$$U_2 = \frac{C}{R_2}$$

$$= \frac{1.443}{1.0} = 1.443 \text{ m/s}$$

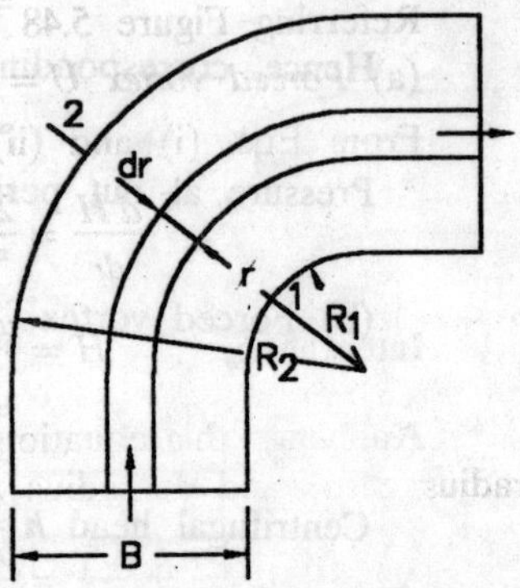

FIG. 5.47. EXAMPLE 5.29

Since the flow is irrotational (free vortex), Bernoulli's equation can be used.

Applying Bernoulli's equation, between inner and outer walls at 1 and 2,

$$\frac{p_1}{w} + \frac{U_1^2}{2g} + z_1 = \frac{p_2}{2} + \frac{U_2^2}{2g} + z_2$$

Since

$$z_1 = z_2,$$

$$\left(\frac{p_2 - p_1}{w} \right) = \left(\frac{U_1^2 - U_2^2}{2g} \right)$$

$$= \frac{(2.886)^2 - (1.443)^2}{2 \times 9.81}$$

$$= 0.3184 \text{ m}$$

5.30 An impeller 0.3 m in diameter rotating concentrically about a vertical axis inside a closed cylinder 0.6m diameter, produces a circular vortex motion in water with which the cylinder is completely filled. This motion takes the form of a forced vortex inside the impeller and a free vortex in the annular space between the impeller and casing; the velocity in the forced and free vortices being equal at the impeller edge. The pressure head at the impeller centre is equal to 1.5 m. Find the pressure head at the casing when the speed of the impeller is 1200 rev./min. (fig. 5.48).

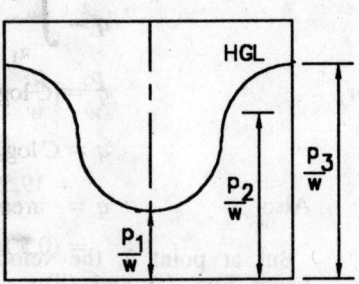

FIG. 5.48. EXAMPLE 5.30

Solution

For 2-D flow, the rate of change of total head is given by Eq. 5.98b

$$\frac{dH}{dr} = \frac{U}{g}\left(\frac{U}{r} + \frac{dU}{dr}\right) \quad ...(i)$$

where $H = p/w + U^2/2g$

Referring Figure 5.48

(a) *Forced vortex* $U = \omega r$ ...(ii)

From Eqs. (i) and (ii)

$$\frac{dH}{dr} = \frac{2\omega^2 r}{g}$$

Integrating, $\quad H = \frac{\omega^2 r^2}{g} + \text{constant}$

Applying this equation between two points 1 and 2, *i.e.* at the centre (radius zero) and at radius r

$$\frac{p_1}{w} + \frac{U_1^2}{2g} = \frac{p_2}{w} + \frac{U_2^2}{2g} - \frac{\omega^2 r_2^2}{g} \quad ...(iii)$$

From Eqs. (ii) and (iii)

$$\frac{p_1}{w} + \frac{\omega^2 r_2^2}{2g} = \frac{p_2}{\omega} \quad \text{Sicne } U_1 = \omega r_1 = 0 \quad ...(iv)$$

Substituting the values in Eq. (iv)

$$\frac{p_2}{w} = 1.5 + \frac{(2\pi \times 1200/60)^2 (0.15)^2}{2g}$$

$$= 19.59 \text{ m} \quad ...(v)$$

(b) *Free vortex* Since for irrotational vortex $dH = 0$, therefore, from Eq. (i)

$$\frac{dU}{U} + \frac{dr}{r} = 0 \quad ...(vi)$$

Integrating, Eq. (vi) $Ur = C$ ...(vii)

Since $\quad dH = 0$, $H_2 = H_3$,

$$\frac{p_2}{w} + \frac{U_2^2}{2g} = \frac{p_3}{w} + \frac{U_3^3}{2g}$$

$$\frac{p_2}{w} + \frac{C^2}{2g} \frac{1}{r_2^2} = \frac{p_3}{w} + \frac{C^3}{2g} \frac{1}{r_3^2} \qquad \text{Using Eq. (vii)}$$

or

$$\frac{p_3}{w} = \frac{p_2}{w} + \frac{C^2}{2g} \left(\frac{1}{r_2^2} - \frac{1}{r_3^2} \right)$$

$$= 19.59 + \frac{C^2}{2g} \left(\frac{1}{0.15^2} - \frac{1}{0.3^2} \right) \qquad \text{...(viii)}$$

But at point 2, the velocity should remain same, therefore,

$$U = \omega \, r_2 = C/r_2$$

$$C = \omega \, r_2^2 = \left(2 \times \pi \times \frac{1200}{60} \right) (0.15)^2$$

$$= 2.826 \qquad \text{...(ix)}$$

Hence from Eqs. (viii) and (ix)

$$p_3/w = 33.156 \ \text{m}$$

5.31 Water flows upwards through a vertical pipe 300 mm diameter and then flows out radially into atmosphere between two parallel circular plates of 800 mm diameter kept 10 mm apart. If the pressure at A is 25 kN/m² gauge, find the discharge through the system shown in the figure.

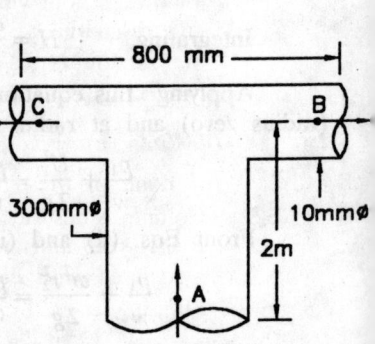

FIG. 5.49. EXAMPLE 5.31

Solution

Using continuity equation

$$(U_A A_A) = (U_B A_B)$$

$$\frac{\pi}{4} (0.3)^2 U_A = \pi \times 0.800 \times 0.01 \times U_B \qquad \text{...(1)}$$

$$U_A = 0.355 \, U_B$$

Apply Bernoulli's theorem between A and B,

$$\frac{p_A}{w} + z_A + \frac{U_A^2}{2g} = \frac{p_B}{w} + z_B + \frac{U_B^2}{2g}$$

assuming, no loss of energy between A and B

$$\frac{25 \times 1000}{9810} + 0 + \frac{(0.355 \, U_B)^2}{2g} = 0 + 2.0 + \frac{U_B^2}{2g}$$

Sovling it, $\qquad U_B = 3.51 \ \text{m/s}$

and $\qquad U_A = 0.355 \, U_B = 1.246 \ \text{m/s}$

$$Q = \pi/4 \times (0.3)^2 \times 1.246$$

$$= 0.088 \ \text{m}^3/\text{s}$$

Objective Questions

5.1 The assumptions about flow required in deriving the equation $gz + U^2/2g + \int dp/\rho$ =constant are that it is

    (a) steady, frictionless, incompressible, along a streamline

    (b) uniform, frictionless along a streamline, ρ a function of p

    (c) steady, uniform, incompressible along a streamline

    (d) steady, frictionless, ρ a function of p along a streamlie

    (e) none of these answers

5.2 The work that a liquid is capable of doing by virtue of its sustained pressure in joule per newton, is

    (a) z (b) p (c) p/w (d) $U^2/2g$ (e) $\sqrt{2gH}$

5.3 The velocity head is

    (a) $U^2/2g$ (b) z (c) U

    (d) $\sqrt{2gH}$ (e) none of these answers

5.4 If a fluid of specific weight w (and specific mass ρ) flows through a flow section with average velocity U, pressure p, elevation head z and discharge Q, then the total energy of the fluid flowing through the section is

    (a) $wQ(p/w + z + U^2/2g)$ (b) $\rho Q(p/w + z + U^2 2g)$

    (c) $(p/w + z + U^2/2g)$ (d) $Q(p/w + z + U^2/2g)$

    (e) none of these answers

5.5 Column A describes the various forms of the Bernoulli's equation whereas B lissts the units which pertains to one of these forms. Match the unit associated with each of the equations

Column A	Column B
(a) $p/w + z + U^2/2g$	(i) total energy per unit volume
(b) $p/\rho + gz + U^2/2$	(ii) total energy per unit mass
(c) $p + wz + \rho U^2/2$	(iii) total energy per unit weight

5.6 The total energy is usually represented by the Bernoulli's equation as $p/w + z + U^2/2g$. The unit, in which the total energy is represented, is

    (a) Nm/m   (b) Nm/N   (c) Nm²/s

    (d) Nm/s   (e) none of these answers

5.7 The kinetic energy correction factor α is expressed as

    (a) $\dfrac{1}{A} \int_A (u /\!/ U)^2 \, dA$ (b) $\dfrac{1}{A} \int_A (u/U)^3 \, dA$

    (c) $\dfrac{1}{A} \int_A (u/U) \, dA$ (d) none of these answers

5.8 The energy correction factor for a triangular velocity distribution with zero velocity at one of the wall is

(a) 0   (b) 1

(c) 1.33   (d) 2   (e) none of these answers

5.9 The energy correction factor for a velocity distribution obtained in a circular pipe of radius R, given by $u/U_m = (1 - r^2/R^2)$ is

(a) 1.01   (b) 2.0

(c) 1.75   (c) 1.75   (d) none of these answers

5.10 The momentum correction factor β is expressed by

(a) $\dfrac{1}{A} \int_A (u/U)\, dA$ (b) $\dfrac{1}{A}(u/U)^2\, dA$

(c) $\dfrac{1}{A} \int_A (u/U)^3\, dA$ (d) $\dfrac{1}{A} \int_A (u/U)^4\, dA$

(e) none of these answers

5.11 The velocity over one third cross section is zero and is uniform over the remaining two thirds of the area. The momentum correction factor is

(a) 1   (b) 1.334   (c) 1.5

(d) 2.20   (e) none of these answers

5.12 While applying momentum equation to a control volume, which of the following assumption is required ?

(a) velocity constant over the cross section

(b) steady flow   (c) uniform flow

(d) compressible fluid   (e) frictionless fluid

5.13 A 30 cm diameter 90° elbow carries water with average velocity of 5 m/s and pressure intensity of $-$ 4 kPa. The force component in the direction of incoming velocity to hold the ellow in place in kN, is

(a) $-$ 5.15   (b) 10.30   (c) 60.21

(d) 0.92   (e) none of these answers

5.14 The thickness of a wall for a penstock is determined by the consideration of

(a) circumferential pipe wall tensile strength

(b) force exerted by the dynamic action at bend

(c) force exerted by static and dynamic action at bends

(d) axial tensile strength

(e) temperature stresses

5.15 When a steady jet impinges on a fixed inclined plate

(a) the velocity is reduced for that portion of the jet which has turned through more than 90° and increased for other portion

(b) the momentum in the direction of the incoming velocity is unchanged

(c) no force is exerted on the jet by the vane

(d) the flow is divided into parts proportional to their angle of deflection

(e) momentum component remains unchanged parallel to the surface

5.16 The pressure intensity at the summit of a siphon for an ideal fluid

(a) will be a minimum

(b) depends upon the height of summit above upstream reservoir only

(c) is independennt of liquid density

(d) is independent of discharge

(e) is independent of downstream leg

5.17 The change in angular momentum of fluid flowing in a curved path results in

(a) a change in its total energy

(b) a change in kinetic energy

(c) a change in pressure   (d) a torque

(e) a dynamic force passing through its centre of curvature

5.18 Select the correct statement

(a) Bernoulli's equation relates various forces involved in the problem

(b) Bernoulli's equation relates various formsof energy

(c) Bernoulli's equation relates various forces with the change in momentum

(d) Bernoulli's equation torque to changes in angular momentum

5.19 When a liquid rotates at constat angular velocity about a vertical axis as a rigid body, the pressure intensity

(a) decreases with the radial distance

(b) increases linearly with the radial distance

(c) increases gradually with the radial distance

(d) none of these answers

5.20 A closed cubical box 1 m on each edge is half filled with water, the other half with oil of specific gravity 0.8. When accelerated vertically upward at the rate of 5 m/s² the pressure difference between bottom and top in *kPa* is

(a) 12.05   (b) 13.32   (c) 14.81

(d) 8.83   (e) none of these answeres

5.21 When the above tank is accelerated uniformly in a horizontal direction parallel to one side at 4.9 m s² the slope of interface is

(a) 0.0   (b) 0.5

(c) 0.75   (d) 1.0   (e) none

5.22 The pressure difference between two points can be determined using Bernoulli's equation for

(a) free vortex flow   (b) forced vortex flow

(c) radial flow   (d) none

5.23 The continuity equation in ideal fluid flow

(a) states that the net rate of inflow into any small volume must be zero

(b) applies to irrotational flow only

(c) implies the existence of velocity potential

(d) none of these answers

5.24 Select the type of vortex motion

(a) flow around a pipe bend

(b) occurrence of a cyclone

(c) flow in the impeller of a centrifugal pump

(d) whirling motion in a river

(e) flow in the volute chamber of a centrifugal pump

(f) flow out of the drain of a wash basin

Problems

5.1 Oil of specific gravity 0.87 is flowing in a 150 mm diameter pipe. At a certain section in the pipe, the pressure is 190 *kPa* and the total energy relative to datum plane 3 m below is 200 joule per newton. Find the discharge in the pipe.

5.2 If each gauge, in Fig. 5.50, shows the same reading for a flow rate of 0.35 m³/s , what is the diameter of the constriction?

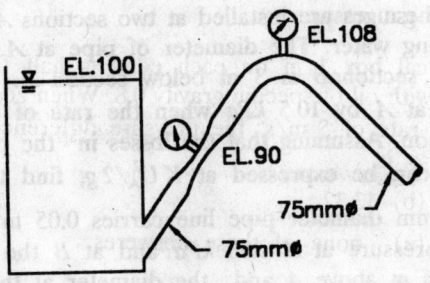

FIG. 5.50 PROBLEM 5.2

5.3 Calculate the diameter, d of the pipe for the two gauges to read the same-value (Fig. 5.51).

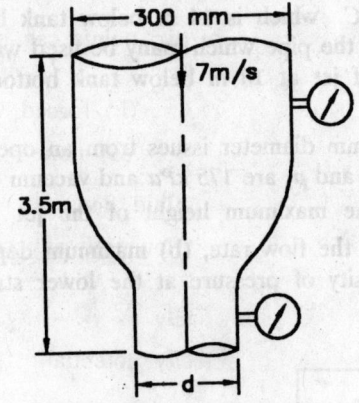

FIG. 5.51 PROBLEM 5.3

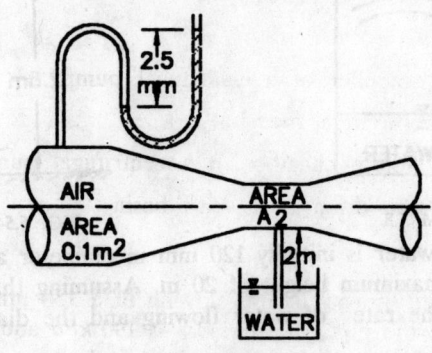

FIG. 5.52 PROBLEM 5.4

5.4 For a flow rate of $2 \, m^3/s$ of air($w = 1.29 \, kg/m^3$) what is the largest value of A_2, which a will cause water to be drawn up to the piezometric opening? Neglect compressibility effects (Fig. 5.52).

5.5 Pressure gauges are installed at two sections A and B in a vertical tapered pipe carring water. The diameter of pipe at A is 15 cm and thatat B is 7.5 cm. The sectionn$B$ is 3 m below section A. The pressure at $B$is greater than that at A by 10.5 kPa when the rate of flow is 0.03 m^3/s in the upward direction. Assuming that the losses in the pipe between the two sections A and$B$ can be expressed at $K U_A^2/2g$, find the value of K.

5.6 A 150 mm diameter pipe line carries 0.05 m^3/s of oil of specific gravity 0.95; the pressure at A is80 kPa and at B the pressure is 25 kPa. The section B is 6 m above A and the diameter at this sectionis 300 mm. Determien the direction of flow and the loss of head.

5.7 A tank contains water to a depth of 7 m. A small opening of 10 cm diameter is drilled at the bottom to which a pipe 28 m long is 7.5 cm diameter and 1 m length is fitted. Calculate the pressure at the entry B to the pipe and at C which is 14 m below tank bottom. Also calculate the maximum length of the pipe which many be used without cavitation. What will be the diameter of jet at 10 m below tank bottom if there is no pipe attached to it?

5.8 A jet of 25 mm diameter issues from an opening as shown in Fig. 5.53. If the pressures p_1 and p_2 are 175 kPa and vaccum of 300 mm of mercury respectively, what is the maximum height of the jet?

5.9 Calculate (a) the flow rate, (b) maximum depth upstream of sluice gate and (c) the intensity of pressure at the lower stagnation point in Fig. 5.54.

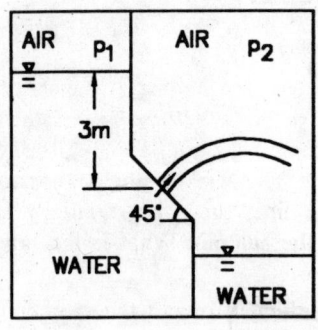

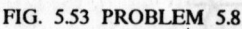

FIG. 5.53 PROBLEM 5.8

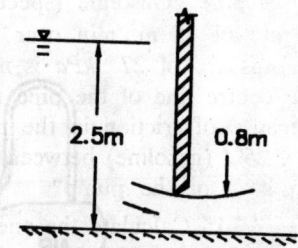

FIG. 5.54 PROBLEM 5.9

5.10 A jet of water is initially 120 mm in diameter and when directed upwards reaches a maximum height of 20 m. Assuming that the jet remains circular, determine the rate of water flowing and the diameter of jet at a height of 10 m.

5.11 The centre line of a tapered pipe AB carrying petrol (sp. gr. 0.74) slopes upwards from A to B at an angle of 30° to the horizontal. The distance A is 5 m and the diameter increase from 100 mm at A to 150 mm at B. The pressure gauges are installed at A and B. Find (a) the flow rate when the reading on the pressure gauges are equal, (b) the pressure difference across AB for the same rate of flow when the direction of taper is reversed.

5.12 A 20 mm diameter pipe draws water from a 600 mm diameter main in which the pressure is maintained at 105 kPa The 20 mm pipe serves a tap which is 7.2 m higher than the junction with the main. If the tap is fully open and no other tappings are taken from the main, determine (a) the pressure in the 20 mm pipe just before the tap, (b) the velocity in the main, (c) the velocity in 20 mm pipe and (d) the discharge from the tap. Neglect all losses.

5.13 During a flow of 6 m^3/s water through a hydraulic turbine (Fig. 5.55), the pressure indicated by gauge A is 9 kPa. What should the gauge B read if the turbine is delivering 400 kW at 75% efficiency ?

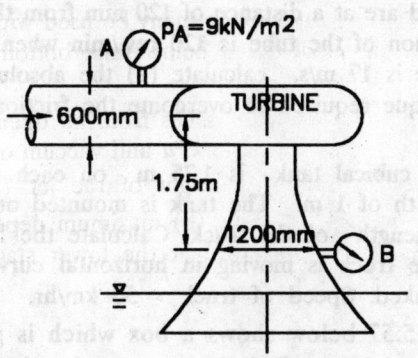

FIG. 5.55 PROBLEM 5.13

5.14 Gasoline (specific gravity 0.67) from a reservoir is pumped at a rate of 45 m^3/min over hill through a pipe line 750 mm in diameter. A pressure of 27 kPa is maintained in the pipe line at the summit where the centre line of the pipe is 100 m above the free surface in the reservoir. Because of friction in the pump and the pipe line, there is an energy loss of 2.25 J (gasoline) between the reservoir and the summit. What is the power (in kW) of the pump?

5.15 Calculate the energy correction coefficient α and the momentum correction factor β for a velocity distribution in a circular pipe given by $(u/U_o) = (y/R)^{1/n}$ where u is the velocity at a distace y from the wall of the pipe, U_o is the centreline velocity, R the radius of the pipe and n is an exponent.

5.16 What propulsive force is exerted on the car shown in Fig. 5.56 ? What is the efficiency of this jet as a propulsive device?

5.17 Water flows at the rate of 0.75 m³/s through the pipe transition 1 m × 0.7 m . If the pressure of the centreline of 1 m section is 100 kPa, what will be the pressure at the centre line of 0.7 m section ? What force will be exerted by the flowing water on the transition ? Also calculate the force acting on the transition if no flow occurs through this transition.

5.18 Thirty five cubic metre per minute of water flows through a 300 mm diameter pipe line that contains 60° bend. The pressure intensity at the entrance to the bend is 25 kPa. Determine the force componnents parallel and normal to the approach velocity required to hold the bend in place.

5.19 Oil of specific gravity 0.75 flows through an expanding end that turns the liquid 120° . The upstream diameter is 600 mm and downstream diameter is 750 mm. The flow through the bend is 2.5 m³/sec . Neglecting energy losses though the bend, determine force components necessary to support the bend. Take inlet pressure = 70 kPa

5.20 A lawn sprinkler consists of a horizontal tube with nozzle at each end normal to the tube but inclined upwards at 40° to the horizontal. A central bearing incorporates the inlet for the water supply. The nozzle are 3 mm in diameter and are at a distance of 120 mm from the central bearing. If the speed of rotation of the tube is 120 rev./min when the velocity of jet relative to the nozzle is 17 m/s, calculate (a) the absolute velocity of jet, and (b) the total torque required to overcome the frictioal resistance of the tube and bearing.

5.21 An open cubical tank is 1.75 m on each side and is filled with water to a dpeth of 1 m. The tank is mounted on a truck with one side parallel to the length of the truck. Calculate the force on each side of the tank when the truck is moving in horizontal curve of 70 m radius. The road is not banked. Speed of truck = 50 km/hr.

5.22 The Fig. 5.57 below shows a box which is given acceleration $a_x = 4.9 \text{ m/s}^2$ and $a_y = 3.0 \text{ m/s}^2$ find the pressure intesity at points B and C in kPa. Each side of box = 1.5m.

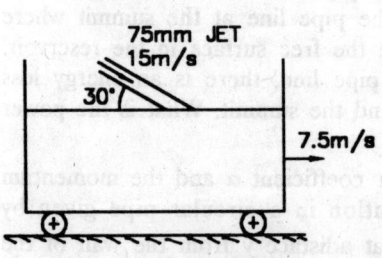
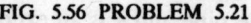
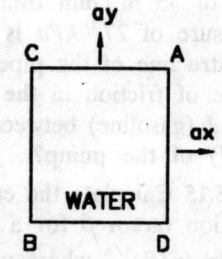

FIG. 5.56 PROBLEM 5.21   FIG. 5.57 PROBLEM 5.22

5.23 An open cylindrical tank, 1.2 m diameter and 1.8 m high, is rotated about a vertical axis at 60 rpm. If it is filled with water to a depth of 0.8 m, determine the pressure intensity at the bottom and sides.

If the tank is now completely filled with water how much water is spilled out and how much depth of water remains at the centre.

5.24 A cylindrical vessel 1 m diameter and 3 m high is filled with water to a depth of 1.2 m. The pressure in the tank at its top is raised to 140 kPa. If the tank is rotated at 200 rpm, calculate the pressure at the wall on the top and the bottom of the tank.

5.25 There is a 90° bend in the horizontal plane in a pressure tunnel of rectangular section 1.5 m wide and 1 m deep. The internal radius of the bend is 1 m. The velocity at the centre line of conduct is 3.5 m/s and the pressure on the base at the centre line is 140 kPa. Calculate the pressure on the roof of the bend in kPa at (i) the outer wall and (ii) inner wall.

5.26 A 4 cm diameter, 1.5 m long pipe is just filled with oil of specific gravity 0.822 and then capped. It is placed in horizontal position and is rotated at 27.5 rad/s about a vertical axis 300 mm from one end. What pressure in kPa is developed at the far end of pipe ?

5.27 A vertical U tube with two legs 2 m apart is filled with water and rotated about a vertical axis 0.5 m from one leg. Determine the difference in elevation of the water levels in the two legs when the speed of rotation is 150 rpm.

6

Dimensional Analysis and Similitude

6.1 INTRODUCTION

The most simple and desirable method in the analaysis of any fluid flow problem is its direct mathematical solution. But the exact solution of all the fluid problems can not be found by direct mathematical methods. Often, some simpler assumptions are made to solve the complex fluid problems. In most of the problems, there are so many variables involved in the differential equations that a direct analytical solution is not possible. In these problems, dimensional analysis can be used to great advantage in obtaining a number of non-dimensional groups among various variables involved. Thus dimensional analysis is a mathematical technique which makes use of the study of dimensions as an aid to the solution of various engineering problems.

The main advantage of a dimensional analysis is to reduce the number of variables in the problem by combining dimensional variables to form "non-dimensional parameters". It should be well understood that dimensional analysis is not a tool to solve all engineering problems but simply a convenient method in obtaining a partial solutions to certain problems.

6.2 DIMENSIONS

Various physical quantities are used to describe the physical phenomenon. These quantities can be described by a set of 'fundamental (primary or basic) units or dimensions'. These primary dimensions are mass (M), length (L) and time (T). Sometimes force (F) is used instead of mass (M), which is interconnected to mass by Newton's second law of motion. The dimensions of other quantities are derived from primary dimensions and hence are known as 'secondary or derived dimensions'. The expression for a derived dimension in terms of primary dimensions is called 'dimension of the physical quantity' and the equation is known as the 'dimensional formula', e.g. $[A] = [M^a L^b T^c]$, where a, b and c are indices which can be evaluated by the principle of dimensional homogeneity. The square bracket is used to indicate that the dimension of A is being considered.

In Table 6.1, the derived dimensions and units of various physical quantities have been given.

(a) *Dimensionless constant.* These are the quantities which do not have any dimensions and remain constant for all system of measurement, e.g. coefficient of discharge C_d .

(b) *Dimensional constant.* Those are quantities which remain constant in particular system of measurement, e.g. gas constant R.

(c) *Independent variable*. These variables which affect the value of the quantity or variable to be determined.

(d) *Dependent variable*. It is the one, whose value is required to be determined, e.g.

$$h_f = \frac{fL}{D} \frac{U^2}{2g} \qquad \qquad ...(6.1 \ a)$$

Here h_f is to. be determined for the given value of f, L, D and g. Hence h_f is dependent on all the variables mentioned and is then known as dependent variable whereas one can assign any value to other variables. These variables, f, L, D and g are then known as independent variable, When Eq. 6.1 a is written as

$$f = h_t \frac{D}{L} \frac{2g}{U^2} \qquad \qquad ...(6.1 \ b)$$

f is known as dependent variable and all others are known as independent variables.

6.3. PRINCIPLE OF DIMENSIONAL HOMOGENEITY

The principle of dimensional homogeneity was given by Fourier which states that an equation expressing a physical relationship between various quantities must be dimensionally homogeneous, *i.e.*, the dimensions of both sides of the equation should be the same. Examples of dimensionally homogeneous equations are

$$t = 2\pi \sqrt{l/g} \qquad \qquad ...(6.2 \ a)$$

$$Q = Cd \, a \sqrt{2gh} \qquad \qquad ...(6.2 \ b)$$

1. Characteristics of dimensionally homogenous equations

Following are some of the characteristics of dimensional homogeneous equations.

(a) These can be written in terms of dimensionless groups.

(b) Two dimensionally homogeneous equations should not be added or subtracted from each other, otherwise resulting equation may not be dimensionally homogeneous.

(c) Two such equations can be multiplied or divided by each other.

(d) Dimensionless group can be multiplied by a numerical constant.

(e) Any dimensionless constant can be added to the dimensionally homogeneous equation.

2. Application of the principle of dimensional homogeneous equation

The principle of dimensional homogeneity can be put into the following uses.

(a) To determine the dimensions of various physical quantities.

(b) To check whether a given equation is dimensionally homogeneous, if not, to modify it to be used in other system of measurement.

(c) To convert the units of physical quantities from one system in to another system of measurement.

(d) To form the basis of dimensional analysis.

The uses of the principle of dimensional homogeneity are illustrated by an example henceafter.

Example

There are several equations in the mechanics which are not dimensionally homogeneous and hence can not be used in the system of units other than for which these have been derived, e.g. Manning's equation, Chezy's equation, expression for specific speed of hydraulic machines, etc. In general, the dimensions of various quantities are substituted in the given equation and checked whether the given equation is dimensionally homogeneous or not. Otherwise, it can be modified to be used in other system of units. As an illustration, Manning's equation in F.P.S. system is written as

$$U = \frac{1.486}{N} R^{2/3} S^{1/2} \qquad \qquad ...(6.3)$$

where U is the velocity of flow and is measured in feet per second and R is the hydraulic radius and is measured in feet. Substituting the dimensions of various terms, one gets,

$$[L/T] = \left[\frac{1.486}{N}\right] [ft]^{2/3} [ft/ft]^{1/2}$$

In this equation, N is known as Manning's roughness coefficient and is characteristic of surface and as such should be a dimensionaless quantity. Hence, it is seen that the above equation is not a dimensionally homogeneous equation. The dimension of multiplying constant $[1.486/N]$ should be $L^{1/3}/T$

That means the unit for this multiplying constant in FPS unit should be $[L\,ft]^{1/3}/[T\,sec]$. To use this equation in MKS system of units, the units of various terms in *FPS* units should be converted into MKS units.

$$\left[\frac{1.486}{N}\right] = \frac{[L \times 0.3048 \text{ metre}]^{1/3}}{[T\,sec]}$$

$$= 0.6729\,[L\,metre]^{1/3}/[T\,sec] \qquad ...(6.4)$$

This means that the conversion coefficient is 0.6729. Hence, Eq. 6.3 in MKS units should be written as

$$U = \left[\frac{1.486}{N}\right] \times 0.6729 \times [R]^{2/3} [S]^{1/2}$$

$$U = \frac{1}{N} \times R^{2/3} S^{1/2} \qquad ...(6.5)$$

In the same way, the units of various physical quantities can be converted from one system into another.

6.4. METHODS OF DIMENSIONAL ANALYSIS

There are two methods of dimensional analysis.

(1) Rayleigh's method
(2) Buckingham's π -method

1. Rayleigh's method

This method is more convenient to use when the number of variables involved in the fluid flow phenomenon is limited to four or five. The method may be well understood by an illustration.

Flow over a rectangular weir depends upon the head H, acceleration due to gravity g, viscosity μ , mass density ρ and a characteristic length of weir L.

$$Q = f((\rho, gH, \mu, L) \qquad ...(6.6 \text{ a})$$

Substituting the dimensions of vaious terms on both sides,

$$[Q] = f[\rho, g, H, \mu, L]$$

It is assumed that Q is related to these variables by the following relation.

$$[Q] = f[\rho^a][g^b][H^e][\mu^d][L^e]$$

where a, b, c, d and e are unknown indices. These indices are determined with the help of the principle of dimensional homogeneity. Therefore, the dimensions of various terms are substituted.

$$[L^3/T] = f[M/L^3]^a [L/T^2]^b [L]^c [M/L\,T]^d [L]^e$$

For the equation to be dimensionally homogeneous, the indices of M, L and T on both sides should be equal.

$$M : 0 = a + d \qquad ...(i)$$
$$L : 3 = -3a + b + c - d + e \qquad ...(ii)$$
$$T : -1 = -2b - d \qquad ...(iii)$$

It is seen that the number of equations are limited by the number or primary dimensions involved *i.e.* 3, whereas the number of variables invovled are five. Hence these equations are solved in terms of certain important variables. It is purely a guess work and hence some insight into the problem is required. As a guide, these equations are solved in terms of indices of the fluid properties like mass density ρ , kinematic viscosity ν , compressibility E_v and/or surface tension σ . The solution of these equations, generally, yield well known dimensionless group, e.g. Reynolds number, Frouds number, etc.

The above equations, Eqs. (i), (ii) and (iii), for example, are solved for a, b and c (*i.e.* in terms of indices d and e of viscosity μ and length L respectively). Hence,

$$a = -d$$
$$b = (1 - d)/2$$
$$c = (5/2 - 3d/2 + e)$$

The expression for discharge Q flowing over the weir, therefore becomes

$$Q = f[\rho^{-d} g^{(1-d)/2} H^{(3/2 - 3d/2 - e)} \mu^d L^e]$$

Rearranging the terms,

$$Q = g^{1/2} H^{5/2} f \left[\left\{ \mu / g^{1/2} H^{3/2} \rho \right\}^d , (L/H)^e \right]$$

$$\frac{Q}{g^{1/2} H^{5/2}} = f \left[\left(\frac{\mu}{\rho H \sqrt{gH}} \right)^{d/2} , (L/H)^e \right]$$

The term on left hand side $Q/H^2 \sqrt{gH}$ is coefficient of discharge C_d

Therefore, $\qquad C_d = f [(Re)^{d/2} , (L/H)^e]$

The variation of C_d with Reynods number R_e and dimensionless length L/H can, now, be studied experimentally and the exact relationship may be determined.

2. Buckingham's π–method

When the number of variables involved in the fluid flow phenomenon is more than four or five. It is more convenient to determine various dimensionless groups, known as π-terms.

Buckingham's π-method states that if the given equation is dimensionally homogeneous and contains 'n' number of dimensionless variables which are completely described by 'm' number of dimensions (e.g. M, L and T), then these may be grouped into $(n-m)$ number of dimensionless terms. Each π-term is an independent dimensionless parameter. Mathematically, if any variable x_1 (say) depends on $x_2, x_3, x_4 \ldots x_n$, independent varibles, then the functional relationship among them can be written as

$$x_1 = f[x_2, x_3, x_4 \ldots x_n] \qquad \qquad ...(6.7\ a)$$
$$f = f_1 (x_1, x_2, x_3, x_4, \ldots x_n) = C , \quad \text{a constant} \qquad ...(6.7\ b)$$

The various variables of Eq. 6.7b can be grouped into a number of π-terms. Thus

$$\pi_1 = x_1^{a1} x_2^{b1} x^{c1} \ldots x_r^{r1} \qquad \qquad ...(6.7\ c)$$
$$\pi_2 = x_1^{a2} x_2^{b2} x_3^{c2} \ldots x_r^{r2} \qquad \qquad ...(6.7d)$$
$$\pi_{m-n} = x_1^{am-n} x_2^{bm-n} x_3^{cm-n} x_1^{rm-n} \qquad ...(6.7c)$$

Since the π term is a dimensionless group of variables, the indices of corresponding primary dimensions should be the same on both sides of each equation, Eq. 6.7c to e. This means that the indices of mass term on left hand side of an equation should be equal to the indices of mass terms on right hand side. Similarly, the indices of length and time on both sides of each equation are equated. The resultant algebraic equations are, then, solved to determine various π-terms i.e. π_1 , $\pi_2 \ldots \pi_n$

3. Repeating and non-repeating variables

(a) *Repeating variables* . These are the variables which are repeated in each π-term like x_2, x_3, x_4, etc. in Eq. 6.7c, d and e; their number is equal to the primary dimensions involved in the flow phenomenon.

(b) *Non-repeating variables* These are the variables which appear only once in each π-group like x_r in Eq. 6.7c to e, their number is equal to $(n - m)$. Hence, the number of π-terms obtained in a flow phenomenon is also equal to $(n - m)$.

Thus the Buckingham's π-method consists of forming a number of π-terms; each π-term consists of a number of repeating variables (equal to m) and anyone of the remaining $(n - m)$ non-repeating variables. Each π-group is then determined using the principle of dimensional homogeneity. Finally, the dependent variable π_1 is expressed as a function of dependent variables π_2, π_3 etc.

For proper choice of repeating variables, the following guide lines should be followed.

(1) The number of repeating variables is equal to the number of primary dimensions involved.

(2) The repeating variables should include all the primary dimensions describing the fluid problem.

(3) The chosen repeating variables should not form a dimensionless group among themselves.

(4) As far as possible, a dependent variable should not be selected as repeating variable.

(5) While selecting repeating variables, a geometric characteristic, a flow characteristic and a fluid property are good choice.

Geometric characteristics may include some characteristic length L, breadth B and head or height H, diameter D, thickness t, etc. Kinematic characteristics may include some form of linear velocity U, angular velocity ω, speed N and acceleration a, etc. Dynamic characteristics may be fluid mass density ρ, viscosity μ, weight density w, pressure p etc. The method is illustrated by means of an example.

Example

The flow of liquid of mass density ρ through a pipe of length, experiences pressure drop Δp . Other variables affecting the flow are viscosity μ, elastic modulus E, surface tension σ, velocity of flow U and characteristic lengths l_1 and l_2 . Express the pressure difference in terms of dimensionless group.

Solution

$$\Delta p = f(\rho, g, \mu, E, \sigma, U, 1, l_1, l_2) \qquad ...(6.8a)$$

Here number of variables invovled are $n = 10$. The phenomenon is completely described by three primary dimensions M, L and T or F, L and T, so that $m = 3$

Hence there will be $(n - m)$ dimensionless π- terms,

i.e. $\qquad (n - m) = 10 - 3 = 7$

$$f(\pi_1, \pi_2 \ldots \ldots \pi_7) = C$$

Let l, U and ρ be chosen as repeating variables then the various π-terms are written as

$$\pi_1 = [\rho^{a1} U^{b1} l^{c1} g^1]$$

$$\pi_2 = [\rho^{a2} U^{b2} l^{c2} \mu^1]$$

$$\pi_3 = [\rho^{a3} U^{b3} l^{c3} E^1]$$

$$\pi_4 = [\rho^{a4} U^{b4} l^{c4} \sigma^1]$$

$$\pi_5 = [\rho^{a5} U^{b5} l^{c5} \Delta p^1]$$

$$\pi_6 = [\rho^{a6} U^{b6} l^{c6} l^1 i]$$

$$\pi_7 = [rho^{a7} U^{b7} l^{c7} l_2^1]$$

Since each π – term is a dimensionless number, each of exponents of M, L and T in it is zero. Let us now take one of the π – terms, say, π_2

$$[\pi_2] = [\rho]^{a2} [U]^{b2} [L]^{c2} [\mu]^1$$

Substitute the dimensions of each term on both sides

$$[M^0 L^0 T^0] = [M/L^3]^{a2} [L/T]^{b2} [L]^{c2}[M/LT]^1$$

Equate the exponents of M, L and T of various terms on left side to that on right hand side,

$$M : 0 = a_2 + 1$$

$$L : 0 = -3a_2 + b_2 + c_2 - 1$$

$$T : 0 = -b_2 - 1$$

Solving these equations,

$$a_2 = -1 \; , \; b_2 = -1 \; \text{and} \; c_2 = -1 \; ,$$

Then,

$$\pi_2 = \left[\frac{\rho\, U L}{\mu} \right]^{-1} = R_e^{-1} = \text{Reynolds number}$$

Similarly,

$$\pi_1 = \frac{U^2}{g L} \doteq N_F^2 = (\text{Froude number})^2$$

$$\pi_3 = \rho\, U^2 / E = N_M^2 = (\text{Mach number})^2$$

$$\pi_4 = \rho\, U^2 L / \sigma = N_w^2 = (\text{Weber number})^2$$

$$\pi_5 = \Delta p / \rho\, U^2 = N_E^2 = (\text{Euler number})^2$$

$$\pi_6 = 1/l_1 = \text{dimensionless length}$$

$$\pi_7 = l/l_2 = \text{dimensinless length}$$

Therefore, $f(\pi_1, \pi_2 \ldots \pi_7) = C$

$$\pi_5 = f(\pi_1, \pi_2, \ldots \pi_7)$$

$$\Delta p / \rho\, U^2 = f[R_e, N_F, N_M, N_w, l/l_1, l/l_2] \qquad \ldots(\text{i})$$

These are various dimensionless groups of variables which have much importance in fluid mechanics. A detailed study about these numbers is given in section 6.9.

In case viscosity μ is only the important variable affecting the pressure drop besides characteristic length l_1 (taken as diameter D), ρ, U and pipe length, l, Eq. (i) reduces to

$$\Delta p / \rho \, U^2 = C f_1 (R_e, L/D)$$

It can be rearranged as

$$\frac{\Delta p}{\rho g} = 2 C \frac{U^2}{2g} \frac{L}{D} f_1 (R_e)$$

$$h_f = 2 C \frac{U^2}{2g} \frac{L}{D} f_1 (R_e)$$

Writing $2 C f_1 (R_e)$ as the characteristics of the pipe surface and assuming it to be f

$$h_f = f \frac{L}{D} \frac{U^2}{2g} \qquad \qquad ...(6.8b)$$

It is known as Darcy Weisbach equation of head loss and f is known as Darcy roughness coefficient.

6.5 SUPERFLUOUS AND OMITTED VARIABLES

A number of variables affect a fluid flow phenomenon. To make the dimensional analysis of fluid flow phenomenon, it is necessary to collect all pertinent variables. There is no hard and fast rule to determine such variables. It is purely a guesswork. Moreover, some insight into the problem (or its knowledge) should be known which helps in the proper selection of all the pertinent variables.

While making the list of variables affecting the flow, often a few such variables are chosen which really are not pertinent to the flow phenomenon. Such variables are known as 'superfluous variables'. To determine the superfluous variables, the procedure given here may be followed. Let us consider the flow through pipe. The pressure drop Δp depends on fluid properties; mass density ρ and dynamic viscosity μ; flow characteristic; flow velocity U and pipe geometric dimensions; pipe length L, pipe diameter D and equivalent sand roughness k. In addition, let acceleration due to gravity g also affect the pressure drop p. Hence

$$\Delta p = f [\rho, U, D, L, \mu, k \, g]$$

By dimensional analysis

$$\frac{\Delta p}{\rho \, U^2} = f \left[\frac{\rho \, U D}{\mu}, \frac{L}{D}, \frac{k}{D}, \frac{U^2}{g D} \right]$$

A number of experiments are now performed and results analysed. The non dimensional group $[\Delta p / \rho \, U^2]$ is plotted against $[\rho \, U D / \mu]$ for various values of $[U^2/g D]$. At the same time, other π terms, L/D and k/D are kept constant. It is observed that all the points fall on a single curve whatever may be the value of $[U^2/g\,D]$. It means $[U^2/g\,D]$ does not affect the relationship between $[\Delta p/\rho\,U^2]$ and $[\rho\,UD/\mu]$. Since in the non dimensional group $[U^2/2g\,D]$, g is a non repeating variable, it can be concluded that g is superfluous variable. Alternatively, $[U^2/g\,D]$ may be varied and plotted against $[\Delta p/\rho\,U^2]$. It is observed that $[U^2/g\,D]$ is plotted as a straight line parallel

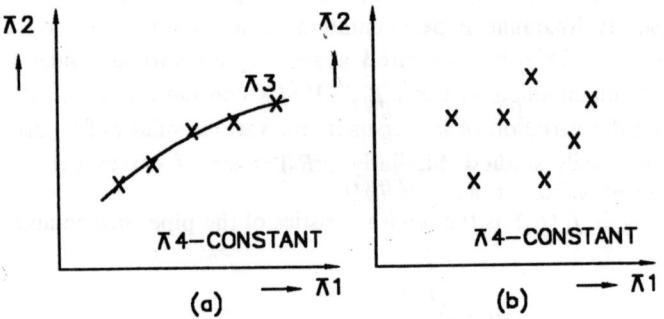

FIG. 6.1. SUPERFLUOUS & OMITTED VARIABLES

to $[U^2/g\,D]$ axis. This means, whatever the value of $[U^2/g\,D]$, the term $[\Delta p/\rho\,U^2]$ does not vary. Therefore, it can be concluded that g is a superfluous variable.

On the other hand, while preparing the list of variables, some pertinent variables may be left out in the beginning. Such variables are known as 'omitted variables'. The conclusions derived from the analysis of such functional relationships are often found incomplete or erraneous. If the hydraulic experiments are done and results are presented in graphical form, the points will appear scattered and no definite relationship is obtained. Even if a curve is obtained, the results would be erraneous. For example, in the above illustration, the fluid viscosity μ is left out from the list of variables. Then,

$$\frac{\Delta p}{\rho\,U^2} = f(L/D, k/D)$$

The plots of $[\Delta p/\rho\,U^2]$ versus $[k/D]$ for various values of L/D will show a lot of scatter and the conclusions derived will be altogether erraneous. Hence, a search is made for some pertinent variable affecting the flow phenomenon. Once the pertinent variable is also included, the final result should yield definite relationship between various $\pi-terms$.

It is to be noted that there are some parameters which have a constant value and when combined with other variables form a new variable. For example, the acceleration due to gravity 'g' when combined with head H or some other linear dimension form a parameter having the dimensions of (velocity). Alternatively the product gH represents the work done/unit mass. As such, this parameter gH is one of the important variable to be used with hydraulic machine problems. It is common mistake to omit g or such variables. Hence, a care should be taken to include such variables.

6.6 PRESENTATION OF EXPERIMENTAL RESULTS

When the number of variables are small, they can easily be represented on two axes X and Y. But if the number of variables are more, say 7, it is cumbersome to present experimental results. The number of variables are then grouped into a number of dimensionless groups by the procedure outlined above. And the affect of variation in different π terms is then studied. For examle $\pi_1 (= \Delta p / \rho U^2)$, say is a function of $\pi_2 (= \rho U D / \mu)$, $\pi_3 (= k/D)$ and $\pi_4 (= L/D)$. By hydraulic experimentation, a set of values of π_1, π_2, π_3 and π_4 are obtained. Then π_1 is plotted against π_2 for various values of π_3 (say a, b, c etc.), maintaining π_4 (*i.e.* L / D) as constant. Thus, a set of curves representing the variation of π_1 versus π_2 for various values of π_3 are obtained, these can be easily studied. Similarly, another set of curves can be obtained for a different value of π_4 (*i.e.* L/D).

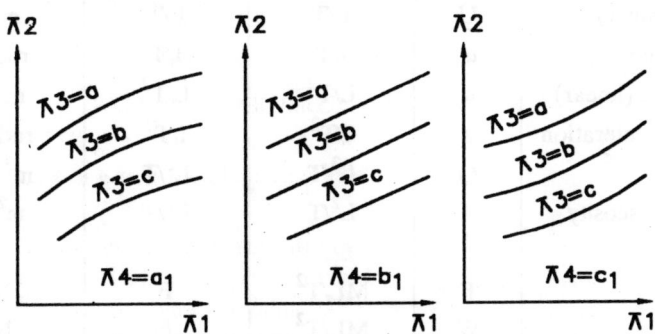

FIG. 6.2. ANALYSIS OF EXPERIMENTAL DATA

This way, for various value of π_3 and π_4 , the relationship between π_1 and π_2 could be established. Thus, dimensional analysis simplifies the presentation of experimental results and defintie results could be derived easily.

6.7. SIMILITUDE

Model studies of proposed hydraulic structures and machines are frequently undertaken as an aid to the designer. They permit the prior knowledge of the hydraulic behaviqr of the proposed structure or machine, e.g. efficiencies and capacities of pumps and turbines, the mechanical energy losses associated with the given flow, the forces acting on a weir, the behaviour change in the rivers due to construction of brides, weirs or the power required to drag an oil tanker through an ocean. Moreover, in the field where calculations are made on the basis of simplfied theory, a model adds to the certainty to the design which can never be obtained from calculations alone. Generally, the models are made of smaller size as compared to the size of original body and hence cost very little. They lead to savings many times lager than their own cost. Many times a full size model or a model larger than its prototype has also been used to study flow phenomena of some small flow systems.

TABLE 6.1 DIMENSIONS OF SOME PHYSICAL QUANTITIES

Quantity	Symbol	Dimensions terms of		Unit of measurement
		M.L.T.	F.L.T.	S.I. Units
GEOMETRIC				
Length	L	L	L	m
Area	A	L^2	L^2	m^2
Volume	V	L^3	L^3	m^3
Slope	S	$M° L° T°$	$F° L° T°$	m/m
KINEMATIC				
Time	T	T	T	s
Velocity (linear)	U	L/T	L/T	m/s
Angular velocity	ω	I/T	I/T	rad/s
Acceleration(linear)	α	L/T^2	L/T^2	m/s^2
Angular Acceleration	a	I/T^2	I/T^2	rad/s^2
Discharge	Q	L^3/T	L^3/T	m^3 /s
Kinematic viscosity		L^2/T	L^2/T	m^2/s
DYNAMIC				
Force	F	ML/T^2	F	N
Weight	W	ML/T^2	F	N
Specific mass	ρ	M/L^2	FT^2/L^4	kg/m^3
Specifie weight	w	M/L^2T^2	F/L^3	N/m^3
Pressure intensity	p	M/LT^2	F/L^2	N/m^2
Shear stress	τ	ML/T^2	F/L^2	N/m^2
Dynamic viscosity	μ	M/LT^2	FT/L^2	Ns/m^2
Surface tension	σ	M/LT	F/L	N/m
Modulus of elasticity	E	M/T^2	F/L^2	N/m^2
Impulse momentum	I,M	M/LT^2	FT	N/s
Work, Energy	W,E	ML/T	FL	Nm
Power	P	ML^2/T^3	FL/T	Nm/s
Torque	T	ML^2/T^3	FL	Nm
MISCELLANEOUS				
Moment of inertia	I	L^4	L^4	m4
Temperature	Y	θ	θ	°C
Heat	H	ML^2/T^2	FL	KCal

In fact, a model may be regarded as a mechanical analogue for solving differential equations of fluid motions with a given set of a rather complicated boundary conditions. Its main function is to obtain useful quantitative and qualitative information which can be safely transferred to its prototype. A thorough knowledge of principles of model similitude is, therefore, necessary for the proper design, construction and operation of model and then the interpretation of model tests. It should be remembered that the art of engineering has to be practised with experience, judgement, ingenuity, and patience for obtaining useful results. These are then correctly interpreted and performance of prototype rightly predicted.

6.8 SIMILARITY IN MODELS

For the given fluid motion, the possible form of equation is derived by the method of dimensional analysis. The experiments are then conducted on the model and the performance of prototype is predicted. For this purpose, model and prototype must be completely similar. This requires that two systems should bear geometrical, kinematical and dynamical similarity.

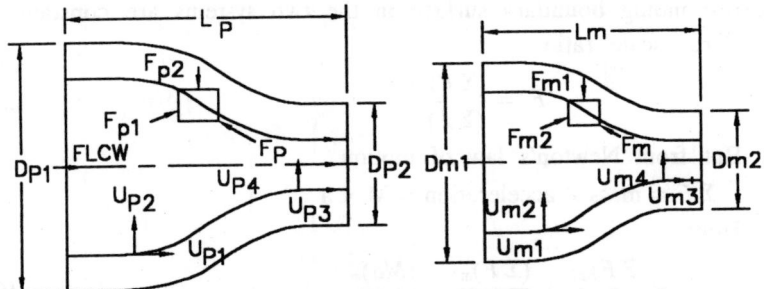

FIG. 6.3. SIMILARITY BETWEEN MODEL AND PROTOTYPE

1. Geometrical similarity

It implies similarity of shape. All parts of the model must bear a constant ratio with corresponding part of the prototype. The length scale ratio L_r is given by

$$L_r = L_m/L_p$$

Similarly,

$$L_r = \frac{B_m}{B_p} = \frac{H_m}{H_p} = \frac{D_m}{D_p} \ , \ etc, \qquad \qquad ...(6.9)$$

Another important factor in maintaining a complete geometrical similarity between two systems is that these should have similar type of surface roughness. A smaller size model will have smoother surface which may result in a model with distorted scales.

2. Kinematic similarity

It is the similarity of motions. As both model and prototype must undergo similar time rate of change of motion, the flow pattern in the two systems must be geometrically similar and the ratios of corresponding velocities and accelerations must be equal.

Velocity scale ratio

$$U_r = \frac{U_{m1}}{U_{p1}} = \frac{U_{m2}}{U_{p2}} \qquad ...(6.10)$$

In the same way, acceleration ratio

$$a_r = \frac{a_{m1}}{a_{p1}} = \frac{a_{m2}}{a_{p2}} \qquad ...(6.11)$$

The discharge scale ratio

$$Q_r = \frac{Q_{m1}}{Q_{p1}} = \frac{Q_{m2}}{Q_{p2}} \qquad ...(6.12)$$

Many more scale ratio's can be derived in this way.

3. Dynamic similarity

It means the similarity of force. The model is said to be similar to its prototype if the ratios of all forces acting on the corresponding fluid particles or corresponding boundary surface in the two systems are constant.

Force scale ratio

$$F_r = \frac{(\Sigma F)_{m1}}{(\Sigma F)_{p1}} \qquad ...(6.13)$$

But from Newton's law of motion,

$$\Sigma F = \text{mass} \times \text{acceleration} = M \times a$$

Hence,

$$F_r = \frac{\Sigma F)_{m1}}{(\Sigma F)_{p1}} = \frac{(\Sigma F)_{m2}}{(\Sigma F)_{p2}} = \frac{(Ma)_m}{(Ma)_p} \qquad ...(6.14a)$$

In any flow system, the term 'Ma' represents the inertia force acting on the flow system and ΣF represents the vectorial summation of all the external forces acting on the fluid particle. These external forces may be either one or more of the following : (i) viscous force F_v (ii) gravity force F_g (iii) comressibility force F_e (iv) surface tension force F_s and (v) pressure force F_p . Besides these forces many more forces may be acting in the complicated systems of flow.

Therefore,

$$\frac{(Ma)_m}{(Ma)_m} = \frac{(\Sigma F)_m}{(\Sigma F)_p} = \frac{(F_v + F_g + F_e + F_s + F_p)_m}{(F_v + F_g + F_e + F_s + F_p)_p} \qquad ...(6.14b)$$

At the same time the ratio of inertia force acting in the model and prototype should be same as the ratio of individual force F_v or F_g or F_e , etc. acting for the two systems.

$$\frac{(F_i)_m}{(F_i)_p} = \frac{(F_v)_m}{(F_v)_p} \qquad ...(6.14c)$$

$$\frac{(F_i)_m}{(F_i)_p} = \frac{(F_g)_m}{(F_g)_p} \qquad ...(6.14d)$$

$$\frac{(F_i)_m}{(F_i)_p} = \frac{(F_c)_m}{(F_c)_p} \qquad ...(6.14e)$$

$$\frac{(F_i)_m}{(F_i)_p} = \frac{(F_s)_m}{(F_s)_p} \qquad ...(6.14f)$$

$$\frac{(F_i)_m}{(F_i)_p} = \frac{(F_p)_m}{(F_p)_\mu} \qquad ...(6.14g)$$

For complete similarity between model and prototype, Eqs. 6.13 and 6.14 should be satisfied simultaneously which is almost impossible (except when the model scale ratio is unity). Fortunately, in most of the engineering problems either one or two forces act predominantly and others (i) may not act (ii) may be of negligible magnitude or (iii) may oppose other forces in such a way that the effect of both is reduced.

6.9 DIMENSIONAL NUMBERS

The various forces can be expressed by the following dimensional equations.

Inertia force F_i = mass × acceleration

$$= [\rho L^3 \times U/T] = [\rho L^2 U^2]$$

$$= [\rho A U^2] \qquad ...(6.15a)$$

Viscous force F_v = shear stress × area

$$= [\tau \times A] = [\mu \times U/L \times L^2] = [\mu U L] \qquad ...(6.15b)$$

Gravity force F_g = mass × acceleration due to gravity

$$= [\rho L^3 g] \qquad ...(6.15c)$$

Pressure force F_p = pressure intensity × area

$$= [p \times A]$$

$$= [p \times L^2] \qquad ...(6.15d)$$

Compressibility force F_e = volume modulus of elasticity × area

$$= [K \times A]$$

$$= [K \times L^2] \text{ or } [E_v \times L^2] \qquad ...(6.15e)$$

Surface tension force F_s = surface tension force/unit length × length

$$= [\sigma L] \qquad ...(6.15f)$$

The ratio of inertia force to one of the various forces is a non- dimensional number. For example

$$\frac{F_i}{F_v} = \frac{\rho L^2 U^2}{\mu U L} = \frac{\rho U L}{\mu}$$

This ratio is a dimensional number and is known as Reynolds number,

$$R_e = \frac{\rho U L}{\mu} \qquad ...(6.16)$$

Similarly from Eqs. 6.14d to 6.14g, other dimensional numbers can be determined

$$\frac{F_i}{F_g} = \left[\frac{U^2}{gL}\right]$$

Froud's number $N_F = \sqrt{U^2/gL}$

$$N_F = U/\sqrt{gL} \qquad \qquad ...(6.17)$$

Mach number $N_M = \sqrt{F_i/F_e}$

$$N_M = \sqrt{\rho L^2 U^2/E_v L^2}$$

$$N_M = \frac{U}{\sqrt{E_v/\rho}} \qquad \qquad ...(6.18)$$

when E_v represents the bulk modulus of elasticity. The ratio

$\dfrac{U^2}{E_v/\rho}$ is known as 'Cauchy's number'.

Weber number $N_W = \sqrt{F_1/F_s}$

$$N_W = \sqrt{\rho L^2 U^2/\sigma L}$$

$$N_W = \frac{U}{\sqrt{\sigma/\rho L}} \qquad \qquad ...(6.20)$$

Euler number $N_E = \sqrt{F_1/F_p}$

$$N_E = \sqrt{\rho L^2 U^2/p L^2}$$

$$N_E = U/\sqrt{p/\rho} \qquad \qquad ...(6.21)$$

6.10 MODEL LAWS

1. Froude model law

Owing to the preponderance of free surface flows, the Froude law is more widely used than any other law. The problems involving mainly inertia and gravity forces are governed by Froude law. It means that Froude number should be maintained same in the model flow as in the prototype flow for achieving complete dynamic similarity.

$$(N_F)_m = (N_F)_p$$

$$\frac{U_m}{\sqrt{g_m L_m}} = \frac{U_p}{\sqrt{g_p L_p}}$$

$$\frac{U_m}{U_p} = \sqrt{\frac{g_p}{g_m}\frac{L_m}{L_p}}$$

Velocity scale ratio $U_r = \sqrt{g_r L_r}$

$$U_r \approx \sqrt{L_r} \qquad \text{Since } g_m \approx g_p \qquad ..(6.22a)$$

Time scale ratio $T_r = L_r/U_r$

$$T_r = \sqrt{L_r} \qquad \qquad ...(6.22b)$$

Similarly, the scale ratios for various hydraulic quantities can be determined and are given in Table 6.2

TABLE 6.2 SCALE RATIOS OF VARIOUS TERMS BASED ON FROUDE AND REYNOLDS LAWS

Item	Symbol	Scale ratio	
		Froude law	Reynolds law
Length	L_r	L_r	L_r
Area	A_r	L_r^2	L_r^2
Volume	V_r	L_r^3	L_r^3
Specific weight	w_r	$\rho_r\, g_r$	$\rho_r\, g_r$
Mass	m_r	$\rho_r L_r^3$	$\rho_r L_r^3$
Velocity	U_r	$\sqrt{g_r L_r}$	$v_r L_r^3$
Time	T_r	$\sqrt{L_r/g_r}$	L_r^2/v_r
Acceleration	a_r	g_r	v_r^2/L_r^3
Force	F_r	$w_r L_r^3$	$\rho_r v_r^2$
Pressure intensity	p_r	$w_r L_r$	$\rho_r v_r^2/L_r^2$
Energy work, Torque	E_r	$w_r L_r^4$	$\rho_r L_r v_r^2$
Power	p_r	$\rho_r g_r^{3/2} L_r^{7/2}$	$\rho_r v_r^3/L_r$
Momentum	M_r	$\rho_r L_r^{3/2}/g_r^{1/2}$	$\rho_r v_r L_r^2$

Some of the examples of such flows where Froude law is applicable are (i) flow over spillways, weirs, sluices, etc; (ii) motiom in river, ocean, etc. where waves are likely to be formed, (iii) flow of jets from an orifice and (iv) flow of one fluid past another fluid of different density.

2. Reynolds model law

The problem involving mainly inertia and viscous force are governed by the Reynolds model law. It means that the same Reynolds number should be maintained in the model flow as in the prototype flow.

$$(R_e)_m = (R_e)_p$$

$$\frac{\rho_m U_m L_m}{\mu_m} = \frac{\rho_u U_p L_p}{\mu_p}$$

$$\frac{\rho_r U_r L_r}{\mu_r} = 1$$

Velocity scale ratio $U_r = v_r/L_r$ ...(6.23a)

Time scale ratio $T_r = L_r/U_r$

$$= L_r^2/v_r \qquad \qquad ...(6.23\ b)$$

Discharge scale ratio $Q_r = A_r U_r$

$$= L_r^2 \frac{v_r}{L_r}$$

$$= L_r v_r \qquad ...(6.23c)$$

The scale ratio for other hydraulic quantities are given in Table 6.2. Some of the examples of flows where this law is applicable are (i) flow of incompressible fluid in closed conduits, (ii) motion of bodies fully submerge in the fluid, e.g. aeroplane, submarines, etc. and (iii) flow around hydraulic structures like bridge piers, etc.

3. Mach model law

When the forces involved in the flow are mainly inertia and compressibility, the flow is governed by Mach's model law. It stipulates the equality of Mach number for both model flow and prototype flow

$$(N_M)_m = (N_M)_p$$

$$\frac{U_m}{\sqrt{E_{vm}/\rho_m}} = \frac{U_p}{\sqrt{E_{v\mu}/\rho_p}} \qquad ...(6.24a)$$

$$\frac{U_m}{U_p} = \sqrt{\frac{E_{vm}}{E_{vp}} \frac{\rho_p}{\rho_m}}$$

Velocity scale ratio $U_r = \sqrt{E_{vr}/\rho_r}$ $\qquad ...(6.24b)$

Time scale ratio $T_r = L_r/U_r$

$$= \frac{L_r \sqrt{\rho_r}}{\sqrt{E_{vr}}} \qquad ...(6.24c)$$

The scale ratios for other fluid mechanics quantities can be derived in a similar manner. Motion of bodies (planes, rockets, satellites, etc.) at high velocity (velocity of sound) and unsteady flow through pipes (water hammer) are some of the applications of this law.

4. Weber's model law

In the flow problems involving the predominance of surface tension force besides inertia force are governed by Weber's model law. It implies the equivalence of Weber's number for model flow and prototype flow

$$(N_W)_m = (N_W)_p$$

$$\frac{U_m}{\sqrt{\sigma_m/\rho_m L_m}} = \frac{U_p}{\sqrt{\sigma_p/\rho_p L_p}}$$

$$U_r = \sqrt{\sigma_r/\rho_r L_r} \qquad ...(6.25a)$$

Time scale ratio $T_r = L_r/U_r$

$$= \frac{L_r^{3/2} \rho_r^{1/2}}{\sigma_r^{1/2}} \qquad ...(6.25b)$$

Acceleration scale ratio $= a_r = U_r/T_r$

$$= \frac{\sigma_r}{\rho_r L_r^2} \qquad ...(6.25c)$$

Force scale ratio $= m_r a_r$

$$= (\rho_r L_r^3 \sigma_r)/(\rho_r L_r^2)$$

$$= \sigma_r L_r \qquad \qquad ...(6.25d)$$

The examples of flow making use of this law are (a) when the flow occurs over a weir or notch at low head, (b) capillary flow taking place through the soil and (c) capillary waves formed in the channel.

5. Other dimensionless numbers

There are some additional parameters which are useful in hydraulic model testing, for example, cavitation number, roughness number, etc. Cavitation number serves as an index by which the experimenter can predict the onset of cavitation in the prototype.

$$\sigma = \frac{p_a - p_v}{0.5 \rho U^2} \qquad \qquad ...(6.26)$$

where p_a and pv are atmospheric pressure and vapour pressure and U is the average velocity of fluid. Similarly, roughness number offers a means of establishing the same type of roughness action both in the model and prototype and is useful in the design of river models.

6.11 MODEL TECHNIQUE

For model testing of any given flow problem, the following steps should be followed.

(1) By dimensional analysis, the various variables affecting flow problem are grouped into dimensionless numbers. Mostly these groups are well known non-dimensional numbers, e.g. R_e, N_F, N_M, etc.

(2) A completely similar model is constructed as mentioned in the above section 6.8. Then the scheme of running the model test is planned.

Following geometrical scale have been widely used.
(a) Spillways for large dams   1:30 to 1:1000
(b) Canal structures, valves, gates,   1:5 to 1:25
(c) River models,   1:100 to 1:1000
Further, there is a minimum size of these models
(a) Spillways : Minimum head   ≮ 75 mm
(b) Canal structures : Minimum bottom width   ≮ 100 mm
(c) Valves, gates or conduits   ≮ 100 mm
Thus a model is constructed having geometrical similarity within the constraints of available fund, space available in the laboratory, the discharge available in the laboratory and the available time for running the model.

(3) The model is now run for preliminary tests. If some discrepencies are found, these should be corrected at this stage. The type of flow in model should be the same as in the prototype. Usually, minor alterations in the model design are indicated, such as shifting of or addition to the measuring equipment, a change in erodible material or the partial redesign of a model component.

(4) This calibrated model is then run and the requisite information is collected. The results are then analysed to get the performance of the prototype. Given below is an example which will be helpful in understanding the procedure.

Example

A prototype rating curve is desired for a 2.5 m needle valve operating at maximum head of 0.75 m. A 150 mm model valve is available for this purpose. The coefficient of discharge for the needle valve for the completely open position is approximaely 0.6 in the expression $Q = C_d A \sqrt{2gH}$, where H is the total head measured one diameter upstream from the valve. The kinematic viscosity $v = 1.0 \times 10^{-6}$ m^2/sec . (a) compute the model discharge required to satisfy the Reynolds law for the maximum flow condition, (b) what would be a reasonable maximum model valve discharge ?

Solution

$$\text{Area of valve} = \pi/4 \times D^2 = 4.91 \text{ sq.m}$$

Maximum prototype discharge

$$= 0.6 \times 4.91 \times \sqrt{2 \times 9.81 \times 75}$$
$$= 113 \text{ m}^3/\text{s}$$

The length scale ratio $L_r = 0.15/2.50 = 1/16$

According to Reynolds law $Q_r = v_r L_r$

But same fluid is used in model and prototype so that

$$v_m/v_p = v_r = 1.0$$

Hence $\quad Q_m = L_r \times Q_p$
$$= 1/16 \times 113$$
$$= 7.06 \text{ m}^3/\text{sec}$$
$$U_m = Q_m/A_m$$

and
$$A_m = \pi/4 \times 0.15^2 = 0.0176 \text{ m}^2$$

Therefore, $\quad U_m = 7.66/0.0176$
$$= 399.5 \text{ m/s at the upstream flange}$$

The Reynolds number in the model and prototype

$$= (399.5 \times 0.15)/(1 \times 10^{-6})$$
$$= 59.93 \times 10^6$$

It is seen that the design of model for this high Reynolds number will be too costly. Alternatively, the model is redesigned to operate at low Reynolds number ($\approx 1.5 \times 10^6$).

Therefore, $1.5 \times 10^6 = \dfrac{U_m \times 0.15}{1 \times 10^{-6}}$

$$U_m = 10 \text{ m/sec}$$

Also $\quad Q_m = U_m \times A_m$
$$= 10 \times 0.0176 = 0.176 \text{ m}^2/\text{sec}$$

Head required $= Q^2/(Cd^2 \times Am^2 \times 2g)$

$$= 0.176^2/(0.6^2 \times 0.0176^2 \times 2 \times 9.81)$$

$$= 14.15 \text{ m}$$

Thus the model is to be run at 14.15 m. In general, the closed conduit models should be operated at the highest available head in the laboratory.

6.12 DYNAMIC SIMILARITY (Special cases)

It is seen in section 6.10 that for true or complete similarly, one of the forces which is predominant is considered and corresponding law (Reynolds law or Froude law etc.) is used. But in certain problems more than one force might be of equal importance. For example, consider motion of a body on the free furface where both viscous and gravitational forces may be equally important.

According to Reynolds law $U_r = v_r/L_r$

According to Froude law $U_r = \sqrt{g_r L_r}$

Hence $\qquad v_r/L_r = \sqrt{g_r L_r}$

$$L_r = v_r^{2/3}/g r^{1/3}$$

$$\approx v_r^{2/3} \qquad \qquad ...(6.27)$$

From Eq. 6.27 it is seen that scale ratio is fixed by the ratio of v_m/v_p . When same fluid is used in the model and prototype $L_r = 1$.

Alternatively, v_r is determined for the predecided L_r

For example, $L_r = 1/50$ will require $v_r = 1/350$, or $v_m = v_p/350$

It is impossible to get such a fluid. In such cases, special model techniques are used; for example in case of ship model testing.

6.13 SHIP MODEL TESTING

The resistance to the motion of a ship is due to frictional resistance on its wetted surface and due to the wave and wake resistance. The latter will depend on the shape of ship and can be reduced by making the body streamlined. The energy utilised in the formation of surface waves is known as 'wash'. The best form of ship can be determined only by experiments, i.e., model testing. Thus,

Total resistance $R =$ Viscous resistance $R_f +$ Wave resistance R_W

$$...(6.28).$$

The total resistance R will depend on length of the ship, its speed U besides fluid properties ρ, μ , etc.

The functional relationship may be written as

$$R = f(\rho, U, L, \mu, g)$$

By dimensional analysis

$$\frac{R}{\rho L^2 U^2} = f\left[\frac{\rho U L}{\mu}, \frac{U}{\sqrt{Lg}} \right] \qquad ...(6.29)$$

For complete similarity of model and prototype,

$$\left(\frac{\rho \, U L}{\mu}\right)_m = \left(\frac{\rho \, U L}{\mu}\right)_p \qquad \qquad ...(6.30a)$$

Also

$$\left(\frac{U}{\sqrt{gL}}\right)_m = \left(\frac{U}{\sqrt{gL}}\right)_p \qquad \qquad ...(6.30b)$$

Then

$$\left(\frac{R}{\rho \, L^2 \, U^2}\right)_m = \left(\frac{R}{\rho \, L^2 \, U^2}\right)_p \qquad \qquad ...(6.30c)$$

Eqs. 6.30a and 6.30b may be used to determined various scale ratios. These scale ratios may then be used to solve Eq. 6.30c to determine the required resistance to the prototype ship. The equation such as Eqs. 6.30a and 6.30b are known as 'design equation' and Eq. 6.30c in known as 'prediction equation' Eq. 6.30c may also be written as

$$R_p = R_m \left(\frac{\rho_p}{\rho_m} \times \frac{L_p^2}{L_m^2} \times \frac{U_p^2}{U_m^2}\right) \qquad \qquad ...(6.30d)$$

The bracketed term in Eq. 6.30d known as 'the prediction factor'.

For the prediction of resistance to the ship the following procedure is followed.

(a) As both Reynolds law and Froude law cannot be simultaneously satisified, the frictional resistance for the model and prototype ships, r_f and R_f respectively, are determined by the following expressions. It was suggested by Froud from his experimental study that

$$R_f = f_p \times A_p \times U_p^2 \qquad \qquad ...(6.31)$$

$$r_f = f_m \times A_m \times U_m^2 \qquad \qquad ...(6.32)$$

Here, f_m and f_p are frictional resistance for unit wetted surface area of model and ship respectively at unit velocity.

(2) Model is then run in a water tank at various velocities and total resistance r experienced by it is measured.

(3) The wave resistance r_w is given as

$$r_w = (r - r_f) \qquad \qquad ...(6.33a)$$

and the wave resistance to the prototype is then determined as

$$R_w = (R - R_f) \qquad \qquad ...(6.33b)$$

Also from Eq. 6.30c wave resistance r_w and R_w can be expressed as

$$\frac{r_w}{\rho_m L_m^2 U_m^2} = \frac{R_w}{\rho_p L_p^2 U_p^2}$$

Therefore,

$$R_w = (r - r_f) \times \frac{\rho_p}{\rho_m} \times \frac{L_p^2}{L_m^2} \times \frac{U_p^2}{U_m^2}$$

$$R_w = (r - r_f) \times \frac{1}{\rho_r L r^3} \qquad \qquad ...(6.34)$$

Since the speed of the model is given by Eq. 6.30b

$$U_m = U_p \sqrt{L_r} \qquad \qquad ...(6.30)$$

(4) The total resistance R can be determined from Eqs. 6.28, 6.31, 6.32 and 6.34

$$R = (R_f + R_w) \qquad \qquad ...(6.28)$$

From Eq. 6.31, & 6.32, $R_f = r_f \times f_p/f_m \times 1/L_r^3$

From Eq. 6.34, $R_w = \dfrac{r - r_f}{\rho_r L_r^3}$

$$\therefore \qquad R = [(r_f \times f_p)/(f_m L_r^3) + (r - r_f)/\rho_r L_r^3]$$

If same fluid is used, $\rho_r = 1.0$,

$$R = \left[\frac{r_f f_p}{f_m L_1^3} + \frac{r - r_f}{L_r^3} \right]$$

$$R = \left(1/L_r^3 \right) \left[r + r_f \left(f_p/f_m - 1 \right) \right] \qquad ...(6.35a)$$

If the surface of the model is made of the same meterial as that of ship so that $f_m = f_p$

Then $\qquad R = r/L_r^3 \qquad \qquad ...(6.35b)$

Alternatively, with ships of similar form and of the same surface area, R may also be expressed as

$$R = f' L^2 U^2 + CL^2 U^2 \qquad \qquad ...(6.36)$$

where C is a coefficient depending on the shape form and L is the linear dimension.

Power required $= R \times U$ kW $\qquad \qquad ...(6.37a)$

where R is in kilo newton and U is in metre per second.

Power $= (f' + C) L^2 U^3 = KL^2 U^3 \qquad \qquad ...(6.37b)$

where K is a constant for the type of ship. The value of K can be determined from a plot (straight line) between P and $L^2 U^3$. These data can be obtained from the ships of similar type and made up of same material.

6.14 SCALE EFFECTS IN THE MODELS

(a) The models are designed and operated only for the predominant force whereas other secondary forces influencing the phenomenon are left out. This creates the descripencies in the predicted results and are conventionally known as 'scale effect'.

(b) Many times the material of required roughness (as per the model laws), may not be available and this will also cause scale effect.

(c) Consider flow of water from a tank filled to a height H above the centre line of an orifice at its bottom. A pipe of diameter D is fixed to the orifice. Dynamical similar model of this tank contains water to a height h above the centre of orifice of diameter d. Here the requirements of dynamical similarity is $\dfrac{p_p}{p_m} = \dfrac{wH}{wh} = \dfrac{D^2}{d^2}$ (Reynolds law). But geometrical similarity requires

$H/h = D/d$. These two requirements are opposed to each other and thus

$$\frac{Q}{q} = \frac{H^{3/2}}{h^{3/2}}$$

cannot be satisfied which will cause 'scale effect'.

(d) Similarly in case of turbines, it is quite impracticable to test model turbines under the enormous heads that the model analysis will require. Instead of doing so, the models are tested at some convenient lower head and later the test results are corrected for the 'scale effect'. L.F. Moody has given the relationship for turbines

$$\frac{1 - \eta_m}{1 - \eta_p} = \left(\frac{1}{L_r}\right)^3 \qquad \qquad ...(6.38)$$

where $\qquad\qquad L_r = \dfrac{\text{diameter of model runner}}{\text{diameter of prototype runner}}$

(i) Generally, the models are constructed at different scale ratios and the results are predicted. A plot between scale ratios and corresponding predicted results is prepared. The plot is extended to $L_r = 1$, which will then indicate the corrected result.

(ii) Sometimes the scale effect can be eliminated by using two fluids of different kinematic viscosity, e.g. water and air. The kinematic viscosity of air can be varied by altering its pressure. Hence, a suitable pressure is chosen and then the model will simulate almost exactly the performance of its full scale prototype.

6.15 DISTORTED MODELS

The long horizontal stretches of rivers, harbours, estuaries, etc, are requried to be modelled. A geomaterical similar model will yield a very small depth of flow and the flow in them will not be dynamical similar. Moreover, the forces which will be negligible (e.g. surface tension and other similar forces) in prototype may be large enough to influence the flow in model. Also, the space and fund restrict the size of the model. In such cases, the models are constructed with larger vertical scale than horizontal scale and are known as 'distorted models'. In a similar way, other types of distoritions need to be introduced which will be discussed in section 6.16.

(a) *Necessity of distorted model.* The distorted models are needed

(1) To maintain the accuracy in the vertical measurement.

(2) To obtain similar flow in the model (viz. turbulent).

(3) To obtain suitable bed material movement.

(4) To obtain suitable roughness of the material.

(5) To accommodate model within available space and fund.

(b) *Merits of distorted models.* The following are some of the merits of distorted models.

(1) Vertical exaggeration results in steeper water surface slope, greater wave height and hence accuracy in vertical measurement.

(2) Increased Reynolds number are obtained for higher velocity and, in turn, cause less viscous resistance along the surface of the model.

(3) Sufficient tractive force is available to simulate the prototype conditions (e.g. movement of bed material).

(4) Smaller size model needed and hence less cost.

(c) *Demerits*. The distorted model has the following demerits.

(1) Pressure and velocity distribution are seriously distorted due to varying horizontal and vertical scale ratios.

(2) Types of wave formed may be different due to difference in the depth of water.

(3) Steep side slopes are needed for distorted models.

(4) Bad psychological effect is caused by the distorted model to the observer.

6.16 TYPES OF DISTORTION

Distortion in the model may be of

(1) Geometrical distortion

(2) Material distortion and

(3) Distertion of hydraulic quantities.

(a) *Geometric distortion*. It can be of geometric dimensions (different scale ratios for horizontal and vertical dimensions) or of configuration wherein the model slope is changed to have sufficient amount of sediment moving on the bed and proper type of flow of water is achieved, etc. The first one is known as 'vertically exaggerated model' and latter one as the 'titled model'.

(b) *Material distortions* Many a times it becomes impossible to obtain the model material of suitable density, roughness, or size to simulate the prototype conditions. In such cases, some lighter material like coal dust, pumice stone, plastic blocks, etc., are used; thus introduing the material distortion.

(c) *Distortion of hydraulic quantities*. When it is desired to test a flow problem having long time period, (say 100 years), it is difficult to wait for corresponding time period (t_m). At the same time, the flood wave may bring huge amount of water alongwith it, which is difficult to be reproduced in the laboratory within permissible space and time constraints. Hence, it is required to be tested with available discharge and within allowable time period, causing the distortion in the predicted results. For illustration, the cases of fixed bed channels and movable bed channels are discussed hereafter.

6.17 FIXED BED CHANNELS

Problems involving relatively long stretches of either a canal or a river wherein actual change in bed configuration are not critical are usually studied in fixed bed channels with different scales for vertical and horizontal dimensions.

The influence of bed and wall roughness is of major importance and hence Manning's formula can be used.

$$U_r = \frac{1}{n_r} \times R_r^{2/3} S_r^{1/2} \qquad ...(6.39)$$

where U_r, R_r and S_r represent the velocity, hydraulic radius and bed scale ratios respectively. By Froud's model law

$$U_r = \sqrt{D_r}$$

Also $\qquad S_r = D_r/L_r \qquad ...(6.40)$

Substituting the value of U_r and S_r in Eq. 6.39

$$\sqrt{D_r} = \frac{R_r^{2/3} \times D_r^{1/2}/L_r^{1/2}}{n_r} \qquad ...(6.40a)$$

$$\frac{D_r}{L_r} = \frac{n_r^2 \times D_r}{R_r^{4/3}} \qquad ...(6.40b)$$

Now there are two possible alternatives. Firstly. If n is known for model and prototype, i.e. n_r is known, the exaggeration D_r/L_r can be computed for the given depth D and hydraulic radius R. Such models are known as the 'vertically exaggerated models'. In models for which i.e. 'slope distortion' is dictated by other cosiderations, an adjustment of model roughness is required to duplicte prototype conditions and can be found from Eq. 6.40.

$$n_r = R_r^{2/3}/\sqrt{L_r}$$

For very wide channels $R_r \approx D_r$

$$n_r = D_r^{2/3}/\sqrt{L_r} \qquad ...(6.41)$$

The required roughness for the model can be achieved by using materials such as coal dust, saw dust, plexiglass, pumice stone, etc. For geometrically similar models, Eq. 6.40b reduces to

$$n_r = L_r^{1/6} \qquad ...(6.42)$$

6.18 MOVABLE BED MODELS

There are many open channel problems invovling scour, tranportation and deposition of channel bed material through the action of flowing water. Such problems are usually studied by means of 'movable bed models'. The general design approach is that of selecting scales and bed materials which will result in bed movement of a nature, generally, similar to that in the prototype for various discharges flowing in it. Distortion (D_r/L_r) may vary from 2 to 7. The design and operation of these movable bed model involve trial and error processes. For this purpose sufficient data, collected in the past for silting and scouring at a various discharges should be available. After preparing the model to the chosen scale, it is 'calibrated or verified' to reproduce the past results with respoect to the discharges at various stages, movement of bed material, etc. Once the model is verified, the model is ready to predict the results for future. For correctly interpreting the model results, rich experience in the movable bed modelling is necessary. The model can be used to forecast the results only for those events for which it has been verified.

6.19 HYDRAULIC MACHINERY MODELS

Performance tests are required to be carried out for hydraulic machines like pumps and turbines for the following purposes.

(1) To guide and verify theoretical development in design.

(2) To evaluate performance under special conditions such as cavitation.

(3) As an aid in evaluating hydrodynamic loading for use in mechanical design.

(4) To perform acceptance tests on competitive deisgn in lieu of full scale tests.

Flow in hydraulic machinery is closely similar to flow Q in a closed conduit and depends on rotor diameter D, its speed N, shaft work gH, fluid density ρ, fluid viscosity μ and bulk modulus of elasticity E_v

$$Q = f(D, g, H, N, \rho, \mu, E_v) \qquad ...(6.43a)$$

It reduces to four dimensionless groups.

$$\pi_1 = Q/ND^3, \quad \pi_2 = gH/N^2 D^2 \quad \pi_3 = \mu/\rho\, N D^3, \pi_4 = Ev/\rho N^2 D^2 \quad ...(6.44)$$

Therefore,

$$\frac{Q}{ND^3} = f\left[\frac{gH}{N^2 D^2}, \frac{\mu}{\rho\, N D^3}, \frac{E_v}{\rho\, N^2 D^2}\right] \qquad ...(6.44b)$$

The principle action in a hydraulic machine is the dynamic transfer of energy between rotating element and the moving fluid. For kinematic similarity the ratio of fluid velocity Q/D^2 and peripheral velocity, ND in model and prototype must be the same,

$$\frac{Q_r}{N_r D_r^3} = 1$$

In addition to this condition, the complete similarity of flow requires the equality of Reynolds number and relative roughness of the surfaces in the model and prototype. In practice, it is not possible to satisfy these conditions but they are approached by making model surfaces smooth and by operating the models (especially pump models) at prototype velocities. Another significant parameter which is used widely in the design of hydraulic machines is ts specific speed.

For pump $\qquad N_s = \dfrac{N\sqrt{Q}}{H^{3/4}}$

For turbines $\qquad N_s = \dfrac{N\sqrt{P}}{H^{5/4}}$

When this condition is satisifed, the previously stated requirement is also satisfied.

Examples 6.1-6.29

6.1 If the critical depth y_c in a right angled triangular channel depends on the discharge Q and acceleration due to gravity g, obtain an expression for y_c.

Solution :

There are in all three variables involved so that $n = 3$

$$y_c = f(Q, g)$$

$$f(y_c, Q, g) = C$$

The primary dimensions involved are only two, *i.e.* L and T so that $m = 2$

Number of π - groups $= (n - m) = 1$

Then

$$\pi_1 = f_1 (Q, g, y_c)$$

$$= f_1 [Q]^a [b]^b [y_c]^1$$

Substitute the dimensions of various quantities

$$M^0 L^0 T^0 = [L^3/T]^a [L/T^2]^b [L]^1$$

Equate the indices of M, L and T on both sides

$$L : 0 = 3a + b + 1$$

$$T : 0 = -a - 2b$$

which gives a $= -2/5$ and $b = 1/5$

Hence $Q^{-2/5} g^{1/5} y_c = C$

$$y_c = C (Q^2/g)^{1/5}$$

The constant C is to be determined experimentally.

6.2 The discharge Q of a liquid flowing over a V-notch of angle θ depends on the upstream head H over its vertex. In addition, it also depends on g, kinematic viscosity v and velocity of approach U_a. Determine the discharge equation of the V-notih.

Solution

The fluid flow problem can be expressed functionally as

$$f(Q, H, g, U_a, \theta, v) = 0$$

Total number of variables, $n = 6$

Total number of primary dimensions involved, $m = 2$

Number of π groups $= (n - m) = 4$

Repeating variables are selected as H and g

Hence $\pi_1 = (g, H, Q)$

$$\pi_2 = (g, H, U_a)$$

$$\pi_3 = (g, H, Q)$$

$$\pi_4 = (g, H, \mathcal{E})$$

Sovling, $\pi_1 = Q/g^{1/2} H^{5/2}$

$$\pi_2 = U_a/\sqrt{gH} , \ \pi_3 = \theta$$

$$\pi_4 = g^{1/2} H^{3/2}/\nu$$

Hence $f\left[\dfrac{Q}{H^2 \cdot \sqrt{gH}} , \dfrac{U_a}{\sqrt{gH}} , \theta , \dfrac{H\sqrt{gH}}{\nu} \right] = C$

$$Q = CH^2 \sqrt{gH} \, f\left[\dfrac{U_a}{\sqrt{gH}} , \theta , \dfrac{H\sqrt{gH}}{\nu} \right]$$

The bracked term is the coefficient of discharge C_d. It shows the dependence of C_d on velocity of approach, angle of V-notch and fluid viscosity.

6.3 Show that the viscous force F exerted by a fluid on a sphere of diameter D, in which it is moving with velocity U, is given by

$$F = \rho D^2 U^2 f (\rho DU/\mu)$$

Solution

$$F = f (\rho , D , U , \mu)$$

In other words, $f(F, \rho , D , U , \mu) = C$

Here total number of variables $= 5$

and total number of primary dimensions involved, $m = 3$

Therefore, number of π -groups $= (n - m) = 2$

Choosing D, U *and* ρ *as the repeating variables,*

$$\pi_1 = f_1 (\rho , D , U , F)$$

$$\pi_2 = f (\rho , D , U , \mu)$$

Now take up first π-group

π_1 : $\quad [M^0 L^0 T^0] = [\rho]^{a_1} [D]^{b_1} [U]^{c_1} [F]^1$

$\qquad\qquad = [M/L^3]^{a_1} [L]^{b_1} [L/T]^{c_1} [ML/T^2]^1$

Equating the indices of M, L and T,

M : $\qquad 0 = a_1 + 1$

L : $\qquad 0 = -3a_1 + b_1 + c_1 + 1$

T : $\qquad 0 = -c_1 - 2$

Solving for a_1, b_1 and c_1

$$\pi_1 = f_1 [F/\rho D^2 U^2]$$

Similarly for second π -group

π_2 : $\quad [M^0 L^0 T^0] = [\rho]^{a_2} [D]^{b_2} [U]^{c_2} [\mu]^1$

$\qquad\qquad = [M/L^3]^{a_2} [L]^{b_2} [L/T]^{c_2} [M/LT]^1$

M : $\qquad 0 = a_2 + 1$

L : $\qquad 0 = -3a_2 + a_2 + b_2 + c_2 - 1$

T : $\qquad 0 = -c_2 - 1$

Solving, $\qquad \pi_2 = f_2 \left[\dfrac{\rho D U}{\mu} \right]$

Combining the π -terms,

$$\frac{F}{\rho D^2 U^2} = f\left(\frac{\rho D U}{\mu}\right)$$

or
$$F = \rho D^2 U^2 f\left(\frac{\rho D U}{\mu}\right)$$

6.4 Using Buckingham's pi theorem, show that velocity through a circular orifice is given by

$$U = \sqrt{2gH} f[D/H, \mu/\rho UH]$$

where f represents some function and H, D, μ, ρ and g are respectively the head causing the flow, the diameter of the orifice, the coefficient of viscosity, the mass density and the acceleration due to gravity.

Solution

The functional relationship for velocity is written as

$$U = f(H, D, \mu, \rho, g)$$

The functional relationship is

$$f(U, H, D, \mu, \rho, g) = C$$

Here $n = 6$ and number of primary dimensions $m = 3$

Therefore number of π-terms $= (6 - 3) = 3$

Choosing H, g and ρ as repeating variables,

$$\pi_1 = f_1(H, g, \rho\, U)$$
$$\pi_2 = f_2(H, g, \rho, D)$$
$$\pi_3 = f_3(H, g, \rho, \mu)$$

Solving in the same way, as above

$$\pi_1 = U/\sqrt{gH}$$
$$\pi_2 = H/D$$
$$\pi_3 = \rho H \sqrt{gH}/\mu$$

Hence $f[U/\sqrt{gH}, H/D, \rho H \sqrt{gH/\mu}] = C$

Rearranging various terms,

$$U = C_1 \sqrt{2gH} f[H/D, \rho H \sqrt{gH}/\mu]$$

where C_1 equal to $\sqrt{2} C$ is a constant to be determined experimentally.

6.5 Assuming that rate of discharge Q of a centrifugal pump is dependent upon ρ, N, D, Δp and μ with the usual notations, show, using Buckingham's π-theorem, that

$$Q = ND^3 f[gH/N^2 D^2, v/ND^2]$$

where H is the head generated by the centrifugal pump and v is kinematic viscosity of fluid.

Solution

$$Q = f(\rho, N, D, \Delta p, \mu)$$

where $\quad \Delta p = wH = $ pressure drop

$$f(Q, \rho, N, D, \Delta p, \mu) = C$$

Here $n = 6$, $m = 3$, $n - m = $ number of π -groups $= 3$

Choosing D, N, ρ as repeating variables,

$$\pi_1 = (\rho, N, D, Q)$$
$$\pi_2 = (\rho, N, D, \Delta p)$$
$$\pi_3 = (\pi, N, D, \mu)$$

Take π_1 –group

π_1 :
$$[M^0 L^0 T^0] = f_1 [\rho, N, D, Q]$$
$$= f_1 [\rho^{a1} N^{b1} D^{c1} Q^1]$$
$$= f_1 [M/L^3]^{a1} [1/T]^{b1} [L]^{e1} [L^3/T]^1$$

Therefore M : $\quad 0 = a_1$

$\quad\quad\quad L$: $\quad 0 = -3a_1 + c_1 + 3$

$\quad\quad\quad T$: $\quad 0 = -b_1 - 1$

Solving, $\quad a_1 = 0$, $b_1 = -1$, $c_1 = -3$

Hence $\quad \pi_1 = f_1 [Q/ND^3]$

Similarly $\quad \pi_2 = f_2 [\rho, N, D, \Delta p]$

$$M^0 L^0 T^0 = f_2 [\rho]^{a2} [N]^{b2} [D]^{c2} [\Delta p]^1$$
$$= f_2 [M/L^3]^{a2} [1/T]^{b2} [L]^{c2} [M/LT^2]^1$$

M : $\quad 0 = a_2 + 1$

L : $\quad 0 = -3a_2 + c_2 - 1$

T : $\quad 0 = -b_2 - 2$

Solving and rearranging the terms

$$\pi_2 = f_2 \left[\frac{\Delta p}{\rho N^2 D^2} \right]$$

Similarly $\quad \pi_3 = f_3 [\rho, N, D, \mu]$

$$= f_3 [\rho]^{a3} [N]^{b3} [D]^{c3} [\rho]^1$$
$$= f_3 [M/L^3]^{a3} [1/T]^{b3} [L]^{c3} [M/LT]^1$$

Solving, $\quad \pi_3 = f_3 \left[\frac{\mu}{\rho N D^2} \right]$

Hence $\quad f \left[\frac{Q}{ND^3}, \frac{\Delta p}{\rho N^2 D^2}, \frac{\mu}{\rho N D^2} \right] = C$

But $\quad \Delta p = \rho g H$

Therefore, $\quad \dfrac{Q}{ND^3} = Cf \left[\dfrac{gH}{N^2 D^2}, \dfrac{\mu}{\rho ND^2} \right]$

or
$$Q = C \times ND^3 f \left[\frac{gH}{N^2 D^2}, \frac{v}{ND^2} \right]$$

6.6 Obtain the relationship for water turbines

$$P = \rho D^5 N^3 f \left[\frac{D}{B}, \frac{\rho N D^2}{\mu}, \frac{ND}{\sqrt{gH}} \right]$$

wherr D is the diameter of runner of width B, running at N r.p.m. and working under a head H in a fluid of mass density ρ and dynamic viscosity μ. Therefrom, derive an expression for the torque produced by the turbine.

Solution

$$P = f(\rho, B, D, \mu, N, g, H)$$

or
$$f[P, B, D, \mu, N, g, H) = C$$

In this problem, $n = 8$, $m = 3$

Number of π -terms $= (n - m) = 5$

Select D, N and ρ as repeating variables

Then
$$\pi_1 = f_1 [\rho, D, N, P]$$
$$\pi_2 = f_2 [\rho, D, N, B]$$
$$\pi_3 = f_3 [\rho, D, N, \mu]$$
$$\pi_4 = f_4 [\rho, D, N, g]$$
$$\pi_5 = f_5 [\rho, D, N, H]$$

π_1 : $[\pi_1] = [\rho]^{a1} [D]^{b1} [N]^{c1} [P]^1$

$[M^0 L^0 T^0] = [M/L^3]^{a1} [L]^{b1} [1/T]^{c1} [ML^2/T^3]^1$

Note : Power $=$ Work done/sec $= [FL/T]$

$$M : 0 = a_1 + 1$$
$$L : 0 = 3a_1 + b_1 + 2$$
$$T : 0 = -c_1 - 3$$

Solving
$$\pi_1 = P/\rho D^5 N^3$$

π_2 : $[\pi_2] = [\rho]^{a2} [D]^{b2} [N]^{c2} [B]^1$

$$M : 0 = a_2$$
$$L : 0 = -3a_2 + b_2 + 1$$
$$T : 0 = c_2$$

Solving
$$\pi_2 = f_2 [B/D]$$

π_3 : $[\pi_3] = f_3 [\rho]^{a3} [D]^{b3} [N]^{c3} [\mu]^1$

$$M : 0 = a_3 + 1$$
$$L : 0 = -3a_3 + b_3 - 1$$
$$T : 0 = -c_3 - 1$$

Solving,
$$\pi_3 = f_3 [\mu/\rho D^2 N]$$

π_4 : $[\pi_4] = [\rho]^{a4} [D]^{b4} [N]^{c4} [g]^1$

$$[M^0 L^0 T^0] = f_4 [M/L^3]^{a_4} [L]^{b_4} [1/T]^{c_4} [L/T^2]^1$$

$$M : 0 = a_4$$

$$L : 0 = -3a_4 + b_4 + 1$$

$$T : 0 = -c_4 - 2$$

Solving $\quad \pi_4 = f_4 [g/N^2 D]$

$$\pi_5 : [\pi_5] = f_5 [\rho]^{a_5} [D]^{b_5} [N]^{c_5} [H]^1$$

Since H has length dimension, $\pi_5 = f_5 [H/D]$

Hence $f[P/\rho D^5 N^3, B/D, \mu/\rho D^2 N, g/N^2 D, H/D] = C$

or $P = C \rho D^5 N^3 f[B/D, \mu/\rho D^2 N, g/N^2 D, H/D]$

Now power $=$ torque $\times$ angular velocity

$$= T \times \omega$$

$$= T \times 2\pi N/60$$

That means $\quad P = C_1 \times T \times N$

or $\qquad T = P/C_1 N$

Hence $\qquad T = C_2 \rho D^5 N^2 f[B/D, \mu/\rho D^2 N, g/N^2 D, H/D]$

6.7 Show by the method of dimensions that for a screw propeller the relation between the thrust F, torque, T, diameter D, speed of travel U, speed of rotation N, density ρ and viscosity μ may be put in the form

$$F = \rho D^2 U^2 \theta \left[\frac{\rho D^3 U^2}{T}, \frac{DN}{U}, \frac{\rho UD}{\mu} \right]$$

Solution

Let the functional relationship be

$$F = f(\overset{*}{\rho}, D, U, N, T, \mu)$$

$$f(F, \rho, D, U, N, T, \mu) = 0 \qquad \qquad \text{...(i)}$$

Here $n = 7$, $m = 3$, therefore, number of π - groups $(n - m) = 4$

Selecting ρ, D, U as respeating variables,

$$\pi_1 = f_1 (\rho, D, U, F) \qquad \qquad \text{...(ii)}$$

$$\pi_2 = f_2 (\rho, D, U, N) \qquad \qquad \text{...(iii)}$$

$$\pi_3 = f_3 (\rho, D, U, T) \qquad \qquad \text{...(iv)}$$

$$\pi_4 = f_4 (\rho, D, U, \mu) \qquad \qquad \text{...(v)}$$

$$\pi_1 : \pi_1 = f_1 (\rho, D, U, F) \qquad \qquad \text{...(vi)}$$

$$[M^0 T^0 L^0] = f_1 [M/L^3]^a [L]^b [L/T]^c [ML/T^2]^1$$

$$M : 0 = a + 1$$

$$L : 0 = -3a + b + c + 1$$

$$T : 0 = -c - 2$$

Solving these equations, $\pi_1 = [F/\rho D^2 U^2] \qquad \qquad \text{..(ii)}$

$$\pi_2 : \pi_2 = f_2 (\rho, D, U, N)$$

$$[M^0 L^0 T^0] = f_2 (M/L^3)^a [b]^b [L/T]^c [1/N]^1$$

Equating the index of M, L and T on both sides and solving,

$$\pi_2 = \left[\frac{DN}{U} \right] \qquad \text{...(iii)}$$

$$\pi_3 : \pi_3 = f_3 [\rho, D, U, T]$$

$$[M^0 L^0 T^0] = f_3 [M/L^3]^a [L]^b [L/T]^c [ML^2/T^2]^1$$

Equate the index of M, L and T on both sides and solve

$$[\pi_3] = f_3 [T/\rho D^3 U^2] \qquad \text{...(iv)}$$

$$\pi_4 : \pi_4 = f_4 [\rho, D, U, \mu]$$

$$[M^0 L^0 T^0] = f_4 [M/L^3]^a [L]^b [L/T]^c [M/LT]^1$$

Solving in the same way

$$\pi_4 = \left[\frac{\rho U D}{\mu} \right] \qquad \text{...(v)}$$

The term on right hand side is known as Reynold's number R_e. Substituting the values of π_1, π_2, π_3 and π_4 in Eq. (i)

$$f[\pi_1, \pi_2, \pi_3, \pi_4] = 0$$

$$\pi_1 = f_5 [\pi_2, \pi_3, \pi_4]$$

$$\frac{F}{\rho D^2 U^2} = f_s \left[\frac{DN}{U}, \frac{T}{\rho D^3 U^2}, \frac{\rho U D}{\mu} \right]$$

$$F = \rho D^2 U^2 f_5 \left[\frac{DN}{U}, \frac{T}{\rho D^3 U^2}, \frac{\rho U D}{\mu} \right]$$

6.8 A projectile fired at an angle θ with initial velocity U. Find the range R in the horizontal plane, assuming it is a fnction of U, θ and g.

Solution

$$R = f(U, g, \theta) \qquad \text{...(i)}$$

Putting the dimensions of various quantities,

$$[L]^1 = f \left[\frac{L}{T} \right]^a \left[\frac{L}{T^2} \right]^b \qquad \text{...(ii)}$$

Since θ is a dimensinless, it does not appear in Eq. (ii).

Solving for a and b,

$$a = 2 \text{ and } b = -1$$

$$\therefore \qquad R = f(U^2/g)$$

$$= C U^2/g$$

This shows that C is a constant and will depend on θ, which is unsatisfactory information as it lacks the designation of θ.

However, if one consider the components of velocity, u and v, in the X and Y direction respectively, then,

$$R_x = f(u, v, g, \theta)$$

Putting L_x and L_y as the length dimensions in X and Y direction respectively,

$$\left[L_x\right]^1 = f \left[\frac{L_x}{T}\right]^a \left[\frac{L_y}{T}\right]^b \left[L_y/T^2\right]^c$$

which gives, L_x : $a = 1$

L_y : $b + c = 0$

T : $-a - b - 2c = 0$

Solving $a = 1$, $b = 1$ and $c = -1$

Hence, $R_x = f[u\, v/g]$

$$= C \left[\frac{u}{U} \times \frac{v}{U} \times \frac{U^2}{g}\right]$$

$$= C\,[\cos\theta \sin\theta]\, U^2/g$$

$\therefore$ $R = C \sin 2\theta . U^2/2g$

6.9 Show that the capilliary rise in a small diameter tube, partly immersed in a liquid is given by

$$\frac{h}{d} = f\left(\frac{\sigma}{w\,d^2}\right)$$

where h is capillary rise, d is the tube diameter and σ is the coefficient of surface tension.

Solution

$$h = f(d, w, \sigma)$$

$$f(h, d, w, \sigma) = 0$$

In this problem, $n = 4$, and $m = $ number of primary dimensions involved i.e., 2 and are taken as F and L,

$\therefore$ $n - m = 4 - 2 = 2$

The specific weight of liquid w and tube diameter d are selected as repeating variables

$$f(\pi_1, \pi_2) = 0$$

where $\pi_1 = f(d, w, \sigma)$

and $\pi_2 = f(d, w, h)$

Solving for

$$\pi_1 = (d, w, \sigma)$$

Putting the dimensions,

$$[M^0 L^0 T^0] = [L]^a [F/L^3]^b [F/L]^1$$

$$F : \quad 0 = b + 1$$

$$T : \quad 0 = a - 3b - 1$$

Solving, $a = -2$, $b = -1$

$$\pi_1 = [\sigma / w \, d^2]$$

Solving for

$$\pi_2 = (d, w, h)$$

$$[F^\circ L^\circ T^\circ] = [L]^a \, [F/L^3]^b \, [L]^1$$

Solving, $\qquad a = -1 \, , \, b = 0$

$$\pi_2 = (h/d)$$

Hence $f(\sigma / w \, d^2, \, h/d) = 0$

or $\qquad\qquad h/d = f(\sigma / w \, d^2)$

6.10 : The efficiency η of a geometrically similar model fan depend on P, μ, N (rev./s), diameter of blades D, and discharge Q. Perform dimensional analysis.

Solution :

$$\eta = f(\rho, \mu, N, D, Q)$$

or $\qquad f(\eta, \rho, \mu, N, D, Q) = 0$

In this problem, $n = 6, \quad m = 3$

Number of pi−terms $= (n-m) = 3$

or $\qquad f(\pi_1, \pi_2, \pi_3) = 0$ ...(i)

Select ρ, N and D as repeating variables.

Then, $\qquad \pi_1 = f_1[\rho, N, D, \eta]$

$$\pi_2 = f_2[\rho, N, D, \mu]$$

$$\pi_3 = f_3[\rho, N, D, Q]$$

Now π_1 : $\pi = f_1[\rho, N, D, \eta]$

$\qquad\qquad = f_1[\eta]$, since η is dimensionless parameter ...(ii)

π_2 : $\quad \pi_2 = f_2[\rho, N, D, \mu]$

$$M^\circ L^\circ T^\circ = f_2 \left[M/L^3 \right]^{a_2} \left[\frac{1}{T} \right]^{b_2} \left[\frac{1}{L} \right]^{c_2} \left[\frac{M}{L_T} \right]^1$$

M : $\quad 0 = a_2 + 1$

L : $\quad 0 = -3a_2 - c_2 - 1$

T : $\quad 0 = -b_2 - 1$

Solving, $\qquad a_2 = -1, b_2 = -1, c_2 = 2$

$$\pi_2 = f_2[\rho^{-1}, N^{-1} D^{-2} \mu]$$

$$= f_2 \left[\frac{\mu}{\rho N D^2} \right]$$ ...(iii)

π_3 : $\quad \pi_3 = f_3[\rho, N, D, Q]$

$$M^\circ L^\circ T^\circ = f_3 \left[\frac{M}{L^3} \right]^{a_3} \left[\frac{1}{T} \right]^{b_2} [L]^{c_3} \left[\frac{L^3}{T} \right]^1$$

M : $\quad 0 = -a_3$

$$L: \quad 0 = -3a_3 + c_3 + 3$$

$$T: \quad 0 = -b_3 - 1$$

Solving, $\quad a_3 = 0, b_3 = -1, \ c_3 = -3$

$$\therefore \qquad \pi_3 = f_3 \left[\frac{Q}{ND^3} \right] \qquad \qquad \text{...(iv)}$$

Substituting in Eq.(i) from Eqs. (ii) to (iv)

$$f \left[\eta, \frac{\mu}{\rho \, N \, D^2}, \frac{Q}{ND^3} \right] = 0$$

$$\eta = f \left[\frac{\mu}{\rho \, N \, D^2}, \frac{Q}{ND^3} \right]$$

6.11 : A metallic spherical ball of diameter D and mass density $\bar{\rho}_s$ moves slowly at terminal velocity U in a fluid of mass density ρ_f. The dynamic viscosity of fluid is μ. Derive a functional relationship for terminal velocity U.

Solution :

In this case, the motion of ball is influenced by viscous and gravity forces, hence

$$U = f \left[\rho_f, D, \mu, \rho_s, g \right]$$

or $\quad f \left[U, \rho_f D, \mu, \rho_s, g \right] = 0$

In this problem, $n = 6, m = 3$

Number of $\pi-$ terms $= (n - m) = 3$

$\therefore \quad f \left[\pi_1, \pi_2, \pi_3 \right] = 0$

Selecting $\quad \rho_f, g, D$ as repeating variables,

$$\pi_1 = f_1 \left(\rho_f, g, D, U \right]$$

$$\pi_2 = f_2 \left[\rho_f, g, D, \mu \right]$$

$$\pi_3 = f_3 \left[\rho_f, g, D, \rho_s \right]$$

$\pi_1 : \qquad \pi_1 = f_1 \left[\rho_f, g, D, U \right]$

$$M^\circ L^\circ T^\circ = f_1 \left[\frac{M}{L^3} \right]^{a_1} \left[\frac{L}{T^2} \right]^{b_1} [L]^{c_1} \left[\frac{L}{T} \right]^1$$

$M : \qquad 0 = a_1$

$L : \qquad 0 = -3a_1 + b_1 + c_1 + 1$

$T : \qquad 0 = -2b_1 - 1$

$$a_1 = 0, b_1 = -1/2, c_1 = -1/2$$

$$\pi_1 = f_1 \left[\rho_f^0 g^{1/2} D^{-1/2} U \right] = \frac{U}{\sqrt{gD}}$$

$\pi_2 : \qquad \pi_2 = f_2 \left[\rho_f, g, D, \mu \right]$

$$M^\circ L^\circ T^\circ = f_2 \left[\frac{M}{L^3} \right]^{a_2} \left[\frac{L}{T^2} \right]^{b_2} [L]^{c_2} \left[\frac{M}{LT} \right]^1$$

$M : \qquad 0 = a_2 + 1$

$$L: \qquad 0 = -3a_2 + b_2 + c_2 - 1$$
$$T: \qquad 0 = -2b_2 - 1$$
$$a_2 = -1, \qquad b_2 = -1/2, \quad C_2 = -3/2$$
$$\therefore \qquad \pi_2 = f_2\,[\rho_f^{-1}, g^{-1/2}, D^{-3/2}, \mu]$$
$$= f_2\left[\frac{\mu}{\rho_f D \sqrt{g\,D}}\right]$$

$\pi_3:$
$$\pi_3 = [\rho_f, g, D, \rho_s]$$
$$\pi_3 = [\rho_f/\rho_f]$$

Since non-repeating variable ρ_s forms a dimensionless group with repeating variable ρ_f, i.e. ρ_s/ρ_f; there is no need to write π_3 equation. Similarly, whenever, non repeating variable is velocity or length, such a method may be used to write down non dimensionless group.
$$\therefore \qquad f[\pi_1, \pi_2, \pi_3] = 0$$
Substituting the values of π_1 to π_3,
$$\frac{U}{\sqrt{gD}} = f\left[\frac{\mu}{\rho_f D \sqrt{gD}}, \frac{\rho_s}{\rho_f}\right]$$

6.12 : The time period T of water surface waves depends on depth of flow D, fluid density ρ, surface tension σ, acceleration due to gravity g, besides waves length λ. Derive the functional relationship by dimensional analysis.

Solution :
$$T = f[\rho, D, \sigma, g, \lambda]$$
$$f(T, \rho, D, \sigma, g, \lambda] = 0$$
Here $n = 6$, $m = 3$,
Number of $\pi-$ groups $= (n - m) = 3$
Seleating $\rho, g,$ and ρ as repeating variables.
$$\pi_1 = f_1[\rho, g, \lambda, T]$$
$$\pi_2 = f_2[\rho, g, \lambda, D]$$
$$\pi_3 = f_3[\rho, g, \lambda, \sigma]$$

$\pi_1:$
$$\pi_1 = f_1[\rho, g, \lambda, T]$$
$$M^\circ L^\circ T^\circ = f_1\left[\frac{M}{L^3}\right]^{a1}\left[\frac{L}{T^2}\right]^{b1}[L]^{c1}[t]^1$$

$M:$
$$0 = a_1$$
$L:$
$$0 = -3a_1 + b_1 + c_1$$
$T:$
$$0 = -2b_1 + 1$$

Solving $a_1 = 0$, $b_1 = 1/2, c_1 = -1/2$
$$\pi_1 = f_1[\rho^0 g^{1/2} \lambda^{-1/2} T]$$
$$= f_1[T\sqrt{g/\lambda}]$$

π_2 : $\qquad \pi_2 = f_2 [\rho, g, \lambda, D]$

$M^\circ L^\circ T^\circ \qquad = f_2 \left[\dfrac{M}{L^3} \right]^{a_2} \left[\dfrac{L}{T^2} \right]^{b_2} [L]^{c_2} [L]^1$

$M:$ $\qquad\qquad 0 = a_2$

$L:$ $\qquad\qquad 0 = -3a_2 + b_2 + c_2 + 1$

$T:$ $\qquad\qquad 0 = -2b_2$

Solving, $a_2 = 0, b_2 = 0, c_2 = -1$

$\qquad\qquad\qquad \pi_2 = f_2 [\rho^\circ g^\circ \lambda^{-1} D]$

$\qquad\qquad\qquad\quad = f_2 [D/\lambda]$

π_3 : $\qquad \pi_3 = f_3 [\rho, g, \lambda, \sigma]$

$M^\circ L^\circ T^\circ \qquad = f_3 \left[\dfrac{M}{L^3} \right]^{a_3} \left[\dfrac{L}{T^2} \right]^{b_3} [L]^{c_3} \left[\dfrac{M}{T^2} \right]^1$

Here dimension of σ should be noted, i..e

$$[\sigma] = [F/L] = \left[\dfrac{ML}{T^2} \times \dfrac{1}{L} \right] = \left[\dfrac{M}{T^2} \right]$$

$M:$ $\qquad\qquad 0 = a_3 + 1$

$L:$ $\qquad\qquad 0 = -3a_3 + b_3 + c_3$

$T:$ $\qquad\qquad 0 = -2b_3 - 2$

Solving, $\qquad\qquad a_3 = -1, b_3 = -1, c_3 = -2$

$$\pi_3 = b_3 [\rho^{-1} g^{-1} \lambda^{-2} \sigma]$$

$$= b_3 \left[\dfrac{\sigma}{\rho g \lambda^2} \right]$$

Hence $f [\pi_1^c, \pi_2, \pi_3] = 0$

$$f \left[T \sqrt{\dfrac{g}{\lambda}}, \dfrac{D}{\lambda}, \dfrac{\sigma}{\rho g \lambda^2} \right] = 0$$

$$T \sqrt{\dfrac{g}{\lambda}} = f \left[\dfrac{D}{\lambda}, \dfrac{\sigma}{\rho g \lambda^2} \right]$$

6.13 A model of torpedo is to be tested in a towing tank at a velocity of 24 m/s. The prototype is expected to attain a velocity of 6m/s in 15.6° C water. (a) What model scale has been used ? (b) What would be the model speed, if tested in a wind tunnel under a pressure of 20 bar and at constant temperature of 20° C ?

Solution :

(a) Let the model scale be x, $\therefore$ $L_m = x L_p$

From Reynolds law,

$$\dfrac{U_m L_m}{\nu_m} = \dfrac{U_p L_p}{\nu_p}$$

$$\frac{24 \times x L_p}{v} = \frac{6 \times L_p}{v} \qquad \text{(Since } v_m = v_p = v\text{)}$$

$$x = 1/4$$

The model scale is 1 : 4

(b) For air, $\mu_a = 18.15 \times 10^{-6} \, N \, s/m^2$ at 20°C

$$\rho_a = p/RT = \frac{20 \times 10^5}{287 \times (273 + 20)} = 23.78 \, kg/m^3$$

and v (water) $= 1.008 \times 10^{-6} \, m^2/s$ at 20° C

From Reynold's law

$$\frac{U_m L_m}{v_m} = \frac{U_p L_p}{v_p}$$

$$\frac{U_m L_p/4}{18.15 \times 10^{-6}/23.78} = \frac{6 \times L_p}{1.008 \times 10^{-6}}$$

Solving, $U_m = 18.17$ m/s

6.14. A centrifugal pump was tested in a laboratory by constructing a 1 : 10 scale geometrically similar model. The test gave the following information. Power consumed is 5 kW, head = 5 m, speed of pump = 500 rpm. If the prototype is to work under a head of 100 m, determine the corresponding information for the prototype.

Solution

For model tests on pumps, the following relationship is obtained by dimensional analysis.

$$\left[\frac{P}{\rho D^5 N^3}\right] = f\left[\frac{D}{B}, \frac{\rho D N}{\mu}, \frac{ND}{\sqrt{gH}}\right] \qquad \text{...(i)}$$

For completely similar machines,

$$\frac{P_r}{\rho D_r^5 N_r^3} = 1 \qquad \text{...(ii)}$$

$$D_r/B_r = 1 \qquad \text{...(iii)}$$

$$\frac{\rho_r D_r^2 N_r}{\mu_r} = 1 \qquad \text{...(iv)}$$

and $$\frac{N_r D_r}{\sqrt{g_r H_r}} = 1 \qquad \text{...(v)}$$

From Eq. (v)

$$N_r \approx \sqrt{H_r}/D_r \text{ Since } g_r = 1.0$$

$$N_r = \frac{(5/100)^{1/2}}{(1/10)} = 2.236$$

$$N_p = \frac{N_m}{N_r} = \frac{500}{2.236}$$

$$= 223.6 \text{ r.p.m.} \approx 224 \text{ r.p.m.}$$

From Eq. (ii),

$$\frac{P_r}{\rho_r D_r^5 N_r^3} = 1$$

$$P_r = D_r^5 N_r^3 \qquad\qquad \text{Since } \rho_r = 1$$

$$= (1/10)^5 (2.236)^3$$

$$= 1/8945$$

$$P_p = P_r . P_m = 8945 \times 5$$

$$= 44.726 \text{ kW}$$

6.15 A model is to be built of flow phenomenon which is dominated by the action of gravity and surface tension. Show that the length scale ratio which will ensure complete hydraulic similitude between model and prototype is

$$L_r = \sqrt{\sigma_r/\rho_r}$$

where σ_r and ρ_r are the ratios, model to prototype of surface tension and density of fluids.

Solution

When gravity force is predominant, Froude law is applicable.

$$\frac{U_r}{\sqrt{g_r L_r}} = 1 \qquad\qquad\qquad ...(i)$$

When surface tension force is predominant Weber's law is applicable.

$$\frac{U_r}{\sqrt{\sigma_r/\rho_r L_r}} = 1 \qquad\qquad\qquad ...(ii)$$

Equating Eqs. (i) and (ii)

$$\frac{U_r}{\sqrt{\sigma_r/\rho_r L_r}} = \frac{U_r}{\sqrt{g_r L_r}}$$

$$L_r = \sqrt{\sigma_r/\rho_r g_r}$$

$$L_r \approx \sqrt{\sigma_r/\rho_r} \qquad\qquad \text{(as } g_r \approx 1.0)$$

6.16 A 1 : 25 scale geometrically similar model of a spillway has been prepared in the laboratory following Froude law. Determine

(i) rate of flow over the model to simulate 6250 m³/s in the prototype.

(ii) the velocity in the prototype corresponding to a velocity of 1.6 m/s observed in the model at a section, and

(iii) the energy dissipated by the hydraulic jump in the prototype corresponding to 0.3 kW in the model.

Solution

$$L_r = 1/25 \text{ (given)}$$

(i) According to Froude law

$$U_r \approx \sqrt{L_r} = 1/5$$

Therefore
$$Q_r = A_r U_r$$
$$= L_r^2 \sqrt{L_r}$$
$$= (1/25)^{5/2}$$

$$Q_m = (1/5)^5 Q_p$$
$$= 6250 (1/5)^5$$
$$= 2.0 \ \text{m}^3/\text{s}$$

$$U_p = U_m/U_r$$
$$= \frac{1.6}{1/5}$$
$$= 8.0 \ \text{m/s}$$

(iii) Energy dissipated/sec = work done/sec
$$= (\rho_r L_r^3 a_r) L_r/T_r$$

But
$$T_r = L_r/U_r$$
$$= \frac{L_r}{\sqrt{L_r}} = \sqrt{L_r}$$

and
$$a_r = U_r/T_r$$
$$= \sqrt{L_r}/\sqrt{L_r} = 1.0$$

Assuming same fluid is used in model and prototype
$$\rho_r = 1.0$$
$$E_r = L_r^{7/2}$$
$$= (1/5)^{7/2}$$

Therefore
$$E_p = 0.3/(1/5)^{7/2} = 83.35 \ \text{kW}$$

6.17. A 10 m model of an ocean tanker 500 m long is dragged through fresh water at 3 m/s with a total measured resistance of 0.105 kN. The surface drag coefficient C_f for model and prototype are 25×10^{-6} and 15×10^{-6} respectively in the equation $R = C_f A U^2$ and R is measured in kN. The wetted surface area of the model is 20 m^3. Find the total drag F of the tanker and power required at the propeller shaft assuming the efficiency 90% for the propeller.

Solution
$$L_r = 10/5000 = 1/50$$
$$R_{tm} = C_r AU^2$$
$$R_{tm} = 25 \times 10^{-6} \times 20 \times 3^2 = 0.0045 \ \text{kN}$$

According to Froude law, $U_r \approx \sqrt{L_r}$

Also
$$\frac{R_{fm}}{R_{fp}} = \frac{C_{fm} A_m U_m^2}{C_{fp} A_p U_n^2}$$

$$\frac{R_{fm}}{R_{fp}} = \frac{25 \times 10^{-6} L_r^2 \times (\sqrt{L_r})^2}{15 \times 10^{-6}}$$

$$= 1.67 L_r^3$$

$$R_{fp} = R_{fm}/1.67 \cdot L_r^3$$

$$= 0.0045/1.67 \ (1/50)^3$$

$$= 336.826 \ kN$$

Furthermore, wave resistance is given by dimensional analysis as

$$\frac{(R_w)_m}{\rho_m U_m^2 L_m^2} = \frac{(R_w)_p}{\rho_p U_p^2 L_p^2}$$

$$(R_w)_p = (R_w)_m \frac{\rho_p}{\rho_m} \frac{U_p^2}{U_m^2} \frac{L_p^2}{L_m^2} \quad (\text{Since } R_{wm} = R_m - R_{fm})$$

$$= (0.105 - 0.0045) \ 1.0256/1.000 \times (1/\sqrt{L_r^2}) \ (1/L_r)^2$$

$$= 12884.1 \ kN$$

Total resistance $R_p = R_{fp} + R_{wp}$

$$= (336.826 + 12884.1)$$

$$= 13220.926 \ kN$$

6.18 If the resistance of 1 : 10 model of an air ship when tested in water at 15 m/sec is 0.250 kN what will be resistance to the prototype in air at the corresponding speed ? It is known that kinematic viscosity for air = 13 times kinematic viscosity of water and $\rho_a = 1.234 \ kg/m^3$

If the air ship is tested in a wind tunnel with air under pressure at 20 atmosphere as a fluid medium, what would be speed and resistance of the model corresponding to that found above ?

Solution

In this flow problem, the air ship will remain fully submerged and hence, Reynolds law will be applicable.

$$U_m L_m/\nu_m = U_p L_p/\nu_p \quad \text{Since } L_m/L_p = 1/10 \ \text{and}$$

$$\nu_p = 13 \nu_m$$

$$15 \times L_m/\nu_m = U_p \times 10 L_m/13 \nu_m$$

$$U_p = 19.5 \ m/sec$$

The resistance R to the motion of an air ship can be expressed as

$$R/\rho L^2 U^2 = f(Re)$$

Maintaining equality of Reynolds number in the model and prototype will yield.

$$\frac{R_m}{\rho_m L_m^2 U_m^2} = \frac{R_p}{\rho_p L_p^2 U_p^2}$$

$$\frac{0.25}{1000 \times L_m^2 \times (15)^2} = \frac{R_p}{1.234 (10 L_m)^2 (19.5)^2}$$

$$R_p = 0.0521 \text{ kN}$$

In the second case, model is tested in a wind tunnel. According to Boyle's law

$$p/\rho = p_1/\rho_1$$

$$\frac{p_{atm}}{1.234} = \frac{20\,p_{atm}}{\rho_1}$$

$$\rho_1 = 24.68 \text{ kg/m}^3$$

The dynamic viscosity of fluid μ is not influenced by the pressure, *i.e.* $\mu_m = \mu_p$. Therefore, Reynolds law yield

$$\frac{\rho_m U_m L_m}{\mu_m} = \frac{\rho_p U_p L_p}{\mu_p}$$

$$\frac{24.68\, U_m L_m}{\mu_m} = \frac{1.2345 \times 10\, L_m \times 19.5}{\mu_m}$$

$$U_m = 9.75 \ \text{m/s}$$

and

$$R_m = R_p \times \frac{\rho_m}{\rho_p} \times \left(\frac{L_m}{L_p}\right)^2 \times \left(\frac{U_m}{U_p}\right)^2$$

$$= 0.0521 \times \frac{24.68}{1.234} \times (1/10)^2 \,(9.75/19.5)^2$$

$$= 0.0026 \ \text{kN}$$

6.19 A flowmeter when tested in a pipe carrying water yields a differential pressure of 53.2 kPa. The power absorbed in the meter was 0.134 kW. What differential pressure would the flowmeter indicate if atmospheric air flows through the system at dynamically same conditions and what would be the corresponding power loss in the meter ? Given that water is 50 times more viscous and 800 times more dense than air.

Solution

For dynamical similarity, the Reynolds number of two flows should be equal.

$$\frac{\rho_a U_a L_a}{\mu_a} = \frac{\rho_w U_w L_w}{\mu_w}$$

$$\frac{U_a}{U_w} = \frac{\rho_w}{\rho_a} \times \frac{L_w}{L_a} \times \frac{\mu_a}{\mu_w}$$

In this case, $\quad L_w = L_a$, $\rho_w = 800\,\rho_a$, $\mu_w = 50\,\mu_a$

Substitute these values,

$$U_a/U_w = 800 \times 1 \times 1/50 = 16$$

$$U_a = 16\, U_w$$

Now prediction equation is used.

$$\frac{(\Delta p)_a}{\rho_a U_a^2} = \frac{(\Delta p)_w}{\rho_w U_w^2}$$

$$= \frac{1}{800} \times (16)^2$$

The loss of power in the meter is caused due to pressure drop. Therefore,

$$\frac{P_a}{P_w} = \frac{(\Delta p)}{(\Delta p)_w} \times \frac{A_a}{A_w} \times \frac{U_a}{U_w}$$

$$= \frac{(16)^2}{800} \times 1 \times 16$$

$$P_a = 0.134 \times \frac{(16)^3}{800}$$

$$= 0.686 \text{ kW}$$

6.20. A distorted model is to be made with a horizontal scale of 1:500 and a vertical scale of 1:30. Find the ratio of discharges of the prototpe and the model using first principle and assuming that the gravity forces are predominating.

Solution

In this case, Froude law is applicable.

Velocity scale ratio $\quad U_r \approx \sqrt{D_r}$

Discharge scale ratio $Q_r = L_r D_r \sqrt{D_r}$

$$= L_r D_r^{3/2}$$

$$= (1/500) \times (1/30)^{3/2}$$

Hence $\qquad Q_v/Q_m = 82158.35$

6.21. A spillway model is to be built to a geometrically similar scale of 1:50 across a flume of 60 cm width. The prototype is 15 m high and the maximum head on it is expected to be 1.5 m.

(i) What height of model and what head on the model should be used.

(ii) If the flow over the model at the particular head is 12 lit/sec., what flow per metre length of the prototype is expected ?

(iii) If the negative pressure in the model is 200 mm, what is the negative pressure in the prototype ?

Solution

For undistorted geometrically similar model

$$L_r = H_m/H_p$$
$$H_m = L_r H_p$$
$$= 1.5/50 = 0.03 \text{ m}$$

Similarly $(H_t)_m = L_r (H_s)_p$

$$= (1/50) \times 15 = 0.3 \text{ m}$$

(iii) Accoring to Fround's law $U_r \approx L_r$

$$Q_r = L_r^{5/2}$$
$$Q_p = Q_m/L_r^{5/2}$$
$$= 12/(1/50)^{5/2} = (12 \times 50)^{5/2} \text{ lit/sec}$$

But $B_p = B_m/L_r$

$$= 0.60/\frac{1}{50} = 30 \text{ m}$$

Hence Q_p per unit width $= Q_p/B_p = \dfrac{12\,(50)^{5/2}}{30}$ lit/s

$$= 7.67 \text{ m}^3/\text{s}$$

(iii) Now $\dfrac{(\Delta p)_m}{(\Delta p)_p} = \dfrac{w_m H_m}{w_p H_p}$

But $w_m = w_p$

$$\left(\frac{\Delta p_m}{\Delta p_p}\right) = \frac{H_m}{H_p}$$

$$(\Delta p_m/\Delta p_p) = 1/50$$

Hence $\Delta p_p = -0.2 \times 50$

$$\Delta p_p = -10.0 \text{ metre.}$$

It is not practicable as it will initiate cavitation.

6.22 A river model has a horizontal scale of 1/1000 and a vertical scale of 1/100. (i) What Q_m corresponding to $Q_p=4000 \text{ m}^3/\text{s}$ in the river is expected ? (ii) If the time of travel of flood peak through 100 m in the model is 1 hour, how much time would the flood peak take to travel the corresponding distance in the river ? (iii) If the Manning's n for the river material is 0.03, calculate the 'n' required for the model material.

Solution

$$L_r = 1/1000 \ , \ D_r = 1/100$$

Flow in the river is governed by Froud's law,
Velocity scale ratio $U_r \approx \sqrt{D_r}$

$$Q_r = A_r U_r$$

$$= L_r D_r \times \sqrt{D_r}$$

$$= L_r D_r^{3/2}$$

$$Q_r = (1/1000) \times (1/100)^{3/2}$$

$$= 10^{-6}$$

$$Q_m = Q_r \times Q_p$$

$$= 10^{-6} \times 4000 \text{ m}^3/\text{s}$$

$$= 0.004 \text{ m}^3/\text{s or 4 lit/sec}$$

(ii) For the given $L_m = 100$ metre, time taken by flood peak in the model is $T_m = 1 \, hr$

So that $U_m = \dfrac{100}{60} = 1.67 \text{ m/min}$

Then $\qquad U_p = \dfrac{U_m}{\sqrt{D_r}} = \dfrac{1.67}{\sqrt{1/100}} = 16.7 \text{ m/min}$

Also $\qquad L_r = L_m/L_p$

$\qquad\qquad = 100/(1/1000) = 10^5$

$\qquad T_p = L_p/U_p$

$\qquad\qquad = (10^5/16.7) \times 1/60$

$\qquad\qquad = 99.8 \text{ hours}$

(iii) Manning equation for distorted model can be written as

$$U_r = (1/n_r) R_r^{2/3} S_r^{1/2}$$

For very wide channels,

$$R_r = A_r/P_r \approx D_r$$

and $\qquad\qquad S_r = D_r/L_r$

Hence $\qquad n_r = \dfrac{D_r^{2/3} (D_r/L_r)^{1/2}}{\sqrt{D_r}}$

$$= \dfrac{D_r^{2/3}}{\sqrt{L_r}}$$

$$= \dfrac{(1/100)^{2/3}}{(1/1000)^{1/2}} = 1.4677$$

Then $\qquad n_m = n_r \times n_p$

$$= 1.4677 \times 0.003$$

$$= 0.044$$

6.23 A certifugal pump is used to supply fluid at 15° C ($v = 1.14 \times 10^{-4} \text{ m}^2/\text{s}$) while rotating at 1500 r. p. m. A model pump using air at 20°C ($v = 1.46 \times 10^{-5} \text{ m}^2/\text{s}$) is to be tested. If the diameter of the model is 4 times the diameter of prototype, determine the corresponding speed for the model pump.

Solution

By dimensional analysis the discharge through the pump can be expressed as

$$\dfrac{Q}{ND^3} = \varphi \left[\dfrac{gH}{N^2 D^2}, \dfrac{v}{ND^2} \right]$$

For dynamically similar model,

$$\left[\dfrac{v}{ND^2} \right]_m = \left[\dfrac{v}{ND^2} \right]_p$$

$$N_m = \dfrac{v_m}{v_p} \times \dfrac{D_p^2}{D_m^2} \times N_p$$

$$= \frac{1.4 \times 10^{-5}}{1.14 \times 10^{-6}} \times \left(\frac{1}{4}\right)^2 \times 1500$$

$$= 1200.6 \text{ r.p.m.}$$

6.24 A 1 : 20 scale model of a turbine is found to develop 2.24 kN with a discharge of 0.25 m³/s under a head of 1.6 m while it rotates at 400 r.p.m. The diameter of the prototype is 6.0m. Calculate corresponding power, discharge, head and speed of prototype. Neglect friction.

Solution

For a hydraulic machine, the power developed can be expressed as

$$\left[\frac{P}{\rho D^5 N^3}\right] = \varphi \left[\frac{D}{B}, \frac{\rho D^2 N}{\mu}, \frac{ND}{\sqrt{gH}}\right]$$

(i) For geometric similarity

$$(D/B)_m = (D/B)_p$$

$$D_m = D_p \times \frac{B_m}{B_p}$$

$$= 6 \times 1/20 = 0.3$$

(ii) Also

$$\frac{D_m}{D_p} = \frac{H_m}{H_p}$$

$$H_p = H_m \times D_p/D_m$$

$$= 1.6 \times 20 = 32 \text{ metre}$$

(iii) For dynamic similarity the design equation is

$$\left(\frac{ND}{\sqrt{gH}}\right)_m = \left(\frac{ND}{\sqrt{gH}}\right)_p$$

$$N_p = N_m \times \frac{D_m}{D_p} \times \frac{H_p^{1/2}}{H_m^{1/2}}$$

$$= 400 \times 1/20 \times \sqrt{20}$$

$$= 89.44 \text{ r.p.m.}$$

(iv) Prediction Eq. is

$$\left(\frac{P}{\rho D^5 N^3}\right)_p = \left(\frac{P}{\rho D^5 N^3}\right)_m$$

$$P_p = P_m \times \rho_p/\rho_m \times (D_p/D_m)^5 (N_p/N_m)^2$$

$$P_p = 2.24 \times 1 \times 20^5 \times (1/\sqrt{20})^3 = 179.67 \text{ kW}$$

(v) The discharge can be expressed in dimensionless form as

$$\left(\frac{Q}{ND^3}\right)_p = \left(\frac{Q}{ND^3}\right)_m$$

$$Q_p = Q_m \times \frac{N_p}{N_m} \times \frac{D_p^3}{D_m^3}$$

$$= 0.25 \times (1/\sqrt{20}) (20)^3$$

$$= 447.22 \text{ m}^3/\text{sec}$$

6.25 The pressure at the entrance to the impeller of a large water pump is expected to be 30 kPa. A 1 : 20 scale model is used to investigate the possibilities of cavitation occuring inside the pump. The speed scale is assumed to be 1 : 5. Determine the required pressure at the entrance of the model pump. Take vapour pressure for water at working temperature as 5 kPa absolute. The effect of viscosity may be neglected.

Solution

For cavitation studies, the cavitation number of model and prototype flows should be equal.

$$\sigma = \left(\frac{p - p_v}{\rho U^2/2} \right)_m = \left(\frac{p - p_v}{\rho U^2/2} \right)_p$$

Assuming $(p_v)_m = (p_v)_p = 5$ kPa,

$$\frac{p_m - 5}{0.5 \rho_m U_m^2} = \frac{30 - 5}{0.5 \rho_m (5 U_m)^2}$$

Since $\rho_m = \rho_p$ and $U_m/U_p = 1/5$

Solving, $p_m = 6$ k Pa

6.26 : A torpedo-shaped object 900 mm diameter is to move in air at 60 m/s and its drag has to be estimated from tests in water on a half scale model. Determine the necessary speed of the model and the drag of the full scale object if that of model is 1140 N. Given $\mu_{air} = 1.86 \times 10^{-5}$ Pas, $\mu_{water} = 1.01 \times 10^{-5}$ Pas, $\rho_{air} = 1.2$ kg/m^3 and $\rho_{water} = 1000$ kg/m^3.

Solution :

The drag of an object F depends on fluid density ρ, viscosity μ, diameter D and velocity U By Buckingham's π-theorem,

$$\frac{F}{\rho U^2 D^2} = f \left[\frac{\rho U D}{\mu} \right]$$

Since the object remains fully submerged while in motion, Reynolds model law is applicable.

$$[Re]_m = [Re]_p$$

$$\frac{\rho_m U_m D_m}{\mu_m} = \frac{\rho_p U_p D_p}{\mu_p}$$

$$U_m = U_p \left(\frac{\rho_p}{\rho_m} \frac{D_p}{D_m} \frac{\mu_m}{\mu_p} \right)$$

Using values of air for prototype with suffix p and that of water for model with suffix m,

$$\frac{D_m}{D_p} = L_r = \frac{1}{2} \text{ (Given)}$$

$$U_m = 60 \times \frac{1.2}{1000} \times \frac{2}{1} \times \frac{1.01 \times 10^{-3}}{1.86 \times 10^{-5}}$$

$$= 7.82 \text{ m/s}$$

Therefore, $\dfrac{F_m}{\rho_m U_m^2 D_m^2} = \dfrac{F_p}{\rho_p U_p^2 D_p^2}$

$$F_p = F_m \times \frac{\rho_b}{\rho_m} \times \frac{U_p^2}{U_m^2} \times \frac{D_p^2}{D_m^2}$$

$$= 1140 \times \frac{1.2}{1000} \times \left(\frac{60}{7.82}\right)^2 \times (2)^2$$

$$= 322.13 \text{ N.}$$

6.27 : A 1:5 scale model of a car is tested in a wind-tunnel to ascertain the drag and power required to overcome the drag of prototype. The prototype moves at a velocity of 80 km/h. The experiments showed that model car experiences a drag of 250 N. Determine the drag and power required for prototype. The properties of air for model and prototype are assumed to remain same.

Solution :

The car moves fully submerged in air.

∴ $(Re)_m = (Re)_p$

$$\frac{\rho_m U_m L_m}{\mu_m} = \frac{\rho_p U_p L_p}{\mu_p}$$

Since air properties remains same, $\rho_m = \rho_p, \mu_m = \mu_p$

$$\frac{U_m}{U_p} = \frac{L_p}{L_m}$$

$$U_m = U_p \cdot \frac{L_p}{L_m}$$

Given $\dfrac{L_m}{L_p} = \dfrac{1}{5}$, $U_p = 80 \text{ km/hr} = 22.22 \text{ m/s}$

$$U_m = 22.22 \times \frac{5}{1} = 111.11 \text{ m/s}$$

For equality of Reynolds model law (Table 6.2)

Force scale ratio $F_r = \rho_r \gamma_r^2$

$$\frac{F_m}{F_p} = \frac{\rho_m}{\rho_p} \cdot \frac{\gamma_m^2}{\gamma_p^2}$$

Since $\rho_m = \rho_b, \gamma_m = \gamma_p,$

$$F_m = F_p = 250 \text{ N}$$

Power required to overcome this drag $= P_p$

$$= 250 \times 22.22 \text{ W}$$
$$= 5.555 \text{ kW}$$

6.28 : A river carries a discharge of 15000 m³/s at 7.5 m depth. The width of stream is 400 m and its bed slope is 0.0025. A model study is to be done for 15 km of this river in a laboratory having 25 m floor area and 0.25 m³/s as maximum available discharge. Determine the following information for model (i) horizontal and vertical scales, (b) slope required for model and (c) roughness scale for the material to be used in the model if river carries a sand with $n_p = 0.01$.

Solution:

Initially an undistorted model is planned.

Required horoizontal scale ratio (L_r) and vertical scale ratio (D_r) are given by

$$L_r = \frac{L_m}{L_p} = \frac{25}{15 \times 1000} = \frac{1}{600}$$

$$Q_r = \frac{Q_m}{Q_p} = \frac{0.25}{15000} = \frac{1}{60000}$$

Also, $Q_r =$ Area × velocity

$$= L_r D_r \times \sqrt{D_r}$$
$$= L_r D_r^{3/2}$$

$$\frac{1}{60000} = \frac{1}{600} \times D_r^{3/2}$$

$$D_r^{3/2} = \left(\frac{1}{100}\right)$$

$$D_r = \frac{1}{21.54} = \frac{1}{25} \text{ (say)}$$

$$D_m = \frac{D_p}{25} = \frac{7.5}{25} = 0.3 \text{ m}$$

In order to modify the distribution, one may ensure a minimum depth of flow of 15 cm (say)

$$\frac{D_m}{D_p} = \frac{0.15}{7.50} = \frac{1}{50}$$

$$U_p = \frac{Q_p}{a_p}$$

$$= \frac{15000}{400 \times 7.5} = 5 \text{ m/s}$$

$$U_r = \sqrt{D_r}$$

$$\frac{U_m}{U_p} = \sqrt{1/50} = \frac{1}{7.07}$$

$$U_m = \frac{U_p}{7.07} = \frac{5}{7.07}$$

$$= 0.707 \text{ m/s}$$

$$h_m = \frac{7.5}{50} = 0.15 \text{ m}$$

$$(Re)_m = \frac{\rho_m U_m L_m}{\mu_m}$$

$$= \frac{0.707 \times 0.15}{10^{-6}}$$

$$(\because \gamma_m = 10^{-6} \text{ m}^2/\text{s for water })$$

$$= 106050 > 2000$$

Hence the flow remains turbulent in the model.

(b)

$$S_r = \frac{D_r}{L_r}$$

$$= \frac{1/50}{1/600}$$

$$S_m = S_p \times \frac{600}{50}$$

$$= 0.0025 \times \frac{600}{50} = 0.03$$

(c)

$$U_r = \frac{1}{n_v} \cdot R_r^{2/3} S_r^{1/2}$$

$$n_r = \frac{R_1^{2/3} S_r^{1/2}}{U_r}$$

Sulestituting $R_r \approx D_r$ (wide river)

$$U_r = \sqrt{L_r} \quad \text{(Froude model law)}$$

$$S_r = D_r/L_r$$

$$n_r = \frac{D_r^{2/3} \left(\dfrac{D_r}{L_r}\right)^{1/2}}{D_r^{1/2}} = \frac{D_r^{2/3}}{L_r^{1/2}}$$

$$n_m = n_p \cdot D_r^{2/3}/L^{1/2}$$

$$= \frac{0.01 (1/60)^{2/3}}{(1/600)^{1/2}}$$

$$= 0.01 \times \frac{24.495}{15.347} = 0.016$$

Adopt $\qquad L_r = 1/600,\ D_r = 1/60,\ S_m = 0.03,\ n_m = 0.016$

6.29 A tidal model of a river estuary has a horizontal scale A and vertical scale B. Derive an expression for ratio between (a) tidal period and (b) the rate of fall of silt for the model and prototype. Discuss critically e assumptions made.

Solution

The river estuary is affected by viscous and gravity forces. Therefore the resistance R can be expressed functionally as

$$R = f[\rho, U, D, \mu, g]$$

By dimensional analysis, the equation can be rewritten as

$$R = \rho\, U^2 D^2 f\left[\frac{\rho\, U D}{\mu}, \frac{U^2}{g D}\right] \qquad \text{...(i)}$$

Here D is the characteristic length. In most instances the flow in estuary is turbulent and hence viscous force is not of much significance. Therefore, gravity force is predominant and Froud's model law should be used, *i.e.*

$$U = \sqrt{gD} \qquad \text{...(ii)}$$

Also $\qquad A = L_m/L_p$, or $L_p = L_m/A$ $\qquad$ ...(iii)

and $\qquad B = D_m/D_p$ or $D_p = D_m/B$ $\qquad$ ...(iv)

(a) The tidal period for model

$$T_m = \frac{L_m}{U_m} = \frac{L_m}{\sqrt{D_m}} \qquad \text{...(v)}$$

and for prototype

$$T_p = \frac{L_p}{U_n} = \frac{L_p}{\sqrt{D_p}}$$

$$T_p = \frac{L_m}{A} \times \frac{\sqrt{B}}{\sqrt{D_m}} \qquad \text{...(vi)}$$

From Eqs. (v) and (vi)

$$\frac{T_m}{T_p} = \frac{L_m}{\sqrt{D_m}} \times \frac{A\sqrt{D_m}}{L_m\sqrt{B}}$$

$$\frac{T_m}{T_p} = \frac{A}{\sqrt{B}}$$

(b) The rate of fall of sediment ω will depend on the work done by the tides on the bed of estuary, *i.e.*,

$$W \alpha R \times U$$

But from Eqs. (i), $R \alpha \rho\, U^2 D^2$

For distorted model, $R \alpha \rho\, U^2 LD$

Hence $\qquad \dfrac{W_m}{W_p} = \dfrac{(\rho\,L\,D\,U^3)_m}{(\rho\,L\,D\,U^3)_p}$

Substitute the value of U from Eqs. (ii) and ρ_m is equal to ρ_p

$$\frac{W_m}{W_p} = \frac{L_m\,D_m^{5/2}}{L_p\,D_p^{5/2}}$$

Substitute the value of L_p and D_p from Eqs. (iii) and (iv)

$$\frac{W_m}{W_p} = \frac{L_m\,D_m^{5/2}}{L_m/A \times (D_m/B)^{5/2}}$$

$$\frac{W_m}{W_p} = A\,B^{5/2}$$

Objective Question

6.1 Select the dimensionless parameter from the following

    (a) specific weight   (b) specific mass
    (c) kinematic viscosity   (d) specific gravity
    (e) angular velocity   (f) Darcy's friction coefficient
    (g) none of these

6.2 The following quantities in column 'A' are given in units indicated against them. The column B describes the conversion factor to convert them in SI units but these are not in proper order. Match the correct conversion factor for each quantity

Column A	Column B
(a) pressure (lb/sq. in to N/cm^2)	(i) 9.81
(b) specific weight (kgf/m^3 to kN/m^3)	(ii) 9.81
(c) dynamic viscosity (poise to N s/m^2)	(iii) 10^{-4}
(d) kinematic viscosity (stokes to m^2/s)	(iv) 0.6986
(e) power (horse power to kW)	(v) 0.735
(f) surface tension (kgf/cm to N/m)	(vi) 0.1

6.3 The dimensions of following quantities of column A are given in column B. Choose the correct dimensions for each parameter of column A from column B

Column A	
(a) Dynamic viscosity	(i) F/L
(b) Chezy's C	(ii) FT/L^2
(c) Discharge constant C_1 for rectangular weir in $Q = C_1\,L\,H^{3/2}$	(iii) $L^{5/2}/T$
(d) Bulk modulus of elasticity E_y	(iv) $L^{1/2}/T$
(e) Energy E	(v) F/L^2
(f) Surface tension σ	

6.4 Determine whether the following equations are dimensionally homogeneous

(a) $Q = 1.84 (L - 0.2H) H^{1.5}$

(b) $\sigma = 500 (h\, r / \cos \theta)$

(c) $N_s = N \sqrt{Q} / H^{3/4}$

(d) $U = C \sqrt{RS}$

(e) $h_f = f L\, Q^2 / (12.1\, D^5)$

(f) $P = w Q H / 75$

6.5 Which of the following group could be π parameter of the function $f(Q, H, g, v, \theta) = 0$. when Q and g are taken as repeating variables?

(a) $Q^2 / g H^4$ (b) $Q^2 / g \theta^2$ (c) $Q / \sqrt{g H}$

(d) $v Q^7 / 5 / g^{1/5}$ (e) none of these

6.6 A dimensionless combination of $\Delta p, \rho, l$ and Q is

(a) $\sqrt{\dfrac{\Delta p}{\rho}} \times \dfrac{Q}{l^2}$ (b) $\dfrac{\rho Q}{\Delta p\, l^2}$

(d) $\dfrac{\Delta p\, l\, Q}{\rho}$ (e) $\sqrt{\dfrac{\rho}{\Delta p}} \times \dfrac{Q}{l^2}$

6.7 Reynolds number may be defined as the ratio of

(a) viscous to inertia force

(b) viscous force to gravity force

(c) gravity force to inertia force

(d) elastic force to inertia force

(e) none of these

6.8 The Table A indicates various dimensionless numbers often used in fluid flow analysis. Indicate their correct definition from Table B.

Table A	Table B
(a) Froude number	(i) surface tension to inertia force
(b) Mach number	(ii) pressure to inertia force
(c) Euler number	(iii) gravity to inertia force
(d) Weber number	(iv) compressibility to inertia force

6.9 Select the situation in which Froude model law is applicable.

(a) flow through an orifice   (b) compressible flow

(c) pipe flow   (d) fully submerged objects

(e) flow through an half opened valve

6.10 Kinematic similarity between model and prototype is

(a) the similarity of streamline pattern

(b) use of same model scale throughout

    (c) the similarity of force influencing the flow

    (d) the similarity of discharge

    (e) none of these

6.11 Dynamic similarity between model and prototype is

    (a) the model and prototype are geometrically similar

    (b) the velocities in model and prototype are similar at corresponding points

    (c) the forces acting at corresponding locations are same

    (d) the forces acting are similar

    (e) none of these

6.12 The scale ratios for some of the quantities have been determined using Froud's model law. Identify them for the list enclosed

    (a) acceleration   (i) $w_r L_r^4$

    (b) angular acceleration   (ii) $w_r L_r^{3/2}/g^{1/2}$

    (c) angular velocity   (iii) $\rho_r g_r^{3/2}/L_r^{7/2}$

    (d) momentum   (iv) g_r

    (e) power   (v) $1/T_r$

    (f) energy   (vi) $1/T_r^2$

6.13 The height of a hydraulic jump in a stilling pool was found to be 15 cm in a model when model scale ratio is 1 : 30.

The prototype jump height in metre is

    (a) 0.45   (b) 4.5   (c) 200   (d) 1/200   (e) none

6.14 A 1 : 15 scale model of a projectile has a drag coefficient 3.5 at $N_m = 2.0$. How many times greater would the prototype resistance be when fired at the same Mach number in air of the same temperature and one half of density ?

    (a) 3.12   (b) 12.5   (c) 25   (d) 100   (e) none

Problems

    6.1 In terms of M,L,T, determine the dimensions of radians, angular velocity, power, work, torque, impulse and momentum.

    6.2 The stagnation pressure at a stagnation point in an air stream depends on the pressure p_o , density ρ_0 and velocity U_0 in the free stream. Determine a dimensionless parameter on which parameter p_s/p_0 depends.

    6.3 The drag F_D of an aeroplane wing is affected by the area A of the wing, the angle of attack α , the velocity U of the flight, the viscosity μ and mass density ρ of air and speed of compression wave in air c. Determine an expression for F_D by the method of dimensional analysis.

    6.4 A surface ship of length L and draft y moves at a speed U through sea water of mass density ρ , viscosity μ and surface tension σ. By dimensional analysis derive an expression for the drag F_0 of the ship. The gravitation force also affects the drag of the ship.

6.5 The capillary rise h of a liquid in a round tube of diameter D depends on the surface tension σ and specific weight w of liquid. Use Rayleigh's method to derive a formula for h.

6.6 If the discharge Q through a mouthpiece is a function of pressure p causing flow, the density ρ and viscosity μ, show that

$$Q = Cd^2 \sqrt{p/\rho}$$

where C is some function of the non-dimensional number.

6.7 A compressor of diameter D, rotating at an angular velocity ω, handles a rate of flow Q of a fluid of density S and viscosity μ. Using dimensional analysis, derive an expression for power P required in terms of these variables.

6.8 Determine the formula for the velocity of a solid particle which settles in a still liquid. It is known that velocity is affected by linear dimension b of the container fluid, properties ρ and μ, solid particle diameter and mass density d and ρ respectively and acceleration due to gravity g.

6.9 The diffusion characteristic of turbulent fluid jet are dependent on jet diameter d, length of jet l, jet velocity U, fluid characteristics ρ_1 and μ_1 and the characteristics of stationary surrounding fluid ρ_2 and μ_2. Derive a dimensional equation for the same.

6.10 Explain the following terms
(a) Design equations and prediction equations
(b) True model   (c) Hydraulic similitude
(d) Prediction factor

6.11 A model is to be built of a flow phenomenon which is dominated by action of gravity and surface tension. Show that the length scale ratio that will ensure complete hydraulic similitude between model and prototype is

$$L_r = \sqrt{\sigma_r/\rho_r}$$

where σ_r and ρ_r are scale ratios for surface tension and mass density.

6.12 To determine the wind force on a suspension bridge, a scale model is tested in a wind tunnel at velocity of 200 km/hr. Calculate (a) the wind velocity in order to ensure dynamic similarity between the model and its prototype (b) ratio of wind forces on the model to prototype. The temperature for both model and prototype are made same.

6.13 Show that the total resistance R of a floating ship is given by the expression

$$R = 1/L_r^3 [r + r_f (f_p/f_m - 1)]$$

where L_r is the scale ratio, and other notations are as usual. Same fluid is used for testing model as used in prototype.

6.14 A 1 : 25 geometrically similar model of a spillway has been prepared in a laboratory following Froud's law. Determine (a) the rate of flow over the model to simulate at actual flow of 6.25 m³/sec in prototype (b) the corresponding velocity of 1.6 m/s observed in the model section (c) the energy dissipated in the prototype corresponding to 0.3 kW in the model.

6.15 The losses at a T junction in a 1.0 diameter duct system carrying air of density 41 kg/m^3 , viscosity 0.002 N s/m^2 and velocity 25 m/s are to be determined by model testing using water. The test facility include the maximum water discharge of 360 m^3/hr . Determine the model scale to be used.

6.16 A model turbine has a runner of 0.6 m and delivers 50 kW, under a head of 30 m at a speed of 4000 r.p.m. If this model is 1 : 2 scale reduction of actual turbine to run at 36 m head, determine its speed and shaft horse power.

6.17 In a test on a centrifugal pump it was found that the discharge was 2.75 m^3/s and the total pressure was 63.5 mm of water column. The shaft power was 1.7 kW. If a geometrically similar fan having dimensions 25% smaller but having twice the rotational speed was used. calculate the output, pressure generated and shaft power required.

6.18 A 20 km length of river is to be modelled in a laboratory having only 12.5 m of available length. The river discharge is known to be in the range of 400-500 m^3/s and the average length and width are 3.5 m and 5.5 m respectively. Propose suitable scales. Also calculate the ratio of time in model to prototype. Take T_p = 12.4 hr.

6.19 A 1.2 m diameter pipe is to transport castor oil (specific gravity 0.96 and dynamic viscosity 98 $\times$ 10^{-5} Ns/m^2) at a rate of 0.4 m^3/s . In order to determine head loss in pipe, it was decided to conduct a model test on small pipe of 15 cm diameter using water at 20° C as the model fluid (v = 0.0131 stokes). Calculate the discharge required in the model. If the head loss in 50 m length of model pipe is 7.75 m/metre length of pipe, determine the pressure drop in 10 km length of prototype ? Also calculate Darcy's f for prototype.

6.20 A distorted model is made of a rectangular channel of test section of horizontal scale ratio, prototype to model, of α_H and vertical scale ratio of α_v . Obtain the design conditions and deduce expression for prediction factor and the prediction equation for velocity in prototype. Use Manning's equation.

7

Laminar Flow

7.1. INTRODUCTION

In this chapter, the flow of real fluid is studied. The flow of real fluid differs from that of an ideal fluid due to its viscosity. The ideal fluid experiences no resistance to its motion and, hence, uniform velocity distribution is obained as shown in Fig. 7.1a. In case of real fluid, the velocity remains zero at the stationary wall and increases asymtotically to free steam velocity U_0 away from the wall, Fig. 7.1b. The real fluid acquires the velocity of the surface of contact due to the viscous action and there is no slip between the contact surface and the fluid layer adjacent to the wall. This 'no' slip condition' is an important condition of the flow of real fluid which was first proposed by L. Prandtl.

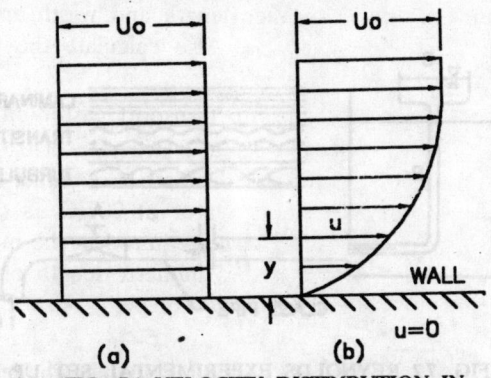

FIG. 7.1 VELOCITY DISTRIBUTION IN
(a) IDEAL FLUID (b) REAL FLUID

Basically, there are two broad classes of flows (i) external flows and (ii) internal flows. The flows around bodies such as airfoils, rockets, surface vessels are termed as external flows. On the other hand, flows which are enclosed by boundaries of interest are termed as internal flows. Examples of internal flows include the flows through pipes, ducts and nozzles.

7.2 REGIMES OF FLOW

All the flows in nature can be classified into two types or regimes. These are, (i) laminar flows and (ii) turbulent flows.

Laminar flow. It is a well ordered pattern of flow, in which fluid motion occurs in layers, one layer gliding smoothly over the adjacent layer, without mixiing with each other. Any tendency towards instability is damped out by viscous forces, that also resist relative motion of adjacent layers.

Turbulent flow. It is an irregular pattern of flow in which the fluid particles move in an disorderly and random fashion. The lumps of fluid particles intermix with each other and in the process interchange their momentum.

7.3. REYNOLDS EXPERIMENT AND ITS SIGNIFICANCE

Osborne Reynolds conducted a classic experiment to demonstrate the various regimes of flow. Water was allowed to flow from a tank through a well mouthed glass pipe, the flow being controlled by valve A (Fig. 7.2). A thin tube, B, leading from a container of dye, C, had its opening within the entrance of the glass pipe. Reynolds discovered that, for low velocities of flow in the glass pipe, a thin filament of dye issuing from the tube did not diffuse but was maintained intact throughout the pipe, forming a thin straight line parallel to the axis of pipe. As the valve was opened, and greater velocities were attained, the dye filament oscillated and broke, diffusing through the flowing water in the pipe. Reynolds found that the mean velocity at which the filament of dye began to break up (termed critical velocity) was dependent on the degree of quiescence of water in the tank, higher critical velocities being obtained with increased quiescence.

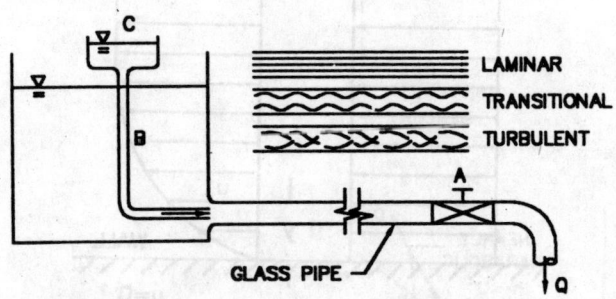

FIG. 7.2 REYNOLDS EXPERIMENTAL SET UP

Since intermingling of fluid particles during flow would cause diffusion of the dye filament, Reynolds deduced from his experiments that at low velocities, this intermingling was absent and that fluid particles moved in parallel layers, or laminae, sliding past adjacent laminae but not mixing with them; this is the regime of laminar flow. Since at higher velocities the dye filament diffused through the pipe, it was apparent that intermingling of fluid particles was occurring, or in other words, the flow was turbulent. It was also noticed that laminar flow broke down to turbulent flow at some higher critical velocity than the one at which turbulent flow was restored to the laminar conditions; the former velocity is known as upper critical velocity and the latter, the lower critical velocity.

The existence of two flow regimes may be deduced from another simple experiment, shown in Fig. 7.3a. The apparatus consists of a long straigth pipe with a U-tube connected to pressure tappings on the pipe. The difference of pressure between two points, L distant apart, is measured by a U-tube manomenter. Let the reading be h_f and the mean velocity of flow through the pipe be U. The fall of pressure h_f is correleted with velocity U in Fig. 7.3b. For the small values of U a plot of h_f against U will be found to yield a straight line $(h_f < \alpha U)$, but at higher values of U a nearly parabolic curve $(h_f \; \alpha U_n)$ will result ; the value of n varying from 1.7 to 2.0 Evidently, the flow is laminar in the first case and turbulent in the second. Between two regimes lies a transition region; as U increases the experimental data follow OABCD but with diminishing U will follow DBAO. From these results it may be deduced that points B and C define the lower and upper critical velocities respectively.

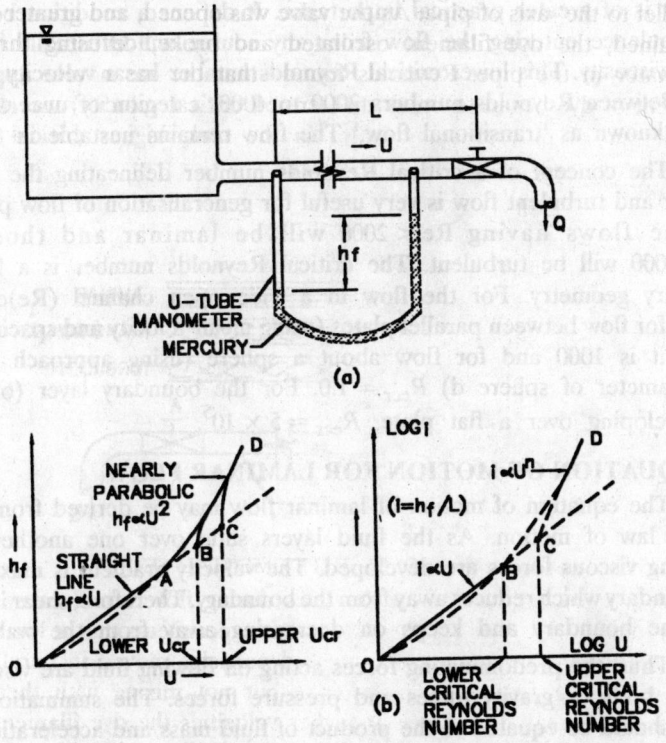

FIG. 7.3 COMPARISON OF RATES OF ENERGY
LOSS IN LAMINAR AND TURBULET FLOW

Reynolds generalised his experimental conclusions by means of a dimensionless number, later called Reynolds number R_e. It was defined as.

$$R_e = \frac{\rho \, UD}{\mu} \qquad \qquad ...(7.1)$$

in which U is the mean velocity of flow, D is the diameter of the pipe and ρ and μ the mass density and visocsity of the fluid flowing therein. The Reynolds number corresponding to lower critcal velocity was defined as " lower critical

Reynolds number" and that corresponding to upper critical velocity as "Upper critical Reynolds number".

The upper limit of Reynolds number was found to vary from 12000 to 14000 and this uppper critical Reynolds number is indefinite. It depends on several incidental conditions such as (1) initial quiescence of the fluid, (2) shape of pipe entrance and roughness of pipe. Ekman repeated the Reynolds experiment taking all necessary precautions and obtained even higher value of (Re)cr, equal to 40,000. These higher values are, however, of little practical interest. An engineer may take the upper limit of laminar flow between 2700 to 4000.

The lower limit of turbulent flow, defined by lower critical Reynolds number is of greater practical importance. It defines a condition below which all turbulence entering the flow from any source will eventually be damped out by viscosity. This lower critical Reynolds number has a value approximately 2000. Between Reynolds numbers 2000 to 4000, a region of uncertainty exists and is known as 'transitional flow.' The flow remains unstable in this region.

The concept of a critical Reynolds number delineating the regimes of laminar and turbulent flow is very useful for generalisation of flow phenomena. All the flows having Re < 2000 will be laminar and those having Re > 4000 will be turbulent. The critical Reynolds number is a function of boundary geometry. For the flow in a wide open channel (Re)er is equal to 500, for flow between parallel plates (using mean velocity and spacing between them) it is 1000 and for flow about a sphere (using approach velocity U and diameter of sphere d) $R_{ecr} = 1.0$. For the boundary layer (of thickness δ) developing over a flat plate, $R_{ecr} \approx 5 \times 10^5$.

7.4. EQUATION OF MOTION FOR LAMINAR FLOW

The equation of motion of laminar flow may be derived from Newton's second law of motion. As the fluid layers slide over one another, whereby opposing viscous forces are developed. The velocity gradient is maximum near the boundary which reduces away from the boundary. Therefore, shear is maximum near the boundary and keeps on decreasing away from the wall.

Thus, the predominating forces acting on flowing fluid are viscous forces besides body or gravity forces and pressure forces. The summation of these forces should be equated to the product of fluid mass and acceleration brought in by these forces. Considering unit volume of fluid, the equation of motion in X-direction may be written as

$$\rho\, a_x = f_x + f_{px} + f_{vx} \qquad \text{...(7.2 a)}$$

Similar equation in Y and Z direction may also be writien.

$$\rho a_y = f_y + f_{py} + f_{vy} \qquad \text{...(7.2b)}$$

$$\rho a_z = f_z + f_{pz} + f_{vz} \qquad \text{...(7.2c)}$$

where f_x, f_y and f_z are body forces, f_{px}, f_{py} and f_{pz} are pressure forces and f_{vx}, f_{vy} f_{vz} are viscous forces per unit volume acting in the three co-ordinate directions.

Simplifying,

$$\left(\frac{\partial u}{\partial t} + u \frac{\partial u}{\partial x} + v \frac{\partial u}{\partial y} + w \frac{\partial u}{\partial z} \right) = \left[X - \frac{1}{\rho} \frac{\partial p}{\partial x} + \right.$$
$$\left. v \left(\frac{\partial^2 u}{\partial x^2} + \frac{\partial^2 u}{\partial y^2} + \frac{\partial^2 u}{\partial z^2} \right) \right] \qquad ...(7.3a)$$

$$\left(\frac{\partial v}{\partial t} + u \frac{\partial v}{\partial x} + v \frac{\partial v}{\partial y} + w \frac{\partial v}{\partial z} \right) = \left[Y - \frac{1}{\rho} \frac{\partial p}{\partial y} \right.$$
$$\left. + v \left(\frac{\partial^2 v}{\partial x^2} + \frac{\partial^2 v}{\partial y^2} + \frac{\partial^2 v}{\partial z^2} \right) \right] \qquad ...(7.3b)$$

$$\left(\frac{\partial w}{\partial t} + u \frac{\partial w}{\partial x} + v \frac{\partial w}{\partial y} + w \frac{\partial w}{\partial z} \right) = \left[Z - \frac{1}{\rho} \frac{\partial p}{\partial z} \right.$$
$$\left. + v \left(\frac{\partial^2 w}{\partial x^2} + \frac{\partial^2 w}{\partial y^2} + \frac{\partial^2 w}{\partial z^2} \right) \right] \qquad ...(7.3c)$$

Here u, v and w are velocity components in the three co-ordinate diections; X, Y and Z represent body forces per unit mass in the corresponding directions. Eqs. 7.3a to 7.3c, are known as 'Navier Stokes equations' of laminar flow. The left hand side of these equations is known as total derivaive or substantive derivative and is expressed as D/Dt. Three terms on the extreme right of each equation are known as Laplacian of u, v and w.

Eqs. 7.3a to 7.3b may be written as

$$\frac{D\overline{U}}{Dt} = F_B - \frac{1}{\rho} \frac{\partial p}{\partial s} + v \nabla^2 \overline{U} \qquad ...(7.4)$$

Here

$$\overline{U} = i\overline{u} + j\overline{v} + k\overline{w} \qquad ...(7.5)$$

and

$$F_B = iX + jY + kZ \qquad ...(7.6)$$

For detailed derivation of Eqs. 7.3a to 7.3c, refer to Appendix 1.

7.5. FLOW BETWEEN TWO PARALLEL PLATES

There are two possible flow cases, (i) both plates remaining stationary and (ii) one of the plate is moving. This latter type of flow is known as "coutte flow".

1. Both plates remaining stationary

(a) *Velocity distribution*. Consider that the steady laminar flow occurs between two stationary parallel plates, situated 'B' distance apart in Fig. 7.4. The plates are assumed sufficiently wide to make the edge effects negligible. Consider a small fluid element of length dx and area of cross section $dy \times 1$; unit width is assumed normal to the plane of paper. The forces acting on this fluid element are pressure and viscous forces only. Since the flow is steady and uniform, the acceleration is zero. Therefore, for static equaibrium of fluid element, the summation of all the forces in the direction of motion should be zero.

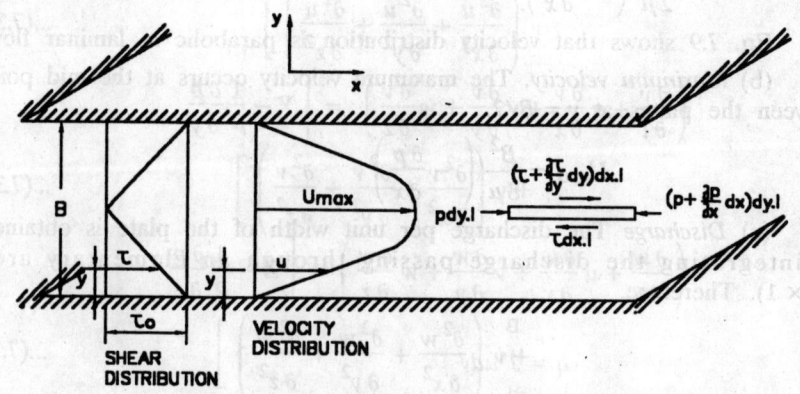

FIG. 7.4 FLOW BETWEEN PARALLEL PLATES

$$pdy - (p + \frac{\partial p}{\partial x} dx) dy - \tau dx + (\tau + \frac{\partial \tau}{\partial y} dy) dx = 0$$

Simplifying, $\frac{\partial p}{\partial x} = \frac{\partial \tau}{\partial y}$ ...(7.7)

From Eq. 1.8c, $\tau = \mu \frac{\partial u}{\partial y}$ ...(7.8)

Then, Eq. 7.7 becomes,

$$\frac{\partial^2 u}{\partial y^2} = \frac{1}{\mu} \frac{\partial p}{\partial x}$$

Integrating with respect to y

$$\frac{\partial u}{\partial y} = \frac{1}{\mu} \left(\frac{\partial p}{\partial x} \right) y + C$$ ...(7.8 a)

Integrating it again with respect to y

$$u = \frac{1}{\mu} \left(\frac{\partial p}{\partial x} \right) \frac{y^2}{2} + Cy + D$$ ...(7.8 b)

The two constants of integration C and D may be evaluated by means of two known boundary conditions.

(i) at $y = 0$, $u = 0$ and (ii) at $y = B, u = 0$

Substituting these boundary conditions in Eq. 7.8b yields

$$D = 0$$

$$C = \frac{B}{2\mu} \left(-\frac{\partial p}{\partial x} \right)$$

Substituting the values of C and D in Eq. 7.8b, the velocity at any point, y distant from the wall is obtained.

$$u = \frac{1}{2\mu} \left(-\frac{\partial p}{\partial x} \right) (By - y^2) \qquad ...(7.9)$$

Eq. 7.9 shows that velocity distribution is parabolic in laminar flow.

(b) *Maximum velocity*. The maximum velocity occurs at the mid point between the plates at $y = B/2$.

$$U_{max} = \frac{B^2}{8\mu} \left(-\frac{\partial p}{\partial x} \right)$$

(c) *Discharge* The discharge per unit width of the plate is obtained by integrating the discharge passing through an elementary area $(dx \times 1)$. Therefore.

$$q = \int_0^B u \, dy$$

$$= \int_0^B \left[\frac{1}{2\mu} \left(-\frac{\partial p}{\partial x} \right) (By - y^2) \right] dy$$

Solving it, $\qquad q = \frac{B^3}{12\mu} \left(-\frac{\partial p}{\partial x} \right) \qquad ...(7.10)$

(d) *Average velocity*. The average velocity U is obtained from continutiy equation.

$$U = \frac{q}{B}$$

$$= \frac{B^2}{12\mu} \left(-\frac{\partial p}{\partial x} \right) = \frac{2}{3} U_{max} \qquad ...(7.11)$$

(e) *Pressure drop*. Rearranging Eq. 7.11, the pressure drop $\dfrac{\partial p}{\partial x}$ is given

by

$$-\partial p = \frac{12\mu U}{B^2} \partial x$$

Integrating it between two sections, L distance apart,

$$\int_1^2 -dp = \int_0^L \frac{12\mu U}{B^2} dx$$

Partial derivative are changed to full derivative since p varies with x only.

$$p_1 - p_2 = \frac{12\mu UL}{B^2} \qquad ...(7.12a)$$

Dividing by specific weight w on both sides, the head loss h_f is obtained.

$$h_f = \frac{p_1 - p_2}{w} = \frac{12 \mu \, UL}{wB^2} \qquad ...(7.12b)$$

(f) *Shear distribution and maximum shear.* From Eqs. 1.8c and Eqs. 7.9.

$$\tau = \mu \frac{\partial u}{\partial y} = \mu \frac{\partial}{\partial y} \left[\frac{1}{2\mu} \left(-\frac{\partial p}{\partial x} \right) (By - y^2) \right]$$

$$\tau = \left(-\frac{\partial p}{\partial x} \right) (B/2 - y) \qquad ...(7.13)$$

Eq. 7.13 shows that shear stress varies linearly with y across the cross section of the parallel plates. The maximum value of shear stress occurs at the wall $(y = 0)$ and is known as wall shear stress τ_0.

$$\tau_0 = - \left(\frac{\partial p}{\partial x} \right) \frac{B}{2} \qquad ...(7.14)$$

2. Inclined parallel plates

When the flow takes place between two inclined parallel plates, the pressure gradient $(-\partial p/\partial x)$ should be replaced by piezometric gradient $-\partial (p + wz)/\partial x$. In this expression, z represents the datum head aboue an arbitrary datum. The analysis is otherwise, carried out in the same manner as is done for horizontal parallel plates in Sec. 7.5.1 above.

3. Coutte flow

When the flow takes place between two parallel plates. one remaining stationary and other moving with velocity U_0, the flow is known as 'general coutte flow. The analysis of coutte flow is used in the theory of lubrication. Let the coutte flow take place between two parallel plates, the lower plate remaining stationary and the upper plate moving with a velocity U_0.

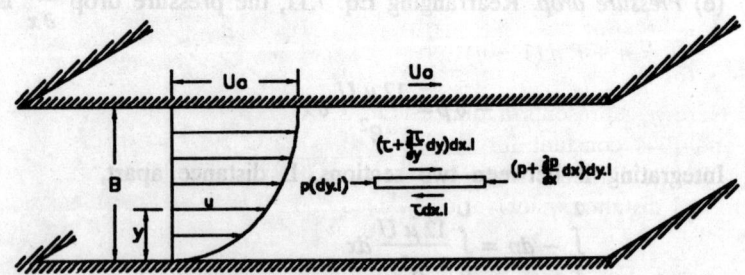

FIG. 7.5 GENERAL COUTTE FLOW

(a) *General form of velocity distribution.* The velocity distribution between two parallel plates is given by Eq. 7.8b.

358 Fluid Mechanics, Fluid Machines and Hydraulics

$$u = \frac{1}{\mu}\left(\frac{\partial p}{\partial x}\right)\frac{y^2}{2} + Cy + D \qquad ...(7.8b)$$

The constants of integration C and D are to be determined with a new boundary conditions applicable to coutte flow, i.e.

(i) at $y = 0$, $u = 0$ and (iii) at $y = B$, $u = U_0$

Substituting these boundary conditions in Eq. 7.8b

$$D = 0 \qquad ...(7.15a)$$

and

$$C = \frac{U_0}{B} - \frac{B}{2\mu}\left(\frac{\partial p}{\partial x}\right) \qquad ...(7.15\ a)$$

Hence, the velocity distribution for general coutte flow is obtained as

$$u = \frac{U_0 y}{B} - \frac{1}{2\mu}\left(\frac{\partial p}{\partial x}\right)(By - y^2) \qquad ...(7.16a)$$

Eq. 7.16a shows that velocity u at any point in the courtte flow depends upon the velocity of the upper plate U_0 and pressure gradient $\partial p/\partial x$. If the pressure gradient $\partial p/\partial x$ in the flow is zero, it becomes a plane coutte flow or simple shear flow. From Eq. 7.16a.

$$u = U_0 y/B \qquad ...(7.17)$$

Similarly, if the velocity of upper plate is zero, i.e. both plates are stationary, it reverts back to the previous flow case (sec. 7.5.1) i.e. flow between two stationary plates.

(b) *Non-dimensional form*. The general equation of coutee flow, Eq. 7.16a, can also be expressed in non-dimensional form,

$$\frac{u}{U_0} = \frac{y}{B} - \frac{B^2}{2\mu U_0}\left(\frac{\partial p}{\partial x}\right)\left(1 - \frac{y}{B}\right)\frac{y}{B} \qquad ...(7.16b)$$

Substituting $\eta = y/B$ and $P = \frac{B^2}{2\mu U_0}\left(-\frac{\partial p}{\partial x}\right)$.

$$\frac{u}{U_0} = \eta + P\eta(1 - \eta) \qquad ...(7.16c)$$

Here η represents a dimensionless distance from the lower stationary plate and P is constant for the given flow case. Eq. 7.16c may be plotted in Fig. 7.6. as a family of curves between nondimensional velocity and non-dimensional distance η for various values of P. There are three possible flow cases.

Case 1: For $P = 0$, pressure gradient is zero, hence it becomes a plane shear flow and is shown plotted in Fig. 7.6 by a straight line

$$u/U_0 = \eta \qquad ...(7.17)$$

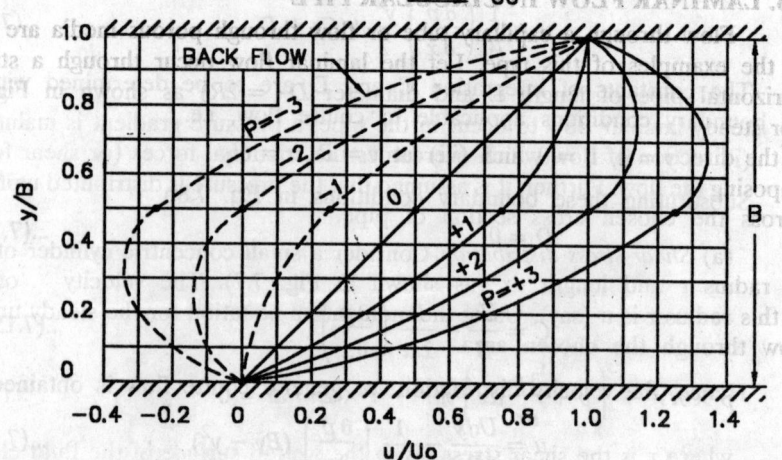

FIG. 7.6 NON–DIMENSIONAL VELOCITY DISTRIBUTION FOR COUTTE FLOW

Case 2 : For $P > 0$, the flow should have negative value of pressure gradient (i.e. $\frac{\partial p}{\partial x} < 0$). Such a flow is known as accelerating flow. The velocity distribution is shown plotted as on the right side of straight line (for P equal zero) in Fig. 7.6.

Case 3 : $P < 0$ or negative, means $(\partial p / \partial x)$ for the fow is positive (also termed as adverse pressure gradient). Such types of flows are known as decelerating flows, since the pressure should increase in the direction of flow. The velocity distribution for decelerating flow is shown plotted in Fig. 7.6 by dotted lines on left side of (P equal to zero) line. It is to be observed from these curves that for certain negative value of P, backflow may take place between the plates (i.e, the direction of velocity is reversed in the vicinity of stationary plate; see Fig. 7.6).

(c) *Discharge.* The volume rate of flow or discharge occurring across an elementary area $dA \ (= dy \times 1)$ is given by

$$dQ = u \ (dy \times 1) \ = U_0 \left[\frac{y}{B} - \frac{B^2}{2\mu U_0} \left(\frac{\partial p}{\partial x} \right) \times \left(1 - \frac{y}{b} \right) \frac{y}{B} \right] dy$$

Integrating it with respect to y,

$$Q = \int dQ = \int U_0 \left[y/B - \frac{B^2}{2\mu U_0} (\partial p / \partial x) \times (1 - y/B) \, y/B \right] dy$$

Solving it

$$Q = \left[U_0 \frac{B}{2} - \frac{B^3}{12 \mu} \frac{dp}{dx} \right] \qquad \ldots (7.18)$$

7.6. LAMINAR FLOW IN CIRCULAR PIPE

Flow through a capillary tube or flow through porous media are some of the examples of this type. Let the laminar flow occur through a straight horizontal pipe of length L and diameter $D(= 2R)$ as shown in Fig. 7.7. For steady laminar flow to occur in the pipe, a pressure gradient is maintained in the direction of flow which overcomes the frictional forces (or shear forces) opposing the flow. Further, it is assumed that the pressure is distributed uniformly across the chosen cross section of pipe.

(a) *Shear stress distribution.* Consider a small concentric cylinder of fluid of radius r and length dx (as shown in Fig. 7.7). The velocity of flow at this radius r is u (say). Using the momentum equation for the steady uniform flow through the chosen area.

$$p \times \pi r^2 - \left(p + \frac{\partial p}{\partial x} dx \right) \pi r^2 - \tau \times 2\pi r\, dr = 0 \qquad ...(7.19a)$$

where τ is the shear stress along the wetted surface of the fluid element and p as well as $\left(p + \frac{\partial p}{\partial r} dr \right)$ are the pressure intensities acting at the two ends of the fluid element.

$$\tau = \left(\frac{-\partial p}{\partial x} \right) \frac{r}{2} \qquad ...(7.19b)$$

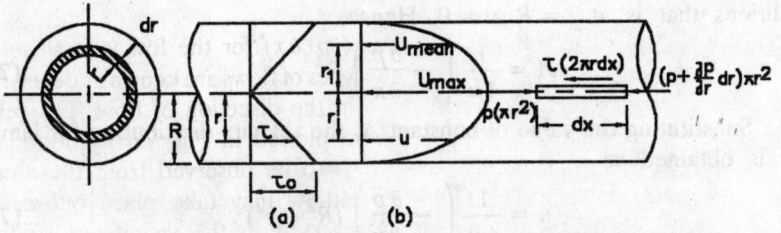

FIG. 7.7 – FLOW THROUGH A CIRCULAR PIPE

(a) SHEAR DISTRIBUTION (b) VELOCITY DISTRIBUTION

It is known that the pressure gradient $\partial p / \partial x$ in the direction of flow depends on x only for any given case of laminar flow and the nagative sign indicates that pressure decreases in the direction of flow.

Eq. 7.19b gives the shear stress distribution across the cross section of pipe. The shear stress varies linearly with radius r of the pipe. It is zero at the centre of pipe $(r = 0)$ and is maximum i.e. τ_0, at the wall of the pipe $(r = R)$. Eq. 7.19b is valid both for laminar and turbulent flows, since no specific condition of flow has been used in its derivation. Thus

$$\tau\, (at\, r = R) = \tau_0 = \left(\frac{-\partial p}{\partial x} \right) \frac{R}{2} \qquad ...(7.19c)$$

(b) *Velocity distribution.* The shear is also expressed by Newton's law of viscosity, Eq. 1.8c, as

$$\tau = \mu \frac{\partial u}{\partial y} \qquad ...(1.8)$$

But
$$y = (R - r), \text{ i.e. } dy = - dr \qquad ...(7.20)$$

From Eqs. 7.19 and 7.20

$$\tau = - \mu \frac{\partial u}{\partial r} = \left(-\frac{\partial p}{\partial x} \right) \frac{r}{2}$$

$$\frac{\partial u}{\partial r} = - \frac{1}{\mu} \left(-\frac{\partial p}{\partial x} \right) \frac{r}{2}$$

Multiplying by ∂r on both side and converting partial derivative into full derivative.

$$du = - \frac{1}{\mu} \left(-\frac{\partial p}{\partial x} \right) \frac{r}{2} dr$$

Integrate it with respect to r

$$\int du = \int - \frac{1}{\mu} \left(\frac{\partial p}{\partial x} \right) \frac{r}{2} dr$$

$$u = - \frac{1}{4\mu} \left(\frac{-\partial p}{\partial x} \right) r^2 + A \qquad ...(7.21)$$

The constant of integration is determined from the known boundary conditions that is at $r = R, u = 0$. Hence,

$$A = \frac{1}{4\mu} \left(-\frac{\partial p}{\partial x} \right) R^2 \qquad ...(7.22)$$

Substituting the value of constant A, the velocity distribution for laminar flow is obtained as

$$u = \frac{1}{4\mu} \left(-\frac{\partial p}{\partial x} \right) (R^2 - r^2) \qquad ...(7.23)$$

Eq. 7.23 shows that the velocity variation for laminar flow is parabolic and it is shown plotted in Fig. 7.7

(c) *Maximum velocity*. The maximum velocity, obviously occurs at the centre of the pipe, i.e. at $r = 0$, and is given by

$$U_{max} = \frac{1}{4\mu} \left(-\frac{\partial p}{\partial x} \right) R^2 \qquad ...(7.24)$$

(d) *Discharge*. The discharge flowing through a concentric annular space of radii r and r + dr respectively is dQ. It is given by

$$dQ = u \times 2\pi r \, dr$$

The total discharge Q is obtained by integrating over the whole area of cross section of pipe.

$$Q = \int dQ = \int_0^R u \times 2\pi r \, dr$$

$$Q = \int_0^R 2\pi r \left[\frac{1}{4\mu} (-\partial p/\partial x)(R^2 - r^2) \right] dr$$

$$Q = \frac{1}{8\mu} (-\partial p/\partial x)\pi R^4 \qquad \qquad ...(7.25)$$

(e) *Average or mean velocity.* The mean velocity of flow U through the pipe is obtained from continuity equation.

$$U = \frac{Q}{\pi R^2}$$

$$U = \frac{1}{8\mu} \left(-\frac{\partial p}{\partial x} \right) R^2 \qquad \qquad ...(7.26)$$

Let the average velocity U occur at a radius r_1, hence equate $u(r = r_1)$ to U.

$$\frac{1}{8\mu} (-\partial p/\partial x) R^2 = \frac{1}{4\pi} (-\partial p/\partial x)(R^2 - r_1^2)$$

Simplifying $r_1 = 0.707 R$ \qquad \qquad ...(7.27)

This means that the average velocity occurs at a radius of 0.707 R.

(f) *Head loss.* Rearranging the terms of Eq. 7.26, the pressure drop is given by

$$\left(\frac{-\partial p}{\partial x} \right) = \frac{8\mu U}{R^2}$$

Dividing by specific weight w on both sides, the head loss occurring in the pipe length L is given by

$$\frac{p_1 - p_2}{wL} = \frac{8\mu U}{wR^2}$$

$$h_f = \frac{8\mu UL}{wR^2}$$

$$h_f = \frac{32\mu UL}{wD^2} \qquad \qquad ...(7.28a)$$

$$h_f = \frac{128\mu QL}{w\pi D^4} \qquad \qquad ...(7.28b)$$

Eq. 7.28 a is known as 'Hagen Poiseulli's equation' for laminar flow. It is to be noted that Eq. 7.28a or 7.28b is valid for fully established laminar flow, i.e. sufficiently away from the entrance of pipe.[*] Secondly, the roughness

---

[*] At the entrance to the pipe the boundary layer just starts developing and the flow is slowed down at the pipe wall. The flow is not fully developed at the entrance and requires a certain length of pipe to become fully developed. Refer chapter 8 on boundary layer for further details.

of the pipe surface does not enter in the Eq. 7.28a or 7.28b. Alternatively, the velocity distribution in Eq. 7.23 may be derived by solving Navier Stokes equations, Eqs. 7.3a to 7.3c

(g) *Relationship between Darcy's friction coefficient f and Re.* The head loss caused due to the fluid flow in the circular pipe of diameter D and length L is given by Darcy Weisbach equation, Eq. 6.8b.

$$h_f = \frac{fLU^2}{2gD} \qquad \qquad ...(6.8b)$$

Comparing Eqs. 7.28a and 6.8b

$$h_f = \frac{32\mu\,UL}{wD^2} = \frac{fLU^2}{2gD}$$

Simplifying $\qquad f = \dfrac{64}{Re}$

(h) *Relationship between shear stress and Darcy's coefficient f.* Wall shear stress τ_0 is given by Eq. 7.19c, i.e.

$$\tau_0 = \left(-\frac{\partial p}{\partial x} \right) \frac{D}{4}$$

$$\tau_0 = \frac{whf}{L}\frac{D}{4}$$

Substiuting the value of h_f from Eq. 6.8b.

$$\tau_0 = \frac{wD}{4L} \times \frac{fLU^2}{2gD}$$

$$\tau_0/\rho = \frac{U^2 f}{8}$$

Taking square root on both sides,

$$\sqrt{\tau_0/\rho} = U_* = U\sqrt{f/8}$$

Since the expression $\sqrt{\tau_0/\rho}$ is having the dimension of velocity, hence it is known as 'shear velocity or frictional velocity' and is written as U_*; this velocity has no physical meaning.

7.7 FLOW THROUGH AN ANNULAR SPACE BETWEEN TWO CON- CENTRIC TUBES

Consider two concentric cylinders of radii r_1 and r_2 respectively, as shown in Fig. 7.8. The laminar flow occur through the annular space between these concentric tubes. Consider a small concentric sleeve of radius r and length dx in the annular space (Fig. 7.8). The forces acting on the fluid element are pressure force and shear force. Applying momentum equation to the fluid in the sleeve,

$$p \times 2\pi r\, dr - \left(p + \frac{\partial p}{\partial x} dx \right) 2\pi r dr + \tau \times 2\pi r dx$$

$$- (\tau + \frac{\partial \tau}{dr} dr) 2\pi\,(r + dr)dx = 0$$

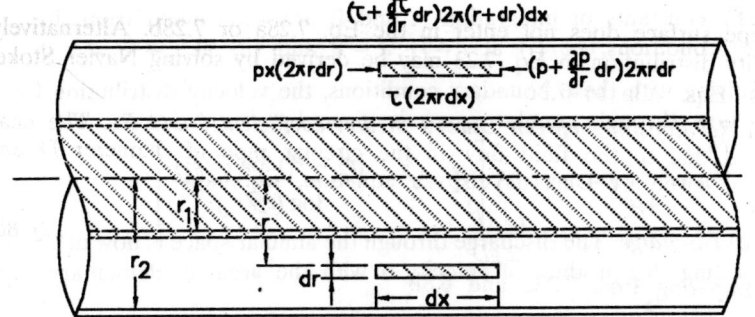

FIG. 7.8 FLOW THROUGH AN ANNULAR SPACE

Simplifying,

$$-\frac{\partial p}{\partial x} \times r - \tau - \frac{\partial \tau}{\partial r} \times r - \frac{\partial \tau}{\partial r} \times dr = 0 \qquad \text{...(7.31a)}$$

The fourth term is of higher order (i.e. product of two smaller eqantities) and hence can be dropped. Rearranging the terms.

$$-\frac{\partial p}{\partial x} - \frac{1}{r}\frac{\partial}{\partial r}(\tau r) = 0 \qquad \text{...(7.31b)}$$

(a) *Velocity distribution.* From Newton's law of viscosity,

$$\tau = \mu \frac{\partial u}{\partial y} = -\mu \frac{\partial u}{\partial r}$$

Hence $-\dfrac{\partial p}{\partial x} - \dfrac{1}{r} \times \dfrac{\partial}{\partial r}\left(-\mu \dfrac{\partial u}{\partial r} \times r\right) = 0 \qquad \text{...(7.32)}$

Multiply on both sides by r dr.

$$-\frac{\partial p}{\partial x} \times r\, dr + \mu \frac{\partial}{\partial r}\left(r \frac{\partial u}{\partial r}\right) dr = 0 \qquad \text{...(7.33)}$$

Integrating it with respect to r,

$$\left(-\frac{\partial p}{\partial x}\right)\frac{r^2}{2} + \mu r \frac{\partial u}{\partial r} = A \qquad \text{...(7.34)}$$

Since the pressure gradient is independet of r and varies only in X-direction and hence can be taken as constant.

Again multiply Eq. 7.34 on both sides by dr/r,

$$\left(-\frac{\partial p}{\partial x}\right)\frac{r}{2}\, dr + \mu \frac{\partial u}{\partial r}\, dr = A\, dr/r \qquad \text{...(7.35)}$$

Integrating with respect to r.

$$\left(-\frac{\partial p}{\partial x}\right)\frac{r^2}{4} + \mu u = A \log r + B \qquad \text{...(7.36)}$$

The constants of integration A and B are determined from the given boundary conditions, i.e (i) at $r = r_1, u = 0$ and (ii) at $r = r_2, u = 0$

Solving with these boundary conditions, the velocity distribution for the laminar flow through annular space is given by

$$u = \frac{1}{4\mu}(-\partial p/\partial x)\left[r_2^2 - r^2 + \frac{(r_2^2 - r_1^2)\log(r/r_2)}{\log(r_2/r_1)}\right] \qquad ...(7.37)$$

(b) *Discharge*. The discharge through the annular space is now determined by integrating the product of velocity u with the area of elementary sleeve.

$$Q = \int_{r_1}^{r_2} u \times 2\pi r\, dr$$

Substituting the value of u from Eq. 7.35 and simplifyting

$$Q = \frac{\pi}{8\pi}(-\partial p/\partial x)\left[r_2^4 - r_1^4 - (r_2^2 - r_1^2)/\left(\log\frac{r_2}{r_1}\right)\right] \qquad ...(7.38)$$

(c) *Shear distribution*. The shear distribution across the space is determined from Newton's law of viscosity, i.e. Eq. 1.8

$$\tau = -\mu\frac{\partial u}{\partial r}$$

Substituting the value of u and solving it.

$$\tau = \frac{1}{4\mu}(-\partial p/\partial x)\left[2r + \frac{(r_2^2 - r_1^2)}{r\log(r_2/r_1)}\right] \qquad ...(7.39)$$

7.8. LAMINAR FLOW OF FLUID IN AN OPEN CHANNEL

Consider a wide open channel in which steady, uniform laminar flow is occurring. Let the depth of flow be d and the bed slope of the channel $S_0 = -dz/dx = \sin\theta$. Take a fluid volume bounded by two section 1 and 2, L distance apart. Since the depth of flow be same at both the sections, therefore, no pressue gradient is available to maintain the flow. The force causing the flow is due to change in potential energy caused due to the slope of the channel. It is expressed as $w S_0 = (w\, dz/dx)$ per unit volume of the fluid. The force resisting the flow is expressed as $(\partial\tau/\partial y)$ per unit volume of the fluid (see Eq. 7.7)

$$w\frac{\partial z}{\partial x} = \frac{\partial\tau}{dy} \qquad ...(7.40)$$

$$w\frac{\partial z}{\partial x} = \mu\frac{\partial^2 u}{\partial y^2} \qquad \text{Using } \tau = \mu\frac{\partial u}{\partial y}$$

$$\therefore \qquad \frac{\partial^2 u}{\partial y^2} = \frac{w}{\mu}\frac{\partial z}{\partial x} \qquad ....(7.41)$$

Since the flow is uniform, $\left(\dfrac{\partial z}{\partial x}\right)$ is independent of y. Integrating Eqs. 7.41 with respect to y.

$$\frac{\partial u}{\partial y} = \frac{w}{\mu} \frac{\partial z}{\partial x} \cdot y + A \qquad \qquad ...(7.42)$$

Again integrating with respect to y,

$$u = \frac{w}{\mu} \frac{\partial z}{\partial x} \cdot \frac{y^2}{2} + Ay + B \qquad \qquad ...(7.43 \text{ a})$$

Here A and B are constants of integration which can be determined by applying known boundary conditions.

(i) At $y = 0$, the velocity at the bed of the open channel is $u = 0$,

$$\therefore \qquad\qquad B = 0$$

(ii) At $y = d$, the velcoity is maximum therefore $\partial u / \partial y = 0$
Substituting this condition in Eq. 7.42.

$$A = \frac{w}{\mu}\left(-\frac{\partial z}{\partial x}\right) d = \frac{wS_0 d}{\mu} \qquad \left(\text{since } S_0 = \frac{-\partial z}{\partial x}\right) \qquad ...(7.43 \text{ b})$$

The velocity distribution in an open channel is given by

$$u = \frac{w}{\mu}\frac{\partial z}{\partial x}\frac{y^2}{2} - \frac{w}{\mu}\left(\frac{\partial z}{\partial x}\right) . d \times y$$

$$u = \frac{w}{\mu}\left(-\frac{\partial z}{\partial x}\right)\left(yd - y^2/2\right) \qquad \qquad ...(7.43 \text{ c})$$

This is a quadratic equation in y, which shows that the velocity distribution is parabolic in a wide open channel.

Average Velocity : The average velocity is obtained by dividing the discharge by the area of cross section of the channel. For obtaining the discharge, integrate the above equation for depth y varying from 0 to d.

$$\therefore \qquad U = \frac{\text{discharge/unit width}}{d} = \frac{q}{d}$$

$$= \frac{\displaystyle\int_0^d udy}{d}$$

$$= \frac{w}{\mu d}\left(-\frac{\partial z}{\partial x}\right)\int_0^d (yd - y^2/2)\, dy$$

$$= \frac{wS_0 d^2}{3\mu} \qquad \qquad ...(7.44)$$

And the discharge flowing per unit width q is given by

$$q = Ud = \frac{w S_0 d^3}{3\mu} \qquad \ldots(7.45)$$

Rearranging the terms, the head loss or drop in potential energy is given by

$$S_0 = \left(-\frac{dz}{dx}\right) = \frac{3\mu q}{w d^3}$$

If the datum head at two section 1 and 2 above arbitrary datum be z_1 and z_2

$$\frac{z_1 - z_2}{L} = \frac{3\mu q}{w d^3}$$

$$h_f = (z_1 - z_2) = \frac{3\mu q L}{w d^3} \qquad \ldots(7.46)$$

Here h_f represents the head loss between two sections.

Shear Stress. The shear stress distribution can be determinated from Newton's law of viscosity and from Eq. 7.42.

$$\tau = \mu\left(\frac{\partial u}{\partial y}\right) = w\left(-\frac{\partial z}{\partial x}\right)(d - y)$$

$$= w S_0 (d - y) \qquad \ldots(7.47)$$

It shows that the shear stress distribution is linear. It is zero at the free surface and $\tau = \tau_0$ at the bed of the open channel.

$$\tau_0 = w S_0 d \qquad \ldots(7.48)$$

7.9 LAMINAR FLOW THROUGH POROUS MEDIA

Flow through porous media also exhibits the characteristics of laminar flow. The porous media consists of number of interstices or pores through which the water (or any other liquid) flows. These interistices may be assumed as little straight conduit and the flow passage is bounded by the impervious sand grains.

Consider a circular pipe of length L and cross sectional area A. It is compeltely filled with porous material, grain size (diameter) ds. Let Q be the discharge flowing through the pipe. Then the superficial (or apparent) velocity of flow is given Q/A. Since the part of the cross sectional area is blocked by the impervious sand grains, the actual area of flow A_f will be less than A. If the ratio of the actual area of flow to the total area of cross section be n .

$$A_f = n A$$

The actual mean velocity of flow will be $U_f = \dfrac{Q}{n A} = \dfrac{U}{n}$. It is obvious that actual velocity of flow U_f is more than appearent velocity of flow. The

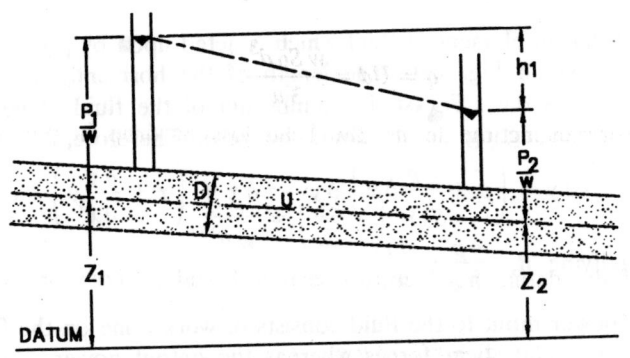

FIG. 7.9 FLOW THROUGH POROUS MEDIA

average size of the pores is assumed to be proportional to the grain diameter d_s.

From Eqs. 7.12 and 7.28, it is seen that the head loss due to laminar flow is given by

$$h_f \ \alpha \ \frac{\mu \, U L}{w \, D^2}$$

For the determination of head loss due to laminar flow through porous media mean velocity U is replaced by U/n and the diameter D is replaced by d_s

$$h_f = k \frac{\mu \, U L}{w \, n \, d_s^2}$$

Rearranging the terms

$$U = \frac{w \, n \, d_s^2 \, h_f}{k \, \mu \, L}$$

$$= K \, i \qquad\qquad ...(7.49)$$

Here 'i' is the hydraulic gradient ($= h_f / L$) and K is known as the coefficient of permeability. It has the dimensions of velocity. Eq. 7.49 is known as Darcy's law, named after Henry Darcy's, a French engineer who first presented it in 1856. Darcy's law has many practical applications. For example, the flow through ground water, flow through embankment dam and design of tube wells. It should be noted that Darcy's law is applicable upto Reynolds number

$$\frac{U \, ds}{v} \ \le 1 \, ; \ (\, R_e \le 1.0 \,)$$

7.10 WORK DONE BY VISCOUS FRICTION

An expression for the rate of conversion of mechanical energy into thermal energy is developed for one dimensional laminar flow, in which the equation of motion and principle of work and energy are utilised.

Consider an element of fluid which is acted upon by pressure and shear forces, as shown in Fig. 7.10. The length of the horizontal edge is δx and that of vertical is δy. For static equilbirium of the fluid element, the sum of all the forces acting on it should be zero. Therefore,

$$p\,\delta y - \left(p + \frac{\partial p}{\partial x}\delta x\right)\delta y - \tau\,\delta x + \left(\tau + \frac{\partial \tau}{\partial x}y\right)\delta x = 0$$

Simplifying it, $\quad \dfrac{\partial p}{\partial x} = \dfrac{\partial \tau}{\partial y}$ $\qquad\qquad$ ...(7.50)

The power input to the fluid consists of work done on the fluid element by the pressure and shear forces whereas the output power consists of the

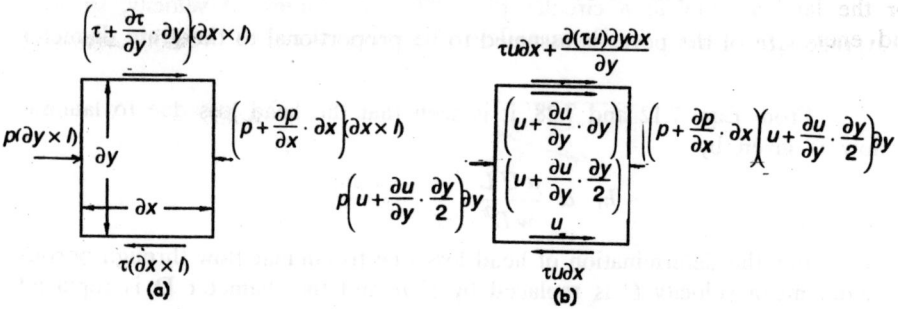

FIG. 7.10 (a) FORCES ACTING AT AN ELEMENT OF FLUID

(b) WORK DONE BY THE FORCES ACTING ON THE FLUID ELEMENT

work done by the fluid element on the surrounding fluid. Hence, the net work done per unit time consists of,

$$p\left(u + \frac{\partial u}{\partial y}\frac{\delta y}{2}\right)\delta y - \left(p + \frac{\partial p}{\partial y}\delta y\right)\left(u + \frac{\partial u}{\partial y}\frac{\delta y}{2}\right)\delta y$$

$$+ \tau u\,\delta x + \frac{\partial}{\partial y}(\tau u)\delta y \ \delta x - \tau u\,\delta x \qquad\qquad ...(7.51a)$$

Substituting for $(\partial \tau/\partial y)$ from Eq. 7.50, and simplifying, net power input per unit volume $= \tau\,(\partial u/\partial y)$ $\qquad\qquad$ ...(7.51b)

From Eq. 1.8c, $\quad \tau = \mu\,(\partial u/\partial y)$

Hence net power input per unit volume,

$$= \frac{\tau^2}{\mu} = \mu\left(\frac{\partial u}{\partial y}\right)^2 \qquad\qquad ...(7.52)$$

Eq. 7.52 is the power used by viscous friction to convert mechanical work into thermal energy.

Consider the laminar flow occurring between two parallel plates, B distant apart. Let the length of the plate be 'L'. Consider a small strip of width dy and length L. Integrating Eq. 7.52.

$$\text{Net power input} = \int_{-B/2}^{B/2} \mu \left(\frac{\partial u}{\partial y} \right)^2 L\, dy$$

$$= \left(\frac{B^3 L}{12\mu} \right) \left(\frac{\partial p}{\partial x} \right)^2$$

But from Eq. 7.10,

$$q = (B^3/12\mu)\,(-\,\partial p/\partial x)$$

Hence, net power input $= qL\,(-\,\partial p/\partial x) = Q \times \Delta p$ ...(7.53)

where Δp is the pressure difference caused in a length L. Eq. 7.53, of course, derived for the flow between parallel plates, is also found to be applicable for the laminar flow in a circular pipe. The distribution of velocity, shear and energy pissipation in laminar flow is shown in Fig. 7.11.

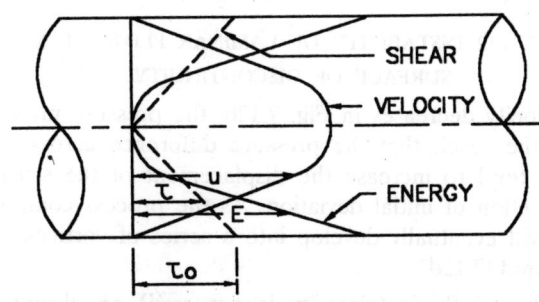

FIG. 7.11 DISTRIBUTION OF SHEAR, VELOCITY AND
ENERGY ACROSS A PIPE CROSS SECTION

7.11 INSTABILITY OF LAMINAR FLOW

In the previous section, the study was made of the laminar flow. The term laminar is applied to the flow because the stream lines (rather surfaces) appear to divide the entire region of flow into orderly series of fluid laminae, generally conformining to the boundary conditions. The viscous flows are governed mainly by two types of forces, viz. inertia forces and viscous forces and hence by Reynolds law of similarity. Local disturbances, whatever may be the cause, are always existing in every flow. But in case of laminar flow, any local fluctuations in velocities are damped by the viscoucs stresses and the flow remains laminar. When the viscous forces are not sufficient to quell such fluctuations, the local disturbances, once started, spread throughout the flow and the flow is said to be turbulent. The inertial tendency of any fluid to cause amplification of the local disturbance is shown in Fig. 7.12 for two layers of non-viscous fluid (ideal fluid).

The streamline at the velocity discontinuity in Fig. 7.12a begins to deviate from a straight line due to local disturbance (or due to some other cause), as shown in Fig. 7.12. The velocity will decrease if the neighouring streamlines diverge and will increase if they converge.

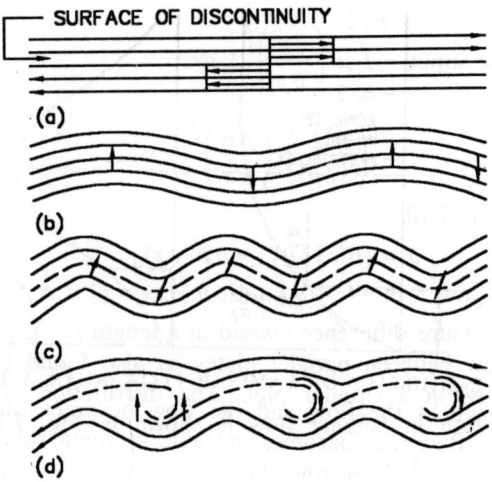

FIG. 7.12 INSTABILITY OF LAMINAR FLOW AT A
SURFACE OF DISCONTINUITY

As the velocity decreases in Fig. 7.12b, the pressure must increase and vice versa, with the result that the pressure difference across the surface of discontinuity will tend to increase the displacement of the streamlines at all points in the direction of initial deviation. As the process continues, the zone of discontinuity will eventually develop into a series of vortices of finite sizes; see Figs. 7.12c and 7.12d.

In case of real fluids (viscosity is not zero) an abrupt discontinuity of the velocity distribution will not be possible. But steeper the local velocity distribution, the more nearly the conditions of instability (shown in Fig. 7.13) are approached. Similarly, other characteristics of fluid as well as of flow (e.g. density, viscosity, proximity of the boundary) decide whether the initial disturbances exisiting in the flow will be amplified or damped. Hunter Rouse combined all these factors into a dimensionless number, viz. stability parameter χ (chi).

$$\chi = \frac{y^2 \rho \, du/dy}{\mu} \qquad ...(7.54)$$

It is seen from above Eq. 7.54 that 'greater the numerator', the greater will be the tendency towards local 'instability of the flow', whereas 'greater the denominator', the greater is the' stability of flow' due to large viscous forces. The parameter is necessarily zero near the boundary ($y = 0$) and at the greater distance from the boundary ($\partial u/\partial y = 0$) . At some intermediate distance, however, it will attain a maximum value which is the zone where the eddies are expected to occur, if the flow is disturbed in any way. The critical value of χ has been found experimentally and is nearly 500. If this value of χ exceeds for any flow and additionally, some local disturbance exists in the flow, eddies will develop in the flow. These eddies are then amplfied

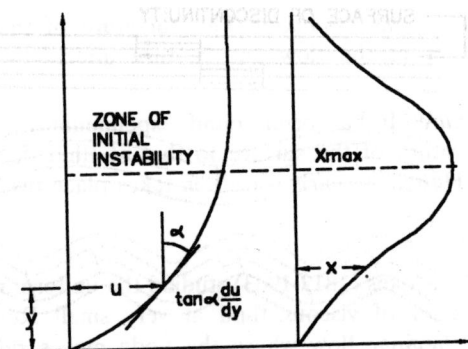

FIG. 7.13 INSTABILITY OF LAMINAR FLOW NEAR A BOUNDAR

and spread throughout the flow and the flow becomes turbulent. It should be noted that the flow first becomes unstable at some value of χ and if this critical value is exceeded slightly, the instability of flow leads to transition of flow and finally to turbulent flow.

7.12 TRANSITION FROM LAMINAR TO TURBULENT FLOW

As has been discussed earlier, the flow remains laminar at small Reynolds number due to the predominance of viscous forces When the Reynolds number is increased, the flow becomes unstable and finally becomes turbulent flow at $R_e = 12000$ or so. This is the upper cricital Reynolds number and its value depends on the initial disturbances present in the flow. For practical purposes, the transition from laminar to turbulent flow (in a circular pipe) may be assumed to take place at lower critical Reynolds number* ($2000 < (Re)_{er} < 4000$). The flow definitely becomes turbulent at $R_e > 4000$. For Re values between 2000 and 4000, a region of uncertainty of flow exists. However, it is to be emphasized that the critical value of Reynolds number is a function of boundary geomety also. For example, $(Re)_{er} = 1000$, for the flow between parallel plates, 'd' distance apart; $(Re)er = 500$ for the flow in a wide open channel and $(Re)_{er} = 1.0$ for the flow around a sphere of diameter D and moving with approach velocity U_t . It is advisable that such values of $(Re)_{er}$ for any flow should be determined by experiments because of obscure origin of turbulence.

The factors affecting the transition from laminar to turbulent flow are discussed below.

(a) *Initial disturbance.* The free stream turbulence prevailing in the incoming fluid (due to pipe entry, vibration in the flow, etc.) increases the Reynolds number of flow, approaching its critical value.

(b) *Roughness of the surface.* Roughness of the boundary increases the Reynolds number of the flow.

(c) *Pressure gradient.* The positive or adverse pressure gradient ($\partial p/\partial x > 0$) for a flow causes the transition of flow to occur at lower critical Reynolds number whereas negative pressure graident ($\partial p/\partial x < 0$) causes the transition to occur at higher critical Reynolds number.

(d) *Curvature of the boundary.* The curvature of the boundary affects the pressure gradient of the flow and in turn affects the critical value of Reynolds number.

(e) *Temperature.* It has been found expeimentally that increasing the ratio of the temperature of the surface to that of fluid decreases the critical Reynolds number. Hence, an early transition takes place over a heated surface.

7.13 STOKES LAW

Sir George G. Stokes (1819-1903) studied the uniform motion of a sphere through a large extent of viscous fluid at very small Reynolds number. It is another type of laminar flow where the body moves relative to the fluid medium. The following assumptions were made by him.

(1) The inertia forces are negligible in comparison to viscous forces.

(2) The fluid is of large extent, hence the walls of the container do not affect the flow around the sphere.

(3) The velocity of fluid layer adjacent to the rigid boundary of the sphere is the same as that of sphere itself.

He showed that the viscous resistance F_D experienced by the sphere of diameter D moving with a velocity U is given by

$$F_D = 3 \pi D \mu U \qquad ...(7.55)$$

The effective weight of the sphere overcomes the viscous resistance and is given by,

Effective weight = weight of sphere − buoyant force due to the fluid

$$W_e = \frac{\pi D^3}{6} (w_s - w) \qquad ...(7.56)$$

where w_s and w are the specific weights of material of the sphere and the liquid.

Equating Eq. 7.55 and Eq. 7.56

$$3 \pi D \mu U = (\pi D^3/6) (w_s - w)$$

Simplifying, $\qquad U = (D^2/18 \mu) (w_s - w) \qquad ...(7.57)$

The viscous resistance (or drag force) experienced by the sphere is generally expressed

$$F_D = C_D \frac{\rho U^2}{2} A \qquad ...(7.58)$$

where A is the area of cross section of the moving body normal to the direction of motion and C_D is known as the coefficient of drag.

Equating Eq. 7.55 and Eq. 7.58,

$$C_D = \frac{24}{R_e} \qquad ...(7.59)$$

Eqs. 7.55 and 7.57 are valid for $R_e \le 0.2$. For larger value of Reynolds number C_D cannot be expressed analytically. Moveover, Eq. 7.55 has been derived for a single sphere falling in the infinite extent of fluid. As the concentration of particles increases, the falling velocity of the individual particle reduces. The above equations, Eqs. 7.55 and 7.57 are a useful tool in analysing such problems as settling of small silt particles in water or falling of mist particles in air.

7.14 DETERMINATION OF VISCOSITY

The instruments used for the determination of viscosity are known as 'viscometers' or 'viscosimeters'. The following methods are used to determine the viscosity of the fluid in the laboratory.

(1) Rotating cylinder method

(2) Falling sphere method

(3) Capillary tube method

Besides these methods; the viscosity of the fluid may also be determined by industrial viscosimeters, e.g. Saybolt viscometer.

1. Rotating cylinder method

This method is based on the Newton's law of viscosity and is also known as 'coutte method'. It consists of two concentric cylinders mounted on the same axes (Fig. 7.14). The annular space between them is filled with liquid whose viscosity is to be determined. The outer cylinder, radius r_2, is mounted on a shaft and is rotated at known speed N r-p.m. The inner cylinder, radius r_1, remains stationary and is suspended by a torsion wire to a rigid surface. The torsion wire is precalibrated, (i.e. the relationship between torque and angular rotation is known). The height of both cylinders is h (say). When the outer cylinder is rotated with an angular speed ω $(= 2\pi N/60$), the liquid in the annular space transmits the torque to the inner cylinder and a velocity gradient is set up in the annular space. The magnitude of the torque is determined from the calibration chart for the known angle of rotation of the outer cylinder. This torque is related to the fluid viscosity as discussed below.

Let the clearance between the walls of the cylinders be 'a'. Since 'a' is small, the variation of velocity in the space is assumed linear. The rate of angular deformation or the velocity gradient is given by

$$\frac{du}{dy} = \frac{\omega\, r_2}{a} \qquad \qquad ...(7.60)$$

The shearing stress developed in the fluid between the cylindrical surfaces

$$\tau = \mu \frac{\partial u}{\partial y}$$

$$= \mu\, \omega\, r_2/a \qquad \qquad ...(7.61)$$

Therefore, the torque exerted on the surface of inner cylinder,

$T_c = $ shearing force $\times r_1$

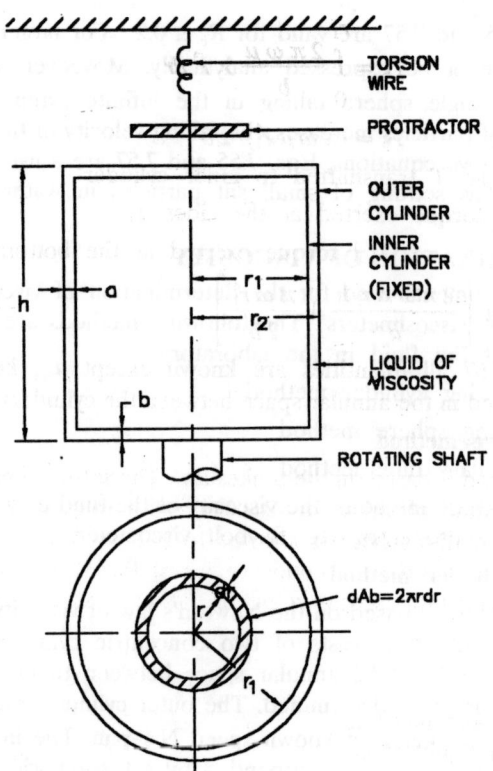

FIG. 7.14 ROTATING CYLINDER VISCOMETER

$T_c = \tau \times$ area of contact $\times r_1$

$T_c = (\mu \, \omega \, r_2/a) \, (2 \pi \, r_1 \, h) \, r_1$

$T_c = 2 \mu \, \pi \, \omega \, r_1^2 r_2 \, h/a$ \hfill ...(7.62)

Let the clearance between the surface at bottom of two cylinders be b. Since the shear stress between the bottom of two cylinders varies linearly in the radial direction, it is computed by integrating the torque exerted on the elementary fluid surface area dA_b. Consider a concentric elementary area of radius r and width dr. (see Fig 7.13).

Shear stress $= \tau_b = \mu \, \omega \, r/b$ \hfill ...(7.63)

Shear forces exerted $= \tau_b \times A_b = \dfrac{\mu \, \omega \, r}{b} \times 2 \pi \, r \, dr$ ...(7.64)

Torque exerted at the bottom

$$T_b = \left(\dfrac{\mu \, \omega \, r}{b} \times 2 \pi \, r \, dr \right) \times r \hfill ...(7.65)$$

Integrating it over the whole area of the bottom,

$$T_b = \int_0^{r_1} \frac{2\pi\omega\mu}{b} \times r^3 \, dr$$

Solving it, $\qquad T_b = (\pi\omega\mu\, r_1^4)/2b$ ...(7.66)

Now torque T transmitted to inner cylinder

$\qquad$ = torque exerted at the sides T_c

$\qquad\qquad\qquad$ + torque exerted at the bottom T_b

$$T = \mu \left[\frac{2\pi\omega\, r_1^2 r_2 h}{a} + \frac{\pi\omega\, r_1^4}{2b} \right] \qquad ...(7.67)$$

In Eq. 7.67 all quantities are known except μ, hence the viscosity μ of the fluid filled in the annular space between the cylinders can be computed.

2. Falling sphere method

This method is based on the Stokes law. The set-up consists of a container filled with the liquid of unknown viscosity and a valve is fitted at its bottom (Fig. 7.15). A metallic sphere is allowed to fall steadily in the liquid through a distance L. Let it take t seconds to travel this distance with its terminal velocity* U_0. Then, the viscosity μ of the liquid is determined from Eq. 7.57.

$$\mu = \frac{D^2}{18U_0}(w_s - w) \quad ...(7.57)$$

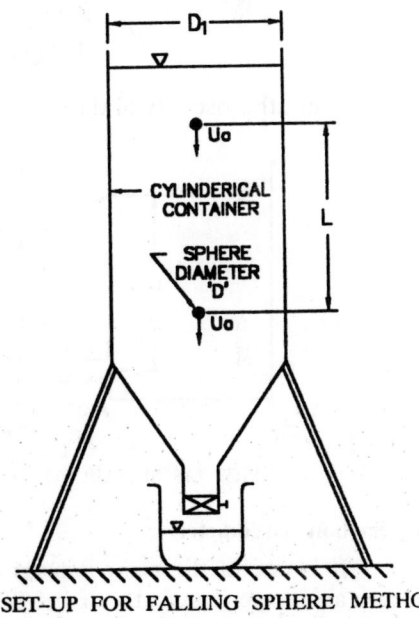

Since Stokes law has been derived for liquid of infinite extent, the above equation Eq. 7.57 needs correction for wall constraint (on account of finite extent of liquid).

The wall correction depends on the ratio of diameter D of the sphere to the diameter D_1 of the container. The actual velocity U_0 is now computed by Eq. 7.68.

$$\frac{U_a}{U_0} = \left[1 + \frac{9D}{4D_1} + \left(\frac{9D}{4D_1} \right)^2 \right] \quad ...(7.68)$$

FIG. 7.15 SET-UP FOR FALLING SPHERE METHOD

---

*Terminal velocity is the maximum velocity acquired by the body while the accelerating force due to gravity acting over it equalises the resisting force due to viscosity.

and the viscosity μ of the liquid at the room temperature is given by

$$\mu = \frac{D^2(w_s - w)}{18\,U_0\left[1 + \dfrac{9D}{4D_1} + \left(\dfrac{9D}{4D_1}\right)^2\right]} \qquad \ldots(7.69)$$

3. Capillary tube method

This method is based on the Hagen Poiseulli's law, Eq. 7.28. This method is also known as transpiration method. The set-up consists of a thin tube connected to reservoir filled with the liquid of viscosity μ (unknown) as shown in Fig. 7.16. A piezometric tube is connected to the this tube AB at point C, to measure the head loss occurring due to the flow in the segment CB. The location of point C is judiceously so selected that the laminar flow has been fully established at this location and it lies sufficiently away from the entrance to the thin tube AB. A regulating value is fitted at other end of tube AB, *i.e.* at B. When the discharge Q flows through the tube of diameter D, under a constant head H (in the reservoir), let the head loss measured by the piezometric tube be h_f. Then, from Eq. 7.28,

$$\mu = \frac{w\,\pi\,D^4\,h_f}{128\,Q\,L} \qquad \ldots(7.28)$$

Thus, the viscosity of the liquid at room temperature can be determined.

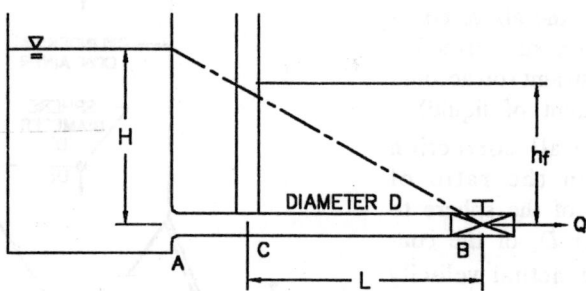

FIG. 7.16 SET–UP FOR CAPILLARY TUBE METHOD

4. Saybolt viscometer

It is one of the many industrial viscometers. It consists of an oil tube, a constant temperature bath, a receiver, a thermometer, a timer and a withdrawal tube or short capillary tube, Fig. 7.17. The diameter of the tube may be between 0.75 cm to 0.178 cm and its length 1.215 cm to 1.235 cm. The time required for the flow of 60 cm^3 of liquid through the capillary tube under a falling head is measured by the timer. This time in seconds is the Saybolt reading. The device measures the kinematic viscosity using Hagen Poiseulli's equation, Eq. 7.28. Rearranging the terms of Eq. 7.28,

$$\frac{\mu}{\rho_t} = \frac{g h \pi D^4}{128 \, (\text{voulume}) \, L} = C_1 \qquad ...(7.70)$$

in which L is the length of capillary tube, D is the diameter and h is the difference between the initial and final level of the liquid in the oil tube. Thus, it is seen that the right hand side is a constant for a particular instrument and is written as C_1. The kinematic viscosity of the liquid v is

$$v = C_1 t \qquad ...(7.71)$$

which shows that v varies directly with time t. Since the capillary tube is quite short, the velocity distribution is not established. The flow tends to enter uniformly, and then, owing to the viscous drag at the walls, slows down there and speeds up in the centre region. A correction is, therefore, needed which is of the form C_2/t ; hence

$$v = C_1 t + C_2/t \quad ...(7.72)$$

The relationship between viscosity and Saybolt seconds is expressed by

$$v = 0.0022 \, t - \frac{1.80}{t} \quad ...(7.73)$$

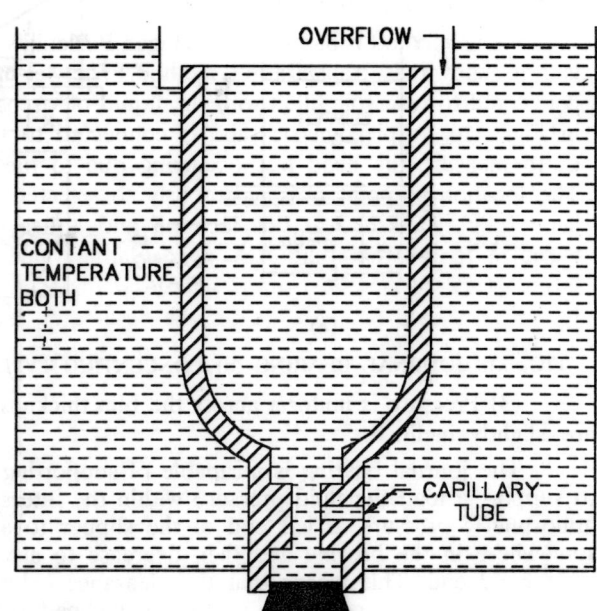

FIG. 7.17 SAYBOLT VISCOMETER

in which v is in stokes and t in secends.

Besides this instrument, there are many other industrial methods that generally have to be calibrated for each case to convert to the absolute units.

7.15 REYNOLDS THEORY OF LUBRICATION

The concentric journal bearing may be simulated (if the clearance is small) by an idealized model in the form of a slipper or sliding block moving over a stationary bearing plate. In order to simplify the analysis, the principle of relative motion is applied to entire system to bring the slipper at rest while the bearing plate moves past it with a constant velocity U_0 which is equal and opposite to that originally possessed by the slipper, as shown in Fig. 7.18. The flow is identical to coutte flow, section 7.5.3. The following assumptions are made.

(1) The surface are of infinite extent in a direction normal to both the film thickness and the direction of motion; *i.e.* the theory is two dimensional.

(2) Viscous forces predominate, *i.e.* the inertia forces are neglected.

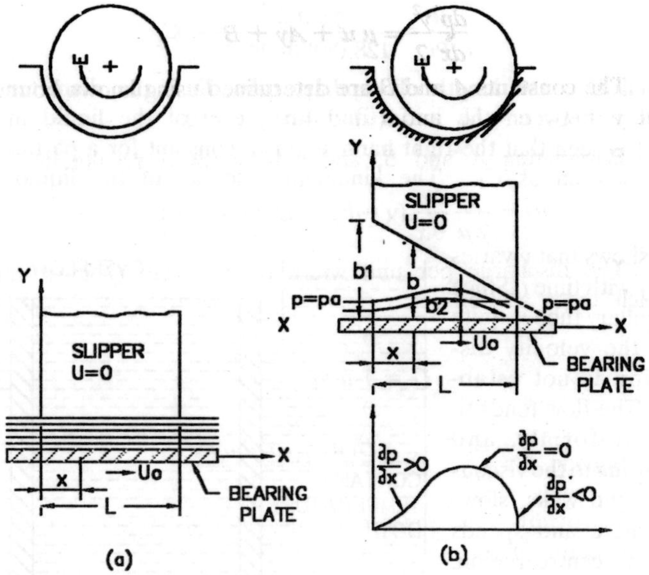

FIG. 7.18 JOURNAL BEARING (a) CONCENTRIC TYPE (b) ECCENTRIC TYPE

(3) Pressure is uniform across the film thickness even when the surfaces are slightly inclined.

The journal bearing is incapable of supporting any load. For a bearing to support a load the fluid pressure within the interspace must increase from atmospheric pressure at left end of the slipper to a certain maximum value somewhere in the bearing and then decrease to atmospheric pressure at the right hand end. This means that the clearance b between the surfaces must be a function of x or upper surface is inclined relative to the lower one. Again, the slipper is assumed stationary while the bearing plate moves with a constant velocity U_0.

The laminar flow equations are used to develop the theory of lubrication. Additional assumptions are made that (i) the velocity distribution is the same as if the plates were parallel and (ii) no flow takes place out of the bearing normal to the plane of Fig. 7.18.

Substituting Eq. 1.18 into Eq. 7.7

$$\frac{dp}{dx} = \mu \frac{d^2 u}{d y^2} \qquad \ldots(7.74)$$

Since p is independent of y, dp/dx is constant ; integrate Eq. 7.74 with respect to y.

$$\frac{dp}{dx} \int dy = \mu \int \frac{d^2 u}{dy^2} dy + A$$

$$\frac{dp}{dx} y = \mu \frac{du}{dy} + A \qquad \ldots(7.75)$$

Again integrate with respect to y .

$$\frac{dp}{dx}\frac{y^2}{2} = \mu u + Ay + B \qquad ...(7.76)$$

The constants A and B are determined using known boundary conditions,
(i) at $y = 0$, $u = U_0$ and (ii) $y = b$, $u = 0$

Eliminating A and B, and solving for u results in

$$u = \frac{y}{2\mu}\frac{\partial p}{\partial x}(y - b) + U_0(1 - y/b) \qquad ...(7.77)$$

The discharge per unit width of the plate Q must remain the same at each cross section.

$$Q = \int_0^b u\, dy$$

Solving, $\qquad Q = \frac{U_0 b}{2} - \frac{b^3\, dp/dx}{12\mu} \qquad ...(7.78)$

The width b at any section distant x from left end may be expressed as a function of x .

$$b = b_1 - \alpha x \qquad ...(7.79a)$$
and $\qquad \alpha = (b_1 - b_2)/L \qquad ...(7.79b)$

Substituting the value of b in Eq. 7.78,

$$dp/dx = 6\mu\, U_0/(b_1 - \alpha x)^2 - 12\mu\, Q/(b_1 - \alpha x)^3$$

Integrating with respect to x,

$$p = \frac{6\mu\, U_0}{\alpha(b_1 - \alpha x)} - \frac{6\mu\, Q}{\alpha(b_1 - \alpha x)^2} + C \qquad ...(7.80)$$

The unknown quantities Q and C may be determined from the known end conditions. Since the pressure intensity is same, say, zero at the ends of the bearing ; namely,

(i) at $x = 0$, $p = 0$ and (ii) $x = L$, $p = 0$

$$Q = \frac{U_0 b_1 b_2}{(b_1 + b_2)}$$

and $\qquad C = - \frac{6\mu\, U_0}{\alpha(b_1 + b_2)} \qquad ...(7.81)$

Thus pressure intensity p is given by

$$p = \frac{6\mu\, U_0 x(b - b_2)}{b^2(b_1 + b_2)} \qquad ...(7.82)$$

Eq. 7.82 shows that p is positive between $x = 0$ and $x = L$, provided $b > b_2$. The pressure distribution is shown plotted in Fig. 7.18b.

The local force P that the bearing is able to sustain is determined by integrating Eq. 7.80 and substituting the value of b from Eq. 7.79a

$$P = \int_0^L p\,dx = \frac{6\mu U_0}{(b_1 + b_2)} \int_0^L \frac{x(b - b_2)}{b^2}\,dx$$

$$= \frac{6\mu U_0 L^2}{(b_1 + b_2)^2}\left[\log_e(b_1/b_2) - 2\frac{(b_1 - b_2)}{b_1 + b_2}\right] \qquad ...(7.83)$$

The drag force required to move the lower surface at velocity U_0 is,

$$D = \int_0^L \tau_0\,dx = \int_0^L \left(-\mu \frac{du}{dy}\right)_{y=0} dx \qquad ...(7.84)$$

Introducing $\dfrac{du}{dy}$ from Eq. 7.77 for $y = 0$,

$$\frac{du}{dy} = \frac{-b}{2\mu}\frac{dp}{dx} - \frac{U_0}{b} \qquad ...(7.85)$$

Solving Eq. 7.84 alongwith 7.85,

$$D = \frac{2\mu U_0 L}{(b_1 - b_2)}\left[2\log_* \frac{b_1}{b_2} - 3\frac{(b_1 - b_2)}{(b_1 + b_2)}\right] \qquad ...(7.86)$$

The maximum load P is computed when $b_1 = 2.2\,b_2$ (a condition when dp/dx is zero).

$$P_{max} = \frac{0.16\mu U L^2}{b_2^3} \quad \text{and} \quad D_{max} = \frac{0.75\mu U_0 L}{b_2} \qquad ...(7.87)$$

The ratio of P_{max} to D_{max} is

$$P_{max}/D_{max} = 0.21\,L/b_2 \qquad ...(7.88)$$

Since b_2 is small, the ratio can be very large.

Examples 7.1 - 7.21

7.1 The space between two square flat plates is filled with oil. Each side of the plate is 60 cm. the thickness of the film is 12.5 mm. The upper plate, which moves at 2.5 m/s, requires a force of 0.01 kN to maintain the speed. Determine (i) the dynamic viscosity of oil, and (ii) and kinematic viscosity of oil, if the specific gravity of the oil is 0.95.

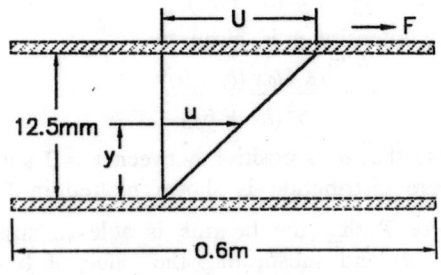

FIG. 7.19 EXAMPLE 7.1

Solution

Two square flat plates, placed 0.0125 m apart, are shown in Fig. 7.19. The lower plate is stationary whereas the upper plate moves with a velocity of 2.5 m/s.

Shearing force $F=$ shear stress $\times$ area in contanct of liquid

$$\tau = 0.01 \times 1000/(0.6 \times 0.6) = 27.7 \, \text{N/m}^2$$

From Eq. 1.8, $\tau = \mu \dfrac{\partial u}{\partial y} = \mu \dfrac{U}{Y}$

$$\mu = \frac{\tau Y}{U} = \frac{27.7 \times 0.0125}{2.5} \, \text{Ns/m}^2$$

(i) $\qquad \mu = 1.39 \times 10^{-1} \, \text{Ns/m}^2$,

(ii) $\qquad v = \dfrac{\mu}{\rho} = \dfrac{1.39 \times 10^{-1}}{0.95 \times 1000} = 1.46 \times 10^{-4} \, \text{m}^2/\text{s}$

7.2 A pipeline, 10 cm diameter, carries glycerine (sp. gr. = 1.3 and dynamic viscosity = 0.7 Ns/m² . If the maximum shear stress at the pipe wall is measured as 0.2 kN/m² , calculate (i) pressure gradient along the flow, (ii) discharge (iii) Reynolds number of flow and (iv) velocity and shear stress at a radius of 2.5 cm from the pipe centre.

Solution

(i) From Eq. 7.19b,

$$\tau = \left(-\frac{\partial p}{\partial x} \right) \frac{r}{2}$$

At the pipe wall, $\tau = \tau_0$ and $y = R$,

$$\tau_0 = \left(-\frac{\partial p}{\partial x} \right) \times R/2$$

Substituting the values,

$$(-\partial p/\partial x) = \frac{0.2 \times 2}{0.05} = 8 \, \text{k N/m}^2/\text{m} \text{ length} \qquad \ldots \text{(i)}$$

(ii) From Eq. 7.23,

$$u = \frac{1}{4\mu} \left(\frac{-\partial p}{\partial x} \right) (R^2 - r^2)$$

At $r = 0$; $u = U_{\text{max}} = \dfrac{1}{4\mu} \left(\dfrac{-\partial p}{\partial x} \right) R^2$

From Eq. 7.26,

$$U = U_{\text{max}}/2 = \frac{1}{8\mu} (-\partial p/\partial x) R^2 \text{ m/s}$$

Therefore, $Q = A U$

$$Q = \frac{\pi}{4}(0.1)^2 \times \frac{1}{8 \times 0.7} \times 8 \times 1000 \times (0.05)^2$$

Solving it, $\quad Q = 0.028 \text{ m}^2/\text{s}$

(iii) $\quad\quad\quad R_e = \frac{\rho\, U D}{\mu}$

Since $\rho = 1.3 \times 1000 \text{ kg/m}^3$

$$R_e = \frac{1300 \times 3.56 \times 0.1}{0.7} = 661 < 2000$$

The flow is laminar

(iv) From Eq. 7.23,

$$u = \frac{1}{4\mu}(-\partial p/\partial x)(R^2 - r^2)$$

Substituting the values,

$$u = \frac{1}{4 \times 0.7} \times (8 \times 1000)(0.05^2 - 0.025^2) = 5.36 \text{ m/s}$$

Shear stress at $r = 2.5$ cm,

$$\tau = \tau_0 \times \frac{r}{R} = 0.2 \times \frac{0.025}{0.050} = 0.1 \text{ kN/m}^2$$

7.3 Crude oil of viscosity 0.15 N s/m^2 and specific gravity 0.9 flows through a 20 mm diameter vertical pipe. Two pressure gauges have been fixed at 20 m apart; the pressure gauge fixed at higher level reads 20 kPa and that at lower level reads 60 kPa. Find the direction and rate of flow of crude oil through the pipe.

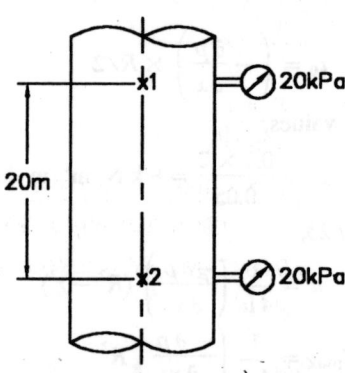

FIG. 7.20 EXAMPLE 7.3

Solution

Let the oil flow from 1 to 2. Applying Bernoulli's theorem between 1 and 2,

$$\frac{p_1}{w} + z_1 + \frac{U_1^2}{2g} = \frac{p_2}{w} + z_2 + \frac{U_2^2}{2g} + h_f$$

$$h_f = \frac{20}{w} + 20 - \frac{60}{w} = 15.922 \text{ m}$$

The oil flows in the upward direction.

Using Eq. 7.28b

$$Q = \frac{w \pi D^4 h_f}{128 \mu L}$$

Substituting the values

$$Q = \frac{9.81 \times \pi (0.02)^4 \times 15.922 \times 1000}{128 \times 0.15 \times 20}$$

$$= 0.000204 \text{ m}^3/\text{s} = 0.204 \text{ l/s}$$

7.4 Oil of specific gravity 0.82 is pumped through a horizontal pipe line 15 cm in diameter and 3 km long, at the rate of 900 lit/min. The pump has efficiency of 65% and requires 7.5 kW to pump the oil. Determine the μ of the oil in kg/m s and also verify whether the flow is laminar.

Solution

(i) Power output $P = w Q h_f$ kW

Power input $P_1 = $ Output/Efficiency $= \dfrac{w Q h_f}{\eta}$ ...(i)

From Eq. 7.28b,

$$h_t = \frac{128 \times \mu Q L}{w \pi D^4} \qquad \text{...(ii)}$$

From Eqs. (i) and (ii)

$$P_1 = \frac{w Q}{\eta} \times \frac{128 \mu Q L}{w \pi D^4}$$

$$\mu = \frac{P_1 \eta \pi D^4}{128 Q^2 L}$$

$$= \frac{(7.5 \times 1000) \times 0.65 \times \pi \times (0.15)^4}{128 \times (0.9/60)^2 \times 3000}$$

$$= 0.08973 \text{ N s/m}^2 = 0.8973 \text{ poise}$$

(ii) $$R_e = \frac{\rho U D}{\mu}$$

$$U = \frac{Q}{\pi D^2/4} = \frac{900}{60 \times 1000} \times \frac{1}{0.785 (0.15)^2} = 0.849 \text{ m/s}$$

$$Re = \frac{0.82 \times 1000 \times 0.849 \times 0.15}{0.08973}$$

$$= 1163.8 < 2000$$

Since the Reynolds number is less than 2000, the flow is laminar.

7.5 A 15 cm diameter vertical cylinder rotates concentrically inside another cylinder of diameter 15.1 cm. Both cylinders 25 cm high. The space between cylinders is filled with a liquid whose viscosity is not known. If the torque 15Nm is required to rotate the inner cylinder at 100 rpm, determine the viscosity of liquid.

Solution

Since the inner cylinder is moving and outer one is stationary, maximum shear stress τ_o will occur at the outer cylinder. Torque T required to rotate the inner cylinder is given by

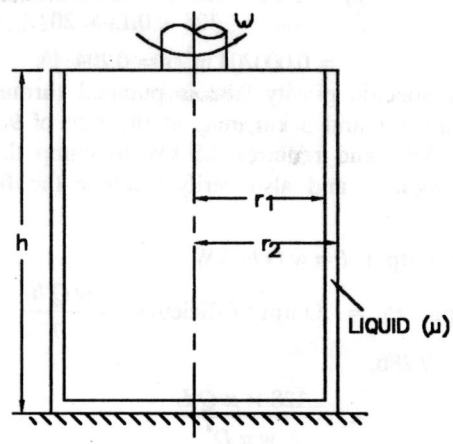

FIG. 7.21 EXAMPLE 7.5

$$T = \tau A r_2 \qquad ...(i)$$

Assuming linear variation of velocity in the gap between two cylinders,

$$\tau = \mu \frac{\partial u}{\partial y} = \mu \frac{U}{(r_2 - r_1)} \qquad ...(ii)$$

From Eqs. (i) and (ii)

$$\mu = \frac{T(r_2 - r_1)}{A r_2 U} = \frac{T(r_2 - r_1)}{\pi r_2^2 r_2 U}$$

Since
$$U = \omega r_1 = 2\pi r_1 N/60$$

$$= \frac{2 \times 3.14 \times 0.15 \times 100}{60 \times 2}$$

$$= 0.785 \text{ m/s}$$

$$\mu = \frac{15(0.151 - 0.150)/2}{\pi (0.151/2)^3 \times 0.785}$$

$$= 93.89 \text{ N s/m}^2$$

7.6 The lower end of a vertical shaft rests in a foot step bearing. Assuming that the end of the shaft and the surface of bearing are both flat and are separated by an oil film of 0.5 mm thickness, find the torque required to rotate the shaft at 750 rpm. The diameter of the shaft is 100 mm and μ of oil is 1.5 poise.

Solution

Consider a small concentric annular ring of radius r and thickness dr. The shearing force acting at this radius r is

$$F = \tau A = \tau\, 2\pi r\, dr$$

But

$$\tau = \mu \frac{\partial u}{\partial y}$$

The outer cylinder rotates at ω rad/sec, therefore,

$$\tau = \frac{\mu \omega r}{b}$$

Hence

$$F = \frac{2\mu \omega}{b} \pi r^2\, dr$$

The torque exerted at the bottom at radius r is

$$dT = Fr$$

$$= \frac{2\mu \omega \pi}{b} r^3\, dr$$

The torque exerted over the whole area of the bottom is

$$T = \int_0^R dT = \int_0^R \frac{2\mu \omega \pi}{b} \times r^3\, dr$$

$$= \left[\frac{2\mu \omega \pi}{b} \times \frac{R^4}{4} \right]$$

$$= \frac{\mu \pi^2 N}{60\, b} R^4 \qquad (\text{ Since } \omega = 2\pi N/60 \text{ })$$

Substituting the values,

$$T = \frac{0.15 \times \pi^2 \times 750}{60 \times 0.5 \times 10^{-3}} \times (0.1/2)^4$$

$$T = 0.233 \text{ N m } (\because\ 1 \text{ poise} = 0.1 \text{ N s/m}^2)$$

7.7 With a free body, as in Fig. 7.22, for uniform laminar flow of a thin sheet of liquid down an inclined plane, show that the discharge per unit width is

$$q = \frac{w}{3\mu} b^2 \sin \theta$$

Solution

Consider the fluid element of length ds and thickness y. The forces acting on it are shear stress τ on its lower surface and its own weight. For static equilibrium, $\Sigma F_s = 0$

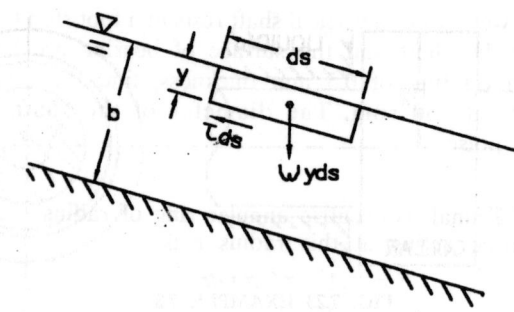

FIG. 7.22 EXAMPLE 7.7

$w\,y \times ds \sin\theta - \tau\,ds = 0$

$$\tau = w\,y \sin\theta \qquad\qquad\text{...(i)}$$

Also $\qquad\qquad \tau = \mu\,(\partial u/\partial y) \qquad\qquad\text{...(ii)}$

Equating Eqs. (i) and (ii)

$$\mu\frac{\partial u}{\partial y} = w\,y \sin\theta$$

Integrating, $\qquad u = \dfrac{1}{\mu} \times \dfrac{w\,y^2}{2}\sin\theta + A$

From the known boundary condition, *i.e.*, $y = b$, $u = 0$

$$A = -\frac{1}{2\mu}\,w\,b^2 \sin\theta$$

Hence $\qquad\qquad u = \dfrac{w\sin\theta}{2\mu}(b^2 - y^2)$

The discharge per unit width, q is given by

$$q = \int_0^d u\,dy$$

$$= \int_0^d \frac{w\sin\theta}{2\mu}(b^2 - y^2)\,dy$$

Solving, $\qquad\qquad q = \dfrac{w\,b^3 \sin\theta}{3\mu}$

7.8 A collar bearing having external and internal diameters 15 cm and 10 cm respectively is used to take the thrust of a shaft. An oil film of thickness 0.025 cm is maintained between the collar surface and bearing. Find the torque and H.P. lost in overcoming the viscous resistance of the oil when the shaft is running at 250 r.p.m. Take $\mu = 0.9$ poise.

Solution

Consider an elementary circular ring of radius r and width dr of the bearing surface, a is the spacing between the collar and shaft. The torque dT required to overcome the viscous resistance is given by

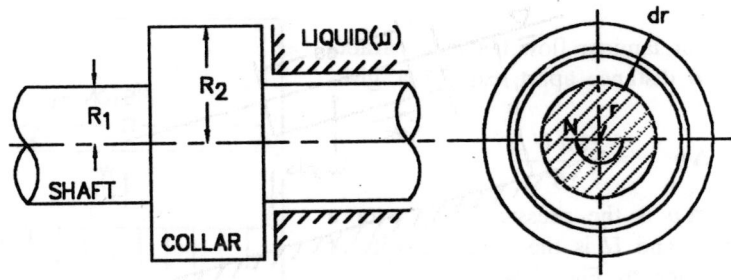

FIG. 7.23 EXAMPLE 7.8

$$dT = F \times r$$

$$= \tau \times 2\pi r \times r$$

$$= \mu \frac{\partial u}{\partial y} \times 2\pi r^2 dr$$

But
$$u = \frac{2\pi r N}{60}$$

$$dT = \frac{4\mu \pi^2 N r^3 dr}{60\, a}$$

Integrating over the whole area of contact of collar of radius R_1 to R_2 ,

$$T = \int_{R_1}^{R_2} \frac{4\mu \pi^2 N r^3 dr}{60\, a}$$

$$= \frac{\mu \pi^2 N}{60\, a} (R_2^4 - R_1^4)\, Nm \qquad \qquad ...(i)$$

Power absorbed in overcoming the viscous resistance

$$= T \times \omega / 1000 \text{ kW}$$

$$= \frac{2\mu \pi^3 N^2 (R_2^4 - R_1^4)}{(60)^2 \times a \times 1000} \text{ kW} \qquad \qquad ...(ii)$$

$$\text{Power absorbed} = \frac{2 \times (0.9 \times 0.1)\, \pi^3 \times (250)^2 \,(0.075^4 - 0.05^4)}{(60)^2 \times (0.025 \times 10^{-2}) \times 1000}$$

$$= 0.000612 \text{ kW}$$

7.9 A piston 7.5 cm diameter and 10 cm long moves vertically in an oil dashpot, the uniform clearance between piston and dashpot wall being 1.25 mm. Under its own weight the piston falls with uniform speed through 2.5 cm in 50 seconds. With an extra load (weight) of 1N on top of the piston it falls through 2.5 cm with uniform speed in 40 seconds. Find the value of the coefficient of viscosity of the oil in poise.

Solution

For laminar flow between parallel plates, B distance apart, Eq. 7.12a, gives Δp

$$\Delta p = \frac{12\,\mu\,U L}{B^2}$$

where Δp is the pressure drop over a length L and U is the mean velocity of flow, Refer to Fig. 7.24

Let W = total weight at the piston

D = piston diameter

W_1 = weight of the piston

U_1 = velocity of piston

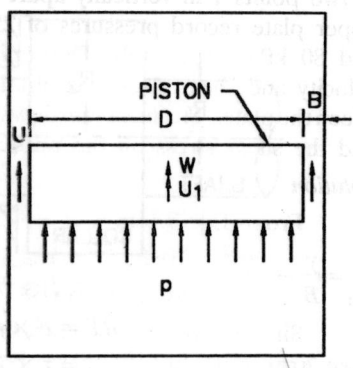

FIG. 7.24 EXAMPLE 7.9

Now

$$Q = \frac{\pi D^2}{4} U_1 = \pi\,D\,B\,U$$

$$U = \frac{D}{4B} U_1 \qquad \qquad \text{...(ii)}$$

From Eqs. (i) and (ii)

$$\Delta p = \frac{4W}{\pi D^2} = \frac{12\,\mu\,L}{B^2} \times \frac{D\,U_1}{4B}$$

i.e.,

$$\mu = \frac{4 B^3 W}{3 \pi\,U_1 D^3 L} \qquad \qquad \text{...(iii)}$$

When $W = W_1$, $U_1 = 1/2000$ m/s, therefore from Eq. (iii)

$$\mu = \frac{4 B^3}{3 \pi D^3 L} \times 2000\,W_1 \qquad \qquad \text{...(iv)}$$

When $W = W_1 + 1$, $U_1 = 2.5/(40 \times 100) = 1/1600$ m/s, therefore,

$$\mu = \frac{4 B^3}{3 \pi D^3 I} \times 1600\,(W_1 + 1) \qquad \qquad \text{...(v)}$$

From Eq. (iv) and (v) $2000\,W_1 = 1600\,(W_1 + 1)$

Solving $W_1 = 4\,N$

Substituting the value of W_1 in Eq. (iv)

$$\mu = \frac{4\,(1.25 \times 10^{-3})^3}{3 \pi\,(7.5 \times 10^{-2})^3 \times 0.1} \times 2000 \times 4$$

$$= 0.157\ \text{N s/m}^2 = 1.57\ \text{poise}$$

7.10 Laminar flow of a fluid of viscosity 0.9 N s/m^2 and specific gravity 1.26 occurs between a pair of plates of extensive width, inclined at 45° to the horizontal, the plates being 10 mm apart. The upper plate moves with a velocity of 1.5 m/s relative to the lower plate and in a direction opposite to the fluid flow. Pressure gauges mounted at two points 1 m vertically apart on the upper plate record pressures of 250 kPa and 80 kPa respectively. Determine the velocity and shear stress distribution between the plates, the maximum flow velocity and the shear stress on the upper plate.

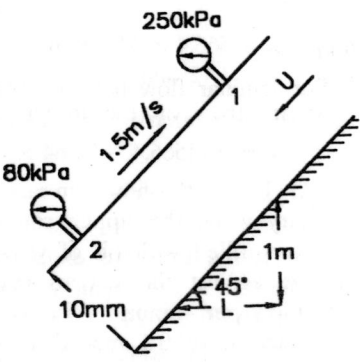

FIG. 7.25 EXAMPLE 7.10

Solution

From Eq. 7.16b,

$$\frac{u}{U_0} = \frac{y}{B} - \frac{B^2}{2\mu U_0}\frac{\partial p}{\partial x}\left(1 - \frac{y}{B}\right)\frac{y}{B}$$

Since the plate is inclined, the pressure gradient should be replaced by piezometric gradient $\partial(p + wz)/dx$

Let the flow takes place from 1 to 2. The energy $(p_1 + wz_1)$ at 1 is

$$= 250 + 9.81 \times 1.26 \times 1 = 262.36 \text{ kPa}$$

Similarly energy at $2 = (p_2 + wz_2)$

$$= (80 + 0) = 80 \text{ kPa}$$

as $z_2 = 0$ if datum is taken at point 2

Flow is down slope and upper plate moves 'up slope'

Pressure gradient $-\left(\dfrac{\partial px}{\partial x}\right) = -\dfrac{(262.36 - 80)}{1 \times \sqrt{2}}$

$$. = 128.95 \text{ kPa per metre, } dx = 1 \times \sqrt{2} \text{ m}$$

From Eq. 7.16b

$$u = U_0\frac{y}{B} - \frac{1}{2\mu}\frac{\partial p_x}{\partial x}(yB - y^2)$$

where $U_0 = -1.5$ m/s, $B = 0.01$ m and u is the local velocity at a point y m above the lower plate. Thus the velocity profile is

$$u = -1.5 \times \frac{y}{0.01} + \frac{1}{2 \times 0.9} \times 128.95 \times 10^3 \times (0.01y - y^2)$$

$$= 566.4y - 71.64 \times 10^3 y^2$$

Shear stress distribution is given by

$$\tau = \mu\,(\partial u/\partial y)$$

$$= 0.9\,[566.4 - 71.64 \times 10^3 \times 2y]$$

Maximum velocity occurs where $du/dy = 0$

or $y = 566.4/(143.28 \times 10^3) = 3.95 \times 10^{-3}$ m

Then
$$U_{max} = 566.4 \times 3.95 \times 10^{-3} - 71.64 \times 10^3 \times (3.95 \times 10^{-3})^2$$
$$= 1.12 \text{ m/s}$$

Shear stress on the upper plate
$$\tau = 0.9 [566.4 - 71.64 \times 2 \times 10^3 \times 0.01] = -0.78 \text{ kPa}$$

7.11 Fig. 7.26 shows an assembly of two plates, the lower of which is stationary while the upper rotates co-axially with it. The space between them is kept filled with oil of viscosity 0.05 poise. Calculate the work done per minute against the viscous resistance when the upper plate rotates at 60 revolution per minute. Also compare the result with the work done if the clearance were 0.1 mm throughout.

Solution

From Eq. 1.8c;
$$\tau = \mu \, (\partial u / \partial y) = \mu \, (U / 2 \, h)$$

But
$$U = \frac{2 \pi r N}{60}$$

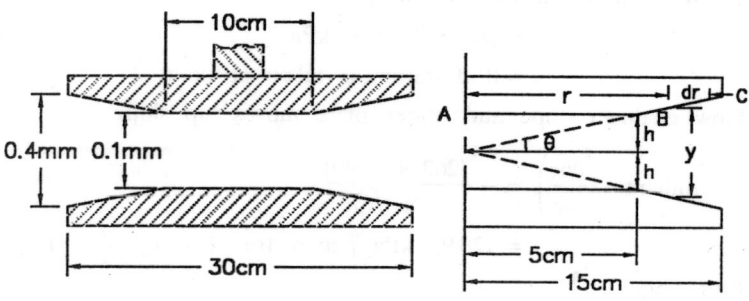

FIG. 7.26 EXAMPLE 7.11

$$\tau = \mu \frac{2 \pi r N}{60 \times 2 h} = \frac{\mu \pi r N}{60 \, h} \qquad \qquad ...(i)$$

But $\qquad r/h = 0.05/(0.05 \times 10^{-3}) = 1000$

Therefore $\qquad \tau = (50/3) \, \mu \, \pi \, N$

For part BC

Consider a small elementary area at radius r

Area of elementary ring at radius r
$$= 2 \pi r \, dr \sec \theta$$
$$\approx 2 \pi r \, dr$$

Tangential force on the ring $= \tau \times$ area
$$= (50/3) \, \mu \, \pi \, N \times 2 \pi r \, dr$$
$$= (100/3) \, \mu \, \pi^2 \, N \, r \, dr$$

Viscous torque on the ring $= F \times r$

$$= (100/3)\, \mu\, \pi^2 N\, r^2\, dr$$

Therefore, viscous torque for part BC

$$= \int_{0.05}^{0.15} \frac{100}{3} \mu\, \pi^2 N\, r^2\, dr$$

$$= (0.0361\, \mu\, \pi^2 N)\ \text{N m} \qquad \qquad ...(ii)$$

For part AB, $h = 0.05 \times 10^{-3}$ m

Therefore from Eq. (i)

$$\tau = \frac{\mu\, \pi\, N}{60} \times \frac{r}{0.05 \times 10^{-3}} = \frac{1000}{3} \mu\, \pi\, Nr$$

Tangential force on the ring $= \tau \times$ area

$$= (1000/3)\, \mu\, \pi\, Nr \times 2\, \pi\, r\, dr$$

$$= (2000/3)\, \mu\, \pi^2 Nr^2\, dr$$

Torque for surface of radius R , *i.e.*

$$AB = \int_0^R \frac{2000}{3} \mu\, \pi^2 N\, r^3\, dr$$

$$= \frac{2000}{3} \mu\, \pi^2 N \left[\frac{r^4}{4} \right]_0^R$$

$$= \frac{500}{3} \mu\, \pi^2 N R^4 \qquad \qquad ...(iii)$$

When $\qquad\qquad R = 0.05$ m, torque $= (500/3)\, \mu\, \pi^2 N\, (0.05)^4$

$$= 0.00104\, \mu\, \pi^2 N \qquad \qquad ...(iv)$$

Therefore, total torque for given plates $=$ Eq. (ii) $+$ Eq. (iv)

$$= (0.0361 + 0.00104)\, \mu\, \pi^2 N$$

$$= 0.03714\, \mu\, \pi^2 N\ \ \text{N} - \text{m}$$

Work done/min $=$ Torque $\times$ angular velocity

$$= 0.03714\, \mu\, \pi^2 N \times 2\, \pi\, N$$

$$= 0.07428 \times (0.5 \times 0.1)\, \pi^3 \times (60)^2$$

$$= 41.456\ \text{N-m}$$

(b) When surface are parallel, from Eq. (iii)

Torque $= (500/3)\, \mu\, \pi^2 N R^4$

Here R is equal to 0.15 m,

Torque $= (500/3)\, \mu\, \pi^2 N\, (0.15)^4 = 0.08436\, \mu\, \pi^2 N\ \ \text{N} - \text{m}$

$$\text{Work done/min} = 00.8436 \, \mu \, \pi^2 N \times 2 \, \pi \, N$$
$$= 0.16872 \, \mu \, \pi^3 \, N^2$$
$$= 0.16872 \times (0.05 \times 0.1) \, \pi^3 \, (60)^2$$
$$= 94.278 \, \text{N} - \text{m}$$

7.12 Kerosence oil flow upwards through inclined parallel plates at the rate of 3 l/s per meter width. The plates are inclined at 30° with the horizontal and the gap between the plates is 12 mm. Determine the difference of pressure between two section 10 m apart. Take specific weight of K. Oil 7845 N/m³ and $\mu = 2 \times 10^{-3}$ kg/ms.

Solution

The mean velocity of fluid $U = \dfrac{q}{B}$

$$U = \frac{3 \times 10^{-3}}{12 \times 10^{-3}} = 0.25 \text{ m/s.}$$

The head loss h_f between parallel plates is given by

$$h_f = \frac{12 \, \mu \, U \, L}{w \, D^2}$$

$$= \frac{12 \times 2 \times 10^{-3} \times 0.25 \times 10}{7845 \times (0.012)^2}$$

$$= 0.0531 \text{ m}$$

But
$$hf = (p_1/w + z_1) - (p_2/w + z_2)$$
$$= (p_1/w - p_2/w) + (z_1 - z_2)$$
$$\left(\frac{p_1}{w} - \frac{p_2}{w} \right) = h_f - (z_1 - z_2)$$
$$= 0.0531 - (-10 \sin 30)$$

$$(\because \, z_2 - z_1 = 10 \sin 30°)$$

$$= 5.0531 \text{ m}$$
$$(p_1 - p_2) = 5.0531 \times 7845$$
$$= 39641.57 \text{ N/m}^2$$

7.13 Determine the optimum diameter of the pipe required to carry 0.15 m³/s of crude oil. Also determine the power required for supplying it over one kilometer. Take $\rho = 950$ kg/m³ and $\mu = 8 \times 10^{-2}$ kg/ms and the flow through the pipe is assumed as laminar.

Solution

$$R_e = \frac{\rho \, U \, D}{v} = \frac{4 \rho \, Q}{\pi \, D \, \mu}$$

$$= 4 \times 950 \times 0.15 / (\pi \times D \times 8 \times 10^{-2})$$

For the laminar flow, $R_e = 2000$

$$\therefore \qquad D = \frac{4 \times 950 \times 0.15}{\pi \times 8 \times 10^{-2} \times 2000} = 1.13 \text{ m}$$

From Eq. 7.28b

$$h_f = \frac{128 \mu \, Q \, L}{w \, \pi \, D^4}$$

$$\therefore \qquad w \, h_f = \frac{128 \times 8 \times 10^{-2} \times 0.15 \times 1000}{3.14 \times (1.13)^4}$$

$$\Delta p = 300 \text{ N/m}^2$$

Power required to supply the crude oil

$$= \Delta p \times Q$$
$$= 300 \times 0.15$$
$$= 45 \text{ W}$$

7.14 For the determination of viscosity of a fluid by falling sphere viscosmeter, it is observed that the spherical steel ball, 1 cm in diameter, travels a distance of 525 cm in 100 seconds. If the specific mass of the oil be 0.95, determine the viscosity of the oil. Take specific mass of steel ball as 8000 kg/m³

Solution

From Eq. 7.57

$$\mu = \frac{D^2}{18 \, U_0} (w_s - w)$$

Here
$$U_0 = 525/100 = 5.25 \text{ cm/s}$$
$$= 0.0525 \quad \text{m/s}$$

Substituting the value in the above equation

$$\mu = \frac{(0.01)^2}{18 \times 0.0525} (8000 \times 9.81 - 0.95 \times 1000 \times 9.81)$$

$$= 7.31 \text{ Ns/m}^2$$

Check for the value of Re

$$R_{R_e} = \frac{\rho \, U_0 D}{\mu}$$

$$= \frac{0.95 \times 1000 \times 0.0525 \times 0.01}{7.31}$$

$$= 0.068 < 1.0$$

Hence, the Stokes law is applicable.

7.15 Determine the viscosity of crude oil using capilliary tube apparatus. The diameter and length of the capillary are 2 mm and 0.5 m respectively.

The following observations were made, head loss = 0.25 m, volume of oil collected = 200 cc. and time of collection oil = 100 seconds. The mass density of oil is taken as 850 kg/m³

Solution

From Eq. 7.28,

$$\mu = \frac{\pi w D^4 h_f}{128 Q L}$$

Substituting the values.

$$\mu = \frac{3.14 \times 850 \times 9.81 \times (2 \times 10^{-3})^4 \times 0.25}{128(200 \times 10^{-6}/100) \times 0.5}$$

$$= 8.18 \times 10^{-4} \, \text{Ns/m}^2$$

7.16 Determine the kinetic energy and momentum correction factor α and β for laminar flow through a circular pipe.

Solution

From Fig. 5.27

$$\alpha = \frac{\int_0^R u^3 \, dA}{U^3 A} \qquad \qquad \text{...(i)}$$

From Eq. 7.23,

$$u = \frac{1}{4\mu} \left(-\frac{\partial p}{\partial x} \right) (R^2 - r^2) = C(R^2 - r^2) \qquad \text{...(ii)}$$

Also from Eq. 7.26,

$$U = \frac{1}{8\mu} \left(-\frac{\partial p}{\partial x} \right) R^2 = \frac{C}{2} R^2 \qquad \qquad \text{...(iii)}$$

Subitituting from Eq. (ii) and (iii) into Eq. (i)

$$\alpha = \frac{\int_0^R \left\{ C(R^2 - r^2) \right\}^3 2\pi r \, dr}{\left\{ \frac{C}{2} R^2 \right\}^3 \pi R^2}$$

$$= \frac{2\pi C^3 \int_0^R (R^6 - 3R^4 r^2 + 3R^2 r^4 - r^6) r \, dr}{\frac{\pi C^3}{8} R^8}$$

$$= \frac{16}{R^8} \left[R^6 \frac{r^2}{2} - 3R^4 \frac{r^4}{4} + 3R^2 \frac{r^6}{6} - \frac{r^8}{8} \right]_0^R$$

$$= \frac{16}{R^8} \left[R^8 \left(\frac{1}{2} - \frac{3}{4} + \frac{3}{6} - \frac{1}{8} \right) \right]$$

$$= 2.0$$

From Eq. 5.52,

$$\beta = \frac{\int_0^R u^2 \, dA}{U^2 A}$$

$$= \frac{\int_0^R \left\{ C(R^2 - r^2) \right\}^2 2\pi r \, dr}{\left(\frac{C}{2} R^2 \right)^2 \pi R^2}$$

$$= \frac{2\pi C^2 \int_0^R (R^4 r - 2R^2 r^3 + r^5) \, dr}{\frac{\pi C^2 R^6}{4}}$$

$$= \frac{8}{R^6} \left[R^4 \frac{r^2}{2} - 2R^2 \frac{r^4}{4} + \frac{r^6}{6} \right]_0^R$$

$$B = \frac{8}{R^6} \left[R^6 (\frac{1}{2} - \frac{1}{2} + \frac{1}{6}) \right]$$

$$= 1.33$$

7.17 A tank contains oil to a depth of 60 cm above its bottom, A vertical pipe of 2 cm diameter and 50 cm length is connected at its bottom and dischages oil at its outlet. Calculate the discharge through this pipe. Take density of oil as 850 kg/m^3 and its viscosity as 1.6 poise.

Solution.

Applying Bernoulli's theorem between 1 and 2,

$$\frac{p_1}{w} + z_1 + \frac{U_1^2}{2g} = \frac{p_2}{w} + z_2 + \frac{U_2^2}{2g} + hf$$

Given $p_1 = 0$, $p_2 = 0$,

$z_2 - z_1 = (0.60 + 0.5) = 1.1$ m

$U_1 = 0$ at liquid surface

$$0 + z_1 + 0 = 0 + z_2 + \frac{U_2^2}{2g} + h_f$$

$$h_f = (z_1 - z_2) - \frac{U_2^2}{2g}$$

$$= 1.1 + \frac{U_2^2}{2g} \qquad ...(i)$$

The head loss through circular pipes is given by Eq. 7.28a,

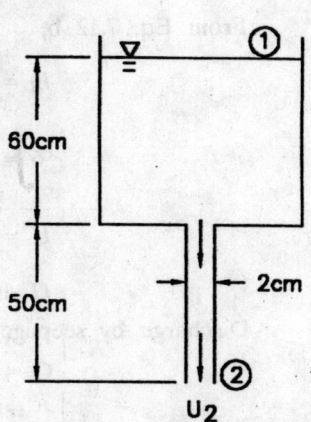

FIG. 7.27 EXAMPLE 7.17

$$h_f = \frac{32\,\mu\,U_2 L}{w\,D^2}$$

Here $L = 0.50$ m, $D = 0.02$ m, $w = 850 \times 981 = 8338.5 \, N/m^3$

$$h_f = \frac{32 \times (1.6 \times 0.1)\, U_2 \times 0.5}{8338.5 \times (0.02)^2}$$

$$h_f = 0.7675\ U_2$$

From Eq. (i) and (ii)

$$1.1 + \frac{U_2^2}{2g} = 0.7675\ U_2$$

Solving, $U_2 = 1.317$ m/s

Discharge through pipe,

$$Q = \frac{\pi}{4} \times (0.2)^2 \times 1.317$$

$$= 0.04135 \text{ m}^3/\text{s}$$

$$= 41.35 \text{ L/s}$$

7.18 A water tank contains water to a depth of 6 m and has got 0.60 m thick wall. A horizontal crack of 5 m long and 0.12 mm thickness was observed in the vertical wall of tank (near its bottom) which extended throughout its thickness. The water seeps through this crack into atmosphere. Assuming kinetic viscosity of water as 10^{-2} m²/s, compute the loss of water by seepage.
Solution.

The horizontal crack may be assumed two parallel plates through which water flows (seeps) with a velocity U.

Given $L = 0.6$ m, $h_f = 6$ m, $B = 0.12 \times 10^{-3}$ m and $\nu = 10^{-6}$ m²/s

$\therefore$ $\mu = 1000 \times 10^{-6}$ Pas

From Eq. 7.12 b,

$$h_f = \frac{12\,\mu\,U L}{w\,B^2}$$

$$6 = \frac{12 \times (1000 \times 10^{-6}) \times U \times 0.6}{9810 \times (0.12 \times 10^{-3})^2}$$

$$U = \frac{6 \times 9810 \times (0.12 \times 10^{-3})^2}{12 \times 1000 \times 10^{-6} \times 0.6}$$

$$U = 0.11772 \text{ m/s}$$

Discharge by seepage $Q = AU$

$$Q = 5 \times (0.12 \times 10^{-3})^2 \times 0.11772$$

$$= 7.06 \times 10^{-5} \text{ m}^3/\text{s}$$

$$= 0.25 \text{ m}^3/\text{hr.}$$

7.19 Two parallel plates are placed 1.5 cm apart. Oil of mass density 900 kg/m³ and dynamic viscosity 0.95 poise flows between them with a mean velocity of 1.25 m/s. Compute (a) velocity distribuition between the plates (b) maximum velocity (c) wall shear stress, (d) velocity and shear stress at 0.25 cm from the plates and (e) the head loss in a length of 30 m.

Solution:

Given ρ = 900 kg/m³, μ = 0.95 poise = 0.095 N/m³

B = 1.5 × 10⁻² m, U = 1.25 m/s

Also from Eq. 7.9,

$$u = \frac{1}{2\mu}\left(\frac{-\partial p}{\partial x}\right)(By - y^2) \qquad \text{(ii)}$$

From Eq. 7.11

$$U = \frac{1}{12\mu}\left(\frac{-\partial p}{\partial x}\right) \times B^2 \qquad \text{(i)}$$

From Eqs. (i) and (ii)

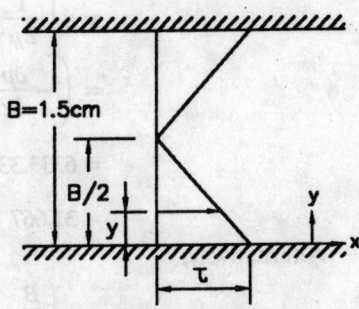

FIG. 7.28 EXAMPLE 7.19

$$\frac{u}{U} = \frac{\dfrac{1}{2\mu}\left(-\dfrac{\partial p}{\partial x}\right)(By - y^2)}{\dfrac{1}{12\mu}\left(\dfrac{-\partial p}{\partial x}\right)B^2}$$

$$= \frac{6(By - y^2)}{B^2}$$

$$u = \frac{6U}{B^2}(By - y^2)$$

$$u = \frac{6 \times 1.25}{(1.5 \times 10^{-2})^2}\left[1.5 \times 10^{-2}y - y^2\right]$$

$$u = 3.33 \times 10^4 [1.5 \times 10^{-2}y - y^2] \qquad \text{(iii)}$$

It is the required velocity distribution.

(b) From Eq. 7.11

$$U = \frac{1}{12\mu}\left(\frac{-\partial p}{\partial x}\right)B^2 = \frac{2}{3}U_{max} \qquad \text{(iii)}$$

$$U_{max} = \frac{3}{2}.U$$

$$= \frac{3}{2} \times 1.25 = 1.875 \text{ m/s} \qquad \text{(iv)}$$

(c)

$$U = \frac{1}{12\mu}\left(-\frac{\partial p}{\partial x}\right)B^2$$

$$\left(-\frac{\partial p}{\partial x}\right) = \frac{12\mu U}{B^2}$$

$$= \frac{12 \times 0.95 \times 0.1 \times 1.25}{(1.5 \times 10^{-2})^2} = 6333.33$$

Also

$$\tau_0 = \left(\frac{-\partial p}{\partial x} \right) \frac{B}{2}$$

$$= 6333.33 \times \frac{1.5 \times 10^{-2}}{2}$$

$$= 47.5 \ \text{N/m}^2 \ \text{at the wall}$$

(d)   u at $y = 0.25 \times 10^{-2}$ m,

$$u = 3.33 \times 10^4 [1.5 \times 10^{-2} \times 0.25 \times 10^{-2} - (0.25 \times 10^{-2})^2]$$

$$= 3.33 \times 10^4 [0.3125 \times 10^{-4}] = -1.04 \ \text{m/s}$$

τ at $y = 0.25 \times 10^{-2}$ m,

$$\tau = \mu \frac{du}{dy}$$

$$= \mu \left[\frac{1}{2\mu} \left(-\frac{\partial p}{\partial x} \right) (B - 2y) \right]$$

$$= \left(-\frac{\partial p}{\partial x} \right) \left(\frac{B}{2} - y \right)$$

$$= 6333.33 \left[\frac{1.5 \times 10^{-2}}{2} - 0.25 \times 10^{-2} \right]$$

$$= 31.667 \ \text{N/m}^2$$

Alternatively,

$$\frac{\tau}{\tau_0} = \frac{\left(\frac{B}{2} - y \right)}{B}$$

$$\tau = \frac{47.5 \times 1.5 \times 10^{-2}}{(1.5 - 0.25) \times 10^{-2}} = 31.667 \ N/m^2$$

(e) From Eq. 7.12 b,

$$h_f = \frac{12 \, U v L}{w B^2}$$

$$h_f = \frac{12 \times (0.95 \times 0.1) \times 1.25 \times 30}{(900 \times 9.81) \times (1.5 \times 10^{-2})^2}$$

$$= 21.52 \ \text{m}$$

7.20 Derive the expression for head loss for laminar flow through a convergent pipe of length L. Assume inlet and outlet diameters as D_1 and D_2 ($D_1 > D_2$).

Solution:

Consider an elementary length dx of convergent pipe at x metre from inlet

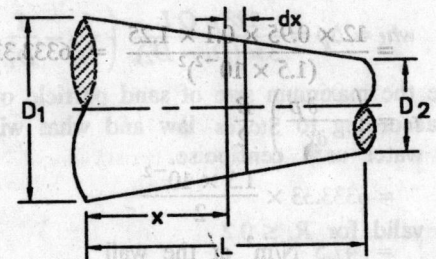

FIG. 7.29 EXAMPLE 7.20

From Eq. 7.12 b,

$$dh_f = \frac{32 \mu U \Delta x}{D^2}$$

It can be written as

$$dh_f = \frac{32 \mu \cdot \left(Q / \frac{\pi D^2}{4} \right) \Delta x}{w D^2}$$

$$= \frac{128 \mu Q \Delta x}{w \pi D^4} \qquad \text{(i)}$$

where

$$D = \left[D_2 + \frac{(D_1 - D_2) \times (L - x)}{L} \right]$$

Differenting w.r. to x,

$$\frac{dD}{dx} = \left[0 + \frac{D_1 - D_2}{L} \times (-1) \right]$$

$$dx = \left(\frac{-L}{D_1 - D_2} \right) dD$$

Substituting in Eq (i)

$$dh_f = \frac{128 \mu Q}{w \pi} \cdot \left(\frac{-L}{D_1 - D_2} \right) \frac{dD}{D^4}$$

Integrating w.r. to D,

$$\int dh_f = \frac{-128 \mu Q L}{w (D_1 - D_2)} \int_{D_1}^{D_2} \frac{dD}{D^4}$$

$$h_f = \frac{-128 \mu Q L}{w \pi (D_1 - D_2)} \left[\frac{D^{-3}}{-3} \right]_{D_1}^{D_2}$$

$$h_f = \frac{128 \mu Q L}{3 w \pi (D_1 - D_2)}, \left[\frac{1}{D_2^3} - \frac{1}{D_1^3} \right]$$

$$wh_t = \Delta p = \frac{128 \mu Q L}{3 \pi (D_1 - D_2)} \left(\frac{1}{D_2^3} - \frac{1}{D_1^3} \right)$$

7.21 Determine the maximum size of sand particle of sp. gr. 2.65 that will settle in water according to Stokes law and what will be its terminal velocity. Take μ for water as 1 centipoise.

Solution:

Stoke's law is valid for $R_e \leq 0.2$

$$R_e = \frac{\rho U D}{\mu}$$

$$0.2 = \frac{1000 \times U \times D}{10^{-3}} \qquad \left(\because \mu = \frac{1}{100} \text{ poise} \right)$$

$$= 10^{-3} \text{ Ns/m}^2$$

$$U = \frac{0.2 \times 10^{-6}}{D} \qquad \qquad \text{(i)}$$

Also from Eq. 7.57

$$U = \frac{D^2}{18 \mu} (w_s - w)$$

$$= \frac{D^2}{18 \times 10^{-3}} [2.65 \times 9810 - 9810]$$

$$= \frac{1.65 \times 9810}{18 \times 10^{-3}} D^2 \qquad \qquad \text{(ii)}$$

From Eqs. (i) and (ii)

$$\frac{0.2 \times 10^{-6}}{D} = \frac{1.65 \times 9810}{18 \times 10^{-3}} D^2$$

$$D^3 = \frac{0.2 \times 18 \times 10^{-9}}{1.65 \times 9810}$$

$$D = 0.061 \times 10^{-3} \text{ m} = 0.061 \text{ mm}$$

From Eq. (i)

$$U = \frac{0.2 \times 10^{-6}}{0.061 \times 10^{-3}}$$

$$= 3.28 \times 10^{-3} \text{ m/s} = 3.28 \text{ mm/s}$$

Objective Questions

7.1 The lower limit of critical Reynolds number (below which all the disturbances are damped by viscous action) in pipe flow is

    (a) 1   (b) 500   (c) 1000

    (d) 2000   (e) 12000

7.2   The upper critical Reynolds number is

(a) about 2000   (b) important from a design point of view
(c) the number at which turbulent flow changes to laminar flow
(d) of no practical importance to laminar flow
(e) none of these answers

7.3   The Reynolds number of pipe flow is given by

(a) UD/ν (b) $UD\mu/\rho$ (c) $\rho UD/\nu$
(d) UD/μ (e) none of these answers

7.4   The shear stress in a fluid flowing in a circular pipe

(a) is constant over the cross section
(b) is zero at the wall and increase linearly to the centre
(c) varies parabolically across the section
(d) is zero at the centre and varies linearly with the radius
(e) none of these answers

7.5   In laminar flow through a circular pipe the discharge varies

(a) linearly as the viscosity
(b) as the square of the radius
(c) inversely as the pressure drop
(d) inversely as the viscosity
(e) as the cube of the diameter

7.6   The shear stress in a fluid flowing between two fixed parallel plates

(a) is constant across the section
(b) is zero at the plates and increases linearly to the mid point
(c) varies parabolically across the section
(d) is zero at the mid plane and varies linearly with distance
(e) none of these answers

7.7   The discharge between two parallel plates, distant B apart, when one moves with a velocity U_0 and other is stationary, is given by any one of the formula. The pressure gradient is assumed zero

(a) $U_0 B/2$ (b) $U_0 B/3$ (c) $\frac{2}{3} U_0 B$
(d) $U_0 B$ (e) none of these answers

7.8   The expression for power input per unit volume to a fluid in laminar motion in the X-direction is

(a) τ/μ^2 (b) $\mu \, du/dy$ (c) $\tau \, (du/dy)$
(d) $\tau \, (du/dy)^2$ (e) none of these answers

7.9 The terminal velocity of a small sphere settling in a viscous fluid is

(a) $\dfrac{D^2 \mu}{18} (w_s - w)$ (b) $\dfrac{\mu}{18 D^2} (w_s - w)$ (c) $\dfrac{D^2}{18 \mu} (w_s - w)$

(d) $\dfrac{D}{18 \mu} (w_s - w)$ (e) none of these answers

7.10 A 10 cm diameter shaft rotates at 250 rpm in a bearing with a radial clearance of 0.15 mm. The shear stress in an oil film of $\mu = 0.1$ poise, in kN/m^2 is

(a) 0.0151 (b) 0.0873 (c) 8.73

(d) 50.3 (e) none of these answers

7.11 A viscometer of the Saybolt was used to determine the viscosity of liquid which took 97 seconds for 60 c.c. of liquid to flow. Determine the kinematic viscosity; assume $C_1 = 0.0022$ and $C_2 = 1.8$

7.12 In laminar flow through a circular tube, the Darcy Weisbach friction factor is related to Reynolds number by

(a) $f = \dfrac{16}{R_e}$ (b) $f = \dfrac{64}{R_e}$ (c) $f = \dfrac{1}{R}$

(d) $f = \dfrac{0.316}{(R_e)^{0.25}}$ (e) none of these answers.

Problems

7.1 A steady flow of water occurs in a 15 cm diameter straight pipe which is inclined at 60° with the horizontal, in a downward direction. If the pressure drop in the direction of flow is 3.5 kPa per 50 m of pipe line, what is the shear stress at the pipe wall?

7.2 Two large plane surfaces are placed parallel to each other at a distance of 12.5 mm. The space between them is filled with glycerine at 20° C . A 2.5 mm plate of $0.2 \, m^2$ is being towed in glycerine by a constant force of 0.01 kN. The plate remains equidistant from the two fixed surface. Calculate the towing speed of the plate.

7.3 Two parallel plates are placed horizontally with 7.5 mm space between them. A liquid of viscosity $0.02 \, N \, s/m^2$ is filled in the space. The bottom plate is fixed and top plate moves with a velocity of 0.5 m/s. What shear stress corresponds to the condition of zero discharge between them ? What is the shear stress at each plate ?

7.4 At what slope should fixed parallel plates be placed so that liquid flows between them without change in pressure intensity? The distance between them is 25 mm, sp. wt $= 0.9 \, k \, N/m^3$, viscosity $\mu = 0.07 \, N \, s/m^2$ and $Q = 0.1 \, m^3/s$ per metre width.

7.5 A certain lubricating oil is pumped at a rate of $0.025 \, m^3/s$ through 500 m length of pipe; diameter being 15 cm. The dynamic viscosity and specific weight of oil are $8 \, kN/m^3$ and $0.1 \, Ns/m^2$ respectively. Calculate the pressure drop (a) if the pipe is horizontal (b) if the pipe is inclined at 10° with the horizontal and the flow is in the upward direction and (c) if the pipe is inclined at 10° with the horizontal and the flow is in the downward direction.

7.6 The tank with the slender outlet tube shown in the accompanying sketch Fig. 7.30 is used to measure the viscosity of liquids. What viscosity would be indicated by a flow of $2 \times 10^{-5} \, m^3$ of liquid in 40 seconds under the given head if the specific gravity, of oil is 0.9 ?

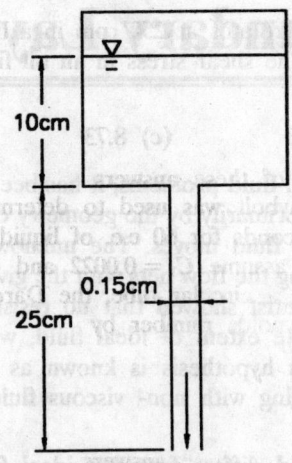

10cm

0.15cm

25cm

FIG. 7.30 PROBLEM 7.6

7.7 The viscous flow takes place in the annular space between two concentric pipes of radii R_1 and R_2 $(R_1 < R_2)$. Derive an expression for the velocity distribution and therefrom show that maximum velocity occurs at radius R given by

$$R = R_1 \sqrt{(a^2 - 1)(2 \log_e a)}$$

where $a = R_2/R_1$

7.8 Oil of sp. gr. 0.9 and viscosity 0.1 N s/m² is pumped through a 75 mm diameter pipe 1000 m long at the rate of 0.03 kN/sec. If the critical Reynolds number is 2000, show that the critical velocity is not exceeded and calculate the pressure required at the pump and the power required.

7.9 The thrust at the lower end of a vertical shaft is taken by a flat disc 10 cm diameter, separated from a flat housing by an oil film of 0.25 mm thick. If the shaft rotates at 1000 rpm and the viscosity of oil is 0.13 N s/m², calculate the power absorbed by the fluid friction.

7.10 A 10 cm journal rotates concentrically in a bearing of 10.05 cm diameter and length 15 cm. The annular space between the journal and bearing is filled with oil and it takes 1 kW to drive the journal at 2400 rev/min. Find the viscosity of oil.

7.11 Oil of sp. gr. 0.87 and viscosity 0.52 poise, flows through an annulus with $R_1 = 1.25$ cm and $R_2 = 0.5$ cm. When the shear at the outer wall is 0.1 kN/m², calculate, (a) the pressure drop per metre for a horizontal system (b) the discharge and (c) the axial force exerted on the inner tube per metre length.

8

Boundary Layer Theory

8.1 INTRODUCTION

In the analysis of ideal fluid problems, it has been found that the pattern of fluid motion is governed primarily by the geometry of the boundary between which or around which the fluid moves. The unknown flow parameters can be determined by constructing the flow nets with the given boundary conditions. D'Alembert, a French scientist showed that no resistance is experienced by a body moving in the infinite extent of ideal fluid, which is in contradiction of experimental results. His hypothesis is known as D'Alembert's paradox. The branch of science dealing with non- viscous fluid is known as classical theory of hydrodynamics.

The flow of real fluid differs from an ideal fluid in certain aspects. The particles of fluid adher to the surface on which (or around which) they are moving and acquire the velocity of the surface and hence the 'condition of no slip' prevails at the surface. The viscosity of fluid, thus, resists the motion of fluid and modifies the configuration over and around the boundary. The viscous resistance extends to the whole fluid boundary. This fact was first recognised by the German scientist Prandtl in 1904 and is known as Prandtl's theory of boundary layer. According to Prandtl's hypothesis, the fluid (of small viscosity) flowing along a solid wall may be divided into two independent regions, (1) fluid within a thin region in the negihbourhood of the solid surface and (2) fluid outside this region. The first region is known as bounary layer and the latter as main flow.

There is, however, no sharp division between these two regions, viz. boundary layer and main flow. Most of the velocity variation takes place in the vicinity of the wall and thereby the viscous resistance is predominant in this region. Outside the boundary layer, the velocity approaches the free stream velocity U_0 (also known as ambient or potential velocity). In this region the flow may be regarded practically as irrotational so that ideal fluid theories, including flownet method, may be used to analyse the flow pattern.

The concept of boundary layer is most significant contribution to the development of fluid mechanics. The theory has been successful in giving the physical picture of the role of viscosity in the fluid flow problems and also in predicting the drag force exerted on various shaped bodies, e.g. ships, submarines or bridge piers, etc.

8.2 BOUNDARY LAYER FLOW OVER A FLAT PLATE

Consider a flat plate of width B placed at zero incidence (or parallel to) in an infinite extent of fluid. The uniform velocity of the free stream approaching the flat plate is U_0 (Fig. 8.1). As soon as the fluid comes in contact with the plate at its leading edge, the velocity reduces to zero in accordance with the 'no slip condition'. The velocity changes rapidly from zero at the plate to free stream velocity U_0 within a very short distance normal to the plate causing a large velocity gradient to develop in the boundary layer. As a result of this large velocity gradient, large shear resistance develops along the plate [$\tau = \mu\,(\partial u/\partial y)$]. Thus, even if the viscosity of the fluid may be small (e.g. air and water), large shear resistance is developed over the plate and thereby a sufficiently thick boundary layer is formed along the plate. As the flow proceeds in the downstream direction, more and more fluid is retarded in the lateral direction and hence boundary layer grows in the direction of flow.

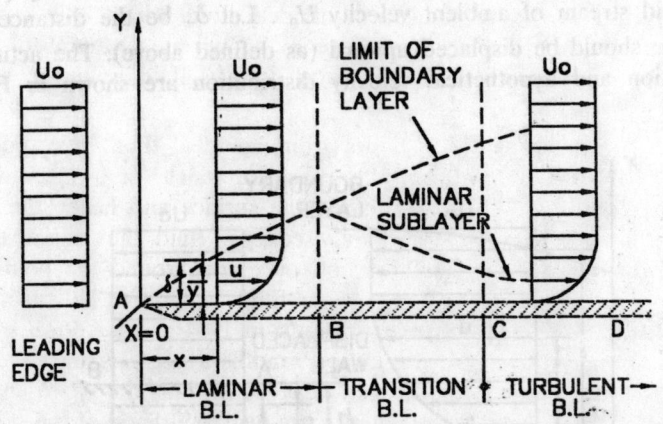

FIG. 8.1 GROWTH OF BOUNDARY LAYER OVER A FLAT PLATE

Near the leading edge of the plate, the flow within boundary layer remains laminar. As the boundary layers grows thicker, more fluid is decelerated from its original uniform motion. The 'laminar boundary layer' flow becomes unstable and finally changes into 'turbulent boundary layer' flow. The transformation from laminar to turbulent takes place gradually through a transition zone called 'transition boundary layer'. The flow in transition boundary layer is partly laminar and partly turbulent in nature; in fact it fluctuates from one to the other. Even within the turbulent region, the flow at a vertical section remains laminar in the immediate vicinity of the plate, passes through transition zone and finally develop into turbulent in nature (Fig. 8.1). The boundary layer developing over a surface is found to be of a few millimeters in thickness.

8.3 BOUNDARY LAYER THICKNESS

The velocity of fluid layer becomes zero at the stationary wall and becomes equal to the free stream velocity U_0 at certain distance normal to the plate.

The variation in velocity takes place asymptotically in vertical direction and hence the distance required will be too large to acquire velociy U_0. Therefore, the boundary thickness is defined in many ways.

(1) *Normal boundary layer thickness* δ. It is defined as the distance normal to the wall where the velocity differs by 1 percent from the free stream velocity U_0. In othe words, $u = 0.99\ U_0$ at $y = \delta$

(2) *Displacement thickness* δ_*. It is defined as the distance normal to the wall by which the actual boundary (or wall) should be shifted in order that actual discharge (volume rate of flow per unit time) would be the same as that of ideal fluid past the displaced boundary. In fact, the displacement boundary layer thickness indicates the distance by which the ambient flow (of velocity U_0) is displaced from the wall due to the growth of boundary layer.

Consider a flat plate of width B (normal to the plane of paper) placed in a fluid stream of ambient velocity U_0. Let δ_* be the distance by which the plate should be displaced upward (as defined above). The actual velocity distribution and hypothetical velocity distribution are shown in Fig. 8.2.

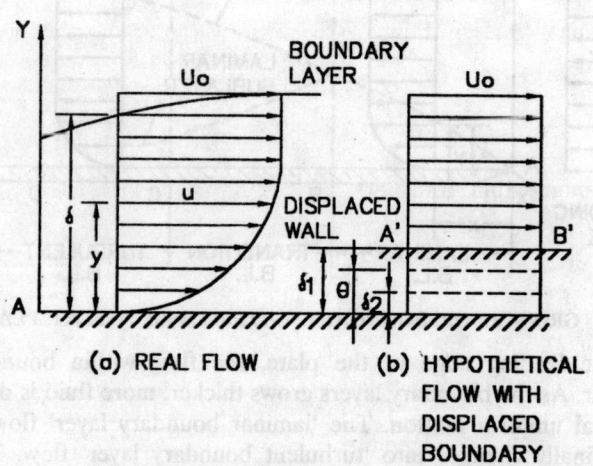

(a) REAL FLOW (b) HYPOTHETICAL FLOW WITH DISPLACED BOUNDARY

FIG. 8.2 BOUNDARY LAYER THICKNESSES

The actual volume of flow across a vertical section, (considering the formation of boundary layer).

$$\int_0^\infty u\,B\,dy = \int_0^\delta u\,B\,dy + \int_\delta^\infty U_0\,B\,dy \qquad ...(i)$$

The total volume of flow, if there would have been no boundary layer.

$$\int_0^\infty U_0\,B\,dy = \int_0^\delta U_0\,B\,dy + \int_\delta^\infty U_0\,B\,dy \qquad ...(ii)$$

From Eqs. (i) and (ii),

The reduction in the flow rate due to the formation of boundary layer

$$= B \int_0^\delta (U_0 - u) \, dy \qquad \text{...(iii)}$$

The total volume of ideal flowing across δ_* with velocity U_0

$$= U_0 B \delta_* \qquad \text{...(iv)}$$

By defintion,

$$U_0 B \delta_* = \int_0^\delta (U_0 - u) \, dy$$

$$\delta_w = \int_0^\infty (1 - u/U_0) \, dy \qquad \text{...(8.2)}$$

(3) *Momentum thickness* θ . It is defined as the distance normal to the boundary by which it is to be shifted such that the momentum flux through this distance θ is equal to the deficiency in the momentum flux caused due to the formation of boundary layer.

The mass rate of flow of real fluid across a vertical section in the boundary layer

$$= \int_0^\delta \rho u B \, dy \qquad \text{...(i)}$$

The momentum transport rate in the boundary layer

$$= \int_0^\delta \rho u^2 B \, dy \qquad \text{...(ii)}$$

The momentum transport rate for the same mass as in Eq. (i) but with velocity U_0

$$= \int_0^\delta (\rho u B \, dy) \, U_0 \qquad \text{...(iii)}$$

Therefore, momentum deficiency caused due to the formation of boundary layer

$$= B \int_0^\delta \rho u \, (U_0 - u) \, dy \qquad \text{...(iv)}$$

Momentum transport rate of ideal fluid across the vertical distance

$$\theta = \rho B \theta U_0^2 \qquad \text{...(v)}$$

From Eqs. (iv) and (v)

$$\rho B \theta U_0^2 = B \int_0^\delta \rho u \, (U_0 - u) \, dy$$

$$\theta = \int\limits_0^\delta (1 - u/U_0)\,(u/U_0)\,dy \qquad \qquad ...(8.3)$$

(4) *Energy thickness* δ_2 . It is also defined in the same manner. It is the distance (normal to the wall) by which the actual wall or boundary be shifted in order that the energy flux of an ideal fluid (moving with velocity U_0) through this distance is equal to the deficiency caused in the energy due to the formation of boundary layer.

The kinetic energy of the real fluid flowing across a vertical section

$$= \int\limits_0^\delta (\rho\,u\,B\,dy)\,u^2/2 \qquad \qquad ...(i)$$

The kinetic energy of the ideal fluid flowing across the vertical section and moving with velocity U_0

$$= \int\limits_0^\delta (\rho\,B\,dy\,u)\,U_0^2/2 \qquad \qquad ...(ii)$$

The deficiency caused in kinetic energy due to the development of boundary layer

$$= \frac{B}{2} \int\limits_0^\delta \rho\,u\,(U_0^2 - u^2)\,dy \qquad \qquad ...(iii)$$

The kinetic energy of ideal fluid passing across an area $B\,\delta_2$

$$= \rho\,B\,\delta_2\,U_0^3/2 \qquad \qquad ...(iv)$$

Equating Eqs. (iii) and (iv)

$$\delta_2 = \int\limits_0^\delta (1 - u^2/U_0^2)\,(u/U_0)\,dy \qquad \qquad ...(8.4)$$

8.4 CHARACTERISTICS OF BOUNDARY LAYER

Consider a flat plate AB placed in a fluid stream of velocity U_0 , the stream lines being parallel to the plate. The boundary layer exhibits the characteristics of laminar boundary layer flow in the region AC, of transitional boundary layer flow in the region CD and of turbulent boundary flow in the region DB in Fig. 8.1. Some of the main characteristics of boundary layer are discussed below.

(1) The boundary layer grows thicker in the direction of flow, *i.e.* $\delta \alpha x$.

(2) The flow of viscous fluid results in a thicker boundary layer, *i.e.* $\delta \alpha \mu$.

(3) The boundary layer remains thin in a high velocity stream, *i.e.* $\delta \alpha 1/U_0$.

(4) As the boundary layer grows thicker the wall shear stress decreases in the direction of flow.

Since $\qquad \tau_0 = \mu \dfrac{\partial u}{\partial y}$,

and ∂y increases and τ_0 decreases in the direction of flow, *i.e.* $\tau \alpha \, 1/x$

(5) It is known that the fluid in the boundary layer is subjected to a pressure gradient from outside the layer. If the pressure decreases in the direction of flow (as happens in contracting channel or pipe), it increases the momentum of the fluid in the boundary layer which results in a thinner boundary layer. If the pressure increases in the direction of flow (flow through a divergng channel, draft tube, etc.), the positive or adverse pressure gradient hastens the growth of boundary layer and a thicker boundary is obtained at the given section.

8.5. BOUNDARY LAYER EQUATIONS

The equations of motion, Eqs. 5.8a and 5.8b alongwith continuity equation, Eq. 4.23c, are sufficient to solve two dimensional fluid flow problems. These equations for steady flow are

$$u \frac{\partial u}{\partial x} + v \frac{\partial u}{\partial y} = -\frac{1}{\rho} \frac{\partial p}{\partial x} \qquad \qquad ...(5.8a)$$

$$u \frac{\partial v}{\partial x} + v \frac{\partial v}{\partial y} = -\frac{1}{\rho} \frac{\partial p}{\partial y} \qquad \qquad ...(5.8b)$$

$$\frac{\partial u}{\partial x} + \frac{\partial v}{\partial y} = 0 \qquad \qquad ...(4.23)$$

These equations have been derived for a ideal fluid but in case of boundary layer flow the viscous forces are also significant and therefore should be considered in the equation of motion. The body forces are not considered to be important in such flows and hence, these have been dropped from Eqs. 5.8a and 5.8b.

Consider a parallelopiped of lengths dx, dy and dz in the three co-ordinate directions respectively (see Fig. 5.1).

The viscous force acting on its lower face $ABCD = \tau \, , dx \, dz$

The viscous force acting on its upper face EFGH

$$= \left(\tau + \frac{\partial \tau}{\partial y} dy \right) dx \, dz$$

Net viscous force acting in X-direction on this pair of faces per unit volume $= \dfrac{\partial \tau}{\partial y}$ $\qquad \qquad ...(8.5a)$

From Eq. 1.8c,

$$\tau = \mu \frac{\partial u}{\partial y}$$

Hence viscous force/unit volume

$$f_{vx1} = \frac{\partial^2 u}{\partial y^2} \qquad \qquad ...(8.5b)$$

It is to be emphasized that there will be another component of shear forces acting on ABHE and BCGF in X-direction (see Fig. 5.1). Therefore, the net viscous force acting in X-direction will be the summation of the two terms.

$$f_{vx} = \mu \left(\frac{\partial^2 u}{\partial x^2} + \frac{\partial^2 u}{\partial y^2} \right) \qquad ...(8.5c)$$

Therefore, the complete equation of motion for 2-D steady flow becomes

$$u \frac{\partial u}{\partial x} + v \frac{\partial u}{\partial y} = -\frac{1}{\rho} \frac{\partial p}{\partial x} + \gamma \left(\frac{\partial^2 u}{\partial x^2} + \frac{\partial^2 u}{\partial y^2} \right) \qquad ...(8.6a)$$

$$u \frac{\partial v}{\partial x} + v \frac{\partial v}{\partial y} = -\frac{1}{\rho} \frac{\partial p}{\partial y} + \gamma \left(\frac{\partial^2 v}{\partial x^2} + \frac{\partial^2 v}{\sigma y^2} \right) \qquad ...(8.6b)$$

$$\frac{\partial u}{\partial x} + \frac{\partial v}{\partial y} = 0 \qquad ...(8.6c)$$

These equations, Eqs. 8.6a to 8.6c are known as the 'Navier Stokes' equations for 2-D viscous flow; the body forces being not included in it. The solution of these equations yield the velocity distribution in X and Y directions. The pressure is supposed to be impressed on the boundary layer flow from outside it (see Eq. 8.8) and can be determined from irrotational fluid flow theory (*i.e.* by the use of Bernoulli's equation). Using the known velocity and pressure distributions, the resisting force (or drag) on any object immersed in the fluid may now be determined. The solution of the equations, Eqs. 8.6a to 8.6c (which are non-homogeneous, non-linear partial differential equations) is too much involved. Therefore, the following assumptions are made in solving the above equations.

(1) The boundary layer theory is essentially developed for flows at high Reynolds number. This means the boundary layer thickness is too small in comparison to any characteristic dimension of boundary surface; $\delta \leq L$

. (2) The viscosity and density of the fluid are assumed to remain constant and the isothermal conditions prevail in the flow.

(3) The boundary surface is streamlined so that the flow pattern and pressure determined by ideal fluid theory are accurate.

The above assumptions result in the following approximations.

(1) The pressure does not vary across any given section of boundary layer. Therefore, the pressure determined by the ideal fluid theory at the edge of the boundary layer holds within the boundary layer also.

(2) The flow in the boundary layer is essentially parallel and viscous (shear) stresses are determined by Newton's law of viscosity. The turbulent shear stresses are negligible as the velocity fluctuations die out near the boundary surface.

(3) The curvature of the boundary is gentle and therefore the co-ordinate axes are taken as X in the direction of flow and Y in the direction normal to the boundary wall.

The following boundary conditions should be satisfied to solve the above equations, Eqs. 8.6a to c.

(1) The condition of 'no slip' at the boundary, *i.e.* at $y = 0$, $u = 0$ and $v = 0$

(2) The velocity u approaches the free stream velocity U_0 at the outer edge of the boundary layer.

(3) The application of Bernoulli's equation to the flow in the boundary layer yields

$$p + \frac{1}{2}\rho U_0^2 = \text{constant}$$

The equation of motion are simplified by writing the order of magnitude of various terms and then dropping the terms of very small order of magnitude. In this way, Eqs. 8.6a to 8.6c reduce to

$$u\frac{\partial u}{\partial x} + v\frac{\partial u}{\partial y} = -\frac{1}{\rho}\frac{\partial p}{\partial x} + v\frac{\partial^2 u}{\partial y^2} \qquad ...(8.7a)$$

$$\frac{\partial u}{\partial x} + \frac{\partial v}{\partial y} = 0 \qquad ...(8.7b)$$

Eq. 8.6b reduces to

$$-\frac{1}{\rho}\frac{\partial p}{\partial y} = 0 \qquad ...(8.8)$$

Eq. 8.8 shows that the pressure in the boundary layer does not vary in the normal direction. The above two relations, Eqs. 8.7a and 8.7b are known as 'Prandtl's boundary layer equations'. These equations can now be solved easily alongwith Eq. 8.8 to determine the unknown velocity components u and v; p is assumed to be known from ideal fluid theory or by the of Bernoulli's equation.

8.6 MOMENTUM INTEGRAL EQUATION

A complete solution of boundary layer equation for a given body is very complex and too much time consuming. Also, many times one is interested in the quantities of integral nature such as total resisting force or drag, etc. For this purpose, Theodore Von Karman obtained integral equation in 1921. The momentum integral method is an approximate method and yields accurate results for simple problems of boundary layer. It is applicable for both laminar and turbulent boundary layer flows.

The Von Karman momentum integral equation of the boundary layer represents the relation between the rate of change of momentum across a section of boundary layer and the surface forces due to the wall shearing stress and pressure gradient.

Consider a control volume ABECD of the fluid of unit width normal to the plane of paper as shown in Fig. 8.3. Let the boundary layer thickness developing over a flat plate be δ and $\delta + \Delta\delta$ at two vertical section AB and CD respectively. The horizontal distance between these two sections is Δx The pressure acting on fluid element *ABCD* varies in the longitudinal direction from p to $p + \Delta p$. Thus pressure acting on BE is average of these two values, *i.e.* $(p + \Delta p/2)$

Applying momentum equation in X-direction to the control volume ABECD.

ΣF_x= Rate of change of momentum in X-direction

= [Rate of momentum outflow − Rate of momentum inflow]   ...(8.9a)

The mass of fluid entering through AB

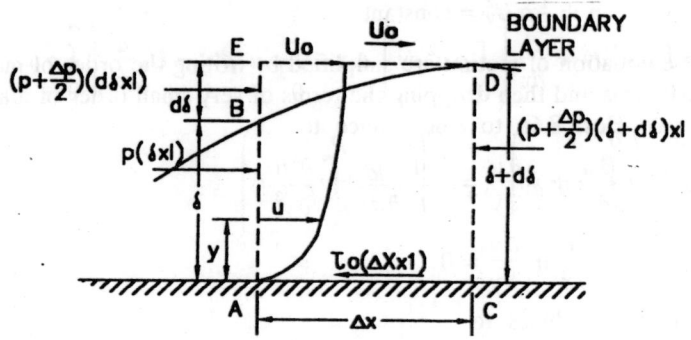

FIG. 8.3 MOMENTUM INTEGRAL EQUATION

$$= \int_0^\delta \rho\, u\, dy \qquad \qquad ...(i)$$

The mass of fluid going out through CD

$$= \int_0^\delta \rho\, u\, dy + \frac{d}{dx}\left(\int_0^\delta \rho\, u\, dy \right) \Delta x \qquad ...(ii)$$

Since no flow takes place through AC, the difference of two mass rate enters into control volume through its face BD.

The mass of fluid entering through *BD*

$$= \frac{d}{dx}\left(\int_0^\delta \rho\, u\, dy \right) \Delta x \qquad ...(iii)$$

The momentum of fluid entering through *AB*

$$= \int_0^\delta \rho\, u^2\, dy \qquad \qquad ...(iv)$$

The momentum of fluid going out through *CD*

$$= \int_0^\delta \rho\, u^2\, dy + \frac{d}{dx}\left(\int_0^\delta \rho\, u^2\, dy \right) \Delta x \qquad ...(v)$$

The momentum brought in by the fluid entering through face BD which was moving with ambient velocity U_0

$$= U_0 \frac{d}{dx} \left(\int_0^\delta \rho u \, dy \right) \Delta x \qquad \text{...(vi)}$$

From Eqs. (iv) to (vi)

The rate of change of momentum

$$= \int_0^\delta \rho u^2 \, dy + \frac{d}{dx} \left(\int_0^\delta \rho u^2 \, dy \right) \Delta x - \int_0^\delta \rho u^2 \, dy - U_0 \frac{d}{dx} \left(\int_0^\delta \rho u \, dy \right) \Delta x$$

$$= \frac{d}{dx} \left(\int_0^\delta \rho u^2 \, dy \right) \Delta x - \left(U_0 \frac{d}{dx} \int_0^\rho \rho u \, dy \right) \Delta x \qquad \text{...(vii)}$$

The forces acting on the fluid in the control volume ABECD are (i) pressure forces acting on faces AB , BE and CD and (ii) shear force τ_0 acting along the wall. Since the velocity gradients are practially zero at the edge of boundary layer and hence no shear stress acts along this surface, therefore,

$$\Sigma F_x = p \, (\delta \times 1) + (p + \Delta p/2) \, (\Delta \delta \times 1)$$
$$- (p + \Delta p) \, (\delta + \Delta \delta) \times 1 - \tau_0 \, (\Delta x \times 1)$$

Simplifying

$$\Sigma F_x = - (\Delta p \, \delta + \tau_0 \Delta x) \qquad \text{...(viii)}$$

neglecting second order terms.

Substituting the valuces in Eq. 8.9

$$\tau_0 = U_0 \frac{d}{dx} \left(\int_0^\delta \rho u \, dy \right) - \frac{d}{dx} \left(\int_0^\delta \rho u^2 \, dy \right) - \delta \frac{dp}{dx} \qquad \text{...(8.9b)}$$

(a) The first bracketed term in right hand side may be written as

$$U_0 \frac{d}{dx} \left(\int_0^\delta \rho u \, dy \right) = \frac{d}{dx} \left(\int_0^\delta \rho u \, dy \right) (U_0)$$

$$- \left(\int_0^\delta \rho u \, dy \right) \frac{d U_0}{dx} \qquad \text{...(ix)}$$

(b) The ambient pressure p can be determined by Bernoulli's equation

$$p + \frac{\rho U_0^2}{2} = C \qquad \text{...(x)}$$

Differenting with respect to x on both sides

$$\frac{dp}{dx} = -\rho \, U_0 \frac{d \, U_0}{dx} \qquad \qquad ...(xi)$$

(c) The boundary layer thickness δ may be written as

$$\delta = \int_0^{\delta} dy \qquad \qquad ...(xii)$$

Substituting the vlaues of various terms from (ix) to (xii) into Eq. 8.9b

$$\tau_0 = \frac{d}{dx}\left(\int_0^{\delta} \rho \, u \, dy\right)(U_0) - \left(\int_0^{\delta} \rho \, u \, dy\right)\left(\frac{d \, U_0}{dx}\right)$$

$$- \left(\frac{d}{dx}\int_0^{\delta} \rho \, u^2 \, dy\right) + \left(\int_0^{\delta} dy\right)\left(\rho \, U_0 \frac{d \, U_0}{dx}\right)$$

$$\tau_0 = \frac{d \, U_0}{dx}\left(\int_0^{\delta} \rho \, (U_0 - u) \, dy\right) + \frac{d}{dx}\left(\int_0^{\delta} \rho \, u \, (U_0 - u) \, dy\right)$$

From Eqs. 8.2 and 8.3

$$\delta_* \, U_0 = \int_0^{\delta} (U_0 - u) \, dy$$

and

$$\theta \, U_0^2 = \int_0^{\delta} (U_0 - u) \, u dy$$

Substituting these values of δ_* and θ

$$\frac{\tau_0}{\rho} = \delta_* \, U_0 \frac{d \, U_0}{dx} + \frac{d}{dx}(\theta \, U_0^2)$$

Simplifying,

$$\frac{\tau_0}{\rho} = U_0 \, (\delta_* + 2 \, \theta) \frac{dU_0}{dx} + U_0^2 \frac{d \, \theta}{dx} \qquad \qquad ...(8.10)$$

Eq. 8.10 is known as momentum integral equation or Von Karman's integral equation. This equation can be used to determine the wall shear stress at any section or wall. For this purpose, the velocity distribution must be known so as to compute δ_* and θ (from Eqs. 8.2 and 8.3). If the velocity distribution is accurate enough, the resulting shear stress obtained from Eq. 8.10 matches with the result obtained by exact solutions of boundary layer equations. For the flow over a flat plate with no pressure gradient ($\partial p/dx = 0$) in the direction of flow, Eq. 8.10 reduces to

$$\frac{\tau_0}{\rho} = U_0^2 \frac{d \, \theta}{dx} \qquad \qquad ...(8.11)$$

The method involves the following steps.

(1) Obtain velocity profiles at various sections in the longitudinal direction

(2) Compute the momentum thickness θ from Eq. 8.3.

(3) Draw a plot between θ versus x .

(4) The product of the slope of this curve at any given section, distant x from leading edge and ρU_0^2 is equal the shear stress at this section. U_0 is the ambient or free stream velocity and ρ is the specific mass of the fluid is which the plate is placed.

8.7 LAMINAR BOUNDARY LAYER

As discussed earlier, the flow in the initial stages of boundary layer development exhibts the characteristics of laminar motion. The laminar motion is characterised by low Reynolds number of flow, which is defined as

$$R_e = \frac{U_0 x}{v}$$

In this expression, x denotes the distance measured from the leading edge of the plate, U_0 is the ambient or free stream velocity and v is the kinematic viscosity of the fluid.

It is obvious that viscous forces are predominant inside the boundary layer whereas the inertia forces are predominant outside it. Therefore, it is reasonable to assume that both viscous and inertia forces will be of the same order of magnitude at the edge of boundary layer. Dimensions of f_i and f_v may, now be written down.

The viscous forces per unit volume

$$f_v = \frac{\partial \tau}{\partial y} \qquad \qquad ...(8.5a)$$

$$= \mu \frac{\partial^2 u}{\partial y^2} \approx \mu \frac{\partial}{\partial y} \left(\frac{\partial u}{\partial y} \right)$$

$$= [\mu U_0/\delta^2] \qquad \qquad ...(i)$$

The inertia forces per unit volume

$$f_i = \rho \, a_x$$

$$= \rho u \frac{du}{dx}$$

$$= [\rho U_0^2/x] \qquad \qquad ...(ii)$$

From Eqs. (i) and (ii)

Inertia force = O (viscous force)

$$[\rho U_0^2/x] = k \, [\mu U_0/\delta^2]$$

Solving it, $\qquad \delta/x = k/\sqrt{R_e} \qquad \qquad ...(8.13)$

where k is a constant and should be determined either experimentally or analytically.

Exact solution. Blasius solved the boundary layer equations for 2-D flows developing over a flat plate placed at zero incidence. The pressure gradient for the flow in normal direction ($\partial p/\partial y = 0$) was assumed to be zero. Blasius assumed that the velocity profiles through the boundary layer remained geometrically similar along the whole length of the laminar section. This may be expressed as

$$\frac{u}{U_0} = f(y/\delta) = f(\eta) \qquad \qquad ...(8.14)$$

But from Eq. 8.13 $\delta \alpha \sqrt{vx/U_0}$

Therefore $\qquad \eta = y/\delta = y \sqrt{U_0/vx} \qquad \qquad ...(8.15)$

Blasius transformed the partial differential boundary layer equations, Eqs. 8.7a and 8.7b into differential equations and obtained the solution of these equations in the form of power series expansion. The values of non-dimensional velocity u/U_b versus y/δ have been tabulated. According to the definition of boundary layer thickness, $u = 0.99 U_0$ at the edge of boundary layer. The value of y/δ ($= y \sqrt{U_0/vx}$) corresponding to $u/U_0 = 0.99$ is found to be equal to 4.91. Thus, from Eq. 8.14,

$$y \sqrt{U_0/vx} = 4.91 \text{ at } y = \delta$$

Rearraning the terms

$$\frac{\delta}{x} = \frac{4.91}{\sqrt{Re_x}} \qquad \qquad ...(8.16a)$$

The value of constant of proportionality equal to 4.91 in Eq. 8.13 has been found for the flow of zero pressure gradient. If the flow is not uniform but U_0 varies with x so that there exists a longitudinal pressure gradient in the flow, the value of constant k also varies. Many authors use a value of k as 5 instead of 4.91. Thus the ratio of δ to x is also written as,

$$\frac{\delta}{x} = \frac{5}{\sqrt{Re_x}} \qquad \qquad ...(8.16b)$$

Table 8.1 gives the value of δ and drag coefficient C_f for various velocity distirubitons obtained in laminar boundary layer.

Using the value of u/U_0 from the table of power series expansion, Blasius obtained the following relationship

$$\delta_* = \int_*^\delta (1 - u/U_0)\, dy = 1.729\, x/\sqrt{Re_x} \qquad \qquad ...(8.17)$$

$$\theta = \int_0^\delta (1 - u/U_0)\, u/U_{04}\, dy = 0.664\, x/\sqrt{Re_x} \qquad \qquad ...(8.18)$$

The velocity gradient at the wall is given by

$$\left(\frac{\partial u}{\partial y}\right)_{y=0} = 0.332\, U_0 \sqrt{Re_x/x} \qquad \qquad ...(8.19)$$

The shear stress τ_0 at the wall can be computed using Eq. 1.8c.

$$(\tau_0)_{y-0} = 0.332 \frac{\mu U_0}{x} \sqrt{Re_x} \qquad ...(8.20)$$

Table 8.1

Velocity distribution	δ	C_f
(a) $\dfrac{u}{U_0} = 2\left(\dfrac{y}{\delta}\right) - \left(\dfrac{y}{\delta}\right)^2$	$5.48/\sqrt{Re_x}$	$1.46/\sqrt{Re_x}$
(b) $\dfrac{u}{U_0} = \dfrac{3}{2}\left(\dfrac{y}{\delta}\right) - \dfrac{1}{2}\left(\dfrac{y}{\delta}\right)^3$	$4.56/\sqrt{Re_x}$	$1.292/\sqrt{Re_x}$
(c) $\dfrac{u}{U_0} = 2\left(\dfrac{y}{\delta}\right) - 2\left(\dfrac{y}{\delta}\right)^3 + \left(\dfrac{y}{\delta}\right)^4$	$5.853/\sqrt{Re_x}$	$1.371/\sqrt{Re_x}$
(d) Exact solution of BL Eqs. (Blasius)	$5/\sqrt{Re_x}$	$1.328/\sqrt{Re_x}$

Usually the ratio of τ_0 to dynamic pressure of the free stream $\rho\, U_0^2/2$ is defined as the local drag coefficient c_f or local skin friction coefficient c_f.

$$c_f = \frac{\tau_0}{\frac{1}{2}\rho\, U_0^2} = \frac{0.664}{\sqrt{Re_x}} \qquad ...(8.21)$$

The local skin friction coefficient c_t is a function of longitudinal distance x and decreases in the direction of flow for negative pressure gradient flow $(\partial p/\partial x < 0)$. The total resisting force or drag F_D over a flat plate of length L and width B (normal to the direction of flow) may now be determined by summing up the shear stress acting over its whole length.

$$F_D = \int_0^L \tau_0 B\, dx \qquad ...(8.22)$$

The average drag coefficient C_f is similarly defined as

$$C_f = \frac{F_D/A}{0.5\rho\, U_0^2} = \frac{1.328}{\sqrt{Re_L}} \qquad ...(8.23a)$$

or $$F_D = C_f A \rho\, U_0^2/2 \qquad ...(8.23b)$$

$$= \frac{1.328}{\sqrt{Re_L}} A \left(\frac{\rho\, U_0^2}{2}\right) \qquad ...(8.23c)$$

where A is the wetted area of the plate and R_{eL} is known as 'plate Reynolds number'. Thus it is seen that the characteristic of laminar boundary layer flow is dependent on Reynolds number of flow Re_x or in other words on the velocity profile. The velocity distribution in laminar boundary layer is parabolic in nature. There may be a number of velocity distributions describing the flow in the laminar boundary layer. But all such velocity distributions should satisfy the following essential boundary conditions.

(a) At $y = 0$, $u = 0$ \qquad ...(i)

(b) At $y = \delta$, $u \to U_0$

$$\frac{\partial u}{\partial y} \to 0 \qquad \qquad ...(iii)$$

$$\partial^2 u / \partial y^2 \to 0 \qquad \qquad ...(iv)$$

Some of the velocity profiles satisfying above conditions are of the form

(a) $\qquad u/U_0 = a + by + cy^2 \qquad \qquad ...(8.24a)$

(b) $\qquad u/U_0 = ay + by^3 \qquad \qquad ...(8.24b)$

8.8 TRANSITIONAL BOUNDARY LAYER

If the plate is of sufficient length, the eddies are developed in the flow which give rise to turbulence with in the bondary layer. The critical vlaue of Reynolds number Re_{cr} signifying the transormation of flow in the boundary layer from laminar to turbulent may range from 3×10^5 or 6×10^5. Indeed, the R_{ecr} depends on many factos. Some of the important ones are (i) Reynolds number of flow, (ii) free stream turbulence, (iii) roughness of the plate (iv) curvature of the plate and (v) pressure gradient in the flow.

The effect of Reynolds number of the value of critical Reynolds number R_{eer} is clearly seen from Hansen's experimental data for boundary layer flow occurring over a smooth plate, being plotted in Fig. 8.4. The effect of free stream turbulence on R_{eer} can be studied by plotting percentage of turbulence in the flow against Reynolds number.

$$\% \text{ turbulence} = (u'/U_0) \times 100 \qquad \qquad ...(8.25)$$

where u' is the fluctuating velocity in the direction of flow and is equal to the difference between instantaneous velocity u and time average velocity $\bar{u}$. The data of Schubauer et. al. are shown plotted in Fig. 8.5 which show that transition takes place once the turbulence exceeds 0.15%.

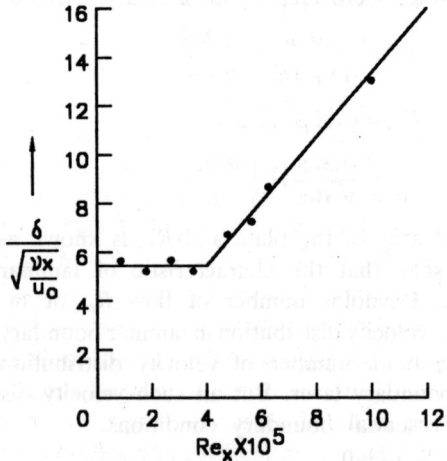

FIG. 8.4 VARIATION OF BOUNDARY LAYER THICKNESS
WITH REYNOLDS NUMBER OF FLOW

The boundary roughness near the leading edge hastens the transition from laminar to turbulent boundary layer. Similarly if the pressure gradient

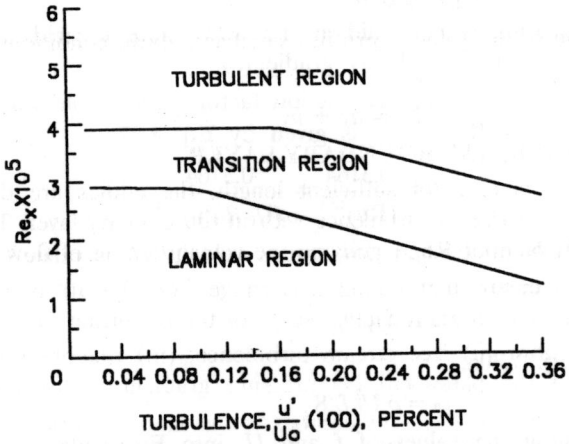

FIG. 8.5 VARIATION OF BOUNDARY LAYER THICKNESS
WITH PERCENTAGE OF TURBULENCE

in the flow is positive (flow occurring in a diverging channel), a lower R_{eer} is expected. Actually, the critical Reynolds number R_{eer} oscillates within a range of Reynolds number. For R_{ex} equal to 10^5, the lamianr boundary layer is very much stable but becomes unstable at R_{ex} equal to 2×10^5. Indeed, the transition may take place within the range of Re_x equal to 2×10^5. In practice, an average value of R_{eer} based on distance x (from the leading edge) is taken as 5×10^5 at which the boundary layer definitely becomes turbulent.

8.9 TURBULENT BOUNDARY LAYER

The presence of turbulence in the boundary layer considerably modifies the velocity distribution and the bondary layer grows at faster rate in the direction of flow. The turbulent boundary layer is distinguished from laminar boundary layer by its larger thickness. The process of transverse mixing tends to made the boundary layer flow more uniform throughout the cross section (resulting in logarithmic velocity distribution) except in the immediate vicinity of the boundary layer. This means a rapid change in velocity (from zero to U_0) takes place in the small distance near the wall, thereby giving a high value of velcity gradient. This in turn gives a larger wall shear stress ($\tau \propto \partial u / \partial y$) at a section as compared to laminar boundary layer.

The turbulent flow parameters could be computed provided the wall shear stress is known in terms of time averaged mean velocity, i.e. turbulent shear stress must be included alongwith viscous shear stress. Such a relation is too much complex. Hence an approximate solution could be obtained using momentum integral equation, provided a reasonable velocity profile for turbulent flow is assumed. In addition some relation for shear stress should also be assumed. For example, the 'one seventh power law' for velocity distribution in smooth pipe is found to be valid for the flow over flat plate.

$$(u/U_0) = (y/\delta)^{1/7} \qquad \qquad ...(8.26)$$

This equation is not valid at the wall where it yields an impossible value of infinity for the velocity gradient.

The Blasius equation for friction factor f applicable within the range of R_e equal to 5×10^5 to 10^7 is given by Eq. 8.27,

$$f = \frac{0.3164}{(\text{Re})^{1/4}} = \frac{0.3164}{(U_0 R_0/v)^{1/4}} \qquad ...(8.27)$$

For a fully established flow, mean velocity U_0 is related to maximum velocity at the centre line.

$$U_0 = 0.8\, U_{max}$$

From Eq. 7.30a,

$$\tau_0 = \rho\, U_0^2 f/8 \qquad \qquad ...(7.30a)$$

Substituting the values of f and U_0 into Eq. 7.30a,

$$\tau_0 = \frac{\rho}{8} (0.8\, U_{max})^2 \times 0.3164 / \left(\frac{0.8\, U_{max} R_0}{v} \right)^{1/4}$$

$$= 0.0225\, \rho\, U_{max}^2 \left(\frac{v}{U_{max} R_0} \right)^{1/4} \qquad ...(8.28)$$

The above equation applicable to pipe flow can also be used to flat plate if it is assumed that a pipe is made by wrapping a flat plate. In that case at $R_0 = \delta$, $U_{max} = U_0$, i.e. free stream velocity.

Hence $\qquad \tau_0 = 0.0225\, \rho\, U_0^2 (v/U_0 \delta)^{1/4} \qquad ...(8.29)$

The momentum thickness θ can be computed by Eq. 8.3 for the assumed 'one seventh power law' of velocity distribution.

$$\theta = \int_0^\delta (1 - u/U_0)\, u/U_0 \; dy = \int_0^\delta [1 - (y/\delta)^{1/7}] \, (y/\delta)^{1/7} \, dy$$

$$= (7/72)\, \delta \qquad \qquad ...(8.30)$$

Substituting the values of τ_0 and θ from Eqs. 8.29 and 8.30 into Eq. 8.11

$$0.0225 \left(\frac{v}{U_0 \delta} \right)^{1/4} = \frac{7}{72} \frac{d\delta}{dx}$$

$$\delta^{1/4} \, d\delta = 0.232\, (v/U_0)^{1/4} \, dx \qquad ...(8.31a)$$

Solving it for whole turbulent boundary layer with the known boundary condition, $\delta = 0$ at $x = 0$ (i.e. at leading edge of the plate) yields

$$\frac{\delta}{x} = \frac{0.37}{(R_{ex})^{1/5}} \qquad \text{...(8.31b)}$$

Similarly other relationships can be derived. These are

$$\frac{\delta_*}{x} = \frac{0.046}{(R_{ex})^{1/5}} = \frac{1}{8}\frac{\delta}{x} \qquad \text{...(8.32)}$$

$$\frac{\theta}{x} = \frac{0.036}{(R_{ex})^{1/5}} = \frac{7}{72}\frac{\delta}{x} \qquad \text{...(8.33)}$$

$$c_f = \frac{\tau_0}{0.5\,\rho\,U_0^2} = \frac{0.059}{(R_{ex})^{1/5}} \qquad \text{...(8.34)}$$

$$C_f = \frac{F_D/A}{0.5\,\rho\,U_*^2} = \frac{0.074}{(R_{ex})^{1/5}} \qquad \text{...(8.35)}$$

It should be noted that these equations are valid for R_e varying within the range of 5×10^5 to 10^7 and for the given one seventh law of velocity distribution. If any other velocity distribution is used, the resulting relation will also be different. Schlichting used logarithmic velocity distribution for turbulent flow which is valid for R_e varying in the range of 5×10^5 to 10^9

The average drag coefficient C_f is then given by

$$C_f = \frac{F_D/A}{0.5\,\rho\,U_0^2} = \frac{0.455}{(\log_{10} R_{eL})^{2.58}} \qquad \text{...(8.36)}$$

Usually the boundary layer develping over a solid boundary remains laminar over the forward portion of the plate and changes to turbulent flow further downstream. The drag or resisting force F_D due to the growth of lamianr boundary layer over x distance in the forward portion of the boundary is given by Eq. 8.23.

$$(F_D)_{lam} = C_f A \rho\, U_0^2/2 = \frac{1.328}{\sqrt{R_{ecr}}} B \times \rho\, U_0^2/2 \qquad \text{...(8.27)}$$

The drag on the remaining rear portion of the plate over which the turbulent boundary layer is formed can be computed by first assuming the turbulent flow to occur over the entire length of the boundary and then substracting the drag due to turbulent boundary layer on the forward portion of the plate. Therefore,

$$(F_D)_{turb} = \left[\frac{0.074\,BL}{(R_{eL})^{1/5}} - \frac{0.074\,Bx}{(R_{ex})^{1/5}} \right] \frac{\rho\, U_0^2}{2} \qquad \text{...(8.38)}$$

The sum of Eqs. 8.37 and 8.38 gives the total drag on the entire plate

$$F_D = \left[\frac{1.328\,Bx}{\sqrt{R_{ecr}}} + \frac{0.074\,BL}{(R_{eL})^{1/5}} - \frac{0.074\,Bx}{(R_{ex})^{1/5}} \right] \frac{\rho\, U_0^2}{2} \qquad \text{...(8.39)}$$

Hence, the average drag coefficient C_f is given by

$$(C_f)_{total} = \left[\frac{1.328\,x/L}{\sqrt{R_{eer}}} + \frac{0.074}{(R_{eL})^{1/5}} - \frac{0.074\,x/L}{(R_{ex})^{1/5}} \right] \qquad \text{...(8.40)}$$

Also $\dfrac{x}{L} = \left[\dfrac{\rho\,U_0 x}{\mu}\right) \Big/ \left(\dfrac{\mu}{\rho\,U_0 L}\right) = \dfrac{(R_{ex})_{er}}{(R_{eL})^{1/5}}$ ...(8.41)

Eq. 8.40 modies to

$$(C_f)_{total} = \dfrac{0.074}{(R_{eL})^{1/5}} - \dfrac{1}{(R_{eL})}\,(0.074\,R_{ex}^{4/5} - 1.328\,R_{ex}^{1/2})$$ ...(8.42)

Substituting R_{ex} equal to 5×10^5,

$$C_f = \left[\dfrac{0.074}{(R_{eL})^{1/5}} - \dfrac{1700}{R_{eL}}\right]$$ ...(8.43)

. Eq. 8.43 is valid for R_e varying from 5×10^5 to 10^7 . The numerical constant 1700 in Eq. 8.43 depends on critical Reynolds number R_{ecr}[1]. To determine C_f for higher range of R_{eL}, Eq. 8.36 should be used in Eq. 8.38 which is valid for value of R_e upto 10^9. Fig. 8.6 shows the variation of C_f with R_{eL}. Also the the Table 8.2 gives the values of numerical constant (for Eq. 8.43) corresponding to various values of $(R_{ex})_{er}$

Table 8.2

$(R_{ex})_{er}$	3×10^5	5×10^5	10^6	3×10^6
Constant	1050	1700	3300	8700

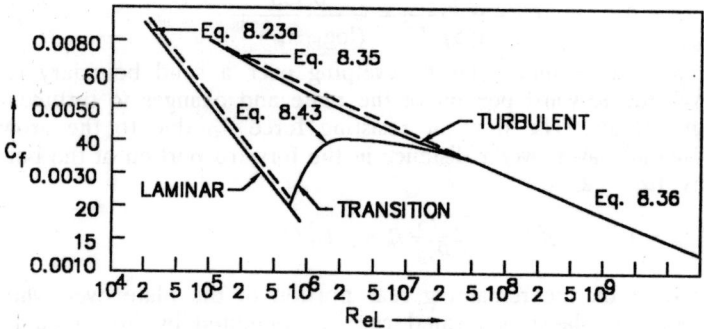

FIG. 8.6 VARIATION OF C_f with R_{eL}

8.10 LAMINAR SUBLAYER

Even in the case of turbulent boundary layrer the flow in the immediate vicinity of smooth boundary exhibits the characteristics of lamianr flow. This narrow region is known as 'laminar sublayer δ' (see also Fig. 8.1). Experimental results have shown that δ' is given by

$$\delta' = 11.6\,v/U_*$$ ...(8.44)

where U_* equal to $\sqrt{\tau_0/\rho}$ is known as shear or friction velocity and τ_0 is the wall shear stress.

---

1. Refer Table 8.2

8.11 ESTABLISHMENT OF FLOW

While the simple illustration of flow along a flat plate has been used to introduce the concept of boundary layer, the boundary layer phenomenon plays an important role in practically every case of flow over various forms of boundary. When the flow enters the inlet pipe from a reservoir, a laminar boundary layer is developed from its leading edge or entrance. Thickening of boundary layer causes the decrease in core area or higher core velocity. This fact also causes the reduced velocity gradient (or decreasing rate of shear stress) at the wall. The gradually expanding boundary layear finally meets at the centre line approximately at a distance x given by

$$\frac{x}{D} = 0.07 \frac{U_0 D}{v} = 0.07 R_0 \qquad \qquad ...(8.45)$$

(Eq. 8.45 has been suggested by Hunter Rouse). Thereafter the laminar flow is fully established and parabolic velocity distrubution describes the laminar motion. The length x required for the establishment of lamianr flow in the pipe depends on many factors; some of them being the shape of entrance and initial turbulence present in the flow.

If the Reynolds number of flow is sufficiently high, the lamianr boundary layer becomes unstable and thereafter transforms into turbulent boundary layer. A fully developed turbulent flow is established approximately at a distance x given by Eq. 8.46.

$$x \approx 50 D \qquad \qquad ...(8.46)$$

where D is the diameter of the pipe and is measured from the entrance section. In the fully turbulent region, the flow is described by logarithmic

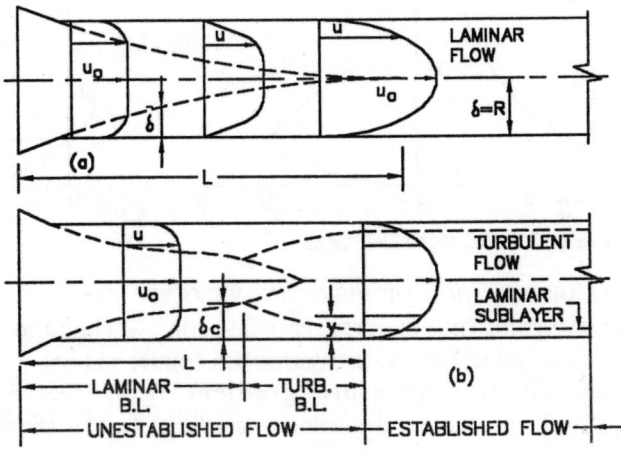

FIG. 8.7 ESTABLISHMENT OF FLOW (a) LAMINAR B.L. (b) TURBULENT B.L. velocity distrubution. The wall shear is also found more inthe region of turbulent flow.

8.12 FLOW UNDER PRESSURE GRADIENT

In the previous sections, the boundary layer flow under zero pressure gradient has been described. Outside the boundary layer, the Prandtl's boundary layer equations, Eqs. 8.7 and 8.8 reduce to

$$U_0 \frac{\partial U}{\partial x} = -\frac{1}{\rho} \frac{\partial p}{\partial x} \qquad \ldots(8.47)$$

and

$$\frac{\partial p}{\partial y} = 0 \qquad \ldots(8.8)$$

which indicates that the outside pressure p is transmitted without any change through the boundary layer to the surface. At the wall, (where $y = 0$) velocity components u and v are zero and hence boundary layer equation, Eq. 8.7a becomes

$$\mu \frac{\partial^2 u}{\partial y^2} = \frac{\partial p}{\partial x} \qquad \ldots(8.48)$$

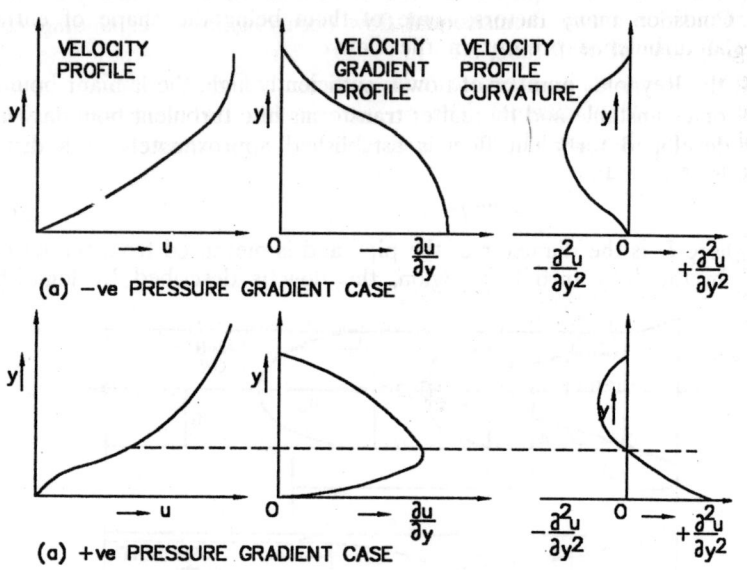

FIG. 8.8 DISTRIBUTION OF VELOCITY, VELOCITY GRADIENT AND
CURVATURE OF VELOCITY PROFILE FOR –ve PRESSURE
GRADIENT, & +ve PRESSURE GRADIENT FLOWS

In case of zero pressure gradient flow, Eq. 8.48 yields $(\partial^2 u / \partial y^2)_{y=0} = 0$ and hence the velocity gradient $\partial u / \partial y$ should decrease steadily from a postiive value at the wall to zero at the outer edge of the boundary layer (Fig. 8.8). It means the velocity profile must have a steadily decreasing form, i.e. it should have no inflection point. In case of negative pressure gradient flow, Eq. 8.48 results in $\partial^2 u / \partial y^2 < 0$ near the boundary. As one moves across a vertical section, the velocity approaches the free stream velocity asymptotically and therefore $\partial u / dy$ should decreases continuously at a slower rate. This means that $(\partial^2 u / \partial y^2)_{y=0}$ is always negative near the outer edge of the boundary layer. In case of positive pressure gradient flow (adverse pressure gradient flow), above equation, Eq. 8.48 yields positive curvature of streamlines near the boundary ($\partial^2 u / \partial y^2 > 0$). However, near the outer edge, still the previous argument of negative curvature of streamlines holds good. This means that there should be a point of inflection in the velocity profile as shown in Fig. 8.8. The positive pressure gradient flow is being maintained by inertia force whereas it is being resisted by viscous resistance as well as adverse pressure gradient force. These resisting forces cause the rapid grwoth of boundary layer and sometimes result in the separation of boundary layer. There are numerous examples of positive pressure gradient flows, e.g. flow in a diverging cone of venturimeter, draft tube, flow around sharp corners and bridge piers, etc.

8.13 SEPARATION OF BOUNDARY LAYER

Consider a two diemsnsional flow occurring in an expanding channel (diverging cone of draft tube, etc.) in Fig. 8.9. The pressure gradient is negative on the left side (*i.e.* the pressure reduces in the direction of flow) and positive on the right side of channel. The pressure variation and velocity distribution describing the flow are shown in Fig. 8.9b and 8.9a respectively. As the flow proceeds from left to right side of the channel, the velocity increases and pressure decreases in the direction of flow. The pressure gradient becomes zero at O, thereafter the pressure gradient becomes positive. The positive pressure gradient decelerates the flow and causes the thicker boundary layer. The resisting forces increasingly distort the velocity distribution and decrease the momentum of the flow in the boundary layers. If the resisting forces, viz. viscous shear and longitudinal adverse pressure gradient, act over a sufficient distance the boundary layer comes to rest just as at point A in Fig. 8.9a.

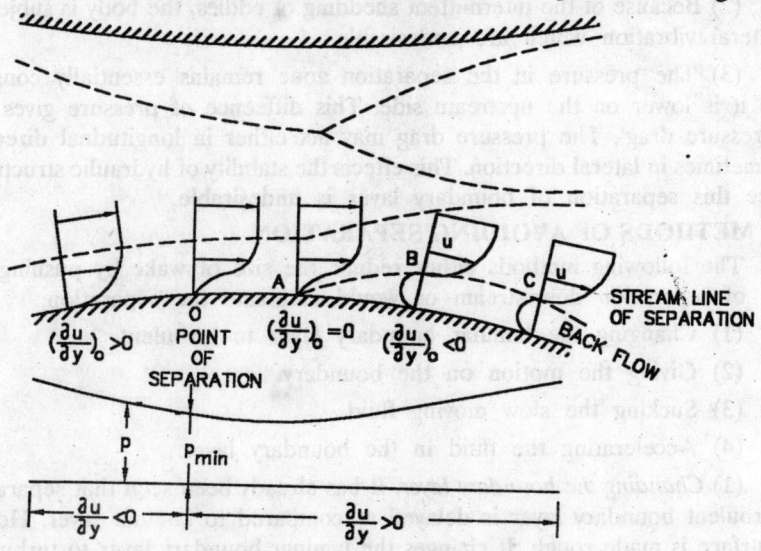

FIG. 8.9 SEPARATION OF BOUNDARY LAYER
(a) VELOCITY DISTRIBUTION (b) PRESSURE VARIATION

The velocity gradient at the wall $(\partial u/\partial y)_{y=0}$ reduces to zero at the point of separation. Further downstream the streamlines are displaced from the wall and back flow starts in the wake, the region downstream of point A. This phenomenon is known as separation of boundary layer. If all the points, below which the reverse flow takes place, are joined by a smooth curve ABC, it is termed as 'streamline of separation'. However, such a streamline is difficult to be located in the flow. This streamline oscillates and does not remain stationary. Its location depends on the form of boundary, Reynolds number of flow and roughness of the boundary.

The laminar boundary layer are more susceptible to separation at some earlier point in the flow than turbulent flow. This happens because the velocity distribution is parabolic for laminar flow and logarithmic for turbulent flow. Thus the velocity is more uniformly distributed across a section in turbulent flow as compared to laminar flow. It is also to be emphasized that laminar flow velocity distribution is inherently unstable. It is usually observed that the transition to turbulent boundary layer takes place before laminar boundary can separate. Under these circumstances, the turbulent boundary layer flow is maintained and separation of flow from the wall is delayed. But this does not mean that laminar separation never occurs.

The separation of flow is not desirable because of the following reasons.

(1) Downstream of the point of separation, the back flow starts near the surface with the formation of large turbulent eddies. These eddies persist for quite some distance downstream until these are damped out by the viscous action of the fluid. Thus the kinetic energy of the eddies is converted into heat and is lost to the surroundings.

(2) Because of the intermittent shedding of eddies, the body is subjected to lateral vibration which are undesirable.

(3) The pressure in the separation zone remains essentially constant while it is lower on the upstream side. This difference of pressure gives rise to 'pressure drag'. The pressure drag may act either in longitudnal direction or sometimes in lateral direction. This effects the stability of hydraulic structures. Hence this separation of boundary layer is undesirable.

8.14. METHODS OF AVOIDING SEPARATION

The following methods either reduce the size of wake by pushing the point of separation downstream or would eliminate the separation.

(1) Changing the laminar boundary layer to turbulent.

(2) Giving the motion on the boundary.

(3) Sucking the slow moving fluid.

(4) Accelerating the fluid in the boundary layer.

(1) *Chanding the boundary layer.* It has already been seen that separation of turbulent boundary layer is delayed as compared to laminar layer. Hence, the surface is made rough. It changes the laminar boundary layer to turbulent. The size of wake is reduced and this in turn causes less drag, Fig. 8.10a.

(2) *Streamlining the bodies*. The bodies are designed to follow the streamlines, *i.e.* they are streamlined. This means that the body curvature is less and the designed body is elongated. Since the body curvature is small, the laminar bundary layer is maintained over the surface of the object. As has been discussed earlier, the skin friction exerted over the surface will be less in case of laminar boundary layer, Fig. 8.10b.

(3) *Giving the motion to the boundary* While the flow takes place over a surface, it acquires the velocity of the boundary. If the boundary is made to move, the slow moving fluid will be accelerated causing lesser viscous resistance, Fig. 8.10c.

(4) *Suction*. Many a times, a few slots are made in the body of the object or its surface is made porous and the slow moving fluid is sucked in by means of pumps. This removes the slow moving fluid. The method sustains the laminar boundary layer over the boundary. Fig. 8.10d.

(5) *Acceleration*. Another method is to pump out more fluid in the boundary layer. This fluid speeds up slow moving fluid which is more resistant to adverse pressure gradient. This method is more effective for the wing of aeroplane of large angles of attack for which separation occurs early. This method creates more turbulence in the flow which accelerates the formation of turbulent boundary layer. Fig. 8.10e.

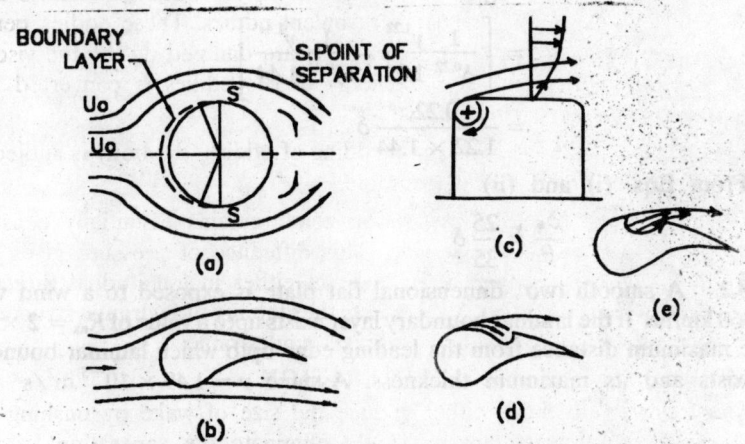

FIG. 8.10 METHODS OF CONTROLLING SEPARATION

Examples 8.1-8.15

8.1 The velocity distribution in the boundary layer over a high spillway surface was found to be

$$\frac{u}{U_0} = \left(\frac{y}{\delta}\right)^{0.22}$$

Express the ratio between momentum thickness θ and displaceent thickness δ_*

Solution

From Eq. 8.2,

$$\delta_* = \int_0^\delta \left(1 - \frac{u}{U_0}\right) dy$$

$$= \int_0^\delta [1 - (y/\delta)^{0.22}] \, dy \qquad ...(i)$$

$$= \frac{0.22}{1.22} \delta$$

From Eq. 8.3

$$\theta = \int_0^\delta \left(1 - \frac{u}{U_0}\right) \frac{u}{U_0} \, dy$$

$$= \int_0^\delta [1 - y/\delta)^{0.22}](y/\delta)^{0.22} \, dy$$

$$= \int_0^\delta [(y/\delta)^{0.22} - (y/\delta)^{0.44}] \, dy$$

$$= \left[\frac{1}{\delta^{0.22}} \frac{y^{1.22}}{1.22} - \frac{1}{\delta^{0.44}} \frac{y^{1.44}}{1.44}\right] \qquad ...(ii)$$

$$= \frac{0.22}{1.22 \times 1.44} \delta$$

From Eqs. (i) and (ii)

$$\frac{\delta_*}{\theta} = \frac{25}{35} \delta$$

8.2 A smooth two dimensional flat plate is exposed to a wind velocity of 360 km/hr. If the laminar boundary layer exists upto a value of $R_{ex} = 2 \times 10^5$, find the maximum distance from the leading edge upto which laminar boundary layer exists and its maximum thickness. Assume $v = 1.49 \times 10^{-5} \, \text{m}^2/\text{s}$

Solution

Let the boundary layer remains laminar for a distance x from the leading edge.

$$R_{ex} = \frac{\rho U_0 x}{\mu} = \frac{U_0 x}{v}$$

$$2 \times 10^5 = \frac{100 x}{14.9 \times 10^{-5}} \quad \text{(Since } U_0 = 360 \text{ km/hr)}$$

$$= \frac{360 \times 1000}{3600} \text{ m/s} = 100 \text{ m/s}$$

Solving, $\qquad x = 2.98$ cm

From Eq. 8.16a

$$\frac{\delta}{x} = \frac{4.91}{\sqrt{R_{ex}}}$$

$$\delta = \frac{4.91 \times 2.98 \times 10^{-2}}{\sqrt{2 \times 10^5}} \text{ m}$$

Solving $\qquad \delta = 0.327$ mm

8.3 Calculate shape factor H, i.e. ratio of displacement thickness and momentum thickness for the following velocity distribution

(a) $\qquad \dfrac{u}{U_0} = \dfrac{y}{\delta}$

(b) Turbulent flow on a flat plate,

$$\frac{u}{U_0} = \left(\frac{y}{\delta}\right)^{1/7}$$

(c) Laminar flow in a pipe,

$$\frac{u}{U_0} = \frac{1}{4\mu}\left(-\frac{\partial p}{\partial x}\right)(R^2 - r^2)$$

Solution

(a) $\qquad \dfrac{u}{U_0} = \left(\dfrac{y}{\delta}\right)$

From Eq. 8.2,

$$\delta_* = \int_0^\delta \left(1 - \frac{u}{U_0}\right) dy$$

$$= \int_0^\delta \left[1 - \frac{y}{\delta}\right] dy$$

$$= \left[y - \frac{1}{\delta} \times \frac{y^2}{2}\right]_0^\delta$$

$$= \left[\delta - \frac{\delta}{2}\right] = \frac{\delta}{2}$$

From Eq. 8.3

$$\theta = \int_0^\delta \left(1 - \frac{u}{U_0}\right)\frac{u}{U_0} dy$$

$$= \int_0^\delta \left[1 - \frac{y}{\delta} \right] \frac{y}{\delta} \, dy$$

$$= \int_0^\delta \left[\frac{y}{\delta} - \left(\frac{y}{\delta} \right)^2 \right] dy$$

$$= \left[\frac{1}{\delta} \frac{y^2}{2} - \frac{1}{\delta^2} \frac{y^3}{3} \right]_0^\delta$$

$$= \left[\frac{\delta}{2} - \frac{\delta}{3} \right] = \frac{\delta}{3}$$

$$H = \frac{\delta_*}{\theta}$$

$$H = \frac{\delta/2}{\delta/3} = \frac{3}{2} = 1.5$$

(b) For turbulent flow

$$\frac{u}{U_0} = \left(\frac{y}{\delta} \right)^{1/7}$$

From Eq. 8.2,

$$\delta_* = \int_0^\delta \left(1 - \frac{u}{U_0} \right) dy$$

$$= \int_0^\delta \left[1 - \left(\frac{y}{\delta} \right)^{1/7} \right] dy$$

$$= \left[y - \frac{1}{\delta^{1/7}} \cdot \frac{y^{8/7}}{8/7} \right]_0^\delta$$

$$= \left[\delta - \frac{7}{8} \cdot \delta \right] = \frac{\delta}{8}$$

$$\theta = \int_0^\delta \left(1 - \frac{u}{U_0} \right) \frac{u}{U_0} \, dy$$

$$= \int_0^\delta \left[1 - \left(\frac{y}{\delta} \right)^{1/7} \right] \left(\frac{y}{\delta} \right)^{1/7} dy$$

$$= \int_0^\delta \left[\left(\frac{y}{\delta} \right)^{1/7} - \left(\frac{y}{\delta} \right)^{2/7} \right] dy$$

$$= \left[\frac{1}{\delta^{1/7}} \cdot \frac{y^{8/7}}{8/7} - \frac{1}{\delta^{2/7}} \cdot \frac{y^{9/7}}{9/7} \right]$$

$$= \left(\frac{7}{8} \delta - \frac{7}{9} \delta \right) = \frac{7}{72} \delta$$

$$H = \frac{\delta_*}{\theta}$$

$$= \frac{\delta/8}{7/72 \, \delta} = 1.286$$

(c) For laminar flow in a pipe, velocity distribution is given by

$$u = \frac{1}{4\mu} \left(\frac{-\partial p}{\partial x} \right) (R^2 - r^2) \qquad \text{...(i)}$$

Also from Eq. 7.24

$$U_m = \frac{1}{4\mu} \left(\frac{-\partial p}{\partial x} \right) R^2 \qquad \text{...(ii)}$$

Therefore

$$u = U_m \left(1 - \frac{r^2}{R^2} \right) \qquad \text{...(iii)}$$

The definition of displacement thickness may be extended to axisymmetrical flow. In other words, the deficiency in mass flow caused due to formation of B.L. is equated to the mass flow rate of ideal fluid through an annular ring of radii R and $(R - \delta_*)$. (Refer Sec. 8.3).

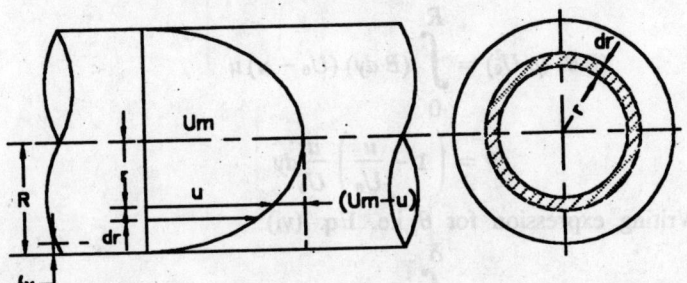

FIG. 8.11 EXAMPLE 8.3

From Eq. 8.2

$$\left(B \, \delta_* \right) \rho \, U_0 = \int_0^\delta \rho \, (B \, dy) \, (U_0 - u)$$

$$\delta_* = \int_0^\delta \left(1 - \frac{u}{U_0}\right) dy$$

Therefore,

$$\left[\rho \pi R^2 \cdot U_m - \rho \pi (R - \rho_*)^2 U_m\right] = \int_0^R (2\pi r \, dr) \, \rho (U_m - u) \qquad \ldots\text{(iv)}$$

$$\rho \pi U_m \left[R^2 - R^2 + 2R\delta_* - \delta_*^2\right] = 2\pi \rho \int_0^R (U_m - u) r \, dr$$

Neglect δ_*^2 on L.H.S. and substituting the value of u

$$R\delta_* U_m = \int_0^R \left[U_m - U_m\left(1 - \frac{r^2}{R^2}\right)\right] r \, dr$$

$$= \int_0^R U_m \frac{r^3}{R^2} \, dr$$

$$\delta_* = \frac{R}{4}$$

In the same way, the momentum thickness θ may be determined, From Eq. 8.3,

$$(B\,\theta)(\rho \, U_0^2) = \int_0^R (B \, dy)\,(U_0 - u)\, u \qquad \ldots\text{(vi)}$$

$$\theta = \left(1 - \frac{u}{U_0}\right) \frac{u}{U_0} dy \qquad \ldots\text{(vii)}$$

Writing expression for θ i.e. Eq. (vi)

$$(2\pi R\,\theta)\rho \, U_m^2 = \int_0^\delta \rho \,(2\pi r \, dr)\,(U_m - u)\, u$$

$$R\,\theta = \int_0^\delta \frac{u}{U_m}\left(1 - \frac{u}{U_m}\right) r \, dr$$

Substitute the value of u/U_m from Eq. (iii)

$$R\theta = \int_0^\delta \left(1 - \frac{r^2}{R^2}\right)\left(\frac{r^2}{R^2}\right) r\, dr$$

Solving $$R\theta = \left(\frac{R^2}{4} - \frac{R^2}{6}\right)$$

$$\theta = \frac{R}{12}$$

Hence $$H = \frac{\delta_*}{\theta}$$

$$H = \frac{R/4}{R/12} = 3$$

8.4 Oil with a free stream velocity of 3 m/s flows over a thin plate 1.25 m wide and 2 m long. Determine the boundary layer thickness and the shear stress at mid length and calculate the double sided resistance of the plate. Assume mass density $\rho = 860\ kg/m^3$ and kinematic viscosity $= 10^{-5}\ m^2/s$

Solution

R_{ex} at the mid length $x = 1$ m is,

$$R_{ex} = \frac{Ux}{v} = \frac{3 \times 1}{10^{-5}}$$

$$= 3 \times 10^5 < 5 \times 10^5$$

R_{ex} is low enough to allow the laminar boundary to survive over this length of the plate.

From Eq. 8.20

$$\tau_0 = 0.332\,\mu\,(U_0/x)\,\sqrt{R_{ex}}$$

$$= 0.332 \times 860 \times 10^{-5} \times (3/1) \times \sqrt{3 \times 10^5}$$

$$= 4.691 \times 10^{-5}\ N/m^2$$

Resisting force on both sides of the plate is given by

$$F_D = 2\,(0.5\,C_f\,A\,\rho\,U_0^2) = C_f\,\rho\,BL\,U_0^2$$

From Eq. 8.23,

$$C_f = \frac{1.328}{\sqrt{R_{eL}}}$$

$$= \frac{1.328}{\sqrt{3 \times 2/10^{-5}}} = 0.00171$$

$$F_D = 0.00171 \times 860 \times 1.25 \times 2 \times 3^2$$

$$= 33.08\ N$$

8.5 A flat plate, 1 m long and 0.8 m wide, is placed in a stream of water ($\mu = 0.01$ poise) flowing along with a velocity of 0.15 m/s. Determine

(i) boundary layer thickness at the end of plate (ii) shear drag on one side of the plate, and (iii) coefficient of drag.

Solution

The Reynolds number at the end of the plate is given by

$$R_{eL} = \frac{\rho U L}{\mu}$$

$$R_{eL} = \frac{1000 \times 0.15 \times 1}{(0.01 \times 0.1)} \qquad (\because 1 \text{ poise } = 0.1 \text{ N s/m}^2)$$

$$R_{eL} = 1.5 \times 10^5$$

Since the laminar boundary exists over the plate, the formulas applicable for laminar boundary layers are used.

(i) From Eq. 8.16, $\dfrac{\delta}{x} = \dfrac{4.91}{\sqrt{R_{ex}}}$

$$\delta = \frac{4.91 \times 1}{\sqrt{1.5 \times 10^5}} \text{ m}$$

$$\delta = 1.27 \text{ cm}$$

(ii) Drag on one side of the plate is given by Eq. 8.23c

$$F_D = \frac{1.328}{\sqrt{R_{eL}}} A \, (\rho \, U_0^2/2)$$

$$= \frac{1.328}{\sqrt{1.5 \times 10^5}} \times 1 \times 0.8 \times \frac{1000 \times (0.15)^2}{2}$$

$$= 0.0308 \text{ N}$$

(iii) The coefficient of drag is given by Eq. 8.23a

$$C_f = \frac{1.328}{\sqrt{1.5 \times 10^5}}$$

$$= 0.00343$$

8.6 Air flows over a flat plate 2 m long at a velocity of 20 m/s. Assuming laminar boundary layer to develop over the plate with velocity distribution

$$\frac{u}{U_0} = \left(\frac{y}{\delta}\right)$$

Determine the rate of flow (per unit width of plate) across vertical sections at the leading edge and trailing edge.

Solution

Consider a control volume ABCD. The boundary layer thickness δ at $x = L = 2$ m can be computed by Eq. 8.16 b.

For laminar B.L., from Eq. 8.16b,

$$\frac{\delta}{x} = \frac{5}{\sqrt{R_{ex}}}$$

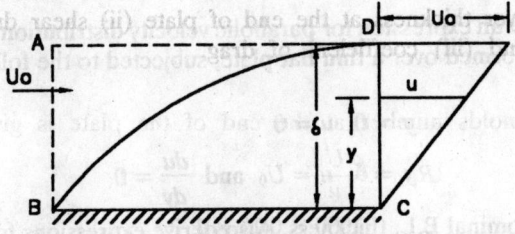

FIG. 8.12 EXAMPLE 8.6

At C, $\qquad x = L = 2 \ \text{m}$

$$\frac{\delta}{L} = \frac{5}{\sqrt{\dfrac{U_0 L}{\nu}}}$$

$$\delta = \frac{5 \times 2}{\sqrt{\dfrac{20 \times 2}{10^{-6}}}} \qquad \text{[for water } \nu = 10^{-6} \ \text{m}^2/\text{s}]$$

$$= \frac{10 \times 10^{-3}}{\sqrt{40}} \text{m} = 1.581 \ \text{mm}$$

Discharge/unit width across $AB = Q_{AB}$

$$Q_{AB} = (1.581 \times 10^{-3} \times 1) \times 20$$

$$= 31.62 \times 10^{-3} \ \text{m}^3/\text{s}$$

Also $\qquad\qquad Q_{CD}$ = area × average velocity across CD

Since $\qquad\qquad \dfrac{u}{U_0} = \dfrac{y}{\delta}$

Average velocity $= \dfrac{U_0}{2} = \dfrac{20}{2} = 10 \ \text{m/s}$

Hence $\qquad\qquad Q_{CD} = (1.581 \times 10^{-3}) \times 10$

$$= 15.81 \times 10^{-3} \ \text{m}^3/\text{s}$$

For given control volume ABCD,

Inflow = Outflow

$$Q_{AB} = Q_{CD} + Q_{BD}$$

$$Q_{BD} = (Q_{AB} - Q_{CD})$$

$$= (31.62 \times 10^{-3} - 15.81 \times 10^{-3}) \ \text{m}^3/\text{s}$$

$$= 15.81 \times 10^{-3} \ \text{m}^3/\text{s}$$

This problem illustrates that (i) the flow is retarded along the plate and (ii) there exists transverse flow across the boundary layer BD. There is no flow across BC (or the solid plate surface).

8.7 Derive an expression for parabolic velocity distribution across a laminar boundary layer formed over a thin flat plate, subjected to the following boundary conditions.

At $\qquad y = 0, \; u = 0$

At $\qquad y = \delta, \; u = U_0 \text{ and } \dfrac{du}{dy} = 0$

where δ is the nominal B.L. thickness. Also derive expressions for B.L. thickness δ_*, θ and wall shear stress τ_0 at a section x from leading edge and also coefficient of drag.

Solution

(a) Assume velocity distribution for laminar boundary layer as

$$\frac{u}{U_0} = a + b\left(\frac{y}{\delta}\right) + c\left(\frac{y}{\delta}\right)^2$$

$$= a + b\,\eta + c\,\eta^2 \qquad\qquad \text{...(i)}$$

Differentiating Eq. (i) w.r. to y

$$\frac{1}{U_0}\frac{du}{dy} = \frac{b}{\delta} + \frac{2c\,y}{\delta} \qquad\qquad \text{...(ii)}$$

Substituting B.C.'s

(i) At $\qquad y = 0, \; \eta = 0 \,;\, u = 0$

(ii) At $\qquad y = \delta, \eta = 1, u = U_0 \text{ and } \dfrac{du}{dy} = 0$

$$a = 0 \qquad\qquad \text{...(iii)}$$

$$a + b + c = 1 \qquad\qquad \text{...(iv)}$$

$$\frac{b}{\delta} + \frac{2c}{\delta}.\eta = 0$$

or $\qquad b + 2c = 0 \qquad\qquad \text{...(iv)}$

Solving Eqs. (iii), (iv) and (v) for unknowns a, b, c.

$$a = 0$$

$$b = 2$$

$$c = -1$$

Hence, velocity distribution is

$$\frac{u}{U_0} = 2\left(\frac{y}{\delta}\right) - \left(\frac{y}{\delta}\right)^2$$

$$\frac{u}{U_0} = 2\eta - \eta^2$$

(a) Now, $\qquad \delta_* = \displaystyle\int_0^\delta \left(1 - \frac{u}{U_0}\right) dy$

$$= \int_0^\delta \left[1 - \left\{ 2\left(\frac{y}{\delta}\right) - \left(\frac{y}{\delta}\right)^2 \right\} \right] dy$$

$$= \left[y - \frac{2}{\delta} \cdot \frac{y^2}{2} + \frac{1}{\delta^2} \cdot \frac{y^3}{3} \right]_0^\delta$$

$$= \left[\delta - \delta + \frac{\delta}{3} \right] = \frac{\delta}{3}$$

and

$$\theta = \int_0^\delta \left(1 - \frac{u}{U_0} \right) \frac{u}{U_0} \, dy$$

$$= \int_0^\delta \left[1 - \left\{ 2\left(\frac{y}{\delta}\right) - \left(\frac{y}{\delta}\right)^2 \right\} \right] \left\{ 2\left(\frac{y}{\delta}\right) - \left(\frac{y}{\delta}\right)^2 \right\} dy$$

$$= \int_0^\delta \left[\left(\frac{y}{\delta}\right) - 5\left(\frac{y}{\delta}\right)^2 + 4\left(\frac{y}{\delta}\right)^3 - \left(\frac{y}{\delta}\right)^4 \right] dy$$

$$= \left\{ \frac{2}{\delta} \cdot \frac{y^2}{2} - \frac{5}{\delta^2} \cdot \frac{y^3}{3} + \frac{4}{\delta^3}\frac{y^4}{4} - \frac{1}{\delta^4} \cdot \frac{y^5}{5} \right\}_0^\delta$$

$$= \left[\delta - \frac{5}{3}\delta + \delta - \frac{\delta}{5} \right] = \frac{2}{15}\delta$$

(c) From Eq. 8.11,

$$\frac{\tau_0}{\rho} = U_0^2 \frac{d\theta}{dx}$$

$$= U_0^2 \cdot \frac{d}{dx}\left(\frac{2}{15}\delta \right)$$

$$= \frac{2\,U_0^2}{15}\frac{d\delta}{dx} \qquad\qquad ...(vii)$$

From Eq. 1.8 c,

$$\left(\tau_0 \right)_{y=0} = \mu \left(\frac{\partial u}{\partial y} \right)_y$$

$$= \mu\,U_0 \left[\frac{\partial}{\partial y}\left\{ 2\left(\frac{y}{\delta}\right) - \left(\frac{y}{\delta}\right)^2 \right\} \right]_{y=0}$$

$$= \mu\,U_0 \cdot \left[\frac{2}{\delta} - \frac{1}{\delta^2} \cdot 2y \right]_{y=0}$$

$$= \frac{2\mu U_0}{\delta} \qquad \qquad ...(viii)$$

Substituting in Eq. (vii) from Eq. (viii)

$$\frac{2\mu U_0}{\rho \delta} = \frac{2 U_0^2}{15} \frac{d\delta}{dx}$$

$$\delta \, d\delta = \frac{15\mu}{\rho U_0} dx$$

Integrating w.r. to x,

$$\frac{\delta^2}{2} = 15 \frac{\mu}{\rho U_0} . x + C$$

When $\qquad x = 0, \ \delta = 0$

$$C = 0$$

Hence $\qquad \dfrac{\delta^2}{2} = 15 \dfrac{\mu x}{\rho U_0}$

Rearranging terms,

$$\frac{\delta^2}{x} = 30 \frac{\mu}{\rho U_0}$$

$$\frac{\delta^2}{x^2} = \frac{30}{\rho U_0 x / \mu}$$

$$\frac{\delta}{x} = \frac{5.477}{\sqrt{R_{ex}}} \qquad \qquad \text{(See Table 8.1)}$$

Substituting the value of δ in Eq. (vii)

$$\frac{\tau_0}{\rho} = 2 \frac{U_0^2}{15} . \frac{d}{dx} \left(\frac{5.477 \, x}{\sqrt{R_{ex}}} \right)$$

$$\frac{\tau_0}{\rho U_0^2} = \frac{2}{15} \times 5.477 \frac{d}{dx} \left(\frac{x}{\sqrt{\dfrac{\rho U_0 x}{\mu}}} \right)$$

$$= 0.730 \frac{d}{dx} \left(\frac{\mu \sqrt{x}}{\sqrt{\rho U_0}} \right)$$

$$= 0.730 \sqrt{\frac{\mu}{\rho U_0}} \times \frac{1}{2} x^{-1/2}$$

$$= 0.365 \sqrt{\frac{\mu}{\rho U_0 x}} = \frac{0.365}{\sqrt{R_{ex}}}$$

Rearranging terms,

$$\frac{\tau_0}{\rho U_0^2 / 2} = c_f = \frac{0.365}{\sqrt{R_{ex}}} \times 2$$

$$c_f = \frac{0.730}{\sqrt{R_{ex}}}$$

(d) Drag force on one side of plate

$$F_D = \int_0^L (\tau_0)_x \times B\, dx$$

$$= \int_0^L \frac{0.365\, \rho\, U_0^2}{\sqrt{\rho\, U_0 x/\mu}}\, B\, dx$$

$$= \frac{0.365\, B\, \rho\, U_0^2}{\sqrt{\rho\, U_0/\mu}} \int_0^L \frac{1}{\sqrt{x}}\, dx$$

$$= \frac{0.365\, B\, \rho\, U_0^2}{\sqrt{\rho\, U_0/\mu}} \left[\frac{x^{1/2}}{1/2} \right]_0^L$$

$$= \frac{0.730\, B\, \rho\, U_0^2}{\sqrt{\rho\, U_0/\mu}} \sqrt{L}$$

$$F_D = \frac{0.730\, B\, (\rho\, U_0^2)}{\sqrt{\rho\, U_0 L/\mu}} \times L$$

$$\frac{F_D/B\,L}{\rho\, U_0^2/2} = \frac{0.730 \times 2}{\sqrt{R_{eL}}}$$

$$C_f = \frac{1.46}{\sqrt{R_{eL}}} \qquad \text{(See Table 8.1)}$$

8.8 For the velocity profile given by

$$\frac{u}{U_0} = \frac{3}{2}\left(\frac{y}{\delta}\right) - \frac{1}{2}\left(\frac{y}{\delta}\right)^3$$

for the laminar boundary layer, determine the expressions for boundary layer thickness, wall shear stress and coefficient of drag in terms of Reynolds number.

Solution

(i) From Eqs. 8.11 and 8.3

$$\frac{\tau_0}{\rho} = U_0^2 \frac{d\theta}{dx} \qquad \qquad ...(8.11)$$

$$\theta = \int_0^\delta \left(1 - \frac{u}{U_0}\right)\frac{u}{U_0}\, dy \qquad \qquad ...(8.3)$$

Substituting the value of u/U_0 in Eq. 8.3.

$$\theta = \int_0^\delta \left[1 - \frac{3}{2}(y/\delta) + \frac{1}{2}(y/\delta)^3 \right]$$

$$\left[\frac{3}{2}(y/\delta) - \frac{1}{2}(y/\delta) \right]$$

$$= \int_0^\delta \left[\frac{3}{2} (y/\delta) - \frac{1}{2} (y/\delta)^3 - \frac{9}{4} (y/\delta)^2 \right.$$

$$\left. + \frac{3}{4} (y/\delta)^4 + \frac{3}{4} (y/\delta)^4 - \frac{1}{4} (y/\delta)^6 \right] dy$$

$$= \int_0^\delta \left[\frac{3}{2} (y/\delta) - \frac{9}{4} (y/\delta)^2 - \frac{1}{2} (y/\delta)^3 \right.$$

$$\left. + \frac{3}{2} (y/\delta)^4 - \frac{1}{4} (y/\delta)^6 \right] dy$$

$$= \left[\frac{3}{2\delta} \frac{y^2}{2} - \frac{9}{4\delta^2} \frac{y^3}{3} - \frac{1}{2\delta^3} \frac{y^4}{4} \right.$$

$$\left. + \frac{3}{2\delta^4} \frac{y^5}{5} - \frac{1}{4\delta^6} \frac{y^7}{7} \right]$$

$$= \left[\frac{3}{4} - \frac{9}{12} - \frac{1}{8} + \frac{3}{10} - \frac{1}{28} \right] = \frac{39}{280} \delta$$

Shear stress τ_0 is given by Eq. 8.11

$$\tau_0 = \rho U_0^2 \frac{d\theta}{dx}$$

$$= \rho U_0^2 \left(\frac{39}{280} \frac{d\delta}{dx} \right) \qquad \text{...(i)}$$

From Eq. 1.8c

$$(\tau_0)_{y=0} = \mu \left(\frac{\partial u}{\partial y} \right)_{y=0}$$

$$(\tau_0)_{y=0} = \mu \frac{\partial}{\partial y} \left\{ \frac{3}{2} \frac{y}{\delta} - \frac{1}{2} \frac{y^3}{\delta^3} \right\} U_0$$

$$= \mu U_0 \left\{ \frac{3}{2\delta} - \frac{3}{2\delta^3} y^2 \right\}_{y=0}$$

$$= \frac{3}{2} \frac{\mu U_0}{\delta} \qquad \text{...(ii)}$$

Equating two values of τ_0 from Eqs. (i) and (ii)

$$\frac{39}{280} \rho U_0^2 \frac{d\delta}{dx} = \frac{3}{2} \frac{\mu U_0}{\delta}$$

$$\delta \, d\delta = \frac{3}{2} \times \frac{280}{39} \frac{\mu}{\rho U_0} dx = \frac{420}{39} \frac{\mu}{\rho U_0} dx$$

Integrating,

$$\frac{\delta^2}{2} = \frac{420}{39} \frac{\mu}{\rho U_0} x + C$$

When $\quad x = 0$, $\delta = 0$,

$$C = 0$$

Hence $\qquad \dfrac{\delta^2}{2} = \dfrac{420}{39} \dfrac{\mu\,x}{\rho\,U_0}$

Simplifying $\qquad \delta = 4.64 \sqrt{\dfrac{\mu\,x}{\rho\,U_0}}$

or $\qquad \dfrac{\delta}{x} = \dfrac{4.64}{\sqrt{R_{ex}}}$

(ii) Substituting the values of δ into Eq. (i)

$$\tau_0 = \dfrac{39}{280} \rho\,U_0^2 \dfrac{d}{dx}\left(4.64 \sqrt{\dfrac{\mu}{\rho\,U_0}} \sqrt{x}\right)$$

$$\tau_0 = \dfrac{39 \times 4.64}{280 \times 2} \dfrac{\rho\,\mu\,U_0^{3/2}}{\sqrt{x}}$$

Rearranging terms

$$\tau_0 = 0.323 \dfrac{\mu\,U_0}{x}\sqrt{R_{ex}}$$

$$\dfrac{\tau_0}{\rho\,U_0^2} = \dfrac{0.323}{\sqrt{R_{ex}}}$$

(iii) From Eq. 8.22

$$F_D = \int\limits_0^L \tau_0\,B\,dx$$

$$= \int\limits_0^L 0.323 \dfrac{\mu\,U_0}{x}\sqrt{R_{ex}}\,B\,dx$$

$$= 0.323\,\mu\,U_0\,B \int\limits_0^L \sqrt{\dfrac{\rho\,U_0}{\mu}} \times \dfrac{\sqrt{x}}{x}\,dx$$

$$= 0.323\,\rho^{1/2}\,U_0^{3/2}\,B\,\mu^{1/2}\int\limits_0^L \dfrac{1}{\sqrt{x}}\,dx$$

Solving, $\qquad F_D = 0.646\,\mu\,U_0\,B \sqrt{\dfrac{\rho\,U_0\,L}{\mu}}$

$$C_f = \dfrac{F_D}{0.5\,\rho\,U_0^2\,BL} = \dfrac{1.292}{\sqrt{R_{eL}}}$$

8.9 Assuming velocity distribution in laminar boundary layer

$$\dfrac{u}{U_0} = \sin\left(\dfrac{\pi\,y}{2\,\delta}\right)$$

Determine boundary layer thickness δ, and drag coefficient in terms of nominal BL thickness δ.

Solution

From Eq. 8.11 and 8.3

$$\frac{\tau_0}{\rho} = U_0^2 \frac{d\theta}{dx}$$

$$\theta = \int_0^\delta \left(1 - \frac{u}{U_0}\right) \frac{u}{U_0} \, dy$$

Substituting the value of $\dfrac{u}{U_0}$ in Eq. 8.3,

$$\theta = \int_0^\delta \left(1 - \sin\frac{\pi y}{2\delta}\right) \sin\frac{\pi y}{2\delta} \, dy$$

$$= \int_0^\delta \left(\sin\frac{\pi y}{2\delta} - \sin^2\frac{\pi y}{2\delta}\right) dy$$

$$= \int_0^\delta \left[\sin\frac{\pi}{2}\frac{y}{\delta} - \frac{1}{2}\left\{1 - \cos 2\left(\frac{\pi}{2}\frac{y}{\delta}\right)\right\}\right] dy$$

$$= \left\{\frac{-\cos\frac{\pi}{2}\cdot\frac{y}{\delta}}{\frac{\pi}{2}\cdot\frac{1}{\delta}}\right\}_0 - \frac{1}{2}\left\{y - \frac{\sin 2\left(\frac{\pi}{2}\cdot\frac{y}{\delta}\right)}{2\cdot\frac{\pi}{2}\cdot\frac{1}{\delta}}\right\}_0^\delta$$

$$= \left[\left\{0 + \frac{1}{\pi/2\delta}\right\} - \frac{1}{2}\left\{\delta - 0\right\} - \left\{0 - 0\right\}\right]$$

$$= \left(\frac{2\delta}{\pi} - \frac{\delta}{2}\right) = \frac{(4 - \pi)}{2\pi}\delta$$

From Eq. 8.11,

$$\frac{\tau_0}{\rho U_0^2} = \frac{d\theta}{dx}$$

$$= \frac{d}{dx}\left(\frac{4 - \pi}{2\pi}\right)\delta$$

$$= \left(\frac{4 - \pi}{2\pi}\right)\frac{d\delta}{dx} \qquad \ldots\text{(i)}$$

Also from Eq. 1.8 c, at $y = 0$

$$\left(\tau_0 \right)_{y = 0} = \mu \frac{du}{dy}$$

where

$$u = U_0 \sin \left(\frac{\pi}{2} \frac{y}{\delta} \right)$$

$$\left(\tau_0 \right)_{y = 0} = \mu U_0 \frac{d}{dy} \left(\sin \frac{\pi}{2} \frac{y}{\delta} \right)$$

$$= \mu U_0 \cos \left(\frac{\pi}{2} \frac{y}{\delta} \right) \times \frac{\pi}{2\delta}$$

$$= \frac{\pi \mu U_0}{2\delta} \cos \left(\frac{\pi}{2} \frac{y}{\delta} \right)$$

$$\left(\tau \right)_{y = 0} = \frac{\pi \mu U_0}{2\delta} \qquad \qquad \text{...(ii)}$$

Equating Eqs. (i) and (ii)

$$\frac{4 - \pi}{2\pi} \cdot \rho U_0^2 \frac{d\delta}{dx} = \frac{\pi \mu U_0}{2\delta}$$

Separating variables,

$$\delta \, d\delta = \frac{\pi \mu U_0}{2\rho} \times \frac{2\pi}{(4 - \pi) \rho U_0^2} \cdot dx$$

$$= \left(\frac{\pi^2}{4 - \pi} \frac{\mu}{} \right) \rho U_0 \, dx$$

Integrating w.r. to x,

$$\frac{\delta^2}{2} = \left(\frac{\pi^2}{4 - \pi} \right) \frac{\mu}{\rho U_0} \cdot x + c$$

At
$$x = 0, \delta = 0$$
$$c = 0$$

(i) Hence,
$$\frac{\delta^2}{2} = \frac{\pi^2}{(4 - \pi)} \frac{\mu x}{\rho U_0}$$

$$\frac{\delta^2}{x} \cdot \frac{1}{x} = \frac{2\pi^2}{(4 - \pi)} \cdot \frac{\mu}{\rho U_0} \cdot \frac{1}{x}$$

$$\frac{\delta}{x} = \sqrt{\frac{2\pi^2}{4 - \pi}} \frac{1}{\sqrt{\rho U_0 x / \mu}} \qquad \qquad \text{...(iii)}$$

$$\frac{\delta}{x} = \frac{4.788}{\sqrt{R_{ex}}}$$

(ii) From Eqs. (ii) and (iii)

$$\tau_0 = \frac{\pi \mu U_0}{2\delta}$$

$$= \frac{\pi \mu U_0}{2} \times \frac{\sqrt{R_{ex}}}{4.788 x}$$

$$= 0.328 \frac{\mu U_0}{x} \sqrt{R_{ex}} \qquad \ldots(iv)$$

Rearranging terms,

$$\frac{\tau_0}{\frac{\rho U_0^2}{2}} = c_f = \frac{0.328}{\frac{\rho U_0^2}{2}} \cdot \frac{\mu U_0}{x} \sqrt{R_{ex}}$$

$$c_f = \frac{0.656}{\sqrt{R_{ex}}}$$

(iii) Drag force $F_D = \displaystyle\int_0^L \tau_0 \times B \times dx$

$$= \int_0^L 0.328 \frac{\mu U_0}{x} \cdot \sqrt{R_{ex}} . B \, dx$$

$$= 0.328 \, \mu \, U_0 B \int_0^L \frac{1}{x} . \sqrt{\frac{\rho U_0 x}{\mu}} . dx$$

$$= 0.328 \, \mu \, U_0 B \sqrt{\frac{\rho U_0}{\mu}} . \int_0^L \frac{1}{\sqrt{x}} \, dx$$

$$= 0.328 \, B \sqrt{\rho \mu U_0^3} \left[\frac{x^{1/2}}{1/2} \right]_0^L$$

$$= 0.656 \, B \sqrt{\rho U_0^3 \mu} \, L^{1/2}$$

Rearranging terms,

$$\frac{F_D / B L}{\frac{\rho U_0^2}{2}} = \frac{0.656 \, B . \sqrt{\rho U_0^3 \mu L}}{B L \rho U_0^2 / 2}$$

$$C_f = \frac{1.312}{\sqrt{R_{eL}}}$$

8.10 A submarine of cylindrical shape with rounded front portion, is 50 m long and 5.0 m diameter. It cruises in sea at 7.5 m/s. Determine the power needed to overcome boundary friction. Assume for sea water $\rho = 1025$ kg/m³ and $\mu = 10^{-3} \, P_a \, s.$

Solution

Reynolds number $R_e = \dfrac{\rho\,U_0\,L}{\mu}$

$$= \frac{1025 \times 7.5 \times 50}{10^{-3}} = 3.84 \times 10^8$$

For the length of plate over which laminar B.L. will develop, assume

$$R_{ecr} = 5 \times 10^5 = \frac{1025 \times 7.5 \times x}{10^{-3}}$$

$$x = \frac{5 \times 10^5 \times 10^{-3}}{1025 \times 7.5} = 0.065 \ \text{m}$$

It is quite small and it may be assumed that turbulent B.L. develops over whole plate.

Now since $R_e > 10^7$, it is better to use Eq. 8.36

$$C_f = \frac{0.455}{\left(\log_{10} R_{eL} \right)^{2.58}}$$

$$= \frac{0.455}{\left(\log_{10} 3.84 \times 10^8 \right)^{2.58}} = 1.77 \times 10^{-3}$$

$$\text{Wetted Area} = \pi D L$$

$$= \pi \times 5 \times 50 = 785 \ \text{m}^2$$

$$F_D = C_f\, A\, \rho\, \frac{U_0^2}{2} = C_f\, \pi\, D\, L\, \frac{\rho\, U_0^2}{2}$$

$$= 1.77 \times 10^{-3}\,(785) \left(\frac{1025 \times 7.5^2}{2} \right)$$

$$= 40055.2 \ \text{N}$$

$$\text{Power} = \frac{F_D \times U}{1000} \ \text{kW}$$

$$= \frac{40055.2 \times 7.5}{1000}$$

$$= 300.414 \ \text{kW}$$

8.11   A smooth flat plate 1 m wide and 3 m long moves through stationary air of specific weight $0.0115 \ \text{kN/m}^3$ at 1 m/s. Calculate the drag force on one side of the plate when (i) the boundary layer is entirely laminar (ii) when the boundary layer is entirely turbulent. What is the thickness of the boundary layer at the trailing edge for both cases ? Take $\nu = 1.5 \times 10^{-5} \ \text{m}^2/\text{s}$

Solution

$$R_{eL} = \frac{U_0\, L}{\nu}$$

$$= \frac{1 \times 3}{1.5 \times 10^{-5}} = 2 \times 10^5$$

(i) When the boundary layer is entirely laminar and assuming it follows Blasius results.

$$F_D = \frac{1.328}{\sqrt{R_{eL}}} \frac{\rho \, BL \, U_0^2}{2}$$

$$F_D = \frac{1.328}{\sqrt{2 \times 10^5}} \times \frac{0.0115}{9.81} \times \frac{1 \times 3 \times (1)^2}{2}$$

$$= 0.52 \times 10^{-5} \text{ kN}$$

(ii) For turbulent boundary layer, assuming the velocity distribution to be one seventh power law,

$$F_D = \frac{0.072}{(R_{eL})^{1/5}} \frac{\rho \, BL \, U_0^2}{2}$$

$$= \frac{0.072}{(2 \times 10^5)^{1/5}} \times \frac{0.0115}{9.81} \times \frac{1 \times 3 \times (1)^2}{2}$$

$$= 1.07 \times 10^{-5} \text{ kN}$$

(iii) The thickness of laminar boundary layer for the velocity distribution used above is given by Eq. 8.16b

$$\frac{\delta}{x} = \frac{5}{\sqrt{R_{eL}}}$$

$$\delta = \frac{5x}{\sqrt{R_{eL}}} = \frac{5 \times 3}{\sqrt{2 \times 10^5}} \text{ m}$$

$$= 0.0335 \text{ m}$$

The thickness of turbulent boundary layer is given by Eq. 8.31a

$$\frac{\delta}{x} = \frac{0.37}{(R_{eL})^{1/5}}$$

$$\delta = \frac{0.37 \times 3}{(2 \times 10^5)^{1/5}}$$

$$\delta = 0.0966 \text{ m}$$

It is evident that the thickness of turbulent boundary layer should be more as compared to laminar boundary layer.

8.12 Water is flowing over a thin smooth plate of length 5 m and width 2 m at a velocity of 1.0 m/s. If the boundary layer flow changes from laminar to turbulent at a Reynolds number of 5×10^5, find (i) the distance from leading edge upto which boundary layer is laminar, (ii) thickness of boundary layer at transition point and (iii) drag force on one side of the plate. Assume $\mu = 0.01$ poise.

Solution

(a) Let the boundary layer remain laminar for distance x from the leading edge.

$$R_{ex} = \frac{\rho U x}{\mu}$$

$$5 \times 10^5 = \frac{1000 \times 1 \times x}{(0.01 \times 0.1)} \qquad (\because 1 \text{ poise} = 1 \text{ N s/m}^2)$$

$$x = 0.5 \text{ m} \qquad \text{...(i)}$$

(b) From Eq. 8.16a

$$\frac{\delta}{x} = \frac{4.91}{\sqrt{R_{ex}}}$$

$$\delta = \frac{4.91}{\sqrt{5 \times 10^5}} \times 0.5 \text{ m}$$

$$\delta = 0.347 \text{ cm} \qquad \text{...(ii)}$$

(c) Drag on one side of the plate = Drag due to laminar boundary layer on x metre + Drag due to turbulent boundary layer on the remaining $(L - x)$ metre

From Eq. 8.23a

$$C_f = \frac{1.328}{\sqrt{R_{eL}}}$$

$$= \frac{1.328}{\sqrt{5 \times 10^5}} = 0.001878 \qquad \text{...(iii)}$$

Drag due to laminar boundary layer

$$C_{flam} \times A \frac{\rho U_0^2}{2} = 0.001878 \,(0.5 \times 2)\, \frac{(1000 \times 1^2)}{2} N$$

$$= 0.000939 \text{ kN} \qquad \text{...(iv)}$$

From Eq. 8.35

$$(C_f)_{tur} = \frac{0.074}{(R_{eL})^{1/5}} = \frac{0.074}{(\rho UL/\mu)^{1/5}}$$

$$= \frac{0.074}{\left[\dfrac{1000 \times 1 \times 5}{0.01 \times 0.1}\right]^{1/5}} = 0.00338 \qquad \text{...(v)}$$

If the boundary layer happens to be turbulent for the whole length

$$(F_D)_{tur} = C_{ftur} \frac{A \times \rho U_0^2}{2}$$

$$= 0.00338 \times (5 \times 2) \times \frac{1000 \times 1^2}{2} N$$

$$= 0.0169 \text{ kN} \qquad \text{..(vi)}$$

Drag due to turbulent boundary layer developing over a distance $\dot{x}\, (= 0.5\ \text{m})$,

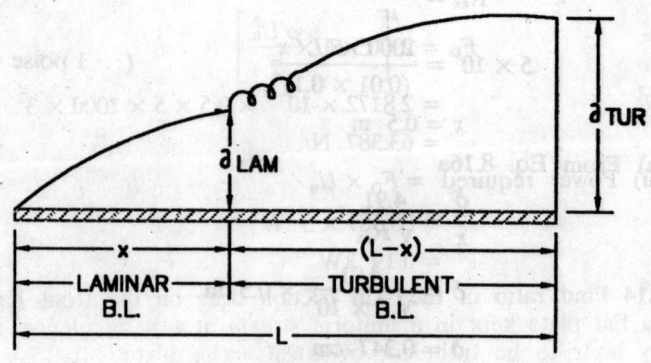

FIG. 8.13 EXAMPLE 8.12

$$F_D = C_f\, tur\, \frac{A_1 \rho\, U_0^2}{2}$$

$$= 0.00338 \times (0.5 \times 2) \times \frac{(1000 \times 1^2)}{2}\ \text{N}$$

$$= 0.00169\ \text{kN} \qquad\qquad \text{...(vii)}$$

From Eqs. (iv), (vi) and (vii)

Drag over the plate = Drag due to laminar boundary for 0.5 m + Drag due turbulent boundary layer for 5 m − Drag due to turbulent boundary on 0.5 m

$$F_D = 0.000939 + 0.0169 - 0.00169$$

$$= 0.01615\ \text{kN}$$

8.13 The drag coefficient due to boundary layer for a flat plate is given by

$$C_r = 0.455/(log_{10} R_{eL})^{2.58}$$

where R_{eL} is the Reynolds number based on length. If a plate 50 cm wide and 5 m long is kept parallel to the flow of water with free stream velocity of 3 m/s. (i) calculate the drag force on both sides of the plate. Take $v = 10^{-6}\ \text{m}^2/\text{s}$ (ii) determine the power required to tow the plate at 3 m/s in the stationary fluid.

Solution

$$R_{eL} = \frac{U_0 L}{v}$$

$$= \frac{3 \times 5}{10^{-6}} = 1.5 \times 10^7$$

(i)
$$C_f = \frac{0.455}{(\log_{10} 1.5 \times 10^7)^{2.58}}$$

$$= 2.8172 \times 10^{-3}$$

From Eq. 8.23a

$$F_D = 2 \left[C_f B L \frac{\rho U_0^2}{2} \right]$$

$$= 2.8172 \times 10^{-3} \times 0.5 \times 5 \times 1000 \times 3^2$$

$$= 63.387 \text{ N}$$

(ii) Power required $= F_D \times U_0$

$$= 63.387 \times 3 \text{ W}$$

$$= 0.19 \text{ kW}$$

8.14 Find ratio of the skin friction drag on the front half and rear half of a flat plate kept in a uniform stream at zero incidence. Assume the boundary layer to be turbulent over the entire plate.

Solution

$$C_f = \frac{0.074}{R_e^{1/5}}$$

For the front half length,

$$R_{eL} = \frac{U_0 (0.5 L)}{v} = \frac{0.5 U_0 L}{v}$$

F_D on the front half portion of the plate

$$F_{D1} = C_f A \frac{\rho U_0^2}{2}$$

$$= \frac{0.074}{\left(\dfrac{0.5 U_0 L}{v} \right)^{1/5}} \times B \times 0.5 L \times \frac{\rho U_0^2}{2}$$

$$= \frac{0.074 \times 0.5}{(0.5)^{1/5}} \times \frac{BL}{R_{eL}^{1/5}} \frac{\rho U_0^2}{2}$$

$$= 0.0425 \, BL \, \rho \, U_0^2 / (2 \times R_{eL}^{1/5}) \qquad \qquad ...(i)$$

F_D on the whole length of the plate

$$F_D = \frac{0.074}{\left(\dfrac{U_0 L}{v} \right)^{1/5}} BL \times \frac{\rho U_0^2}{2} \qquad \qquad ...(ii)$$

Therefore drag on the rear half portion of the plate

$$F_{D2} = F_D - F_{D1}$$

$$= \left[0.074 - \frac{0.074 \times 0.5}{(0.5)^{1/5}} \right] \times BL \times \rho \, U_0^2 / (2 \, R_{eL}^{1/5})$$

$$= 0.0315\, BL \times \rho\, U_0^2 / 2R_{eL}^{1/5} \qquad \text{...(iii)}$$

From Eqs. (i) and (iii)

$$\frac{F_{D1}}{F_{D2}} = \frac{0.0424}{0.0315} = 1.35$$

8.15 Air flows through a converging diverging passage such that the velocity profile at a given section is defined by the following expression. Check whether the flow will remains attached to the wall or separate.

(a) $$\frac{u}{U_m} = \left(1 - \frac{r^2}{R^2} \right)$$

(b) $$\frac{u}{U_0} = \left(y/\delta \right)^{1/7}$$

(c) $$\frac{u}{U_0} = 2\,(y/\delta) - 2\,(y/\delta)^3 + (y/\delta)^4$$

Solution

The necessary condition for the flow to separate is that

(i) pressure gradient should be adverse or $\dfrac{\partial p}{\partial x} > 0$ and

(ii) velocity gradient at the wall or $\left(\dfrac{\partial u}{\partial y} \right)$, at $y = 0$ should be zero

(a) $$\frac{u}{U_m} = \left(1 - \frac{r^2}{R^2} \right) \qquad \text{...(i)}$$

It is the expression for velocity distribution for laminar flow through circular pipe.

If distance y is measured from wall or boundary

$$y = (R - r), \text{ i.e. } r = (R - y)$$

$$\therefore \quad \frac{u}{U_m} = \left[\frac{R^2 - r^2}{R^2} \right]$$

$$= \left[\frac{R^2 - (R - y)^2}{R^2} \right]$$

$$= \frac{2Ry - y^2}{R^2}$$

At the section of separation of flow, the necessary condition is $\left(\dfrac{\partial u}{\partial y} \right) = 0$ at $y = 0$.

$$\therefore \quad \left(\frac{\partial u}{\partial y} \right)_y = \frac{U_m}{R^2} \frac{d}{dy} \left(\{ 2Ry - y^2 \} \right)$$

$$\left(\frac{\partial u}{\partial y} \right)_y = \frac{U_m}{R^2} (2R - 2y)$$

(iii)...

$$\left(\frac{\partial u}{\partial y}\right)_{y=0} = \frac{U_m}{R^2}(2R) = \frac{2U_m}{R}$$

Since it is positive, there is no likelyhood of this flow being separated.

(b)

$$\frac{u}{U_0} = \left(\frac{y}{\delta}\right)^{1/7}$$

The necessary condition is $\left(\dfrac{\partial u}{\partial y}\right)_{y=0} = 0$

$$\left(\frac{\partial u}{\partial y}\right) = \frac{\partial}{\partial y}\left(\frac{y}{\delta}\right)^{1/7}$$

$$\left(\frac{\partial u}{\partial y}\right) = \frac{1}{7} \cdot \frac{1}{\delta^{1/7}} \cdot y^{6/7}$$

$$\left(\frac{\partial u}{\partial y}\right)_{y=0} = 0$$

Since $\left(\dfrac{\partial u}{\partial y}\right)$ is zero at $y = 0$, there is likelyhood of this flow being separated

(c)

$$\frac{u}{U_0} = 2\left(\frac{y}{\delta}\right) - 2\left(y/\delta\right)^3 + \left(y/\delta\right)^4$$

Here

$$\frac{1}{U_0}\frac{\partial u}{\partial y} = \frac{\partial}{\partial y}\left[2\left(\frac{y}{\delta}\right) - 2\left(\frac{y}{\delta}\right)^3 + \left(\frac{y}{\delta}\right)^4\right]$$

$$= \left[\frac{2}{\delta}\times 1 - \frac{2}{\delta^3}\times 3y^2 + \frac{1}{\delta^4}\cdot 4y^3\right]$$

$$\frac{1}{U_0}\left(\frac{\partial u}{\partial y}\right)_{y=0} = \left[\frac{2}{\delta} - 0 - 0\right]$$

$$= \frac{2}{\delta} > 0$$

Since $\dfrac{\partial u}{\partial y} > 0$, there is no likelyhood of this flow being separted from boundary.

Objective Questions

8.1 When the fluid flows along the solid boundary, more and more fluid is retarded in the viscinity of boundary. This retardation of fluid is caused by

(a) high velocity out side the boundary layer

(b) high viscosity of fluid

(c) high velocity gradients existing near the boundary

(d) the assumption of fluid being ideal

(e) none of these answers

8.2 The displacement thickness of boundary layer is

(a) the distance from the boundary affected by boundary shear

(b) the distance by which the main flow is displaced

(c) the distance normal to the plate where $u/U_0 = 0.99$

(d) one half the actual boundary layer thickness

(e) none of these answers

8.3 Match the correct group from column A and column B

Column A   **Column B**

(a) nominal thickness   (i) $\int_0^{\delta}(1 - u/U_0) u/U_0 \, dy$

(b) displacement thickness   (ii) $\int_0^{\delta} (1 - u/U_0) \, dy$

(c) momentum thickness   (iii) $\int_0^{\delta} (1 - u^2/U_0^2) u/U_0 \, dy$

(d) energy thickness   (iv) $y = \delta$ at $u = 0.99 \, U_0$

8.4 Momentum integral equation (for $\partial p/\partial x = 0$) is given by

(a) $\dfrac{\tau_0}{\rho} = U_0 \dfrac{d\delta_*}{dx}$ (b) $\dfrac{\tau_0}{\rho} = U_0^2 \dfrac{d\theta}{dx}$

(c) $\dfrac{\tau_0}{\rho} = U_0 \dfrac{d\theta}{dx}$ (d) $\dfrac{\tau_0}{\rho} = \dfrac{1}{U_0^2} \dfrac{d\theta}{dx}$

(e) none of these answers

8.5 The laminar boundary layer thickness varies as

(a) $x^{1/2}$ (b) $x^{-1/2}$ (c) $x^{1/7}$

(d) $x^{4/5}$ (e) none of these answers

8.6 The turbulent boundary layer thickness varies as

(a) $x^{1/5}$ (b) $x^{-1/5}$ (c) $x^{1/2}$

(d) $x^{4/5}$ (e) none of these answers

8.7 The drag coefficient for a flat plate of unit width is

(a) $\dfrac{2 F_D}{\rho \, U_0^2 L}$ (b) $\dfrac{\rho \, U_0 L}{F_D}$ (c) $\dfrac{\rho \, U_0 L}{2 F_D}$

(d) $\dfrac{\rho \, U_0^2 L}{2 F_D}$ (e) none of these answers

8.8 Which of the following velocity distribution u/U_0 satisfies the boundary conditions for flow along a flat plate ?

(a) $e^{y/\delta}$

(b) $\cos\left(\dfrac{\pi y}{2\delta}\right)$

(c) $\left(\dfrac{y}{\delta}\right) - \left(\dfrac{y}{\delta^2}\right)$

(d) $2\left(\dfrac{y}{\delta}\right) - \left(\dfrac{y}{\delta}\right)^3$

(e) none of these answers

8.9 Separation of boundary layer is caused by

(a) reduction of pressure to vapour pressure

(b) an adverse pressure gradient

(c) reduction of pressure gradient to zero

(d) boundary layer thickness becoming zero

(e) none of theese answers

8.10 Separation occurs when

(a) the boundary layer comes to rest

(b) the pressure intensity reaches a minimum

(c) the velocity gradient at the wall becomes zero

(d) the cross section of the channel reduces to zero

(e) none of these answers

Problems

8.1 Determine the ratio of momentum and displacement thickness to the boundary layer thickness δ when the velocity profile is given by

(a) $u/U_0 = (y/\delta)^{1/2}$

(b) Laminar flow equation

$$u = \frac{1}{2\mu}\,(\partial p/\partial x)\,(R^2 - y^2)$$

(c) $u/U_0 = \sin\left(\dfrac{\pi}{2}\dfrac{y}{\delta}\right)$

8.2 A smooth flat plate 3 m wide and 30 m long is towed through still water at 20°C at a speed of 6 m/s. Determine the total drag on the plate and the drag on the first 3 m of the plate

8.3 A flat plate is drawn submerged through still water at a velocity of 9 m/s. If the plate is 9 m wide and 20 m long, determine the laminar to turbulent transition position and the total drage force acting on the plate. Take water temperature as 20°C   [At 20°C, $v = 10^{-6}$ m^2/s]

8.4 For the velocity distribution given by the following expression for laminar boundary layer, determine boundary layer thickness, wall shear stress and coefficient of drag in terms of Reynolds number, wall shear stress and coefficient of drag in terms of Reynolds number

(a) $u/U_0 = 2(y/\delta) - 2(y/\delta)^3 + (y/\delta)^4$

(b) $u/U_0 = (y/\delta)^{1/n}$

8.5 The velocity profile describing laminar boundary layer given as

$$\frac{u}{U_0} = \sin\left(\frac{\pi}{2} \times \frac{y}{\delta}\right)$$

Show that boundary layer thickness δ, wall shear stress τ_0 and coefficient of drag C_f are given by

$$\delta = \frac{4.795 x}{\sqrt{R_{ex}}} ; \tau_0 = 0.327 \frac{\rho U_0^2}{\sqrt{R_{ex}}} \text{ and } C_f = \frac{1.31}{\sqrt{R_{eL}}}$$

8.6 Find the power required to tow a plate of dimension 1.25 m × 3 m in water with 3 m side in the flow direction at 1 m/s. Make allowance for the fact that boundary layer changes from laminar to turbulent on the plate.

8.7 Find the ratio of friction drag on the front two third length and the rear one third of a flat plate kept in a stream at zero incidence. What will be this ratio for the front and rear halves under similar conditions ?

8.8 A thin plate, 2 m square is towed edgewise in water at 3 m/s. At the trailing edge, the boundary layers both on upper and lower side have the thickness of 5 cm. The velocity distribution within the boundary layer is linear. What is the total drag on the plate ?

8.9. For the turbulent boundary layer on a flat plate the velocity follows the law $u/U_0 = (y/\delta)^{1/9}$. Obtain expressions for δ/x, c_f and C_f. Compare the results with Eqs. 8.31a, 8.34 and 8.35.

8.10 A ship 50 m long and with wetted area 400 m^2 requires 175 kW to overcome the resistance to motion at 7.0 m/s velocity. The total resistance consists of frictional resistance and wave resitance. Determine the frictional resistance and wave resistance. Take $\rho = 1030$ kg/m^3 and $\nu = 0.93 \times 10^{-6}$ m^2/s.

9

Turbulent Flow

9.1 INTRODUCTION

Once the flow of a viscous fluid becomes unstable in any region, the resulting disturbances (eddies) spread over the entire flow section, thereby producing a complex pattern of motion which varies continuously with time. This phenomenon is known as fluid turbulence. The fluid turbulence is similar to macroscopic intermixing of molecules in which bunches of fluid particles move as eddies (*i.e.* macroscopic intermixing). The mixing of fluid particles, in turn, causes more uniform velocity distribution in turbulent flow. Hence, the velocity gradient is much sharp near the boundary. ($\tau_0 = \partial p / \partial x \times y/2$). This means that pressure gradient which is a measure of energy dissipation, is much larger in the turbulent flow.

9.2 TURBULENCE

1. Definition

The best definition of turbulent fluid motion was given by Hinze. Turbulent fluid motion is defined as an irregular condition of flow in which the various quantities like density, velocity, pressure, etc., show a random variation with time and space co-ordinates, so that statistically distinct average values can be discerned.

Since the turbulence is generated by frictinal forces either at the wall or by the flow of layers of fluids with different velocities past or over one another, the kinetic energy of turbulent flow gives rise to the generation of heat. Turbulence by its very nature of origin is dissipative. Hence, if there is no external source of energy to make good the losses due to frictional forces, turbulence will decay. It implies the existence of viscous resistance to motion in a fluid as a necessity. The other functin of viscosity is to spread or diffuse to every part of the flow field.

The fluid turbulence (e.g. fluctuations in velocities, pressure) are the functions of time and spatial co-ordinates. These functions are too complicated and are not known in complete detail. Because of the random nature of the fluid turbulence, the theoretical treatment needs the application of the methods of statistical theory of turbulence which satisfies the equation of motion. Inspite of considerable advancement in this field, the solution of only simplest type of the problem of turbulence have been possible which are termed as 'statistically homogeneous and isotropic turbulence'. Homogeneous turbulence is that turbulence whose statistical average characteristics do not change from point to point. Isotropic turbulence is defined as the turbulence whose statistical parameters and their derivative remain invariant with the rotation and reflection of axes. The turbulent quantities like velocities and pressures can be measured by means of electronic instruments such as hot wire anemometer, laser doppler anemometry, etc.

Consider a typical fluid motion in which the X-component of velocity has been observed over a long period, say, T (Fig. 4.1). The velocity measured at any time instant t is known as instantaneous velocity u. For theoretical study, it is convenient to integrate it over a given time interval (say) T period and obtain the time average velocity $\bar{u}$. Thus the instantaneous velocity u is composed of average velocity $\bar{u}$ and fluctuating component of velocity u'.

$$u = \bar{u} + u' \qquad \qquad ...(9.1a)$$

Similarly, the Y and Z components of velocities and other fluctuating flow parameters can be expressed.

$$v = \bar{v} + v' \qquad \qquad ...(9.1b)$$

$$w = \bar{w} + w' \qquad \qquad ...(9.1c)$$

$$p = \bar{p} + p' \; i.e. \; \text{fluid pressure} \qquad ...(9.1d)$$

The time average quantities are defined as

$$\bar{u} = \frac{1}{T} \int_{t_0}^{t_0+T} u \, dt \qquad \qquad ...(9.2a)$$

$$\bar{v} = \frac{1}{T} \int_{t_0}^{t_0+T} v \, dt \qquad \qquad ...(9.2b)$$

$$\bar{w} = \frac{1}{T} \int_{t_0}^{t_0+T} w \, dt \qquad \qquad ...(9.2c)$$

$$\bar{p} = \frac{1}{T} \int_{t_0}^{t_0+T} p \, dt \qquad \qquad ...(9.2d)$$

Similarly, the time average of the fluctuating components can be determined and these are all equal to zero.

$$\bar{u'} = \frac{1}{T} \int_{0}^{T} u' \, dt = 0 \qquad \qquad ...(9.3a)$$

$$\bar{v'} = \frac{1}{T} \int_{0}^{T} v' \, dt = 0 \qquad \qquad ...(9.3b)$$

$$\bar{w'} = \frac{1}{T} \int_{0}^{T} w' \, dt = 0 \qquad \qquad ...(9.3c)$$

$$\bar{p'} = \frac{1}{T} \int_{0}^{T} p' \, dt = 0 \qquad \qquad ...(9.3d)$$

The sampling time over which the integration is made should be sufficiently large so as to include an adequate number of fluctuations.

2. Intensity of turbulence

The intensity, degree or level of turbulence quantifies how violent these fluctuations are. It is defined as the ratio of 'root mean square values' of fluctuations and time average velocity.

$$I_t = \frac{\sqrt{(\overline{u'^2} + \overline{v'^2} + \overline{w'^2})/3}}{U_0} \qquad ...(9.4)$$

Isotropic turbulence. In case of isotropic turbulence, the root mean square values of the fluctuating velocities in all the three directions are equal.

$$\overline{u'^2} = \overline{v'^2} = \overline{w'^2} \qquad ...(9.5)$$

where

$$\overline{u'^2} = \frac{1}{T} \int_0^T (u')^2 \, dt \qquad ...(9.6)$$

and similarly the expression for $\overline{v'^2}$ and $\overline{w'^2}$ may be written. The degree of turbulence in a laboratory wind tunnel may be controlled by introducing screens of finer mesh in the flow and is defined as

$$I_t \text{ (wind tunnel)} = \frac{\sqrt{\overline{u'^2}}}{U_0} \qquad ...(9.7)$$

3. Scale of turbulence

It is the measure of the average size of the eddies produced in the flow. The eddies vary in size. The smallest eddy exists near the wall and increases in size away from the wall. The largest size of eddy or the largest scale of turbulence is of the order of the scale of flow. In case of boundary layer flow, the largest size of eddies is of the order of the thickness of the boundary layer. Similarly, in case of pipe flow, it may be of the order of pipe diameter. The term 'order of' means that it is nearly of the same size.

4. Kinetic energy of turbulence

The kinetic energy of turbulence is defined by Eq. 9.8.

$$\text{K.E./unit mass} = \frac{(\overline{u'^2} + \overline{v'^2} + \overline{w'^2})}{2} \qquad ...(9.8)$$

9.3 SHEAR STRESS DUE TO TURBULENCE

The mechanism govering the turbulent flow is quite complex. The rapid fluctuations in velocity components in all the three directions cause a turbulent mixing which also results in a transport of momentum from one layer to another. A large number of fluid particles move continuously in a random fashion and intermix with the adjoining fluid layers. Since each layer has different velocity, such intermixing of fluid layers also causes changes in their momentum; this, in turn, results in additional shear stresses and normal stresses of high magnitude. Thus, in turbulent flow, the shear stress at any point is composed of two components; one due to the viscosity of the fluid known as 'viscous shear' and the other due to turbulence present in the flow, known as turbulent shear.

$$\tau = \tau_l + \tau_t \qquad ...(9.9)$$

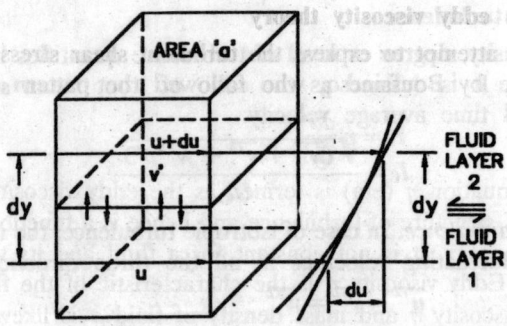

FIG. 9.1 SHEAR STRESS IN TURBULENT FLOW

Consider two fluid layers 1 and 2, which are separted by a small distance dy, in a two dimensional turbulent flow Fig. 9.1. The main flow is in the longitudinal direction only so that $u = u$ (y), $v = 0$, $w = 0$. The time average velocities of 1 and 2 are u_1 and u_2 respectively such that $u_2 > u_1$. In other words, the layer 2 moves in the forward direction with a velocity $u_2 - u_1 = \Delta u$ relative to the lower layer 1. During intermixing, let a small amount of fluid mass be transferred through a small area da between these two layers, with velocity v' (fluctuating compoent of velocity in the normal direction).

The mass of fluid transported $= \rho\, v'\, da$

The layer 2 moves relative to the layer 1 with velocity Δu (which is the same as fluctuating compoennt of velocity u' in the longitudinal direction). Therefore, the rate of change of momentum between these layers

$$= (\rho\, v'\, da)\, u'$$

According to the impulse momentum equation, Eq. 5.58, this causes an additional shear force along an imaginary plane parallel to the main flow.

$$F_t = \rho\, u'\, v'\, da \qquad \qquad ...(9.10a)$$

The turbulent shear stress τ_t is then given by

$$\tau_t = F_t/area = \rho\, u'\, v' \qquad \qquad ...(9.10b)$$

This is known as the Reynolds shear stress. The next problem is to express temporal or fluctuating velocity components in terms of mean velocities. But so far as a workable rational approach based on the statistical mechanics (or average values) is still lacking. For this reason several semi-empirical theories have been proposed.

9.4 SEMI-EMPRICIAL THEORIES

These semi-empirical theories are based on a simplified conceptual model and thus the mathematical formulation is much more simplified. These theories are called semi-empirical because certain numerical values associated with them must be found experimentally to determine the missing physical data.

1. Boussinesq's eddy viscosity theory

The first attempt to express the turbulent shear stress in mathematical form was made by Boussinesq, who followed the pattern of laminar flow,

$$\tau_t = \eta \frac{du}{dy} \qquad ...(9.11)$$

In this equation η (eta) is termed as the eddy viscosity which depends primarily on the structure of turbulence and hence is a function of flow. Unlike the dynamic viscosity, it is not constant for a fluid and its value varies from point to point. Eddy visocsity η is the characteristic of the fluid motion. The ratio of eddy viscosity η and mass density of fluid ρ is likewise termed eddy kinematic viscosity ε .

$$\varepsilon = \frac{\eta}{\rho} \qquad ...(9.12)$$

Eq. 9.9 may now be written in the following form

$$\tau = \tau_{lam} + \tau_{tur} = \mu \frac{\partial \bar{u}}{\partial y} + \eta \frac{\partial \bar{u}}{\partial y} \qquad ...(9.13a)$$

to include the effect of fluid viscosity and fluid turbulence. In turbulent flow, the numerical value of η is too large (several thousand times that of μ). Therefore, the laminar shear term may be neglected for turbulent flow.

$$\tau \approx \bar{\tau}_t = \eta \frac{\partial \bar{u}}{\partial y} \qquad ...(9.13b)$$

For the determination of turbulent shear, a functional relation must be determined between η and $\bar{u}$ but such a relation is not possible to assume as indicated by experimental results.

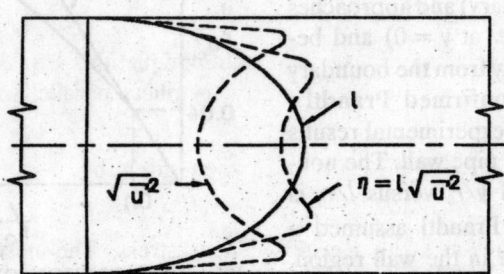

FIG. 9.2 VARIATION OF KINETIC VISCOSITY AND MIXING
LENGTH WITH THE DISTANCE FROM THE WALL

2. Prandtl's mixing length theory

Prandtl succeeded in relating the fluctuating components of the velocities to the general flow characteristics with his theory of mixing length on the concept of mean free path (used in the theory of gases).

In the kinetic theory of gases, it is known that the viscosity μ of a gas depends upon the density of gas, the mean free path of molecules and the mean molecular velocity. If one follows the same analogy between macroscopic molecular motion and macroscopic eddy motion of fluid turbulence, the eddy viscosity should also depend upon the density of the fluid, mean free path traversed by a eddy and some characeristic velocity of eddy motion. Prandtl assumed the most appropriate charactreistic velocity as the root mean square value of temporal velocity $\sqrt{u'^2}$ and characteristic length as mixing length 'l'.

Prandtl defined the mixing length 'l' as the transverse distance normal to the main flow, which the lumps of fluid particles are assumed to traverse in such a way that their original momentum is conserved. By Prandtl's hypothesis, u' has the same magnitude as the difference in the mean velocity (X-direction) between two layers 'l' distance apart* (Fig 9.1)

$$u' = l\frac{du}{dy} \qquad \qquad ...(9.14)$$

Prandtl further assumed that fluctuating compoent of velocity in, Y-direction, v', is of the same order of magnitude as the fluctuating compoent of velocity in X-direction, u', i.e.

$$u' \approx v' \qquad \qquad ...(9.15)$$

Thus Eq. 9.10b becomes

$$\tau = \rho\, u'\, v' = \rho\, l^2 \left(\frac{du}{dy}\right)^2 \qquad \qquad ...(9.16)$$

This is the well known Prandtl's mixing length theory. The variation of l within a round pipe is shown in Fig. 9.3. The major drawback of Eq. 9.16 is that l is a function of y (distance from the rigid boundary) and approaches zero at the wall (i.e. at y = 0) and becomes too large away from the boundary wall. Nikuradse confirmed Prandtl's hypothesis from his experimental results for regions near the pipe wall. The non-dimensional plot of y/r_0 versus l/r_0 is shown in Fig. 9.3. Prandtl assumed a linear variation for l in the wall region.

$$l \,\alpha\, y$$

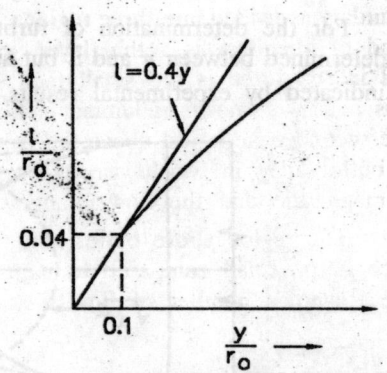

FIG. 9.3 VARIATION OF $\frac{l}{r_0}$ with $\frac{y}{r_0}$

$$l = k\,y \qquad \qquad ...(9.17)$$

* The physical interpretation of it can be seen by multiplying by ρ on both sides of Eq., 9.14.

$$\rho\, u' = l\frac{d\,(\rho\, u)}{dy}$$

i.e., the excess momentum produced in X-direction by instantaneous velocity between two layers 1 and 2 is equal to the quantity of momentum exchanged when the particles move through a distance l.

where k is a constant of proportionality and is known as Karman's universal constant and its value is found to be 0.4 in the region very close to the pipe wall.

3. Von Karman's similarity theory

Von Karman pointed out that l does not directly depend on the distance from the pipe wall y, but on the distribution of the point velocity in the turbulent flow and gave well known "Von karman's similarity theory"[*]

$$I = k \frac{\dfrac{du}{dy}}{\dfrac{d^2u}{dy^2}} \qquad ...(9.18)$$

The limitation of Von Karman's theory is that it leads to zero value of the mixing length at the centre of the pipe, where velocity gradient is zero. The above conclusion is a physical impossible proposition as it leads to zero turbulent shear at the centre which is not correct.

9.5 VELOCITY DISTRIBUTION LAW

As discussed in chapter 8, the fluid layer adjacent to the solid boundary acquires the velocity of the boundary, *i.e.* there is no slip between the fluid and the boundary. It means that the velocity must vary from zero at the rigid stationary boundary to the velocity of turbulent flow; the flow over a solid boundary is divided into three regions. The first zone in the immediate neighour-hood of boundary is a thin layer, in which the viscous force predominates and inertia force is too small (*i.e.* Reynolds number of flow is too small). This region is known as laminar sublayer and the flow in it remains laminar. The second zone is just above the first zone and is known as transition region or buffer zone in which viscous force and inertia force are of same order of magnitude and the flow changes from laminar to turbulent flow.

The region above buffer zone extends into the main flow; the viscous force is too small compared to inertia force and the flow is fully turbulent. The Reynolds number of flow is too high in the turbulent zone.

---

[*]   Karman assumed that the fluctions are statistical and differ from point to point only by time and length scales. He expanded the velocity distribution by Taylor's series.

$$u(y + \Delta y) = u(y) + \frac{du}{dy} \Delta y + \frac{1}{2} \frac{d^2u}{dy^2} (\Delta y)^2 + ...$$

and assumed that mixing length l depends on mean point velocity and it should be a function of

$$\frac{du}{dy}, \frac{d^2u}{dy^2}, etc$$

$$\therefore \qquad 1 \, \alpha \, \frac{(du/dy)}{(d^2u/dy^2)}$$

1. Velocity distribution in the laminar sublayer

The shear stress at the boundary is termed as well shear stress τ_0 (i.e. τ at $y = 0$). From Newton's law of viscosity, it is given by

$$\tau_0 = \mu \left(\frac{\partial u}{\partial y} \right)_{y=0}$$

Dividing by ρ on both sides

$$\frac{\tau_0}{\rho} = v \left(\frac{\partial u}{\partial y} \right)_{y=0} = v \frac{u}{y} \qquad ...(9.19a)$$

Substituting $\tau_0/\rho = U_*^2$ and rearranging terms

$$\frac{u}{U_*} = \frac{U_* y}{v} \qquad ...(9.19b)$$

Eq. 9.19 shows that a linear variation exists between u/U_* and $U_* y/v$. In other words, it shows that velocity varies linearly in the region of laminar sublayer. Experimentally, the following values of $U_* y/v$ have been found for the three regions mentioned above,

Laminar sublayer : $\quad \dfrac{U_* y}{v} \leq 5$ $\qquad ...(9.20a)$

Buffer zone $\quad 5 < \dfrac{U_* y}{v} \leq 70$ $\qquad ...(.20b)$

Turbulent flow $\quad \dfrac{U_* y}{v} > 70$ $\qquad ...(9.20c)$

2. Karman Prandtl's velocity distribution

In the turbulent region ($y > \delta$), the Reynolds shear stress τ_t predominates as compared to viscous forces. From Eq. 9.16,

$$\tau = \rho l^2 \left(\frac{du}{dy} \right)^2 \qquad ...(9.21a)$$

Prandtl assumed that the shear stress remains constant in a thin region near the boundary and is equal to wall shear stress τ_0

$$\tau = \tau_0 = \rho l^2 \left(\frac{du}{dy} \right)^2_{y=0} \qquad ...(9.21b)$$

According to Karman's theory, Eq. 9.17,

$$l \approx k y \qquad ...(9.17)$$

near the solid boundary

Hence, $\qquad \dfrac{\tau_0}{\rho} = k^2 y^2 \left(\dfrac{du}{dy} \right)^2 \qquad ...(9.21c)$

Rearranging the terms and writing U_*^2 in place of τ_0/ρ

$$\frac{du}{U_*} = \frac{dy}{ky}$$

Integrating, $\quad \dfrac{u}{U_*} = \dfrac{1}{k}\log_e y + C \qquad ...(9.22)$

Here C is a constant of integration which should be determined from

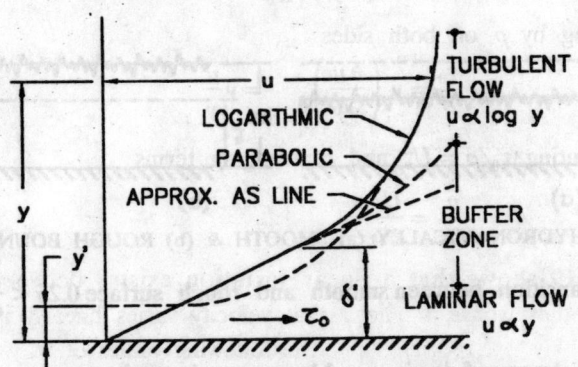

FIG. 9.4 DEFINITION SKETCH – LAMINAR SUB LAYER

known boundary conditions. Eq. 9.22 shows that the velocity distribution is logarithmic · in the turbulent region.

Referring to Fig. 9.4, it is seen that the velocity becomes zero at certain distance, y' from the boundary (for logarithmic velocity distribution in the turbulent region)

This means $\qquad C = \dfrac{-1}{k}\log y'$

The velocity distribution in the turbulent region is then given by,

$$\frac{u}{U_*} = \frac{1}{k}\log_e \frac{y}{y'} \qquad ...(9.23a)$$

The value of Karman's constant is found to be nearly 0.4 near the wall. Hence,

$$\frac{u}{U_*} = 5.75 \log_{10} \frac{y}{y'} \qquad ...(9.23b)$$

3. Hydrodynamically smooth and rough surface

All the physical boundaries have protrusions or projections over them which are irregular in nature. As a matter of fact there is no surface which may be regarded as completely smooth. The terms smooth and rough are relative.

When the turbulent flow takes place over a surface and the thickness of laminar sublayer is relatively large such that the protrusions are completely submerged in it, the surface behaves as a smooth boundary and is thus known as hydrodynamically smooth surface. If the laminar sublayer is thin enough so that the protrusions are projecting out of the laminar sublayer, the surface behaves as a hydrodynamically rough surface, Fig. 9.5. The criterion to determine whether the surface will behave as smooth or rough is

(a) Hydrodynamically smooth surface: $\dfrac{k_s}{\delta'} < 0.25$ ...(9.24a)

(b) Hydrodynamically rough surface: $\dfrac{k_s}{\delta'} > 6$ ...(9.24b)

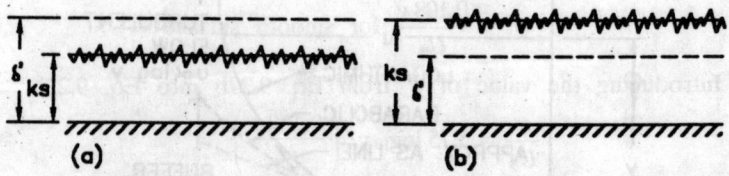

FIG. 9.5 HYDRONAMICALLY (a) SMOOTH & (b) ROUGH BOUNDARIES

(b) Transition between smooth and rough surface $0.25 < \dfrac{k_s}{\delta'} < 6$

...(9.24c)

The thickness of laminar sublayer can be written as

$$\delta' = \frac{cv}{U_*}$$

from Eq. 8.44. Substituting the value of U_* from Eq. 7.30b

$$U_* = U\sqrt{f/8}$$

the dimensionless ratio δ'/D becomes

$$\frac{\delta'}{D} = \frac{c'v}{UD\sqrt{f}} = \frac{14.14}{\text{Re}\sqrt{f}}$$ ...(9.25)

The thickness of laminar sublayer decreases as the Reynolds number of flow is increased; the variation of f is small with change in R_e. Thus, it is seen that the same surface may behave as smooth or rough depending upon the Reynolds number of flow.

4. Velocity distribution over a smooth surface

The distance $y = \delta'$ marks the limit of the stability of laminar sublayer and is represented by χ, Eq. 7.54. Replacing the parabolic segment of velocity profile near the boundary in Fig. 9.4 by a straight line, Eq. 9.19a is written as,

$$\frac{du}{dy} = \frac{\tau_0}{\mu}$$

Therefore, $\chi = \dfrac{y^2\, du/dy}{v}$

$$\chi = \frac{(\delta')^2}{v}\frac{\tau_0}{\mu} = \frac{\delta'^2\, \tau_0}{\rho\, v^2} = C_2$$

So that $\delta' = \dfrac{\sqrt{C_2}\, v}{\sqrt{\tau_0/\rho}} = \sqrt{C_2}\, v/U_* = C_3\, y'$ ...(9.26)

Eq. 9.26 shows the relationship between δ' and y' . This hypothesis has been also verified experimentally by Nikuradse and he obtained the value of constant C_2 and C_3 . Nikuradse obtained.

$$\delta' = 11.6\, v/U_*\qquad\qquad ...(9.27a)$$

and

$$y' = \frac{\delta'}{107}$$

$$y' = \frac{0.108\, v}{U_*}\ \text{for smooth surface}\qquad ...(9.27b)$$

Introducing the value of y' from Eq. 9.27b into Eq. 9.23b,

$$\frac{u}{U_*} = 5.75\log_{10} y/\left(\frac{0.108\, v}{U_*}\right)$$

Simplifying,

$$\frac{u}{U_*} = 5.75\log_{10}\left(\frac{U_* y}{v}\right) + 5.5\qquad ...(9.28)$$

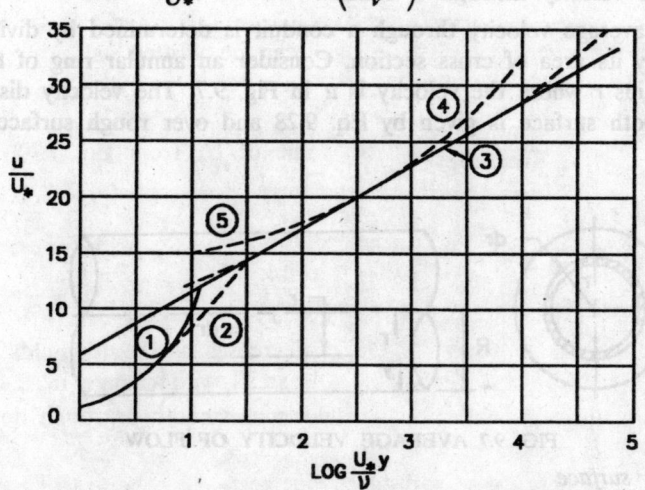

FIG. 9.6 VARIATION OF u/U* with U*y/ν FOR SMOOTH PIPES,

(1) EQ. 9.19b (2) TRANSITION FROM LAMINAR TO TURBULENT

(3) EQ. 9.28 (4) EQ. 9.42 (5) EQ. 9.37 WITH m = 1/10

Eq. 9.28 shows that the non-dimensional velocity u/U_* for turbulent flow (over a smooth surface) depends on non-dimensional parameter $U_* y/u$, a form of Reynolds number as shown in Fig. 9.6.

5. Velocity distribution over a rough boundary

For turbulent flow, the distance y' of Eq. 9.23b is expected to be directly proportional to the average height of protrusions k_s . Nikuradse and many other investigators did experiments on artificially roughened pipes and found that k_s should be greater than $10\,\delta'$. The pipes were made artificially rough by cementing coatings of sand grain of diameter k_s . (It is used as a measure of roughness of commercial pipes). In fact, y' was found to be related with k_s as

$$y' = \frac{k_s}{30} \qquad ...(9.29)$$

for rough pipes.

Introducing this value of y' in Eq. 9.23b,

$$\frac{u}{U_*} = 5.75 \log_{10} \frac{y}{(k_s/30)}$$

Simplifying,

$$\frac{u}{U_*} = 5.75 \log_{10} \frac{y}{k_s} + 8.5 \qquad ...(9.30)$$

Eq. 9.30 shows that the velocity in turbulent flow over rough surface depends only on the parameter y/k_s.

6. Average velocity through a conduit

The average velocity through a conduit is determined by dividing the discharge by its area of cross section. Consider an annular ring of thickness dr at a radius r where the velocity is u in Fig. 9.7. The velocity distribution over a smooth surface is given by Eq. 9.28 and over rough surface by Eq. 9.30.

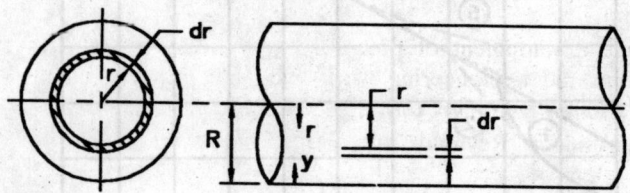

FIG. 9.7 AVERAGE VELOCITY OF FLOW

(a) *Smooth surface*

$$dQ = (2\pi r\, dr)\, u$$

Substituting the value of u from Eq. 9.28 and integrating,

$$Q = \int_0^R 2\pi r\, U_* \left[5.75 \log \frac{U_* (R - r)}{v} + 5.5 \right] dr \qquad ...(9.31)$$

where

$$y = (R - r)$$

The average velocity U is given by

$$U = \frac{Q}{\pi R^2}$$

Simplifying

$$\frac{U}{U_*} = \left[5.75 \log_{10} \frac{U_* R}{v} + 1.75 \right] \qquad ...(9.32)$$

(b) *Rough surface*

$$Q = \int_0^R 2 \pi r \, dr \, U_* \left[5.75 \log_{10} \frac{y}{k_s} + 8.5 \right]$$

and

$$U = \frac{Q}{\pi R^2}$$

Solving these two equations,

$$\frac{U}{U_*} = \left[5.75 \log_{10} \frac{R}{k_s} + 4.75 \right] \qquad \qquad ...(9.33)$$

It is interesting to note that the difference of velocities, *i.e.* $(u-U)/U_*$ versus y is found to be the same for both smooth and rough surface.

From either Eqs. 9.28 and 9.32 or from Eqs. 9.30 and 9.33,

$$\frac{u - U}{U_*} = [5.75 \log_{10} \frac{y}{R} + 3.75] \qquad \qquad ...(9.34)$$

It means that if the shear or friction velocity U_*, defined as $\sqrt{\tau_0/\rho}$ is the same for smooth and rough surface, the velocity u at any elevation y above the solid boundary remains the same.

9.6 OTHER FORMS OF VELOCITY DISTRIBUTION

The velocity distribution for turbulent flow in a closed conduit can also be expressed in other forms.

1. Power law

Before the development of pipe theory by Prandtl, Von Karman and Nikuradse, Blasius did a pioneering work and gave expressions for velocity, wall shear and friction factor for turbulent flow through a smooth pipe. These equations were valid for Reynolds number varying in the range of 3×10^3 to 10^5.

$$f = \frac{0.3164}{(R_e)^{1/4}} \qquad \qquad ...(9.35)$$

Substituting the value of f from Eq. 9.35 into Eq. 7.30b

$$U_* = U \sqrt{f/8}$$

$$\frac{\tau_0}{\rho} = \frac{U^2 f}{8}$$

$$\tau_0 = \frac{\rho U^2}{8} \frac{0.3164 \mu^{1/4}}{(\rho U D)^{1/4}} = 0.0332 \, \mu^{1/4} \, R^{-1/4} \, U^{7/4} \, \rho^{3/4} \qquad ...(9.36)$$

Blasius assumed that the velocity profile for turbulent flow could be approximated by

$$\left(\frac{u}{U_c} \right) = \left(\frac{y}{R} \right)^m \qquad \qquad ...(9.37)$$

where U_c is the maximum velocity occurs at the centre line of the pipe.

The average velocity of flow U through the pipe can now be determined.

$$U = \frac{1}{\pi R^2}\left[\int_0^R u\,(2\pi r\,dr)\right]$$

From Eqs. 9.37 and 9.38

$$U = \frac{1}{\pi R^2}\left[\int_0^R U_c\left(\frac{y^m}{R^m}\right)2\pi r\,dr\right]$$

Solving it,

$$\frac{U}{U_c} = \frac{2}{(m+1)(m+2)} \qquad ...(9.39)$$

Dividing Eq. 9.39 by Eq. 9.37,

$$\frac{U}{u} = \frac{2}{(m+1)(m+2)}\left(\frac{R}{y}\right)^m \qquad ...(9.40)$$

Using this value of U from Eq. 9.40 into Eq. 9.36,

$$\tau_0 = 0.0332\left[\frac{2}{(m+1)(m+2)}\right]^{7/4}\mu^{1/4}R^{7m/4-1/4}\times y^{-7m/4}\rho^{3/4}u^{7/4}$$

$$...(9.41)$$

Blasius reasoned that the wall shear stress could depend upon the velocity profile and physical properties of the fluid but could not depend on the size of the pipe ; hence, the exponent of R must be zero. From this argument, he concluded that the exponent m of the velocity profile must be $1/7$. This hypothesis has been found to agree quite well with the experimental results and is known as 'one seventh root law'.

$$\left(\frac{u}{U_c}\right) = \left(\frac{y}{R}\right)^{1/7} \qquad ...(9.42)$$

Some engineers express the exponent in Eq. 9.37 as $1/n$ instead of m, Indeed, the exponent has been found to depend on the Reynolds number of turbulent flow and may vary up to $1/10$ for Re equal to or more than 2×10^6.

Table 9.1

Re	4×10^3	2.3×10^4	1.1×10^5	1.1×10^6	2×10^6
l/n	6.0	6.6	7.0	8.8	10.0

It is to be noted that both velocity profiles described by Eqs. 9.28 and 9.42 have the defect of non-zero value of du/dy at the centre line of the conduit.

2. Universal velocity distribution

The velocity distribution for the turbulent flow outside the buffer zone is described by Eq. 9.22. The constant of integration C may be determined using alternative boundary condition. At the centre line of the pipe $y = R$ and $u = U_{max}$

Substituting this boundary condition into Eq. 9.22

$$C = \frac{U_{max}}{U_*} - \frac{1}{k} \log_e R \qquad ...(9.23b)$$

Hence, the velocity distribution, Eq. 9.22, becomes

$$\frac{u}{U_*} = \frac{1}{k} \log_e \frac{y}{R} + \frac{U_{max}}{U_*}$$

or

$$\frac{U_{max} - u}{U_*} = 5.75 \log_{10} \left(\frac{R}{y} \right) \qquad ...(9.42)$$

The difference in velocity term $U_{max} - u$ is usually referred as velocity defect and Eq. 9.42 is known as 'velocity defect law' which is applicable to all type of turbulent flow irrespective of the nature of the surface.

3. Von Karman's velocity distribution

Von Karman considered the similarity of turbulent flow pattern (Sec. 9.4.3) and found that shearing stress between any two layers in a turbulent flow is given by

$$\tau = \rho \, l^2 \left(\frac{du}{dy} \right)^2 = \rho \, k^2 \, \frac{(du/dy)^4}{(d^2u/dy^2)^2} \qquad ...(9.43)$$

The shearing stress varies linearly with radius of the pipe.

$$\tau = \tau_* \frac{r}{R} = \tau_0 \, (1 - y/R) \qquad ...(9.44)$$

where y is the distance measured from the pipe wall

Equating Eqs. 9.43 and 9.44, and simplifying

$$\frac{\left(\dfrac{du}{dy} \right)^2}{\dfrac{d^2u}{dy^2}} = \frac{1}{k} \sqrt{\frac{\tau_0}{\rho} \left(1 - \frac{y}{R} \right)} \qquad ...(9.45a)$$

Substituting U_* in place of $\sqrt{\tau_*/\rho}$ and writing the reciprocal of above equation,

$$\left(\frac{du}{dy} \right)^{-2} \frac{d}{dy} \left(\frac{du}{dy} \right) = \frac{k}{U_*} \left(\frac{\sqrt{R}}{\sqrt{R - y}} \right) \qquad ...(9.45b)$$

Integrating it,

$$-\left(\frac{du}{dy} \right)^{-1} = \frac{-2k}{U_*} \sqrt{R} \, (\sqrt{R - y}) + C \qquad ...(9.46)$$

where C is the constant of integration which can be determined by using the known boundary condition, i.e. at $y = 0$, du/dy is too large and hence $(du/dy)^{-1}$ is approximately zero.

$$C = \frac{2kR}{U_*} \qquad \ldots (9.47)$$

Substituting the value of C in Eq. 9.46,

$$-\left(\frac{du}{dy}\right)^{-1} = \frac{-2k}{U_*}\sqrt{R}\sqrt{R-y} + \frac{2kR}{U_*}$$

or

$$\left(\frac{du}{dy}\right) = \frac{U_*}{2kR}\left(\frac{1}{1-\sqrt{1-y/R}}\right) \qquad \ldots (9.48)$$

Eq. 9.48 represents the velocity gradient for the Karman's velocity profile. Putting $(1-y/R) = z^2$, so that $-dy = 2Rz\,dz$

$$du = \frac{U_*}{2kR}\left(\frac{1}{1-z}\right)(-2Rz\,dz)$$

Integrating it,

$$\frac{u}{U_*} = \frac{1}{k}\left[\log_e(1-z) + z\right] + C \qquad \ldots (9.49a)$$

Replacing z by $\sqrt{1-y/R}$

$$\frac{u}{U_*} = \frac{1}{k}\left[\log\left(1-\sqrt{1-y/R}\right) + \sqrt{1-y/R}\right] + C$$

At the centre of pipe, $y = R$, $u = U_{max}$

Therefore $C = U_{max}/U_*$

Hence, Karman's velocity distribution is given by

$$\frac{u - U_{max}}{U_*} = \frac{1}{k}\left[\log(1-\sqrt{1-y/R}) + \sqrt{1-y/R}\right] \qquad \ldots (9.49b)$$

4. Velocity distribution over a flat plate

Sufficiently large experimental data was collected for the flow over flat plate by various investigators. The data was then plotted in the non-dimensional form over a semi-logarithmic graph; u/U_* over simple scale and U_*y/v over log scale. The slope of the straight line fitted to various points in the wall region resulted in the experimental value of Karman's constant for the flow over a flat plate as 0.417 instead of 0.4. The intercept on the u/U_* scale yields the value of the constant C as 5.84, thus the velocity distribution for the flow over flat plate becomes,

$$\frac{u}{U_*} = 5.52\log_{10}\frac{U_*y}{v} + 5.84 \qquad \ldots (9.50)$$

9.7 RESISTANCE LAW

While the real fluid flows through a pipe the energy loss due to friction occurs to the flow. Many empirical formulas have been derived by various investigators. One of the rational formula relating friction loss with average velocity was developed by Darcy in 1854. Simultaneously, Weisbach also developed similar formula. Hence it is known as Darcy Weisbach equation for head loss.

9.8 DARCY WEISBACH EQUATION

Let us consider a fluid of known mass density ρ and dynamic viscosity μ which flows through an inclined pipe of diameter D. Let the length of pipe be L and let it make an angle θ with the vertical direction. The forces causing the flow are the pressures p_1 and p_2 acting at its two ends and the weight component of the fluid acting in the direction of flow. The force resisting the flow is the shear τ_0, (or frictional force) acting along the surface of contact.

$$p_1 \frac{\pi D^2}{4} - p_2 \frac{\pi D^2}{4} + W \cos \theta = \tau_0 \pi D L$$

Since $\cos \theta = dz/dL = (z_1 - z_2)/L$

Simplifying,

$$[(p_1 + w z_1) - (p_2 + w z_2)] D/4L = \tau_0$$

where z_1 and z_2 are the elevations of two ends above an arbitrary datum,

Writing $(p_1 + w z_1) - (p_2 + w z_2) = w h_f$

$\therefore \quad w h_f (D/4L) = \tau_0$

where h_f is the head loss occurring between sections 1 and 2 which are L distance apart.

From Eq. 7.30b, $\tau_0 = f \rho U^2/8$

$$w h_f (D/4L) = f \rho U^2/8$$

Solving it, $h_t = f \dfrac{L}{D} \dfrac{U^2}{2g}$ ...(9.51)

Eq. 9.51 is known as 'Darcy Weisbach equation'. In this equation f is known as Darcy's frictional coefficient which needs to be evaluated for various conditions of flow and varying nature of the surface of contact.

9.9 COEFFICIENT OF FRICTION AND ITS VARIATION

The wall shear stress τ_0 and in turn, Darcy's friction coefficient f depends on the average velocity of flow U, the pipe diameter D, the fluid density ρ, the fluid viscosity μ, and the nature of the surface or the average wall roughness k_s Thus the functional relationship for f may be written as

$$f = \varphi(\rho, U, D, \mu, k_s) \qquad ...(9.52a)$$

By dimensional analysis, the following relationship is obtained.

$$f = \varphi(R_e, k_s/D) \qquad ...(9.52b)$$

Eq. 9.52b shows that f depends on the Reynolds number of the flow and relative roughness of the pipe. The friction factor for flows in two pipes will be the same if these are completely similar geometrically (similarity of k_s/D) and dynamically (similarity of Reynolds number).

9.10 RESULTS OF PIPE FRICTION EXPERIMENTS

The relationship of Eq. 9.52b indicates a convenient means of representing data on friction factor. In 1914, Stanton plotted $\log f$ against $\log R_e$ for various values of k_s/D (termed as relative roughness). Later the results of systematic tests by Nikuradse on turbulent flow in smooth and rough pipes demonstrated a perfect relationship between f, R_e and k_s/D . Fig. 9.8. In these tests the geometric similarity of roughness pattern was obtained by gluing a coating of uniform sand grains to the pipe wall, thus giving an easily measureable index for relative roughness k_s/D ; k_s being the diameter of the uniform size sand grains. Nikuradse's results are accepted today as the basic standards. But these curves are not to be used directly in solving engineering problems of commercial pipes. In the case of artificially roughnened pipes, the roughness is uniform; whereas in commercial pipes it is irregular in size and in distribution.

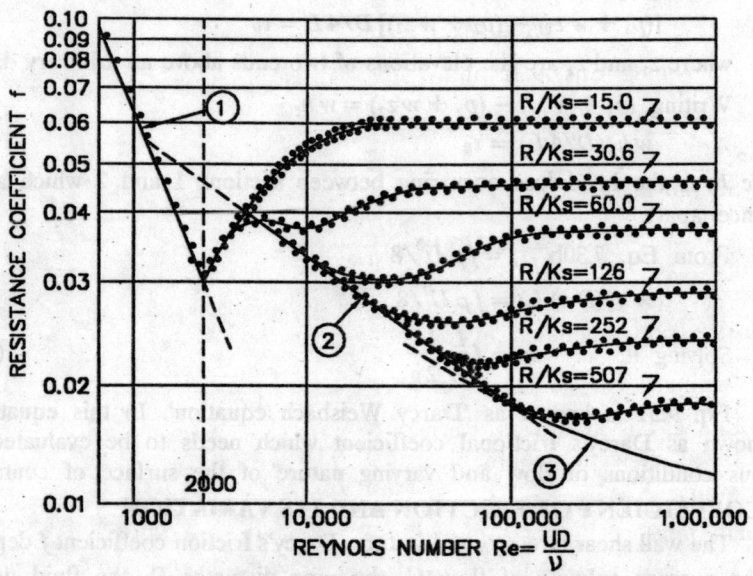

FIG. 9.8 NIKURADSE CURVE – VARIATION OF FRICTION FACTOR
FOR ARTIFICIALLY ROUGHENED PIPES (1) EQ. 7.29,
(2) EQ. 9.35 & (3) EQ. 9.54

It is to be noted that for R_e under 2000, a simple relationship exists betwen f and R_e which is completely independent of roughness of the wall. The relationship described by Eq. 7.29 is plotted as a straight line on log log–scale in Fig. 9.8. For laminar region through pipe, the relationship is

$$f = 64/R_e \qquad \qquad ...(7.29)$$

Beyond the critical range of R_e, a transitional region exists in which the values of f are uncertain and the flow might be either laminar or turbulent.

In turbulent flow, there are three regions - smooth pipe zone of the flow, transition between smooth pipe zone and rough pipe zone and rough pipe zone of the flow. Blasius suggested an empirical equation for the smooth pipe zone which is valid for R_e values upto 10^5

$$f = \frac{0.3164}{R_e^{1/4}} \qquad ...(9.35)$$

9.11 UNIVERSAL RESISTANCE LAWS

1. Smooth pipe

The average velocity for turbulent flow through a smooth pipe is given by Eq. 9.32

$$\frac{U}{U_*} = 5.75 \log_{10} \frac{U_* R}{\nu} + 1.75 \qquad ...(9.32)$$

and the shear velocity U_* is given by Eq. 7.30b

$$U_* = U \sqrt{f/8} \qquad ...(7.30b)$$

Combining Eqs. 9.32 and 7.30b,

$$\frac{U}{U \sqrt{f/8}} = 5.75 \log_{10} \frac{U \sqrt{f/8}\, R}{\nu} + 1.75$$

Simplifying,

$$\frac{1}{\sqrt{f}} = 2.03 \log_{10} \frac{U D \sqrt{f}}{\nu} - 0.91 \qquad ...(9.53)$$

The experimental measurements for flows on smooth pipes follow Eq. 9.53 with slightly modified numerical constants.

$$1/\sqrt{f} = 2 \log_{10} R_e \sqrt{f} - 0.8 \qquad ...(9.54)$$

Eq. 9.54 is known as 'Karman-Prandtl's universal resistance equation' for turbulent flow in smooth pipe. The equation is valid for R_e values up to 3.4×10^6.

2. Rough pipe

The average velocity for turbulent flow in a rough pipe is given by Eq. 9.33

$$\frac{U}{U_*} = 5.75 \log \frac{R}{k_a} + 4.75 \qquad ...(9.33)$$

Combining Eqs. 9.33 and 7.30b,

$$\frac{U}{U \sqrt{f/8}} = 5.75 \log_{10} \frac{R}{k_s} + 4.75$$

Solving it,

$$\frac{1}{\sqrt{f}} = 2.03 \log_{10} \frac{R}{k_s} + 1.68 \qquad ...(9.58)$$

Again, a comparison with Nikuradse's experimental measurements suggests a slightly modified numerical constants

$$\frac{1}{\sqrt{f}} = 2 \log \frac{R}{k_s} + 1.74 \qquad ...(9.56)$$

Eq. 9.56 is known as 'Karman-Prandtl's universal resistance equation' for turbulent flow in rough pipes.

It is to be noted f for turbulent flow in a rough pipe depends only on the relative somoothness R/k_s, of the pipe and is independent of Reynolds number of flow. This is so because in completely rough pipes the fluid resistance is caused due to the pipe roughness (known as form drag) and the laminar sublayer is too thin at high Reynolds number of the flow. Eq. 9.56 is represented by the horizontal segement (on the right) of curve in Fig. 9.8 for varius values of R/k_s .

3. Transition region between smooth and rough pipes

A pipe behaves as a smooth pipe at low Reynolds number of flow and as a rough pipe at high Reynolds number. In the intermediate zone, both viscosity and wall prqtrusions determine the boundary resistance. Thus, the ratio of δ' to k_s , i.e., δ'/k_s should determine the value of f in the transition region. This hypothesis has been verified by plotting $\dfrac{R_e \sqrt{f}}{R/k_s}$ as abcissa and $1\sqrt{f} - 2 \log R/k_s$ as ordinate in Fig. 9.9. In this diagram the middle segment shows the Nikuradse's curve for artificially rough pipes as well as for commerical pipes. The diagram also indicates the range of smooth and rough surface.

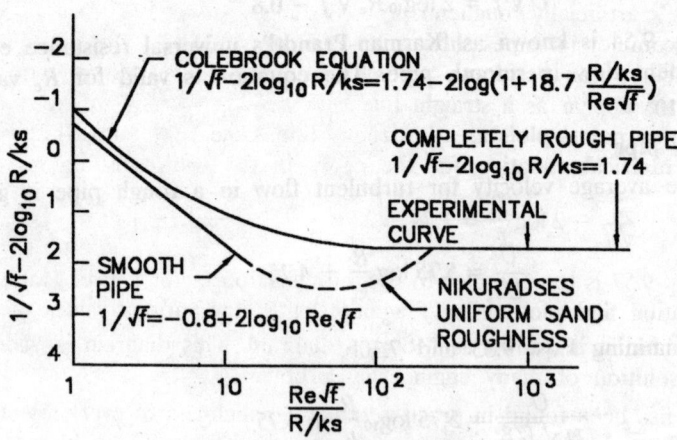

FIG. 9.9 TRANSITION FUNCTION FOR (a) ARTIFICIALLY ROUGH
AND (b) COMMERCIAL PIPE

Smooth surface: $\dfrac{R_e\sqrt{f}}{R/k_s} = 17$

Transitional surface: $17 < \dfrac{R_s\sqrt{f}}{R/k_s} < 400$

Rough surface: $\dfrac{R_e\sqrt{f}}{R/k_s} = 400$

9.12 RESISTANCE OF COMMERCIAL PIPES

Nikuradse's curve in Fig. 9.8 cannot be directly used to evaluate the coefficient of resistance for commercial pipes. It is obvious that irregularities on the boundary of commercial material such as metal, wood and concrete vary considerably in the average height, form and pattern so that it is impossible to describe wall irregularities in terms of a single length dimention, i.e. sand grain diameter. However, the eqlvalent sand roughness of a commercial pipe may be determined from the following procedure.

(1) Experimentally determine f, using Darcy;s Eq. 9.51, for various values of R_e .

(2) Plot $\log f$ against $\log R_e$.

(3) Read the value of f corresponding to the horizontal portion of the $\log f - R_e$ curve for the wholly rough region of turbulent flow.

(4) Compute relative smoothness R/k_s from Eq. 9.56, and thereby ti.. equivalent sand roughness. k_s for the commercial pipe.

In the transition region (between smooth pipe flow and rough pip flow), the friction factor depends on the wall roughness and Reynolds numbr and hence the results obtained for commercial pipes are expected to diff from those of uniform size sand roughened pipes. In Fig. 9.9 C.F. Colebroo' experimental data for commercial pipes have been superimposed over thε Nikuradse's artificially roughend pipes in the transition region. It is seen that data for commercial pipes show a lot of scatter but as a first approximation, a single curve can be drawn through all these points. In the smooth pipe region, data appear as a straight line with a slope 2.0 and in the rough pipe region, these points plots as a horizontal line. Colebrook and White proposed a semi empirical equation for the curve in the transition region.

$$\frac{1}{\sqrt{f}} - 2\log\frac{R}{k_s}' = 1.74 - 2\log\left(\frac{1 + 18.7\,R/k_s}{R_e\sqrt{f}}\right) \qquad ...(9.57)$$

Eq. 9.57 is too complex to solve for friction factor f. L.F. Moody solved this equation and plotted $\log f$ against $\log R_e$ for various values of R/k_s in Fig. 9.10 and it is known as Moody's diagram. This diagram is widely used for the solution of many engineering problems.

It has been found in practice that the roughness of every material usec for commercial pipe increases in due course of time. The values of k_s used in Fig. 9.10 are for new pipes and need revision from time to time whilε

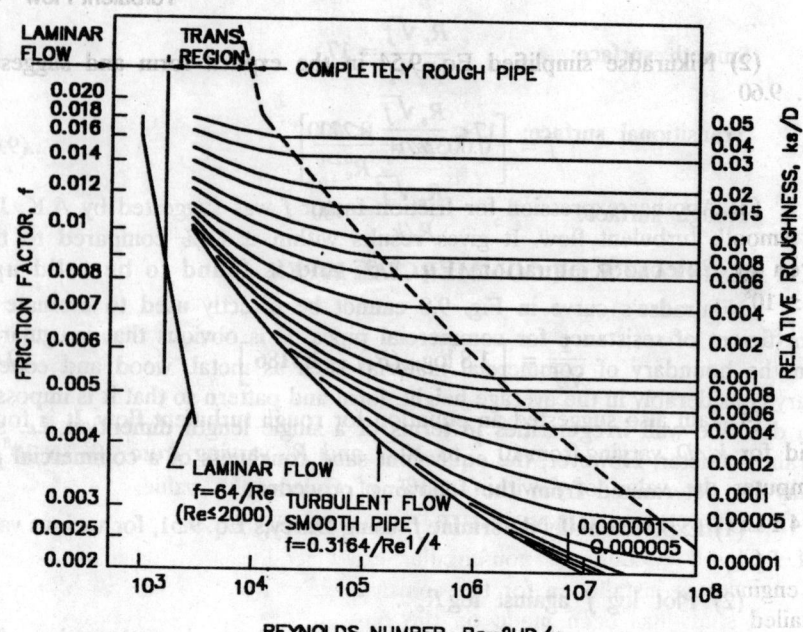

FIG. 9.10 MOODY'S DIAGRAM FOR DETERMINING FRICTION
FACTOR FOR COMMERCIAL PIPES

the pipes are in use. Colebrook and White have shown that the boundary
roughness increases to k_o after a lapse of time t and is given by

$$k_0 = k_s + \alpha t \qquad \qquad ...(9.58)$$

where α is time rate of change of roughness. A fair estimate of α can be
made by taking resistance measurements at different times for future variation
in pipe capacity.

9.13 EXPLICIT EQUATION FOR FRICTION FACTOR

Many times the value of f required for the computation of head loss
for the flow through pipes lies in the transition region; for which Colebrook
expression, Eq. 9.57, is applicable. This equation is implicit in nature and
f appears on both sides of the equation. The solution of such an equation
needs trial and error procedure for the evaluation of f. For this reason,
some explicit formulae are required which contain f only on one side of the
equation. There are various formuale suggested by reseachers, some of which
are discussed below.

(1) Blasius suggested Eq. 9.35 for smooth turbulent flow. This equation
is valid for R_e value upto 10^5

$$f = \frac{0.3164}{R_e^{1/4}} \qquad \qquad ...(9.59)$$

(2) Nikuradse simplified Eq. 9.54 in the explicit form and suggested Eq. 9.60

$$f = \left[0.00332 + \frac{0.221}{R_e^{0.237}} \right] \qquad ...(9.60)$$

(3) Another expression for friction factor f was suggested by A.K. Jain for smooth turbulent flow. It gives results within $\pm 1\%$ compared to that given by Colebrook equation, Eq. 9.57 and is found to be valid upto $R_e \leq 10^8$

$$\frac{1}{\sqrt{f}} = \left[1.8 \log_{10}(R_e) - 1.5186 \right] \qquad ...(9.61)$$

(4) Jain also suggested an equation for rough turbulent flow. It is found valid for k_s/D varying from 10^{-6} to 10^{-2} and R_e varying from 10^3 to 10^8. It computes the value of f within $\pm 1\%$ of Colebrook's value.

9.14 FLOW THROUGH NON-CIRCULAR PIPES

Closed conduits of non-circular cross section are frequently used in an engineering installation for the conveynance of fluids. However, not much detailed study has been made on the flow of fluids through non-circular pipes.

Velocity distribution patterns for turbulent flows in rectangular, triangular and trapezoidal section were obtained by Nikuradse, Schiller and Prandtl. In contrast to circular cross section, the existence of secondary motion was reported by Nikuradse, Prandtl and others. The secondary flow is superimposed over longitudinal flow of the fluid particles and in this process the secondary motion transports momentum from rest of the fluid towards the corners. Therefore, comparatively large longitudinal velocities are found at the corners. In Fig. 9.11 the lines of equal velocities in the two cross-sections of the conduits are shown.

The relationship for resistance to fluid at any section can be obtained by integrating Eq. 9.28 for smooth section to obtain average velocity of flow. The shear velocity U_* is expressed in terms of average velocity and friction factor f by Eq. 7.30b. Similar procedure may be followed for rough conduits using Eq. 9.30. Since the section is different than circular, different numerial constants are obtained in the expression for f.

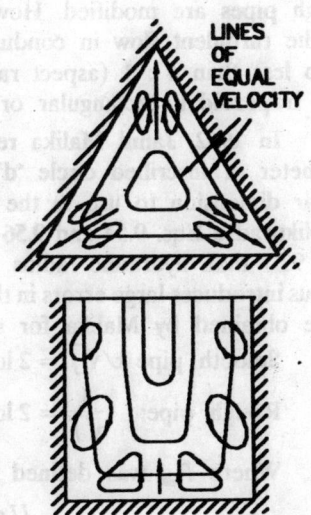

LINES OF EQUAL VELOCITY

FIG. 9.11 VELOCITY DISTRIBU-TION AND SECONDARY FLOW THROUGH NON–CIRCULAR CONDUITS

Smooth: $\qquad \dfrac{1}{\sqrt{f}} = 2.03 \log \left(\dfrac{2BU}{\nu} \sqrt{f} \right) - 0.47 \qquad$ ...(9.62)

Rough: $\qquad \dfrac{1}{\sqrt{f}} = 2.03 \log \left(\dfrac{B/2}{k_s} \right) + 2.11 \qquad$ ...(9.63)

In Eq. 9.62, B is width of cross section or spacing between the boundries. The constants of integration need to be modified as to satisfy the experimental data. Unfortunately, not much experimental data are available for non-circular sections. The assumption of similar velocity distribution is questionable for non-circular sections. Moreover, the wall shear stress τ_0 is also not expected same at all points of the boundary. Hence, the results of above equations are of qualitative nature.

It is a common practice to use hydraulic radius R in place of diameter D of the pipe in the earlier derived resistance equations. The hydraulic radius is defined as the ratio of cross sectional area of the flow to the wetted perimeter

$$R = \frac{A}{P} = \frac{D}{4} \quad \text{for circular cross section} \qquad ...(9.64)$$

Hence, the Darcy's Eq. 9.51 for non-circular section is modified as

$$h_f = f \frac{L}{4R} \frac{U^2}{2g} \qquad ...(9.65)$$

Similarly, other resistance equations for evaluation of f for smooth and rough pipes are modified. However, the validity of such method is limited to the turbulent flow in conduits of such cross sections which have aspect ratio less than 4 : 1 (aspect ratio is the ratio of longer side to small side) like trapezoidal, rectangular or elliptical, etc.

In 1962, Jamil Malika reported from his experimental study that the diameter of inscribed circle 'd' (to the given cross-section) is a far better linear dimension to use in the Reynolds number and roughness parameters of Nikuradse Eqs. 9.54 and 9.56 and Colebrook and White resistance equation Eq. 9.57 than hydraulic radius. He further noticed that the use of hydraulic radius introduces large errors in the estiamted value of 'f'. The following equations were obtained by Malika for smooth and rough pipes.

Smooth pipe $1/\sqrt{f} = 2 \log_{10} R_{ed} \sqrt{f} - 0.8 \qquad$ ...(9.66)

Rough pipe: $\qquad \dfrac{1}{\sqrt{f}} = 2 \log_{10} \dfrac{d}{2 k_s} + 1.74 \qquad$ ...(9.67)

Where R_{ed} was defined as

$$R_{ed} = \frac{Ud}{\nu}$$

d being the diameter of the inscribed circle.

Example 9.1-9.18

9.1 If the velocity distribution a pipeline is given by

$$\frac{u}{U_m} = \left[1 - \left(\frac{r}{R} \right)^n \right]$$

where U_m is maximum velocity at the centre and n is the velocity at a distance r from the centre in a pipeline of radius R, determine average velocity U, energy correction factor α and momentum correction factor β.

Solution

Considering small annular ring at a radius r and thickness dr

$$dQ = 2 \pi r \, dr \times u$$

Integrating,

$$Q = \int_0^R 2 \pi u \, r \, dr$$

$$= 2 \pi \int_0^R U_m \left\{ 1 - \left(\frac{r}{R} \right)^n \right\} r \, dr$$

$$= 2 \pi U_m \int_0^R \left(r - \frac{r^{n+1}}{R^n} \right) dr$$

$$= 2 \pi U_m \left[\frac{r^2}{2} - \frac{1}{R^n} \cdot \frac{r^{n+2}}{n+2} \right]_0^R$$

$$= 2 \pi U_m \left[\frac{R^2}{2} - \frac{1}{R^n} \cdot \frac{R^{n+2}}{n+2} \right]$$

$$= 2 \pi U_m \left[\frac{R^2}{2} - \frac{R^2}{n+2} \right]$$

$$= 2 \pi U_m \left(\frac{n R^2}{2 (n+2)} \right)$$

$$= \pi R^2 U_m \left(\frac{n}{n+2} \right)$$

Average velocity $U = \dfrac{Q}{\pi R^2}$

$$= \frac{\pi R^2 U_m n/(n+2)}{\pi R^2} = \left(\frac{n}{n+2} \right) U_m \quad \text{...(i)}$$

From Eq. 5.27,

$$\alpha = \frac{\int u^3 \, dA}{U^3 A}$$

Substituting value of u,

$$\alpha = \frac{\int_0^R U_m^3 \left(1 - \frac{r^n}{R^n}\right)^3 2\pi r \, dr}{U^3 . \pi R^2}$$

$$= \frac{2 U_m^3}{U^3 R^2} \int_0^R \left[1 - \frac{3 r^n}{R^n} + \frac{3 r^{2n}}{R^{2n}} - \frac{r^{3n}}{R^{3n}}\right] r \, dr$$

$$= \frac{2}{R^2} \left(\frac{U_m}{U}\right)^3 \int_0^R \left[r - \frac{3}{R^n} . r^{n+1} + \frac{3}{R^{2n}} . r^{2n+1} - \frac{1}{R^{3n}} . r^{3n+1}\right]$$

$$= \frac{2}{R^2} \left(\frac{U_m}{U}\right)^3 \left[\frac{r^2}{2} - \frac{3}{R^n} \frac{r^{n+2}}{n+2} + \frac{3}{R^{2n}} . \frac{r^{2n+2}}{2(n+1)} - \frac{1}{R^{3n}} . \frac{r^{3n+2}}{3n+2}\right]_0^R$$

$$= \frac{2}{R^2} . \left(\frac{U_m}{U}\right)^3 . \left[\frac{R^2}{2} - \frac{3}{n+2} . R^2 + \frac{3}{2(n+1)} . R^2 - \frac{1}{3n+2} . R^2\right]$$

$$= 2 \left(\frac{U_m}{U}\right)^3 \left[\frac{1}{2} - \frac{3}{n+2} + \frac{3}{2(n+1)} - \frac{1}{3n+2}\right]$$

$$= 2 \left(\frac{U_m}{U}\right)^3 \left[\frac{3n^3}{2(n+1)(n+2)(3n+2)}\right]$$

Substitute for $\left(\frac{U_m}{U}\right)$ from Eq. (i)

$$\alpha = \frac{2 (n+2)^3}{n^3} \left[\frac{3n^3}{2(n+1)(n+2)(3n+2)}\right]$$

$$= \frac{3(n+2)^2}{(n+1)(3n+2)}$$

For turbulent flow (n = 2),

$$\alpha = 2.0$$

From Eq. 5.59,

$$\beta = \frac{\int\limits_{A} u^2 \, dA}{U^2 A}$$

$$= \frac{\int\limits_{0}^{R} U_m^2 \left(1 - \frac{r^n}{R^n}\right)^2 . 2\pi r \, dr}{U^2 . \pi R^2}$$

$$= \left(\frac{U_m}{U}\right)^2 . \frac{1}{R^2} \int\limits_{0}^{R} \left(1 - \frac{2r^n}{R^n} + \frac{r^{2n}}{R^{2n}}\right) r \, dr$$

$$= \frac{2}{R^2} \left(\frac{U_m}{U}\right)^2 . \int\limits_{0}^{R} \left\{r - \frac{2}{R^n} . r^{n+1} + \frac{1}{R^{2n}} r^{2n+1}\right\} dr$$

$$= \frac{2}{R^2} \left(\frac{U_m}{U}\right)^2 \left[\frac{r^2}{2} - \frac{2}{R^n} . \frac{r^{n+2}}{n+2} + \frac{1}{R^{2n}} . \frac{r^{2n+2}}{2n+2}\right]_0^R$$

$$= \frac{2}{R^2} \left(\frac{U_m}{U}\right)^2 \left[\frac{R^2}{2} - \frac{2}{n+2} . R^2 + \frac{1}{2n+2} . R^2\right]$$

$$= 2 \left(\frac{U_m}{U}\right)^2 \left[\frac{1}{2} - \frac{2}{n+2} + \frac{1}{2n+2}\right]$$

$$= 2 \left(\frac{U_m}{U}\right)^2 . \frac{n^2}{2(n+1)(n+2)}$$

Substitute for $\dfrac{U_m}{U}$ from Eq. (i)

$$\beta = \frac{(n+2)^2}{n^2} . \frac{n^2}{(n+1)(n+2)}$$

$$= \left(\frac{n+2}{n+1}\right)$$

For turbulent flow (n = 2)

$$\beta = \frac{2+2}{2+1} = 1.33.$$

9.2 For a turbulent flow in pipes determine the distance from the wall where point velocity is equal to the mean velocity of flow

Solution

From Eq. 9.34,

$$\frac{u - U}{U_*} = \left[5.75 \log_{10} y/R + 3.75 \right]$$

But as the required, point velocity $u = U$

$$\therefore \qquad \left[5.75 \log y/R + 3.75 \right] = 0$$

Solving, $\qquad y = 0.2227 \, R$

9.3 From the equations for velocity distribution in smooth and rough pipes, show that

$$U_m/U = \left[1.325 \sqrt{f} + 1.0 \right]$$

Solution

From Eq. 9.34

$$\frac{u - U}{U_*} = \left[5.75 \log_{10} y/R + 3.75 \right]$$

At $\qquad y = R \, , \, u = U_m$

$$\frac{U_m - U}{U_*} = 3.75 \qquad \qquad ...(i)$$

From Eq. 7.30 b,

$$U_* = U \sqrt{f/8} \qquad \qquad ...(ii)$$

From Eqns. (i) and (ii)

$$\frac{U_m - U}{U \sqrt{f/8}} = 3.75$$

$$\frac{U_m}{U} = \left[3.75 \sqrt{f/8} + 1 \right]$$

$$\frac{U_m}{U} = \left[1.325 \sqrt{f} + 1 \right]$$

9.4 Design the diameter of a steel pipe to carry water having kinematic viscosity $v = 10^{-6} \, m^2/s$ with a mean velocity of 1 m/s. The head loss is limited to 50 cm per 100 m length of pipe; consider height of the equivalent sand roughness of pipe $k_s = 45 \times 10^{-4}$ cm. Assume that Darcy–Weishbach friction factor over the whole range of turbulent flow can be expressed as

$$f = 0.0055 \left[1 + \left(20 + 10^3 \, ks/D + 10^6/R_e \right)^{1/3} \right]$$

where D is the diameter of pipe and R_e is the Reynolds number of flow.

Solution

For the pipe, the trial method of design is used.

Trial 1. Assume $D = 1$ m as a first trial.

$$R_e = \frac{\rho U D}{\mu} = \frac{U D}{v}$$

$$= \frac{1 \times 1}{10^{-6}} = 10^6$$

$$f = 0.0055 \left[1 + \left(20 \times 10^3 \times 45 \times \frac{10^{-4}}{1.0} + 10^6/1 \times 10^6 \right)^{1/3} \right]$$

$$= 0.03$$

$$h_{f1} = f \frac{L}{D} \frac{U^2}{2g}$$

$$= 0.03 \times \frac{100}{1} \times \frac{(1)^2}{2 \times 9.81}$$

$$= 0.153 < 0.5 \ \text{m}$$

Trial 2 To increase the head loss, assume a smaller diameter 0.5 m for the pipe.

$$R_e = \frac{UD}{v} = \frac{1 \times 0.5}{10^{-6}} = 5 \times 10^5$$

$$f = 0.0055 \left[1 + \left(20 \times 10^3 \times 45 \times \frac{10^{-4}}{0.5} + 10^6/5 \times 10^5 \right)^{1/3} \right]$$

$$= 0.005 \, [1 + 5.65] = 0.0366$$

$$h_{f2} = 0.0366 \times \frac{100}{0.5} \times \frac{(1)^2}{2 \times 9.81} = 0.373 \, m < 0.5$$

Trial 3 It is still less than 0.5 m, hence assume a still samller diameter of the pipe as 0.3 m.

$$R_e = \frac{UD}{v} = \frac{1 \times 0.3}{10^{-6}} = 3 \times 10^5$$

$$f = 0.0055 \left[1 + \left(20 \times 10^3 \times \frac{45 \times 10^{-4}}{0.3} + \frac{10^6}{3 \times 10^5} \right)^{1/3} \right]$$

$$= 0.0055 \, [1 + 6.72] = 0.0425$$

$$h_{f3} = 0.0425 \times \frac{100}{0.3} \frac{(1)^2}{2 \times 9.81} = 0.721 \, m > 0.5 \ \text{m}$$

Trial 4 Another trial should be made with $D = 0.4$ m

$$R_e = \frac{UD}{v} = \frac{1 \times 0.4}{10^{-6}} = 4 \times 10^5$$

$$f = 0055 \left[1 + \left(20 \times 10^3 \times \frac{45 \times 10^{-4}}{0.4} + \frac{10^6}{4 \times 10^5} \right)^{1/3} \right]$$

$$= 0.0055 \, [1 + 6.105] = 0.039$$

$$hf_4 = 0.039 \times \frac{100}{0.4} \times \frac{(1)^2}{2 \times 9.81} = 0.498 \, m = 0.5$$

In case, it is found still different than the required 0.5 m, a plot may be made between h_f and D. From this plot, required diameter is obtained corresponding to given value of hf.

Diameter of pipe required = 0.4 m

9.5 Determine the size of the steel pipe required to carry 35 lps. The head loss is expected to be 50 m per kilometer of pipe length. The average height of pipe wall projection may be taken as 0.045 mm and viscosity of water as 1 centi poise.

Solution

$$h_f = \frac{fl Q^2}{12.1 \, D^5}$$

$$D^5 = \frac{fl Q^2}{12.1 \, h_f}$$

$$= \frac{f \times 1000 \times (0.035)^2}{12.1 \times 50}$$

$$= 0.0020248 \, f$$

$$R_e = \frac{UD}{v} = \frac{4 \rho Q}{\pi D v}$$

$$= \frac{4 \times 1000 \times 0.035}{3.14 \, D \times 1 \times 10^{-2} \times 0.1} \qquad \left(\text{Since 1 poise} = 0.1 \, \frac{Ns}{m^2} \right)$$

$$= 44585.98/D \qquad \qquad \text{...(ii)}$$

Further $\qquad \dfrac{k_s}{D} = \dfrac{0.045 \times 10^{-3}}{D} \qquad \qquad$ ...(iii)

Assume $\qquad f = 0.025$

$$D^5 = 0.0020248 \times 0.025$$

$$D = 0.1383 \, m$$

∴ $\qquad R_e = 3.22 \times 10^5$

and $\qquad \dfrac{k_s}{D} = 3.26 \times 10^{-4}$

From Moody's diagram the value of f can be read corresponding to $R_e = 3.22 \times 10^6$ and $\dfrac{k_s}{D} = 3.26 \times 10^{-4}$

∴ $\qquad f = 0.0170$

It is the first trial value of f which is further improved

From Eq. (i) $D^5 = 0.002048 \times 0.0170$

From Eq. (ii) $R_e = 44585.98/0.1280$

$$= 3.483 \times 10^5$$

From Eq. (iii) $\dfrac{k_s}{D} = \dfrac{0.045 \times 10^{-3}}{0.1280}$

$$= 3.51 \times 10^{-4}$$

$$k_s = 0.045 \times 10^{-3} \text{ m}$$

From Moody's diagram, $f = 0.0165$

For this value f , $D^5 = 0.002048 \times 0.0165$

$$D = 0.127 \text{ m}.$$

Since the value is not much different than 0.128 m, hence no further improvement is needed.

Further $\qquad \tau_0 = \left(\dfrac{\partial p}{\partial x} \right) \dfrac{D}{4}$

$$= \dfrac{w \, h_f}{L} \dfrac{D}{4} = \dfrac{9810 \times 50}{1000} \times \dfrac{0.127}{4}$$

$$= 15.57 \text{ N/m}^2$$

$$U_* = \sqrt{\tau_0/\rho}$$

$$= \sqrt{15.57/1000}$$

$$= 0.1248 \text{ m/s}$$

$$\delta' = \dfrac{11.6 \times (1 \times 10^{-2} \times 0.1)}{1000} \times \dfrac{1}{0.1248} \qquad \ldots(9.24)$$

$$= 9.29 \times 10^{-5} \text{ m}$$

$\therefore \qquad \dfrac{k_s}{\delta'} = \dfrac{0.045 \times 10^{-3}}{9.29 \times 10^{-5}} = 0.484 > 0.25$

Since $k_s/\delta' > 0.25$ and $k_s/\delta' < 6$, the surface behaves as a transition between smooth and rough surfaces.

9.6 A smooth pipe carries a discharge of 0.4 m^3/s of water and the head loss is 20 m in 500 m length of pipe. If the kinematic viscosity of water at 20° C is $10^{-6} \, m^2/s$, compute the size of the pipe.

Solution

$$R_e = \dfrac{4Q}{\pi D v}$$

$$= \dfrac{4 \times 0.4}{3.14 \times D \times 10^{-6}} = 5.095 \times 10^5/D \qquad \ldots(i)$$

Also $\qquad h_f = \dfrac{f \, l \, Q^2}{12.1 \, D^5}$

$$20 = \frac{f \times 500 \times (0.4)^2}{12.1 \, D^5}$$

$$D^5 = 0.3305 f \qquad \qquad ...(ii)$$

Assume $\qquad f = 0.02$

$$D^5 = 6.61 \times 10^{-3} \text{ , so that } D = 0.366 \text{ m}$$

Then $\qquad R_e = \dfrac{5.095 \times 10^5}{D}$

$$= 1.390 \times 10^6$$

Since the pipe acts as a smooth pipe, from Eq. 9.60.

$$f = 0.0032 + \frac{0.221}{(R_e)^{0.237}} \qquad \qquad ...(9.60)$$

$$= 0.01093$$

From Eq. (ii), $\quad D^5 = 0.3305 \times 0.01093 = 0.003614$

$$D = 0.3248 \text{ m}$$

From Eq. (i), $\quad R_e = 5.095 \times 10^5 / 0.3248$

$$= 1.568 \times 10^6$$

Recalculation of f from Eq. 9.60 yields

$$f = 0.0032 + \frac{0.221}{(1.568 \times 10^6)^{0.237}}$$

$$= 0.01071$$

Since the value of f is approximately the same as the previously found value of f, no further trial is required.

Size of pipe = 0.3248 m

9.7 In a laboratory experiment on a 30 cm diameter pipeline carrying water gave mean and velocity gradient as 2 m/s and 12.5 per second at a point 2.5 cm from the pipe wall. Assume rough turbulent flow, determine (i) friction velocity, (ii) average height of roughness, (iii) Darcy's friction coefficient and (iv) flow rate in the pipeline.

Solution

For turbulent flow, Eq. 9.16,

(i) $\qquad \tau = \rho \, l^2 \left(\dfrac{du}{dy} \right)^2$, where $\quad l = k \, y = o.4 \, y$

$$= 1000 \times (0.4 \, y)^2 \, (12.5)^2 = 25000 \times (2.5/100)^2$$

$$= 15.625 \text{ N/m}^2$$

$$\tau_0 = \tau \frac{R}{(R - y)}$$

$$= 15.625 \times \frac{0.15}{(0.15 - 0.025)}$$

$$= 18.75 \text{ N/m}^2$$
$$U_* = \sqrt{\tau_0/\rho}$$
$$= \sqrt{18.75/1000}$$
$$= 0.137 \text{ m/s}$$

(ii) From Eq. 9.30,

$$\frac{u}{U_*} = \left[5.75 \log y/k_s + 8.5\right]$$

$$\frac{2}{0.137} = \left[5.75 \log \frac{0.025}{k_s} + 8.5\right]$$

$$\log \frac{(0.025)}{k_s} = \frac{1}{5.75}\left(\frac{2}{0.137} - 8.5\right)$$

$$= 1.0619$$

$$k_s = 2.17 \text{ mm}$$

From Eq. 9.33

$$\frac{U}{U_*} = \left[5.75 \log R/k_s + 4.75\right]$$

$$\frac{U}{0.137} = \left[5.75 \log \frac{0.15}{2.17 \times 10^{-3}} + 4.75\right]$$

Solving, $U = 2.10$ m/s

$\therefore$ $Q = \pi/4 \times (0.3)^2 \times 2.10 = 0.148 \text{ m}^3/\text{s}$

Also $U_* = U\sqrt{f/8}$

$$f = 8 (U_*/U)^2$$
$$= 8 \times (0.137/2)^2$$
$$= 0.0341$$

9.8 A pipeline of one meter diameter carries oil at the rate of 1.1 m^3/s . If the specific gravity of oil is 0.80 and kinematic viscosity is equal to 0.025 stokes, determine the permissible height of protrusions so as to cause minimum loss of enery. Also determine the height of protrusions beyond which the pipe acts as rough.

Solution

(i) $$U = \frac{1.1}{\pi/4 \times (1)^2} = 1.40 \text{ m/s}$$

$$R_e = \frac{UD}{\nu}$$

$$\frac{1.40 \times 1.0}{0.025 \times 10^{-4}} = 5.605 \times 10^5$$

For minimum energy loss, pipe should act as smooth.

$$f = \left[0.0032 + \frac{0.0221}{(R_e)^{0.237}}\right]$$

$$= \left[0.0032 + \frac{0.221}{(5.605 \times 10^5)^{0.237}} \right]$$

$$= 0.01279$$

The criterion for smooth pipe is

$$\frac{R_e \sqrt{f}}{R/k_s} = 17$$

$$R/k_s = \frac{R_e \sqrt{f}}{17} = \frac{5.605 \times 10^5 \sqrt{0.01279}}{17}$$

Solving, $\quad R/k_s = 3729.25$

$$k_s = \frac{0.5}{3729.25}$$

$$= 0.134 \times 10^{-3} \text{ m or } 0.134 \text{ mm}$$

(ii) The pipe will act as rough when

$$\frac{R_e \sqrt{f}}{R/k_s} \geq 400$$

$$\sqrt{f} \geq \frac{400 \, R/k_s}{R_e}$$

$$\geq \frac{400 \, R/k_3}{5.605 \times 10^5}$$

Also for rough turbulent flow,

$$\frac{1}{\sqrt{f}} = [2 \log (R/k_s) + 1.74]$$

$$\frac{5.605 \times 10^5}{400 \, (R/k_s)} = [2 \log (R/k_s) + 1.74]$$

Solving by trial, $R/k_s = 218$

$$k_s = \frac{0.5}{218} = 2.29 \times 10^{-3} \text{ m or } 2.29 \text{ mm}$$

Hence the pipe will behave as rough pipe when the height of protrusions is equal to or greater than 2.29 mm.

9.9 Seven hundred liters of water flows per minute through a pipeline 10 cm in diameter and 5.5 km long. Taking the pipe as smooth, calculate Darcy's friction factor, frictional head loss, wall shear stress, centreline velocity, shear stress and velocity at 2 cm from the centre line. Also determine the thickness of laminar sublayer. Take kinetic viscosity of water $v = 0.0195$ stokes.

Solution

The mean velocity is given by $U = \dfrac{Q}{(\pi/4) \, d^2}$

$$U = \frac{700}{1000 \times 60} \times \frac{1}{\pi/4 \times (0.1)^2} = 1.486 \text{ m/s}$$

$$R_e = \frac{UD}{\nu}$$

$$= \frac{1.486 \times 0.1}{0.195 \times 10^{-4}}$$

$$= 776237 < 10^5$$

(i) For smooth pipe, Blasius equation, Eq. 9.35 is applicable

$$f = \frac{0.3164}{(R_e)^{1/4}}$$

$$= \frac{0.3164}{(76237)^{1/4}}$$

$$= 0.019$$

(ii) From Eq. 7.30b

$$U_* = U\sqrt{f/8}$$

$$= 1.486\sqrt{0.019/8}$$

$$= 0.0724 \text{ m/s}$$

(iii) From Eq. 9.51

$$h_f = f\frac{L}{D}\frac{U^2}{2g}$$

$$= 0.019 \times \frac{5500}{0.10} \times \frac{(1.486)^2}{2 \times 9.81} = 117.61 \text{ m}$$

(iv)

$$\tau_0 = \rho\, U_*^2$$

$$= 100 \times (0.0724)^2$$

$$= 5.24 \text{ N/m}^2$$

(v) The velocity distribution in a smooth pipe is defined by Eq. 9.28

$$\frac{u}{U_*} = \left[5.75 \log_{10}\frac{U_* y}{\nu} + 5.5\right]$$

At the centre of the pipe, $y = R$, $u = U_c$

$$\frac{U_c}{0.0724} = \left[5.75 \log_{10}\frac{0.0724 \times 0.05}{0.0195 \times 10^{-4}} + 5.5\right]$$

$$U_c = 0.0724\,(24.29) = 1.759 \text{ m/s}$$

(vi) The velocity at $r = 0.02$ m or $y = (0.05 - 0.02) = 0.03$ m

$$u = 0.0724\left[5.75 \log_{10}\frac{0.0724 \times 0.03}{0.0195 \times 10^{-4}} + 5.5\right]$$

$$= 0.0724\,[23.0192] = 1.67 \text{ m/s}$$

(vii) The shear stress at $r = 0.02$ m is given by

$$\tau = \tau_0\,(r/R)$$

$$= 5.24 \times (0.02/0.05)$$
$$= 2.096 \text{ N/m}^2$$

(viii) The thickness of laminar sublayer is given by Eq. 9.27a

$$\delta' = 11.6 \, v/U_*$$
$$= (11.6 \times 0.0195 \times 10^{-4}/0.0724) \, m$$
$$= 0.312 \text{ mm}$$

9.10 A rough pipe (height of roughness projection $= 2.5$ mm) of 100 cm diameter and 1000 m length carries water such that a pitot tube records a velocity of 70.8 cm/s at a distance of 25 cm from the centre line. Calculate the friction velocity U_*, head loss hf and the discharge flowing through it. Also verify that the flow is a rough turbulent flow.

Solution

The velocity is given at a distance r from the centre line

$$\therefore \qquad y = (R - r) = (0.5 - 0.25) = 0.25 \text{ m}$$

(i) Shear velocity (from Eq. 9.30)

$$u/U_* = [5.75 \log_{10} y/k_s + 8.5]$$
$$0.708/U_* = [5.75 \log_{10}(0.25/2.5 \times 10^{-3}) + 8.5]$$
$$= 20$$
$$U_* = 0.708/20 = 0.0354 \text{ m/s}$$

(ii) Mean velocity (from Eq. 9.33)

$$U/U_* = [5.75 \log_{10}(R/k_s) + 4.75]$$
$$U/0.0354 = [5.75 \log_{10}(0.5/2.5 \times 10^{-3}) + 4.75]$$
$$= 17.98$$
$$U = 17.98 \times 0.0354$$
$$= 0.636 \text{ m/s}$$

(iii) Discharge

$$Q = A \, U$$
$$= \pi/4 \, (1)^2 \times 0.636$$
$$= 0.5 \text{ m}^3/\text{s}$$

(iv) Friction factor
From Eq. 7.30 b,

$$U_* = U \sqrt{f/8}$$
$$f = 8 \cdot (U_*/U)^2$$
$$= 8 \, (0.636/0.0354)^2$$
$$= 0.0247$$

(v) Head loss

$$h_f = f \frac{L}{D} \frac{U^2}{2g}$$

$$= 0.0247 \times \frac{1000}{1} \times \frac{(0.636)^2}{2 \times 9.81}$$

$$= 0.512 \text{ m}$$

9.11 Two reservoirs with water surface difference of 20 m are to be connected by a pipe, 1 m diameter 6 km long. What will be the discharge when a C.I. pipe of $k_s = 0.3$ mm is used ? What will be the increase in discharge if C.I. pipe is replaced by a steel pipe of $k_s = 0.1$ mm ? Neglect minor losses.

Solution

(i) From Eq. 9.56

$$1/\sqrt{f} = \left[2 \log_{10} R/k_s + 1.74 \right]$$

Substituting the values of R and k_s

$$\frac{1}{\sqrt{f}} = \left[2 \log_{10} \frac{0.5}{0.3 \times 10^{-3}} + 1.74 \right]$$

$$f = 0.01493$$

From Eq. 9.51

$$h_f = \frac{fL Q_1^2}{12.1 D^5}$$

$$Q_1 = \sqrt{\frac{12.1 h_f D^5}{fL}}$$

$$Q_1 = \sqrt{\frac{12.1 \times 20 \times (1)^5}{0.01493 \times 6000}} = 1.637 \text{ m}^3/\text{s}$$

(ii) In the second case, $k_s = 0.1 \times 10^{-3}$ m

$$\frac{1}{\sqrt{f}} = \left[2 \log_{10} \left(\frac{0.5}{0.1 \times 10^{-3}} \right) + 1.74 \right]$$

Solving, $f = 0.01198$

Then $$Q_2 = \sqrt{\frac{12.1 \times 10 \times (1)^5}{0.01198 \times 6000}} = 1.827 \text{ m}^3/\text{s}$$

% increase in discharge $= \dfrac{Q_2 - Q_1}{Q_2}$

$$= \frac{1.827 - 1.637}{1.827} \times 100$$

$$= 10.42 \%$$

9.12 If sand grains of 0.076 cm diameter are cemented on the inner surface of a 10 cm diameter pipe for test purposes, at what velocity of water will the surface roughness just begin to disturb the laminar sublayer ? At what velocity will the pipe wall behave as rough ? Take $v = 10^{-6} \text{ m}^2/\text{s}$

Solution

(i) The limiting condition is $k_s/\delta' = 0.25$

$$\delta' = k_s/0.25 = 0.076 \times 10^{-2}/0.25 \text{ cm}$$

$$= 0.304 \times 10^{-2} \text{ m}$$

Also, from Eq. 9.27 a

$$\delta' = 11.6 \, v/U_*$$

$$0.304 \times 10^{-2} = \frac{11.6 \times 10^{-6}}{U_*}$$

Sovling, $\qquad U_* = 3.82 \times 10^{-3} \text{ m/s}$

From Eq. 9.32, for smooth turbulent flow,

$$U/U_* = [5.75 \log_{10} (U_* R/v) + 1.75]$$

$$U = 3.82 \times 10^{-3} \left[5.75 \log_{10} \left(\frac{3.82 \times 10^{-3} \times 5 \times 10^{-2}}{10^{-6}} \right) + 1.75 \right]$$

$$= 0.0568 \text{ m/s}$$

(ii) For given value of R and k_s , the friction factor is computed from Eq. 9.56,

$$1/\sqrt{f} = [2 \log_{10} R/k_s + 1.74]$$

$$\frac{1}{\sqrt{f}} = \left[2 \log_{10} \left(\frac{5 \times 10^{-2}}{0.076 \times 10^{-2}} + 1.74 \right) \right] = 5.3752$$

Solving, $\qquad f = 0.0346$

For rough turbulent flow,

$$k_s/\delta' = 6$$

or $\qquad k_s = 6 \delta' = 6 \times 11.6 \, v/U_*$

or $\qquad U_* = \frac{6 \times 11.6 \times 10^{-6}}{0.076 \times 10^{-2}} = 9.15 \times 10^{-2} \text{ m/s}$

From Eq. 9.33 for rough turbulent flow

$$U/U_* = [5.75 \log_{10} (R/k_s) + 4.75]$$

$$= \left[5.75 \log \left(\frac{0.05}{0.076 \times 10^{-2}} \right) + 4.75 \right] = 15.20$$

$$U = 15.20 \times 9.15 \times 10^{-2} = 1.39 \text{ m/s}$$

9.13 A 60 cm diameter pipe carries oil with centre line velocity of 4.5 m/s. If the velocity at a radial distance of 10 cm from pipe axis is found to be 4.2 m/s, calculate the discharge in the pipe.

Solution

From Eq. 9.42,

$$\frac{U_m - u}{U_*} = 5.75 \log_{10} \left(\frac{R}{y} \right)$$

$$\frac{4.50 - 4.2}{U_*} = 5.75 \log \frac{0.30}{(0.30 - 0.10)}$$

$$\frac{0.3}{U_*} = 1.01252$$

$$U_* = 0.2963 \text{ m/s}$$

From Eq. 9.34,

$$\frac{U_m - U}{U_*} = 3.75$$

$$\frac{4.5 - U}{0.2963} = 3.75$$

$$U = 3.389 \text{ m/s}$$

Discharge $\qquad Q = \frac{\pi}{4} D^2 . U$

$$= \frac{\pi}{4} (0.6)^2 \times 3.389$$

$$= 0.9577 \text{ m}^3/\text{s}$$

9.14 A 20 cm diameter pipe carries water. A velocity profile traversed by a pitot tube and it was observed that velocity increased by 15 % as the pitot moved from a point 1.5 cm away from the wall to a point 4.0 cm away from wall. Extimate the relative roughness and friction factor f for the pipe.

Solution

Since the flow is in region of rough turbulent, use Eq. 9.30,

$$\frac{u}{U_*} = 5.75 \log \frac{y}{k_s} + 8.5$$

Hence $\qquad \dfrac{u_1}{U_*} = 5.75 \log \dfrac{y_1}{k_s} + 8.5 \qquad \qquad ...(i)$

$$\frac{u_2}{U_*} = 5.75 \log \frac{y_2}{k_s} + 8.5 \qquad \qquad ...(ii)$$

From Eqs. (i) and (ii)

$$\frac{u_2 - u_1}{U_*} = 5.75 \log_e \frac{y_2}{y_1}$$

Since $\qquad u_2 = 1.15\,u_1 , y_1 = 0.015\,m , y_2 = 0.040 \text{ m},$

$$\frac{1.15\,u_1 - u_1}{U_*} = 5.75 \log \frac{0.040}{0.015}$$

$$\frac{u_1}{U_*} = \frac{5.75}{0.15} \log \frac{0.040}{0.015} = 16.329$$

Also from Eq. (i)

$$\frac{u_1}{U_*} = 5.75 \log \frac{y_1}{k_s} + 8.5$$

$$16.329 = 5.75 \log \frac{0.015}{k_s} + 8.5$$

$$\log \frac{0.015}{k_s} = \frac{16.329 - 8.5}{5.75} = 1.3615$$

$$\frac{0.015}{k_s} = 22.99$$

$$k_s = \frac{0.015}{22.99} = 6.52 \times 10^{-4} \text{ m}$$

Hence relative roughness $= k_s/D$

$$\frac{k_s}{D} = \frac{6.52 \times 10^{-4}}{20 \times 10^{-2}} = 3.26 \times 10^{-3}$$

From Eq. 9.56,

$$\frac{1}{\sqrt{f}} = 2 \log \frac{R}{k_s} + 1.74$$

$$= 2 \log \frac{D}{2k_s} + 1.74$$

$$= 2 \log \left(\frac{1}{2} \times \frac{1}{3.26 \times 10^{-3}} \right) + 1.74$$

$$= 2 \times 2.1857 + 1.74 = 6.1115$$

$$f = 0.0268$$

9.15 In a meteorological laboratory, wind velocity measurements gave velocities of 4.0 m/s and 5.0 m/s at a height of 3.0 m and 6.0 m. What should be velocity at a height of 20 m above the ground. Assume similar atmospheric conditions to prevail at this height.

Solution

From Eq. 9.23b,

$$\frac{u}{U_*} = 5.75 \log \frac{y}{y'} \qquad \qquad ...(i)$$

Given $\quad u_1 = 4$ m/s, $u_2 = 5$ m/s, $y_1 = 3.0$ m., $y_2 = 6$ m,

$$\frac{4}{U_*} = 5.75 \log \frac{3}{y'} \qquad \qquad ...(ii)$$

$$\frac{5}{U_*} = 5.75 \log \frac{6}{y'} \qquad \qquad ...(iii)$$

Subtracting Eq. (iii) from Eq. (ii)

$$\frac{5 - 4}{U_*} = 5.75 \log \frac{6}{3}$$

$$\frac{1}{U_*} = 1.731$$

$$U_* = 0.577 \text{ m/s}$$

At an elevation of y_3 $(= 20$ m$)$ above G. L.

$$\frac{u_3}{U_*} = 5.75 \log \frac{20}{y'} \qquad \text{...(iv)}$$

From Eqs. (ii) and (iv)

$$\frac{u_3 - 4}{U_*} = 5.75 \log \frac{20}{3}$$

$$\frac{u_3 - 4}{U_*} = 4.7374$$

$$u_3 = 4.7374\, U_* + 4$$

$$u_3 = 6.737 \text{ m/s}$$

9.16 A 20 cm diameter pipe is found to have friction factor f as 0.025 after 5 years of its use and 0.030 after 10 years of its use. What should be the friction factor after 15 years of its in service.

Solution

From Eq. 9.56

$$\frac{1}{\sqrt{f}} = 2 \log \frac{R}{k_s} + 1.74$$

At $t = 5$ years, $f_1 = 0.025$, $R = 0.1$ m,

$$\frac{1}{\sqrt{0.025}} = 2 \log \frac{0.1}{k_s} + 1.74$$

$$2 \log \frac{0.1}{k_{s1}} = \left(\frac{1}{\sqrt{0.025}} - 1.74\right)$$

$$= 4.5845$$

$$k_{s1} \, 5.1021 \times 10^{-4} \text{ m}$$

$$\approx 0.51 \text{ mm}$$

At $t = 10$ yrs., $f_2 = 0.03$, $R = 0.1$ m

$$\frac{1}{\sqrt{0.03}} = 2 \log \frac{0.1}{k_{s2}} + 1.74$$

$$5.7735 = 2 \log \frac{0.1}{k_{s2}} + 1.74$$

$$k_{s2} = 9.6216 \times 10^{-4} \text{ m} \approx 0.962 \text{ mm}$$

From Eq. 9.58,

$$k_{s2} = k_{s1} + \alpha t$$

$$0.962 \times 10^{-3} = 0.510 \times 10^{-3} + \alpha (10 - 5)$$

$$\alpha = (0.962 \times 10^{-3} - 0.510 \times 10^{-3})/5$$

$$= 0.0904 \times 10^{-3} \text{ m/yr.}$$

At $t = 15$ years

$$k_{s3} = k_{s1} + \alpha (t_3 - t_1)$$

$$= 0.510 \times 10^{-3} + 0.0904 \times 10^{-3} (15 - 5)$$

$$= 1.414 \times 10^{-3} \text{ m} = 1.414 \text{ mm}$$

From Eq. 9.56,

$$\frac{1}{\sqrt{f_3}} = 2 \log \frac{R}{k_{s3}} + 1.74$$

$$= 2 \log \left(\frac{0.1}{1.414 \times 10^{-3}} \right) + 1.74$$

$$f_3 = 0.0338$$

9.17 A 200 mm diameter pipe with equivalent roughness $k_s = 0.01$ mm. carries water over a length of 125 mm. It is observed that the pressure drops in this length by 15.25 kN/m². Find whether the pipe behaves as smooth or rough. Also determine centre line velocity and discharge through the pipe.

Solution

(a) From Eq. 7.19c,

$$\tau_0 = -\frac{dp}{dx} \cdot \frac{R}{2}$$

$$\tau_0 = \frac{15.25 \times 1000}{125} \times \frac{(0.2/2)}{2} = 6.1 \text{ N/m}^2$$

$$U_* = \sqrt{\frac{\tau_0}{\rho}}$$

$$= \sqrt{\frac{6.1}{1000}} = 0.078 \text{ m/s}$$

From Eq. 9.27a,

$$\delta' = 11.6 \, \nu/u_*$$

$$= \frac{11.6 \times 10^{-6}}{0.078} = 1.485 \times 10^{-4} \text{ m}$$

(Assume $\nu = 10^{-6}$ m²/s)

$$\frac{k_s}{\delta'} = \frac{0.01 \times 10^{-3}}{1.485 \times 10^{-4}}$$

$$\frac{k_s}{\delta'} = 0.067 < 0.25$$

Hence the pipe surface behaves as a smooth surface

(b) From Eq. 9.28,

$$\frac{u}{U_*} = \left[5.75 \log \frac{U_* y}{\nu} + 5.5 \right]$$

At
$$y = R = 0.1 \text{ m}, u = U_m$$

$$\frac{U_m}{0.078} = \left[5.75 \log \frac{0.078 \times 0.1}{10^{-6}} + 5.5 \right]$$

$$= (22.3795 + 5.5) = 27.8795$$

$$U_m = 2.175 \text{ m/s}$$

(c) From Eq. 9.33

$$\frac{u}{U_*} = \left[5.75 \log \frac{U_* R}{\nu} + 1.75 \right]$$

$$\frac{U}{0.078} = \left[5.75 \log \frac{0.078 \times 0.1}{10^{-6}} + 1.75 \right] = 24.1295$$

$$U = 1.882 \text{ m/s}$$

Discharge $\qquad = \dfrac{\pi}{4} (0.2)^2 \times 1.882$

$$= 0.059 \text{ m}^3\text{/s}$$

9.18 A 25 diameter pipeline carries water at 20° C at a velocity of 4 m/s. If friction factor f for the pipeline is assumed as f = 0.030 (a) what should be wall shear stress (b) Compute shear stress, velocity and velocity gradient at 7.5 cm from pipe axis (c) also determine maximum velocity and at what distance from pipe surface, is average velocity obtained.

Solution

(a) From Eq. 9.56 for rough turbulent flow,

$$\frac{1}{\sqrt{f}} = 2 \log R/k_s + 1.74$$

$$\frac{1}{\sqrt{0.030}} = 2 \log \left(\frac{R}{k_s} \right) + 1.74$$

$$2 \log \left(R/k_s \right) = \frac{1}{\sqrt{0.030}} - 1.74 = 4.0335$$

$$\left(\frac{0.125}{k_s} \right) = 103.932$$

$$k_s = 1.202 \times 10^{-3} \text{ m} = 1.202 \text{ mm}$$

From Eq. 7.30 b,

$$U_* = \sqrt{\tau_0/\rho} = U \sqrt{f/8}$$

$$\tau_0 = \rho U^2 f/8$$

$$= \frac{1000 \times 4^2 \times 0.03}{8} = 60 \text{ N/m}^2$$

Corresponding shear velocity can now be computed.

$$U_* = \sqrt{\tau_0/\rho}$$

$$= \sqrt{60/1000}$$

$$= 0.245 \text{ m/s}$$

(b) Since variation of shear stress is linear with τ_0 at wall and zero at centre line,

$$\tau = \tau_0 \left(1 - y/R\right)$$

At $r = 7.50$ cm,

$$y = (R - r) = (12.5 - 7.5) = 5 \text{ cm or } 0.05 \text{ m}$$

$$\tau = 60 \left(1 - \frac{0.05}{0.125}\right)$$

$$= 36 \text{ N/m}^2$$

From Eq. 9.30,

$$\frac{u}{U_*} = \left[5.75 \log\left(y/k_s\right) + 8.5\right]$$

$$= \left[5.75 \log\left(\frac{0.05}{1.202 \times 10^{-3}}\right) + 8.5\right]$$

$$= 17.81$$

$$u = 17.81 \times 0.245$$

$$= 4.363 \text{ m/s}$$

Also

$$\frac{u}{U_*} = [5.75 \log_{10}\left(y/k_s\right) + 8.5]$$

$$= [2.5 \log_e\left(y/k_s\right) + 8.5]$$

Differentiating w.r. to y

$$\frac{1}{U_*}\frac{du}{dy} = \frac{2.5}{\left(y/k_s\right)} \times \frac{1}{k_s}$$

$$\frac{du}{dy} = \left(\frac{2.5\, U_*}{y}\right)$$

$$= \frac{2.5 \times 0.245}{0.05}$$

$$= 12.25 \text{ s}^{-1}$$

(c) At $y = R, u = U_m$

$$\frac{U_m}{U_*} = 5.75 \log \frac{R}{k_s} + 8.5$$

$$= \left(5.75 \log \frac{0.125}{1.202 \times 10^{-3}} + 8.5\right)$$

$$= 11.5978 + 8.5 = 20.0978$$

$$U_m = 20.0978 \times 0.245$$

$$= 4.924 \text{ m/s}$$

(d) From Eq. 9.34,

$$\frac{u - U}{U_*} = 5.75 \log_{10} \frac{y}{R} + 3.75$$

Let $u = U$ at a distance y from wall,

$$5.75 \log_{10}\left(y/R\right) + 3.75 = 0$$

$$\log_{10}\left(y/R\right) = -\frac{3.75}{5.75} = -0.6522$$

$$y = 0.2227 \text{ R}$$

$$= 0.2227 \times 0.125 = 0.0278 \text{ m}$$

$$= 2.78 \text{ cm from pipe surface}$$

OBJECTIVE QUESITONS

9.1　Prandtl defined the mixing length as the distance traversed by the main flow through which

　　(a) The energy of the fluid particles remains constant.
　　(b) The momentum of the fluid particles remains constant.
　　(c) The turbulent shear remains constant.
　　(d) None of the these answers.

9.2　The causes of turbulence in the fluid flow may be

　　(a) High Reynolds number
　　(b) Critical Reynolds number
　　(c) Abrupt discontinuity in velocity distribution
　　(d) Existence of velocity distribution without abrupt discontinuity.
　　(e) None of these answers

9.3　Intensity of turbulence is

　　(a) Average kinetic energy of turbulence.
　　(b) The frequency of turbulent fluctuations.
　　(c) Measured by the root mean square value of velocity fluctuations.
　　(d) Average momentum of turbulence.
　　(e) None of these answers.

9.4　Which of the following terms represents the turbulent shear stresses

　　(a) $-\rho u'^2$　　(b) $-\rho v^2$　　　　　　　　　(c) $-\rho v'^2$
　　(d) $-\rho u' w'$　(e) $-\rho w'^2$

9.5　The velocity distribution for turbulent flows follow

　　(a) Parabolic law　(b) Logarithmic law
　　(c) Hyperbolic law　(d) Linear law　　(e) None of these.

9.6　The velocity distribution in rough pipes being dependent on the relative roughness may be expressed as

　　(a) $u/U_* = [5.75 \log U_* y/\nu + 5.5]$
　　(b) $u/U_* = [5.75 \log R/k_s + 8.5]$
　　(c) $u/U_* = [5.75 \log R/k_s + 4.75]$
　　(d) None of the above.

9.7   For a hydrodynamically smooth surface

(a) $ks/\delta' > 6$ (b) $ks/\delta' > 2.5$

(c) $R_e \sqrt{f}/(R/k_s) < 17$ (d) $R_e \sqrt{f}/(R/k_s) = 400$

(e) None of these answers.

9.8   The friction factor f in turbulent flow in smooth pipes depends upon the following.

(a) U, D, ρ, L, μ (b) Q, L, μ, ρ

(c) U, D, ρ, p, u (d) U, D, μ, p

(e) p, L, D, Q, U

9.9   In the completely turbulent zone (rough pipes)

(a) Rough pipes and smooth pipes have the same friction factor.

(b) The friction factor depends upon Reynolds number only

(c) The head loss varies as the square of the velocity.

(d) The friction factor is independent of relative roughness.

(e) The laminar film covers the roughness projections.

9.10   Identify the Karman Prandtl resistance equation for turbulent flow in smooth pipes :

(a) $f = 0.3164/(R_e)^{0.25}$

(b) $1/\sqrt{f} = 2 \log R_e \sqrt{f} - 0.8$

(c) $f = 64/R_e$

(d) $1/\sqrt{f} = 2 \log R/k_s + 1.74$

PROBLEMS

9.1 Describe Prandtt's mixing length theory. Mention also the underlying assumptions made.

9.2 Describe Nikuradse's curve and with the help of his experimental curves, explain the resistance behaviour of pipes of different roughnesses and at different values of Reynolds number.

9.3 A velocity traverse was carried out in a pipeline of 30 cm diameter with a Pitot tube. Following readings were observed: velocity at centre 6.5 m/s, velocity at 6 cm from the pipe wall 5 m/s. Calculate (i) the mean friction velocity, (ii) mean velocity of flow, and (iii) Darcy's friction coefficient.

9.4 Rough turbulent flow occurs in a pipeline 30 cm diameter conveying water. The mean velocity and velocity gradient at 2 cm from the wall of pipe are found to be 2.13 m/s and 13.5 s^{-1}. Determine (i) the average height of roughness projections(ii) wall shear stress, and (iii) Darcy's friction factor.

9.5 Show that for smooth and rough turbulent flows, the following velocity distribution is applicable.

$$(u - U)/U_* = (3.75 + 5.75 \log_{10} y/R)$$

Therefore, derive the expressions for mean velocity U ,
$$U/U_{max} = 1/(1 + 1.43 \sqrt{f})$$
where U_{max} is center line velocity, f is *Darcy's friction factor* and U_* is the *shear or friction velocity.*

9.6 In order to determine the discharge of water through a round pipe, the Prandtl's tubes are installed at mid point and at the quarter point of 20 cm diameter pipe .What discharge is indicated by the simultaneous readings of 1.85 m/s and 1.65 m/s at these two points ? Also, determine the value of f and the equivalent sand roughness k_s

9.7 A smooth brass pipeline 7.5 cm diameter and 900 m long carried water at the rate of 7 litres per second. If kinematic viscosity of water is 0.0195 stokes, calculate the loss of head, wall shearing stress, maximum velocity, shear stress and velocity at 2.5 cm from the centreline and the thickness of laminar sublayer. Take $\rho = 1000 \, kg/m^3$

9.8 Obtain the velocity distribution for turbulent flow through pipe, using Karman's similarity hypothesis. Assume $\tau = \tau_0$ for small values of y . The two boundary conditions are (i) du/dy very large as $y \to 0$ and (ii) at $y = R$, $u = U_{max}$

9.9 A pipe 150 mm in diameter with $k_s = 0.01$ mm carries water at 20°C cover a length of 100 m with a pressure difference of 26.613 kN/m². State whether ther pipe will behave as smooth or rough. Also. determien the maximum velocity, average velocity and discharge.

9.10 A pipe 100 mm diameter which acts as rough pipe yielded the values of f as 0.026 and 0.030 after five years and 10 years of use. Estimate the value of friction factor after 15 years of service.

9.11 Sand grains of uniform size (average diameter 0.76 mm) were cemented to the inner surface of a 100 mm diameter pipe carrying water. Determine the type of flow and f if (i) $Q = 14.89$ litres per minute, (ii) 1507 litres per minute.

9.12 Obtain an expression for f if the velocity distribution is given by
$u/U_* = 8.74 \, (U_* y/v)^{1/7}$

10

Pipe Flow

10.1 INTRODUCTION

A pipe is a closed conduit through which the fluid flows under pressure. Hence, it is also known as pressure flow. Mostly, the pipes are circular in shape. but in some special cases, non- circular pipes may be used. Essentially, the pipe should run full, that is, there exists no free surface in the pipes. In case the pipe runs partially full as in the sewerage lines.the air will enter into the pipe and there will exist a free surface. Such fluid flow problems are treated with laws of open channed flow (chapter 12). The flulid flow is always resisted by viscous forces, at the boundary as well as between adjacent fluid layers. This viscous resistance is overcome by the drop in the total energy line in the direction of flow. That is, a portion of total energy is lost in the direction of flow. The fluid resistance depends on the type of flows. Separate laws govern the frictional resistance to laminar and turbulent flows. These are discussed in this chapter. Besides frictional resistance, the energy loss also occurs due to non uniformity of flow caused due to various pipe fittings (e.g.sudden expansion, valves, etc.) and are described below. A few problems of turbulent flow through pipe are also dealt with hereinunder.

10.2 LAWS OF FLUID FRICTION

As stated earlier, the friction resistance offered to the flow depends on the type of flow, i.e. it is different for laminar and turbulent flow. On the basis of experimental observations, the following laws of fluid resistance are summarised below:

1. Fluid friction laws for laminar flows

(a) The fluid resistance is directly proportional to the velocity of flow.

(b) It is proportional to the area of contact surface.

(c) It is independent of the nature of the contact surface.

(d) It is independent of the pressure.

(e) It greatly varies with the temperature.

The fluid resistance for laminar flow is independent of the nature of the contact surface since a film of stationary liquid in contact with the surface is formed. In case of laminar flow, the fluid resistance is entirely due to viscosity of the fluid, such flows are also known as viscous flows. Moreover, the viscosity is greatly affected by the temperature, thereby the fluid resistance to the laminar flow also varies with temperature.

2. Fluid friction laws for turbulent flows.

(a) The fluid resistance is proportional to (velocity)^n

(b) It is proportional to the area of the contact surface.

(c) It is proportional to the nature of the contact surface.

(d) It is independent of the pressure.

(e) It is proportional to the density of the fluid.

(f) The fluid resistance slightly varies with the temperature.

Mostly, the flow through pipes is turbulent. Hence, in the various problems dealt in this chapter, turbulent flow is assumed to occur and the fluid resistance laws for turbulent flow are used.

10.3 FROUDE'S EXPERIMENT

W.Froude conducted a series of experiments to determine the frictional resistance of wooden surface moving in water. The experiments were done in a tank 100 m (300 ft.) long, 11 m (33 ft) wide and 3 m (10 ft) deep. Thin wooden boards 5 mm thick, 7.5 cm wide and 60 cm to 15 m long were towed endwise over the water surface and were connected to a carriage. Two rails were fitted over the top edge of the tank and the carriage was hauled along at speeds varying from 30 m to 300 m per minute. A wire rope was fixed to the carriage which passed around a drum and the force required to tow the board was measured. The boards remained completely submerged in the water while moving. The surface of the board was coated by varnish, tinfoil, calico and sand, in turn to change their surface roughness.

From the result of these experiments, Froude concluded :

(1) The frictional resistance varies approximately with the square of the velocity.

(2) The frictional resistance varies with the nature of the surface.

(3) The frictional resistance varies with the per square metre of the surface, and decreases as the length of the board increases. But it is constant for long lengths.

Let f be frictional resistance per square per square metre of a given surface at unit velocity. A be the area of the watted surface (m^2), U be the velocity of surface (m/s)

The frictional resistance F is given by

$$F = f' A U^n$$

Assuming the index n = 2,

$$F = f' A U^2$$

In this equation except f' all quantities are known and hence f' can be calculated.

10.4 DARCY-WEISBACH EQUATION

The head loss due to friction in pipes was derived by Darcy and Weisbach simultaneously and it is known as Darcy-Weisbach equation.

Consider a horizontal pipe of diameter D, length L between two sections 1 and 2. The pressure and datum head corresponding to section 1 are p_1 and z_1 whereas corresponding to section 2 are p_2 and z_2.

Applying Bernoulli's equation between 1 and 2.

$$\frac{p_1}{w} + z_1 + \frac{U_1^2}{2g} = \frac{p_2}{w} + z_2 + \frac{U_2^2}{2g} + h_f$$

Since pipe is of uniform diameter, $U_1 = U_2$ and for horizontal pipe $z_1 = z_2$

$$h_f = \left(\frac{p_1 - p_2}{w} \right) \qquad \text{...(10.3)}$$

Thus, the difference of pressure head between section 1 and 2 is equal to the head loss due to friction.

From Eq. 10.3, the force resisting the flow is due to friction alone. Let A be the area of cross section. P be the wetted perimeter and f' be the frictional resistance per unit area per unit velocity

The resisting force $F = f' \, PL \, U^2$ ...(i)

The force causing the flow $= (p_1 - p_2) A$ ...(ii)

Equating Eqns. (i) and (ii)

$$(p_1 - p_2) A = f' \, PL \, U^n$$

Writing, $(p_1 - p_2) = w \, h_f$

$$w \, h_f A = f' \, PL \, U^n$$

$$h_f = \frac{f'}{w} \, \frac{P}{A} \, . \, LU^n$$

The ratio of A/P is known as hydraulic radius or hydraulic mean depth R.

For circular pipe. $R = \dfrac{A}{P} = \dfrac{D}{4}$

Assuming index $n = 2$

$$h_f = \frac{f'}{w} \, . \, \frac{4}{D} \, . \, LU^2 \qquad \text{...(10.4)}$$

Multiply and divide by 2 g on right hand side

$$h_f = \frac{8gf'}{w} \, \frac{U^2}{2g} \, \frac{L}{D}$$

Putting $\dfrac{8gf'}{w} = f$

$$h_f = f \frac{L}{D} \frac{U^2}{2g} \qquad \text{...(10.5)}$$

where f is known as the Darcy's friction coefficient or coefficient of friction and U is the mean velocity of flow. Eq. 10.5 is known as Darcy-Weisbach equation. It is commonly used to determine the head loss due to friction. It should be noted well that f is not a constant but varies with Reynolds number (Re) and the nature of the surface (Refer section 9.9).

10.5 OTHER FORMULAE FOR HEAD LOSS DUE TO FRICTION

1. Chezy's Formula

From Eq. 10.4,

$$\frac{h_f}{L} = \frac{f'}{w} \cdot \frac{P}{A} \cdot U^n$$

The ratio h_f/L is the slope of hydraulic gradient line and is written as S or i, Assuming n = 2.

$$S = \frac{f'}{w} \cdot \frac{1}{R} U^2$$

$$U = \sqrt{\frac{w}{f'}} \sqrt{RS}$$

Putting $\sqrt{w/f'} = C = $ Chezy's coefficient,

$$U = C\sqrt{RS} \qquad \qquad ...(10.6)$$

Eq. 10.6 is known as Chezy's equation where C is known as Chezy's coefficient of friction. It is not much used for pipe flow problems but is widely used for flow through open channels. The value of C can be obtained either from experimental results or from tables.

2. Manning's Formula

Similar to Chezy's formula, it is also widely used for flow through open channels but rarely used for pipes.

$$U = \frac{1}{n} \cdot R^{2/3} S^{1/2} \qquad \qquad ...(10.7)$$

where n is known as Manning's rugosity coefficient and depends on the nature of the surface. For different surfaces, the value of n can be referred from Table 12.2. It should be noted that S is the slope of hydraulic gradient line, (= hf/L), R is the hydraulic radius and U is the mean velocity of flow.

3. Hazen William's Formula

Another very useful formula is Hazen William's formula which is widely used in the design of water supply mains.

$$U = 0.85 \, C_1 \, R^{0.63} \, S^{0.54} \qquad \qquad ...(10.8)$$

where C_1 is a coefficient and its value depends on the nature of the boundary, U- is the mean velocity of flow, R is hydraulic radius and S is the slope of hydraulic gradient line for uniform diameter pipe. Some of the values of coefficient C_1 are given below.

TABLE 10.1

Type of Surface	Value of C_1
1. Extremely smooth and straight, like steel (new surface)	140
2. Very smooth surface, lime concrete (new surface)	130
3. Smooth masonry surface	120
4. Cast iron (old), moderately corrugated.	100
5. Old rivetted steel	95

10.6 MINOR LOSSES

The dissipation of energy of flow in a pipe line consists of loss due to frictional resistance and loss due to local disturbance. Conventionally, the former is termed as major loss and the latter as minor loss. The minor losses may be due to sudden contraction, sudden enlargement, valves, elbows, etc., fitted in a pipe line. The term minor loss is a misnomer, because in many situations they are more important than frictional losses, e.g. in the case of the suction pipe of a pump along with its strainer and foot valve, the loss of head at entrance may be very much greater than the friction loss in the short length of suction pipe.

In general the minor losses result from changes in velocity of flow-either a change in its magnitude or its direction or a change in both. Whenever, a weak disturbance occurs in a pipe line, eddy currents are set up in the flow (because of separation of flow) which cause more turbulence in the flow as compared to normally present in the flow. The eddying turbulence persists for considerable length downstream and is eventually damped out by the fluid viscosity. The eddy motion derives the energy from the main flow which is finally dissipated as viscous resistance and thus a portion of useful energy is lost, The magnitude of this localised loss is proportional to the abruptness of the velocity change. Though the disturbing effect is usually confined to a very short length of path, the effects may not disappear for a considerable distance downstream. Moreover, if the transitions are carefully streamlined, the flow separation may be avoided and thus the resulting loss of energy may be minimum.

The minor losses are found to very approximately linearly with the velocity head, that is,

$$h_L = K_L \frac{U^2}{2g} \qquad \qquad ...(10.9)$$

The term K_L is known as energy loss coefficient. Except the loss of head caused due to sudden enlargement, most of the minor losses are determined experimentally.

The loss coefficient K_L depends upon (i) flow geometry, (ii) becomes constant at high Reynolds number and (iii) increases with increase in roughness as well as with decreasing Reynolds number.

For convenience, minor losses are also expressed in terms of equivalent length l_e of the pipe that would cause the same amount of energy loss.

$$K_L \frac{U^2}{2g} = f \frac{l_e}{D} \frac{U^2}{2g} \qquad \qquad ...(10.10)$$

The minor losses caused due to following transitions are discussed henceafter

(1) Loss due to sudden enlargement.

(2) Loss due to sudden contraction.

(3) Loss at entrance.

(4) Loss at exit.

(5) Loss at bend.

(6) Loss due to pipe fittings.

1. Loss of head due to enlargement

(a) Sudden Enlargement : The flow pattern in a sudden enlargement is shown in Fig. 10.1 along with hydraulic gradient and total energy lines. It is seen from Fig. 10.1 that a rise in pressure is caused due to decrease in velocity in the larger pipe. At the same time, a state of excessive turbulence exists from sections C to F (in a distance of 50 D or so) beyond which the flow becomes more smooth along the wall than at the centre line of the pipe.

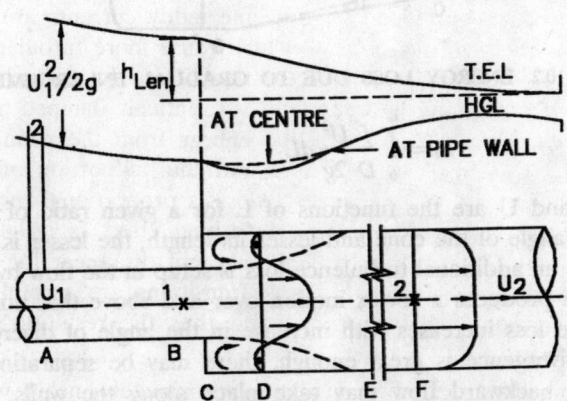

10.1. ENERGY LOSS DUE TO SUDDEN ENLARGEMENT

The energy loss due to sudden enlargement can be determined by Borda-Carnot's formula, Eq. 5.62.

$$h_{L_{enl}} = (U_1 - U_2)^2 / 2g \qquad \qquad ...(5.62)$$

where U_1 is the velocity in the smaller diameter pipe and U_2 is the velocity in the larger diameter pipe.

(b) Gradual Enlargement : In order to reduce the above mentioned loss, the area of cross section should be reduced gradually as shown in Fig. 10.2. It is known as diffuser, which may either be a frustrum of a cone or whose surface may be given a curved outline. The loss of head will be a function of the angle of divergence and also the ratio of the two areas, the length of the diffuser being determined by these two variables. Diffusers are very useful pressure recovery devices such as draft tube used in turbines, diffuser passage for centrifugal pump and similar other practical applications.

It is seen that for a given angle α the loss in the diffuser increases with increase in the ratio of D_2/D_1, owing to greater length of CD. Similarly, for a given ratio D_2/D_1, the length of CD decreases and the loss of energy increases. In fact, the loss in a diffuser may be considered as made up of two factors, i.e. the friction loss and the turbulence loss. The friction loss is given by.

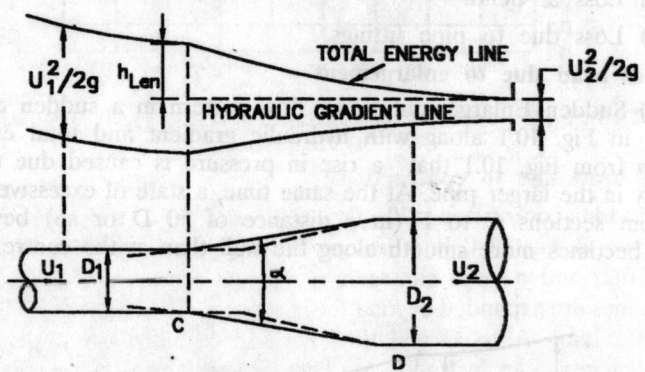

FIG. 10.2. ENERGY LOSS DUE TO GRADUAL ENLARGEMENT

$$h_f = \int_0^L \frac{f}{D} \frac{U^2}{2g} \, dL \qquad \ldots(10.11)$$

in which f,D and U are the functions of L for a given ratio of areas A_2/A_1, the larger the angle of the cone and lesser its length, the lesser is pipe friction loss. However, an additional turbulence loss is setup in the flow by the induced currents which produces a vortex motion over and above that normally exists. The turbulence loss increases with increase in the angle of divergence. If the ratio of the divergence is great enough, there may be separation of flow at the walls and backward flow may take place along the walls. It has been found experimentally that the combined effect of friction and turbulence (or eddies) is minimum at an angle of 6° for very smooth boundaries. If the bounding surface are rough, the optimum cone angle found 7°. The loss coefficient is higher for a gradual divergence due to the combined effects. Hence it is better to use a sudden enlargement than a diffuser of cone angle other than optimum. In general, the loss of head due to gradual enlargement is expressed as

(b) Gradual Enlargement : To reduce the above mentioned loss, the area of cross section should be enlarged gradually as shown in Fig.

$$h_L = K_{L1} \frac{(U_1 - U_2)^2}{2g}$$ ...(10.12)

where K_{l1} is the loss coefficient and is expressed as a function of the angle of divergence and is shown in Fig 10.3.

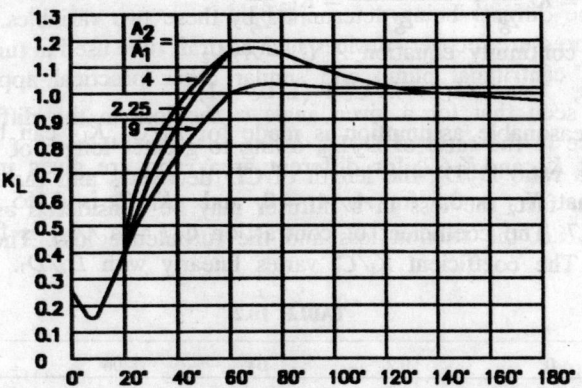

FIG. 10.3. RELATION BETWEEN LOSS COEFFICIENT AND THE ANGLE OF DIVERGENCE

2. Loss of head due to contraction

(a) Sudden contraction : The flow pattern through an abruptly contracting pipe is shown in Fig 10.4. It is observed that the streamlines are contracted at the junction and a vena contracta is formed in the small diameter pipe. The streamlines are expanded beyond the section of vena contracta. The pressure drops from section A to C and then rises on the downstream side due to change of velocity. The hydraulic gradient line and total energy line are also shown in Fig 10.4. The energy loss or head loss due to sudden contraction

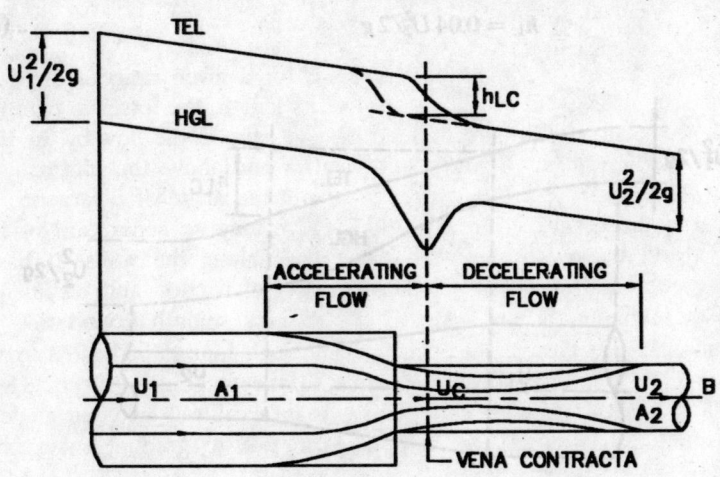

FIG. 10.4. ENERGY LOSS DUE TO SUDDEN CONTRACTION

is supposed to be made up of two portion, viz.loss of head due to friction in the region of accelerating flow from A to C and turbulence loss beyond section C. Thus

$$h_{Lc} = K_f \frac{U_c^2}{2g} + \frac{(U_c - U_2)^2}{2g} = K_{L2} \frac{U_2^2}{2g} \qquad \qquad ...(10.13)$$

From continuity equation $A_c U_c = A_2 U_2$

Hence, $k_{L2} = k_f/C_c^2 + (1/C_c - 1)^2$ ...(10.14)

If a reasonable assumption is made for K_f/C_c^2, K_{L2} can be estimated. The value of K_{L2} and K_f/C_c^2 for different area ratio are given in Table 10.2. It is seen that K_{L2} is 0.5 for $A_2/A_1 = 0$, and K_f/C_c^2 is 0.155 as the value of C_c is 0.617. The coefficient of contraction C_c (= A_c/A_2) is found related with A_2/A_1. The coefficient K_f/C_c^2 varies linearly with D_2/D_1.

TABLE 10.2

A_2/A_1	0	0.2	04	06	08
C_c	0.617	0.63	0.66	0.71	0.81
K_f/C_c^2	0.115	0.075	0.040	0.018	0.005
K_{L2}	0.5	0.41	0.30	0.18	0 .06

(b) **Gradual contraction.** In order to reduce the head loss due to sudden contraction, the abrupt changes in the cross section should be avoided. A thin boundary layer is developed along the wall of the contraction and the flow is irrotational outside it and hence the loss of head through a reducer is almost negligible. If the contraction is too long, the frictional loss may be high due to higher average velocity in the reducer than a larger diameter straight pipe. An angle of 20° to 40° is appropriate to give minimum loss of energy due to contraction which is mainly due to friction (Fig 10.5)

$$h_L = 0.04 \, U_2^2/2g \qquad \qquad ...(10.15)$$

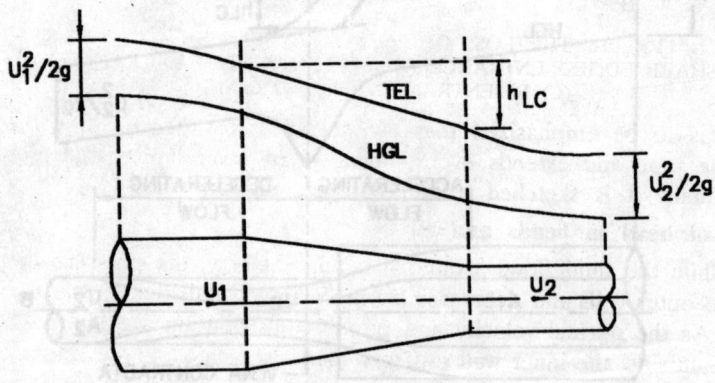

FIG. 10.5. TEL AND HGL FOR GRADUAL CONTRACTION

3. Loss of energy at entrance

The flow pattern at entrance is a limiting case of sudden contraction with $A_2/A_1 = 0$ and the energy loss at entrance can be determined accordingly. The energy loss at entrance depends on the shape of the entrance. In Fig. 10.6, the fluid flowing through various shaped entrance is shown. The head loss at sharp edged entrance for highly turbulent flow is given by

$$h_{Lent} = 0.5 \frac{U_2^2}{2g} \qquad \ldots(10.16)$$

For bell mouthed entrance, loss of head is reduced substantially. Hamilton has shown that if the radius of the rounding is greater than 0.14 diameter, the formation of vena contracta is prevented and this eliminates the loss of head. The nominal value of loss coefficient for bell mouthed entrance is 0.1

$$H_{Lent} = 0.1 \frac{U_2^2}{2g} \qquad \ldots(10.17)$$

and so the loss coefficient for bell mouthed entrance, K_{L3} is 0.1.

A pipe projecting into the tank is known as "re-entrant" type entrance. If the pipe wall is very thin and the plane of opening is more than one diameter upstream from the reservoir wall, the loss coefficient is very high and is nearly 0.8. This high value is caused due to small vena contracta and consequent large decelerating loss. For thick walled pipes larger vena contracta is formed and correspondingly the loss coefficient is smaller and it approaches a value for square edged entrance.

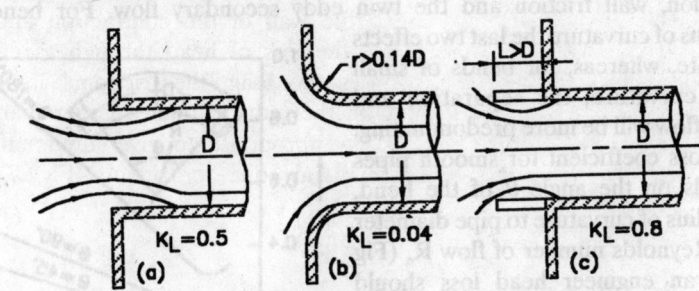

FIG. 10.6. THE LOSS OF ENERGY AT THE ENTRANCE
(A) SHARP EDGED ENTRANCE (B) BELL MOUNTED ENTRANCE AND (C) RE-ENTRANT TYPE ENTRANCE

It is to be emphasized that the entrance loss occurs after the fluid enters the pipe and extends over a distance of several pipe diameters, but conventionally it is sketched at the entrance section.

4. Loss of head in bends and elbows

While the fluid flows around a bend or elbow, the pressure increases along the outer wall and decreases along the inner wall due to the curvature of flow. As the normal velocity and pressure distribution are approached on downstream side, the inner wall pressure must rise again. As the velocity along the surface is zero, it cannot decrease to provide for a pressure increase and hence there may be separation from the inner wall. The result of this unbalanced condition is to produce a secondary flow. This motion combined with axial velocity forms a double spiral flow which persists for some distance downstream (Fig. 10.7).

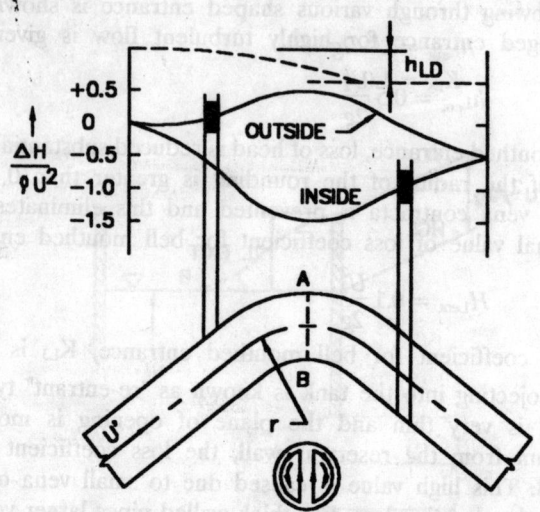

FIG. 10.7. VARIATION OF HEAD AT BEND

Loss of head in smooth pipe bends are caused by the combined effects of separation, wall friction and the twin eddy secondary flow. For bends of larger radius of curvature the last two effects predominate, whereas, for bends of small radius of curvature, the separation and secondary flow will be more predominating. Thus the loss coefficient for smooth pipes K_L depends on the angle θ of the bend, ratio of radius of curvature to pipe diameter R/D and Reynolds number of flow R_e (Fig 10.8). To an engineer head loss should be minimum for given R/D so as to provide an efficient pipe design. The value of K_L for smooth bend (at $R/D = 0$) is found experimentally equal to 1.1 Such bends are known as metre bends. Sometimes guide vanes are provide at the corner of bend to avoid secondary flow and separation of flow.

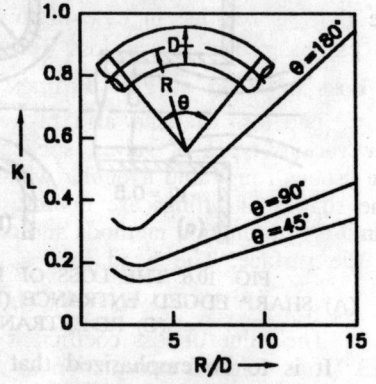

FIG. 10.8. COEFFICIENT OF LOSS AT SMOOTH BEND

Installation of vanes break up the spiral motions, improves the velocity distribution and thus reduces the head loss to $0.2\, U^2/2g$, i.e. $K_{L_4} = 0.2$.

5. Loss of head at the exit

When a fluid with a velocity U is discharged from the end of a pipe into a tank or reservoir Fig. 10.9, whole of its kinetic energy is dissipated in the formation of eddies and high turbulence. Applying Bernoulli's theorem between A and C.

$$h_{L_{exit}} = U^2/2g \qquad ...(10.8)$$

and thus $K_{L5} = 1.0$

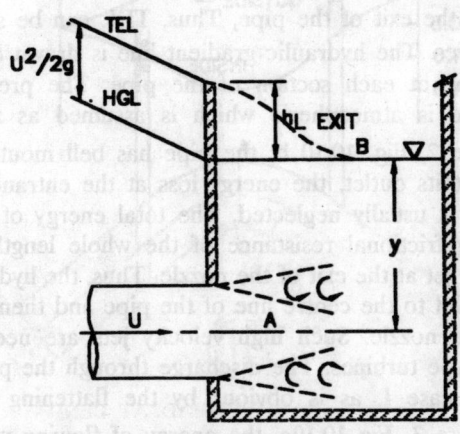

FIG. 10.9. ENERGY LOSS AT EXIT

The large amount of energy loss at exit could be reduced by diverging the pipe as is done in case of draft tube (used with the turbines). It must be emphasized that exit loss occurs after the fluid leaves the pipe.

6. Loss of Head at Pipe Fittings.

The loss of head also takes place at different shapes of pipe fitting like various types of valves, sockets, etc., The inner surface of such fittings are usually rough and irregular which produce excessive large scale turbulence. The shapes of fittings are mainly governed by structural properties, ease of handling, production methods and other practical requirement than smoothness of the surface. The head loss is given by

$$h_{L0} = K_{L6} (U^2/2g) \qquad ...(10.9)$$

The value of loss coefficient for different fittings is given in the Table 10.3 More detailed information about minor losses has been compiled in the handbook of hydraulics by Kings.

TABLE 10.3

Globe valve	10.0	1/2 open	5.0
Angle valve	5.0	1/4 open	24.0
Gate valve		Return bend	2.2
Fully open	0.10	90° bend	0.90
3/4 open	1.15	45° bend	0.42

10.7. ANALYSIS OF FLOW THROUGH PIPE SYSTEM

When the fluid through a pipe system under a head H (say), the energy of flowing water is lost in overcoming the frictional resistance besides minor losses occurring in the flow due to the change of section. In Fig. 10.10, four different flow cases are shown. In each case, the total energy line and hydraulic gradient line are also shown. In the first case. Fig 10.10 a, the energy of water in the reservoir, i.e. head H, is used (a) to overcome entrance loss h_{L_e} (b) in overcoming frictional losses and (c) in imparting the velocity energy $U^2/2g$ to the water at the exit of the pipe, Thus. TEL can be sketched easily depicting all these losses. The hydraulic gradient line is drawn $U^2/2g$ ordinate below total energy line at each section of the pipe. The pressure head at the outlet of the pipe is atmospheric which is assumed as zero.

In the flow case 2, Fig. 10.10 b, the pipe has bell mouthed entry and a nozzle is attached at its outlet. the energy loss at the entrance to the pipe will be too small and is usually neglected. The total energy of flowing water is used in overcoming frictional resistance of the whole length of pipe and forming a high velocity jet at the exit of the nozzle. Thus, the hydraulic gradient line initially runs parallel to the centre line of the pipe and then drops sharply at the entrance to the nozzle. Such high velocity jets are needed to rotate the wheels of pelton type turbines. The discharge through the pipe is reduced as compared to flow case I, as is obvious by the flattening of HGL line.

For the flow case 3, Fig 10.10c, the energy of flowing water,H (which will be the difference in water levels of two reservoirs) is dissipated in (a)

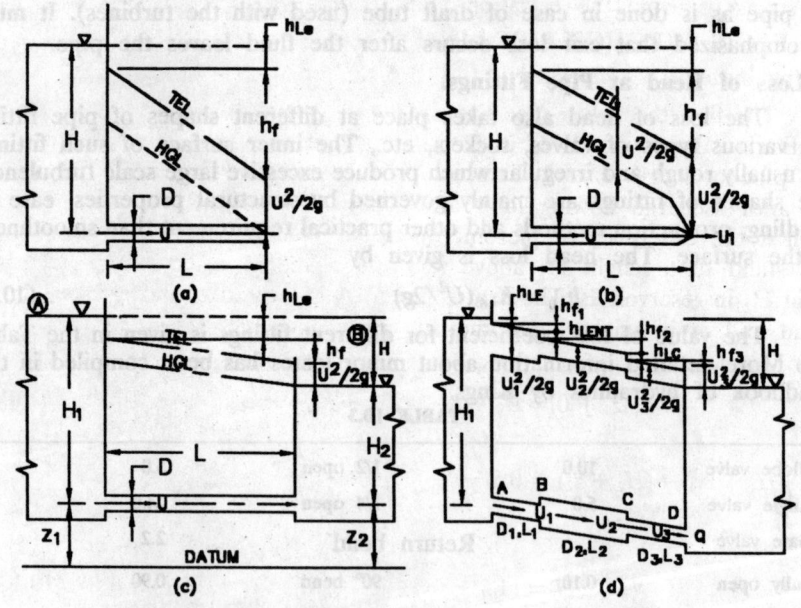

FIG. 10.10 ANALYSIS OF FLW THROUGH PIPE SYSTEM

the loss at entry (b) pipe friction and (c) conversion into velocity energy (or exit loss), which is subsequently lost in eddying in the downstream reservoir. The TEL and HGL runs parallel to each other and are shown in the diagram. If the length of pipe line is sufficiently large, the difference in elevations between these two lines (which is equal to the velocity energy) become smaller and smaller. Hence sometimes in practical problems involving long pipes, only single energy line is drawn, although it is theoretically not a correct procedure.

Case 4, Fig 10.10d, shows different diameter pipes joining two reservoirs. The total energy line drops continuously in the direction of flow due to frictional resistance being experienced by the flowing water. The total energy of water, H, is dissipated in (a) overcoming the entrance loss at A (b) frictional loss in pipe AB, (c) sudden enlargement loss at B, (d) frictional loss in the pipe BC (e) sudden contraction loss at C (f) frictional loss in the pipe CD and (g) exit loss at D. The HGL lies below TEL by an amount equal to velocity energy appropriate at the given section. It is seen from Fig. 10.10d, that HGL rises in the pipe segment BC as compared to AB or CD due to higher pressure existing in the larger diameter pipe BC.

Many a times the pipe connecting two reservoirs is not straight bur bends so as to cross a mount or high elevation ground (Refer to Fig. 5.6), such a pipe behaves as a siphon. In this case the HGL lies below the centre line of the pipe and hence the pressure at any point in the segment CD remains lower than atmospheric pressure. The lowest pressure occurs at the apex of the pipe line. In the design of pipe line system, it is ensured that the pressure does not fall below vapour pressure ar any point of the pipe line so as to avoid the caviation phenomenon to occur in it.

10.8 FLOW THROUGH PIPE LINE

1. Pipe outlet is Submerged

The flow through a pipe line can be determined by applying Bernoullis equation to the two ends of it. Consider two reservoirs A and B connected by a pipe of length L and diameter D in Fig 10.10c. The mean velocity of flow and discharge flowing in it are U and Q respectively under head H which is the difference of piezometric heads at its two ends. Let the water level stand to a height H_1 above the centre line in reservoir A and to a height H_2 in reservoir B. The centre line at A is located z_1 above an arbitrary datum and at a height z_2 at another end.

Applying Bernoulli's theorem between the two ends of pipeline,

$$H_1 + z_1 + 0 = H_2 + z_2 + h_{L_{ent}} + h_{f_{AB}} + h_{L_{exit}} \qquad ...(10.10a)$$

or $$(H_1 + z_1) - (H_2 + z_2) = 0.5\frac{U^2}{2g} + f\frac{L}{D}\frac{U^2}{2g} + \frac{U^2}{2g}$$

or $$H = (1.5 + f\frac{L}{D})\frac{U^2}{2g} \qquad ...(10.10c)$$

or
$$U = \sqrt{\frac{2gH}{(1.5 + fL/D)}} \qquad ...(10.10c)$$

From continuity equation

$$Q = AU = \frac{\pi D^2}{4} \sqrt{\frac{2gH}{1.5 + fL/D}} \qquad ...(10.11)$$

If the length of the pipe is small, full equation, Eq, 10.10a or 10.11 should be used. If the length of the pipe is sufficiently large, the frictional losses are much larger as compared to minor losses and hence the term 1.5 may be dropped.

2. Pipe Outlet is Free

If the pipe discharges freely into atmosphere, Eq. 10.10a modifies to

$$H_1 + z_1 = z_2 + 0.5 \frac{U^2}{2g} + f \frac{L}{D} \frac{U^2}{2g} + \frac{U^2}{2g}$$

or
$$H_1 + z_1 - z_2 = H = \left(1.5 + f\frac{L}{D}\right) \frac{U^2}{2g} \qquad ...(10.12)$$

where H is the height of liquid level in the reservoir A above the outlet of the pipe at its other end.

10.9 TRANSMISSION OF POWER THROUGH PIPE LINE

The water stored in a reservoir under a gross head H_1 is conveyed to powerhouse by means of pipe lines or penstocks to run the turbines and produce power. The energy of flowing water is used mainly to overcome the frictional losses and to generate either a high velocity jet under atmospheric pressure (or a low velocity stream under pressure) at its exit end; the minor losses are of less significance. Thus, the head of water available at discharging end of pipe is the difference of gross head H_1 and frictional and other losses hf, i.e. net head H.

$$H = H_1 - h_f$$

But
$$h_f \propto Q^2$$

$$h_f = kQ^2$$

Thus
$$H = H_1 - kQ^2 \qquad ...(10.13)$$

The power transmitted at the discharging end is given by

$$P = w\,QH \qquad ...(10.14)$$

where Q is the discharge flowing in the pipe line.

It is seen from Eq. 10.13 that maximum net head H will be available if the frictional losses hf are minimum. This means that Q is zero, but it gives zero power. Similarly, the value of H will be minimum or zero when Q is maximum. Since P is the product of Q and H, the maximum power will be transmitted to the turbine at the outlet for intermediate value of discharge Q.

From Eqs. 10.13 and 10.14

$$p = wQ(H_1 - h_f)$$

$$P = waU\left(H_1 - f\frac{L}{D}\frac{U^2}{2g}\right) \qquad \qquad ...(10.15)$$

where U is the average velocity of water flowing in the pipe line. Differentiating Eq. 10.15 with respect to U,

$$\frac{dP}{dU} = \frac{d}{dU}\left[wa\left(H_1 U - f\frac{L}{D}\frac{U^3}{2g}\right)\right]$$

$$= wa\left[H_1 - 3f\frac{L}{D}\frac{U^2}{2g}\right]$$

$$= wa\left[H_1 - 3h_f\right]$$

For maximum power $\dfrac{dP}{dU} = 0$

or $\qquad H_1 = 3h_f$

or $\qquad h_f = H_1/3 ...(10.16)$

Efficiency of transmission $= \dfrac{wQH}{wQH_1}$

$$= (1 - h_f/H_1)$$
$$= 2/3 \text{ or } 66.67\% \qquad \qquad ...(10.17)$$

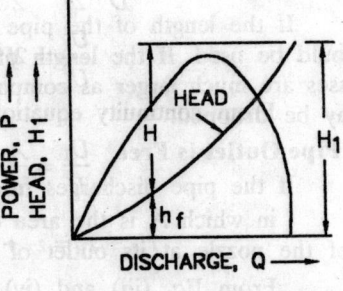

FIG. 10.11. HEAD AND POWER DELIVERED BY A PIPE

Thus it is seen that maximum power is transmitted through a pipe line, if the head loss is limited to one third of the head available at its inlet. It is to be emphasized that the above result has been derived on the basis of Darcy's formula for head loss caused to the turbulent flow. In case any other formula is used for the computation of h_f the result will be slightly different.

10.10 FLOW OF LIQUID THROUGH NOZZLE

In case of certain machines (impulse turbine), a high velocity jet is needed to rotate the wheel. The high velocity is produced by fixing a nozzle (tapering pipe) at the outlet end of the pipe.

Usually, the nozzle discharges into atmosphere and the proportion of energy of flowing water which is converted into high velocity energy (or kinetic energy) at the outlet of the nozzle depends on the ratio of the nozzle diameter d to pipe diameter D; the nozzle losses being neglected. Let the velocity of flowing water in the pipe be U.

From Eq. 10.16 for maximum transmission of power.

$$h_f = \frac{H_1}{3} \qquad \qquad ...(10.16)$$

Also $\qquad H = H_1 - h_f = 2/3\,H_1$

Thus $\qquad h_f = H/2 \qquad \qquad ...(i)$

Let the jet discharge into atmosphere with a velocity U_1, therefore,

$$H = 0 + U_1^2/2g \qquad \qquad ...(ii)$$

From Eqs. (i) and (ii)

$$h_f = \frac{1}{2} (U_1^2/2g)$$

Substituting the value of h_f, from Darcy's formula Eq. 10.5

$$f \cdot \frac{L}{D} \cdot \frac{U^2}{2g} = \frac{1}{2} \frac{U_1^2}{2g}$$

$$\frac{U_1^2}{U^2} = 2f \frac{L}{D} \qquad \qquad ...(iii)$$

From continuity equation,

$$\frac{U_1}{U} = \frac{A}{a} . \qquad \qquad ..(iv)$$

in which A is the area of the pipe of diameter D and a is the area of the nozzle at its outlet of diameter d.

From Eq. (iii) and (iv).

$$A/a = \sqrt{2fL/D}$$

Solving $\qquad d/D = (D/2fL)^{1/4} \qquad \qquad ...(10.18)$

Effeciency of transmission

The power transmitted through the nozzle is the ratio of the output power to input power.

$$\eta = \frac{U_1^2/2g}{H}$$

$$= (U_1^2/2g H) \qquad \qquad ...(10.19)$$

10.11 ECONOMICS OF PIPE LINES

The head loss and consequently the power lost due to friction in conveyance of liquids depends directly on the size (diameter) of the pipe; larger the size, the less is the power lost. But the larger diameter of pipe costs more. Thus the most economical size of the pipe will be that for which the sum of the cost of pipe and the value of the power lost is a minimum.

Let the water flow in a pipe of diameter d, wall thickness t, length L under a pressure p. The volume rate of flow per second is Q. The frictional resistance to the flow of water may be computed by Darcy's formula, Eq. 10.5. The power lost in conveyance is given by

$$P_1 = \frac{w Q h_f}{1000} kW$$

and $\qquad \qquad h_f = \frac{f L Q^2}{12.1 D^5}$

Thus, cost of power lost $\propto f/D^5$

or $\qquad \qquad C_1 = A/D^5 \qquad \qquad ...(i)$

The constant of proportionality A depends on length of the pipe L, cost of unit power, the specific weight of the fluid and the frictional resistance of the surface.

The hoop stress f_t in the material of the pipe is given by Eq. 2.21b.

$$f_t = \frac{pd}{2t} \qquad \qquad \text{...(2.21b)}$$

It is seen from Eq. 2.22b, that for given f_1 (permissible) and p, the wall thickness of the pipe will increase with increase in its diameter. This, in turn, will increase the weight and cost of the pipe. Hence, the fixed annual cost of the pipe can be approximately expressed as the square of the diameter.

$$\text{Fixed cost of pipe } \propto \text{ unit cost } \times \frac{D^2}{4} \times L$$

$$C_2 \propto BD^2 \qquad \qquad \text{...(ii)}$$

where B depends on the unit cost, diameter and length of the pipe. Thus, the total cost (computed on the annual basis) is the sum of the two costs.

$$C = C_1 + C_2$$

$$C = \frac{A}{D^5} + BD^2 \qquad \qquad \text{...(iii)}$$

For minimum cost, $\dfrac{dC}{dD}$ should be zero.

$$\frac{dC}{dD} = -5\frac{A}{D^6} + 2BD$$

Solving $\quad D^7 = \dfrac{5}{2}\dfrac{A}{B} \qquad \text{...(10.20)}$

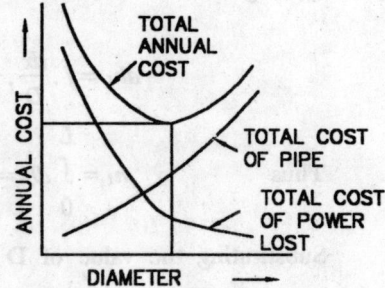

FIG. 10.12. ECONOMICAL SIZE OF THE PIPE

Eq. 10.20 gives the most economical diameter of the pipe on the assumptions that A and B,i.e. annual cost of power lost and annual cost of pipe etc., remains constant, which is strictly is not always true. Fig. 10.12. shows the variation of the cost of the pipe with its diameter. It is to be noted that the most economical diameter, is not always used due to many practical constraints.

10.12 FLOW THROUGH A TAPERING PIPE

Fig.10.13 shows a tapering pipe AB whose diameter varies from D_1 to D_2 in a length L. It carries a discharge Q. Let us take a small length dx at a distance x from smaller diameter end, and let its diameter at this section be D. The tapered pipe is supposed to be frustum of a cone whose vertex is at O such that $BO = l$

$$\frac{D_1}{D_2} = \frac{L + l}{l}$$

Solving, $\qquad l = \dfrac{LD_2}{(D_1 - D_2)} \qquad \qquad \text{...(10.21a)}$

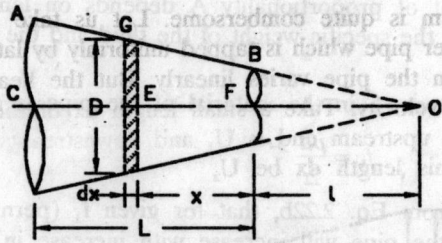

FIG. 10.13. FLOW THROUGH TAPERED PIPE

From similar triangles GEO and BFO

$$\frac{D}{D_2} = \frac{x+l}{l}$$

Solving, $$D = D_2 \frac{(x+l)}{l} \qquad \qquad ...(10.21b)$$

The loss of head occurring through the whole length of pipe is computed by integrating the loss of head caused in the elementary length dx, say, dh_f

$$dh_f = f \cdot \frac{dx}{D} \cdot \frac{U^2}{2g}$$

Thus $$h_f = \int_0^L dh_f = \int_0^L f \frac{dx}{D} \times \frac{U^2}{2g}$$

Substituting the value of D from Eq. 10.21b.

$$h_f = \int_0^L \frac{f}{2g} \frac{dx}{D} \left(\frac{4Q}{\pi D^2} \right)^2$$

$$= \frac{16fQ^2}{2\pi^2 g} \int_0^L \frac{dx}{D^5}$$

$$= \frac{16fQ^2}{2\pi^2 g} \int_0^L \frac{l^5}{D_2^5 (x+l)^5} dx$$

Solving it,

$$h_f = \frac{2fQ^2}{\pi^2 g D^5} \left[\frac{1}{l^4} - \frac{1}{(L+l)^4} \right] \qquad ...(10.22)$$

Eq.10.22 computes the head loss through a tapered pipe where l is given Eq. 10.21a.

10.13 FLOW THROUGH UNIFORMLY TAPPED PIPES

In water supply systems the main pipe is provided with a number of laterals to feed different localities. In such flow case, the discharge and hence the corresponding velocity decreases continuously along the pipe line. The

Usually, the geometrical properties of the pipe net work are known, that means, f_1, L_1, D_1 and f_2, L_2, D_2 are known. Now, if the discharge Q is known one can compute H and vice versa.

If the minor losses are also considered, the Bernoulli's equation between A and B yields,

$$0 + 0 + H = 0 + 0 + 0 + K_{L1}\frac{U_1^2}{2g} + f_1\frac{L_1}{D_1}\cdot\frac{U_1^2}{2g}$$

$$+ \frac{(U_1 - U_2)^2}{2g} + f_2\frac{L_2}{D_2}\frac{U_2^2}{2g} + \frac{U_2^2}{2g} \qquad ...(10.25b)$$

From continuity equation,

$$U_2 = \left(\frac{A_1}{A_2}\right) U_1 = \left(\frac{D_1}{D_2}\right)^2 U_1 \qquad ...(10.26)$$

From equations 10.25b and 10.26.

$$H = \frac{U_1^2}{2g}\left[K_{L1} + f_1\frac{L_1}{D_1} + (1 - D_1^2/D_2^2)^2 + f_2\frac{L_2 D_1^4}{D_2^5} + \left(\frac{D_1}{D_2}\right)^4\right]$$

$$= \frac{U_1^2}{2g}[C_1 + C_2 f_1 + C_2 f_2] \qquad ...(10.27b)$$

where $C_1 = [K_{L1} + (1 - .D_1^2/D_2^2)^2 + D_1^4/D_2^4]$

$C_2 = L_1/D_1$

$C_3 = L_2 D_1^4/D_2^5$

where C_1, C_2 and C_3 are geometric properties of the pipe network and are usually known. Thus, one of the unknown quantity H or Q can be computed from Eq. 10.27b.

(a) Analysis of flow : There are two possibilities (i) when the discharge Q is given, H is required and (ii) when the head difference H is known, Q is to be computed. In the first case, when from the known quantities Q, D_1, D_2 and fluid properties ρ and ν, Reynolds number of the flow is calculated for each pipe.The values of f_1 and f_2 is then read from Moody's diagram, Fig. 9.10. Thus H is computed from Eq. 10.27.

In the second case, initially the values of f_1 and f_2 are assumed (they may be assumed equal in the first instance). With the known value of H, the velocity U_1, and hence the discharge Q is computed from Eq. 10.27. From this value of U_1, the Reynolds number of flow in each pipe is computed and the values of f_1 and f_2 are read from Fig 9.10. A second trial for U_1 is now made using equation 10.27. Since f varies slightly with Reynolds number, the trial solution converges rapidly. i.e. only two or three trials are needed. The same method may be used to more than two pipes connected in series.

(b) Equivalent Pipe Method : Another method of solving the problem is to replace the length of all the pipes in terms of equivalent lengths of any one given pipe size, usually the one which figures predominantly in the system. By equivalent length is meant a length L_e of pipe of certain diameter D_e which carry the same discharge and dissipate same energy or head h_f as the one with length L and diameter D. Thus,

$$h_{fe} = f_e \frac{L_3}{D_e} \frac{U_e^2}{2g} \qquad ...(i)$$

$$h_f = f \frac{L}{D} \frac{U^2}{2g} \qquad ...(ii)$$

From continuity equation

$$A_e U_e = AU \qquad ...(iii)$$

From Eqs. (i) to (iii)

$$h_f = h_{fe}$$

$$L_e = L \frac{f}{f_e} \frac{D_e}{D} \frac{U^2}{U_e^2} = L \frac{f}{f_e} \left(\frac{D_e}{D} \right)^5 \qquad ...(10.28)$$

Thus, the equivalent length of each pipe may be computed. Usually, the minor losses due to pipe fittings are also expressed in terms of equivalent lengths Hence the summation of all the equivalent lengths is determined and equated to the differential head between reservoirs A and B to determine the unknowns.

$$H = f \frac{(L_{e1} + L_{e2} + L_{e3})}{D_e} \frac{U_e^2}{2g} \qquad ...(10.29a)$$

and

$$Q = A_e U_e = \frac{\pi}{4} D_e^2 U_e \qquad ...(10.29b)$$

(c) **Compound Pipe :** It is sometimes required to replace multiple pipes of different diameter D_1, D_2 etc. by a single pipe of uniform diameter D and length L; the discharge Q and head h_f remaining the same. Thus, from Eq. 10.25a.

$$H = (h_{f1} + h_{f2} + ...) \text{ neglecting minor losses.}$$

Substituting the value of head loss, in terms of discharge

$$f \frac{LQ^2}{12.1 D^5} = \frac{fQ^2}{12.1} \left[\frac{L_1}{D_1^5} + \frac{L_2}{D_2^5} + ... \right] \qquad ...(10.30a)$$

or

$$L = D^5 \left[\frac{L_1}{D_1^5} + \frac{L_2}{D_2^5} + ... \right] \qquad ...(10.30b)$$

The diameter of single pipe D can be computed by Eq. 10.30b.

2. Pipe Connected in Parallel

(a) A combination of two or more pipes connected in such a way that the flow is divided into them at certain point A (say) and joins again at point B is known as pipes connected in parallel. This pipe system provides a number of routes for the water to flow from one reservoir into another. The conditions to be satisfied are

$$\left(\frac{p_B}{w} + z_A\right) - \left(\frac{p_b}{w} + z_B\right) = h_{f1} = h_{f2} = h_{f3} \qquad ...(10.31a)$$

and
$$Q = Q_1 + Q_2 + Q_3 \qquad ...(10.31b)$$

where p_A and p_B are the fluid pressure and z_A and z_B are datum heads at A and B respectively and Q is the discharge flowing either in the inlet pipe or in the outlet pipe.

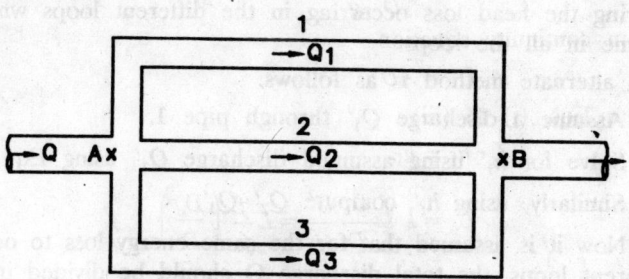

FIG. 10.16. PIPE CONNECTED IN PARALLEL

In this case also two types of the problems are met; (1) The pressure and datum heads at A and B are known; to compute the discharge and (2) the discharge is known; to determine the difference of piezometric head.

Case 1: Since the difference of piezometric head

$$\left(\frac{p_A}{w} + z_A\right) - \left(\frac{p_B}{w} + z_B\right) = h_f \text{ (say)}$$

is known, the discharges flowing in each pipe Q_1, Q_2, Q_3 etc., can be computed from Eq. 10.31a and then added up to determine the total discharge Q.

Case 2. The total discharge Q is given and the head loss and distribution of flow among the circuits are required to be known, The procedure is as follows:

For any one loop.

$$h_f = \left(f\frac{L_1}{D_1} + \Sigma K_L\right)\frac{U^2}{2g} \qquad ...(10.32)$$

where ΣK_L represents minor losses which may be neglected for pipes longer than 1000 times its diameter.

From continuity equation

$$Q_1 = A_1 U_1$$

or
$$Q_1 = A_1 \sqrt{\frac{2gh_f}{fL_1/D_1 + \Sigma K_L}}$$

or
$$Q_1 = C_1 \sqrt{h_f} \qquad ...(10.33)$$

The flow through other pipes can similarly be determined. Then

$$Q = Q_1 + Q_2 + Q_3 + ...$$

$$Q = \sqrt{h_f} \, [C_1 + C_2 + C_3 + \dots] \qquad \dots(10.34)$$

In Eq. 10.34, C_1, C_2 etc., are constant,s The value of friction factor for various pipes is assumed the same as a first trial. Solving Eq. 10.34, h_f is calculated and then distribution of discharge is determined using Eq. 10.33. Knowing trial values of Q_1, Q_2 etc.,. the corresponding R_e and hence f_1 and f_2 are determined for various pipes. The accuracy of the method is checked by comparing the head loss occurring in the different loops which should be the same in all the loops.

The alternate method is as follows:

(1) Assume a discharge Q_1' through pipe 1.

(2) Solve for h_f' using assumed discharge Q_1' using Eq. 10.32

(3) Similarly, using h_f' compute Q_2' Q_3'.

(4) Now it is assumed that for the same energy loss to occur in the three different loops, the total discharge Q should be divided in the same proportion as Q_1', Q_2', Q_3' This means.

$$Q_1 = \left(\frac{Q_1'}{\Sigma Q'}\right) Q \,, Q_2 = \left(\frac{Q_2'}{\Sigma Q'}\right) Q,$$

$$Q_3 = \left(\frac{Q_3'}{\Sigma Q'}\right) Q \qquad \dots(10.35)$$

(5) Check the correctness of the procedure by computing h_{f1}, h_{f2} and h_{f3} for the three different loops which should be the same. Even if there is slight difference, say 1% or so, the solution is taken quite satisfactory.

(b) Compound Pipe : The diameter D of the compound pipe may be determined by Eq. 10.34. Replacing Q by $C\sqrt{h_f}$ and substituting the values of C, C_1, and C_3.

$$C\sqrt{h_f} = \left[C_1 + C_2 + C_2 \right] \sqrt{h_f}$$

$$\frac{D^{5/2}}{L^{1/2}} = \left[\frac{D_1^{5/2}}{L_1^{1/2}} + \frac{D_2^{5/2}}{L_2^{1/2}} + \frac{D_3^{5/2}}{L_3^{1/3}} \right]$$

The minor losses due to pipe fittings, etc. have been neglected.

10.15 FLOW THROUGH A BYE PASS

Sometimes the water is diverted from the main pipe through a diversion pipe either for repair work or to supply some locality in the nearby area. Referring to Fig. 10.17, the water is diverted from section 1 to section 2, the head loss between them is $(H_1 - H_2)$. Let the lengths of main pipe and bye pass be L and I, and their respective diameters be D and d respectively, The head loss at inlet and outlet including any other loss due to valve, etc., in the bye pass be represented as $ku^2/2g$. The velocity of flow in the main pipe is represented by U and that in the bye pass pipe by u, then

$$H_1 - H_2 = f\frac{L}{D}\frac{U^2}{2g} = f\frac{l}{d}\frac{u^2}{2g} + k'\frac{u^2}{2g}$$

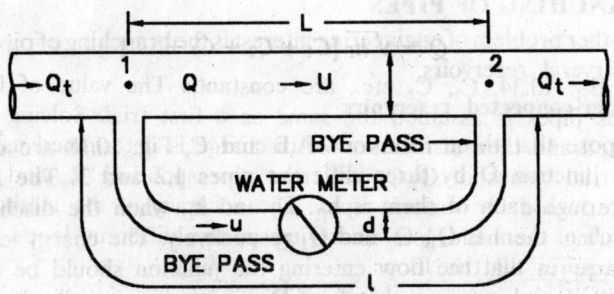

FIG. 10.17. FLOW THROUGH BYE PASS

$$\frac{L\,U^2}{D} = \left(\frac{1}{d}\frac{u^2}{} + k\,u^2\right) \text{ where } k = \frac{k'}{f}$$

$$(U^2/u^2) = \frac{D}{L}\,(l/d + k) \qquad\qquad ...(10.37)$$

$$Q = \frac{\pi D^2}{4}\,U$$

$$q = \frac{\pi d^2}{4}\,u$$

$$\therefore \qquad \frac{Q}{q} = \frac{D^2}{d^2}\cdot\frac{U}{u}$$

$$\frac{Q}{q} = \frac{D^2}{d^2}\sqrt{\frac{D}{L}\left(\frac{l}{d} + k\right)} \qquad\qquad ...(10.38)$$

$$\frac{Q + q}{q} = 1 + \frac{D^2}{d^2}\cdot\sqrt{\frac{D\,(1 + kd)}{Ld}}$$

$$q = \frac{(Q + q)}{1 + \sqrt{\dfrac{D^5}{d^5}\left(\dfrac{1 + kd}{L}\right)}} \qquad\qquad ...(10.39)$$

In the above expression, it is assumed that no water in withdrawn from the bye pass pipe. Further $(Q + q) = Q_t$ total discharge flowing in the main before section 1 or after section 2.

If a watermeter is fixed in the bye pass pipe to measure q and the total discharge is measured by volumetric method (or any other method), the ratio of Q_t to q can be found out.

$$K_d = Q_t/q$$

This ratio K_d is known as discharge constant of bye pass. Thus, it offers another method for measuring discharge through big size mains of water supply scheme where usual method of discharge measurement like watermeter, etc. may not be available or can not be used. The bye pass is calibrated first in the laboratory and thereafter can be used in field.

10.16 BRANCHING OF PIPES

Another problem of engineering interest is the branching of pipes connected between serveral reservoirs.

1.Three inter-connected reservoirs

Suppose that three reservoirs A,B and C, Fig. 10.18 are connected to a common junction D by three different pipes 1,2 and 3. The head loss to the flow through each of them is h_{f1}. h_{f2} and h_{f3} when the discharge flowing through each of them is Q_1, Q_2 and Q_3 respectively. The energy and continuity equation requires that the flow entering the junction should be equal to the flow leaving it and pressure head at D is common to all pipes. The flow must be out from higher reservoir and flow into the lowest; hence either of the two conditions must be satisfied

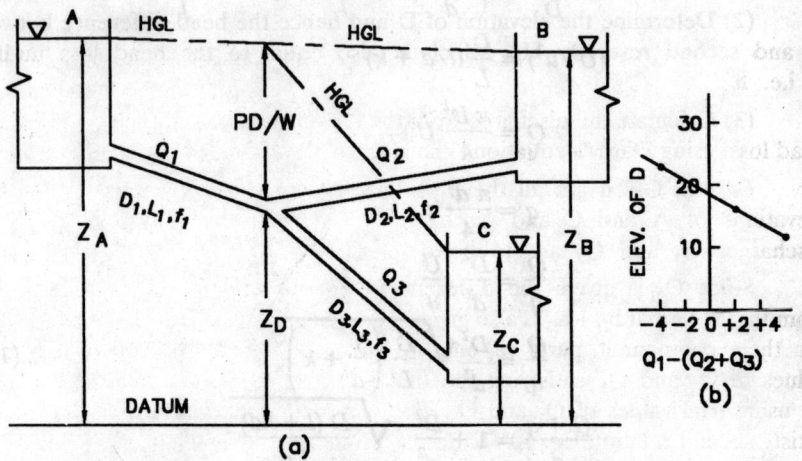

FIG. 10.18 (A) THREE INTER–CONNECTED RESERVOIRS
(B) SAMPEL PLOT BETWEEN $Q_1 - (Q_2 + Q_3)$ VERSUS ELEVATION

$$Q_1 = Q_2 + Q_3 \qquad \qquad ...(10.41a)$$

$$Q_1 + Q_2 = Q_3 \qquad \qquad ...(10.41b)$$

Elevation of D is common to all pipes $\qquad ...(10.41c)$

If the elevation of hydraulic gradient line at the junction is above the elevation of the intermediate reservoir, the flow is into the reservoir, but if the elevation at D is below the intermediate reservoir, the flow is out of it.

Writing the Bernoulli's equation between A and D.

$$z_A = \frac{p_D}{w} + z_D + \frac{U_1^2}{2g} + h_{f1} \qquad ...(10.42a)$$

If the velocity head is small and is neglected.

$$h_{f1} = z_A - \left(\frac{p_D}{w} + z_D\right) \qquad ...(10.42b)$$

Similarly, $$h_{f2} = z_B - \left(\frac{p_D}{w} + z_D\right)$$ ...(10.42c)

and $$h_{f3} = z_c - \left(\frac{p_D}{w} + z_D\right)$$ ...(10.42d)

Three of the several flow problems relating to three reservoirs case are discussed below.

Case 1: Given are all pipe lengths and diameters, surface elevations of any two reservoirs, say, A and B and discharge from any one of the two reservoirs, say Q_1. The elevation of the third reservoir and the discharge Q_2 and Q_3 are to be determined. The solution of the problem is simple.

(1) Assume a proper value of f and calculate h_{f1} for given l_1, D_1 and Q_1.

(2) Determine the elevation of D and hence the head difference between D and second reservoir H_{D2} which is also equal to the head loss in pipe 2, i.e. h_{f2}.

(3) Calculate the discharge from the third reservoir and the corresponding head loss: using Darcy's equation, The surface elevation can then be determined.

Case 2: Given are all the pipe lengths and pipe diameters, the surface elevations of A and C and discharge Q_2, The surface elevation of B and discharges Q_1 and Q_3 are to be determined.

Since Q_2 is given, the difference Q_1-Q_3 is known. Similarly, it is seen from Fig 10.18 that $h_{f1} + h_{f3}$ is also given. These relations are solved simultaneously for their component parts in one of the two ways. (a) Assume successive values of Q_1 and Q_3 satisfying the first relation Eq. 10.41a. Compute h_{f1} and h_{f3} using trial values of Q_1 and Q_3. The computed values of h_{f1} and h_{f3} should satisfy second relation Eq. 10.41c. alternatively (b) assume successive elevation of D satisfying the second relation, determine Q_1 and Q_3 (using Darcy's equation until the first relation is also satisfied.

Case 3: Given all pipe lengths, diameters and elevations of all three reservoirs, find the flow in each pipe. This problems is known as 'three reservoir problem'.

It differs from the earlier two flow cases as it is not evident whether the flow is into or out of the reservoir B. The direction is directly determined by first assuming no flow in pipe 2. In other words the piezometric levels at D and B are assumed at the same level. The head losses h_{f1} and h_{f3} are then used to determine Q_1 and Q_3 by Darcy's equation. If $Q_1 > Q_3$, the flow is going into reservoir B and if $Q_1 < Q_3$ the flow is going out of reservoir B. Once the direction of Q_2 is determined, another trial elevation of piezometric head at D is assumed and h_{f1}, h_{f2}, and h_{f3} computed; Then Q_1, Q_2, and Q_3 are determined and the equation of continuity is satisfied. If the flow into the junction is too great, a higher piezometric head at D is assumed, which will reduce the inflow and increase the outflow.

As an alternate the final piezometric level of D may be determined by making a small plot between $Q_1 - (Q_2 + Q_3)$ versus elevation of D, as shown in Fig. 10.18b.

2. Four reservoirs interconnected with two junctions.

The same procedure is followed with more than three reservoirs. Suppose four reservoirs shown in Fig 10.19, are interconnected in such a way that they have two junction points. In such problems, it is important that only one independent assumption is made otherwise the convergence of the solution would be haphazard. The method involves the following steps:

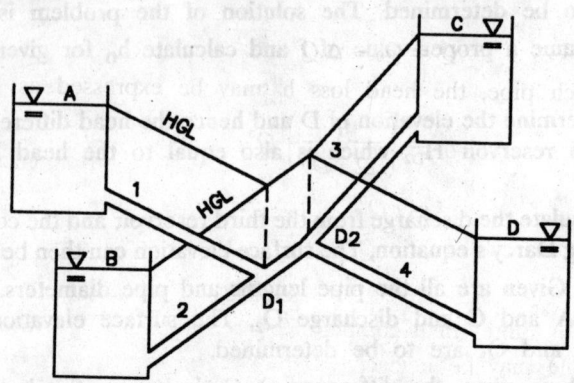

FIG. 10.19, FOUR RESERVOIRS INTER−CONNECTED
WITH TWO JUNCTION POINTS

(1) Assume the elevation of hydraulic gradient line at one junction point D_1 (say)

(2) Determine the flow through pipes 1 and 2 using the three reservoir method and compute the elevation of the hydraulic gradient line of second junction point D_2.

(3) Check whether the flows in pipes 3 and 4 satisfy the continuity at second junction point D_2. If not, a new assumption is made for the elevation of hydraulic gradient line at D_1.

(4) Repeat the procedure until the continuity is satisfied at both junctions D_1 and D_2.

10.17 PIPE NETWORKS

A pipe network is a set of pipes which is interconnected so that flow from a given inlet node or to a given outlet node may come through several different routes. Frequently such pipe networks are encountered in municipal distribution systems. A network may be quite complex but the flow in it must satisfy the basic relations of continuity and energy as given below:

(1) The flow into any junction must equal the flow out of it.

(2) The flow in each pipe must satisfy the pipe friction laws.

(3) The algebraic sum of head losses around any closed circuit must be zero.

It is not practical to solve complicated network analytically, since the equations are non-linear (except for laminar flows), and large number of non-linear simultaneous equations preclude a direct algebraic solution. However, methods are available which successively improve an assumend distribution of flows or heads. The 'Hardy Cross Method' of successive approxmation is one of such methods. The correction applied to flow or head loss at any step is determined by Eqs. 10.43 ot 10.44a.

Let Q be the correct discharge through any pipe, Qo be the assumed discharge and ΔQ be the correction to be applied at any step of approxmation. Therefore,

$$Q = Q_0 - \Delta Q \qquad \qquad ...(10.43)$$

For each pipe, the head loss h_f may be expressed as

$$h_f = \left(\frac{fl}{12.1 D^5} \right) Q^n \qquad \qquad ...(10.44a)$$

$$= r Q^n$$

$$= r (Q_0 + \Delta Q)^n$$

$$= r (Q_0^n + n Q_0^{n-1} \Delta Q + ...) \qquad ...(10.44b)$$

If ΔQ is quite small compared with Q_0, the terms of the series after the second one may be neglected. Now, for a circuit, with ΔQ being the same for all pipes.

$$\Sigma h_f = \Sigma r Q^n = \Sigma r Q_0^n + \Delta Q \Sigma r n Q_0^{n-1} = 0 \qquad ...(10.44c)$$

As the corrections of head loss in all pipes must be summed up arithmetically, ΔQ is given by

$$\Delta Q = \frac{\Sigma r Q_0^n}{\Sigma r n Q_0^{n-1}} \qquad \qquad ...(10.45)$$

From Eq. 10.44a $h_f/Q_0 = r Q_0^{n-1}$

$$\Delta Q = \frac{\Sigma h_f}{n \Sigma (h_f/Q_0)} \qquad \qquad ...(10.46)$$

It must be emphasized that the numerator of Eq. 10.45 or 10.46 must be added algebraically with due account of sign, while the denominator is

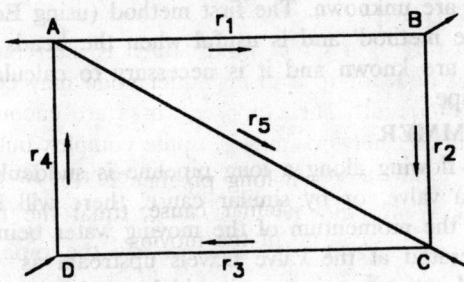

FIG. 10.20. PIPE NETWORKS

summed up arithmetically. Adopt a sign convention that values of h_f and Q are taken as positive in pipes in which the flow is clockwise with regards to the loop under consideration, and negative if anticlockwise. The negative sign of ΔQ of Eq. 10.46 indicates that the positive (clockwise) values of ΔQ are to be reduced and negative (anticlockwise) values are to be increased. When a system has a number of loops, the pipes which are common to two loops will receive corrections for each loop.

Minor losses are generally neglected in pipe networks but may be included simply by adding the equivalent lengths for the minor losses. The method invloves the following steps:

(1) By proper inspection assume the most reasonble distribution of flow that satisfies continuity condition 1,

(2) Write the head loss in the form

$$h_f = r Q^n$$

and compute in each pipe the loss of head hf.

(3) Compute the algebraic sum of the head losses around each elementary circuit,

$$\Sigma h_f = \Sigma r Q^n$$

Consider losses for clockwise flows as positive, and anticlockwise negative.

(4) Also compute in each circuit the sum of quantities nr Q^{n-1} without reference to sign.

(5) Adjust the flow in each circuit by a correction, ΔQ, to balance the head in that circuit and give $\Sigma r Q^n = 0$. The cirrection ΔQ is computed by Eq. 10.45. This is first trial and in most cases, the head lost in the pipe network is not balanced (i.e. $\Sigma Q^n = 0$ is not obtained).

(6) After each circuit is given a first correction, the losses will still not balance because of interaction of one circuit upon another (pipe which are common to two loops receive two independent correction, one for each circuit). The procedure is repeated, arriving ar a second correction, so on, until the corrections become negligible. (Refer Examples 10.18)

The correction ΔQ may also be computed by Eq 10.46. This method is known as 'head balance method' and is useful when the total volume rate of flow through network is known, but the pressures or heads at junctions within the network are unknown. The first method (using Eq 10.45) is known as 'quantity balance method' and is usuful when the heads at various points in a pipe network are known and it is necessary to calculate the quantities flowing in each pipe.

10.18 WATER HAMMER

If the water flowing along a long pipeline is suddenly brought to rest by the closing of a valve, or by similar cause, there will be a sudden rise of pressure due to the momentum of the moving water being destroyed. The high pressure generated at the valve travels upstream as a pressure wave along the pipe and sets up noises in it which are known as knocking. The magnitude of this pressure depends on the length of the pipe. In hydro-electric plants the water is conveyed to turbines by means of penstocks with automatic discharge regualting system. The discharge fed to the turbines varies with the power to be generated. Thus,when no discharge is needed by the turbine, the valve closes suddenly. The sudden rise in pressure in a pipe due to stoppage of flow is known as 'water hammer',

The pressure wave causes shock and noise as it travels backwards and forwards along the pipe. In a long pipe, excessive pressure can be produced which may damage the joints. In such cases. some practical methods are adopted to absorb the energy of the wave such as surge tanks or relief valves.

1. Inertia Pressure due to Gradual Closure

Consider a pipe AB of length L and diameter D connected to a reservoir containing water under a constant head H. A valve is fitted at B (Fig.10.21). For a given valve opening, a constant pressure head 'Ba'will be established at B, and there will be a normal hydraulic gradient line 'oa' falling from A to B. If the valve is closed at a uniform suitalble rate, the pressure at B willl rise by an amount h_i, with corresponding displacement of the hydraulic gradient line from oa to ob. As the valve is closed furhter, the HGL line rises furhter and becomes oc. When the valve is fully closed. HGL drops suddenly to od, (i.e. horizontal line) and pressure head throughout the pipe is stabilized at a value equal to the static head in the reservoir. This additional pressure is known as inertia pressure and equivanent head is the inertia head h_i.

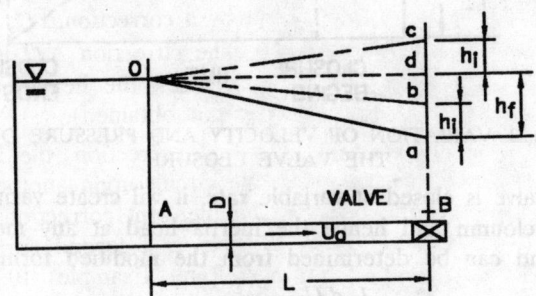

FIG. 10.21. INERTIA PRESSURE DUE TO GRADUAL CLOSURE

It is assumed that the rate of closure is adjusted so as to bring the water column in the pipe to rest (with uniform retardation) from an initial velocity U_0 in time t seconds.

The total mass of liquid in the pipe $= wAL/g$

The rate of retardation of water columm $= U_o/t$

From Newton's equation of motion,

Force $=$ mass $\times$ acceleration

$$F_i = \frac{w}{g} \frac{\pi}{4} . D^2 L \times \frac{U_0}{t}$$

F_i is the inertia force developed in the pipe.

$$p_i \times \frac{\pi}{4} D^2 = \frac{w}{g} \frac{\pi D^2 L}{4} \times \frac{U_0}{t}$$

Solving inertia pressure $p_i = \dfrac{w L U_0}{g t}$ ...(10.47a)

inertia head $\qquad h_f = \dfrac{L U_0}{g t}$ ...(10.47b)

The inertia pressure given by Eq 10.47a is developed at the end of pipe B. At any other point on the pipe, the pressure rise can be determined easily. The maximum pressure from all causes is represented as

$(p_i)_{max}$ = (static pressure + inertia pressure-frictional resistance) (10.48)

It is, obvious, that maximum pressure will be developed in the pipe just before the complete closure of valve, i.e. when the frictional head loss will be minimum. Fig 10.22 shows the variation of velocity and pressure during the valve closure.

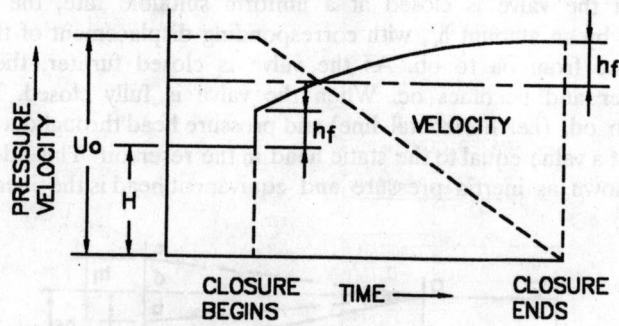

FIG. 10.22. VARIATION OF VELOCITY AND PRESSURE DURING THE VALVE CLOSURE

If the valve is closed at variable rate, it wil create variable retardation to the water cloumn and hence the inertia head at any moment will also be variable and can be determined from the modified form of Eq 10.47b.

$$h_f = \frac{L}{g} \frac{d U_0}{dt}$$ ...(10.47c)

2. inertia pressure due to Instantaneous Closure

Although it is physically impossible to close a valve instantaneously, such a concept is useful as an introduction to the study of real cases. The sequence of enents taking place in a pipe after instantaneous closure is discussed below by means of Fig. 10.23.

(a) Consider a pipe line AB with a valve at its downstream end The valve is suddenly turned off so that the flow of water is stopped.

At the instant of valve closure, the fluid nearest to the valve is compressed, brought to rest and the pipe wall is stretched. As soon as the fluid layer nearest to the valve is compressed, the process is repeated for the layer next to it until other end is reached. The momentum lost is converted into high intertia pressure and elastic energy of pipe. The fluid continues to flow from reservoir A to the pipe. The high pressure wave travels from B to A with the velocity of sound in water, i.e. 'c'.

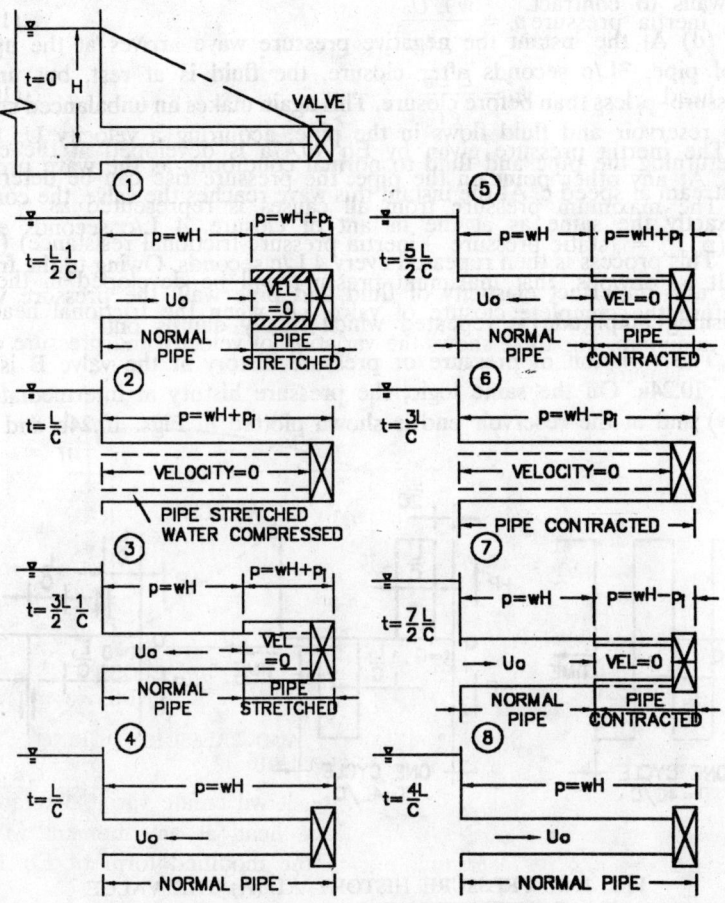

FIG. 10.23. SEQUENCE OF EVENTS FOLLOWING INSTANTANEOUS CLOSURE

(b) As the pressure wave arrives at A after a time interval L/c seconds, an unblanced pressure exists at A but the reservoir contains water under a head H and hence the pressure at A should be wH. Thus the pressure falls to normal at A and this normal pressure wave progresses in the downstream direction with speed c till it arrives ar B. Fig. 10.23d. The fluid starts flowing backwards, beginning at the upstream end A. At the instant 2 L/c, the wave arrives at the valve, pressure are back to normal along the pipe and velocity is everywhere U_o in the backward direction.

(c) Since the valve is closed, no fluid is available to maintain the flow' at the valve and a low pressure $-p_i$ develops such that the fluid is brought to rest (i.e.negative velocity reverts back to zero) in Fig. 10.23e. This low pressure wave travels upstream at speed c and everywhere brings the fluid to rest, causes it to expand due to lower pressure intensity and allows the pipe walls to contract.

(d) At the instant the negative pressure wave arrives at the upstream end of pipe, 3L/c seconds after closure, the fluid is at rest, but uniformly at pressure -p_i less than before closure. This again makes an unbalanced condition at the reservoir and fluid flows in the pipe, acquiring a velocity U_o forward and returning the pipe and fluid to normal conditions as the wave progresses downstream at speed c. At the instant this wave reaches the valve, the conditions are exactly the same as at the instant of closure, 4 L/c seconds earlier.

This process is then repeated every 4 L/c seconds. Owing to the frictional effects and imperfect elasticity of fluid and pipe wall, the pressure wave of diminishing amplitude is repeated which finally damps out.

The variation of pressure or pressure history at the valve B is shown in Fig. 10.24a. On the same logic, the pressure history at intermediate point D (say) and at the reservoir end is shown plotted in Figs. 10.24b and 10.24c.

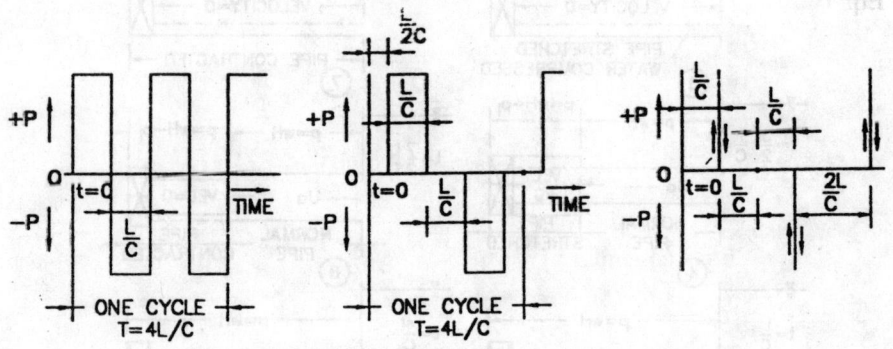

FIG. 10.24. PRESSURE HISTORY AT (A) THE VALUE
(B) AT INTERMEDIATE POINT & (C) RESERVOIR

All the preceeding analysis assumes that the wave of rarefaction will not cause the minimum pressure at any point to drop down to or below the vapour pressure, If it falls below pv, the separation of flow will take place in the pipe which will produce a discontinuity.

The magnitude of inertia pressure is now determinde considering the pipe as rigid and also elastic.

(a) *Pressure rise due to sudden closure.* Let the water flow in a pipe AB with a velocity U_o which is brought to rest by sudden closure of valve at B (Fig 10.23). the pipe is assumed as regid and non-elastic so that there is no radial expansion of its walls. Before closure the water has a kinetic energy due to its velocity; after closure of valve this energy is converted into strain energy due to compression of water. Consider the short length dL of the pipe.

Then loss of kinetic energy of water

$$= w\frac{A\,dL}{g} \times \frac{U_0^2}{2} \qquad \ldots\text{(i)}$$

Strain enrgy = work done by pressure rise

= average pressure × volumetric stain   ...(ii)

Initally the inertia pressure is zero in the pipe. As soon as the valve is closed, it increase from zero to p_i and changes the vloume V by dV. The volumetric stain dV is determined as follows:

$$K = \frac{\text{Stress}}{\text{Volumetric stain}} = \frac{p_i}{dV/V}$$

or

$$dV = \frac{p_i V}{K} \qquad \ldots\text{(iii)}$$

where K is the bulk modulus of elasticity of water.

The strain energy developed in the given volume of water is given by Eq. (iv)

$$\text{Strain energy} = \frac{p_i}{2} \times dV$$

$$= \frac{p_i}{2}\frac{p_i V}{K}$$

$$= \frac{p_i^2}{2K}AdL \qquad \ldots\text{(iv)}$$

From Eqs. (i) and (iv)

$$\frac{wAdL}{g}\frac{U_0^2}{2} = \frac{p_i^2}{2K}AdL$$

Solving it,

$$p_i = U_0\sqrt{\frac{wK}{g}} = U_0\sqrt{\rho K} \qquad \ldots(10.48a)$$

$$h_i = p_i/w = U_0\sqrt{\frac{K}{gw}} \qquad \ldots(10.48b)$$

(b) *Effect of pipe elasticity.* In practice, the long pipe lines carrying water are anchored at regular intervals. Thus the pipe may stretch around its circumference and its length remains rigid between anchors. The change in volume, now, takes place due to the pressing of water cloumn and stretcing of pipe circumference. Let dV_1 be the change in vloume of water due to compression and dV_2 be the change in volume due to stretching of pipe circumference. Then

$$dV = dV_1 + dV_2 \qquad \ldots\text{(i)}$$

The amount of change in volume of water dV_1 is given by

$$\frac{dV_1}{V} = \frac{p_i}{K}$$

or $\qquad dV_1 = \frac{p_i V}{K}$ ...(ii)

Let the pipe diameter D increase by x and let f_t be the hoop stress in the material of the pipe and t be the wall thickness.

From Eq. 1.21b, $f_t = p_i D/2t$ ...(iii)

Also $\qquad E = \text{stress/strain}$

or $\qquad E = \frac{f_t}{x/D}$ ...(iv)

From Eqs. (iii) and (iv)

$$x = (p_i D^2/2t \, E)$$

∴ Increase in the volume dV_2 ...(v)

$$= \left[\frac{\pi}{4} (D + x)^2 - \frac{\pi}{4} D^2 \right] dL$$

$$= \frac{\pi}{4} dL \, (x^2 + 2x \, D)$$

or $\qquad \dfrac{dV_2}{V} = \dfrac{\dfrac{\pi}{4} dL \, (x^2 + 2xD)}{\dfrac{\pi}{4} D^2 \, dL}$;

neglecting x^2/D^2 to be too small ...(iv)

From Eqs. (v) and (vi)

$$dV_2/V = p_i D/t E$$ ...(vii)

Substituting in Eq. (i) from Eqs. (ii) and (vii)

$$dV = \left(\frac{p_i}{K} + \frac{p_i D}{t E} \right) V$$ ...(viii)

$$\frac{dV}{V} = p_i \left(\frac{1}{K} + \frac{D}{t E} \right)$$ ...(viii)

Let the effective bulk modulus of elasticity be K_0, then

$$K_0 = \frac{\text{stress}}{\text{Volumetric strain}}$$

$$K_0 = \frac{p_i}{dV/V} = \frac{p_i V}{dV}$$

Substituting the value of V/dV from Eq. (viii)

$$K_0 = \frac{1}{(1/K + D/t E)}$$

Substituting the value of effective bulk modulus of elasticty into Eq. 10.48a.

$$p_i = U_0 \sqrt{\frac{w K_0}{g}}$$

$$p_1 = U_0 \sqrt{\frac{w}{g\,(1/K + D/t\,E)}} \qquad \text{...(10.49)}$$

Velocity of propagation of pressure wave c is given by

$$c = \sqrt{\frac{K_0\,g}{w}}$$

$$= \sqrt{\frac{g}{w}\,\frac{1}{(1/K + D/tE)}} \qquad \text{...(10.50)}$$

From Eqs. 10.49 and 10.50

$$\frac{p_i}{c} = \frac{w\,U_0}{g}$$

$$p_1 = \rho\,c\,U_0 \qquad \text{...(10.51a)}$$

or $\qquad h_i = \dfrac{U_0\,c}{g} \qquad$ ...(10.51b)

Eq. 10.51. is known as Allevi's equation of water hammer.

3. Rapid Closure of Valve

It is not possible to close the valve instantaneously; the closure of valve may be effected repidly in finite time τ which may be more than zero but less than 2L/c (the required value for the reflected pressure wave to reach the valve). In such cases, the pressure rise in the pipe can be studied by considering the valve to be closed in successive steps. say n small movements after each very small interval of time, of duration τ/n seconds. This means that the valve is closed by a small amount so as to impart a sudden retardation to the flow by dU and in turn generating a pressure rise by dpi. Each such small valve movement will set up a pressure wave, shown in Fig 10.25 as in previous case but of less amptitude. The total inertia pressure at any instant can be found by summing up the individual pressure increments. If the number of steps is infinite (that is too large) the total pressure curve will be smoothened, Fig. 10.25b. If the time of closure is either equal to or less than 2L/c, pressure time diagram as shown in Fig 10.25c will be obtained. Thus it is seen that

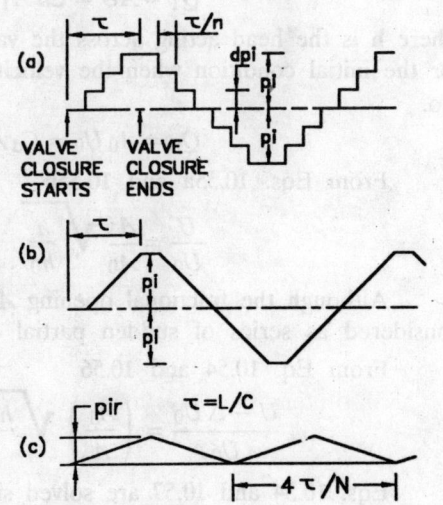

FIG. 10.25. PRESSURE RISE DUE TO RAPID CLOSURE

the hypothetical diagram for instantaneous closure is modified with sides inclined instead of vertical.

In case, the time of closure τ exceeds 2t ($=2L/c$), the reflected wave reaches the valve the magnitude of pressure rise is reduced to p_{ir}. Until the arrival of first pressure wave at the valve, the rate of increase of total inertia pressure at the valve is p_{ir}/τ and therefore, after an interval of 2t, the pressure will have attainted the value $p_{ir} \times 2t/\tau$ which is the maximum value. The inertia pressure, thereafter, diminishes again subsequently fluctuating between p_{ir} and zero with periodicity of 4 t

The pressure rise due to rapaid closure is determined by numercial proces. The rapid closure of valve is considered as if the value is closed in discrete steps with instantaneous partial closure. The pressure rise at each step is given by Eq 10.52.

$$\Delta h = \frac{C \Delta U_0}{g} \qquad ...(10.52)$$

At the instant of complete closure, the rise in inertia pressure is

$$\Sigma \Delta h = \frac{C \Sigma \Delta U_0}{g} = \frac{U_0 C}{g} \qquad ...(10.53)$$

Dividing Δh_0 by initial head h_0 and rearranging the terms of Eq. 10.52

$$\frac{\Delta h_0}{h_0} = \frac{C \Delta U_0}{g h_0} = \frac{CU_0}{g h_0} \cdot \frac{\Delta U_0}{U_0} \qquad ...(10.54)$$

The valve may bc treated as an opening with variable area of cross section A_1 and coefficient of dischanrge C_d. The discharge through the valve at any instant of time t is given by continuity equation.

$$Q_1 = AU = Cd A_1 \sqrt{2gh} \qquad ...(10.55a)$$

where h is the head acting across the valve. Similar equation can be written for the initial condition when the velocity is U_0 and area of the opening is Ao.

$$Q_0 = A_0 U_0 = C_d A_0 \sqrt{2gh_0} \qquad ...(10.55b)$$

From Eqs. 10.55a and 10.55b

$$\frac{U}{U_0} = \frac{A_1}{A_0} \sqrt{\frac{h}{h_0}} \qquad ...(10.56)$$

Although the fractional opening A_1/A_0 is a function of time but it is considered as series of sudden partial closures.

From Eq. 10.54 and 10.56

$$\frac{U - \Delta U_0}{U_0} = \left(\frac{A_1}{A}\right) \sqrt{\frac{h + \Delta h}{h_0}} \qquad ...(10.57)$$

Eqs. 10.54 and 10.57 are solved simultaneously for h/h_0 and U/U_0 at any instant of time t_1. The new values of U, h and A_1/A are then inserted in Eqs. 10.54 and 10.57 and are again solved for h/h_0 and U/U_0.

Summarising above discussion, following characteristics should be noted.

(1) If the pipe is rigid, celerity c of propagation of pressure wave is given by

$$c_d = \sqrt{\frac{K}{\rho}}$$

(2) If the material of pipe is considered elastic,

$$c = \sqrt{\frac{g}{w}} \; \frac{1}{\sqrt{\left(\dfrac{1}{K} + \dfrac{D}{tE}\right)}}$$

$$= \sqrt{\frac{K}{\rho}} \; \frac{1}{\sqrt{1 + DK/tE)}}$$

where t = pipe wall thickness and D is diameter.

(3) The periodicity of pressure wave, i.e time of travel for one complete cycle in a pipe of length L is

$$T = \frac{4L}{c}$$

(4) Critical time 'T_0' is the time taken by pressure wave to travel from valve to inlet and its reflected wave to reach valve

$$T_0 = \frac{2L}{c}$$

(5) If the valve is operated (closed or opened) instantaneously ($t = 0$), the pressure rise pi is computed by Eq. 10.51.

$$pi = \rho c U_0 \hspace{3cm} ...(10.51)$$

(6) Indeed the valve closure or opening takes some finite time. If $T < \dfrac{2L}{c}$, the operation is considered rapid and pressure rise can be considered rapid and pressure rise can be computed by method of sec. 10.18.3. Alternatively

$$pi = \rho c U_0$$

(7) If time of closure (or opening) $T > \dfrac{2L}{c}$, the operation is considered gradual closure and is computed by Eq. 10.47a.

$$pi = \rho L U_0/t$$

Alternatively, pi $\alpha \dfrac{1}{t}$

$$\therefore \quad \frac{(pi)_{grad}}{(pi)_{rapid}} = \frac{T_0}{t}$$

$$(pi)_{:grad} = \frac{T_0}{t}(pi)_{rapid} = \frac{T_0}{t} \times \rho c U_0$$

where t = actual time of closure (or opening) of valve.

(8) If time of operation of valve $T < \dfrac{2L}{c}$, the length x of pipe (from valve end) will experience maximum water hammer pressure.

$$x = \left(L - c\,\frac{T}{2}\right)$$

Examples 10.1 – 1027

10.1. Water flows through a pipe line of 50 cm diameter and 1000 m length between two reservoirs A and B. The difference of water surface between A and B is 40 m. The pipe passes over a summit which is 100 m away from reservoir A and its peak is 2 m avove reservoir A. Determine the maximum discharge through the pipe and the pressure in the pipe at the highest peak. Assume Darcy's f as 0.03 and atmospheric pressure equal to 10 m of water.

Solution

Apply Bernoulli's equation between A and B.

$$\frac{p_1}{w} + z_1 + \frac{U_1^2}{2g} = \frac{p_2}{2} + z_2 + \frac{U_2^2}{2g} + h_{L_{ent}} + h_{f_{AB}}$$

$$0 + 40 + 0 + 0 = 0 + 0 + \frac{U^2}{2g} + \frac{0.5\,U^2}{2g} + f\frac{L}{D}\frac{U^2}{2g}$$

$$40 = \frac{U^2}{2g}\left(1.5 + \frac{0.03 \times 1000}{0.5}\right)$$

Solving $U = 3.57$ m/s

$$Q = AU$$

$$= \frac{\pi}{4}(0.5)^2 \times 3.57$$

$$= 0.7 \text{ cumec}$$

Again applying Bernoulli's eqution between A and the summit C.

$$\frac{p_a}{w} + z_1 + \frac{U_1^2}{2g} = \frac{p_c}{2} + z_2 + \frac{U_2^2}{2g} + h_{L_e} + h_{f_{AC}}$$

$$10 + 0 + 0 = \frac{p_c}{w} + 2 + \frac{U^2}{2g} + 0.5\frac{U^2}{2g} + \frac{0.03 \times 100}{0.5}\frac{U^2}{2g}$$

Solving, $p_c/w = 8 - (1.5 + 6)\,U^2/2g$

$$= 3.52 \text{ m absolute}$$

10.2 A discharge of 50 metres per second flows in pipe line laid with its axis 30° to the horizontal. The pipe line suddenly enlarges from 15 cm to 30 cm diameter. A is a point 1 m away from the enlargement in the 15 cm diameter pipe. B is another point above A 1 m away from enlargement in 30 cm pipe. The pressure gauge fixed at B reads 5 kPa. Find the reading of pressure gauge fixed at A when the water flows from (a) A to B (b)

B to A. Assume coefficient of contraction ($=$area at vena contracta/area of opening) as 0°60

Solution

Area of small pipe $= \dfrac{\pi}{4}(0.15)^2$

$$A_1 = 0.0176 \text{ m}^2$$

Area of large diameter pipe

$$A_2 = \dfrac{\pi}{4} \times (0.3)^2$$

$$A_2 = 0.0707 \text{ m}^2$$

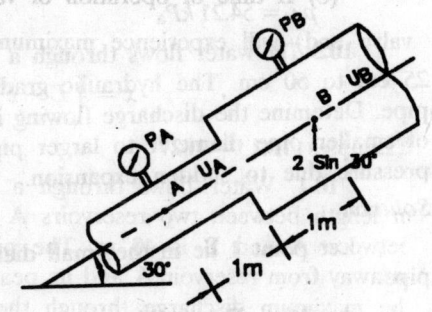

FIG. 10.26. EXAMPLE 10.2

$$U_A = \dfrac{50}{1000 \times 0.0176} = 2.84 \text{ m/s}$$

$$U_B = \dfrac{50}{1000 \times 0.0707} = 0.71 \text{ m/s}$$

(a) Flow from A to B

Applying Bernoulli's equation between A and B.

$$\dfrac{p_A}{w} + z_A + \dfrac{U_A^2}{2g} = \dfrac{p_B}{w} + z_B + \dfrac{U_B^2}{2g} + \dfrac{(U_A - U_B)^2}{2g}$$

$$\dfrac{p_A}{w} + 0 + \dfrac{(2.84)^2}{2g} = \dfrac{5}{9.81} + 2\sin 30° + \dfrac{(0.71)^2}{2g} + \dfrac{(2.84 - 0.71)^2}{2g}$$

$$\dfrac{pA}{w} = \dfrac{5}{9.81} + 1 + \dfrac{(0.71)^2}{2g} + \dfrac{(2.13)^2}{2g} - \dfrac{(2.84)^2}{2g}$$

$$p_A = 58.29 \, kP_A$$

(b) Flow from B to A

Applying Bernoulli's equation from B to A

$$\dfrac{p_B}{w} + z_B + \dfrac{U_B^2}{2g} = \dfrac{p_A}{w} + z_A + \dfrac{U_A^2}{2g} + \dfrac{(U_C - U_A)^2}{2g}$$

From continuity equation

$$U_c = \left(\dfrac{A}{A_c}\right) U = U/C_c$$

$$U_c = U/0.6 = 1.67 \, U$$

Therefore,

$$\dfrac{5}{9.81} + 2\sin 30° + \dfrac{(0.71)^2}{2g} = \dfrac{p_A}{w} + 0 + \dfrac{(2.84)^2}{2g} + \dfrac{(1.67 U_A - U_A)^2}{2g}$$

$$\dfrac{p_A}{w} = \dfrac{5}{9.81} + 1 + \dfrac{(0.71)^2}{2g} - \dfrac{(2.84)^2}{2g} - \dfrac{(2.84)^2}{2g}(0.67)^2$$

$$p_A = 6.1216 - 0.5956$$

$$p_A = 54.21 \ kP_a$$

10.3 The water flows through a pipe line which expands suddenly from 25 cm to 50 cm. The hydraulic gradient line rises by 1.5 cm in the larger pipe. Detemine the discharge flowing in the pipe line. Also compute the ratio of smaller pipe diameter to larger pipe diameter to cause maximum rise of pressure due to sudden expansion.

Solution

Let point 1 lie in the small diameter pipe and 2 in the large diameter pipe.

Applying Bernoulli's equation to sections 1 and 2.

$$\frac{p_1}{w} + z_1 + \frac{U_1^2}{2g} = \frac{p_2}{2} + z_2 + \frac{U_2^2}{2g} + \frac{(U_1 - U_2)^2}{2g}$$

or $\left(\dfrac{p_2}{w} + z_2\right) - \left(\dfrac{p_1}{w} + z_1\right) = \dfrac{(U_1^2 - U_2^2)}{2g} - \dfrac{(U_1 - U_2)^2}{2g}$

or $\qquad h = \dfrac{(U_1^2 - U_2^2) - (U_1^2 - 2\,U_1\,U_2 + U_2^2)}{2g}$

or $\qquad h = \dfrac{2\,U_1\,U_2 - 2U_2^2}{2g} = \dfrac{U_2^2}{g}\left(\dfrac{U_1}{U_2} - 1\right)$ ...(i)

From continuity equation.

$$U_1 A_1 = U_2 A_2$$

$$U_1/U_2 = A_2/A_1 = (0.50/0.25)^2 = 4 \qquad ...(ii)$$

Substituting the values in Eq. (i)

$$0.015 = \frac{U_2^2}{g}(4 - 1)$$

Solving, $\qquad U_2 = 0.221$ m/s

Discharge, $\qquad Q = A_2\,U_2 = \dfrac{\pi}{4}(0.5)^2 \times 0.221$

$$Q = 0.0435 \ \text{m}^3/\text{s}$$

(b) Let the diameter of small pipe be D_1 and that of larger pipe be D_2, so that $D_1/D_2 = \eta$

From Eq. (i), $\qquad h = \dfrac{(U_1\,U_2 - U_2^2)}{g} = \dfrac{U_1^2}{g}\left(\dfrac{U_2}{U_1} - \dfrac{U_2^2}{U_1^2}\right)$

From Eq.(ii) $A_1\,U_1 = A_2\,U_2$

or $U_2/U_1 = A_1/A_2 = D_1^2/D_2^2 = \eta^2$

Therefore, $\qquad h = \dfrac{U_1^2}{g}\,[\eta^2 - \eta^4]$

Differentiating h with respect to η and equating it to zero.

$$dh/d\eta = (U_1^2/g)[2\eta - 4\eta^3]$$

Hence $\qquad \eta = 1/\sqrt{2} = D_1/D_2$

The maximum pressure will be

$$h = (U_1^2/g)\left[\frac{1}{2} - \frac{1}{4}\right] = 0.25\ (U_1^2/g)$$

$\Delta p/\rho\ U_1^2$ = pressure coefficient = 0.25

10.4 Water stands at a constant elevation of + 100m in a tank feeding water into a horizontal compound pipeline. The geometric dimensions are as follows :

i. A sharp entry at its end A, pipe AB 50 m long, 20 cm diameter and f is 0.032;

ii Sudden enlargeme at B, pipe, BC 200 m long, 40 cm diameter and f is 0.04 ;

iii Sudden contraction at C, coefficient of contraction is 0.625, pipe CD 30 m long, 15 cm diameter and f is 0.02;

iv A sharp exit end D into a lower tank.

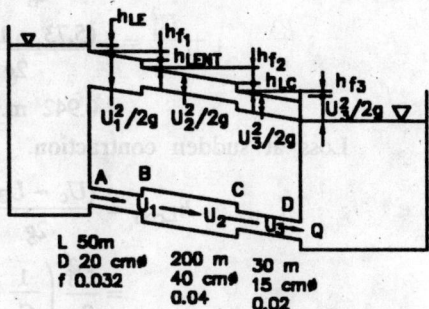

FIG. 10.27. EXAMPLE 10.4

If the flow down the pipe is 0.18 m³/s, (a) find all the losses occuring in the pipe line and draw T.E.L. and H.G.L. for the pipe line. Also determine the elevation of the water level in the lower tank. (b) if the water line in the lower tank stands at an elevation of + 84 m, determine the flow through the pipe line.

Solution

(a) The areas of cross section of various pipe AB, BC and CD and velocity of flow through them are computed below

$$A_1 = \pi\ (0.2)^2/4 = 0.0314\ m^2$$

$$A_2 = \pi\ (0.4)^2/4 = 0.1256\ m^2$$

and $\qquad A_3 = \dfrac{\pi}{4}\ (0.15)^2 = 0.01766\ m^2$

From continuity equation,

$$Q = A_1 U_1 = A_2 U_2 = A_3 U_3$$

$$U_1 = \frac{0.18}{0.0314} = 5.73\ m/s; \quad \frac{U_1^2}{2g} = \frac{(5.73)^2}{2 \times 9.81} = 1.675\ m$$

$$U_1 = \frac{0.018}{0.1256} = 1.433 \text{ m/s} \ ; \ \frac{U_2^2}{2g} = \frac{(1.433)^2}{2 \times 9.81} = 0.1046 \text{ m}$$

$$U_3 = \frac{0.18}{0.01766} = 10.19 \text{ m/s} \ ; \ \frac{U_3^2}{2g} = \frac{(10.19)^2}{2 \times 9.81} = 5.29 \text{ m}$$

The various losses are now determined

Loss at sharp entry at A, $h_{L_e} = 0.5 \, (U_1^2/2g)$

$$= 0.5 \, (1.675) = 0.8375 \text{ m}$$

Loss at sudden enlargement,

$$h_{L_{ent}} = \frac{(U_1 - U_2)^2}{2g}$$

$$= \frac{(5.73 - 1.433)^2}{2g}$$

$$= 0.942 \text{ m.}$$

Loss at sudden contraction.

$$h_{L_{con}} = \frac{(U_c - U_3)^2}{2g}$$

$$= \frac{U_3^2}{2g} \left(\frac{1}{C_c} - 1 \right)^2$$

$$= \frac{(10.19)^2}{2 \times 9.81} \left(\frac{1}{0.625} - 1 \right)^2$$

$$= 1.9044 \text{ m}$$

Loss at the exit.

$$(h_l)_{exit} = \frac{U_3^2}{2g} = \frac{(10.19)^2}{2 \times 9.81}$$

$$= 5.29 \text{ m}$$

The Loss the head due to friction in pipe AB,

$$h_{f_1} = f_1 \frac{L_1}{D_1} \frac{U_1^2}{2g}$$

$$= \frac{0.032 \times 50}{0.2} \times \frac{(5.73)^2}{2 \times 9.81} = 13.4 \text{ m.}$$

The loss of head due to friction in pipe BC,

$$h_{f_2} = f_2 \frac{L_2}{D_2} \frac{U_2^2}{2g}$$

$$= 0.04 \times \frac{200}{0.4} \times \frac{(1.433)^2}{2 \times 9.81} = 2.092 \text{ m}$$

The loss of head due to friction in pipe CD

$$h_{f_3} = f_3 \frac{L_3}{D_3} \frac{U_3^2}{2g}$$

$$= \frac{0.02 \times 30}{0.15} \times \frac{(10.19)^2}{2 \times 9.81} = 21.16 \text{ m}$$

With all the minor and frictional losses being computed, total energy line and hydraulic gradient line can be drawn as shown in Fig. 10.27.

Total head loss $h_L = (h_{L_e} + h_{f_1} + h_{L_{ent}} + h_{f_2} + h_{L_{con}} + h_{f_3} + h_{L_{exit}})$

$$h_L = (0.8375 + 13.4 + 0.945 + 2.092 + 1.9044 + 21.16 + 5.29)m$$

$$h_L = 45.62m$$

The water level in the lower tank will stand at an elevation.

$$= (100 - losses)$$

$$= (100 - 45.62) = 54.38 \text{ m}$$

(b) Water level in the lower tank = + 84m.

Difference in water levels in the two tanks

$$= (100 - 84) \text{ m}$$

$$= 16 \text{ m}$$

Thus, in this case, the total losses should sum up to 16 m only. The losses h_L are directly proportional to the square of the discharge. Therefore,

$$\frac{h_{L_1}}{h_{L_2}} = \frac{Q_1^2}{Q_2^2}$$

or

$$Q_2^2 = Q_1^2 \left(\frac{h_{L_2}}{h_{L_1}} \right)$$

or

$$Q_2 = Q_1 \sqrt{\frac{h_{L_2}}{h_{L_1}}} = 0.18 \sqrt{\frac{16}{45.62}}$$

or

$$Q_2 = 0.1066 \text{ m}^3/\text{s}$$

10.5 The pipe line of Example 10.4 is to be replaced by a single compound pipe of the same length. Determine the diameter of the compound pipe having $f = 0.03$.

Solution

The pipe of different diameters are connected in series, therefore, the total head loss will be the summation of the head losses through the individual pipe.

$$h_f = h_{f_1} + h_{f_2} + h_{f_3}$$

Let the diameter of the compound pipe to replace the existing pipe line be D and its length L is equal to $(L_1 + L_2 + L_3)$.

Substituting the values,

$$\frac{0.03 \times 280}{D^5} = \frac{0.032 \times 50}{(0.2)^5} + \frac{0.04 \times 200}{(0.4)^5} + \frac{0.02 \times 30}{(0.15)^5}$$

Solving, $D = 0.228$ cm ≈ 0.23 cm.

10.6 Two pipes, one of 15 cm diameter, 300 m long and the other of 30 cm diameter and 800 m long are connected in parallel. The total discharge through the pipe system is 0.08 m³/s. Find the discharge through each pipe and the head loss. Assume $f = 0.02$ for 15 cm diameter pipe and $f = 0.03$ for 30 cm diameter pipe.

Solution

Since the two pipe are connected in parallel, between two points A and B the following equations should be satisfied.

$$h_{f_{AB}} = h_{f_1} = h_{f_2} \qquad \text{...(i)}$$

$$Q = Q_1 + Q_2 \qquad \text{...(ii)}$$

From Eq. (i)

$$\frac{f_1 L_1 Q_1^2}{12.1 D_1^5} = \frac{f_2 L_2 Q_2^2}{12.1 D_2^5}$$

$$= \frac{0.02 \times 300 \times Q_1^2}{12.1 (0.15)^5} = \frac{0.03 \times 800 \times Q_2^2}{12.1 (0.3)^5}$$

or $\qquad Q_1 = 0.35 \, Q_2$

From Eq. (ii)

$$0.08 = Q_1 + Q_2 \qquad \text{..(ii)}$$

Solving Eqs. (i) and (ii)

$$0.35 \, Q_2 + Q_2 = 0.08$$

$$Q_2 = 0.059 \text{ m}^3/\text{s}$$

$$Q_1 = 0.021 \text{ m}^3/\text{s}$$

$$h_{f_1} = \frac{0.02 \times 300 \times (0.021)^2}{12.1 \times (0.15)^5} = 2.612 \text{ m}$$

10.7 Three pipes were connected between two points A and B to carry 0.3 cumec. The point A and B lie 30 m and 25 m above a given datum. respectively. The pressure at A is maintained at 600 kPa. The pipe 1 is 100 m long and 0.3 m in diameter, the pipe 2 is 750 m long and 0.2 m is diameter and pipe 3 is 200 m long and 0.4 m is diameter. Assume all the pipes to be smooth. . Determine the flow in each pipe and the pressure at B. Take kinemetic viscosity of water $= 10^{-6}$ m²/s.

Solution

The friction factor for smooth pipe depends upon Reynolds number of flow. Let us assume discharge Q_1' flows through pipe 1 as 0.1 cumec so that $R_{e1} = 0.42 \times 10^6$ and f_1 (from Fig. 9.10) = 0.015.

From Eq. 10.5.

For pipe 1, $\quad h_{f1} = \dfrac{f_1 L_1 Q_1^2}{12.1 D_1^5}$

$$= \frac{0.015 \times 1000 \times (0.1)^2}{12.1 (0.3)^5} = 5.1 \text{ m}$$

For pipe 2, $\quad h_{f2} = \dfrac{f_2 L_2 Q_2^2}{12.1 D_2^5}$

As a first trial, assume same value of f_2 as of f_1

$$5.1 = \frac{0.015 \times 750 \times Q_2'^2}{12.1 \times (0.2)^5}$$

$$Q_2' = \sqrt{12.1 \times 5.1 \times \frac{(0.2)^5}{0.015 \times 750}}$$

$$= 0.0419 \text{ m}^3/\text{s}$$

For pipe 3, $\quad h_{f3} = \dfrac{f_3 L_3 Q_3^2}{12.1 D_3^5}$

Again assume $f_3 = f_1$

$$5.1 = \frac{0.015 \times 1200 \times Q_3'^2}{12.1 (0.4)^5}$$

$$Q_3' = \sqrt{\frac{5.1 \times 12.1 \times (0.4)^5}{0.015 \times 1200}} = 0.1873$$

Thus, the total discharge $Q' = Q_1' + Q_2' + Q_3'$

$$= 0.3293 \text{ m}^3/\text{s}$$

Hence, $\quad Q_1 = \dfrac{Q_1'}{Q'} \times Q = \dfrac{0.1}{0.3293} \times 0.3 = 0.0911$

$$Q_2 = \frac{Q_2'}{Q'} \times Q = \frac{0.0419}{0.3293} \times 0.3 = 0.0382$$

$$Q_3 = \frac{Q_3'}{Q'} \times Q = \frac{0.1873}{0.3293} \times 0.3 = 0.1706$$

For pipe 1, $\quad Q_1 = 0.0911 \text{ m}^3/\text{s}$

$$Re_1 = \frac{4\,Q_1}{\pi\,D_1} = \frac{4 \times 0.0911}{\pi \times 0.3 \times 10^{-6}} = 3.866 \times 10^5$$

From Moody diagram Fig. 9.10

$$f_1 = 0.0135$$

Hence

$$h_{f_1} = \frac{f_1 L_1 Q_1^2}{12.1\,D_1^5}$$

$$= \frac{0.0135 \times 1000 \times (0.0911)^2}{12.1 \times (0.3)^5}$$

$$= 3.81 \text{ m}$$

For pipe 2, $Q_2 = 0.0382 \text{ m}^3/\text{s}$,

$$Re_2 = \frac{4 \times 0.0382}{6 \times 0.2 \times 10^{-6}} = 2.432 \times 10^5$$

$$f_2 = 0.016$$

Hence

$$h_{f_2} = \frac{f_2 L_2 Q_2^2}{12.1\,D_2^5}$$

$$= \frac{0.016 \times 750 \times (0.0382)^2}{12.1\,(0.2)^5}$$

$$= 4.52 \text{ m}$$

For pipe 3, $Q_3 = 0.1706 \text{ m}^3/\text{s}$.

$$Re_3 = \frac{4 \times 0.1706}{\pi \times 0.4 \times 10^{-6}} = 5.430 \times 10^5$$

$$f_3 = 0.0128$$

Hence

$$h_{f_3} = \frac{0.0128 \times 1200 \times (0.1706)^2}{12.1\,(0.4)^5}$$

$$= 3.61 \text{ m}$$

Since h_{f_1}, h_{f_2} and hf_3 are not equal, a second trial has to be made for Q_1', Q_2' and Q_3'. Assume $h_f = 3.8$ m , $Q_1 = 0.09$ m^3/s , $Q_2 = 0.035$ m^3/s and $Q_3 = 0.175$ m^3/s.

The corresponding head losses for the three pipes are $h_{f_1} = 3.78$ m, $h_{f_2} = 4.01$ m and $h_{f_3} = 3.8$ m.

(b) Apply Bernoulli's equation between A and B.

$$\frac{p_A}{w} + z_A + \frac{U_A^2}{2g} = \frac{p_B}{w} + z_B + \frac{U_B^2}{2g} + h_f$$

or

$$\frac{p_B}{w} = \left(\frac{p_A}{w} + z_A - z_B - h_f \right)$$

$$= \left[\frac{600}{9.81} + 30 - 25 - 3.8 \right]$$

$$= 62.36 \text{ m}$$

$$p_B = 611.77 \text{ kPa.}$$

10.8. A pipe line of 0.6 m diameter is 1.5 km long. To augment the discharge, another pipe line of the same diameter is introduced parallel to the first one for the last one kilometer length. Neglecting the minor losses, find the increase in the discharge. The head at inlet is given as 30 m and $f = 0.04$.

Solution

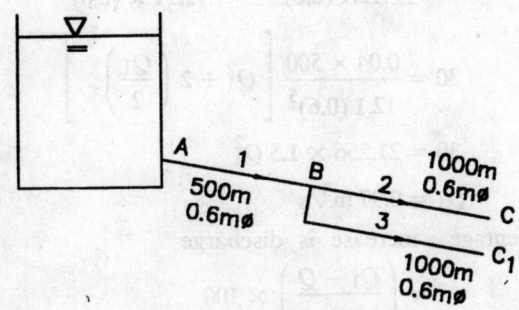

FIG. 10.28. EXAMPLE 10.8

Case I: Only one pipe line supplies the water.

$$h_f = \frac{f L Q^2}{12.1 D^5}$$

$$30 = \frac{0.04 \times 1500 \times Q^2}{12.1 (0.6)^5}$$

$$Q = \sqrt{\frac{30 \times 12.1 \times (0.6)^5}{0.4 \times 1500}}$$

$$= 0.6859 \text{ m}^3/\text{s}$$

Case II: When a parallel pipe line is laid alng with the first one for the last 1000 m, let total discharge be Q_1

$$Q_1 = Q_2 + Q_3 \qquad \qquad ...(i)$$

From continuity equation $Q = AU$

$$A_1 U_1 = A_2 U_2 + A_3 U_3$$

(Since $A_1 = A_2 = A_3$)

or

$$U_1 = U_2 + U_3 \qquad \qquad ...(ii)$$

Also, the head lost through parallel pipes 2 and 3 should be same.

$$h_{f_2} = h_{f_3}$$

$$\frac{f L_2 U_2^2}{2g D_2} = \frac{f L_3 U_3^2}{2g D_3}$$

or $$U_2 = U_3 \qquad\qquad\qquad ...(iii)$$

From Eqs. (ii) and (iii)

$$U_1 = 2U_2 \; ; \; \text{then} \; Q_2 = Q_3 = \frac{Q_1}{2} \qquad ...(iv)$$

Now consider the loop ABC.

$$h_f = h_{f_{AB}} + h_{f_{BC}}$$

or $$30 = \frac{f \times 500 \times Q_1^2}{12.1 \, (0.6)^5} + \frac{f \times 1000 \times (Q_2)^2}{12.1 \times (0.6)^5}$$

or $$30 = \frac{0.04 \times 500}{12.1 \, (0.6)^5} \left[Q_1^2 + 2 \left(\frac{Q_1}{2} \right)^2 \right]$$

or $$30 = 21.256 \times 1.5 \, Q_1^2$$

$$Q_1 = 0.97 \, \text{m}^3/\text{s}$$

Hence percentage increase is discharge

$$= \left(\frac{Q_1 - Q}{Q} \right) \times 100$$

$$\% \text{ increase} = \frac{(0.97 - 0.6859)}{0.6859} \times 100$$

$$\% \, Q = 41.42\%$$

10.9 A set of three parallel pipe, supplies, water at the rate of 0.45 m³/s from resenoir. A to reservoir B. Determine the discharge carried by each pipe. The details, of pipe line are given below.

Solution

Pipe	Length	Diameter	f
1	1200 m	25 cm	0.020
2	1500 m	30 cm	0.015
3	1000 m	20 cm	0.020

This problem is solved using equivalent pipe concept which eliminates the need of making number of trials. It is a simplified procedure

From Eq. 10.36 (sec. 10.14), an equivalent pipe length causes same head loss and carries same discharge as the original pipe (or its fittings)

$$\therefore \quad \sqrt{\frac{D_e^5}{f_e \, L_e}} = \sqrt{\frac{D_1^5}{f_1 \, L_1}} + \sqrt{\frac{D_2^5}{f_2 \, L_2}} + \sqrt{\frac{D_3^5}{f_3 \, L_3}}$$

Here Le, De and Fe are quantities for equivalent pipe.

For example 25 cm diameter pipe is chosen as equivalent pipe. Then find Le for this parallel pipe system

$$\sqrt{\frac{(0.25)^5}{0.02 \times Le}} = \left[\sqrt{\frac{(0.25)^5}{0.02 \times 1200}} + \sqrt{\frac{(0.3)^5}{0.015 \times 1500}} + \sqrt{\frac{(0.2)^5}{0.02 \times 1000}} \right]$$

$$\frac{0.221}{\sqrt{Le}} = [6.379 \times 10^{-3} + 10.39 \times 10^{-3} + 4 \times 10^{-3}]$$

$$\frac{0.221}{\sqrt{Le}} = 20.769 \times 10^{-3}$$

$$Le = 113.28 \text{ m}$$

Corresponding head loss h_f is now computed.

$$h_{fe} = f_e \frac{L_e}{D_e} \frac{U_e^2}{2g} = f_e \frac{L_e}{D_e} \cdot \frac{\left(Q / \frac{\pi}{4} \cdot D_e^2 \right)^2}{2g}$$

$$= \frac{f_e L_e Q^2}{12.09 D_e^5}$$

$$= \frac{0.02}{12.09} \times \frac{113.28}{(0.25)^5} \cdot (0.45)^2$$

$$= 38.858 \text{ m}$$

Also $h_{fe} = h_{f1} = h_{f2} = h_{f3}$

Hence, $h_{f1} = \dfrac{f_1 L_1 Q_1^2}{12.09 D_1^5}$

$$38.858 = \frac{0.02 \times 1200 \times Q_1^2}{12.09 \times (0.25)^5}$$

Solving, $Q_1 = 0.13826 \text{ m}^3$

Similarly, $h_{f2} = \dfrac{f_2 L_2 Q_2^2}{12.09 D_2^5}$

$$38.858 = \frac{0.015 \times 1500 \times Q_2^2}{12.09 \times (0.3)^5}$$

$$Q_2 = 0.22525 \text{ m}^3/\text{s}$$

and $h_{f3} = \dfrac{f_3 L_3 Q_3^2}{12.09 D_3^5}$

$$38.858 = \frac{0.02 \times 1000 \times Q_3^2}{12.09 \times (0.2)^5}$$

$$Q_3 = 0.867 \text{ m}^3 \text{ is}$$

As a check, $Q_1 + Q_2 + Q_3 = (0.13826 + 0.22625 + 0.0867)$

$$= 0.4502 \text{ m}^3/\text{s}.$$

10.10 Two reservoirs are connected by a pipe of 50 cm diameter and 60 mm long $(f = 0.02)$ Determine the discharge supplied to reservoir B if the W.L in reservoir A is kept 200 m above that of B.

During summer, the discharge is increased by 40% by laying a parallel pipe of same diameter for some distance and joining it to main pipe at suitable junction Estimate the length of additional pipe. Also determine the pressure head at the junction.

Solution

Case I : In case I, only one pipe line AB connects two reservoirs. Applying Bernoulli's theorem,

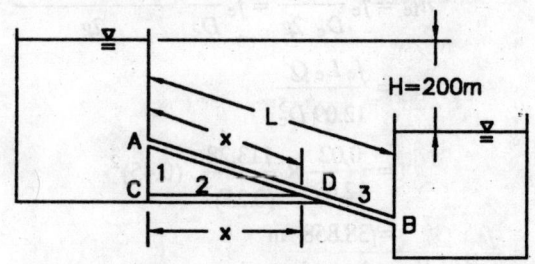

FIG. 10.29. EXAMPLE 10.10

$$H = \left(0.5 \frac{U^2}{2g} + \frac{fL}{2g} \frac{U^2}{D} + \frac{U^2}{2g} \right)$$

$$= \left(1.5 + \frac{fL}{D} \right) \frac{U^2}{2g}$$

$$200 = \left(1.5 + \frac{0.02 \times 60 \times 1000}{0.5} \right) \frac{U^2}{2g}$$

$$200 = (1.5 + 2400) \frac{U^2}{2g}$$

$$U = 1.278 \text{ m/s}$$

(Note : Since minor losses are too small, these can be neglected.)

$$Q = AU$$

$$= \frac{\pi}{4} (0.5)^2 \times 1.278 = 0.25 \text{ m}^3/\text{s}$$

Case II : Additional pipe, CD of length x is laid paralled to main pipe AD.

Increased discharge $Q_3 = 1.4Q$

$$Q_3 = 1.4 \times 0.25 = 0.35 \ m^3/s \text{ is}$$

Also $h_{f_{AD}} = h_{f_{CD}}$ for parallel pipes.

$$f_1 \frac{x}{D_1} \frac{U_1^2}{2g} = f_2 \frac{x}{D_1} \frac{U_2^2}{2g}$$

Since $f_1 = f_2, D_1 = D_2$

$\therefore$ $U_1 = U_2$

and $Q_1 = Q_2$ ...(i)

From continuity principle.

$$Q_1 + Q_2 = Q_3$$ ...(ii)

From Eqs. (i) and (ii)

$$Q_3 = 2Q_1$$ ...(iii)

Now take pipe ADB,

$$h_{f_{AB}} = h_{f_{AD}} + h_{f_{BD}}$$

$$200 = \frac{f_1 x U_1^2}{2g D_1} + \frac{f(L-x) U_3^2}{2g D_3}$$

Writing $U = Q / \frac{\pi}{4} D^2$

$$200 = \frac{f_1 x Q_1^2}{12.09 D_1^5} + \frac{f.(L-x) Q_3^2}{12.09 D_3^5}$$

Substituting   for Q_3 from Eq. (ii)

$$200 = \frac{0.02 \times x \times (Q_3/2)^2}{12.09 (0.5)^5} + \frac{0.02 (L-x) Q_3^2}{12.09 (0.5)^5}$$

$$200 = \frac{0.02 \times Q_3^2}{12.09 \times (0.5)^5} \left[\frac{x}{4} + L - x \right]$$

$$200 = \frac{0.02 \times (0.35)^2}{12.09 \times (0.5)^5} \left[L - \frac{3}{4}x \right]$$

$$= 6.4847 \times 10^{-3} (L - 3/4x)$$

$$\left(L - \frac{3}{4}x \right) = 30841.84 \ m$$

$$x = \frac{4}{3}(60 \times 1000 - 30841.84) = 38877.5 \ m = 38.8775 \ km$$

Head at junction D will be equal to the head loss in pipe 3 of length $(L - x)$ i.e.

$$(L - x) = (60,000 - 38875) = 21122.5 \text{ m}$$

$$H_D = h_{f_3}$$

$$= \frac{fL_3 Q_3^2}{12.09 D_3^5} = \frac{f}{12.09 D_3^5} (L_3 Q_3^2).$$

$$= \frac{0.02}{12.09 (0.5)^5} (L_3 Q_3^2)$$

$$= 0.05294 \times L_3 Q_3^2$$

$$= 0.05294 \times 21122.5 \times (0.35)^2$$

$$= 136.97 \text{ m}$$

[Note : As a check, $h_{f_1} = h_{f_2}$ can be computed and it should be equal to $(200 - 136.97) = 63.03$ m)

10.11. Two pipes of equal length L have respective diameter D and d. If the pipe are arranged in parallel, the loss of head, when the quantity of water flows through them is h. If the pipes are arranged in series and the same quantity of water flows through them, the loss of head is H. If $d = D/2$, find the ratio of H and h, neglecting minor losses and assuming friction factor f to be same for both the pipes.

Solution

(i) Pipes connected in series,

$$H = h_{f_1} + h_{f_2}$$

$$H = \frac{fL Q^2}{12.1 D^5} + \frac{fL Q^2}{12.1 d^5}$$

$$H = \frac{fL Q^2}{12.1} \left(\frac{1}{D^5} + \frac{1}{d^5} \right)$$

$$H = \frac{33}{32} \frac{fL Q^2}{12.1 d^5}$$

(since $D = 2d$) ...(i)

(ii) Pipes connected in parallel.

Let the discharge Q divide into Q_1 through pipe of diameter D and Q_2 through pipe of diameter d.

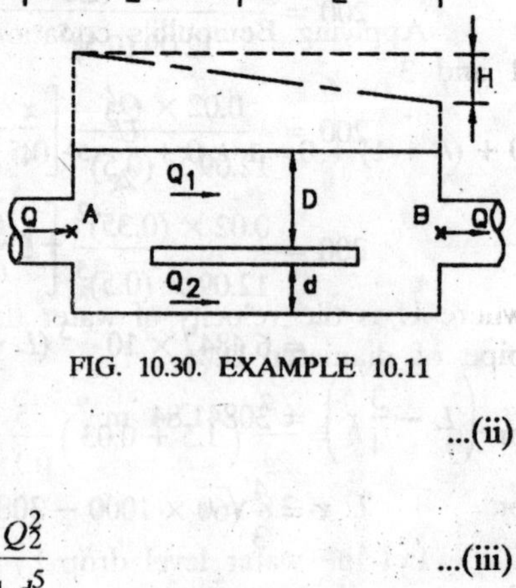

$$Q = Q_1 + Q_2$$ ...(ii)

Also

$$h = h_{f_1} = h_{f_2}$$

$$= \frac{fL Q_1^2}{12.1 D^5} = \frac{fL Q_2^2}{12.1 d^5}$$ ...(iii)

FIG. 10.30. EXAMPLE 10.11

$$Q_1^2 = (D/d)^5 Q_2^2$$
$$= (2d/d)^5 Q_2^2$$
$$Q_1 = \sqrt{32}\, Q_2 \qquad\qquad ...(iv)$$

From Eqs. (ii) and (iv)

$$Q = \left(\sqrt{32}\, Q_2 + Q_2\right)$$

$$Q_2 = \frac{Q}{6.66} \qquad\qquad ...(v)$$

From Eq. (iii)

$$h = (fL/12.1\, d^5)\,(Q/6.66)^2$$

$$h = \frac{1}{44.355}\,\frac{fLQ^2}{12.1\, d^5} \qquad\qquad ...(iv)$$

From Eqs. (i) and (vi)

$$\frac{H}{h} = \frac{33}{32} \times 44.355 = 45.74$$

10.12. An over head tank, 7 m long and 2 m wide and 2 m deep, is to be emptied by a vertical pipe 15 cm diameter fixed at the bottom of the tank. The pipe is 5 m long and at its lower end dips into a sump in which the water level is kept constant 4 m below the bottom of the tank. Assume $f = 0.03$. If the tank is originally full, calculate how much water will escape in one minute after emptying begins. In case, there is no water in the sump, how much time will it take to completely empty the tank ?

Solution

(i) Let the water level in the tank stand at a height h metre above the water level in the sump at time t, Fig. 10.31.

Applying Bernoulli's equation between 1 and 3

$$0 + (h + 1) + 0 = 1 + 0 + \frac{U^2}{2g} + 0.5\,\frac{U^2}{2g}$$
$$+ f\frac{L}{D}\frac{U^2}{2g}$$

where U is the velocity of water through the pipe of diameter D.

or

$$h = \frac{U^2}{2g}\left(1.5 + 0.03\right)\frac{5}{0.15} = 2.5\,\frac{U^2}{2g}$$

or

$$U = 2.8 \sqrt{h}$$

Let the water level drop by dh in the time interval dt so that,

$$A\, dh = -Q\, dt$$

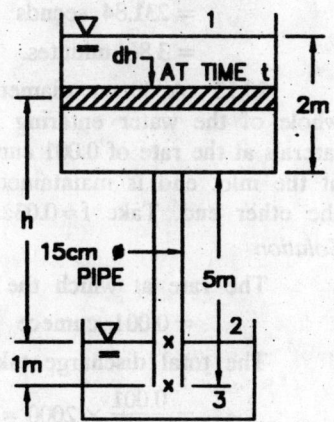

FIG. 10.31. EXAMPLE 10.12

or $\quad\quad dt = -A\,dh/Q$ $\qquad\qquad\qquad$ ..(ii)

Therefore, the time required to drop the water level from h_1 to h_2 is obtained by intergrating Eq.(ii)

$$\int_0^t dt = \int_{h_1}^{h_2} -\frac{Adh}{Q} = \int_{h_1}^{h_2} \frac{7 \times 2 \times dh}{\frac{\pi}{4} \times (0.15)^2 \times U}$$

$$T = \int_{h_2}^{h_1} 282.94\,(dh/\sqrt{h})]$$

$$= 282.94 \times 2\,[\sqrt{h_1} - \sqrt{h_2}] \qquad\qquad ...(\text{iii})$$

But $\qquad\qquad h_1 = 2 + 4 = 6$ m, and $T = 60$ sec,

$$60 = 565.9\,[\sqrt{6} - \sqrt{h_2}]$$

Solving, $h_2 = 5.492$ m above W.L. in the sump.

Quantity of water escaping in 1 minute

$$= 7 \times 2 \times (2 - 1.492)\ \text{m}^3 \qquad (\because\ \text{Water depth} = (h_2 - 4)\ \text{m})$$

$$= 7.112\ \text{m}^3$$

(ii) When no water is in the sump, h is measured above freely discharging end.

From Eq. (iii)

$$T = 565.9\,[\sqrt{h_1} - \sqrt{h_2}]$$

Here $h_1 = 5 + 2 = 7$ and $h_2 = 5$ m above the outlet of pipe.

$$T = 565.9\,[\sqrt{7} - \sqrt{h_2}]$$

$$= 231.84\ \text{secnds}$$

$$= 3.86\ \text{minutes}.$$

10.13 A 30 cm diameter cast iron pipe has a length of 2000 m; the whole of the water entering at one end of it is drained off uniformly by laterals at the rate of 0.001 cumec per 50 metre length of pipe. If the pressure at the inlet end is maintained as 145 kPa, what would be the pressure at the other end. Take f = 0.032.

Solution

The rate at which the water is taken off is.

$$= 0.001\ \text{cumece per 50 metres}.$$

The total discharge taken off is.

$$= \frac{0.001}{50} \times 2000 = 0.04\ \text{cumec}$$

The velocity of water at entrance U

$$= \frac{0.04}{\frac{\pi}{4}(0.30)^2}$$

(ii)
= 0.5652 m/s

Therefore, the discharge entering at the take off point is equal to 0.04 cumec and the discharge at the other end is zero. Then

$$h_f = \frac{1}{3}\left[f\frac{L}{D}\frac{U^2}{2g}\right]$$

$$= \frac{1}{3}\left[0.032 \times \frac{2000}{0.30} \times \frac{(0.5652)^2}{2 \times 9.81}\right]$$

$$= 1.157 \text{ m}$$

Pressure at other end $= [145 - 9.81 \times 1.157]$
$$= 1.33.65 \text{ kPa}$$

10.14 A 20 cm diameter pipe lead from a reservoir to a point 500 m long where it branches into a 10 cm diameter pipe 300 m long with open end and a 15 cm diameter pipe 2000 m long with a 5 cm diameter nozzle at the end. Both branch pipes discharge into atomosphere at point 20 m below the reservoir level. Calculate the flow in each of the branch pipes and the pressure at the junction if it is 12 m below the reservoir level. Take coefficient of discharge for the nozzle as 0.96 and f for all the pipe as 0.04 The minor losses are negligible.

Solution

Let the velocity through pipe AD, DB and DC be U_1, U_2 and U_3, respectively and through the nozzle be U_n

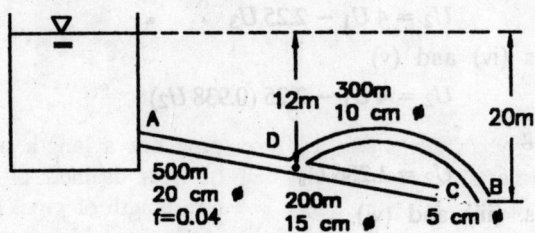

FIG. 10.32. EXAMPLE 10.14

Loss in the nozzle $= (1/C_v^2 - 1) U_n^2/2g$

But $\qquad U_3 A_3 = U_n A_n$

$$U_n = (A_3/A_n) U_3 = (0.15/0.5)^2 U_3 = 9 U_3 \qquad ...(i)$$

$$h_{L_n} = \left[1/0.96^2 - 1\right](9 U_3)^2/2g = 6.89 U_3^2/2g \qquad ...(ii)$$

Applying Bernoulli's theorem between A and B, (following the loop ADB)

$$0 + 20 + 0 = 0 + h_{f_{AD}} + h_{f_{DB}} + U_2^2/2g$$

$$20 = \frac{0.04 \times 500}{0.20} \times \frac{U_1^2}{2g} + \frac{0.04 \times 300}{0.10} \times \frac{U_2^2}{2g}$$

Solving it,

$$5.097 \, U_1^2 + 6.116 \, U_2^2 = 20 \qquad \text{...(iii)}$$

For the pipes DB and DC,

Total loss in pipe DB = total loss is pipe DC

$$h_{f_{DB}} + \frac{U_2^2}{2g} = h_{f_{DC}} + \frac{U_n^2}{2g} + h_{L_n}$$

$$\left(\frac{0.04 \times 300}{0.1} + 1 \right) \frac{U_2^2}{2g} = \left(\frac{0.04 \times 200}{0.15} \right) \frac{U_3^2}{2g} + \frac{U_n^2}{2g} + \left(\frac{1}{0.96^2} - 1 \right) \frac{U_n^2}{2g}$$

$$121 \, U_2^2 = \left[\frac{160}{2} U_3^2 + \frac{1}{(0.96)^2} U_n^2 \right]$$

$$= \left[\frac{160}{3} U_3^2 + \frac{(9 \, U_3)^2}{(0.96)^2} \right]$$

Solving it, $\quad U_3 = 0.938 \, U_2 \qquad \text{...(iv)}$

The discharge through pipe 1 divides into pipes 2 and 3.

$$Q_1 = Q_2 + Q_3$$

$$\frac{\pi}{4} (0.20)^2 \, U_1 = \frac{\pi}{4} (0.10)^2 \, U_2 + \frac{\pi}{4} (0.15)^2 \, U_3$$

Solving,

$$U_2 = 4 \, U_1 - 2.25 \, U_3 \qquad \text{...(v)}$$

From Eqs (iv) and (v)

$$U_2 = 4 \, U_1 - 2.25 \, (0.938 \, U_2)$$

Simplifying

$$U_2 = 1.286 \, U_1$$

From Eqs. (iii) and (vi)

$$5.097 \, U_1^2 + 6.116 \, (1.286 \, U_1)^2 = 20$$

Simplifying;

$$U_1 = 1.147 \ \text{m/s}$$

$$U_2 = 1.474 \ \text{m/s}$$

$$U_3 = 1.353 \ \text{m/s}$$

Corresponding discharges are

$$Q_1 = (\pi/4) \, (0.2)^2 \times 1.147 = 0.0360 \ \text{m}^3/\text{s}$$

$$Q_2 = (\pi/4) \, (0.1)^2 \times 1.474 = 0.0116 \ \text{m}^3/\text{s}$$

$$Q_3 = (\pi/4) \, (0.15)^2 \times 1.353 = 0.0244 \ \text{m}^3/\text{s}$$

Now apply Bernoullis equation to A and D, taking a horizontal plane through D as datum.

$$0 + 12 + 0 = \frac{p_D}{w} + 0 + \frac{U_1^2}{2g} + h_{fAD}$$

or

$$\frac{p_D}{2} = 12 - \frac{U_1^2}{2g} - 0.04 \times \frac{500}{0.2} \times \frac{U_1^2}{2g}$$

$$12 = \frac{(1.147)^2}{2 \times 9.81}\left[1 + 0.04 \times \frac{500}{0.2}\right]$$

$$p_D/w = 6.154 \text{ m guage}$$

10.15 For the distribution main of a town water supply, a 25 cm main is required. As pipes above 20 cm diameter are not available, it is decided to lay n parallel mains of the same diameter. Find the diameter of the parallel mains in terms of n. If n is two, find the diameter of the parallel mains.

Solution

Let D be the diameter of the large pipe which is to be replaced by n parallel pipe of equal diameter d. All the pipes are of equal length l. The head loss in the each of the parallel pipes as well as in the large pipes is hf (say).

$$\therefore \quad h_f = \frac{fLU^2}{2gD}$$

where U is mean velocity of flow through large pipes.

$$U = \sqrt{\frac{2g\,h_f}{f}}\,\sqrt{\frac{D}{L}}$$

The discharge Q through large diameter pipe

$$Q = AU$$

$$= \left(\pi D^2/4\right) . \sqrt{\frac{2g\,h_f}{f}}\,\sqrt{\frac{D}{L}}$$

$$= \left(\pi/4\right) . \sqrt{\frac{2g\,h_f}{f}}\,\sqrt{\frac{D^5}{L}}$$

Similarly, the head loss in each of small pipe.

$$h_f = \frac{fLu^2}{2gd}$$

where u is the mean velocity of flow through small diameter pipe

$$\therefore \quad u = \sqrt{\frac{2g\,h_f}{f}}\,\sqrt{d/L}$$

The discharge through each of small diameter pipe

$$Q_1 = Q_2 = \dots = au$$

$$= \pi d^2/4 \sqrt{\frac{2g\,h_f}{f}} \sqrt{d/L}$$

$$= \pi/4 \sqrt{\frac{2g\,h_f}{f}} \sqrt{d^5/L}$$

But
$$Q = Q_1 + Q_2 + \ldots Q_n$$

$$\frac{\pi}{4} \sqrt{\frac{2g\,h_f}{f}} \sqrt{\frac{D^5}{L}} = \frac{\pi}{4} \sqrt{2g\,h_f/f} \left[\sqrt{\frac{d^5}{L}} + \ldots + n \; terms \right]$$

$$D^{5/2} = n\,d^{5/2}$$

$$d = \frac{D}{n^{2/5}}$$

If
$$n = 2, d = \frac{0.25}{(2)^{2/5}} = 18.95 \; cm$$

Since 18.95 cm is not a standard diameter, therefore it has to be specially manufactured or the next standrad size of 20 cm diamter pipe is to be used.

10.16. Two water mains of length L, identical in all respect convery a total discharge 2 Q from one reservoir to another. The difference between their water levels is being assumed constant as H. Cross connections are provided at L/6 distance apart. If two adjacent cross connections are used to divert the whole flow from the length L/6 to another, so that corresponding length L/6 of the other may be repaired, what would be the percentage reduction in discharge. Neglect minor losses.

Solution

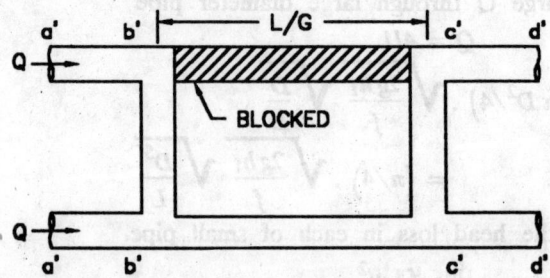

FIG. 10.33. EXAMPLE 10.16

Let the head loss through ab, bc and cd be h_{f_1}, h_{f_2} and h_{f_3}.

The hydraulic gradient in the regments ab, bc and cd will be same,

$$i = h_f/l = \left(h_{f1} + h_{f2} + h_{f3} \right) /L$$

Since $h_f \propto Q^2$ and the section bc will be carrying double the discharge than carried either by ab or cd.

$$\therefore \qquad \frac{h_{f2}}{L/6} \neq 4 \cdot \frac{(h_{f1} + h_{f3})}{(L - L/6)} \qquad \qquad ...(i)$$

That is, the slope of energy line in the segment bc will be four times sharper than in the segments ab or cd.

Since $h = h_{f_1} + h_{f_2} + h_{f_3} =$ total head loss between ends a and c.

$$\therefore \qquad h_{f1} + h_{f3} = (h - h_{f2}) \qquad \qquad ...(ii)$$

Solving Eqs. (i) and (ii)

$$h_{f2} = \frac{4}{9} h \qquad \qquad ...(iii)$$

Initially out of total dischange Q, each pipe carry Q.

$$\therefore \qquad h = f L Q^2 / 12.1\, d^5 \qquad \qquad ...(iv)$$

When segment be is blocked, total dischange is reduced to Q_1

In this case, discharge through bc $= Q_1$

$$\therefore \qquad h_{f2} = \frac{f\,(L/6)\,(Q_1^2)}{12.1\, d^5} \qquad \qquad ...(v)$$

From Eqs. (iii), (iv) and (v)

$$\frac{f\,(L/6)\,Q_1^2}{12.1\, d^5} = \frac{4}{9} \frac{f L Q^2}{12.1\, d^5}$$

$$Q^2 = \frac{3}{8} Q_1^2$$

$$Q_1 = \sqrt{8/3}\ Q$$

Percentage reduction in discharge

$$= \frac{2Q - Q_1}{2Q} \times 100$$

$$= 1 - \frac{\sqrt{8/3}\ Q}{2Q} \times 100$$

$$= 18.35\%$$

10.17 Water is supplied by means of a 60 cm diameter pipe, to a power plant and the head loss due to friction is 27 m. In order to reduce the power consumption, it is proposed to lay another main of appropriate diameter alongside of existing one so that both pipes work in parallel for the entire length and reduce the head loss to 9.6 m. Find the diameter of new pipe which has same value of f and are of same length.

Solution :

Case I : Single pipe of diameter, D_1,

$$h_f = \frac{f L U^2}{2g\, D} = \frac{f L Q^2}{12.09\, D_1^5}$$

$$27 = \frac{fL}{12.09} \cdot \frac{Q^2}{D_1^5}$$

$$= K \frac{Q^2}{D_1^5}$$

$$Q = \sqrt{\frac{27 D_1^5}{K}} \qquad \qquad ...(i)$$

Case II : Two pipes, of diameters, D_1 and D_2

$$h_f = h_{f_1} = h_{f_2}$$

$$9.6 = \frac{fL Q_1^2}{12.09 D_1^5} = \frac{fL Q_2^2}{12.09 D_2^5}$$

$$9.6 = \frac{K Q_1^2}{D_1^5} = \frac{K Q_2^2}{D_2^5} \qquad \qquad ...(ii)$$

$$\left(\frac{Q_1}{Q_2}\right)^2 = \left(\frac{D_1}{D_2}\right)^5 \qquad \qquad ...(ii)$$

$$\frac{Q_1}{Q_2} = \left(\frac{D_1}{D_2}\right)^{5/2} \qquad \qquad ...(iii)$$

Also $\qquad\qquad Q = Q_1 + Q_2 \qquad \qquad ...(iv)$

Substituting value from Eqs. (i), (ii) and (iii)

$$\sqrt{\frac{27 D_1^5}{K}} = \left[\sqrt{\frac{9.6 D_1^5}{K}} + \sqrt{\frac{9.6 D_2^5}{K}} \right]$$

$$\sqrt{9.6 D_2^5} = \left[\sqrt{27 D_1^5} - \sqrt{9.6 D_1^5} \right]$$

$$(D_2)^{5/2} = D_1^{5/2} \left[\sqrt{\frac{27}{9.6}} - 1 \right]$$

$$D_2^{5/2} = 0.6771 D_1^{5/2}$$

$$D_2 = (0.6771)^{2/5} D_1$$

$$= 0.8555 \times 0.6$$

$$= 0.513 \text{ m} = 513 \text{ mm}$$

10.18 Power is to be transmitted hydraulically by means of a number of pipes 8000 m long and 10 cm in diameter, arranged in parallel and laid horizontally. The inlet pressure is 7000 kN/m². Find the minimum number of pipes required for this case to ensure 92% of efficiency of transmission of power. The power required to be delivered at the other is 150 kW. Take $f = 0.03$. Also determine the maximum power than can be transmitted in this case.

The efficiency of transmission η is given by

$$\eta = \frac{H - h_f}{H}$$

where h_f is the head loss in friction.

$$0.92 = \frac{H - h_f}{H} \qquad \text{Since } H = \frac{7000}{9.81} = 713.55 \text{ m}$$

$$h_f = 0.08 \, H = 0.08 \times 713.55 = 57.08 \text{ m}$$

Now

$$h_f = \frac{fL\,U^2}{2gD}$$

$$57.08 = \frac{0.03 \times 8000 \times U^2}{2 \times 9.81 \times 0.10}$$

$$U = \sqrt{\frac{57.08 \times 2 \times 9.81 \times 0.10}{0.03 \times 8000}}$$

$$= 0.683 \text{ m/s}$$

Let n be the number of parallel pipes laid horizontally.

Power delivered $= n\,w\,Q\,(H - h_f)$ watts

$$150 \times 1000 = n \times 9810 \times \pi/4 \,(0.1)^2 \times 0.683 \times (713.55 - 57.08)$$

$$n = \frac{150 \times 1000}{9810 \times \pi/4 \times (0.1)^2 \times 0.683 \times (713.55 - 57.08)}$$

$$= \frac{15 \times 10^4}{9810 \times 0.785 \times 0.01 \times 0.683 \times 656.47}$$

$$= 4.34 = 5$$

For maximum transmission of power.

$$h_f = H/3 = \frac{715.55}{3}$$

$$= 238.51 \text{ m}$$

Now

$$238.51 = \frac{fL\,U^2}{2gD}$$

$$= \frac{0.03 \times 800 \times U^2}{2 \times 9.81 \times 0.1}$$

$$U = \sqrt{\frac{238.51 \times 2 \times 9.81 \times 0.1}{0.03 \times 800}}$$

$$= 1.396 \text{ m/s}$$

$$Q = \pi/4 \,(0.1)^2 \times 1.396 = 0.01096 \text{ m}^3/\text{s}$$

Maximum Power $= n\,w\,Q\,(H - h_f)$ watts

$$= 5 \times 9810 \times 0.01096 \times (713.55 - 238.51) \text{ watts}$$
$$= 256.47 \text{ kW}$$

10.19 A pipe 60 cm diameter 1500 m long conveys water to an impulse turbine. The head at the inlet end is 120 m. A nozzle is fitted at the outlet of pipe to obtain maximum power. Compute the diameter of nozzle and power transmitted. Take $f = 0.025$.

Solution :

From Eq. 10.18.

$$\frac{d}{D} = \left(\frac{D}{2fL} \right)^{1/4}$$

$$= \left[\frac{0.60}{2 \times 0.025 \times 1500} \right]^{1/4}$$

$$= 0.2991$$

$$d = 0.2991 \ D$$

$$= 0.2991 \times 0.6$$

$$= 0.1794 \ \text{m} = 17.94 \ \text{cm}$$

For maximum transmission of power,

$$h_f = \frac{H_1}{3}$$

$$= \frac{120}{3} = 40 \ \text{m}$$

Also,

$$h_f = \frac{fL\,U^2}{2g\,D} = \frac{fL\,Q^2}{12.09\,D^5}$$

$$40 = \frac{0.025 \times 1500 \times Q^2}{12.09 \times (0.6)^5}$$

$$Q = 1.0 \ \text{m}^3/\text{s}$$

Maximum power transmitted $= w\,Q\,H$

$$= 9810 \times 1 \times (120 - 40)$$

$$= 784800 \ W = 784.8 \ \text{kW}.$$

10.20. A reservoir A (Fig 10.34) with its surface 60 m above datum supplies water to a junction D through 30 cm diameter pipe 1500 m long . From the junction, a 25 cm diameter pipe 800 m long feeds reservoir B, in which the suface is 30 m above datum, while another pipe 400 m long and 20 cm diameter feeds another reservoir C. The water level in the reservoir C stands at 15 m above datum. Calculate the discharge to each reservoir. Assume f for each pipe as 0.03.

Solution

By inspection, it is seen that water level elevation of reservoir A is higher then in reservoir B and C. Therefore, it is assumed that water will flow from A to D and then from D to B and from D to C. Assume, the piezometric head at D as 35.0. Then,

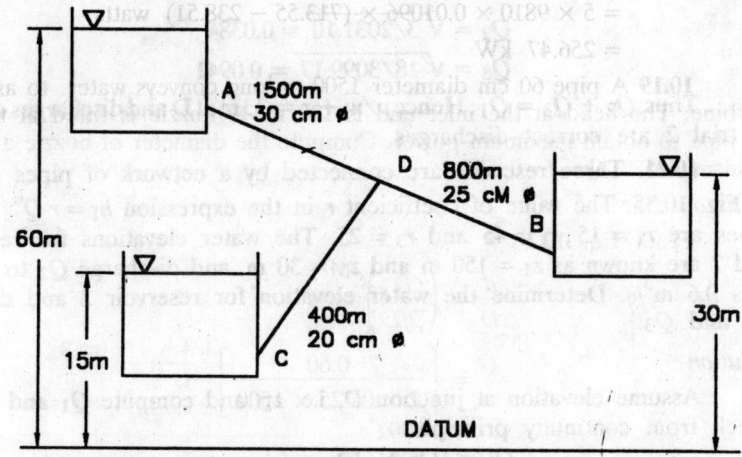

FIG. 10.34. EXAMPLE 10.20

$$H_A - H_D = h_{fAD} = 60 - 35 = 25 \text{ m}$$

$$H_D - H_B = h_{fBD} = 35 - 30 = 5 \text{ m}$$

$$H_D - H_c = H_{fCD} = 35 - 15 = 20 \text{ m}$$

Also

$$h_f = \frac{fLQ^2}{12.1 D^5} = KQ^2$$

For pipe 1, $\quad K_1 = \dfrac{0.03 \times 1500}{12.1 \,(0.3)^5} = 1530.456$

For pipe 2, $\quad K_2 = \dfrac{0.03 \times 800}{12.1 \times (0.2)^5} = 2031.0$

For pipe 3, $\quad K_3 = \dfrac{0.03 \times 400}{12.1 \times (0.2)^5} = 3099.17$

The discharge is computed by Darcy's formula, Eq. 9.51.

$$Q_1 = \sqrt{h_{fAD}/K_1} = \sqrt{25/1530.456} = 0.1278$$
$$Q_2 = \sqrt{h_{fDC}/K_2} = \sqrt{5/2031} = 0.0496$$
$$Q_3 = \sqrt{h_{fDC}/K_3} = \sqrt{20/3099.17} = 0.08033$$

Since $Q_2 + Q_3 > Q_1$, lower value of piezometric head at D should be assumed ; let it be 33 m.

Trial 2. $H_A - H_D = h_{fAD} = 60 - 33 = 27\text{m}$

$$H_D - H_B = h_{fDB} = 33 - 30 = 3 \text{ m}$$

$$H_D - H_C = h_{ffd} = 33 - 15 = 18 \text{ m}$$

then, corresponding discharges are computed.

$$Q_1 = \sqrt{27/1530.456} = 0.138$$

$$Q_2 = \sqrt{3/2031.10} = 0.0384$$

$$Q_3 = \sqrt{18/3099.17} = 0.0941$$

Thus, $Q_2 + Q_3 = Q_1$. Hence $p/w + z = 33$ m at D and discharges computed in trial 2 are correct discharges.

10.21. Three reservirs are connected by a network of pipes of shown in Fig. 10.35. The value of coefficient r in the expression $h_f = r Q^n$ for three pipes are $r_1 = 15$, $r_2 = 45$ and $r_3 = 25$. The water elevations for reservoir 1 and 2 are known as $z_1 = 150$ m and $z_3 = 30$ m, and discharge Q_2 to reservoir 2 is 0.6 m³/s. Determine the water elevation for reservoir 2 and discharges Q_1 and Q_3.

Solution

Assume elevation at junction D, i.e. z_D and compute Q_1 and Q_3, then check from continuity principle.

$$Q_1 = (Q_2 + Q_3)$$

or
$$Q_2 - (Q_1 - Q_3) = 0$$

The computations are made in tabular form Writing $h_f = r Q^2$

or
$$Q_1 = \sqrt{h_f/r_1}$$
$$= \sqrt{\dfrac{(z_1 - z_D)}{r_1}}$$

and
$$Q_3 = \sqrt{\dfrac{z_D - z_3}{r_3}}$$

z_D	$Q_1 = \sqrt{\dfrac{(z_1 - z_D)}{r_1}}$	$Q_3 = \sqrt{\dfrac{z_D - z_3}{r_3}}$	$\left[Q_2 - \lvert Q_1 - Q_3 \rvert \right]$
50	2.582	0.894	− 1.0875
60	2.449	1.094	− 0.7535
70	2.309	1.265	− 0.444
80	2.1602	1.414	− 0.146
85	2.0816	1.483	− 0.0016

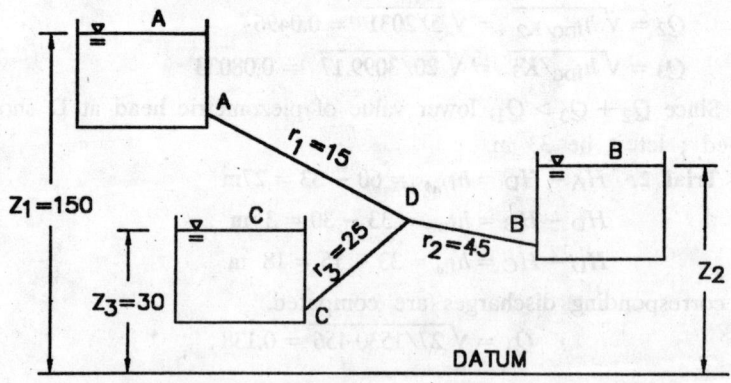

FIG. 10.35. EXAMPLE 10.21

For last trial $\quad Q_1 = 2.0816 \text{ m}^3/\text{s}$

$$Q_3 = 1.483 \text{ m}^3/\text{s}$$

$$Q_2 = 0.6 \text{ m}^3/\text{s} \quad (\text{ given})$$

and

$$z_D = 85 \text{ m}$$

$$h_{f2} = r Q_2^2$$

$$(z_2 - z_D) = 45 Q_2^2$$

$$z_2 - 85 = 45 (0.6)^2$$

$$z_2 = 85 + 16.2$$

$$z_2 = 101.2 \text{ m}$$

10.22 Three reservoirs A, B and C have elevation 40, 35 and 20 metres, respectively. A 30 cm diameter pipe line, 1500 m long, connects two reservoirs A and B while another 20 cm diamter pipe, 2500 m long, connects reservoir A and C. For a distance of 500m from A both the pipe lie side by side upto a junction D where they are inter-connected by a short branch pipe. Assuming that $f = 0.02$ and neglecting minor losses, find (a) the direction of flow with respect to B and (b) the discharge leving A and entering C.

Solution

Inititally, assume there is no flow along DB. The hydraulic gradient line will be as shown in Fig. 10.36a by dotted lines.

For pipe 1.

$$h_{f_1} = \frac{f_1 L_1}{12.1 D_1^5} Q_1^2$$

$$= \frac{0.02 \times 500}{12.1 \times (0.3)^5} (Q_1)^2 = 340.1 Q_1^2 \qquad \text{...(i)}$$

For pipe 4.

$$h_{f_4} = \frac{0.02 \times 500}{12.1 \times (0.2)^5} (Q_4)^2 = 2582.6 Q_4^2 \qquad \text{...(ii)}$$

Since there is no flow through BD, elevation of B and D is same,

$$h_{f_1} = h_{f_4} = (40 - 35) = 5 \text{ m}$$

From Eq. (i) $\quad Q_1 = 0.1212 \text{ m}^3/\text{s}$

From Eq. (ii) $\quad Q_4 = 0.044 \text{ m}^3/\text{s}$

Then $\qquad h_{f_3} = 35 - 20 = \dfrac{0.02 \times 2000 \, Q_3^2}{12.1 \times (0.2)^5}$

$$h_{f_3} = 15 = 1033.6 Q_3^2 \qquad \text{...(iii)}$$

$$Q_3 = 0.0381 \text{ m}^3/\text{s} \qquad \text{...(iv)}$$

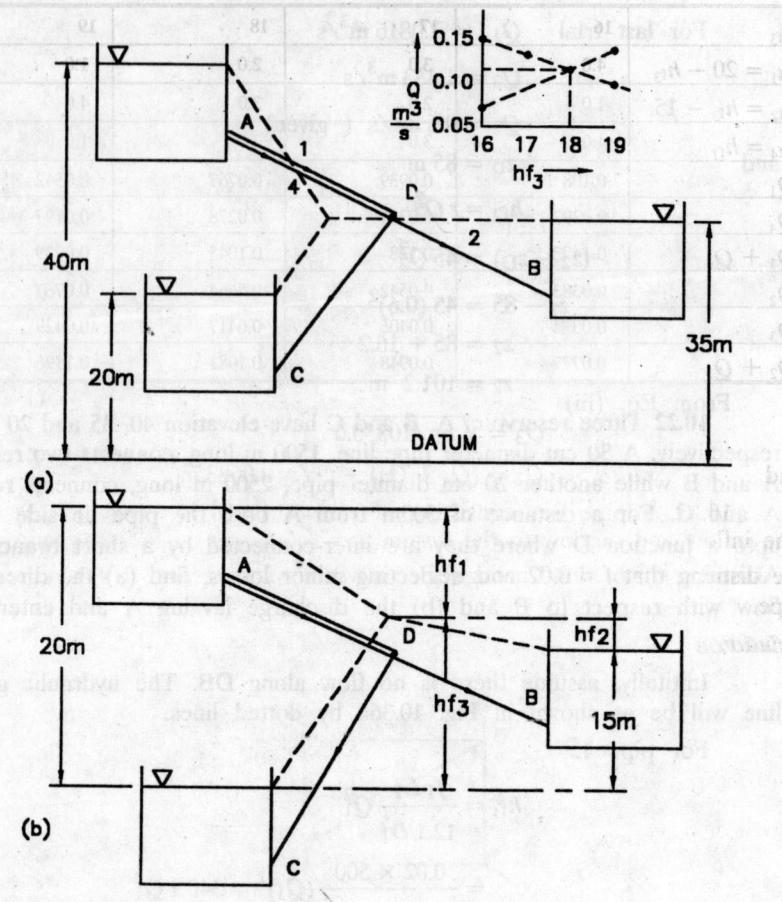

FIG. 10.36(A) & (B) EXAMPLE 10.22

Similarly, $\qquad h_{f2} = \dfrac{0.02 \times 1000 \times Q_2^2}{12.1 \times (0.3)^5}$

$$= 680.2 \, Q_2^2 \qquad \qquad ...(v)$$

Since $Q_1 + Q_4 > Q_3$, the flow is from A to B. Assume the piezometric head at D to be more than h_{f3} or 15 m. The computation is done in a tabular form for various assumed values of piezometric head at D. (see on next page)

Now make plots of $(Q_1 + Q_4)$ versus h_{f3} and $(Q_2 + Q_3)$ versus h_{f3}. (inset of Fig. 10.36). At the point of intersection, $h_{f3} = 18.0$ m and $Q_1 + Q_4 = 0.11$ m³/s which is the discharge leaving the reservoir A.

h_{f_3}	16	17	18	19
$h_{f_1} = 20 - h_{f_3}$	4.0	3.0	2.0	1.0
$h_{f_2} = h_{f_3} - 15$	1.0	2.0	3.0	4.0
$h_{f_4} = h_{f_1}$	4.0	3.0	2.0	1.0
Q_1	0.108	0.0939	0.0767	0.0542
Q_4	0.0393	0.0341	0.0278	0.0197
$Q_1 + Q_4$	0.1473	0.128	0.1045	0.0739
Q_2	0.0383	0.0542	0.0664	0.0767
Q_3	0.0394	0.0406	0.0417	0.0429
$Q_2 + Q_3$	0.0777	0.0948	0.1081	0.1196

From Eq. (iii)

$$Q_3 = \sqrt{h_{f_3}/10330.6}$$

and $\qquad Q_2 = (Q_1 + Q_4) - Q_3 = 0.0683 \text{ m}^3/\text{s}$

10.23 A pipe net consisting of various pipes is shown in Fig 10.37. The inflow and outflow to the system are also shown in the diagram. Obtain the distribution of flow through the network. Assume that $h_f = r Q^2$ for each pipe.

Solution

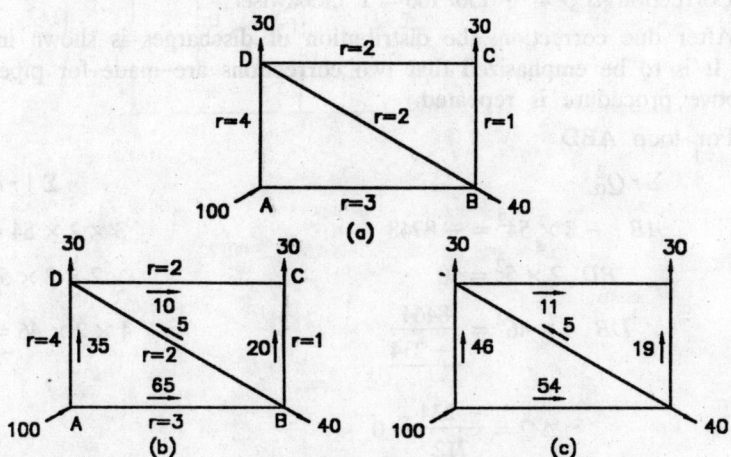

FIG. 10.37. EXAMPLE 10.23

The problem is solved by Hardy Cross method.

(1)   Assume a reasonable distribution of discharge so that the inflow is equal to outflow at each junction.

(2)   Compute the head loss in each pipe by $hf = rQ^2$ with due regard to the sign.

(3)   Obtain correction by Eq. 10.45

$$Q = \frac{\Sigma r Q_o^n}{\Sigma |r n Q_o^{n-1}|}$$

(4)   Adjust the flow in each pipe of the loop.

For the given problem, let us assume the distribution as shown in Fig. 10.37b.

For the loop ABD,

$\Sigma r Q_0^2$ $\hspace{5cm}$ $\Sigma |rn Q_0|$

$AB, -3 \times 6^2 = -12675$ $\hspace{3cm}$ $3 \times 2 \times 65 = 390$

$BD, -2 \times 5^2 = -50$ $\hspace{3.2cm}$ $2 \times 2 \times 5 = 20$

$DA + 4 \times 35^2 = \dfrac{4900}{-7825}$ $\hspace{2.2cm}$ $4 \times 2 \times 35 = \dfrac{280}{690}$

Correction $\Delta Q = -7825/690 = -11$ chokwise.

For the loop BCD,

$\Sigma r Q_0^2$ $\hspace{5cm}$ $\Sigma |rn Q_0|$

$BC, -1 \times 20^2 = -400$ $\hspace{2.7cm}$ $1 \times 2 \times 20 = 40$

$CD, 2 \times 10^2 = 200$ $\hspace{3cm}$ $2 \times 2 \times 10 = 40$

$DB, 2 \times 5^2 = \dfrac{50}{-150}$ $\hspace{2.7cm}$ $2 \times 2 \times 5 = \dfrac{20}{100}$

Correction $\Delta Q = -150/100 = 1$ clockwise.

After due correction, the distribution of discharges is shown in Fig. 10.37c. It is to be emphasized that two corrections are made for pipe BD. The above procedure is repeated.

For loop ABD

$\Sigma r Q_0^2$ $\hspace{5cm}$ $\Sigma |rn Q_0|$

$AB, -3 \times 54^2 = -8748$ $\hspace{2.7cm}$ $3 \times 2 \times 54 = 324$

$BD, 2 \times 5^2 = 50$ $\hspace{3.3cm}$ $2 \times 2 \times 5 = 20$

$DB, 4 \times 46^2 = \dfrac{8464}{-234}$ $\hspace{2.5cm}$ $4 \times 2 \times 46 = \dfrac{368}{712}$

$$\Delta Q = \dfrac{-234}{712} \approx 0$$

For loop BCD

$\Sigma r Q_n$ $\hspace{5cm}$ $\Sigma |rn Q_0|$

$BC, -1 \times 19^2 = -361$ $\hspace{2.7cm}$ $1 \times 2 \times 19 = 38$

$CD\ 2 \times 11^2 = 242$ $\hspace{3.2cm}$ $2 \times 2 \times 11 = 44$

$DB, -2 \times 5^2 = \dfrac{-50}{-169}$ $\hspace{2.5cm}$ $2 \times 2 \times 5 = \dfrac{20}{102}$

$\Delta Q = -169/102 = 1$

Another adjustment may be made to the discharges to obtain accurate result (see Fig. 10.37 c).

10.24 An elastic pressure conduit ($E = 120 \times 10^6$ kPa) of a hydro-electric scheme is 30 cm in diameter and of 2.5 cm wall thickness. It is designed for a maximum hoop stress in the material of the pipe of 2.16×10^4 kPa and is vulnerable to instantaneous closure at its discharge end. Assuming for water $K = 2.1 \times 10^6$ kPa, determine the maximum permissible discharge in the conduit. How long does the pressure wave take to travel 1 km length of this conduit?

Solution

The celerity c of the pressure wave is given by

$$c = \sqrt{K/\rho} \qquad \ldots(i)$$

and the pressure rise is given by Allevi's formula, Eq. 10.51

$$h_i = (U_0 c/g)$$

$$p_i = w h_i = \rho U_0 c \qquad \ldots(i)$$

Also $\qquad f_t = (p D/2 t) \qquad \ldots(ii)$

From Eqs. (i) and (ii)

$$U_0 = (2 t f_t / D \rho c) \qquad \ldots(iii)$$

where c is the celerity of the propagation of pressure wave

$$c = \sqrt{Kg/w} \left[\frac{1}{\sqrt{1 + \dfrac{D}{t} \times \dfrac{K}{E}}} \right]$$

$$= \sqrt{\frac{2.1 \times 10^6 \times 9.81}{9.81}} \left[\frac{1}{\sqrt{\dfrac{0.30}{0.025} \times \dfrac{2.1 \times 10^6}{120 \times 10^6}}} \right] \qquad \ldots(iv)$$

$$= 1317 \text{ m/s}$$

Hence $\qquad U_0 = \dfrac{2 \times 0.025}{0.30} \times \dfrac{2.16 \times 10^4 \times 1000}{1317 \times 1000}$

(Since $\rho = 1000$ kg/m^3)

$$U_0 = 2.73 \text{ m/s}$$

$$Q_0 = \pi/4 \times (0.3)^2 \times 2.73 = 0.193 \text{ m}^3/\text{s}$$

$$t = L/c = 1000/1317$$

$$= 0.76 \text{ sec.}$$

10.25. A C.I. pipe 50 cm diameter 1 km long (wall thickness 15 mm) carries water at a velocity of 4 m/s. A valve fitted at the end is closed in 15 s to stop the flow. (a) what is the maximum rise of pressure due to water hammer at the valve (b) If the closure time is 8s, estimate the pressuere rise (c) Also estimate the length of pipe subjected to maximum pressure is case (a). Take K for water= 2.1×10^6 kPa and $E = 105 \times 10^6$ kPa

Solution

From Eq. 10.50.

$$c = \sqrt{\frac{K_0}{\rho}} = \sqrt{\frac{g}{w} \cdot \frac{1}{\left(\dfrac{1}{K} + \dfrac{D}{tE}\right)}}$$

$$= \sqrt{\frac{K}{\rho}} \sqrt{\frac{1}{\left(1 + \dfrac{DK}{tE}\right)}}$$

$$c = \sqrt{\frac{2.1 \times 10^6 \times 10^3}{1000}} = \sqrt{\frac{1}{\left[1 + \dfrac{0.5 \times 2.1 \times 10^6 \times 10^3}{1.5 \times 10^{-3} \times 105 \times 10^6 \times 10^3}\right]}}$$

$$= 1449.1 \times \sqrt{\frac{1}{1 + 0.6667}}$$

$$= 1449.1 \times 0.7746 = 1122.47 \text{ m/s}$$

Critical time of travel $T_0 = \dfrac{2L}{c}$

$$T_0 = \frac{2 \times 1000}{1122.47} = 1.784 \text{ s}$$

(a) When $T = 1.5 \, (< T_0)$, it is rapid closure.

From Eq. 10.51

$$h_i = \frac{p_i}{w} = \frac{U_0 c}{g}$$

$$pi = \rho c U_0$$

$$= 1000 \times 1122.47 \times 4 \text{ N/m}^2$$

$$= 4489.88 \text{ kN/m}^2$$

(a) When $T = 8\,s \, (> T_0)$, it is gradual closure.

From Eq. 10.47 a,

$$pi = \frac{w}{g} \cdot \frac{L}{T} U_0$$

But $\qquad L = c\,T_0$

$$pi = \frac{T_0}{T} (\rho\, c\, U_0)$$

$$= \frac{1.78}{8} (4489.88) \text{ kN/m}^2$$

$$= 999 \text{ kN/m}^2$$

(c) Length of pipe subjected to maximum pressure (measured from valve end) for case I (a).

$$x = L - c\,\frac{T}{2}$$

$$= \left(1000 - 1122.47 \times \frac{1.5}{2}\right)$$

$$= (1000 - 841.85) = 158.14 \text{ m}$$

10.26 A steel pipe, 400 cm diameter, 200 m long supplies water from a lake to a power plant. The pressure head of the entranc is 120 m. A valve fitted at the exit when operated gradually reduces the velocity from 4 m/s to 1 m/s in 6s. Calculate the pressure at the valve at the end of valve closure. What is maximum time for rapid closure. Given K for water 2100 MPa and E for steel $= 2.1 \times 10^{11} P_a$. Pipe is designed as rigid.

Solution

For rigid pipe $c = \sqrt{\dfrac{K}{\rho}}$

$$= \sqrt{\frac{2100 \times 10^6}{1000}} = 1449.14 \text{ m/s}$$

Critical time $\quad T_0 = \dfrac{2L}{c}$

$$= \frac{2 \times 2000}{1449.14} = 2.76 \text{ s}$$

Since valve reduces velocity from 4 m/s to 1 m/s in $T = 6s\,(> T_0)$, it is gradual closure.

From Eq., 10.47 a

$$pi = -\frac{w}{g}\frac{L}{T}U_0$$

$$p_i = -\frac{w}{g}\cdot\frac{(cT_0)}{T}\cdot U_0 \qquad (\because\ L = CT_0)$$

$$= -\frac{T_0}{T}(\rho\,c\,U_0)$$

$$= -\frac{2.76}{6}(1000 \times 1449.14)\,(4 - 1)$$

$$= -\frac{2.76}{6}(4347.4)$$

$$= 1999.8 \text{ k N/m}^2$$

(a) Pressure at the valve = static pressure + dynamic pressure due to water hammer

$$= 9.81 \times 120 + 1999.8 \text{ kN/m}^2$$

$$= 1177.2 + 1999.8 \text{ kPa}$$

$$= 3177 \text{ kPa}$$

(b) Maximum time for rapid clossure is critical time $T_0 = 2.765$.

i.e if the valve is closed in 2.76 s, the pressure rise is maximum $= \rho c U_0 = 4347.4$ kPa.

10.27 A penstock 60 cm in diameter and 3623 m long supplies water from a reservoir to a power plant at a velocity of 4.0 m/s. Due to fault in power plant the valve at downstream end is closed suddenly. Sketch pressure rise with respect to time (a) at the valve, (b) mid point (c) at inlet and (d) at an intermediate point 725 m from valve where surge tank is located. K for water is 2.1×10^9 kN/m^2

Solution

For rigid pipe $c = \sqrt{\dfrac{K}{\rho}}$

$$= \sqrt{\frac{2.1 \times 10^9}{1000}} = 1449.14 \text{ m}$$

From Eq. 10.51,

Pressure rise $\quad pi = \rho c U_0$

$$= 1000 \times 1449.14 \times 4 = 5796.5 \text{ kN/m}^2$$

Critical time $\quad T_0 = \dfrac{2L}{c}$

$$= \frac{2 \times 3623}{1449.14} = 5 s$$

(a) *Pressure variation at valve.*

As soon as the valve is closed instantaneously the pressure will rise at B. This pressure wave will travel from B to A in time L/c seconds and then reflected wave start from A. It will take L/c seconds to reach B. During this time, pressure will be pi at value B as shown in Fig. 10.38.

Time to travel of +pi wave from B to A$= \dfrac{L}{c} = 2.5 s$

Time to travel of reflected wave from A to B $= \dfrac{L}{c} = 2.5 s$

During this time, 0 to 2.5 s and 2.5 s to 5.0 s, pressure at B=pi
Time of travel of –pi from B to A = 2.5 s
Time of travel of reflected wave from A to B = 2.5 s.

Thus from 5.0 s to 10 s (from initial instant of closure), the pressure at $B = -pi$.

Again, + pi wave will start from B to reach A in 2.5 s and so on. This cycle is repeated. (See Fig. 10.38)

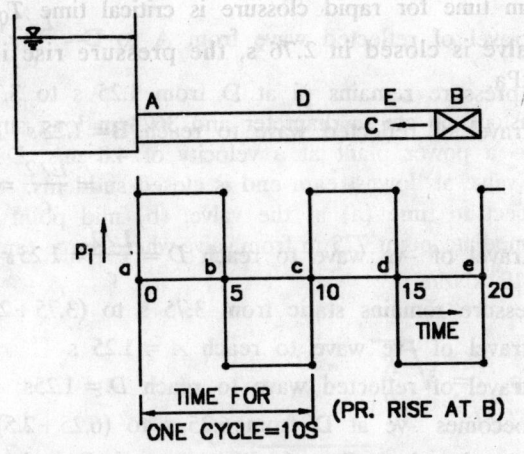

FIG. 10.38. EXAMPLE 10.27

Time for one cycle $= ab + bc$

$$= 5 + 5 = 10s$$

(b) *Pressure rise at mid point*

At $i = 0$, pressure at $D = 0$ (static pressure referred as zero)

At $\cdot t = \dfrac{L/2}{c}$, pressure at $D = $ pi

i.e. time of travel of $+$pi from B to $D = \dfrac{L/2}{c} = 1.25\,s$

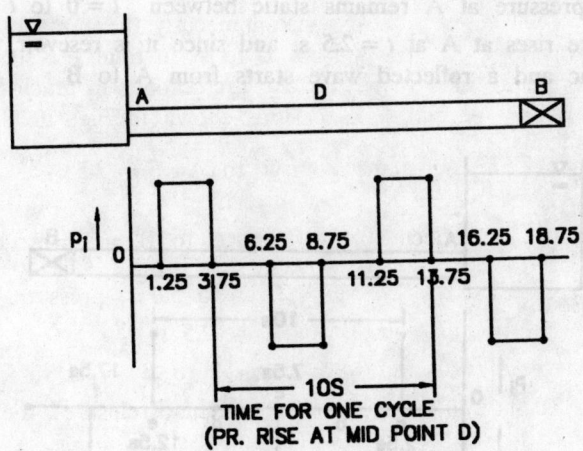

FIG. 10.39. EXAMPLE 10.27

Time of travel of $+$ pi from D to $A = \dfrac{L/2}{c} = 1.25\,s$

Time of travel of reflected wave from A to $D = \dfrac{L/2}{c} = 1.25\,s$

Thus the pressure remains pi at D from 1.25 s to 3.75 s

Time of travel of reflected wave to reach B = 1.25 s

$$= \dfrac{L/2}{c} = 1.25\,s$$

Time of travel of –ve wave to reach $D = \dfrac{L/2}{c} = 1.25\,s$

Hence pressure remains static from 3.75 s to $(3.75 + 2.5) = 6.25\,s$

Time of travel of –ve wave to reach $A = 1.25$ s

Time of travel of reflected wave to reach $D = 1.25s$

Pressure becomes –ve at D from 6.25 s to $(6.25 + 2.5) = 8.75\,s.$

Again, time taken by reflected wave to reach B and + ve wave to reach D $(1.25s + 1.25\,s) = 2.5s.$

Hence, the pressure rises at D from $8.75 + 2.5 = 11.25s$ and remains high for $t = 13.75s$

This way, the cycle is repeated, (see Fig. 10.39)

Time for one complete cycle af or $ck = (11.25 - 1.25) = 10$ s

(c) *Pressure at inlet A*

At $t = 0$, pressure at $A = 0$ (see Fig. 10.40)

Time taken by +ve wave to travel, B to A $= \dfrac{L}{c} = 2.5s$

Thus, pressure at A remains static between $t = 0$ to $t = 2.5$ s

Pressure rises at A at $t = 2.5$ s. and since it is resevoir, immediately becomes static and a reflected wave starts from A to B

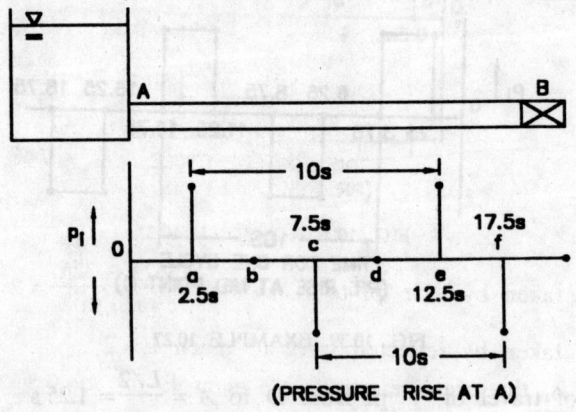

(PRESSURE RISE AT A)

FIG. 10.40. EXAMPLE 10.27

Time taken by reflected wave to reach B $= \dfrac{L}{c} = 2.5 \ s$

Time taken by $-$ve wave to reach A $= \dfrac{L}{c} = 2.5 \ s$

Thus, pressure remains static at A from $t = 2.5 \ s$ to $(2.5 + 5.0) = 7.5 \ s$

As soon as -ve pi reaches A, it reverts back to static pressure.

Time taken by reflected wave to travel from A to B

$$= \dfrac{L}{c} = 2.5 \ s.$$

Time taken by $+$ve wave to travel from B to A $= \dfrac{L}{c} = 2.5 \ s.$

That is, the pressure remains static for $t = 7.5$ s to $12.5 \ s$

At $t = 12.5$s, the pressure rise at A and immediately becomes normal and a reflected wave travels from A to B. (This way, the cycle is repeated)

Time taken by one cycle 'ae' $= (12.5 - 2.5) = 10$s.

(d) *Pressure variation at E.*

At $t = 0$, pressure at E $= 0$ (Fig. 10.41)

Time taken by $+$ve pi to reach E $= \dfrac{x}{c} = \dfrac{725}{1449.14} = 0.5 \ s$

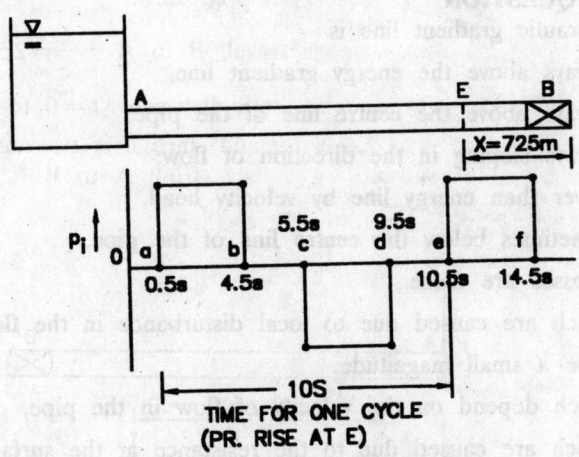

FIG. 10.41. EXAMPLE 10.27

Time taken by $+$ve pi to reach A $= \dfrac{(3623 - 725)}{1449.14} = 2 \ s$

Time taken by reflected wave to reach E $= 2 \ s$

That is, the pressure remains $+$pi at E for $t = 0.5 \, s$ to $4.5 \ s$.

Time taken by reflected wave to reach $B = \dfrac{x}{c} = 0.5$ s

Time taken by –ve pi to reach $E = \dfrac{x}{c} = 0.5$ s

Time taken by -ve pressure wave to reach A and reflected wave to reach
$$E = \frac{2(L-x)}{c} = 4\,s$$

This means, pressure at E remains static between $t = 4.5$ s to $t = 5$ s

The pressue becomes –pi at E at $t = 5.5$ s and remains -ve for an interval of $(2+2 = 4s)$. i.e. $t = 5.5$ s to 9.5 s

Time taken by reflected wave to travel from E to B
$$= \frac{x}{c} = 0.5 \text{ s}$$

Time taken by +ve wave to reach from B to E= 0.5s

This means, pressure rises again at E from $t (= 9.5 + 1) = 10.5$ s and remains so for $\dfrac{2(L-x)}{t} = 4s$.

This way, the cycle of pressure wave is repeated

Time for one cycle, ae $= (10.5 - 0.5) = 10\ s$

OBJECTIVE QUESTION

10.1 The hydraulic gradient line is

    (a) always above the energy gradient line.

    (b) always above the centre line of the pipe.

    (c) always sloping in the direction of flow.

    (d) lower than energy line by velocity head.

    (e) sometimes below the centre line of the pipe.

10.2 Minor losses are those

    (a) which are caused due to local disturbance in the flow.

    (b) have a small magnitude.

    (c) which depend on the velocity of flow in the pipe.

    (d) which are caused due to the resistance at the surface.

    (e) none of these answers.

10.3 For the pipes arranged in series

    (a) the flow is different in different pipes.

    (b) the velocity of flow is same in all the pipes.

    (c) the head loss must be same in all the pipes.

(d) the local head loss per unit length is same for all the pipes.

(e) none of these answers.

10.4 For pipes arranged in parallel

(a) the discharge is same through all the pipes.

(b) the head loss is same through each pipe.

(c) the discharge divides in the ratio of area of the pipe.

(d) the trial solution is required to determine discharge through each pipe.

(e) none of these answers.

10.5 Loss of head due to sudden expansion of a stream in a closed conduit is expressed by

(a) $(U_1^2 - U_2^2)/2g$ (b) $(U_1 - U_2)/2g$

(c) $(U_2^2 - U_1^2)/2g$ (d) $(U_1 - U_2)^2/g$

(e) $(U_1 - U_2)^2/2g$

where U_1 and U_2 are the velocities through smaller diameter and larger diameter pipes respectively.

10.6 The pipe system is said to be equivalent to another pipe when one of the sets of quantities are same

(a) L,Q   (b) hf,Q   (c) f,D

(d) U,D   (e) none of these answers.

10.7 The ratio hf/H for maximum transmission of power through a pipe is

(a) 33.3%   (b) 66.67%   (c) 100%

(d) 0%   (e) none of these answers

10.8 The most economical diameter of the pipe is given by

(a) $(2.5 B/A)^{1/7}$ (b) $(2.5 A/B)^{1/5}$ (c) $(B/A)^{1/7}$

(d) $\left(\dfrac{5}{2} AB\right)^{1/7}$ (e) none of these answers.

where A is the annual cost of power lost and B is the annual cost of pipe.

10.9 In a pipe system, n pipes of equal diameter D are connected in parallel. Assuming that these are similar in all respects, the diameter of compound pipe is given by

(a) $Dn^{2/5}$ (b) $D/n^{1/5}$ (c) D/n

(d) D/n^2 (e) none of these answers.

10.10 In the network of pipes
   (a) the head loss around each loop must be zero.
   (b) the energy loss in all the loops is the same.
   (c) the continuity equation at each junction should be satisfied
   (d) none of these answers.

10.11 To solve a pipe network problem, Hardy Cross method is used. The correction   Q is given by

   (a) $\dfrac{\Sigma\, n\, r\, Q^n}{\Sigma\, |\, n\, Q^{n-1}\, |}$

   (b) $\dfrac{\Sigma\, n\, Q^n}{\Sigma\, |\, r\, n\, Q^{n-1}\, |}$

   (c) $\dfrac{\Sigma\, n\, Q^{n-1}}{\Sigma\, |\, r\, n\, Q^n\, |}$

   (d) none of these answers.

10.12 The speed of a pressure wave depends upon
   (a) the length of the pipe.
   (b) diameter of pipe.
   (c) viscosity of fluid.
   (d) initial velocity of fluid
   (e) none of these answers

10.13 The water hammer is caused due to
   (a) sudden closure of a valve.
   (b) sudden opening of a valve.
   (c) compressibility of water.
   (d) stretching of pipe.
   (e) none of these answers.

10.14 Valve closure is rapid when time of closure t_c is
   (a) $t_c > 2L/c$ (b) $t_c = 2L/c$ (c) $t_c = L/c$
   (d) $t_c = 2L/U_0$ (e) $t_c < L/c$ (f) none of these answers

where L is the pipe length, c is the celerity of pressure wave and U_0 is the initial velocity.

10.15 The maximum pressure rise caused by water hammer phenomenon is .
   (a) $U_0 c/w$ (b) $\rho\, U_0\, c$ (c) $U_0 c/\rho$
   (d) $\rho\, U_0/c$ (e) none of these answers.

10.16 When time of closure of the valve $t_c = L/c$, the portion of the pipe subjected to maximum pressure, expressed in percent, is
    (a) 25   (b) 50   (c) 75
    (d) 100   (e) none of these answers.

10.17 The loss at the exit of a submerged pipe in a reservoir is
    (a) negligible   (b) $0.05\, U^2/2g$ (c) $0.5\, U^2/2g$

    (d) $U^2/2g$ (e) none of these answers.

PROBLEMS

10.1 A siphon pipe to 10 cm diameter is to be used to conduct water over a summit from a tank into another tank at lower level. The rising leg of the siphon is 350 m long and the falling leg is 35 m long. At the peak (highest point) the pipe axis is 2.4 m above the water level in the upstream tank and 15.9 m above the level in the lower tank. Calculate the maximum possible discharge through the siphon. If the pipe line of the same total length is passed through the peak instead of over it, compute the discharge through the pipe of 10 cm diameter. Assume f as 0.03.

10.2 Power is being supplied from a hydroelectric plant to an industry by means of three parallel pipes of 15 cm diameter. The pipe lines are 60 km long and are laid horizontally. The pressure at inlet is maintained as 5000 kPa and the efficiency of transmission obtained is 94%. If one of the pipes becomes unserviceable, what increase in pressure is required at the inlet end of pipe to supply same amount of power and what would be the efficiency of transmission under this condition? Take $f = 0.03$.

10.3 Two reservoirs A and C having a difference of 15 m are connected by a 20 cm diameter pipe. The pipe AB is 300 m long and BC is 150 m from C. When the flow from A to C is 0.05 m³/s, the gauge at B shows the pressure head of 0.5 m of water and loss of head across the valve is 5 m. Determine the maximum rate of flow when the loss of head across valve is 1.3 and it is partially open. Assume that the pipes AB and BC have constant f but BC is slightly rougher than AB. Also draw the hydraulic gradient line for this discharge. Allow for the effect of velocity head in the pipe at exit but neglect loss of head at entry. Point B is 11.8 m above W.S. in C.

10.4 Two reservoirs M and N are connected by a compound pipe ABCDE. The water level in the reservoir M stands at 25 m above the centre line of pipe at A and in the reservoir N at 5 m above the centre line of pipe, at E (Fig. 10.42). Estimate the rate of flow of water from M to N when both valves are fully open. The loss coefficients for the gate valve and glove valve are 0.19 and 10 respectively. Assume $f = 0.02$ for both the pipes. Also draw TEL and HGL for the pipe system.

10.5 It is proposed to transmit oil (specific gravity 0.75 and dynamic viscosity 1.2×10^{-3} kg/m s) through a pipe line. The permissible pressure drop

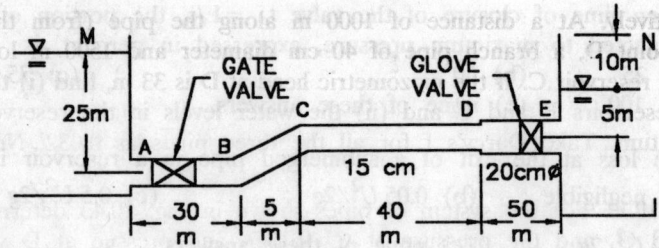

FIG. 10.42. PROBLEM 10.4

for the pipe is 30 kPa per 100 m length. What size of the steel pipe should be used. Assume the pipe to be smooth. Take Q = 25 lit/s.

10.6 Two parallel water mains of length L and identical in all respects convey a total discharge Q from one reservoir to another, the difference in water level being assumed to remain constant. Cross connections are made along the pipe at the distance of L/6 apart. If two adjacent cross connections are used to divert the whole flow through one pipe for a length of L/6, so that the corresponding length L/6 of other pipe may be repaired. What would be the percentage reduction in discharge, neglecting secondary losses?

10.7 Three parallel pipes are connected between two points A and B. At the upstream end A, the pressure is maintained at 800 kPa and its elevation above an arbitrary datum is 35 m whereas the elevation of point B is 20 m. When a total discharge of 0.04 m^3/s is following in the system, determine the flow in each pipe. Pipes have following dimensions.

Pipe 1: $L_1 = 200m$, $D_1 = 7.5m$, $f_1 = 0.018$, minor loss coefficient $K_1 = 12$.

Pipe 2: $L_2 = 150$ m, $D_2 = 5$ cm, $f_2 = 0.011$, $K_2 = 6$

Pipe 3: $L_3 = 300$ m, $D_3 = 10$ m, $f_3 = 0.03$, $K_3 = 16$.

10.8 A horizontal water main comprises 1500m of 15cm diameter pipe followed by 1000m of 10cm pipe($f = 0.025$ for both pipes). All the water is drawn off at a uniform rate per metre length of pipe.

If the total input is 0.25 m^3/s, find the pressure drop along the main, neglecting all the losses except friction. Also draw the HGL taking the pressure at inlet as 60 m.

10.9 The pipe APD is used to supply the water from reservoir A to reservoir B and C. The pipe APD branches off at the junction point D. A pump P is fitted in the pipe AD at an elevation 0.0. The elevation of water surfaces in the reservoirs A,B and C are 10m, 30 m and 50m respectively. The dimensions of various pipes are AP; $L_1 = 300m$, $D_1 = 45cm$, $f = 0.04$; PD,$L_2 = 1500m$, $D_2 = 45cm$, $f = 0.04$; DB,$L_3 = 600m$, $D_3 = 20cm$,$f = 0.02$; and DC, $L_4 = 1000m$, $D_4 = 30cm$ and $f = 0.01$. The pump supplies 0.06m^3/s to the junction D, calculate the discharge supplied to reservoir B and C and also the pressure at point D.

10.10 A pipe of diameter 50cm and length 4000m connects two reservoirs A and B. The water levels in A and B are 40 m and 30 m above the datum respectively. At a distance of 1000 m along the pipe (from the entrance) at a point D, a branch pipe of 40 cm diameter and 1500 m long connects a third reservoir C. If the piezometric head at D is 33 m, find (i) the discharge into reservoirs B and C and (ii) the water levels in the reservoir C above the datum. Take Darcy's f for all the three pipes as 0.032. Neglect minor losses.

10.11 For the system of pipes shown in Fig. 10.43 determine (a) Q_1, Q_2 and Q_3 and the pressure at C, (b) Q_2 and pressue at D when $Q_3 = 0$. Assume for both cases that the pressure at A is 200 kPa and that the discharge at B and C is into atmosphere. All pipes are 0.35 m in diameter and f for all pipes is 0.03.

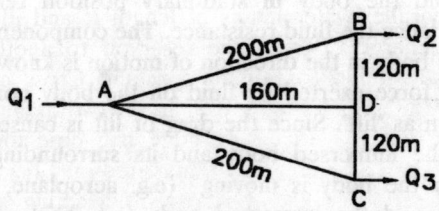

FIG. 10.43. PROBLEM 10.11

10.12 Determine the distribution of flow in the network shown in Fig. 10.44. Assume n = 2.

10.13 The water is flowing with a velocity of 1.5 m/s in a pipe of length

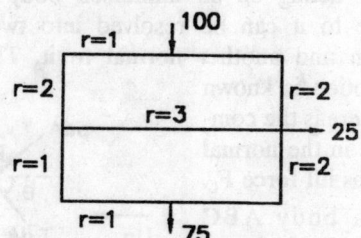

FIG. 10.44. PROBLEM 10.12

2500 m and of diameter 50 cm. The valve fitted at the end of pipe is closed suddenly, find the circumferential and longitudinal stresses developed in the pipe wall. The pipe wall is 1 cm thick, E for pipe material is 200×10^6 kPa. and K for water is 2×10^6 kPa.

10.14 A valve at the end of a pipeline 1200 m long through which water flows at 2.5 m/s is closed in 5 seconds in such a way that the pressure rise on the upstream size of a valve increases at a uniform rate. Assuming that celerity c of the pressure wave = 1500 m/s, find the increase of pressure caused by the valve closure.

11

Flow Around Immersed Bodies

11.1 INTRODUCTION

Flow past bridge piers or tall buildings or an aeroplane flying high in the air are some of the numerous examples of the ' flow around immersed bodies'. Whenever the relative motion occurs between the solid body and the fluid surrounding it, the former experiences the fluid resistance. Thus, a force is required to hold the body in stationary position relative to the moving fluid to counter-balance the fluid resistance. The component of the force exerted by the fluid on the body in the direction of motion is known as 'drag'. Similarly, the component of force exerted by fluid on the body normal to the direction of motion is known as 'lift'. Since the drag or lift is caused due to the relative motion between the immersed body and its surrounding fluid, it makes no difference whether the body is moving (e.g. aeroplane, submarines, etc.) or the fluid flows around the immersed body (e.g. bridge piers, tall buildings, etc.). The knowledge of this force is important in the design of these structures. Similarly, sufficient force produced and supplied by the driving unit of fluid machines (e.g. turbines, wind mills, etc.) must be known in advance.

11.2 DRAG FORCE ON IMMERSED BODIES

The force F acting on an immersed body by a fluid moving with a velocity U_0 relative to it can be resolved into two components; one in the direction of motion and another normal to it. The component of force in the direction of motion is known as drag force F_D whereas the component of the force in the normal direction is known as lift force F_L.

Concider a 'body ABC placed immersed in a fluid of mass density ρ and dynamic viscosity μ. Let the relative velocity of the fluid with respect to the solid body be U_o. Consider an elementary area dA of· the body, on which fluid exerts a force dF. The tangent to the surface makes an angle θ with the direction of motion, as shown in Fig. 11.1. Let the pressure acting normally on ·the elementary area dA (= ds × 1) be p and shear

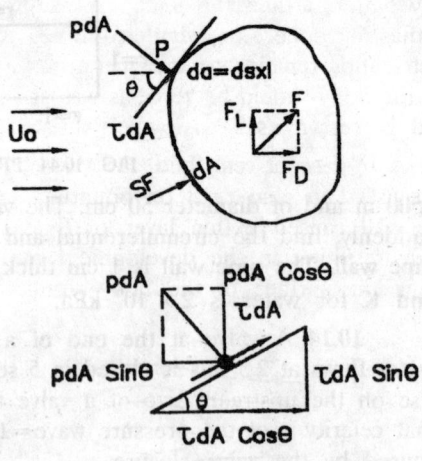

FIG. 11.1 DEFINITION SKETCH

stress acting tangentially to the area be τ.

Resolving the forces in the direction of motion,

$$dF_D = \tau_0 \, dA \cos\theta + p \, dA \sin\theta$$

Summing up the components of shear and pressure acting over the entire surface area of the body,

$$\int_A dF_D = \int_A \tau_0 \, dA \cos\theta + \int_A pd \, A \sin\theta$$

$$F_D = F_{Dv} + F_{Dp} \qquad \qquad ...(11.1)$$

Total drag force = viscous drag + pressure drag.

Similarly, resolving the forces in the normal direction,

$$dF_L = \tau_0 \, dA \sin\theta + p \, dA \cos\theta$$

Summing up all the components of shear and pressure acting over the entire surface area of the body,

$$\int_A dF_L = \int_A \tau_0 \, dA \sin\theta + \int_A pdA \cos\theta$$

$$F_L = F_{L_v} + F_{L_p} \qquad \qquad ...(11.2)$$

The symbol $\int_A$ represents the integration over the entire surface exposed to the flow. The first term in Eqs. 11.1 and 11.2 represents the contribution of viscous force and the second term represents the contribution of pressure force. The relative contribution of each of these forces to the total drag (or total lift) depends to a great extent on the shape of the body and characteristics of fluid and flow.

Type of drag :- The drag force can be obtained by considering the flow pattern around the object. In case of flow of an ideal fluid past asymmetrical bodies like sphere or cylinder, the velocity distribution and hence the pressure distribution remains symmetrical around the body. This means, the force acting on the body should be zero, as was shown by a German scientist D' Alembert and is known as D' Alembert's paradox.

In case of real fluid, the viscosity plays an important role, as has been disscussed in chapter 8 on boundary layer theory. The 'no slip condition'at the wall caused a thin layer of fluid to adher to the surface of the solid body resulting in the development of boundary layer. The fluid is resisted along the surface of the body resulting in 'skin friction drag'.

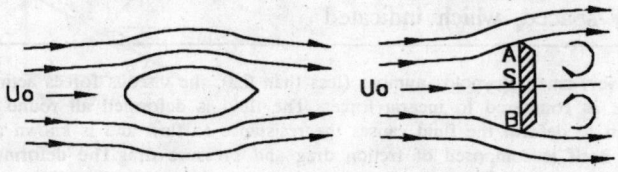

FIG. 11.2 FLOW AROUND OBJECTS WITH DIFFERENT ORIENTATION

Besides viscosity, the velocity and pressure distribution are also affected by the physical presence of the body. The fluid is deformed in the vicinity of the body and the forces of deformation cause the resistance to flow; especially at low Reynolds number of the flow*.

Additionally, when the body is held normal to the flow, a stagnation point exists on the front face of the body (which may even extend into a stagnation region). On the rear face of the body, the flow is separated and a wake is formed as shown in Fig 11.2. For a round shaped body such as sphere or cylinder, the separation point depends on the Reynolds number, roughness of the surface and Turbulence present in the approaching flow. The location of the point of separation also depends on whether the boundary layer is laminar or turbulent. The flow in the wake (at the rear) is highly turbulent and consists of large scale eddies. The flow is reversed in the wake resulting in the formation of vortices. The pressure in the turbulent wake remains more or less constant and is found to be much lower than the pressure at the stagnation point on the front of the body. The differential pressure acting on two faces of the body further increases the drag force and it is known as 'pressure drag'. The degree to which the rear pressure approaches the front stagnation pressure is known as ' pressure recovery'. In case of small wake, the pressure recovery occurs to a large degree and vice versa.

Thus, the total drag acting on a body consists of two components- skin friction drag and pressure drag and is termed as profile drag.

Profile drag = skin friction drag + pressure drag. (11.1)

For a streamlined body, such as shown in Fig. 11.2a, the pattern of streamlines conform very well to the surface configuration of the immersed body so that the region of separation is limited to the rear of the body. In this case, wake formed at the rear is small, the pressure recovery occurs to a large degree and hence the contribution of pressure drag is also small. Similarly, when a flat plate is placed parallel to the flow, the pressure recovery occurs to a large degree and the profile drag is mainly due to friction drag.

When a body with sharp corners, such as a cubical body/flat plate is held normal to the flow, Fig. 11.2b; the separation of flow always occurs at the edges and the wake extends across the full projected width of the body. The total drag or profile drag is entirely due to the pressure difference between upstream and downstream of the flat plate, (i.e. pressure drag) and the skin friction drag is almost equal to zero. The stream line pattern upstream of plate is almost similar to irrotational flow with a stagnation point at the centre of the upstream face of the plate. Near the edges of the plate, the streamlines are closely spaced, which indicated

---

*At very small Reynolds number (less than 0.2), the viscous forces acting on the body are too large as compared to inearia forces. The fluid is deformed all round the body. The force required to deform the fluid causes the resistance to flow and is known as 'deformation drag'; which itself is composed of frction drag and pressure drag.The deformation is felt to a large distance at small Reynolds number and is limited to a smaller distance (i.e. finally to the boundary layer) as the Reynolds number increases.

that the condition of high velocity and low pressure occurs in these regions. As these regions are adjacent to the turbulent wake on the downstream side of the plate, there is sufficient intermixing of flow and correspondingly low pressure. This results in an appreciable difference on two side of the body. In this case, the profile drag is mainly due to pressure drag. The pressure drag is also brown as " Form Drag "

11.3 DIMENSIONAL ANALYSIS FOR DRAG AND LIFT

Let a smooth object having area A move with velocity U_o through a fluid of mass density ρ, viscosity μ and modulus of elastity E. The motion is also affected by acceleration due to gravity g and the shape of the body which is repressednted by a factor ζ. Thus, the functional relationship can be written for drag force F_D and lift force F_L.

$$F_D = f_1 (\rho, \mu, V_0, A, E, g, \zeta) \qquad ...(11.3a)$$

and

$$F_L = f_2 (\rho, \mu, U_0, A, E, g, \zeta) \qquad ...(11.4a)$$

By dimensional analysis Eqs. 11.3a and 11.4a are reduced to

$$F_D = \frac{\rho U_0^2 A}{2} \left(\frac{\rho U_0 D}{\mu}, \frac{U}{\sqrt{g} A^{1/4}}, \frac{U_0}{\sqrt{E/\rho}}, \zeta \right)$$

$$F_D = \frac{\rho U_0^2 A}{2} f_3 (R_e, N_F, N_M, \zeta) \qquad ...(11.3b)$$

Similarly,

$$F_L = \frac{\rho U_0^2 A}{2} f_3 (R_e, N_F, N_M, \zeta) \qquad ...(11.4b)$$

Conventionally, the drag and lift forces acting on solid objects are defined by non-diamenssional coefficients; known as drag coefficient C_D and lift coefficient C_L recpectively. These coefficient are expressed as

$$C_D = \frac{F_D/A}{\rho U_0^2/2} \qquad ...(11.3c)$$

and

$$C_L = \frac{F_L/A}{\rho U_0^2/2} \qquad ...(11.4c)$$

Thus from Eqs. 11.3b, 11.3c

$$C_D = f_3 (R_e, N_F, N_M, \zeta) \qquad ...(11.3d)$$

Similarly, from Eqs. 11.4b and 11.4c

$$C_L = f_4 (R_e, N_F, N_M, \zeta) \qquad ...(11.4d)$$

Eqs. 11.3d and 11.4d indicate that the bodies of the same shape and having the same alignment with the flow (e.g.model and prototype placed with same alignment) possess the same coefficients of drag and lift, provided the various non- dimensional numbers (Reynolds number, Froude number, Mach number and body shape factor ζ) are maintained the same.

In most of the problems of engineering only, one of the force is predominant and others are having low bearing on the phenomenon. If the flow velocities are smaller as compared to the velocity of sound (celerity c), the compressibility effects may be neglected. The gravity force is predominant for the free surface flows or where the density difference between two immiscible fluids is sufficiently large and the motion of the body takes place at the interface of these two fluids. In case of an incompressible fluid without a free surface, the coefficients of drag and lift are functions of Reynolds number and body shape only.

$$C_D = fs\,(R_e, \zeta) \qquad \qquad ...(11.3e)$$

and
$$C_L = fs\,(R_e, \zeta) \qquad \qquad ...(11.4c)$$

The coefficient of drag C_D defined as

$$C_D = \frac{F_D/A}{0.5\rho\,U_0^2} \qquad \qquad ...(11.3c)$$

is modified from of Eular's number N_E

$$N_E = \Delta p/0.5\rho\,U_0^2 \qquad \qquad ...(11.5)$$

The coefficient of drag C_D depends, on the shape of the body and Reynolds number and its variation for different shaped bodies has been studied experimentally as well as theoretically (using methods of hydrodynamics) by many investigators.

11.4 SHAPE OF THE BODY

(a) *Streamlined body.* When the shape of the body is such that separation is either eliminated or is confined in a small rear part of the body, the wake is kept as small as possible. This results in a small pressure drag; (mostly the profile drag is caused due to skin friction). Such a body shape is called streamlined body or well shaped body, e.g.,airfoil.

(b) *Bluff body.* When the body shape is such that flow is separated much ahead of its rear resulting into a larger wake, and there is a higher contribution due to pressure drag. (The contribution of friction drag is small). Such a body shape is known as 'bluff body', e.g. flat plate held normal to the flow or a square body, etc.

The object of streamlining a body is to move the point of separation as far back as possible and thus to produce the minimum size of wake; this way the pressure drag is reduced. But the friction drag is increased by making the body longer to promote gradual increase in pressure along the length of the body. Hence, the optimum amount of streamlining is that, for which, the sum of pressure drag(or form drag) and skin friction drag is minimum.

11.5 FLOW PAST THREE DIMENSIONAL BODIES

1 Flow past a sphere

Consider first the flow around a sphere immersed in a fluid which has been studied extensively.

ᐠ (a) *Flow pattern.* Fig. 11.3a shows the streamline pattern of non-viscous fluid around a sphere which can be constructed by means of flownet theory. The velocity increases untill the vertical axis of symmetry is reached and then decreases in an exactly similar manner. Since the streamlines are symmetrical about the vertical axis, the pressure at corresponding points on the front and rear is also indentical Fig. 11.3a, and therefore, the drag is zero. Fig. 11.3b shows the flow pattern when the real (viscous) fluid flows past the sphere and laminar boundary layer develops on the surface of the sphere. The flow is separated at point s at 80^0 from the front stagnation points. Fig. 11.3c shows the corresponding flow pattern when turbulent boundary layer develops on the surface of sphere. The flow is separated at about 115^0 from front stagnation point and the wake is relatively smaller in size.

(b) *Drag.* Sir G.G. Stokes analysed the laminar flow past a spherical body occurring at low Reynolds number. He assumed that the inertia forces are too small and may be neglected. Therefore, the viscous forces only need to be considered. Hence, for steady laminar flow, the Navier Stokes equations of motions, Eqs. 7.3a to 7.3c may be simplified. The equation of motion in X-direction is

$$\left(u\frac{\partial u}{\partial x} + v\frac{\partial u}{\partial y} + w\frac{\partial u}{\partial z} \right) = \left[\times - \frac{1}{\rho}\frac{\partial p}{\partial x} \right.$$
$$\left. + \nu\left(\frac{\partial^2 u}{\partial x^2} + \frac{\partial^2 u}{\partial y^2} + \frac{\partial^2 u}{\partial z^2} \right) \right] \quad ...(7.3a)$$

Since the inertia terms are too small and no body force is considered, the Eq. 7.3a reduces to

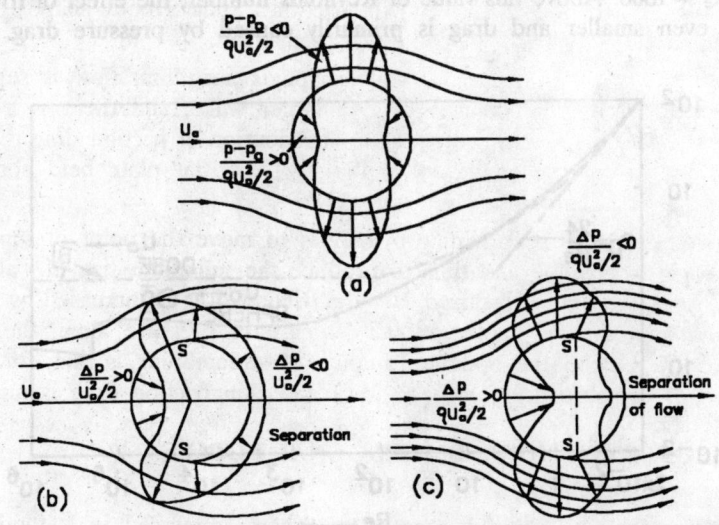

FIG. 11.3 FLOW AROUND A SPHERE (A) FLOW PATTERN AND IRROTATIONAL FLOW (B) LAMINAR BOUNDARY LAYER (C) TURBULENT BOUNDARY LAYER

$$\frac{\partial p}{\partial x} = \mu \left(\frac{\partial^2 u}{\partial x^2} + \frac{\partial^2 u}{\partial y^2} + \frac{\partial^2 u}{\partial z^2} \right) \qquad ...(11.6)$$

The drag force F_D can then be obtained by solving Eq. 11.6, using the boundary condition that the components of velocity, viz. u, v and w, should all be zero at the surface of the sphere. Thus, Stokes obtained Eq. 11.7 for the drag F_D.

$$F_D = 3 \pi D \mu U_0 \qquad ...(11.7)$$

This equation, Eq. 11.7, has been verified by many other investigators. It can also be shown experimentally that total drag F_D consists of one third of the total drag as pressure drag ($= 2 \pi D \mu U_0$).

Equating Eq. 11.3c and 11.7

$$F_D = C_D \times \frac{\rho U_0^2}{2} A = 3 \pi D \mu U_0$$

or
$$C_D = \frac{24}{R_e} \qquad ...(11.8)$$

where A is the area of the object (normal to the direction of flow) and is equal to $\pi D^2 / 4$. Eq. 11.8 also confirms the results of dimensional analysis that the coefficient of drag is a function of Reynolds number. Eq. 11.8 is valid for Reynolds number less than or equal to 0.1. As the Reynolds number is increased to about 10, the flow starts separating and weak eddies begin to form enlarging into a fully developed wake near a Reynolds number of 1000. In the range of Reynolds number, the drag results from a combination of pressure and frictional drag; the contribution of latter decreases to 5% only at $R_e = 1000$. Above this value of Reynolds number, the effect of friction becomes even smaller and drag is primarily caused by pressure drag. The

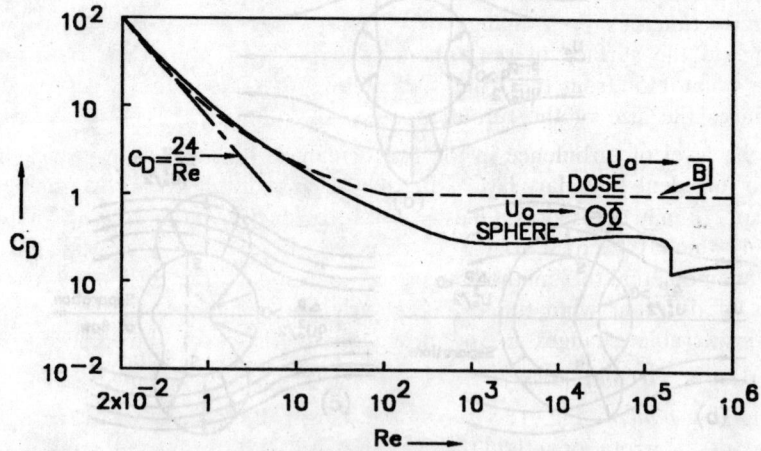

FIG. 11.4. VARIATION OF COEFFICIENT OF DRAG WITH REYNOLDS NUMBER FOR THREE DIMENSIONAL BODIES

plot of experimental results over a large range of Reynolds number for spheres of different sizes tested in various fluids given a single curve for coefficient of drag C_D, Fig. 11.4.

Experimentally it has been shown that if the sphere moves in an infinite fluid contained in a vessel of diameter D_1, the proximity of the walls of the container increases the coefficient of drag. It is given by

$$C_D = \frac{24}{R_e} \left(1 + 2.1 \frac{D}{D_1} \right) \qquad ...(11.9)$$

In 1927, Osean solved Eq. 7.3, considering some of the inertia terms and obtained modified expression for C_D, which is also plotted in Fig. 11.4.

$$C_D = \frac{24}{R_e} \left(1 + \frac{3}{16} R_e \right) \qquad ...(11.10)$$

It is seen from Fig. 11.4 that Eq. 11.10 confirms the experimental results upto Reynolds number of 2.0 and thereafter deviates from the experimental plot.

As the Reynolds number is increased beyonds 1.0, the laminar boundary layer separates from the surface of the sphere, beginning first at the rear of the stagnation point where the adverse pressure gradient is the strongest. The curve of C_D begins to level off as the pressure drag becomes of increasing importance and the drag begins nearly proportional to U^2. With further increase of R_e, the point of separation moves forward on the sphere, increasing the size of the turbulent wake and consequently the proportion of form drag, until at $R_e = 1000$, the point of separation remains fairly stable at 80^0 from the forward stagnation point, Fig. 11.3c. For a considerable range of Reynolds number, the flow conditions remain fairly stable; the laminar boundary layer separating from the forward half of the sphere and C_D remaining fairly constant at about 0.45. At a value of R_e of about 2.5×10^5 for smooth sphere, however, the drag coefficient is suddenly reduced to about 50%, Fig. 11.4. The reason for this reduction lies in a change of laminar boundary layer to turbulent, developing on the surface of the sphere. The point of separation is moved back to a point 115^0 from the front stagnation point. The shift of separation point reduces the size of the turbulent wake and thereby the pressure drag.

If the level of turbulence in the free stream is high, the transition from laminar to turbulent boundary layer will take place at lower Reynolds number. (Thus, a sphere may be used as a measure of turbulence by noting the Reynolds number at which C_D equal to 0.3 is obtained. Before the development of hot wire anemometer, this method was used to compare the turbulence characteristics of different wind tunnels). Similarly, the roughness of the surface causes considerable changes in the drag characteristics of the sphere.

2. Flow past a circular disk

(a) *Flow pattern*. Fig. 11.5 shows the flow pattern past a thin circular disk for two cases–irrotational fluid flow and real fluid flow. In case of irrotational flow past a thin disk held normal to the flow, symmetrical streamline pattern is obtained with a stagnation point at the centre of the plate on the upstream face of the plate. The stream lines have theoretically zero radius of curvature at the edges of the disk and thereby negative infinity pressure intensity. However, such reduction in pressure is physically impossible, the fluid separates at the edge of the plate with increased radius of curvature and correspondingly less extreme pressure at the edges of the disk. The pressure distribution existing on both sides of the plate is also shown in Fig. 11.5.

(b) *Drag*. Experimental data for C_D versus R_e for the flow around a disk is also shown plotted in Fig. 11.4. The drag coefficient for a circular disk held normal to the flow is found to be independent of Reynolds number beyond the range of deformation drag, i.e. $R_e \approx 1000$. The reason is that the separation point is fixed at the edges of the disk and the turbulent wake always extends across the full projected area of the disk, thus resulting in a relatively constant value of C_D, Fig. 11.4.

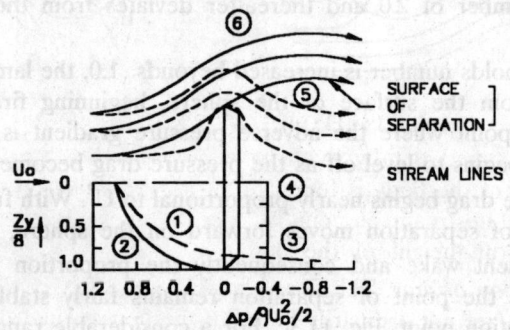

FIG. 11.5. FLOW PAST A CIRCULAR DISK

11.6 FLOW PAST TWO DIMENSIONAL BODIES

1. Flow past a cylinder

(a) *Flow pattern*. The flow pattern and pressure distribution around a cylinder of long length is shown in Fig. 11.6. The flow of incompressible non-viscous fluid gives rise to a symmetrical pressure distribution about the vertical axis of the cylinder, Fig. 11.6a. In a real fluid (viscous fluid), the fluid velocity at the surface must be zero and a boundary layer develops on the surface. The fluid velocity reduces to zero at point S, lying on the forward face of the cylinder. The flow is accelerated from this point S upto another point B, where the flow is separated from the boundary. The location of the point of separation is governed by the condition of flow in the boundary layer at the surface of the cylinder. The boundary layer remains laminar upto Reynolds number of 2.5×10^5 and thereafter the flow becomes turbulent in the boundary layer formed in the front portion of the cylinder. As the turbulent motion extends farther into the regions of higher pressure existing along the curved surface of the cylinder, the point of separation moves further downstream towards the rear of the cylinder (also refer to section 8.12).

Downstream from the point of separation, the flow is characterised by the formation of turbulent eddies and vortices which persist for some distance

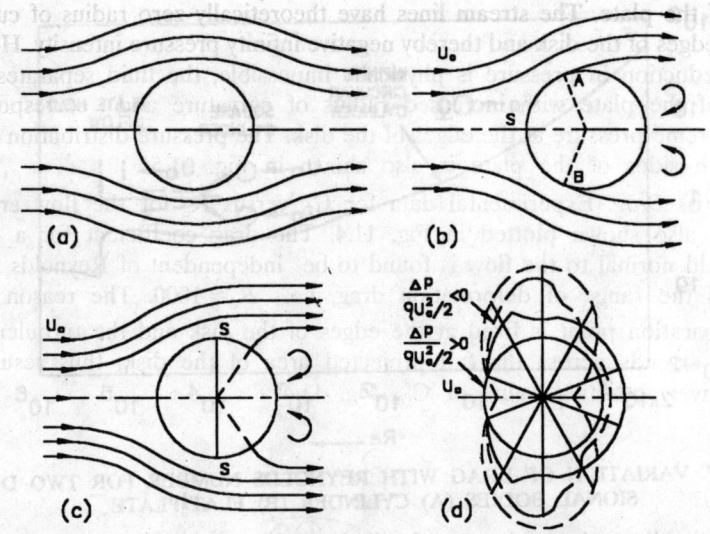

FIG. 11.6. FLOW PAST A CYLINDER

and then are damped out by the viscous action. Therefore, the pressure in the rear portion of the body is found to be too less than on the front portion of the body, i.e. upstream of point B. The lower pressure remains constant throughout the full height of the body.

(b) *Variation of drag.* The flow around a cylinder exhibits some peculiar properties which are not ordinarily found in the flow around three dimensional bodies (like sphere). For Reynolds number less than 1.0, the flow remains completely viscous and the inertia forces are negligible within this range of R_e. The drag is found to be proportional to free stream velocity U_0. In other words, the coefficient of drag C_D varies inversely proportional to the Reynolds number R_0 and is shown plotted by a straight line in Fig 11.7. The major part of the drag is caused due to friction drag. As R_0 is increased from 2 to about 30, the boundary layer separates symmetrically from the two sides and two weak symmetrical eddies are formed. The equilibrium of the eddies is maintained by the flow from the separated boundary layer. The eddies increase in the length with increase in velocity in order to dissipate their rotational energy. These vortices remain stably attached to the rear of the cylinder up to $R_0 \leq 60$. The total drag at this value af R_e, mainly consists of pressure drag and the slope of the curve between C_D and R_e decreases. With further increase of R_e the coefficient of drag further decreases reaching a minimum value of nearly 0.95 at R_e equal to 2000. The value of C_D then increases slightly to a value of 1.2 at R_e value to 5000 and remains the same for R_e value up to 2×10^5. At R_e value of 5000, the characteristics of wakes in the rear of the cylinder change. The point of separation also shifts slightly upstream of vertical diameter. At Reynolds number of 2×10^5, the boundary layer turns turbulent and the readjustment of the point of separation takes place; this

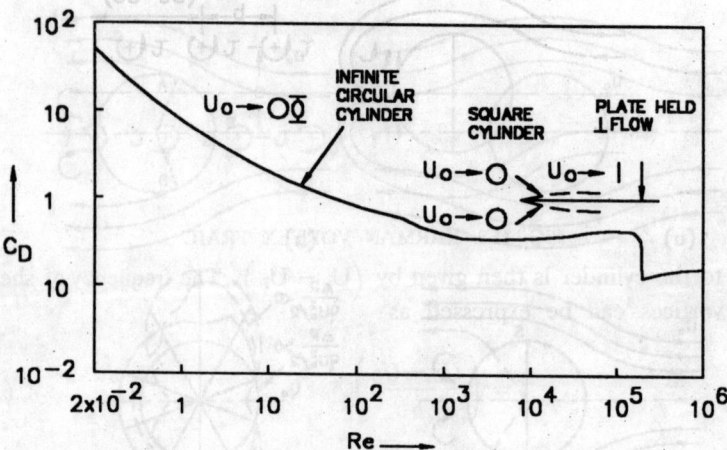

FIG. 11.7. VARIATION OF DRAG WITH REYNOLDS NUMBER FOR TWO DIMEN-
SIONAL BODIES (A) CYLINDER (B) FLAT PLATE

results in smaller wake on the rear of cylinder and hence lower value of coefficient
of drag is obtained.The value of C_D is found as 0.3 at R_e equal to
5×10^5. The experimental data for R_e more than 5×10^5 are scarce but it
appears that C_D is likely to rise to about 0.7 within the reange of R_e varying
from 5×10^5 to 10^7 (Fig 11.7).

117 KARMAN'S VORTEX TRAIL

The vortices formed on the rear of a circular cylinder become unstable
as R_e exceeds 30. The eddies elongate, break off from the body and wash
away with the main flow; and this process continues in the flow past cylinder.
This pattern of vortices is known as "Karman vortex trail". The limiting Reynolds
number at which the eddies break off from the body varies with the shape
of cylinder and also depends on the width of the confining channel and the
turbulence present in the stream. The eddies are shed alternatively from opposite
side, Fig 11.8, upto Reynolds number of 120. This results in a staggered double
row of vortices in the wake behind th cylinder. Karman analysed the flow
around the cylinder and found that there is only one spacing between the
vortices at which the pattern of vortices remains stable. With any other spacing,
the vortices will be unstable. Karman obtained the ratio of a/b, experssed
by Eq. 11.11b

$$\sinh(\pi a/b) = 1 \qquad \qquad ...(11.11a)$$

or $$a/b = 0.281 \qquad \qquad ...(11.11b)$$

The analytical result of Karman, Eq. 11.11b has been confirmed by
many experiments.

It is seen that the entire vortex system moves with respect to the fluid
at a velocity U_e which varies directly as the strength of the vortices and inversely
as the spacing 'b' between them. The relative velocity of the vortex trail with

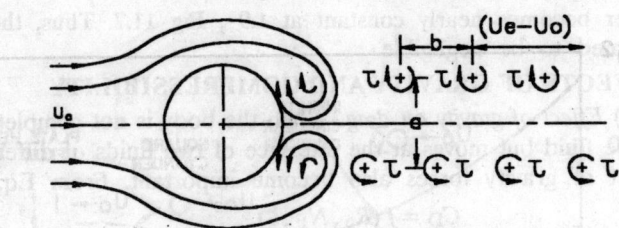

FIG. 11.8. KARMAN VORTEX TRAIL

FIG. 11.8. KARMAN VORTEX TRAIL

respect to the cylinder is then given by $\left(U_e - U_o\right)$. The frequency of shedding of the vortices can be expressed as

$$f = \left(\frac{U_e - U_0}{b}\right) \qquad ...(11.12)$$

Taylor gave Eq. 11.13 for the frequency of the shedding

$$f = 0.198 \frac{U_0}{D}\left(1 - \frac{19.7}{R_e}\right) \qquad ...(11.13)$$

where R_e is the Reynolds number of the flow and the dimensionless number f D/U_o is known as 'Strouhl number's.

The alternate shedding of eddies continues beyond R_e equal to 120. Beyond this value of R_e and upto R_e equal to 2×10^4, the eddies continue to be washed away but their pattern is diffcult to perceive. The corresponding variation of Strouhl number is found between 0.17 to 0.20.

The periodic shedding of vortices behind the cylinder gives rise to lateral thrust on the body of the object or lift which acts normal to the direction of flow. This leads to aerodynamic instability of object such as tall chimneys and suspension bridge when these are exposed to winds. The singing of electric wires while the wind blows across them is also caused on account of sheding of voritices or eddies. The worst condition is reached when the frequency of shedding becomes equal to the natural frequency of the cylinder. Thus, while desiging elastic bodies, these lateral forces should also be considered. The coefficient of drag C_D is related to Strouhl number S by Eq. 11.14

$$S = \frac{0.21}{C_D^{0.75}} \qquad ...(11.14)$$

Flow around a flat plate

In case of flow around a flat plate held normal to the flow the separation points are fixed at its edges, Fig. 11.9. The pressure in the downstream turbulent wake remains nearly constant but much less than the pressure on the point of staignation on the upstream of the plate. The total drag consists of only pressure drag; the friction drag being zero. The drag coffcient C_D for suffciently long plate decreases with Reynolds number until R_e is equal to 1000 and there-after becomes nearly constant at 1.9 , Fig 11.7. Thus, the end effects are assumed to be negligible.

11.8 EFFECTS OF GRAVITY AND COMPRESSIBILITY

(a) *Effect of gravity on drag.* When the body is not completely immersed in a single fluid but moves at the interface of two fluids of different densities, the effect of gravity forces also become important. From Eq. 11.3

$$C_D = f(R_e, N_F, \zeta)$$

neglecting the effects of the forces of compressibility. For examples, a ship floats at the interface of water and air. The resistance to the motion of the ship consists of skin friction drag on its hull and pressure drag from the wake and wave resistance at the prow. Since the ship is a streamlined body,

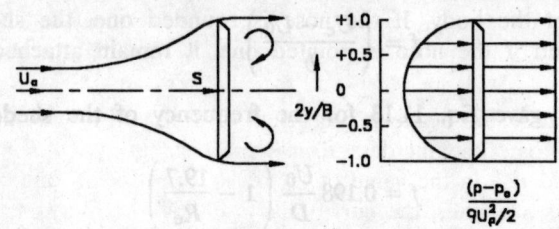

FIG. 11.9. FLOW PAST A TWO DIMENSIONAL FLAT PLATE

the skin friction drag is much larger than pressure drag and can be computed by the methods discussed in chapter 8 on the boundary layer theory. The pressure drag is obtained as the difference of profile drag, determined from the model tests,(similarity of Froude number) and skin friction drag (For complete detail, see section 6.11)

(b) *The effect of compressibility on the drag.* The effect of compressible forces are expressed by another dimensionless parameter or Mach number N_M. It is defined as the ratio of fluid velocity U_0 to the velocity of sound in the fluid medium (since any small disturbance is propagated in the fluid medium with speed of sound c). For example, a disturbance in still air travels outwards as a spherical pressure wave. In subsonic flows, $N_M < 1$, the object causing the disturbance moves with a velosity U_0 less than the speed of sound and hence the pressure wave travels ahead of the of the object. This give the fluid a chance to adjust itself to the oncoming body. For example, a body moves a distance $U_0 t$ from the centre O in time t i.e. distance OP, and the disturbance travels a distance r= c t (Fig 11.10 a). As the body moves ahead, new spherical waves are generated but all such waves are contained within the initial spherical wave. In case of supersonic flows, $N_M > 1$, i.e. $U_0 > c$, the body causing the disturbance moves faster than the pressure wave emitted from it. Thus, a conical shape wave front is formed with vertex at the body. The half angle of this cone is known as ' Mach angle'.

The conical wave front left behind is known as shock wave. The sudden change in velocity and pressure occurs across this wave front.

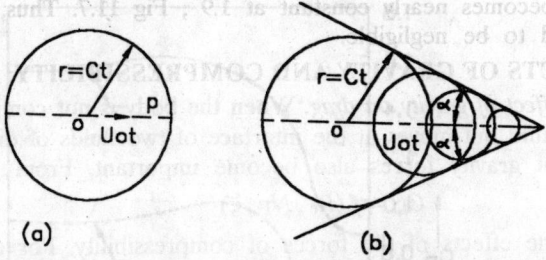

FIG. 11.10 PROPAGATION OF PRESSURE WAVE (A) BODY VELOCITY SUBSONIC
(B) BODY VELOCITY SUPERSONIC

The pattern of shock wave also depends on the geometric configuration of the nose of the body. If the nose is rounded one, the shock wave lies ahead of it and if the nose is pointed one, it remain attached to the nose itself.

The relationship between coefficient of drag and Mach number is shown in Fig. 11.12. Experimental data from drag tests in supersonic wind tunnels indicate a rapid rise in the value of C_D as N_M approaches unity. As the Mach number increases further, the curve falls gradually and approaches a constant value asymptotically. It is to be noted that by the time velocity becomes high enough for compressible effects to become important, the viscous effects become negligible and hence the Reynolds number does not enter the picture. It has been mentioned earlier that streamlined bodies experience minimum drag against

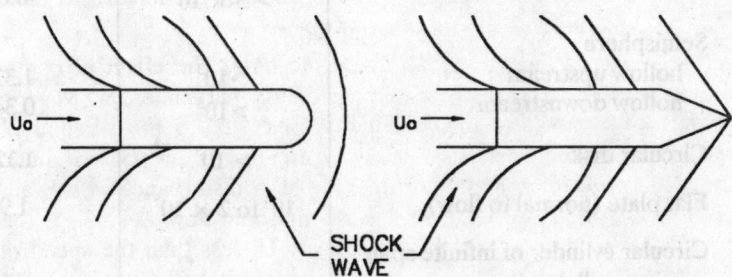

FIG. 11.11. EFFECT OF THE SHAPE OF LEADING EDGE ON THE PATTERN
OF SHOCK WAVE

subsonic flows. In supersonic flows, the best form is a sharp pointed shape. This produces the minimum extent of shock wave. The wake resistance is not important because the low pressure within the wake is limited to absolute zero of vacuum; pressure causing minimum wake resistance.

The coefficient of drag for important shaped bodies are given in Table 11.1

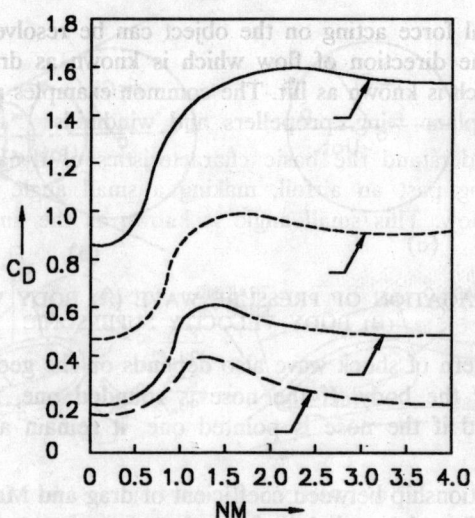

FIG. 11.12 VARIATION OF THE COEFFICIENT OF DRAG WITH
THE MACH NUMBER

TABLE 11.1. DRAG COEFFICIENTS FOR VARIOUS BODY SHAPES

	Form of body	R_e	C_D
1	Sphere	10^4 to 10^5	0.5
		$> 3 \times 10^5$	0.0
2	Semisphere		
	hollow upstream	$>10^3$	1.33
	hollow downstream	$>10^3$	0.34
3	Circular disk	$> 10^3$	1.12
4	Flat plate (normal to flow)	10^4 to 2×10^5	1.9
5	Circular cylinder of infinite span		
	axis parallel to flow		
	axis normal to flow	2×10^4 to 2×10^5	1.2
		$>5 \times 10^5$	0.35
6	Square cylinder		
	side parallel to flow	10^4 to 2×10^5	2.0
	diagonal parallel to flow	10^4 to 2×10^4	1.6
7	Streamlined airfoil	4×10^4	1.07

11.9 PHENOMENON OF DYNAMIC LIFT

As discussed in section 11.1, whenever the fluid flows around an object
which may either be unsymmetrical or makes an angle with the direction of

flow, the total force acting on the object can be resolved into two directions, namely, in the direction of flow which is known as drag and in the normal direction which is known as lift. The common examples making use of dynamic lift are aeroplane wing, propellers and windmills.

To understand the basic characteristics of dynamic lift, consider the flow occurring past an airfoil, making a small angle with the direction of irrotational flow. This small angle is known as the angle of attack α_0. The

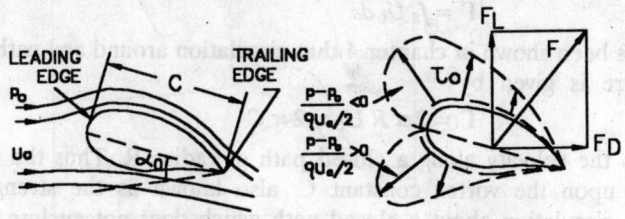

FIG. 11.13. FLOW AROUND AN AIRFOIL (A) DEFINITION SKETCH
(B) PRESSURE DISTRIBUTION

airfoil has 'chord length' C (chord is a straight line joining the centres of curvature of the leading and trailing edges). Since the airfoil is a streamlined body, the separation is limited to a small region near the trailing region. The streamlines in the approaching flow are uniformly spaced at some distance ahead of the leading edge. As the flow approaches the airfoil and passes over it, the spacing of streamlines decreases over the upper surface and increases along the underside (of airfoil). Since the velocity is inversely proportional to the streamline spacing, the velocity of fluid over the upper surface of the airfoil will be greater and on the underside, the velocity of fluid will be lower than the mean velocity U_o of the approaching fluid. According to Bernoulli's theorem, the pressure will be lower on the top surface and higher on the underside. The pressure distribution is shown in Fig. 11.13 which can be integrated over the whole surface area of the airfoil and the resultant force acting on the airfoil can be determined. The component of this force acting normally on the object in the upward direction is known as lift force F_L. If the viscous force acting along the surface of airfoil resisting the flow is also considered, the lift force F_L is given by

$$F_L = \int_A p \, dA \cos \theta - \int_A \tau_0 \, dA \sin \theta \qquad ...(11.2a)$$

in which $\int_A$ designates integration over the whole surface of the object. Usually, the contribution of shear stress is too small, therefore,

$$F_L = \int_A p \, dA \cos \theta \qquad ...(11.2b)$$

which is also expressed in terms of dynamic head.

$$F_L = C_L \frac{\rho U_0^2}{2} A \qquad ...(11.4c)$$

Here A is the projected area of the body normal to the direction of the motion and $\rho U_0^2/2$ is the equivalent pressure of the approaching stream.

11.10 CIRCULATION THEORY AND LIFT

1. Significance of circulation

As discussed in section 4.10, circulation refers to the summation of the product of the tangential velocity U_t and the length of curved path ds.

$$\Gamma = f_s \, U_t \, ds$$

It has been shown in chapter 4 that circulation around any path enclosing vortex centre is given by

$$\Gamma = 2 \pi R \, U_t = 2 \pi \, C$$

where U_t is the velocity along a closed path of radius R. Thus the circulation Γ depends upon the vortex constant C, also known as the strength of the vortex. The circulation about a closed path which does not enclose the vortex centre is found to be zero.

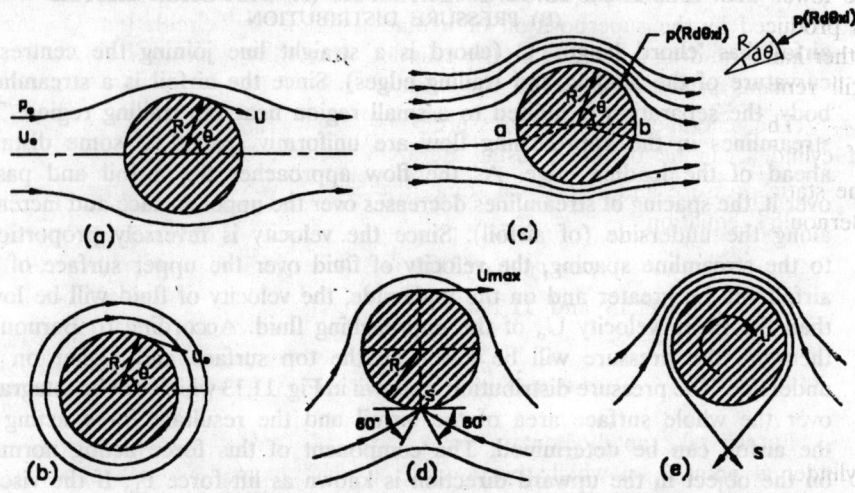

FIG. 11.14. FLOW AROUND A CIRCULAR CYLINDER

(A) IRROTATIONAL FLOW (B) CIRCULATION (C) SUPERIMPOSED FLOW
(D) BOTH SEPARATION POINTS MERGE (E) SEPARATION POINT REMOVED
AWAY FROM CYLINDER

2. Flow about a cylinder

Let us now consider the steady flow of an ideal fluid about a cylinder of long length (in order to consider it as a two- dimensional body) with an ambient velocity U_o, Fig. 11.14a.

From hydrodynamics, one can determine the velocity of fluid at any point P on the periphery of the cylinder.

$$u = 2 U_0 \sin \theta \qquad \qquad ...(11.16)$$

Let the cylinder be imparted a circulation in the clockwise direction (adopting it as the positive direction). The velocity U_0 due to circulation at point P on the periphery of cylinder may be determined as

$$U_0 \sin \theta + \frac{\Gamma}{2\pi R} \qquad ...(11.17)$$

The superposition of irrotational flow with circulatory motion yields the composite flow pattern shown in Fig. 11.14c. The velocity of composite flow at point P may now be obtained as the vectorial sum of the two components of the velocity

$$U = 2 U_0 \sin \theta + \frac{\Gamma}{2\pi R} \qquad ...(11.18)$$

It is seen from Fig. 11.14c that the superposition of the two motions causes higher velocity on the top surface of the cylinder than on the underside of the cylinder. This means that the pressure around the upper portion should be lower than around the lower portion. Therefore, a resultant force or lift is produced by the superposition of irrotational flow and circulation. On the other hand, no drag is exerted on the cylinder, since the composite flow pattern still remains symmetrical about the vertical axis.

The general equation for pressure p acting at any point P on the periphery of cylinder can be obtained, using Bernoulli's equation. Let p_0 and U_0 be the static pressure and velocity at some distance ahead of the cylinder. Using Bernoulli's equation

$$p = p_0 + \rho/2 \, (U_0^2 - U^2) \qquad ...(11.19a)$$

From Eqs. 11.18 and 11.19a

$$p = p_0 + \frac{\rho}{2} \left\{ U_0^2 - \left(2U_0 \sin \theta + \frac{\Gamma}{2\pi r} \right)^2 \right\}$$

Let us take an elementary area dA ($= L R d\theta$) on the periphery of cylinder at point P on which the pressure acting is p and the corresponding lateral force is dF_L. It is given by

$$dF_L = - (p L R d\theta) \sin \theta \qquad ...(11.20)$$

The negative sign is used to indicate that the pressure force always directs towards the surface of cylinder. For positive value of θ, lift force acts downwards.

Integrating Fig. 11.20 over the whole surface.[*]

$$\int dF_L = - \int_0^{2\pi} p_x (L \cdot R \, d\theta) \sin \theta$$

Substituting the value of p and solving the above equation,

$$F_L = \rho U_0 L \Gamma \qquad ...(11.21)$$

Theoretically $\int dF_D = \int_0^{2\pi} p_x (L \cdot R \, d\theta) \cos \theta = 0$. In practice, since the fluid possesses viscosity, there exists some drag which is finite drag and provides for resistance to flow.

Eq. 11.21 is known as the 'Kutta-Joukowski theorem'-named after the two scientists who first developed it. Although this theorem has been developed for a circular cylinder but it is valid for any two dimensional body.

In the derivation of above Eq. 11.21 for lift force, circulatory motion was superimposed over the uniform flow and the cylinder behaves as a vertex. The circulation can also be approximated experimentally by the rotation of the cylinder in a fluid stream. This phenomenon was first observed by German scientist Magnus in 1852 and hence this phenomenon of production of lift force is also referred to as 'Magnus effect'. This phenomenon is also observed in the curved pitch of a baseball.

It is clear from Fig. 11.14c that the points of stagnation shift downward from the horizontal axis but they are still symmetrical about vertical axis. At stagnation point, the velocity on the periphery to cylinder, u, must be zero, Therefore, from Eq.11.18

$$2 U_0 \sin\theta + \Gamma/2\pi R = 0$$

$$\Gamma = -4\pi R U_0 \sin\theta \qquad \qquad ...(11.22)$$

Eq. 11.22 shows that if the angle θ to the point of stagnation is measured and free stream velocity U_o is known, the circulation Γ can be computed.

For $\Gamma < 4\pi R U_0$, $\sin\theta < 1$, the two stagnation points will lie on the opposite side of the vertical axis, Fig. 11.14c. For $\Gamma < 4\pi R U_0$; $\sin\theta < 1$, the stagnation points merge on the negative Y-axis. The two stream lines make an angle of $60°$ with the tangent to the cylinder, Fig. 11.14d. Finally, for $\Gamma < 4\pi R U_0$, the stagnation points will lie as shown in Fig. 11.14e. Since $\sin\theta$ cannot be greater than 1, this is only possible when the stagnation point moves away from the surface of the cylinder. In case $\Gamma < 4\pi R U_0$ the maximum velocity occurs at the top of the cylinder.

$$U_{max} = 2 U_0 + 4\pi R U_0/2\pi R = 4 U_0 \qquad \qquad ...(11.23)$$

This means that the condition of merging of two stagnation points may be obtained by rotating the cylinder in such a way that peripheral velocity u is four times the uniform velocity.

Comparing Eqs. 11.4c and 11.21,

$$C_L = \frac{F_L/A}{\rho U_0^2/2} = \frac{F_L/(L \times 2 R)}{\rho U_0^2/2}$$

$$C_L = \frac{\rho U_0 L \Gamma}{\rho U_0^2 L R} = \frac{\Gamma}{U_0 R}$$

Substituting the value of Γ,

$$C_L = \frac{2\pi U_c}{U_0} \qquad \qquad ...(11.24)$$

Eq. 11.24 shows that the coefficient of lift is a function of U_c/U_o for irrotational flow. But the circulatory motion around a cylinder is usually produced due to existence of viscosity (which causes the development of boundary layer on the surface of cylinder). This causes the discrepancy between the theoretical and experimental results as shown in Fig. 11.15.

11.11 LIFT CHARACTERISTICS OF AIRFOIL

One of the widely used body shape is airfoils which are used in aircraft wings, blades of propellers, turbines, etc. The law of Kutta-Joukowski is applied in the theory of lift for all such bodies. According to the Kutta-Joukowski expression, Eg. 11.21, the production lift requires the superposition of circulation on the uniform velocity. In case of flow past cylinder the circulation may be provided to the cylinder by rotating it, but the airfoils do not rotate. Hence, for the production of circulation around an airfoil, a different mechanism works for the production of circulation. Consider the correction of flow around a typical airfoil of infinite length as it starts to move. The mechanism is explained in steps.

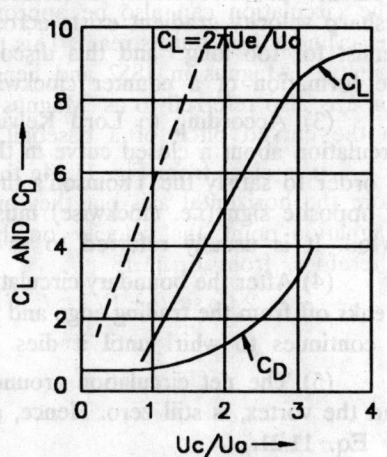

FIG. 11.15. EFFECT OF CIRCULATION VELOCITY ON THE COEFFICIENT OF DRAG AND LIFT

1 Development of lift

(1) Initially the flow pattern ahead of the airfoil is irrotational and the circulation about the airfoil is zero. Hence, the lift acting on the airfoil is also zero, Fig. 11.6a.

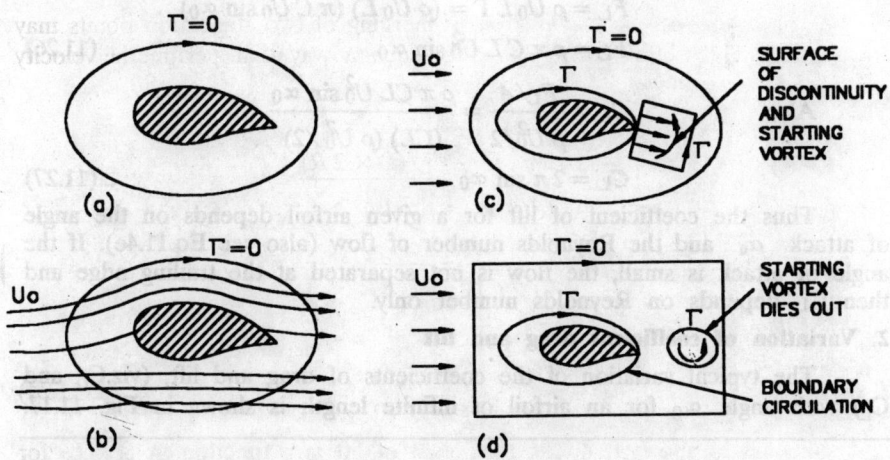

FIG. 11.16. FLOW AROUND AN AIRFOIL OF INFINITE SPAN

(2) As soon as the flow passes over the airfoil (which is slightly inclined to the main flow), the velocities of fluid layers on the top surface remain lower than those of the fluids which are passing underside of the airfoil (velocity is inversely proportional to the spacing of the streamlines), Fig. 11.16b. Thus, a surface of discontinuity is formed at the trailing edge of the airfoil and a sharp velocity gradient exists across this surface. But this condition cannot persist for too long and this discontinuity in velocity distribution promotes the formation of a counter clockwise starting vortex at the trailing edge.

(3) According to Lord Kelvin's theorem of invariant circulation, the circulation about a closed curve in the fluid does not change with time. Thus, in order to satisfy the Thomson's theorem, a circulation of equal strength but of opposite sign (i.e. clockwise) must automatically be generated around the airfoil. It is usually referred to as boundary circulation, Fig. 11.6c.

(4) After the boundary circulation has been generated, the starting vortex breaks off from the trailing edge and is left behind as the airfoil moves forward. It continues to whirl until it dies out from viscous effect.

(5) The net circulation around a curve, including the profile of airfoil and the vortex, is still zero. Hence, a lift is set up on the airfoil as predicted by Eq. 11.21.

(6) When the airfoil comes to rest or changes its angle of attack, new vortices are formed to affect the necessary change in circulation.

The above discussed airfoil with cambering* is known as lifting vane or low drag airfoil. The condition of flow at the trailing edge depends on the magnitude of circulation

$$\Gamma = \pi\, C\, U_0 \sin \alpha_0 \qquad \qquad ...(11.25)$$

where C is the strength of vortex and α_0 is the angle of attack.

Hence, the lift given by Eq. 11.21 modifies to

$$F_L = \rho\, U_0\, L\, \Gamma = (\rho\, U_0\, L)\, (\pi\, C\, U_0 \sin \alpha_0)$$

$$F_L = \rho\, \pi\, C\, L\, U_0^2 \sin \alpha_0 \qquad \qquad ...(11.26)$$

Also

$$C_L = \frac{F_L/A}{\rho\, U_0^2/2} = \frac{\rho\, \pi\, CL\, U_0^2 \sin \alpha_0}{(CL)\, (\rho\, U_0^2/2)}$$

$$C_L = 2\pi \sin \alpha_0 \qquad \qquad ...(11.27)$$

Thus the coefficient of lift for a given airfoil depends on the angle of attack α_0 and the Reynolds number of flow (also see Eq.11.4e). If the angle of attack is small, the flow is not separated at the trailing edge and then C_L depends on Reynolds number only.

2. Variation of coefficient drag and lift

The typical variation of the coefficients of drag and lift, (viz.C_D and C_L) with angle α_0 for an airfoil of infinite length is shown in Fig. 11.17.

---

* Camber line : The centre line of airfoil; camber δ; the maximum distance between camber line and chord. Thus precentage camber is given by 100 δ/c.

The efficiency of an airfoil is usually defined by the ratio of the coefficients of lift and drag, C_L/C_D. The ratio C_L/C_D is found much larger for an airfoil than for a rotating cylinder and, therefore, the airfoil is a much superior lifting device than any other shaped body. Also, as the angle of attack α_0 increases, the lift force produced on the airfoil increases. But at large value of α_0 the flow may separate even at the leading edge and thus reduce its efficiency. This condition of airfoil is known as 'stall' and it is characterised by the highest point on C_L versus α_0 curve. The coefficient curve starts falling after the condition of stall is reached.

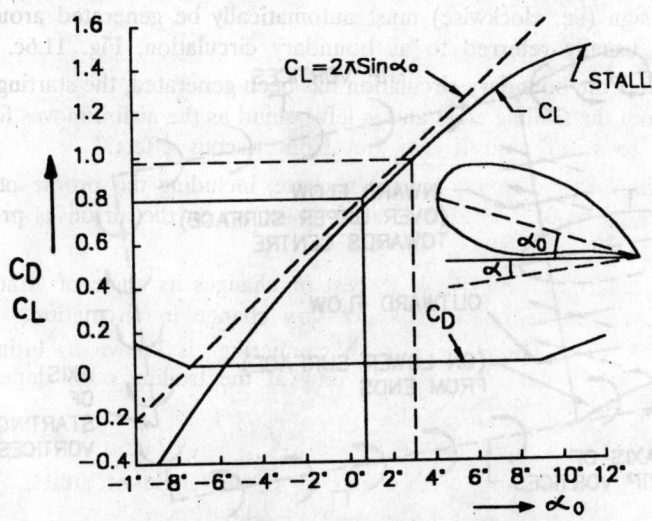

FIG. 11.17. VARIATION OF COEFFICIENTS OF DRAG AND LIFT WITH THE ANGLE OF ATTACK

11.12 FLOW AROUND AN AIRFOIL OF FINITE LENGTH

When the fluid flows about airfoils of finite length, the flow around its two ends affects both lift and drag. Consider an airfoil of finite length L. Let the stream of fluid move past the airfoil with velocity U_0 relative to the airfoil. Since the pressure on the under side of airfoil is greater than that on its top surface, the fluid will escape from below the airfoil at the ends and flow towards the top. This, is turn, distorts the general flow around the airfoil. The fluid moves inwards over the top of the airfoil (towards the centre) and outwards over the bottom (away from the centre) as shown in Fig.11.18. As the streams of fluid merge at the trailing edge, a surface of discontinuity is set up. The inward flow on the top surface and the outward flow at the bottom give rise to the vortices at the ends. A sheet of vortices is developed across the surface of discontinuity. But such a vortex sheet is unstable and hence, the rotary motions contained therein combine to form two large vortices trailing from the two ends of the airfoil. These vortices are known as tip vortices. These are often visible when an airfoil passes through the dust ladden air or when condensation of atmospheric moisture occures on the wings of an aircraft.

It is known from the properties of vortices that their axis can either end at the solid boundaries or it should extend upto infinity or it should form a closed path. The theorem of Lord Kelvin still holds good because the tip vortices are of equal and opposite magnitude; that means the circulation about the closed path should add upto zero. Indeed, the closed path comprises the axis of the airfoil, axis of the tip vortices and axis of starting vortex at the trailing edge (see Fig.11.18). The circulation around this large closed path adds upto zero. Of course, in real fluid, the circulation persists only about

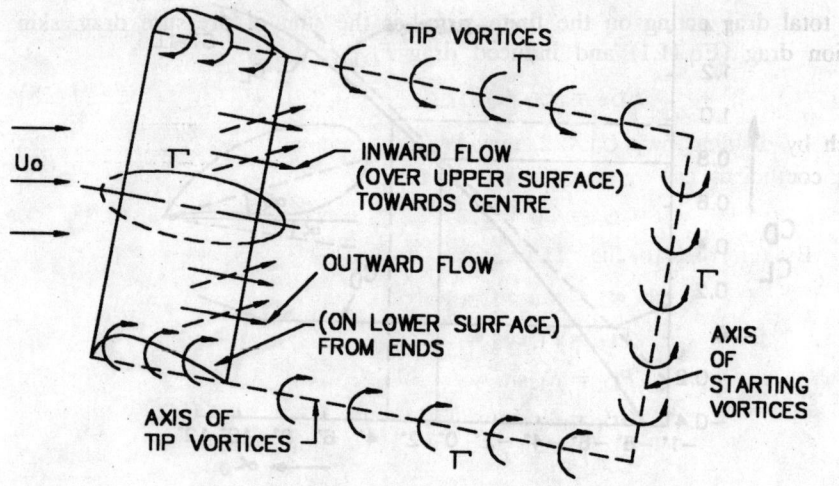

FIG. 11.18. FLOW AROUND AN AIRFOIL FINITE SIZE

the airfoil and the portions of tip vortices soon die out due to visous action.

The tip vortices introduce a velocity in the downward direction to the mainflow; see Fig. 11.19. It is known as 'downwash velocity.' Thus, the velocity of main flow modifies to U_e, which will be the vectorial sum of free stream velocity U_0 and downwash velocity U_i. The angle of attack α_0 also changes to α ($= \alpha - \alpha_1$); which is the angle subtended by the chord of the airfoil with the resultant velocity U_e. The flow around finite airfoil may now be analysed as an infinite airfoil which moves in a fluid stream moving with velocity U_e; the angle of attack being taken as α_0.

The lift force F_L acting on the airfoil of infinite span (normal to the resultant velocity U_e should be resolved into two components, one in the direction of U_0 and is known as induced drag F_{Di} and the other normal to the velocity U_0 and is known as the lift force F_{Le} acting on the finite airfoil.

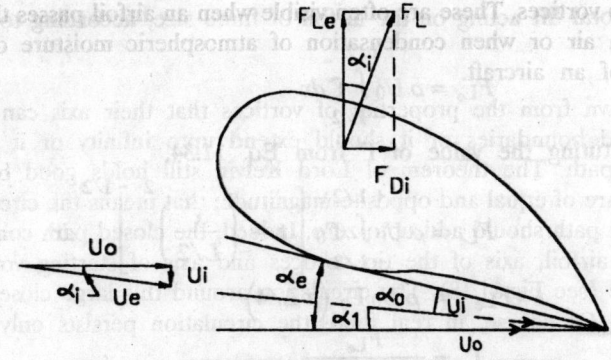

FIG. 11.19. INDUCED DRAG ON THE AIRFOIL

The total drag acting on the finite airfoil is the sum of pressure drag, skin friction drag (Eq.11.1) and induced drag F_{Di} ,

$$F_{De} = F_D + F_{Di} \qquad ...(11.28)$$

which by dividing by $\rho U_0^2 A/2$, may be expressed in terms of dimensionless drag coefficient as

$$C_{De} = C_D + C_{D1} \qquad ...(11.29)$$

By referring to Fig. 11.19, since $\propto_1$ is a small angle,

$$\sin \propto_1 \approx \tan \propto_1 \approx \propto_1 \text{ and } \cos \propto_1 \approx 1$$

$$F_{L0} = F_L \cos \propto_1 \approx F_L \qquad ...(11.30)$$

$$F_{D1} = F_L \sin \propto_1 \approx F_L \propto_1 \qquad ...(11.31)$$

$$\therefore \qquad C_{D1} = U_e \sin \propto_1 \approx U_e \propto_1 \qquad ...(11.32)$$

Also $$U_0 = U_e \, Sin \, \alpha_1 \approx U_e \, \alpha_1 \qquad ...(11.33)$$

Prandtl found the distribution of circulation over the airfoil of span L as semi-elliptical with a maximum value Γ_0 at the centre of the span and reducing to zero at the two ends, Fig.11.20. According to Kutta-Joukowski's theorem, Eq. 11.21, the lift is directly proportional to the length of the airfoil, hence, the distribution of lift across the span is also elliptical. The circulation at distance x from the centre of span of airfoil is given by

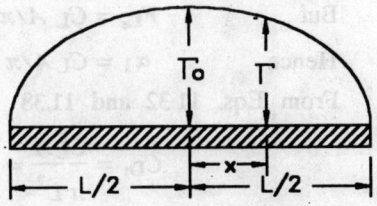

FIG. 11.20. VARIATION OF CIRCULATION ALONG THE SPAN OF AIRFOIL

$$\Gamma = \Gamma_0 \left[1 - \left(\frac{x}{L/2} \right)^2 \right]^{1/2} \qquad ...(11.34)$$

The total lift acting on the airfoil of finite size, according to Eq. 11.21,

$$F_{L_e} = \rho U_0 \int_{-L/2}^{L/2} \Gamma \, dx$$

Substituting the value of Γ from Eq. 11.34,

$$F_{L_e} = \rho U_0 \int_{-L/2}^{+L/2} \Gamma_0 \left[1 - \left(\frac{x}{L/2} \right)^2 \right]^{1/2} dx$$

$$F_{L_e} = \rho U_0 \Gamma_e \left(\pi L/4 \right)$$

$$\Gamma_e = \frac{F_{L_e}}{\rho U_0 \pi L/4} \qquad \qquad ...(11.35)$$

The circulation around an airfoil is the product of the velocity and the length of the path along the closed curve. Prandtl found that the circulation Γ_0 of the boundary vortex at the centre remains constant and is given by

$$\Gamma_0 = 2 L U_1$$

or

$$U_1 = \Gamma_0 / 2L \qquad \qquad ...(11.36)$$

From Eqs. 11.35 and 11.36,

$$U_1 = \frac{F_{L_e}}{(\rho U_0 \pi L/4) \, 2L} = 2 \frac{F_{L_e}}{\pi \rho U_0 L^2} \qquad \qquad ...(11.37)$$

The angle $\propto_1$ between U_0 and U_1 is given by

$$\propto_1 = U_1 / U_0$$

Substituting the value of U_1 from Eq. 11.37.

$$\propto_1 = \frac{F_{L_0}}{\pi \, (\rho \, U_0^2 / 2) \, L^2}$$

But

$$F_{L_e} = C_L \, A / \pi \, L^2 \qquad \qquad ...(11.38)$$

Hence

$$\propto_1 = C_L A / \pi \, L^2 \qquad \qquad ...(11.38)$$

From Eqs. 11.32 and 11.38

$$C_{D_1} = \frac{C_L^2 A}{\pi \, L^2} = \frac{C_L^2}{\pi \, L^2 / A} \qquad \qquad ...(11.39)$$

The ratio L^2/A is known as the aspect ratio (AR). The Eq. 11.39 shows that the induced drag is inversely proportional to the aspect ratio; becoming zero for infinity aspect ratio and increasing as the span and aspect ratio decreases. The practical significance of these expressions, Eqs. 11.38 and 11.39, lies in corelating the experimental data obtained for finite span airfoils.

11.13 POLAR DIAGRAM

A number of tests are conducted on the airfoils in a wind tunnel and a large number of experimental data are collected for lift and drag. The results of such tests may be presented graphically as a plot between lift and drag versus angle of attack. Since the efficiency of the airfoil is measured by the

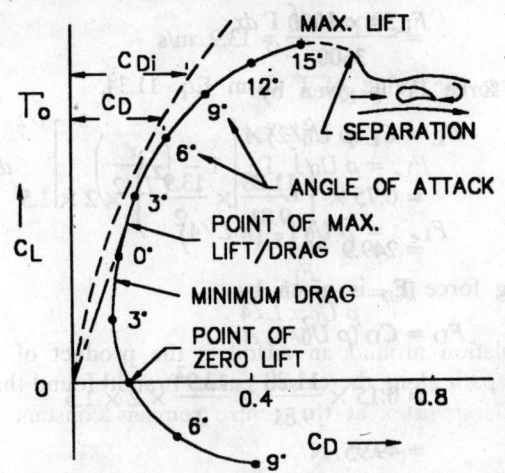

FIG. 11.21. POLAR DIAGRAM FOR THE AIRFOIL OF FINITE SPAN

ratio of lift to drag, generally the coefficients of lift and drag are plotted against angle of attack. Prandtl plotted these three parameters on a single curve which is known as a *polar diagram* C_L on vertical axis, C_D on horizontal axis with $\propto_0$ as third parameter (Fig.11.21). On this diagram, the coefficient of induceddrag C_{Di} is also plotted.

The ratio of lift to drag is simply the slope of the line from the origin to the requisite point on the curve(corresponding to the given angle of attack). The maximum ratio of C_L /C_D is obtained when the line from origin is tangential to the curve. The curve also indicates the point of minimum drag and of zero lift. The lift is seen to increase with the angle of attack upto a certain point, which is known as 'point of stall'; thereafter, the lift decreases with increase in the angle of attack. Beyond the point of stall, the boundary layer along the upper surface separates and a large turbulent wake is formed. This increases the pressure on the upper surface, thereby reducing the lift acting on the airfoil.

The diagram also shows the coefficient of induced drag C_{Di} being plotted against angle of attack α_0 for a given aspect ratio. As the aspect ratio increases the curve moves closer to the vertical axis and correspondingly total drag is reduced.

Examples 11.1-10.19

11.1 A flat plate, 2 m long and 1.5 m wide, moves at 50 km/h in stationary air of specific weight 11.28 N/m³. If the coefficients of drag and lift are 0.15 and 0.75 respectively; determine (a) lift force (b) drag force (c) resultant force and (d) the power required to keep the plate in motion.

Solution

The velocity of the flat plate relative to the air, U_o

$$= \frac{50 \times 1000}{3600} = 13.9 \text{ m/s}$$

(a) The lift force F_L is given by

$$F_L = C_L \,(\rho \, U_0^2/2) \, A$$

$$= 0.75 \times \left(\frac{11.28}{9.81} \times \frac{13.9^2}{2} \right) \times 2 \times 1.5$$

$$= 249.9 \text{ N}$$

(b) The drag force F_D is given by

$$F_D = C_D \,(\rho \, U_0^2/2) \, A$$

$$= 0.15 \times \frac{11.28}{9.81} \times \frac{13.9^2}{2} \times 2 \times 1.5$$

$$= 49.95 \text{ N}$$

(c) Resultant force $F = \sqrt{F_D^2 + F_L^2}$

$$= \sqrt{(249.9)^2 + (49.95)^2}$$

$$= 254.84 \text{ N}$$

(d) Power required to drive the plate through the air

$$= F_D \times U_0/1000 \text{ kW}$$

$$= \frac{49.95 \times 13.95}{1000} kW$$

$$= 0.697 \text{ kW}$$

11.2 A kite weighing 10 N and having an area of 1 m^2 makes an angle of 10^0 to the horizontal when flying in a wind of 36 km/h. If the kite is held by a cord, in which the tension is 50 N, and the cord makes an angle of 45^0 to the horizonal, calculate the drag and lift coefficients. Assume specific weight of air as 12.0 N/m^3.

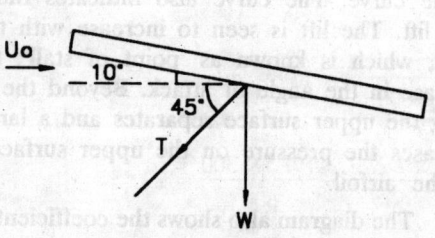

FIG. 11.22. EXAMPLE 11.2

Solution

(a) Resolving the forces in the direction of motion of wind,

$$F_D - T \cos 45° = 0$$

or
$$F_D = T \cos 45°. \qquad ...(i)$$

From Eq. 11.3c

$$T \cos 45° = C_D A \rho \, U_0^2/2$$

$$C_D = \frac{T \cos 45°}{A \rho U_0^2/2}$$

Since
$$U_0 = \frac{36 \times 1000}{3600}$$
$$= 10 \text{ m/s}$$

$$C_D = \frac{50 \times 1 \sqrt{2}}{1 \times 12/9.81 \times (10)^2/2} = 0.578$$

(b) Similarly, resolving the forces in the normal direction to the motion,

$$F_L - T \sin 45° - W = 0$$
$$F_L = 50 \sin 45° + 10$$
$$= 35.36 + 10 = 45.46 \text{ N}$$

Also,
$$F_L = C_L A \rho U_0^2/2$$

or
$$C_L = \frac{F_L/A}{\rho U_0^2/2}$$

$$= \frac{45.46/1}{12.09/9.81 \times (10)^2/2} = 0.743$$

11.3 Two 10 m long rotors, each 1.5m in diameter, are used to propel a ship. Estimate the longitudinal force exerted upon the rotors when the relative wind velocity is 50 km/h (as shown in Fig. 11.23) and the rotors are required to rotate at 300 rpm in the clockwise direction.

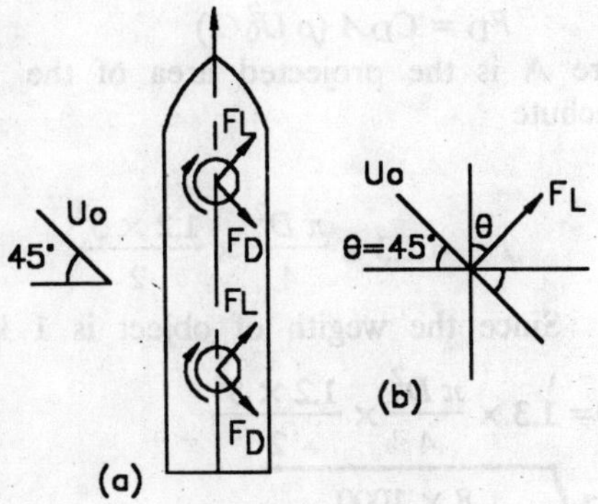

Solution

$U_0 = 50$ km/h

$= \dfrac{50 \times 1000}{3600} = 13.89$ m/s

FIG. 11.23. EXMPLE 11.3

$U_c = \dfrac{\pi DN}{60} = \dfrac{\pi \times 1.5 \times 300}{60} = 23.55$

m/s

$$\frac{U_c}{U_0} = \frac{23.55}{13.89} = 1.695$$

From Fig. 11.15, $C_D = 1.5$ and $C_L = 4.2$

$$F_L = C_L A \rho U_0^2/2 = C_L (LD) \rho U_0^2/2$$
$$= 4.2 \times 10 \times 1.5 \times 1.2 \times (13.89)^2/2 \text{ N}$$
$$= 7292.8 \text{ N}$$

$$F_D = C_D (LD) \rho U_0^2/2 = C_D F_L/C_L$$
$$= (1.5/4.2) \times 7292.8$$
$$= 2604.5 \text{ N}$$

Force required in the direction of motion

$$F = 2 [F_L \cos \theta - F_D \sin \theta]$$
$$F = 2 [F_L \cos 45° - F_D \sin 45°]$$
$$= 2 [7292.8 - 2604.5] \times 1 \sqrt{2}$$
$$= 6629.2 \text{ N}$$

11.4 Calculate the diameter of a parachute to be used for dropping an object weighing 1 kN so that maximum terminal velocity of dropping is 5 m/s. The drag coefficient for the parachute, treated as hemispherical, is 1.3. The mass density of air is 1.2 kg/m³

Solution

The parachute is treated as hemisphere, therefore,

$$F_D = C_D A (\rho U_0^2/2)$$

where A is the projected area of the parachute

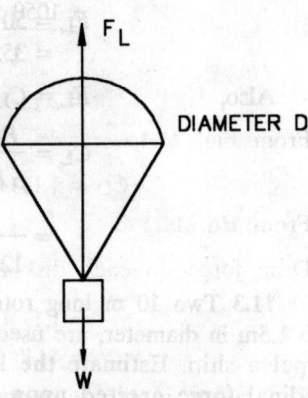

FIG. 11.24. EXAMPLE 11.4

$$F_D = 1.3 \times \frac{\pi D^2}{4} \times \frac{1.2 \times 5^2}{2}$$

Since the wegith of object is 1 kN or 1000 N, hence

$$1000 = 1.3 \times \frac{\pi D^2}{4} \times \frac{1.2 \times 5^2}{2}$$

$$D = \sqrt{\frac{8 \times 1000}{1.3 \pi \times 1.2 \times 25}} = 8.08$$

m

11.5 A mixing device consists of two circular disks, 10 cm in diameter mounted at the ends of a 1 m long horizontal rod. The rod is hung at the centre and rotates at 60 rpm. Determine the power of the motor required to rotate the mixer. Assume ρ for the fluid as 1050 kg/m³ and μ as 1.2×10^{-3} kg/m s.

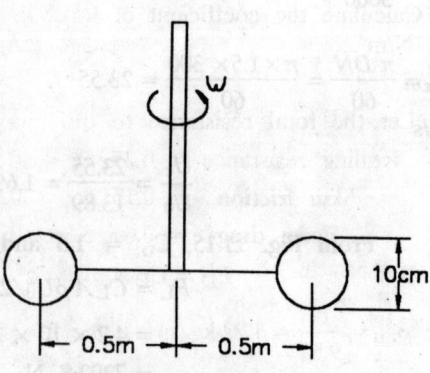

FIG. 11.25 EXAMPLE 11.5

Neglect the resistance of the rods supporting the disks.

Solution

The tangential velocity of rotation U_t is given as

$$U_t = \frac{2\pi Nr}{60} = \frac{2\pi \times 60}{60} \times 0.5$$

$$= 3.14 \text{ m/s}$$

Therefore

$$R_e = \rho U_t D/\mu, \text{ where D-diameter of disk}$$

$$= \frac{1050 \times 3.14 \times 0.10}{1.2 \times 10^{-3}}$$

$$= 2.75 \times 10^5$$

From Fig. 11.4,

$$C_D = 1.1 \text{ for } R_e \text{ equal to } 2.75 \times 10^5$$

From Eq. 11.3 c

Drag force on each disk $F_D = C_D A \rho U_t^2/2$

$$= 1.1. \times \pi/4 . (0.1)^2 \times 1050 \times 3.14^2/2$$

$$= 44.7 \text{ N}$$

The power required to derive the mixer

$$= F_D \times U_t \text{ watts}$$

$$= \frac{44.7 \times 3.14}{1000} kW$$

$$= 0.14 \text{ kW}$$

11.6 A truck having a projected area of 6.5 m² travelling at 80 km/h experiences a total resistance of 2 kN. Out of this, 25% is due to rolling friction, 15% due to surface friction and the remaining 60% due to form drag. Calculate the coefficient of form drag. Assume specific weight of air as 12 N/m³.

Solution

Let the total resistance to the motion of the truck be R.

Rolling resistance = 0.25 R = 0.5 kN

Skin friction = 0.15 R = 0.3 kN

Form drag = 0.6 R = 1.2 kN

But $F_D = C_D A \rho U_0^2/2$

where $\rho_{air} = \dfrac{12}{9.81} = 1.22 \text{ kg/m}^3$, and $U_0 = \dfrac{80 \times 1000}{3600} = 22.2 \text{ m/s}$

$$F_D = 1.2 \times 1000 = C_D \times 6.5 \times 1.22 \times (22.2)^2/2$$

$$C_D = \frac{1200 \times 2}{6.5 \times 1.22 \times (22.2)^2} = 0.163$$

11.7 A jet plane, which weighs 30 kN and has a wing area of 20 m², flies at a velocity of 250 km/h. When the engine delivers 8000 kW, 65% power is used to overcome the drag resistance of the wing. Calculate the coefficient of drag and lift for the wing. Assume specific weight of air as 12 N/m³.

Solution

(a) When the jet plane is flying, the lift force must equal its weight.

$$F_L = W = C_L A (\rho \, U_0^2/2)$$

$$U_0 = \frac{250 \times 1000}{3600} = 264 \text{ m/s}$$

$$\rho = 12/9.81 = 1.22 \text{ kg/m}^3$$

$$C_L = \frac{30 \times 1000}{20 \times 1.22 \times 264^2/2}$$

$$= 0.035$$

(b) The engine has to overcome the resistance to its motion, therefore,

Power needed = $F_D \times U_o$

Since, the efficiency of transmission is 65%

Power to be generated = ($F_D \, U_o/0.65$)

$$F_D = \frac{0.65 \times 8000 \times 1000}{264} \text{ N}$$

$$= 19.696 \text{ kN}$$

(c) $\qquad F_D = C_D A \rho \, U_0^2/2$ ...(i)

$\qquad\qquad F_L = C_L A \rho \, U_0^2/2$ ...(ii)

Dividing Eq. (i) by (ii)

$$C_D = C_L F_D/F_L = 0.035 \times 19.696/30$$

$$= 0.023$$

11.8 A ping pong ball weighing 0.025 N and having a diameter of 3.5 cm is served in such a manner that it moves over the net in a horizontal direction with a velocity of 15 m/s and a forward spin of 90 revolutions/second. Determine the instantaneous magnitude and direction of its acceleration.

Solution

The circulatory velocity U_c is given by

$$U_c = \omega \, r = 2 \pi N r$$

$$= 2 \pi \times 90 \times 1.75/100 = 9.89 \text{m/s}$$

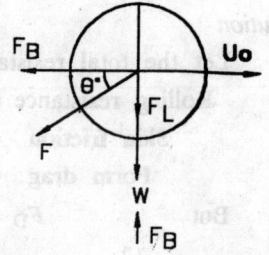

FIG. 11.26. EXAMPLE 11.8

Hence $U_e/U_0 = 9.89/15 = 0.66$

The values of C_D and C_L are read from Fig. 11.15,

$C_D = 1.0$ and $C_L = 0.8$

$F_L = C_L A \rho U_0^2 = 0.8 \times \pi/4 (3.5/100)^2 \times 1.15 \times 15^2/2 = 0.09953$ N

$F_D = C_D F_L/C_L = 1.0 \times 0.09953/0.8 = 0.1244$ N

Therefore, required upward force $= F_B + F_1$

$$F_1 = 0.025 + 0.09953 = 0.1245 \text{N}$$

$$F = \sqrt{F_D^2 + F_1^2} = 0.1593 \text{N}$$

$$\theta = \tan^{-1} F_1/F_D$$

$$= \tan^{-1} (0.1245/0.1244) = 45°$$

The acceleration a of the ball is given by

$$a = \frac{F}{W/g}$$

$$= -\frac{0.1593}{0.025/9.81}$$

$$= 62.5 \text{ m/s/s}$$

11.9 A cylinder whose axis is perpendicular to the stream of air having a velocity of 20 m/s, rotates at 300 rpm. The cylinder is 2 m in diameter and 10 m long. Find (a) the circulation (b) theoretical lift per unit length (c) position of stagnation points and (d) the actual lift, drag and the direction of resultant force. Assume $U_c/U_o = 15.7$, $C_L = 3.4$ and $C_D = 0.65$

Solution

$$U_e = \frac{\pi D N}{60} = \frac{3.14 \times 2 \times 300}{60} = 31.4 \text{ m/s}$$

Hence $U_c/U_o = 31.4/20 = 1.57$

(a) Circulation $\Gamma = 2\pi r U_c$

$$= 2 \times 3.14 \times 2/2 \times 31.4$$

$$= 197.2 \text{ m}^2/\text{s}$$

(b) Theoretional life $F_L = \rho U_e L \Gamma$

$$= 1.2 \times 31.4 \times 10 \times 197.2 \text{N}$$

$$= 74.3 \text{ kN}$$

(c) At the location of stagnation, the velocity u = 0

From Eq. 11.18,

$$u = 2 U_0 \sin\theta + U_c$$

or $u/U_0 = 2 \sin\theta + (U_c/U_0) = 0$

$$\sin\theta = -U_c/2 U_0 = -\frac{1}{2} \times 1.57$$

$$\theta = (180 + 51° 42')$$
$$= 231° 42'$$

(d) Actual lift $F_L = C_L A \rho\, U_0^2/2 = C_L\,(L \times D)\,\rho\, U_0^2/2$

$$= 3.4\,(2 \times 10) \times 1.2 \times (20)^2/2\,N$$
$$= 16.32\ kN$$

Actual drag $\quad F_D = C_D A \rho\, U_0^2 = C_D F_L/C_L$

$$= \frac{0.65}{3.40} \times 16.32$$
$$= 3.12\ kN$$

The resultant force $\quad F = \sqrt{F_D^2 + F_L^2}$

$$\tan\theta = F_L/F_D \text{ with horizontal}$$
$$= 16.32/3.12 = 5.23$$
$$\theta = 79.17°$$

11.10 A $1/20^{th}$ model of an aeroplane wing was tested in a wind tunnel at 400 m/s and mass density of air is 5.2 kg/m^3. The total drag measured was 320 N. If the wind tunnel data refer to an infinite span of the wing, compute the total drag for the full size wing of aeroplane which has a span of 10 m and chord length of 2. m. The aeroplane needs 40 kN of lift force to fly at 360 km/h in the air. The air mass density is 1.2 kg/m^3 and circulation around the wing is assumed as elliptical.

Solution

For model : $\quad C_D = \dfrac{F_D/A}{0.5\,\rho\, U_0^2}$

$$= \frac{320/A_m}{0.5 \times 5.2 \times (400)^2}$$

The area of model $\quad A_m = A_p L_r^2 = 10 \times 2 \times (1/20)^2$

$$= 1/20\ m^2$$

$$C_D = \frac{320}{0.5 \times 5.2 \times (400)^2 \times (1/20)} = 0.015$$

For prototype : $U_0 = \dfrac{360 \times 1000}{36000} = 100$ m/s

$$C_L = \frac{F_L/A}{0.5\,\rho\, U_0^2} = \frac{40 \times 1000/(10 \times 2)}{0.5 \times 1.2 \times (100)^2}$$
$$= 0.33$$

From Eq. 11.39

$$C_{D1} = C_L^2/\pi\ (\text{aspect ratio}) = C_L/\pi\ (L/C)$$

$$= \frac{(6.33)^2}{\pi \times (10/2)} = 0.0069$$

Total drag for full size wing $= F_{D_t}$

$$= C_{D_t} A \rho \, U_0^2/2$$

Here $\qquad C_{D_t} = C_D + C_{D_i}$

$$= 0.015 + 0.0069 = 0.0219$$

$$F_{D_t} = 0.0219 \times (10 \times 2) \times 1.2 \times (100)^2/2$$

$$= 2628 \text{ N}$$

11.11 An aeroplane weighs 24 kN and has an area of 35 m². If the coefficient of lift varies linearly from 0.3 to 0.8 while the angle of attack varies from 0^0 to 8^0, calculate the angle of attack for the aeroplane speed of 150 km/h. Assume $\rho = 1.1 \, kg/m^3$

Solution

Since the weight of aeroplane should be balanced by the lift force,

$$F_L = W = C_L A \rho \, U_0^2/2$$

(Since $\qquad U_0 = \dfrac{150 \times 1000}{3600} = 41.66$ m/s)

or $\qquad 24 \times 1000 = C_L \times 35 \times 1.1 \times 41.66^2/2$

$$C_L = \frac{24000 \times 2}{35 \times 1.1 \times 41.66^2}$$

$$C_L = 0.717$$

Since C_L changes by 0.5 for 8° change in α_0;

Therfore, α_0 by interpolation ,

$$\alpha_0 = 6.67°$$

11.12 Electric transmission towers, 10 m high, are fixed 400m apart to support 10 cables, each of 2 cm diameter. Determine the moment acting at the base of each tower when a wind flows with a velocity of 100 km/h. Assume $\rho_{air} = 1.2$ kg/m³ and μ(air) $= 1.6 \times 10^{-5}$ kg/ms. Also calculate the frequency of vortex shedding.

Solution

$$F_D = C_D A \rho \, U_0^2/2$$

$$R_e = \rho \, U_0 D/\mu$$

(Since $\qquad U_0 = 100 \times 1000/36 = 27.7$m/s)

$$R_e = \frac{1.2 \times 27.7 \times 0.02}{1.6 \times 10^{-5}}$$

$$= 4.1 \times 10^3$$

From Fig 11.7 $C_D = 0.95$ and $A = L \times D = 400 \times 0.02$ m²

Therefore, the drag on each wire 400 m long is

$$F_D = 0.95 \times (400 \times 0.02) \times 1.2 \times 27.7^2/2 \text{ N}$$
$$= 3.5 \text{ kN}$$

Moment at the base $= F_D \times 10/2$
$$= 3500 \times 5 \text{ N m}$$
$$= 17.5 \text{ kN m}$$

The frequency of vorteex shedding is given by, Eq. 11.13, and $R_0 < 10^5$

$$f = 0.198 \frac{U_0}{D} \left(1 - \frac{19.7}{R_e}\right)$$

$$= 0.198 \times \frac{27.7}{0.02} \left(1 - \frac{19.7}{4.15 \times 10^3}\right)$$

$$= 272.9 \text{ Hz}$$

11.13 In a meteorological laboratory an experimental balloon, weight 100 N and filled with gas of mass density 0.2 kg/m^3, is used to collect observations at higher attitude. If the ballon is desired to rise at a terminal velocity of 0.15 m/s. What should be the diameter of balloon. Use $\rho_{air} = 1.21 \text{ kg/m}^3$ and $\nu_{air} = 1.5 \times 10^{-5} \text{ m}^2/\text{s}$.

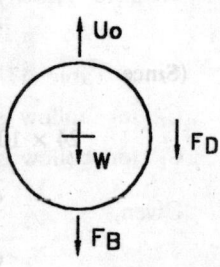

FIG.11.27. EXAMPLE 11.13

Solution

When balloon is rising,

Buoyant force – Weight = Drag force

$$(\rho_a - \rho_g) \times g \frac{\pi D^3}{6} - 100 = C_D . A \frac{\rho_a U_0^2}{2}$$

Assuming $C_D = 0.2$ for spherical bodies for Re $\geq 25 \times 10^5$ (See Fig. 11.4)

$$9.81 (1.21 - 0.22) \frac{\pi D_1^3}{6} - 0.2 \times \frac{\pi D^2}{4} \times 1.2 \times \frac{(1.5)^2}{2} = 100$$

$$5.0826 D^3 - 0.21195 D^2 = 100$$

Solving by trial

$$D = 2.712 \text{ m}$$

$$\text{Re} = UD/\nu$$

$$= \frac{1.5 \times 2.712}{1.5 \times 10^{-5}} = 2.712 \times 10^5 > 2.5 \times 10^5$$

Hence, the assumed $C_D = 0.2$ is correct

Diameter of balloon required = 2.712 m.

11.14 A cup anemometer consists of two hemispherical cups of 100 mm diameter mounted in opposite directions on a horizontal rod (Fig. 11.28) which rotates about a vertical axis at midway. (a) Calculate the speed of rotation of anemometer in a wind of 45 km/hr. (b) what is the torque required at cups to make them stationary in a wind of 45 km/hr.

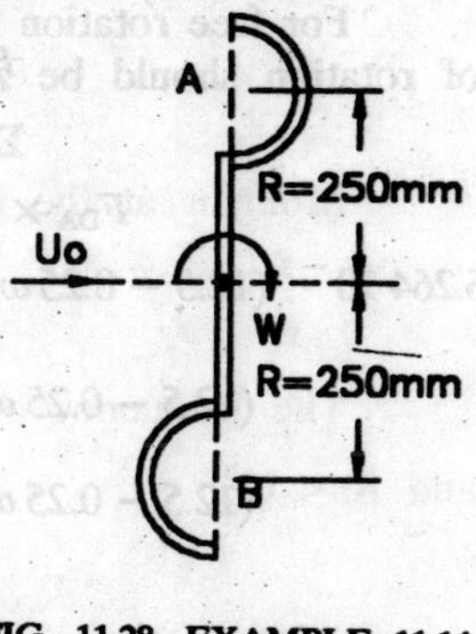

Given $\rho_a = 1.2$ kg/m^3

Solution

Let ω be the speed of rotation of anemometer and U_0 be the wind velocity

FIG. 11.28. EXAMPLE 11.14

Assuming no friction at the bearings and for constant ω.

Relative velocity U_{rA} of concave cup, $A = (U_0 - \omega R)$

Relative velocity U_{rB} of convex cup B,

$$\doteqdot (U_0 + \omega R)$$

From Table 11.1,

C_D for hollow sphere upstream $= 1.33$

C_D for hollow sphere. downstream $= 0.34$

Given, $$U_0 = \frac{45 \times 1000}{3600} = 12.5 \text{ m/s}$$

$$D = 0.1 \text{ m and } R = 0.25 \text{ m}$$

Then $$F_{DA} = \frac{C_D \times A \times \rho \, U_{rA}^2}{2}$$

$$= 1.33 \times \frac{\pi}{4}(0.1)^2 \times 1.2 \frac{(12.5 - 0.25\,\omega)^2}{2}$$

$$= 6.264 \times 10^{-3}(12.5 - 0.25\,\omega)^2$$

$$F_{DB} = C_{DB} A \rho \frac{U_{rB}^2}{2}$$

$$F_{DB} = 0.34 \frac{\pi}{4}(0.1)^2 1.2 \frac{(12.5 + 0.25\,\omega)^2}{2}$$

$$= 1.601 \times 10^{-3}(12.5 + 0.25\,\omega)^2$$

$$F_{DB} = C_{DB} A \rho \frac{U_{rB}^2}{2}$$

$$F_{DB} = 0.34 \frac{\pi}{4}(0.1)^2 \times 1.2 \frac{(12.5 + 0.25\,\omega)^2}{2}$$

$$= 1.601 \, 10^{-3}(12.5 + 0.25\,\omega)^2$$

For free rotation of anemometer, the net torque about the vertical axis of rotation should be zero.

$$\Sigma T = 0$$

$$F_{DA} \times R = F_{DB} \times R$$

$$6.264 \ 10^{-3} (12.5 - 0.25 \, \omega)^2 = 1.601 \times 10^{-3} (12.5 + 0.25 \, \omega)^2$$

$$(12.5 - 0.25 \, \omega) = \left(\frac{1.601}{6.264}\right)^{1/2} (12.5 + 0.25 \, \omega)$$

$$(12.5 - 0.25 \, \omega) = 0.506 \, (12.5 + 0.25 \, \omega)$$

$$\omega = \frac{12.5 \, (1 - 0.506)}{1.25 \times 0.25} = 19.76 \text{ rad /s}$$

Also

$$\omega = \frac{2 \pi N}{60}$$

$$N = \frac{60 \, \omega}{2 \pi} = \frac{60 \times 19.76}{2 \times \pi}$$

Rotational speed $= 188.79$ r.p.m.

(b) To make cups stationary,

Torque at cup A about vertical axis $= F_{DA} \times R$

Torque at cup B about vertical axis $= F_{DB} \times R$

Net° torque required at cups

$$= (F_{DA} \, R - F_{DB} \times R)$$

$$= R \left[C_{DA} A \frac{\rho}{2} U_{rA}^2 - C_{DB} A \frac{\rho \, U_{RB}^2}{2} \right]$$

Since the cups are made stationary and both set of cups are exposed to same wind velocity of 12.5 m/s. (= 45 km/hr)

∴ $\quad U_{RA} = U_{RB} = 12.5$ m/s

∴ Torque required $= RA \dfrac{\rho \, U_0^2}{2} (C_{DA} - C_{DB})$

$$= 0.25 \times \frac{\pi}{4} (0.1)^2 \frac{1.2 \times 12.5^2}{2} (1.3 - 0.34)$$

$$= 0.1766 \text{ Nm.}$$

11.15 A car has a projected area of 2.0 m² and can travel at a maximum speed of 120 km/hr. Calculate the power required to overcome the air resistance, assuming C_D for car $= 0.4$ If a new streamlined model of car is to be manufactured with same power of engine and having $C_D = 0.35$, how much increase in speed of car is expected. Use $\rho_{air} = 1.2$ kg/m³.

Solution

Velocity $\quad\quad U_{01} = 120$ km/hr.

$$= \frac{120 \times 1000}{3600} = 33.33 \text{m/s}$$

(a) Drag force $F_D = \dfrac{C_D \times A . \rho\, U_0^2}{2}$

$$= 0.4 \times 2 \times \frac{1.2 \times (33.33)^2}{2}$$

$$= 533.23 \text{ N}$$

Power required $= F_D \times U_0$

$$= 533.23 \times 33.33 \text{ N m/s}$$

$$= 17.77 \text{ kW}$$

(b) Power of new car $= F_D \times U_0$

$$= C_D . A \rho \frac{U_0^2}{2} \times U_0 = C_D A \rho \frac{U_0^3}{2}$$

$$17.77 \times 1000 = 0.35 \times 2 \times 1.2 \times \frac{U_0^3}{2}$$

$$U_0^3 = \frac{17770 \times 2}{0.35 \times 2 \times 1.2} = 42309.5$$

$$U_0 = 34.87 \text{ m/s} = 125.53 \text{ km/hr}$$

% increase in speed $= \dfrac{(34.87 - 33.33)}{33.33} \times 100$

$$= 4.6 \text{ \%}$$

11.16 An aircraft weighing 1000 kN when empty has a wing area of 226 m². It is to take off at a velocity of 300 km/hr. and a 20° angle of attack. Determine the allowable weight of cargo and power required. Assume $\rho_{air} = 1.2$ kg/m³ and $C_L = 1.42$ for the wing inclined at 20° angle and $C_D = 0.17$

Solution

$$U_0 = 300 \text{ km/hr}$$

$$= \frac{300 \times 1000}{3600} = 83.33 \text{ m/s}$$

Lift force $F_L = C_L A \rho \dfrac{U_0^2}{2}$

$$= 1.42 \times 226 \times \frac{1.2 \times (83.33)^2}{2} \text{ N}$$

$$= 1337.06 \text{ kN}$$

Allowable weight of cargo $= F_L - $ Wt of aircraft

$$= 1337.06 - 1000$$

$$= 337.06 \text{ kN}$$

Drag force $F_D = C_D A \rho \dfrac{U_0^2}{2}$

$$= 0.17 \times 226 \times \frac{1.2 \times (83.33)^2}{2}$$

$$= 160.07 \text{ kN}$$

Power reqd. for engine $= F_D \times U_0$

$$= 160.07 \times 83.33$$

$$= 13338.7 \text{ kW.}$$

11.17 A light aeroplane has wing of span 9 m and chord length 1.5m. It experiences a lift force of 27 kN while moving horizontally in air at 200 km/hr. If lift drag ratio is assumed as 9, (a) what should be the coefficients of lift and drag and (b) the power required to derive the plane.

Solution

$$U_0 = 200 \text{ km/hr}$$

$$= \frac{200 \times 1000}{3600} = 55.56 \text{ m/s}$$

$$F_L = C_L A \rho \frac{U_0^2}{2} = 27 \times 1000 \qquad \text{...(i)}$$

$$F_D = C_D A \rho \frac{U_0^2}{2} \qquad \text{...(ii)}$$

$$\frac{F_L}{F_D} = \frac{27000}{C_D \times (9 \times 1.5) \times \dfrac{(1.2 \times 55.56^2)}{2}} = 9 \qquad \text{(Given)}$$

$$C_D = \frac{27000}{9 \times (9 \times 1.5) \dfrac{(1.2 \times 55.56^2)}{2}} = 0.12$$

From Eqs. (i) and (ii)

$$\frac{F_L}{F_D} = \frac{C_L A \rho \dfrac{U_0^2}{2}}{C_D A \rho \dfrac{U_0^2}{2}}$$

$$9 = \frac{C_L}{C_D}$$

$$C_L = 9 \times 0.12 = 1.08$$

Also $\dfrac{F_L}{F_D} = 9$

$$F_D = \frac{F_L}{9} = \frac{27 \times 1000}{9}$$

$$F_D = 3000 \text{ N}$$

Power required $= F_D \times U_0$

$$= 3000 \times 55.56 \frac{N\,m}{s} \text{ or } W$$

$$= 166.68 \text{ kW.}$$

11.18 An aeroplane has wings, span 8 m and chord length 1.25 m and weighs 10 kN. Assuming that it has characteristics as shown in Fig. 11.21 (a) determine the angle of attack for take off speed of 150 km/hr. (b) Also determine the stall speed   Take $\rho_{air} = 1.2$ kg/m^3

Solution

$$U_0 = 150 \text{ km/hr}$$

$$= \frac{150 \times 1000}{3600} = 41.67 \text{ m/s}$$

(a)

$$F_L = C_L . A \frac{\rho\, U_0^2}{2} = W$$

$$10 \times 1000 = C_L \times 8 \times 1.25 \times \frac{1.2 \times 41.67^2}{2}$$

$$C_L = 0.956$$

Aspect ratio $\qquad = \dfrac{L}{C}$

$$= \frac{8}{1.25} = 6.4$$

For aspect ratio of 6.4, and $C_L = 0.956$, read corresponding α_0 from diagram between C_L vs. α_0 (See. Fig. 11.17)

$$\alpha_0 = 10°$$

Alternatively, from Eq. 11.27,

$$C_L = 2\pi\, Sin\, \alpha_0$$

$$\alpha = Sin^{-1}\left(\frac{C_L}{2\pi}\right)$$

$$= \sin^{-1}\left(\frac{0.956}{2\pi}\right) = 8.76°$$

(b) It is seen from Fig. 11.21, that maximum lift occurs corresponding to $C_L = 1.3$ and thereafter "stall" occurs or lift starts decreasing as α increases.

Let U_0 be the stall speed,

From Eq. (i)

$$10,000 = 1.3 \times (8 \times 1.25) \times \frac{(1.2 \times U_0^2)}{2}$$

$$U_0^2 = \frac{2 \times 10000}{1.3 \times 8 \times 1.25 \times 1.2} = 1282.05$$

$$U_0 = 35.81 \text{ m/s} = 128.9 \text{ km/hr.}$$

11.19 A wing of an aeroplane of 10 m span and 2 m mean chord is to be designed to develop a lift of 50 kN at a speed of 380 km/hr. A $\frac{1}{25}$ scale model when tested in a wind tunnel at speed of 450 m/s. experienced a total drag of 425 N. The pressure of air used in the wind tunnel was compressed to 4.5 times atmospheric pressure. Calculate the total drag experienced by the full size wing, assuming wind tunnel data refer to infinite size of wing. ρ for atmospheric air $\rho_{air} = 1.2$ kg/m^3.

Solution

For model: $L_r = \dfrac{1}{25}$, $A_r = L_r^2 = \dfrac{1}{625}$

$$A_m = \frac{A_p}{625}$$

$$= \frac{10 \times 2}{625} = 0.032 \ \text{m}^2$$

From Boyle's law,

$$\frac{p_a}{\rho_a} = \frac{p_m}{\rho_m}$$

$$\rho_m = \left(\frac{p_m}{p_a}\right) \times \rho_a$$

$$= \left(\frac{4.5 \, p_a}{p_a}\right) \times 1.2 = 5.4 \ \text{kg/m}^3$$

$$\left(F_D\right)_m = C_{Dm} . A_m \frac{\rho_m U_m^2}{2}$$

$$C_{Dm} = \frac{F_{Dm}}{A_m \dfrac{\rho_m U_m^2}{2}}$$

$$= \frac{425}{0.052 \times 5.4 \times \dfrac{(450)^2}{2}} = 0.015$$

For prototype , $U_0 = 380$ km/hr

$$= 105.56 \ \text{m/s}$$

$$F_L = C_L . A . \rho \, U_0^2/2$$

$$50 \times 1000 = C \times (10 \times 2) \times 1.2 \times (105.56)^2/2$$

$$C_L = \frac{50,000 \times 2}{10 \times 2 \times 1.2 \times (105.56)^2} = 0.374$$

Now, assuming elliptical distribution of lift,
From Eq. 11.39,

$$C_{Di} = \frac{C_L^2}{\pi \times \text{(aspect ratio)}} = \frac{C_L^2}{\pi \times L^2/A}$$

where $A = \text{Span} \times \text{mean chord length} = L \times C$

$$= C_{Di} = C_L^2/\pi \, (L/C)$$

$$C_{Di} = \frac{(0.374)^2}{\pi \left(\dfrac{10}{2} \right)} = 0.00891$$

Hence, total drag coefficient C_D is given by

$$C_D = C_{Dp} + C_{Di} \hspace{2cm} \text{(Since } C_{Dm} = C_{Dp}\text{)}$$

$$= 0.015 + 0.00891$$

$$= 0.0239$$

Total drag of wing of prototype,

$$F_D = C_D A \rho \frac{U_0^2}{2}$$

$$= 0.0239 \times (10 \times 2) \times \frac{1.2 \times (105.56)^2}{2}$$

$$= 3197.03 \, N \text{ or } 3.197 \text{ kN}.$$

Objective questions

11.1 The drag force experienced by a body placed immersed in a fluid is

  (a) the horizontal component of resultant force acting over the body

  (b) the component of force acting in the direction of motion

  (c) the component of the force acting in the normal direction of motion

  (d) the component of force acting in the direction of longitudinal axis of the body

  (e) none of these anwwers

11.2 The pressure drag depends on

  (a) the characteristics of approaching flow

  (b) the occurrence of a wake

  (c) the shape of the body

  (d) the type of boundary layer developed around the body

  (e) none of these answers

11.3 The wake

  (a) is a region of high pressure

  (b) always occurs after a separation point

  (c) is the principal cause of skin friction .

(d) is a region of low turbulence

(e) none of these answers

11.4 A streamlined body is such that

(a) it produces no drag for the flow around it

(b) it is symmetrical about the axis along the free stream

(c) separation of flow is avoided along its surface

(d) the shape of the body coincides with the stream surface

(e) none of these answers

11.5 The terminal velocity of a particle settling in a fluid (R_e) varies as

(a) first power of its diameter

(b) inverse of its diameter

(c) the inverse of the difference in specific weight of particle and fluid

(d) inversely poportional to the drag coefficient

(e) none of these answers

11.6 The drag coefficient is defined as

(a) $\dfrac{F_D/A}{\rho U_0^2}$ (b) $\dfrac{F_D/A}{2\rho U_0^2}$ (c) $\dfrac{F_D}{0.5\rho U_0^2}$

(d) $\dfrac{F_D}{0.5\rho U_0^2 A}$ (e) none of these answer

11.7 The drag coefficients for some of the objects of column A are indicated in column B. Match the correct answer

(a) Mini-bus   (i) 1.3

(b) Tall building   (ii) 2.0

(c) Non-streamlined engine   (iii) 0.73

(d) Sign board   (iv) 0.04

(e) Well shaped airfoil   (v) 1.9

11.8 The drag due to ideal fluid flow around a circular cylinder with circulation is

(a) $\rho U_0 \Gamma$ (b) $\rho U_0^2 \Gamma$ (c) $\rho U_0 \Gamma^2$

(d) $\rho U_0^2 A$ (e) none of these answers

11.9 The lift per unit length due to ideal fluid flow around a circular cylinder with circulation is

(a) $(\rho U_0 \Gamma^2)$ (b) $\rho U_0^2 \Gamma$ (c) $\rho U_0 \Gamma$

(d) $\rho U_0/\Gamma$ (e) none of these answers

11.10 In Karman's vortex trail formed at the rear of a long cylinder, the vortices

(a) remain attached to the cylinder

(b) are shed simultaneously from top and bottom of the cylinder

(c) are shed alternatively from top and bottom of the cylinder

(d) none of these answers

11.11 The Strouhl number is used to define the frequency of vortex shedding ($S = fD/U_0$). It varies with Reynolds number. Match the answers

Strouhl number	Reynolds number
(a) 0.20	(i) 2×10^5
(b) 0.12	(ii) 2×10^5
(c) 0.21	(iii) 2×10^6

11.12 The circulation around an airfoil required for the lift to be produced is

(a) by the rotation of airfoil

(b) the airfoil is inclined to the main foil

(c) a surface of discontinuity is formed at its trailling edge

(d) because of tip vortices

(e) none of these answers

11.13 The point of stall is used with reference to an airfoil. It is the point at which

(a) the drag is zero

(b) the lift is zero

(c) the lift is maximum

(d) drag is minimum

(e) none of these answers

11.14 The polar diagram is related to the flow around an airfoil, the maximum efficiency of airfoil is obtained when

(a) the drag/lift is maximum

(b) the drag/lift is minimum

(c) the lift is maximum

(d) the drag is minimum

(e) none of these answers

11.15 Cite some examples where separation is a desirable phenomenon

Problems

11.1 A 90 cm × 120 cm plate moves at 13.5 m/s in still air at an angle of 10^0 with horizontal. Determine the resultant force exerted by the air on the plate and power required to keep the plate moving. Assume $\rho_{air} = 1.2 \, \text{kg/m}^3$ $C_D = 0.17$ and $C_L = 0.70$.

11.2 Calculate the diameter of a parachute to be used for dropping an object weighing 1 kN so that the maximum terminal velocity is 5 m/s. The drag coefficient for the hemi-spherical parachute may be taken as 1.2. The specific weight of air is 11.95 kg/m^3.

11.3 A kite weighing 10 N has an effective area of 1 m^2. It makes an angle of 12^0 to the direction of wind, while the string attached to the kite makes an angle of 45^0 to the horizonal. Find the velocity of wind and the tension in the string. The coefficients of drag and lift are given as 0.65 and 0.85 respectively and specific mass of air is 1.2 kg/m^3.

11.4 Assuming an automobile to have a projected area of 3 m^2, estimate the power required to overcome the wind resistance at a speed of 80 km/h (a) if the car is well streamline and (b) if the car is not well streamlined.

11.5 A cup anemometer used in measuring wind velocity consists of two hollow hemi-spheres mounted in opposite directions at the ends of a horizontal rod which turns freely about a vertical axis. What torque would be required to hold the rotating member stationary in a 50 km/h wind? Take lever arm 0.45 m and cup D as 0.1 m,

11.6 Determine the lift and drag of an aeroplane having a span of 15 m and a chord length of 2 while travelling at a speed of 300 km/h and making such an angle of attack which gives maximum value of lift/drag ratio. What percentage of total drag is due to the finite span of the wing?

11.7 An aeroplane section is tested in a wind tunnel under the conditions simulating an infinite aspect ratio (through use of thin plates mounted parallel to the flow at each end of the section). At an angle of attack of $30°$, the coefficient is determined to be 0.7 and drag coefficient 0.05. What would be the corresponding magnitude of C_{Di} for an aspect ratio of 7 ?

11.8 A circular cylinder, 0.5 m diameter is placed in an irrotational flow with a uniform velocity of 10 m/s. The cylinder has a clockwise free vortex motion around it whose circulation is $\Gamma = 20 \, \text{m}^2/\text{s}$. (a) Locate the stagnation points on the cylinder (b) Calculate the velocities at the two points on the cylinder at $90°$ and $270°$ from the leading edge. $\rho_{air} = 1.2 \, \text{kg/m}^3$.

11.9 For the cylinder of Problem 10.8, compute the circulation of the free vortex motion surrounding the cylinder in order to produce a lift force of 250 N per metre length of the cylinder when it is submerged in air at 20^0 C and atmospheric pressure. Also calculate the maximum and minimum pressure on the cylinder. Neglect the end effects.

11.10 An instrument fitted vertically to a submarine is 0.2 m in diameter and the submarine is travelling at 20 km/h. What is the frequency of vortex shedding and the force per metre length of the instrument? Assume mass density of sea water as 1030 kg/m^3 and kinemetic viscosity of water as $1.25 \times 10^{-2} \, \text{cm}^2/\text{s}$.

12

Open Channel Flow

12.1 INTRODUCTION

Liquids may flow through a pipe or in an open channel. The open channel flow must have a free surface subjected to atomspheric pressure, whereas pipe flow has got no such free surface. Pipe flow, being confined in a closed conduit and running full, exerts no direct atmospheric pressure. The flow in an open channel is caused due to gravity or by its slope whereas the pipe flow takes place under hydraulic pressure. The problem of flow in open channels are more difficult to solve than pipe flow on account of the following reasons.

(i) The location of free surface. The location of free surface varies with time and space co-ordinates (i.e.,it fluctuates at various time and from section to section). (ii) The depth of flow: The discharge and the slope of the channel bottom all are interdependent. Thus the area of cross section, the velocity of flow and other variables do change from from instant to instant. (iii) Shape of channel: The cross section of pipe is generally round whereas the cross section of channel may vary from circular to irregular shape of natural streams. (iv) Roughness: The roughness of interior surface of pipe may vary from a smooth brass or copper pipe to old eroded cast iron or galvanised iron pipe. In case of channels, the roughness may vary from a very smooth glass surface of laboratory flume to very irregular and rough natural stream. Moreover, the free surface itself fluctuate causing variation in roughness. Thus a greater amount of uncertainty is introduced in the estimation of roughness coefficient for given open channel. (v) Hydraulic gradient line: Application of Bernoulli's theorem shows that the ordinate $(p/w + z)$ represent the hydraulic gradient line for the flow in pipe. In case of open channel flow, the piezometric surface is represented by $(y + z)$; y being the depth of flow. Thus the piezometric line coincides with the water surface line. It is to be noted that flow in a closed conduit is not always a pipe flow but it is to be treated as an open channel flow if it flows partially full as is the case with the sewer lines.

12.2 TYPES OF CHANNEL

The open channel may be either natural or artificial. The natual channels are irregular in shape and their size varies from a hilly rivulets to large rivers and tidal estuaries. Artificial channels are those which are constructed and developed by human efforts. Their shape and size depend upon the requirement of the project. Under various circumstances in engineering practice, an artificial channel may be named as canal, flume, chute, drop, culvert and open flow tunnel, etc. The 'canal' is usually a long mild sloped channel built in the

633

ground and may be unlined or lined with stone masonry, concrete, bricks, etc. The 'flume' is a channel built of wood, metal, concrete or masonry usually supported above the surface of the ground. 'Chute' is a channel of steep slope as provided with side channel spillway. The 'drop' is a chute but the slope is effected in à short reach. The culvert is a covered channel of small length and running partially full. It is provided to drain water under the high-way. The 'open flow tunnel' is a long drain through hills to drain water.

12.3 GEOMETRIC ELEMENTS OF OPEN CHANNEL

(1) *Prismatic and non-prismatic channel.* A channel of constant slope and cross section for sufficient length is called a 'prismatic channels.' Mostly, the artificial channels are prismatic channels. Generally, a triangular cross section is adopted for small discharge and trapezoidal section for carrying large discharge. 'Non prismatic channel:' The slopes at various cross sections of all the natural streams do not remain the same throughout a reach. Actually, these channels aie of irregular shape which itself gets changed with time. Such channels are called non-prismatic channels.

(2) *Depth of flow (y).* It is the vertical distance of the lowest point of a channel section from the free surface.

(3) *Depth of flow section (d).* It is the depth of flow normal to the direction of flow. For a channel of longitudinal slope.

$$d = y \cos \theta \qquad \qquad ...(12.1)$$

(4) *Water area (A).* It is the cross sectional area of the flow normal to the direction of flow.

(5) *Top width (T).* It is the width of channel section at the free surface.

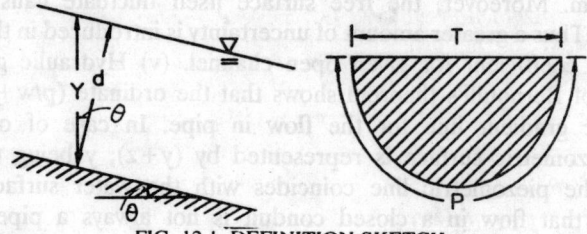

FIG. 12.1. DEFINITION SKETCH.

(6) *Hydraulic depth (D).* It is the ratio of the water area A to the top width T,

$$D = A/T \qquad \qquad ...(12.2)$$

(7) *Wetted perimeter (P).* It is length of the line of intersection of the channel wetted surface with a cross sectional plane normal to the direction of flow.

(8) *Hydraulic radius (R).* It is the ratio of water area A to the wetted perimeter P,

$$R = A/P \qquad \qquad ...(12.3)$$

(9) *Section factor for critical flow (Z)*. It is used for the computation of critical flow and is defined as

$$Z = \sqrt{A^3/T} \qquad \qquad ...(12.4)$$

(10) *Section factor for uniform flow A*. It is defined as

$$Z = A\,R^{2/3} \qquad \qquad ...(12.5)$$

(11) *Conveyance (K)*. It is defined as

$$K = \frac{Q}{\sqrt{S}} = \frac{1}{n} A\,R^{2/3} \qquad \qquad ...(12.6)$$

12.4 CLASSIFICATION OF FLOW

Open channel flow can be classified into many types and described in many ways. The following classification is made according to the change in flow depth with respect to time and space.

1. With respect to time and space

(a) Steady and unsteady flow. Time is the basis. The flow is said to be 'steady' if the depth of flow does not change durring the time interval (or it can be assumed so during the given time interval under consideration). In most of the channels, the behaviour of flow is analysed as steady,

$$\partial y/\partial t = 0 \qquad \qquad ...(12.7a)$$

If the depth of flow changes during the given time interval, it is said to be 'unsteady flow'. Flood waves and surges are practical examples of unsteady flow.

$$\partial y/\partial t \neq 0 \qquad \qquad ...(12.7b)$$

(b) *Uniform and non-uniform flow*. Space is the basis. The flow is said to be 'uniform' if at the given instant of time the depth of flow remains the same at every section of a given channel.

$$\partial y/\partial s = 0 \qquad \qquad ...(12.8a)$$

If the depth of flow varies from section to section at the given instant of time, the flow is said to be 'non-uniform or varied flow'

$$\partial y/\partial s \neq 0 \qquad \qquad ...(12.8b)$$

A uniform flow may be steady or unsteady, depending on whether depth changes with time or not.

(c) *Steady uniform flow*. It is the fundamental type of flow in which the depth of flow does not change along the length of channel during the given interval of time. This means that the depth of flow remains the same at all the cross section of the channel.

(d) *Unsteady uniform flow*. The establishment of unsteady uniform flow would require that the water surface should fluctuate from time to time while remaining parallel to the channel bottom, Obviously, it is practically impossible condition. Therefore, the term 'uniform flow' exclusively refers to steady uniform flow.

TABLE 12.1. GEOMETRIC ELEMENTS OF CHANNEL SECTIONS

SECTION	AREA A	WETTED PERIMETER, P	HYDRAULIC RADIUS, R	TOP WIDTH T	HYDRAULIC DEPTH, D	SECTION FACTOR, Z
RECTANGLE	By	$(B+2y)$	$\dfrac{By}{(B+2y)}$	B	y	$By^{3/2}$
TRAPEZOIDAL	$(B+zy)y$	$B+2y\sqrt{1+z^2}$	$\dfrac{(B+zy)y}{(B+2y\sqrt{1+z^2})}$	$B+2zy$	$\dfrac{(B+zy)y}{(B+2zy)}$	$\dfrac{(B+zy)^{3/2}y^{3/2}}{\sqrt{B+2zy}}$
TRIANGLE	zy^2	$2y\sqrt{1+z^2}$	$\dfrac{zy}{2\sqrt{1+z^2}}$	$2zy$	$\dfrac{y}{2}$	$\dfrac{z y^{5/2}}{\sqrt{2}}$
CIRCLE	$\dfrac{D^2}{8}(\theta-\sin\theta)$	$\dfrac{\theta D}{2}$	$\dfrac{1}{4}\left(1-\dfrac{\sin\theta}{\theta}\right)D$	$D\sin\theta/2$ OR $2\sqrt{y(D-y)}$	$\dfrac{1}{8}\dfrac{(\theta-\sin\theta)}{\sin\theta/2}D$	$\dfrac{\sqrt{2}}{32}\dfrac{(\theta-\sin\theta)^{3/2}}{\sqrt{\sin\theta/2}}D^{5/2}$
PARABOLA	$\dfrac{2}{3}Ty$	$T+\dfrac{8}{3}\dfrac{y^2}{t}$	$\dfrac{2T^2 y}{3T^2+8y^2}$	$\dfrac{3A}{2y}$	$\dfrac{2}{3}y$	$\dfrac{2\sqrt{6}}{9}Ty^{3/2}$

(e) *Steady varied (non-uniform) flow.* This type of flow requires that the depth of flow at a section remains constant with time but varies from section to section. Varied flow may further be classified as 'gradually varied flow' and 'rapidly varied flow'. The flow behind a dam, and at a channel transition, etc., are some of the examples of this class. Hydraulic jump occurring at the foot of a spillway or below a sluice gate and flow at the free overfall are the examples of rapidly varied flow.

(f) *Unsteady varied flow.* This type of flow requires that the depth of flow must vary from section to section as well as it must vary with time. A flood wave travelling in a natural stream is an example of this type. Similarly, the afflux created by a dam produces such type of flow.

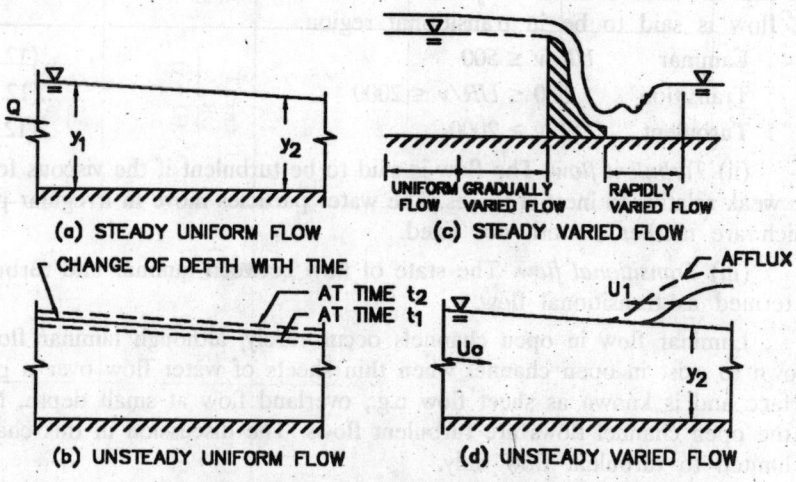

FIG. 12.2. CLASSIFICATION OF FLOW BASED ON TIME
AND SPACE CO-ORDINATES

2. CLASSIFICATION BASED ON FORCES

(a) *Effect of viscous forces.* The state of flow in an open channel is governed by the effects of viscosity and gravity relative to the inertia forces of flow. An open channel flow may be laminar, transitional or turbulent depending on the relative effect of viscosity to the inertia. The Reynolds number of flow in an open channel which is a measure of the effect of viscosity is defined as

$$R_e = \frac{\rho \, U \, (4R)}{\mu} \qquad \qquad ...(12.9)$$

where U is the average velocity of flow, 4 R replaces the diameter of pipe in its earlier definition (Eq. 6.16) and R is the hydraulic radius. For a circular conduit, the hydraulic radius is equal to one fourth of the diameter of conduit.

(b) *Laminar flow.* The flow is said to be laminar if the viscous forces are so strong relative to inertia forces that viscosity plays a significant part in determining flow behaviour. The water particles appear to move in definite smooth paths, or streamlines, and infinitesimally thin layers of fluid seems to slide over adjacent layers.

Laminar flow ceases to exist in pipe when R_e ($= UD/v$) is greater than 2000. Accordingly, critical Reynolds number at which the laminar flow changes from laminar state to turbulent state in channel may be expressed as

$$UR/v = 500 \qquad ...(12.10)$$

Indeed, the experiments in open channel have shown that the flow remains laminar when

$$UR/v \leq 500$$

and that the flow is turbulent when $UR/v > 2000$. In between these two limits, the flow is said to be in transitional region.

Laminar	$UR/v \leq 500$	...(12.11a)
Transition	$500 \leq UR/v \leq 2000$	...(12.11b)
Turbulent	$UR/v \geq 2000$	...(12.11c)

(ii) *Turbulent flow.* The flow is said to be turbulent if the viscous forces are weak relative to inertial forces. The water particles move in irregular paths which are neither smooth nor fixed.

(iii) *Transitional flow.* The state of flow between laminar and turbulent is termed as transitional flow.

Laminar flow in open channels occur rarely, although laminar flow is known to exist in open channel when thin sheets of water flow over a plane surface and is known as sheet flow e.g., overland flow at small depth. Most of the open channel flows are turbulent flows. The discussion in this chapter is limited to turbulent flow only.

(b) *Effect of gravity.* The effect of gravity upon the state of flow is represented by a ratio of gravity forces to intertial forces. This ratio is known as Froude's number and is defined as

$$N_F = U/\sqrt{gL} \qquad ...(12.12)$$

Here U is the average velocity of flow and L is the characteristic length. In open channel flow, L may be replaced by hydralic depth D ($= A/P$), for rectangular channel, the characteristic length is the depth of flow y. When Froude's number is unity, Eq. 12.12 gives

$$U = \sqrt{gD} \qquad ...(12.13)$$

and the flow is known as 'critical' flow. If N_F is less than unity or $U < \sqrt{gD}$, the flow is said to be 'subcritical' or 'tranquil flow'. If N_F is more than one, or $U > \sqrt{gD}$, the flow is known as 'supercritical', 'rapid' or 'shooting' flow.

In shallow water, the momentary change in the local depth of water causes small gravity waves. The velocity of these small waves is known as celerity which is also given by

$$c = \sqrt{gD} \qquad ...(12.14)$$

It is to be noted that the celerity is greater than the velocity of flow in subcritical flow, hence a gravity wave can travel upstream. In case of supercritical flow, the wave cannot travel upstream (which forms when the velocity of flow is affected or controlled by changes occurring at downstream end). The control section for supercritical flows lies at upstream end and for subcritical flows it lies on downstream section.

12.5 REGIMES OF FLOW

The combined effect of viscosity and gravity produces any one of the four regimes of flow.

    (1) Subcritical laminar flow

    (2) Supercritical laminar flow

    (3) Subcritical turbulent flow

    (4) Supercritical turbulent flow

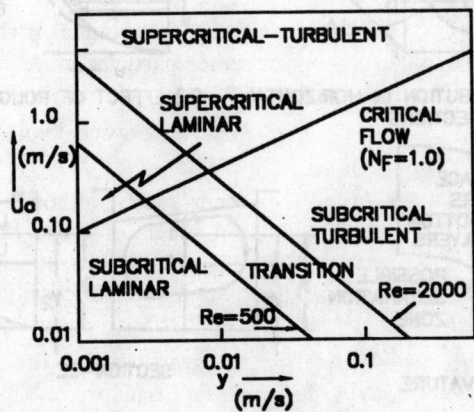

FIG. 12.3. REGIMES OF FLOW

The laminar turbulent band intersects $N_F = 1$ line and thus divides the whole area into four regimes in Fig. 12.3. The first two regimes are of limited interest as in the overland flow, erosion control and hydraulic model studies. The last two flow regimes are discussed in this text.

12.6 VELOCITY DISTRIBUTION

The velocity of flow in an open channel is not uniformly distributed in a channel section. The non-uniform distribution of velocity in an open channel is due to friction along the channel wall and free liquid surface. Fig. 12.4 illustrates a typical velocity distribution over various vertical and horizonal sectionsas represented by isobars or lines of equal velocity in a straight reach of an open channel. The maximum velocity occurs below the free surface at a distance of 0.05 to 0.25 of the depth; closer is the bank, the lower is the muximum value.

The velocity distribution in a channel section depends also on other factors, such as the unusual shape of channel section, the roughness of the channel and the presence of bends. The roughness of the channel causes the curvature of the vertical velocity distribution curve to increase as shown in Fig. 12.4b. On a bend, the velocity increases greatly at the convex side owing to the centrifugal force acting outwardly on the flow, Fig. 12.4c.

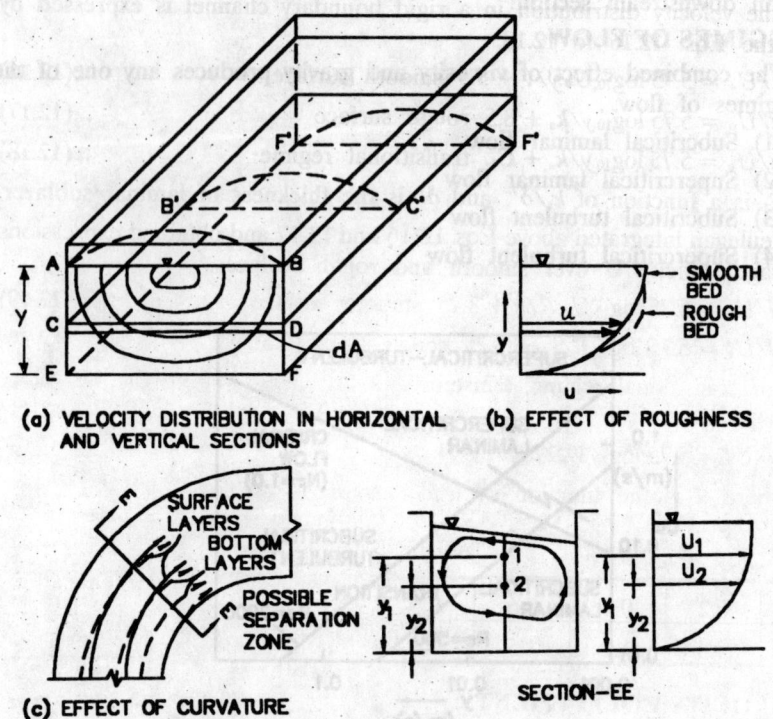

(a) VELOCITY DISTRIBUTION IN HORIZONTAL   (b) EFFECT OF ROUGHNESS
AND VERTICAL SECTIONS

(c) EFFECT OF CURVATURE   SECTION–EE

FIG. 12.4. VELOCITY DISTRIBUTION

From the study of a large number of vertical distribution curves obtained by actual field and laboratory measurements the following observations are made: (i) The mean velocity in a vertical plane normally lies at 0.55 to 0.65 of the flow depth (the depth being measured from water surface). The velocity measured at 0.6 y is taken as the mean velocity which is found to be correct within ± 5% (ii) Alternatively, for more reliable results the velocities measured at $0.2y$ and $0.8y$ are averaged out. It gives mean velocity within ± 2%. (iii) For accurate results, the section should be subdivided into a number of segments, The velocity measured along the vertical line and the velocity profile is plotted. The mean velocity is then determined by integrating, Eq. 12.15.

$$U = \frac{\int (A_1 U_1 + A_2 U_2 + A_3 U_3)}{A} \qquad ...(12.15)$$

These facts form the basis of measuring the discharge of streams. Observation taken in very wide channels have shown that the velocity distribution in the central region of the section is essentially the same as it would be in a rectangular channel of infinite width. In other words, the sides of channel have practically no influence on the velocity distribution in the central region. A wide open channel is defined as a rectangular channel whose width is greater than 10 times the depth of flow.

Following the same procedure as in section 9.5 and using mixing length theory, the velocity distribution in a rigid boundary channel is expressed by one of the Eqs. 12.16 to 12.18.

$$u/U_* = 5.75 \log_{10} U_* y/v + 5.5 \quad \text{smooth surface} \qquad \text{...(12.16)}$$

$$u/U_* = 5.75 \log_{10} y/k_s + 8.5 \quad \text{rough surface} \qquad \text{...(12.17)}$$

$$u/U_* = 5.75 \log_{10} y/k_s + C_1. \quad \text{transitional regime} \qquad \text{...(12.18)}$$

where C_1 is a function of k_s/δ', and δ' is the thickness of laminar sublayer.

Keulegan integrated above Eqs. 12.16 and 12.17 and obtained expressions for average velocity U over smooth and rough surfaces.

$$U/U_* = 5.75 \log_{10} U_* R/v + 3.25 \quad \text{smooth surface} \qquad \text{...(12.19)}$$

$$U/U_* = 5.75 \log_{10} R/k_s + 6.25 \quad \text{rough surface} \qquad \text{...(12.20)}$$

For transitional regime, Einstein and Barbarossa wrote the resistance equation as

$$U/U_* = 5.75 \log_{10} 12.27 R x/v \qquad \text{...(12.21)}$$

where x is the function of ks/δ' and is shown in Table 12.2.

TABLE 12.2

k_s/δ'	0.2	0.4	0.6	0.8	1.0	2.0	4.0	10.0
x	0.8	1.1	1.5	1.58	1.60	1.28	1.1	1.0

12.7 VELOCITY COEFFICIENTS

1. Energy correction coefficient

As discussed above the velocity of flow varies over the cross section, being zero at the boundary and increasing with depth of flow. As a result of this non-uniform distribution of velocity, the kinetic energy per unit mass is greater than $U^2/2g$; U being the mean velocity of flow. The correct value of velocity head or kinetic energy per unit mass is expressed as $\propto U^2/2g$, where $\propto$ is known as 'energy coefficient' or 'Coriolis coefficient' in honour of G. Coriolis.

Consider an elementary area of flow dA out of the whole water area A and the velocity of flow through this area dA is u.

The mass of fluid passing through area $dA = \delta m = (w u dA/g)$

Kinetic energy of fluid mass passing through this elementary strip

$$= \frac{w}{g} u dA \frac{u^2}{2}$$

Hence, the kinetic energy of the whole fluid mass

$$= \int_A \frac{w}{2g} u^3 \, dA \qquad \text{...(i)}$$

Let the average velocity of flow through area A be U.

The kinetic energy of the whole fluid mass

$$= \propto \frac{w}{2g} U^3 A \qquad \text{...(ii)}$$

Equating Eqs. (i) and (ii),

$$\propto = \frac{\int_A u^3 \, dA}{U^3 A} \qquad \text{...(12.22 a)}$$

If the flow is two-dimensional as in a wide rectangular channel,

$$A = BY \text{ and } dA = B \, dy, \text{ and}$$

$$\propto = \frac{1}{Y} \int_A (u/(U)^3 \, dy \qquad \text{...(12.22 b)}$$

where y is the depth of flow section.

2. Momentum correction coefficient

Similarly, as a result of non-uniforminty of velocity distribution the momentum per unit volume is greater than ρU. The correct value of momentum flux is $\beta \rho U$, where β is known as 'momentum correction coefficient' or 'Boussinesq coefficient'.

The momentum flux of water passing through dA per unit time is the product of mass $\rho u \, dA$ and the velocity u. The total momentum flux of whole fluid is the summation of momentum flux passing through elementary area

$$\text{Momentum flux} = \int_A \rho u^2 \, dA \qquad \text{...(i)}$$

The momentum flux of whole fluid may also be written as

$$= \int_A \rho U^2 \, dA \qquad \text{...(ii)}$$

Equating Eqs. (i) and (ii)

$$\beta = \frac{\int_A u^2 \, dA}{U^2 A} \qquad \text{...(12.23a)}$$

For a wide channel, as in case of rectangular channel, A = By

$$\beta = \frac{1}{y} \int_A (u/U)^2 \, dy \qquad \text{...(12.23b)}$$

Alternatively, the velocity profiles are measured and then curves for $u \propto y$; $u^2 \propto y$ and $u^3 \propto y$ are plotted. Therefore, the areas of these curves are measured over the graph paper or measured by means of a planimeter.

$$\text{Average velocity } U = \frac{(\text{area of u} - \text{y curve} \times \text{width of section})}{(\text{area of flow section})}$$

$$\text{...(12.24)}$$

Energy correction coefficinet

$$\alpha = \frac{\text{area of } u^3 - y \text{ curve} \times \text{width of section}}{A\,U^3} \qquad ...(12.25)$$

Momentum correction coefficient

$$\beta = \frac{\text{area of } u^2 - y \text{ curve} \times \text{width of section}}{A\,U^2} \qquad ...(12.26)$$

For approximate values of α and β, the following formulas can be used

$$\alpha = 1 + 3\,\varepsilon^2 - 2\,\varepsilon^3 \qquad ...(12.27a)$$

$$\beta = 1 + \varepsilon^2 \qquad ...(12.12b)$$

where $\varepsilon = U_m/U - 1$; U_m is the maximum velocity and U is the average velocity of flow.

The value of α and β are invariably greater than 1.0. Their values vary between 1.05 to 1.10. In case of irregular channels even higher values of α and β have been reported in the literature. For channels of regular section and fairly strainght alignment, the effect of non-uniform velocity distribution on α and β is small. Therefore the coefficients are often assumed to be unity.

12.8 PRESSURE DISTRIBUTION

1. Effect of curvature of streamlines

The pressure at every point on the cross section of the flow in a channel of small slope can be measured by the height of the water column in a piezometric tube installed at the point. The pressure at any point is directly proportional to the depth of point below free water surface and is equal to the hydrostatic pressure corresponding to this point. Therefore, the water in the piexometric tube rises upto the free water surface. p = w y

This is known as the hydrostatic law of pressure distribution. This law is applicable if the stream lines are parallel or flow is parallel flow or uniform flow. In actual problem, the depth of flow varies slightly in the direction of flow, i.e., it is gradually varied flow. This flow may also be regarded as parallel flow. Hence, the law of hydrostatic pressure may also be applied to this type of flow.

If the curvature of stream lines is appreciable the flow is known as curvilinear flow. The effect of curvature is to produce the centrifugal force in the outward direction. Thus, the pressure distribution deviates from the hydrostatic. In concave flow, the centrifugal force acts in downward direction, Fig. 12.5c and hence the hydrostatic pressure is increased at the given section. In convex flow, the centrifugal force acts in the upward direction against the gravity action and hence the resulting hydrostatic force at any point is less than the pressure in a parallel flow, Fig. 12.5b.

Let the deviation in hydrostatic pressure be c. This can be computed using Newton's second law of motion. Consider a control volume of one square metre of cross sectional area and y metre of depth. The normal acceleration produced in the flow due to curved flow is

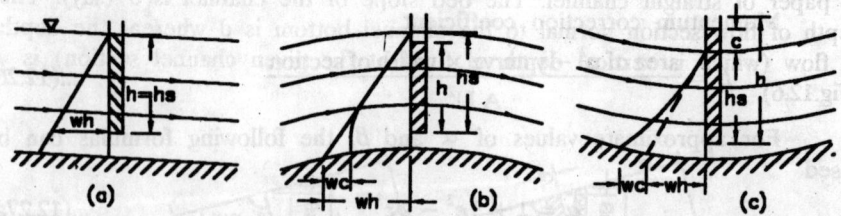

FIG. 12.5. PRESSURE DISTRIBUTION IN AN OPEN CHANNEL (A) PARALLEL FLOW (B) CONVEX FLOW (C) CONCAVE FLOW

$$a_n = U^2/r$$

where r is the radius of curvature of the streamlines and U is the average velocity at the given section. Hence, the deviation (or correction) in pressure distribution, c, is given by,

$$c = \frac{wy}{g} \frac{U^2}{r} \qquad \qquad ...(12.28)$$

The true pressure intensity is then given by

$$h_c = h \pm c \qquad \qquad ...(12.29)$$

The positive sign is to be used for concave flow and negative sign is to be used for convex flow. For practical purposes, where the curvature of streamlines is not appreciable, the value of c is used as unity, e.g., uniform or gradually varied flow in open channel. Whenever the streamlines curvature is appreciable as in case of rapidly varied flow (a hydraulic jump, the flow at free fall, flow through a sluice gate) the true pressure distribution should be corrected for curvature effect.

2. Pressure coefficient

For simplicity, the curvilinear pressure can be determined using pressure coefficient α' or in other words, the curvilinear pressure p_c can be written as

$$p_c = \alpha' wy$$

Consider an elementary element of fluid of area dA and possessing velocity u. The depth of flow normal to the bed is d. Then the total weight of fluid passing through this section is $\int wu\, dA$. If the average velocity of flow is U and the cross sectional area is A the weight of fluid at this section is w Q y. Therefore, the pressure coefficient α' is given by

$$\alpha' = \frac{1}{Qy} \int_A u d\, dA \qquad \qquad ...(12.30)$$

The value of α' is usually greater than 1.0 for concave flow and less than 1.0 for convex flow.

3. Effect of slope on pressure distribution

Consider a prism of length dx and of unit width normal to the plane of paper of straight channel. The bed slope of the channel is θ (say). The depth of flow section normal to the channel bottom is d whereas the depth of flow (which is vertical depth of fluid at the given channel section) is y (Fig.12.6).

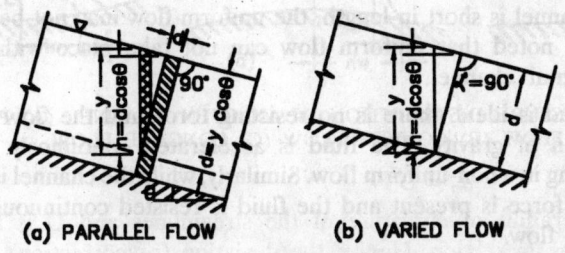

(a) PARALLEL FLOW   **(b) VARIED FLOW**

FIG. 12.6. PRESSURE DISTRIBUTION-EFFECT OF SLOPE

The weight of fluid in the prism is $wd\,(dx \times 1)$ or $w(y \cos \theta)dx$ This cause the hydrostatic pressure at the channel bottom to become

$$P = wd\,dx \cos \theta \qquad \qquad ...(12.31a)$$

$$P = wy\,dx \cos^2 \theta \qquad \qquad ...(12.31b)$$

Therefore, the pressure intensity p or its equivalent water head h is

$$h = d \cos \theta \qquad \qquad ...(12.31c)$$

$$h = y \cos^2 \theta \qquad \qquad ...(12.31d)$$

Thus, it is seen that the depth of flow section y should be multiplied by $\cos^2 \theta$ to correct for steep slope. This means that if the angle θ (bed slope) is small, $\cos \theta$ is nearly unity and no correction is needed. For steep slope (a slope of 1 in 10 or more, i.e., 6° or more) the correction for slope should be applied. These channels are known as channels of large slope. It should be noted that the Eq. 12.31b is not valid for varied flow as seen from Fig. 12.6b.

If the channel of large slope is having appreciable curvature of streamlines, the correction in pressure both for slope as well as curvature should be applied.

$$p = \alpha' \, wy \cos^2 \theta \qquad \qquad ...(12.31e)$$

12.9 UNIFORM FLOW

The uniform flow has two main features, namely (i) the depth, water area, velocity and discharge at every section of the channel remain same and ((ii) the slope of bed S_o, slope of water surface S_W and slope of energy line S_f, remain same and hence, the bed, the water surface and total energy line all remain parallel.

Fig. 12.7 illustrates the establishment of uniform flow in a long reach of a channel. The fluid in the reach is acted upon by gravity force in the direction of flow (causing the flow) and shear force in opposite direction (resisting the flow). While the fluid enters the channel at left end, the gravity forces acting on the fluid body are more than resisting force and, therefore, the body of fluid is accelerated and the flow becomes varied flow. The velocity and resistance gradually increase until a balance between resistance and gravity is reached. From this section downstream, the flow becomes uniform. Towards downstream end also, the resistance may again be exceeded by gravity force and the flow may again become varied. The length of channel required for establishment of uniform flow is known as the transitory zone.

If the channel is short in length, the uniform flow may not be established in it. It can be noted that uniform flow can not take place with ideal fluid or in a horizontal channel.

If the fluid is ideal, there is no resisting force and the flow takes place under the action of gravity. The fluid is accelerated continuosly in the flow direction resulting in a non-uniform flow. Similarly, while the channel is horizontal, no accelerating force is present and the fluid is resisted continuously resulting in non-uniform flow.

12.10 RESISTANCE EQUATION

Most of the formulas for the mean velocity of turbulent uniform flow in an open channel are expressed in the following general form

$$U = C \ R^x S^y \qquad \qquad ...(12.32)$$

The exponents x and y and the constant C have been determined differently by various investigators of open channel flow. Earliest worker in this direction was a French Engineer Antoire Chezy.

1. The Chezy Formula

The Chezy's formula can be derived mathematically from two assumptions which are:

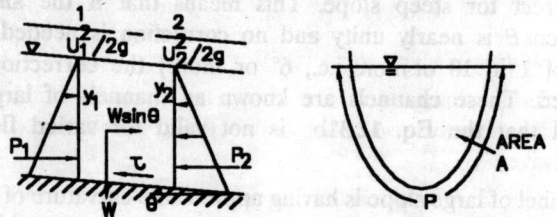

FIG. 12.7. FORCES ACTING ON A CONTROL VOLUME OF FLUID

(1) The force resisting the flow per unit area of channel is proportional to the square of the velocity.

(2) The effective component of gravity force causing the flow must be equal to the total force of resistance.

(a) *Uniform flow.* Consider the body of fluid between sections 1 and 2, distance L apart (Fig.12.7). The force acting on it are (i) hydrostatic force p_1 and p_2, (ii) weight component in the direction of flow, W $\sin \theta$ ($= w \ A \ L \ S_0$) and (iii) shear stress along its wetted surface. Using momentum theorem, Eq. 5.58, summation of all the external forces acting on this water body should be equal to the product of mass and acceleration. In case of uniform flow, the acceleration is zero. Hence, the net sum of all the external forces should be zero.

The force causing the flow = $-W\sin\theta = -wALS_0$

The force resisting the flow = $\tau_0 PL$

The hydrostatic forces p_1 and p_2 are equal in magnitude and act in opposite directions and hence their contribution is zero. Therefore, the summation of these forces should be equated to zero.

$$-wALS_0 - \tau_0 PL = 0$$

$$\tau_0 = -w(A/P)S_0 = -wRS_0 \qquad \qquad ...(12.33)$$

where the slope of bed S_0 is defined as

$$S_0 = \frac{-dz}{dx} \qquad \qquad ...(12.34)$$

and R is the hydraulic radius.

(b) *Non-uniform flow*. Here the depth of flow is changing in the direction of flow. Let the difference in water depth between sections 1 and 2 be dy. Thus the differential (hydrostatic) pressure will be another force causing the force. The magnitude of this force is determined as

$$dP = P_1 - P_2$$

$$= wy_1A_1 - wy_2A_2$$

$$= wA(y_1 - y_2)$$

Since $A_1 \approx A_2$ and dy is the change in the depth of flow from section 1 to 2. distance $dx(=L)$ apart. thus the net force in the direction of flow is

$$-(wALS_0 + wA\,dy) - \tau_0 PL.$$

The velocity is changing in the direction of flow and acceleration is no longer zero. For steady non-uniform flow, only convective acceleration is present and is given by Eq. 4.19a

$$a_s = u(du/dx)$$

Using momentum equation, Eq. 5.58,

$$-(wALS_0 + wA\,dy) - \tau_0 PL = (wAL/g)(u\,du/dx)$$

Simplifying,

$$\tau_0 = -wR\left(\frac{dz}{dx} + \frac{dy}{dx} + \frac{u}{g}\frac{du}{dx}\right)$$

$$= -wR\left[\frac{d}{dx}(y+z) + \frac{u}{g}\frac{du}{dx}\right]$$

$$= -wR\left[\frac{dh}{dx} + \frac{d}{dx}\left(\frac{u^2}{2g}\right)\right]$$

where $\qquad\qquad h = y + z = $ piezometric head

$$= - wR\frac{d}{dx}\left(h + \frac{u^2}{2g}\right)$$

But $H = h + u^2/2g = $ total head

$$\tau_0 = wR\frac{dH}{dx} = wRS \qquad \qquad ...(12.35)$$

Therefore, it is seen that the boundary shear is written as

$$\tau_0 = wRS_t$$

For uniform flow $S = S_o = S_f$ and hence the slope S_f is replaced by S_o.

The slope S_f is defined as

$$S_t = \frac{dH}{dx}$$

Chezy assumed that the resisting force is proportional to the square of the velocity, therefore,

Resisting force $= KU^2 P\,dx$

Hence, resisting force per unit wetted area $= KU^2$ ...(12.36a)

Equating Eqs. 12.33 and 12.36a

$$wRS_f = KU^2$$

which means $U^2 = \sqrt{w/K}\,\sqrt{RS_f}$

Expressing w/K as a factor C.

$$U = C\sqrt{RS_f} \qquad \qquad ...(12.36b)$$

It is well known Chezy's equation for velocity of flow. The factor 'C' is known as Chezy's coefficient in honour of Chezy. It is a measure of the roughness of the boundary. It is believed to depend on hydraulic radius of the section, the channel slope and the boundary roughness. Many attempts have been made in the past to determine the value of C, as discussed henceafter.

2. Ganguillet and Kutter's formula

Based on extensive experimental data, two Swiss engineers Ganguillet and Kutter expressed the value of C in terms of hydraulic radius R, the slope S (i.e. S_o or S_f) and boundary roughness coefficient n.

$$C = \frac{23 + \dfrac{1}{n} + \dfrac{0.0015}{S}}{1 + \left(23 + \dfrac{0.00155}{S}\right)\dfrac{n}{\sqrt{R}}} \qquad \qquad ...(12.37)$$

Here n is known as Kutter's coefficient and its values for different surfaces is tabulated in Table 12.3.

3. Bazin's formula

French hydraulician H. Bazin believed that C is independent of channel slope and depends only on the hydraulic radius. He gave the formula

$$C = \frac{157.6}{1.81 + m/\sqrt{R}} \qquad ...(12.38)$$

In this formula m is known as Bazin's coefficient and its value are given in Table 12.4.

4. Manning's formula

In 1889, an Irish Engineer Robert Manning expressed C as

$$C = \frac{R^{1/6}}{n} \qquad ...(12.39)$$

Substituting this value in Eq. 12.36, the average velocity is writtern as

$$U = \frac{1}{n} R^{2/3} S^{1/2} \qquad ...(12.40)$$

Eq. 12.40 is known as Manning's equation and n is known as Manning's rugosity coefficient or Manning's roughness coefficient.

Manning's formula Eq. 12.40, is dimensionally non-homogeneous and hence it can be used only in the system of units for which it has been derived. Customarily, n is assumed to remain the same in all the systems of units and the constant in the numerator is changed when it is used in another system of units. Owing to its simplicity of form and satisfactory results of practical problems, it is most widely used of all the uniform flow formulas for open channel flow.

(a) **Determination of roughness coefficient.** There is no exact method for the determination of roughness coefficient whether it is Chezy's C, Bazin's m or Manning's n . To select a value of resistance coefficient means to estimate the resistance to flow in a given channel, which is difficult to measure. Its estimation is a matter of sound engineering judgement and experience. As a guide, its value can be obtained by studying the factors affecting it or from Table 12.3. Ven Te Chow has given a set of photographs of typical flow conditions in open channel flow alongwith its 'n' values. One can study these photographs and become acquainted with the variation in the values of n for various surfaces.

(b) **Factors affecting Manning's rugosity coefficient.** The value of n is not constant but depends on a number of factors. Some of these are discussed below.

(1) *Surface roughness.* The surface roughness is represented by the size and shape of the grains of the meterial forming the wetted perimeter. The value of n is low for fine grained surface and high for coarse grained surface.

(2) *Channel irregularity.* The channel irregularity comprises irregularity of wetted perimeter and variations in cross section along its length (its size and shape). Such irregularity may be introduced by the presence of ridges and depressions, humps on channel bed and sand bars, etc. A gradual and uniform change in cross section, size and shape does not introduce much

change in the value of n but abrupt changes cause large change in the value n.

(3) *Channel alignment.* Smooth curvature with large radius will give small value of n whereas sharp curvature with small radius will give large value of n (as in case of meandering channels). It has been found that value of n increases by 0.001 for every 20° of curvature in a 30 m channel.

(4) *Size and shape.* There is no definite evidence that size and shape has direct effect on 'n'. While the channel condition is good, hydraulic radius reduces the value of n whereas if the channel condition is not good, it increases the value of n.

(5) *Vegetation.* Vegetation growing in the channel retards the flow and thereby directly increases the roughness of the channel. The effect depends upon their type, size or height, density and spacing.

(6) *Silting and scouring.* Silting of channel make irregular section regular and smooth and thus reduces its n value. Scouring of bed and bank material causes uneven surface and thus increases its n value.

(7) *Obstruction.* Bridge, piers, logs and such obstruction cause an increase in the value of n. The increase in the value of n depnds on the nature of obstruction, their size, shape and number.

(8) *Stage and discharge.* When the stage is low, the surface irregularities are projected out and affect the flow pronouncedly and hence n value is high. While the discharge is high and stage is high, the value of n is reduced due to diminishing effect of roughness particles. The value of n will increase if banks are rougher than its wetted perimeter.

5. Strickler's formula

When the surface roughness can be represented by an equivelent roughness size k_s (as defined by Nikuradse) and R is defined as hydraulics radius, the Manning's rugosity coefficient may be determined by Strickler's equation developed for rough channels

$$n = \frac{k_s^{1/6}}{25.6} \qquad \qquad ...(12.41)$$

within the range of R/k_s varying from 5 to 700.

Manning n is frequently interpreted as a measure of surface roughness in an open channel similar to k_s in pipe. Therefore, the ratio $R^{1/6}/k_s$ may be taken as a relative roughness parameter comparable to k_s/D. The dimensions of n is, therefore, is length raised to power of one sixth or $\propto k_s^{1/6}$. Thus a thousand fold change in the magnitude of k_s results in about three fold change in the value of n.

Therefore, the error in k_s affects the value of n only slightly.

TABLE 12.3
VALUE OF KUTTER'S OR MANNING'S n

Nature of surface	n
1. Smooth surface	0.010
2. Neat cement surface	0.011
3. Finished concrete, planed wood or steel	0.012
4. Mortar, clay, glazed brick surface	0.013
5. Vitrified clay, surface	0.014
6. Brick surface lined with cement mortar	0.015
7. Unfinished cement surface	0.017
8. Rubble masonry	0.020
9. Earth channel/corrugated metal sheet	0.025
10 Earth channel with dense weeds	0.035
11 Natural channel with clean bottom	0.050
12 Flood plain with dense bush	0.100

TABLE 12.4
VALUES OF BAZIN'S m

Natural of surface	m
Very smooth cement or planed wood surface	0.11
Concrete, good brickwork or unplaned wood surface	0.21
Rubble masonry or poor brick work	0.83
Earth channel : Very good condition	1.54
Fair condition	2.35
Very roguh condition	3.17

12.11 MOST EFFICIENT CROSS SECTION

The discharge through an open channel can be determined using continuity equation alongwith Manning's equation Eq. 12.40a.

$$Q = AU = A \times 1/n \, R^{2/3} S^{1/2} \qquad ...(12.42a)$$

$$= \frac{1}{n} \frac{A^{5/3}}{P^{2/3}} S^{1/2} \qquad ...(12.42b)$$

Thus, it is seen that for given n, S and area of flow, the disharge is maximum when hydraulic radius R is maximum. Such a section is known as the 'most efficient section'. It implies that wetted perimeter P is minimum. Obviously of all the geometric figures, the circle has the least perimeter for the given area of cross section. Semi-circular channels are often built of pressed steel and other forms of metal but for other type of construction such a shape is impracticable. The channels excavated in earth for small discharge may be triangular in shape while for large discharge it may be trapezoidal. The lined channels may be even rectangular in shape. Thus it is a problem of optimisation of given shape to determine best dimensions (of the given shape) of channel. It may be noted that minimum perimeter means minimum cost of lining.

From Eq. 12.42b,

$$P = S^{3/4} A^{5/2} / (n\, Q)^{3/2} = K_1 A^{5/2} \qquad ...(12.43)$$

It shows that minimum perimeter also means minimum area of cross section or minimum cost of excavation. Thus, the most efficient section will carry maximum discharge for a given area of cross section and its cost of excavation and lining will, be minimum, that is to say, it is also the *'most economical section.'* There are many other factors besides hydraulic efficiency which determine the best shape of the channel.

1. Most efficient rectangular section

Consider a rectangular section shown in Fig. 12.8 whose bed width is B and depth of flow in it is y. Let the area of cross section be A and its wetted perimeter be P.

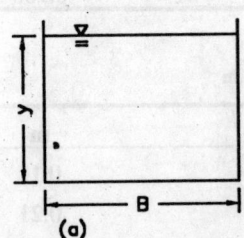 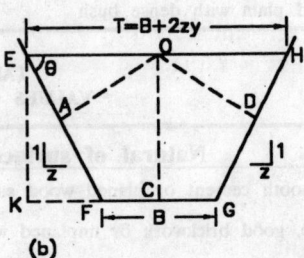

(a) (b)

FIG. 12.8 (A) RECTANGULAR SECTION (B) TRAPEZOIDAL SECTION

(i) Area of flow $A = By$ ...(i)

Wetted perimeter $P = B + 2y$ ...(ii)

From Eqs. (i) and (ii)

$$P = A/y + 2y \qquad ...(iii)$$

For the most efficient section, the perimeter should be minimum.

Therefore, differentiate Eq. (iii) with respect to y and equate it to zero.

$$\frac{dP}{dy} = -\frac{A}{y^2} + 2 = 0$$

Substitute the value of A from Eq. (i) and solve it,

$$B = 2y \qquad ...(12.44a)$$

or $$y = B/2 \qquad ...(12.44b)$$

Thus for a most efficient section, the depth of flow must be half of its bed width.

(ii) The hydraulic radius is given by

$$R = \frac{A}{P} = \frac{By}{B + 2y}$$

Substituting the value of B from Eq. 12.43a

$$R = \frac{2yy}{2y + 2y}$$

$$R = y/2 \qquad \qquad ...(12.45)$$

For the most economical section the hydraulic radius is equal to half the depth of flow.

2. Most efficient trapezoidal section

The given section whose side slope is 1H : z V is shown in Fig. 12.8b. Therefore,

$$A = (B + zy)y \qquad \qquad ...(i)$$

and $$P = (B + 2y\sqrt{1 + z^2}) \qquad \qquad ...(ii)$$

Substitute for B from Eq. (i) into Eq. (ii)

$$B = (A/y - zy)$$

$$P = (A/y - zy + 2y\sqrt{1 + z^2}) \qquad \qquad ...(iii)$$

Differentiate Eq. (iii) with respect to y holding z constant and equating the resulting expression to zero.

$$\frac{dP}{dy} = -\frac{A}{y^2} - z + 2\sqrt{1 + z^2} = 0$$

$$\frac{A}{y^2} + z = 2\sqrt{1 + z^2}.$$

But $$A = (B + zy)y$$

Therefore,

$$\frac{(B + zy)y}{y^2} + z = 2\sqrt{1 + z^2} \qquad \qquad ...(12.46a)$$

Rearranging the terms,

$$\frac{(B + 2z)y}{2} = y\sqrt{1 + z^2} \qquad \qquad ...(12.45a)$$

Top width $$T = B + 2zy \qquad \qquad ...(iv)$$

Length of slopping side $$S = y\sqrt{1 + z^2} \qquad \qquad ...(v)$$

From Eqs. (iv) and (v)

$$T/2 = S \qquad \qquad ...(12.46b)$$

This means that the length of sloping side should be equal to half the width at water surface

(ii) Again differentiate Eq. (iii) with respect to z holding y as constant and set dP/dz equal to zero.

$$\frac{dP}{dz} = -y + 2y \cdot \frac{1}{2\sqrt{1+z^2}} \cdot 2z = 0$$

$$\frac{2z}{\sqrt{1+z^2}} = 1$$

Solving it for z,

$$z = 1\sqrt{3} \qquad \qquad ...(12.47a)$$

$$\tan \theta = 1/z = \sqrt{3}$$

i.e. $\qquad \qquad \theta = 60° \qquad \qquad ...(12.47b)$

This meass that the best section is one half of hexagonal section.

(iii) The hydraulic radius $R = A/P$

$$= \frac{(B + zy)y}{(B + 2y\sqrt{1+z^2})}$$

From Eq. 12.45 a, $B = 2y\sqrt{1+z^2} - 2zy$

Substitute this value of B in the expression for R and solve it.

$$R = y/2 \qquad \qquad ...(12.48)$$

That is, the hydraulic radius is equal to half the depth of flow for most efficient section.

(iv) Further, draw normals from O (middle point of water surface) to the sloping sides and bottom of channel; these are OA, OC and OD. Refer to Fig. 12.8b

In $\quad \Delta EFK$, $\sin \theta = EK/EF$

In $\quad \Delta OAE$, $\sin \theta = OA/OE$

But from Eq. 12.45 b, $OE = EF$, $T/2 = S$

Hence $\qquad OA = EK = y \qquad \qquad ...(12.49a)$

Similarly, $\qquad OD = OC = y \qquad \qquad ...(12.49b)$

Thus a semi circle having its centre in the middle of the water surface and radius equal to the water depth can be inscribed in the most efficient section.

3. Most efficient circular section

Circular conduits are used to carry sewage. They run partially full with a free surface. Flow in such conduits are then governed by the principles of open channel flow. Consider a pipe of radius r carrying water to a depth y, Fig. 12.9.

Area of flow $A = (OACB - OAB)$

If 2θ is the angle subtended at the centre O by water surface, then

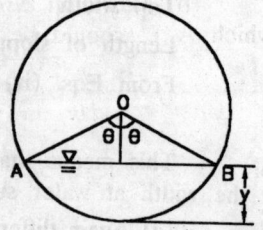

FIG. 12.9. CIRCULAR SECTIONS

$$A = (\pi r^2/2\pi) \times 2\theta - \frac{1}{2} \times 2 \times r \sin \theta \times r \cos \theta$$

$$= [r^2 \theta - (r^2 \sin 2\theta)/2] \qquad \qquad ...(i)$$

Wetted perimeter $P = 2\theta r$ ...(ii)

It is evident that area A and perimeter P are both variable and therefore, maximum velocity and maximum discharge will not occur at the same depth.

From Eq. 12.40

$$U = 1/n \, R^{2/3} \, S^{1/2} = 1/n \, (A/P)^{2/3} \, S^{1/2}$$ ...(12.40)

and $\quad Q = AU = 1/n \, (A^5/P^2)^{1/3} \, S^{1/2}$ ...(12.41)

For maximum velocity the necessary condition can be obtained by differentiating A/P with respect to θ and equating it to zero. For maximum discharge A^5/P^2 should be differentiated and the resulting expression is equated to zero.

(A) *Maximum velocity*. Differentiating A/P with respect to θ

$$\frac{d}{d\theta}(A/P) = \frac{P\dfrac{dA}{d\theta} - A\dfrac{dP}{d\theta}}{P^2} = 0$$

$$P\frac{dA}{d\theta} - A\frac{dP}{d\theta} = 0$$ ...(iii)

Substituting values from Eqs. (i) and (ii)

$$2\theta r \left[r^2 (1 - \cos 2\theta) \right] - r^2 \left[\theta - \left(\frac{\sin 2\theta}{2} \right)(2r) \right] = 0$$

From which $\tan 2\theta = 2\theta$

Solution of above trigonometric equation gives

$$2\theta = 257.5°$$ ...(12.50)

Therefore, depth of water for maximum velocity is

$$y = r - r\cos\theta$$
$$y = r \left(1 - (\cos 257.5°/2) \right)$$
$$y = 1.62 \, r$$ ...(12.51a)

Depth of flow $= 0.81 \, D$ ...(12.51b)

where D is the diameter of the circular pipe.

(b) *Maximum discharge*. Condition for maximum discharge is that for which A^5/P^2 should be maximum, that is

$$\frac{d}{d\theta}(A^5/P^2) = \frac{P^2 \times 5A^4 \, dA/d\theta - A^5 \times 2P \, dP/d\theta}{P^4} = 0$$

or $\quad 5P\dfrac{dA}{d\theta} = 2A\dfrac{dP}{d\theta}$ ...(iv)

Substituting the necessary terms from Eqs.(i) to (ii) in Eq. (iv),

$$5 \, (2r\theta) \, [r^2 (1 - \cos 2\theta)] = 2 \, [r^2 \, (\theta - (\sin 2\theta/2) \, (2r) = 0.$$

or $\quad 3\theta = 5\cos 2\theta - \sin 2\theta$

Solving this trigonometric equation,

$$2\theta = 302.3° \qquad \qquad ...(12.52)$$

Therefore, the depth of flow y for maximum discharge is

$$y = r(1 - \cos\theta) = r(1 - \cos 302.3°/2)$$
$$= 1.876\,r \qquad \qquad ...(12.53a)$$
$$= 0.938\,D \qquad \qquad ...(12.53b)$$

As the depth of water is 0.936 D, even a slight backwater will cause the section to run full.

In addition to these sections (rectangular, trapezoidal and circular) other sections (oval shaped or egg shaped) are also used as sewers. In such cases, the velocity is kept maximum at low depth of flow (or low rate of discharge) so as to prevent deposition of the suspended material and velocity is kept low at high discharge to prevent its excessive wear and tear.

11.12 SECTION OF CONSTANT VELOCITY

Many a times the constant velocity section is required because it is independent of depth. For ordinary channel section (as used for sewers, drains, etc.) the discharge fluctuates within wide range during the year; thereby velocity of flow also varies. While the depth of flow is large, it produces excessive velocity which may damage the channel lining. On the other hand, the velocity may become small if the depth of flow is low, causing deposition of suspended materials. Therefore, the section is to be so designed that it carries no silting, no scouring velocity.

Let the section shown in Fig. 12.10 be a 'constant velocity section' whose shape is to be determined. Take a small strip of fluid of width 2x at a distance y from co-ordinate axis X. The thichness of strip is dy (say). Therefore,

Area of flow of this strip dA = 2x dy

Perimeter of this strip $dP = 2\sqrt{(dx)^2 + (dy)^2}$

Then hydraulic radius . $R = \dfrac{dA}{dP} = \dfrac{xdy}{\sqrt{(dx)^2 + (dy)^2}}$

The velocity of flow is given by eq. 12.36b

$$U = C\sqrt{RS}$$

For given slope S and Chezy's constant C, the velocity will be constant if hydraulic radius is constant.

Therefore,

$$R^2 = \frac{x^2\,dy^2}{(dx^2 + dy^2)}$$
$$x^2(dy)^2 = R^2(dx)^2 + R^2(dy)^2$$
$$(dy)^2(x^2 - R^2) = R^2(dx)^2$$
$$dy/dx = R/\sqrt{x^2 - R^2}$$

Integrating both sides,

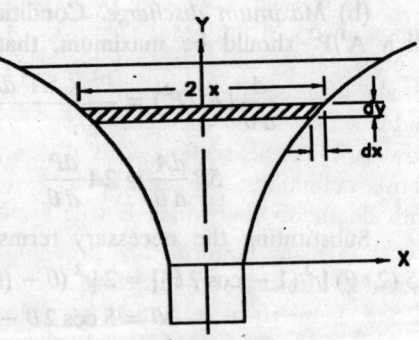

FIG. 12.10. SECTION OF CONSTANT VELOCITY

$$y = R \log_e (x + \sqrt{x^2 - R^2}) + C_1 \qquad \ldots(12.54\overline{a})$$

where C_1 is constant of integration. The 'constant velocity section' is defined by Eq. 12.54a. If its two side curves (catenaries) are extended, they provide a bottomless section. Hence, below the point $y = 0$, the channel section may be either rectangular, trapezoidal or parabolic. Depending upon the shape, slope and other boundary conditions, the constant C_1 is determined and thereby the shape of bottom section is decided.

At $\qquad y = 0, x = R,$

$$C_1 = - R \log_e R$$

Substituting the value of C_1 in Eq. 12.54a,

$$y = R [\log_e (x + \sqrt{x^2 - R^2}) - \log_e R] \qquad \ldots(12.54b)$$

12.13 COMPUTATION OF UNIFORM FLOW

1. Conveyance of a channel section

The discharge of uniform flow in a channel is given by

$$Q = AU$$

$$= A (1/n) R^{2/3} S^{1/2}$$

where the Manning's formula has been used for mean velocity. It can also be expressed as

$$Q = K \sqrt{S} = (1/n) A R^{2/3} S^{1/2} \qquad \ldots(12.55)$$

where K is known as the conveyance of the channel section. It is the measure of carrying capacity of the channel section and is given by

$$K = AR^{2/3}/n \qquad \ldots(12.56)$$

or $\qquad K = 1/n (Z) \qquad \ldots(12.57)$

The term Z equal to $AR^{2/3}$ is known as the section factor for uniform flow which is useful in the computation of uniform flow.

Thus, from Eqs. 12.55 to 12.57

$$AR^{2/3} = n Q/\sqrt{S} \qquad \ldots(12.58a)$$

or $\qquad Z = nK \qquad \ldots(12.58b)$

It is seen from Eq. 12.58 that section factor $(= A R^{2/3})$ depends on the geometry of the area. Therefore, it shows that for given n, Q and S there is only one possible depth for maintaining the uniform flow in the channel. It is known as the 'normal depth' of flow $(= y_n)$. Conversely, for given n and S of a section there can be only one discharge for maintaining uniform flow through the section. This discharge is called 'normal discharge'. In the above definitions, the underlying assumption is that $AR^{2/3}$ always increases with depth of flow which is true for all sections except the circular section.

In many uniform flow problems Q, n and S are given (that is section factor is known) and therefore uniform depth can be determined from Eq. 12.58a. Similarly if n, S and normal depth y are known, the discharge can be determined from Manning's formula.

Alternatively, the dimensionless curves between $AR^{2/3}/B^{8/3}$ and y/B are prepared for various shaped channel sections, $(AR^{2/3}/D^{8/3}$ for circular section). From known values of $Z/B^{8/3}$ the value of normal depth y can be directly read from these curves.

2. Determination of normal depth

(a) *Analytical method.* Determine A, P and R in terms of unknown normal depth y_n. Substitute the values of Q, n, and R in the Manning's formula and then solve the quadratic equation to determine y_n.

(b) *Trial and error method.* From given value of n, Q and S determine Z equal to $nQ/\sqrt{S}$. For various values of y, determine A, R, $R^{2/3}$ and the $AR^{2/3}$. The value of $AR^{2/3}$ corresponding to given $nQ/\sqrt{S}$ is the required normal depth.

(c) *Graphical method.* Instead of making trial, the computations for A, R, $R^{2/3}$ and $AR^{2/3}$ are made in tabular form for various values of y. (i.e. y = 1,2,3 etc) Then a graph is plotted between $AR^{2/3}$ versus y. It is then graph for section factor. From this graph read y_n for given value of $AR^{2/3}$.

12.14 CRITICAL FLOW IN A CHANNEL

1. Specific energy

It is defined as the energy per unit weight of water at any section of a channel measured with respect to the channel bottom. Thus, the specific energy E is expressed as

$$E = d \cos \theta + \alpha\, U^2/2g \qquad \text{...(12.59a)}$$

For a channel of small slope ($\cos \theta \approx 1$), the energy coefficient $\alpha \approx 1.0$ and $y \approx d$. Then

$$E = y + \frac{U^2}{2g} \qquad \text{...(12.59b)}$$

Therefore, the specific energy may be written as the sum of the depth of water and velocity head or in functional form

$$E = y + \frac{Q^2}{2g A^2} \qquad \text{....(12.59c)}$$

The specific energy is a function of y and Q both. Therefore, three different curves can be plotted. (i) E versus y (ii) Q versus y and (iii) E versus Q or q ($= Q/B$).

2. Speciffic energy curve

For given discharge Q, a curve between E and y is plotted which is known as 'specific energy curve'. The specific energy has two components, namely depth y and velocity energy $U^2/2g$. These are plotted as curves I and II in Fig. 12.11. By summing up the ordinates of these two curves, a composite curve is obtained which is the required 'specific energy curve'.

The following characteristics of this curve should be noted.

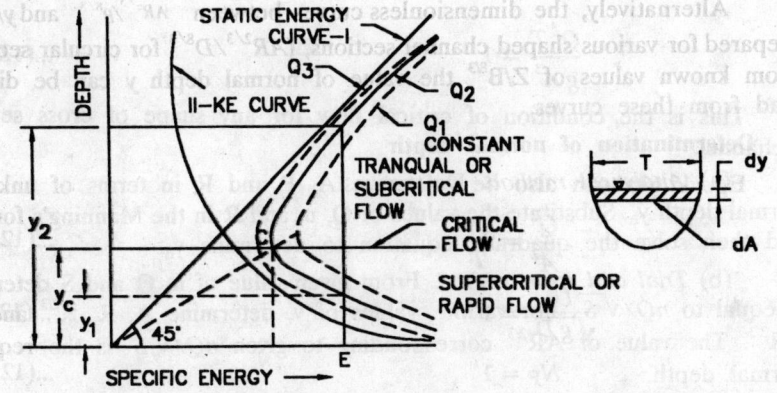

FIG. 12.11. SPECIFIC ENERGY CURVE

(1) The curve is asymptotic to energy line at one end and to a datum energy line at other end(i.e. a line making an angle of 45° with X-axis).

(2) For any given value of E, there are two possible depths which are known as 'alternate depths, y_1 and y_2 respectively.

(3) The specific energy is minimum at point C which is a critical point. The depth corresponding to C is known as 'critical depth y_c.'

(4) When the depth y is more than y_c the flow is known as 'subcritical' or tranquil flow', When the depth is less than critical, the flow is known as 'supercritical', shooting' or 'rapid flow'.

(5) The static energy line makes 45° angle with E axis for small slope channel. For steeper channel, the static energy line will be steeper. For steeper channels, Eq. 12.59a is used to draw specific energy curve instead of Eq. 12.59b.

(6) The above curve has been plotted for constant discharge Q_1. If the discharge Q_2 is more than Q_1 the curve will lie above it. When the discharge Q_3 is less than Q_1, the specific energy curve will lie below it.

(7) To derive the condition for critical state of flow, Eq. 12.59,b. is differentiated with respect to y and equated to zero (to locate the depth at which E is minimum).

$$\therefore \quad \frac{dE}{dy} = 1 + \frac{Q^2}{2g} \times \frac{(-2)}{A^3} \times \frac{dA}{dT} = 0 \qquad ...(12.60)$$

For given cross section of the channel, let the top width at water surface be T. Take an elementary strip of depth dy below it (see inset to Fig. 12.11). Therefore,

$$dA = T \, dy$$

or $$dA/dy = T \qquad ...(12.61)$$

Substituting the value of dA/dy in Eq. 12.60 and simplifying

$$\frac{Q^2 T}{g A^3} = 1 \qquad \qquad ...(12.62a)$$

This is the condition of critical flow for any shape of cross section of channel.

Eq. 12.62a can also be written as

$$\frac{Q^2}{A^2} = \frac{gA}{T} \qquad \qquad ...(12.62b)$$

or

$$\frac{U}{\sqrt{gD}} = 1 \qquad \qquad ...(12.62c)$$

or

$$N_F = 1 \qquad \qquad ...(12.62d)$$

The Froude's number of flow is unity for critical flow. It is less than one for subcritical flow and more than one for supercritical flow. The alternate depths y_1 and y_2 and critical depth y_e may be obtained from Eqs. 12.59b and 12.62 respectively.

3. Relation between discharge and depth of flow

From Eq. 12.59c, the discharge Q is obtained in terms of E and y

$$Q = A \sqrt{2g(E - y)} \qquad ...(12.59c)$$

The plot between Q and y can be plotted for constant value of E. Conventionally, the plot is made between discharge $q(=Q/B=$ discharge per unit width) and y in Fig. 12.12.

It can be observed from q - y curve that there are two depths of flow, y_1 and y_2 for a given discharge Q and given specific energy E. These are alternate depths. The discharge q is maximum at critical depth y_e.

$$Q = \sqrt{2g} \times A \times \sqrt{E - y} \qquad ...(12.59c)$$

Differentiating Eq. 12.59c with respect to y and equating to zero.

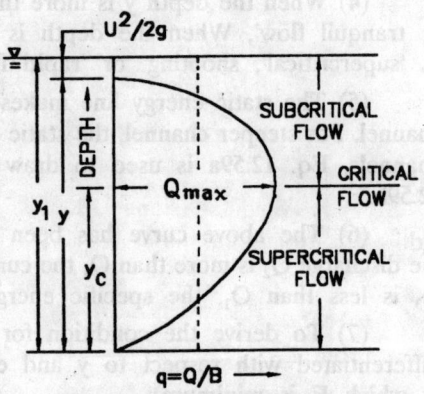

FIG. 12.12 PLOT BETWEEN DISCHARGE PER UNIT WIDTH AND STAGE

$$\frac{dQ}{dy} = \left[A \times \frac{1}{2} \times \frac{1 \times (-1)}{\sqrt{(E - y)}} + \sqrt{(E - y)} \cdot \frac{dA}{dy} \right] = 0$$

Substituting the value of dA/dy = T from Eq. 12.61,

$$2(E - y) T - A = 0$$

From Eq. 12.59c, $(E - y) = Q^2/2g A^2$

Hence,

$$\frac{Q^2 T}{g A^3} = 1$$

or

$$Q/\sqrt{g} = \sqrt{A^3/T} = Z_c \qquad \qquad ...(12.62a)$$

which is the condition of critical flow, Eq. 12.62a. This equation defines the 'section factor for critical flow'.

Thus at critical flow condition (i) the specific energy for given discharge remains minimum, (ii) the discharge for given specific energy is maximum and (iii) the Froude's number is unity.

4. Relation between E and Q

The relation between E and Q (or q) is of least importance. The curve between E and q for given depth of flow is shown in Fig. 12.13. It is evident from Eq. 12.59c that if the specific energy $E < y$, the flow is physically not possible. Even for $E \approx y$, the discharge is zero. At E equal to 1.5y, the critical flow condition exists.

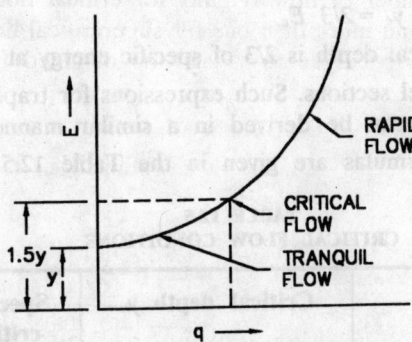

FIG. 12.13. RELATION BETWEEN E AND q FOR CONSTANT y

5. Critical flow

(a) Rectangular channel. Let us consider a rectangular section of bed width B carrying discharge Q at critical depth y_c.

$$A = B \, y_c$$
$$T = B \qquad \qquad ...(12.63)$$

From Eq. 12.62a $Q^2/g = A^3/T$

Substituting the values of A and T

$$B^3 \, yc^3/B = Q^2/g$$

Solving,

$$y_c^3 = \frac{(Q/B)^2}{g}$$

$$y_c = \left(\frac{q^2}{g} \right)^{1/3} \qquad \qquad ...(12.64)$$

where q = discharge/width = Q/B

Eq. 11.62a can also be written as

$$\frac{Q^2}{A^2} = g \frac{A}{T}$$

$$U^2 = \frac{g \, B y_c}{B}$$

$$\frac{U}{\sqrt{g \, y_c}} = 1$$

Solving, $\qquad N_F = 1.0$ $\qquad\qquad$ ....(12.65)

The specific energy E_c for critical flow is written as,

$$E_c = y_c + U^2/2g$$
$$= y_c + y_c/2$$
$$E_c = 1'5 \, E_c \qquad\qquad ...(12.66a)$$

That means, the specific egergy at critical conditions is 1.5 times the critical depth. In other words,

$$y_c = 2/3 \;\; E_c \qquad\qquad\qquad ...(12.66b)$$

That means critical depth is 2/3 of specific energy at critical condition.

(b) Other channel sections. Such expressions for trapezoidal, triangular and parabolic sections can be derived in a similar manner

The resulting formulas are given in the Table 12.5

TABLE 12.5
CRITICAL FLOW CONDITIONS

Channel shape	Critical depth y_c	Specific energy at critical state, E_c
Triangular (side slope 1 : z)	$\left(2 Q^2/g \, z^2\right)^{1/5}$	$5/4 \, y_c$
Trapezoidal (side slope 1:z)	y_c	$\dfrac{y_c \, (3B + 5z \, y_c)}{2 \, (B + 2z \, y_c)}$
Circular (central angle 2θ)	y_c	$\left[y_c + \dfrac{(2\theta - \sin \theta) \, D}{16 \sin \theta} \right]$
Parabolic $T = k \sqrt{y_c}$ $A = \frac{2}{3} T y_c$	$\left(\dfrac{27 \, Q^2}{8g \, k^2} \right)^{1/4}$	$4/3 \, y_c$

12.15. DIMENSIONLESS SPECIFIC ENERGY DIAGRAM

The specific energy in a rectangular channel is given by Eq. 12.59c

$$E = y + \frac{U^2}{2g} = y + \frac{q^2}{2 \, g \, y^2} \qquad\qquad ...(12.59c)$$

The specific energy curve for a constant discharge Q_1 is shown in Fig. 12.11. For a discharge Q_2(more than Q_1) the curve lies above the original curve and for $Q_3(<Q_1)$ the curve lies below it. Thus for different discharges a separate curve is needed. A dimensionless specific energy curve is applicable to all discharges Q through a given channel section of width B.

Divide Eq. 12.59c on both side by y_c,

$$\frac{E}{y_c} = \frac{y}{y_c} + \frac{q^2}{2gy^2 y_c}$$

For critical flow $y_c^3 = q^2/g$

Thus $E/y_c = y/y_c + \frac{1}{2}(y_c/y)^2$ ...(12.67)

Eq. 12.67 is useful for all discharges. A dimensionless specific energy diagram may be plotted between E/y_c and y/y_c. Similarly, a dimensionless discharge curve can also be obtained.

Devide by y_c^3 on both sides of Eq. 12.59c.

$$E/y_c^3 = y/y_c^3 + q^2/(2gy^2 y_c^3)$$

But $y_c^3 = qm^2/g$. Substitute this value of y_c^3 in the last term and multiply by y^2 on both sides where q_m is the value of q corresponding to y_c

$$\frac{E}{y_c^3}\frac{y^2}{y_c^3}y^3 + \frac{1}{2}\left(\frac{q}{qm}\right)^2$$

Further, substitute the value of $E = 3/2 y_c$

Hence $3/2\,(y/y_c)^2 = (y/y_c)^3 + \frac{1}{2}(q/q_m)^2$ ...(12.68)

It is dimensionless discharge equation and the dimensionless plot is drawn between q/q_m and y_c.

12.16 NORMAL, CRITICAL AND CRITICAL NORMAL SLOPE

(a) Normal slope. For given discharge and roughness, the slope of the channel required to maintain a uniform flow in it at normal depth y_n is known as normal slope S_n.

(b) Critical slope. For the given discharge and roughness, the slope of the channel required to maintain a uniform flow at a critical depth y_e is known as critical slope S_e

The smallest value of critical slope for channel of given shape and roughness is called the limit slope S_L

The critical slope is a function of critical depth and varies inversely proportional to depth.

$$Q^2 = K^2 S_c$$

Also $Q^2 = Z_c^2 g$

Eliminating $Q^2, S_c = Z_c^2 g/K^2$

$$= \frac{gA^3}{T}\frac{n^2}{A^2 R^4/3}$$

$$= g\,n^2 A/TR^{4/3}$$

$$= C\,(1/y_c^3)$$ ...(12.69)

The critical slope varies inversely with critical depth.

(c) *Critical slope at normal depth* S_{en}. The channel slope required to obtain a critical flow at the given normal depth by varying descharge flowing in it as well as its slope is known as 'critical slope at normal depth' S_{en}.

12.17 APPLICATION OF SPECIFIC ENERGY

The concept of energy is of great practical importance. Some of its uses are in the design of transitions, for the flow measurement (by venturiflume, standing flume and Parshal flume) and the flow over broad creasted weir.

1. Flow through rectangular channel transition

A channel flowing from its head to tail end has to cross many hydraulic structures like aquaducts, highway culverts, etc. While crossing these structures, the dimensions of channel section need to be changed. The original section is to be joined to the changed section by means of transitions. As an example, a trapezoidal channel section while crossing a highway culvert may be changed to rectangular section for ease of construction (from economy considerations). The transitions may be either gradual or sudden and may be affected either by (i) changing the width of section or by (ii) by raising its bed or (iii) by a combination of both. Only rectangular reducing transitions are discussed here. The expanding transitions and transitions of other shape can be referred to elsewhere.

(a) *Reduction by width*. Consider a rectangular section carrying a discharge Q in Fig. 12.14. The width and depth of flow at section 1 are B_1 and y_1 respectively. The channel section is contracted to B_2 at section 2. Since the section is contracting (and the flow is accelerating) and the length of transition is small, it can safely be assumed that no energy loss takes place between these section 1 and 2. Therefore, the specific energy at sections 1 and 2 remains the same. The approaching flow at section 1 may either be subcritical or supercritical. Let us first consider the case of approaching subcritical flow at section 1 so that $y_1 > y_c$. The discharge per unit width at sections 1 and

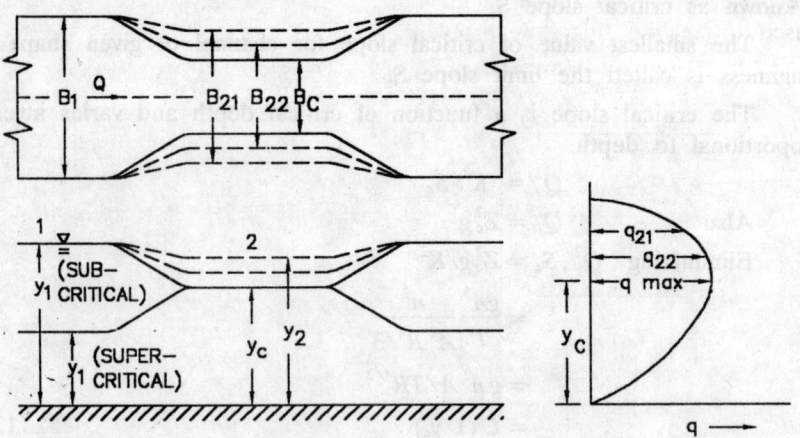

FIG. 12.14. FLOW THROUGH A TRANSITION WIDTH OF CHANNEL REDUCED

2 are q_1 ($= Q/B_1$) and q_2 (Q/B_2) respectively. Since the channel is converging, q_2 is greater than q_1

As the flow proceeds from upstream section to contracting section, the subcritical depth y_1 reduces to y_2; this can be seen from stage- discharge curve, Fig. 12.12. If the width is reduced further, the depth at 2 becomes still smaller. If the reduction in width is continued, the width at downstream section becomes B_c and the flow becomes critical at this section. Thus the depth of flow at 2 becomes critical and equal to y_c whereas the discharge rate (Q/B_c) becomes maximum, that is $q_c = q_{max}$ Further reduction in width of section 2 needs a still large unit discharge $q_2' > q_{max}$ which is physically not. possible with the given upstream specific energy E_1 as is obvious from Fig. 12.12. Therefore, for the flow to continue through contracted section at the critical state with discharge rate q_2' the upstream specific energy has to increase. This causes a rise in upstream water level to y_1' ($> y_1$) or afflux at upstream end, Fig. 12.14.

Similarly, if the approaching flow is supercrittcal the reduction in width at section 2 causes rise in water level at contracted section. When the width of contracted section becomes B_c, the flow becomes critical and y_2 becomes equal to critical depth y_e (Refer to the lower half portion of stage discharge diagram Fig. 12.12). The discharge rate/unit width q_2 acquires its maximum value, i.e. q_{max} with the given upstream specific energy. Further reduction in width of section 2, (say) B_4 requires still larger unit discharge q_2' ($> q_{max}$) which is physically not possible with given E_1. At this stage, radical change takes place on the upstream water surface and a hydraulic jump is formed. between sections 2 and its downstream section.

(b) *Transition: rise in channel bed.* Consider again a rectangular channel carrying a discharge Q, Fig. 12.15. Its bed at section 2 is raised by Δz (say) relative to section 1; width remaining same at both the section 1 and 2. Due to the difference in bed level at sections.1 and 2 the specific energy at these sections does not remain same while the discharge (for constat Q) can be used to analyse this flow problem.

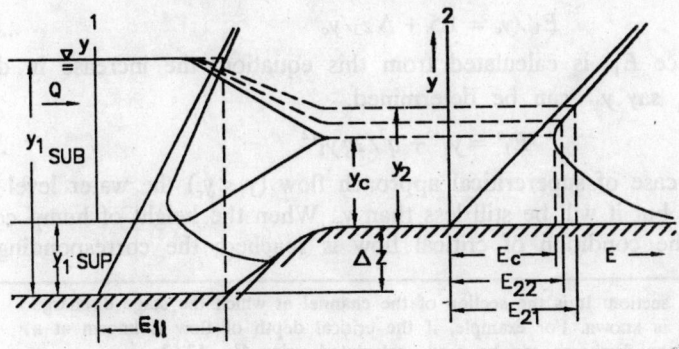

FIG. 12.15. FLOW THROUGH A TRANSITION DEPTH OF FLOW REDUCED

While the height of hump (rise) Δz is small the flow condition shown by dotted line results. The specific energy at 1 and 2 is related by Eq. 12.70.

$$E_1 = E_2 + \Delta z$$

$$y_1 + \frac{q^2}{2gy_1^2} = y_2 + \frac{q^2}{2gy_2^2} + \Delta z \qquad ...(12.70)$$

where y_1 and y_2 are the depths of water at 1 and 2 and q is the discharge per unit width.

Now first consider the subcritical approaching flow ($y_1 > y_e$). As discussed earlier, the water surface drops down at the hump but is still greater than y_e. When the height of hump continues to rise, the condition of critical flow is reached at section 2. The specific energy at section 2 then becomes E_e and the corresponding depth of flow becomes y_e. It is given by

$$E_c = \frac{3}{2} y_c = \frac{3}{2} (q^2/g)^{1/3}$$

The height of jump Δz_2 is given by

$$\Delta z_2 = E_1 - E_2 = E_1 - E_c \qquad ...(12.71)$$

$$= E_1 - 1.5 (q^2/g)^{1/3}$$

Under this condition the section 2 behaves as a control section*. The flow at upstream section 1 is unaffected by the flow at section2.

If the height of hump is raised further, say, $\Delta z_3 (> \Delta z_2)$

Specific energy at section 2 becomes less than E_c.

$$E_2 = E_1 - \Delta z_3 \qquad ....(12.72)$$

Thus the flow cannot take place with the given specific energy E_1 at section 1, as is evident from Fig. 12.15. Therefore, for the flow to occur, the energy E_1 at section 1 should increase to E_1' which is given by Eq. 12.72. The flow condition at 2 still remains critical, $(E_2 = E_e)$.

$$E_1' = E_2 + \Delta z_3 = E_c + \Delta z_3 \qquad ...(12.73a)$$

$$= 1.5 y_c + \Delta z_3$$

$$E_1'/y_c = 1.5 + \Delta z_3/y_c \qquad ...(12.73b)$$

Once E_1' is calculated from this equation, the increase in depth at section 1, say y_1' can be determined.

$$E_1' = y_1' + q^2/2gy_1'^2 \qquad ...(12.64)$$

In case of supercritical approach flow ($y_1 < y_c$) the water level rises at the hump but it will be still less than y_c. When the height of hump continues to rise, the condition of critical flow is reached; the corresponding height

---

* Control section: It is the section of the channel at which the stage discharge relation is known. For example, if the critical depth of flow is known at a section the discharge can be easily calculated using Eq. 12.62a.

of hump is its maximum height, Δz_{max} (say) for the flow to occur with the given E_1, that is

$$E_2 = E_1 - \Delta z_{max}$$
$$= E_c \qquad\qquad ...(12.75)$$

If the height of hump is raised further to $\Delta z_3 (> \Delta z_{max})$, say, the water level at the hump must rise. Since the specific energy at 2 or E_2 becomes less than critical energy E_c, the flow cannot take place through the channel with given E_1.

$$E_2 = E_1 - \Delta z_3$$
i.e. $$E_2 < E_c \qquad\qquad ....(12.76)$$

Therefore, the flow adjusts itself in such a way that the specific energy E_1 increases to E_1' at upstream and a hydraulic jump forms over the hump. (Refer to flow over broad crested weir). The specific energy E_1' is determined from Eq. 12.73b and Eq. 17.67

Alternate treatment of flow through transitions. The total energy at a section, H, of the water flowing in a rectangular channel is given by

$$H = y + z + \frac{q^2}{2gy^2} = E + z \qquad\qquad ...(12.77)$$

Defferentiate it with respect to x, q is assumed as constant

$$\frac{dH}{dx} = \frac{dy}{dx} + \frac{dz}{dx} + \frac{q^2}{2g}(-2y^{-3})\frac{dy}{dx} = 0$$

But $N_F = q/\sqrt{gy^3}$, therefore, rearranging the terms

$$\frac{dy}{dx}(1 - N_F^2) + \frac{dz}{dx} = 0, \text{ assnming H as constant}$$

or $$dz/dx = -dy/dx (1 - N_F^2) \qquad\qquad ...(12.78)$$

For a rise in bed level, dz/dx is positive and hence the product of dy/dx and $(1-N_F^2)$ should be negative to satisfy Eq. 12.78. For subcritical flow, NF < 1, $(1-N_F^2) > 1$ and hence dy/dx will be negative or drop in water level. For supercritical flow, NF > 1, $(1-N_F^2) > 1$, and therefore, dy/dx will be positive or rise in water level. The same arguments can be applied for drop in bed level.

Contraction. In case of contracting channel, the width B is a variable and so also q but z is constant.

Again differentiate Eq. 12.77 with respect to x.

$$\frac{dH}{dx} = \frac{dy}{dx} + \frac{2q}{2gy^2} \times \frac{dq}{dx} - \frac{q^2}{gy^3} \times \frac{dy}{dx} = 0 \qquad\qquad ...(12.79)$$

But $Q = qb$, differentiating with respect to x,

$$\frac{dQ}{dx} = \frac{b\,dq}{dx} + q\frac{db}{dx} = 0, \text{ Since Q is constant.}$$

$$dq/dx = - (q/b)\, db/dx \qquad \qquad ...(12.80)$$

Substituting the value of dq/dx from Eq. 12.80 into Eq. 12.79, and putting N_F equal to $q/\sqrt{gy^3}$

$$\frac{dy}{dx}(1 - N_F^2) - \frac{q}{gy^2} \times \frac{q}{b}\frac{db}{dx} = 0$$

Rearranging the terms:

$$\frac{dy}{dx}(1 - N_F^2) = NF^2 \frac{y}{b}\frac{db}{dx} \qquad \qquad ....(12.81)$$

For contracting channel, db/dx is negative; therefore dy/dx $(1 - N_F^2)$ should also be negative. For subcritical flow NF < 1, $(1 - N_F^2) > 0$ or 'positive; hence dy/dx should be negative or water level should drop at the channel contraction. For supercritical flow NF > 1, $(1 - N_F^2) < 0$ or negative; hence dy/dx should be positive or water level should rise at the channel contraction.

2. Measurement of flow in an open channel

The theory of critical flow can be used for the measurement of flow in an open channel. These devices are known as 'critical flow meters'. Some of them are Venturiflume, standing wave flume, Parshal flume and broad crested weir.

(a) Flow in a Venturiflume. A venturiflume essentially consists of constriction of channel section without any change in bed level. It consists of a converging section, a parallel throat and a gradual diverging channel section made out of concrete, masonry or even metal.

As discussed above, the constriction causes the drop in water level at the throat. This creates a difference $\Delta y'$ (say) in the water level between the section 1 and 2 at the throat. If the throat is designed properly, the critical flow will occur at the throat and the depth of flow will be y_c.

From Eqs. 12.64 and 12.66a

$$y_c = (q^2/g)^{1/3} = [(Q/B_2)^2/g]^{1/3}$$

and
$$E_1 = y_1 + U_1^2/2g = E_c$$

$$= 15\, y_c$$

$$y_1 + U_2^2/2g = 1.5\,[1/g \times (Q/B_2)^2]^{1/3}$$

If the velocity energy $U_1^2/2g$ is neglected.

Solving, $\qquad Q = 0.544\, B_2 \sqrt{g}\, y_1^{3/2}. \qquad ...(12.82)$

It is applicable in S.I. and M.K.S. units. It is observed from Eq. 12.82 that only a single measurement of depth at upstream section is required for the computation of discharge.

If the constriction B_2 (> B_c) is such that critical flow does not occur at section 2, the discharge is given by

$$Q = \frac{B_1 B_2 y_1 y_2 \sqrt{2g(y_1 - y_2)}}{\sqrt{B_1^2 y_1^2 - B_2^2 y_2^2}} \qquad \text{...(12.83a)}$$

Taking into accounts the coefficient of discharge C_d.

$$Q = C_d B_1 B_2 y_1 y_2 \sqrt{2g(y_1 - y_2)} / \sqrt{B_1^2 y_1^2 - B_2 y_2^2} \qquad \text{...(12.83b)}$$

Merits. (i) The energy loss between sections 1 and 2 is relatively too less. (ii) It can be used even for silt ladden water as the bed is at the same level throughout its length.

Demerit. The difference of levels of water is relatively small.

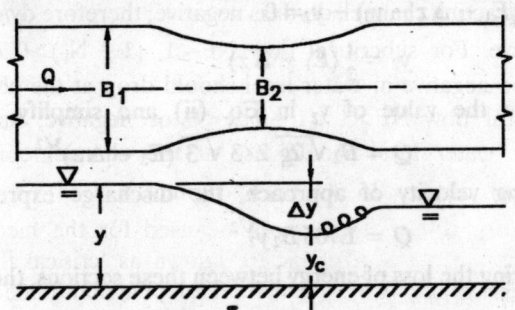

FIG. 12.16. (A) FLOW IN A VENTURIFLUME

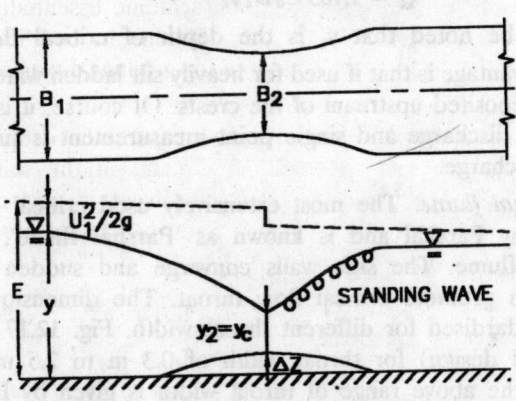

FIG. 12.16. (B) STANDING WAVE FLUME

(b) *Flow in a standing flume.* Another device for the measurement of flow in a channel is standing wave flume. The critical flow condition at section 2 is obtained by raising its bed as well as contracting the width of channel. A standing wave or hydraulic jump is formed downstream of throat section 2. Let the bed be raised at section 2 by Δz relative to section 1. The specific energy at these section is related as

$$E_1 = E_2 + \Delta z \qquad \text{...(i)}$$

$$= y_2 + \frac{Q^2}{2g B_2^2 y_2^2} + \Delta z$$

or
$$Q = \sqrt{2g\, B_2^2 y_2^2\,(E_1 - y_2 - \Delta z)} \qquad \text{...(ii)}$$

For maximum discharge condition occurring at critical state of flow, differentiate Eq (ii) with respect to y_2 and equate it to zero.

$$dQ/dy_2 = \sqrt{2g}\; B_2 \left[y_2 \left\{ \frac{1}{2} \frac{1}{(E_1 - \Delta z - y_2)^{1/2}} \right\} + \sqrt{(E_1 - \Delta z - y_2)}\,(1) \right] = 0$$

$$2\,(E_1 - \Delta z - y_2) - y_2 = 0$$

$$y_2 = \frac{2}{3}\,(E_1 - \Delta z)$$

Substitute the value of y_2 in Eq. (ii) and simplify,

$$Q = B_2 \sqrt{2g}\; 2/3 \sqrt{3}\;(E_1 - \Delta z)^{3/2}$$

Neglecting velocity of approach, the discharge expression becomes

$$Q = 1.705\, B_2 y_2^{3/2} \qquad \text{...(12.84a)}$$

Considering the loss pf energy between these sections, the actual discharge is given

$$Q = 1.705\, C_d\, B_2 y_2^{3/2} \qquad \text{...(12.84b)}$$

It is to be noted that y_2 is the depth of critical flow y_c.

Its disadvantage is that if used for heavily silt ladden water, the suspended material gets deposited upstream of the crests. Of course, it is a simple device to measure the discharge and single point measurement is sufficient for computation of discharge.

(c) *Parshal flume.* The most extensively used critical flowmeter which was designed by Parshal and is known as 'Parshal flume'. It is similar to standing wave flume. The side walls converge and sudden dip in the bed are provided to promote critical flow throat. The dimensions of this flume have been standardised for different throat width. Fig. 12.17 shows a parshal flume (standard design) for throat width of 0.3 m to 2.5 m. The discharge expression for the above range of throat width is given by Eq. 12.85 in FPS units (since all the charts for corrections C, etc., are available in FPS units only)

$$Q = 4B\,H_a \qquad \text{...(12.85a)}$$
$$C = 1.522\, B^{0.026} \qquad \text{...(12.85b)}$$

when the submergence ratio $H_a/H_b < 0.7$., H_a and H_b are the depths of water at sections 1 and 3 and are measured above the upstream bed level. If the ratio H_b/H_a exceeds 0.7, the flow becomes submerged. The effect of submergence is to reduce the discharge. Therefore, a correction is made to the discharge calculated by Eq. 12.85b.

. (d) *Broad crested weir.* As discussed in section 12.17.2b, the height of hump equal to or greater than limiting value of rise in bed creates a state of critical flow at the control section. This fact can be used as a flow measuring device. A broad crested weir should be of sufficient crest width so that the conditions of parallel flow are obtained over it. The pressure distribution at the two ends are assumed hydrostatic and the flow over it is critical. The edges of the weir are made round so as to minimise the loss of energy between entrance section and a section over the crest (otherwise there is likelyhood of the separation of flow at the entrance causing large energy loss). An extensive study of the flow over a broad crested weir has been made by Ranga Raju, *et. al.* They have determined the coefficients of correction for the

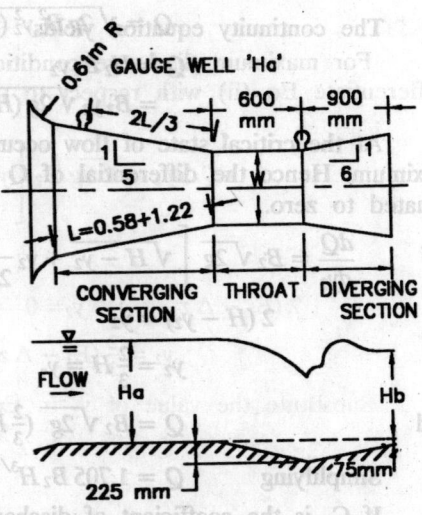

FIG. 12.17 PARSHAL FLUME

effects of surface tension, viscosity, curvature of flow and friction on the discharge passing over the weir.

Consider a broad crested weir of crest height Z and length L in the direction of flow and width B normal to the direction of flow. Let depth of water above the crest at the upstream section 1 be H and above the crest be y_c.

Let the water flow with a velocity U_2 over the weir. Therefore, the energy equation becomes,

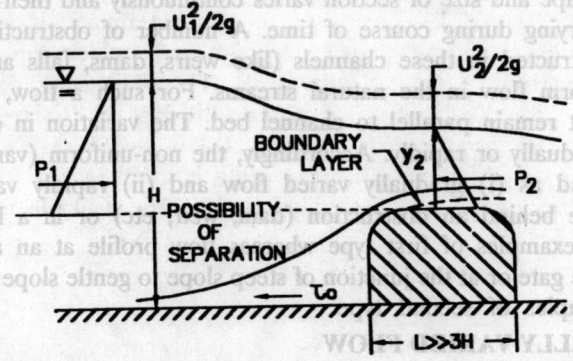

FIG. 12.18. FLOW OVER A BROAD CRESTED WEIR

$$H + U_1^2/2g = y_2 + U_2^2/2g$$

Neglecting the energy loss and velocity(of approach) energy

$$U_2 = \sqrt{2g\,(H - y_2)}$$

The continuity equation yields

$$Q = U_2 B_2 y_2$$
$$= B_2 y_2 \sqrt{2g(H - y_2)}$$

At the critical state of flow occurring over the weir, the discharge is maximum. Hence the differential of Q with respect to depth y_2 should be equated to zero.

$$\frac{dQ}{dy_2} = B_2 \sqrt{2g} \left[\sqrt{H - y_2} + y_2 \frac{1}{2\sqrt{H - y_2}} (-1) \right] = 0$$

$$2(H - y_2) = y_2$$

$$y_2 = \frac{2}{3} H = y_c$$

and
$$Q = B_2 \sqrt{2g} \left(\frac{2}{3} H\right) \left(\frac{1}{3} H\right)^{1/2}$$

Simplifying
$$Q = 1.705 B_2 H^{3/2} \qquad ...(12.86a)$$

If C_d is the coefficient of discharge, the actual discharge is given by

$$Q = 1.705 C_d B_2 H^{3/2} \qquad ...(12.86b)$$

The value of C_d varies from 0.55 to 0.65. The minimum width of crest is given by

$$L/H \geq 3.$$

12.18 NON-UNIFORM FLOW

The uniform flow generally occurs in an artificial channel of constant size, shape and roughness (of its section) laid at a constant bed slope. As a result of it, the water surface remains parallel to its bed. But the flow occurring in natural streams and small flumes is of non-uniform type. In these channels, the shape and size of section varies continuously and their bed slope also goes on varying during course of time. A number of obstructions which are usualy constructed in these channels (like weirs, dams, falls and others) create non-uniform flow in the natural streams. For such a flow, the water surface does not remain parallel to channel bed. The variation in depth may occur either gradually or rapidly. Accordingly, the non-uniform (varied) flows may be classified as (i) gradually varied flow and (ii) rapidly varied flow. The flow profile behind an obstruction (dam, weir, etc) or in a long reach of channel are examples of first type whereas flow profile at an abrupt fall or below a sluice gate or at the junction of steep slope to gentle slope (hydraulic jump) are examples of second type.

12.19 GRADUALLY VARIED FLOW

For the design of open channels and analysis of flow in them, an engineer must be able to predict the form and position of water surface profiles and the extent of their spread. To achieve this objective, a relationship for the change in depth is required. It is known as differential or dynamic equation of gradually varied flow, When this equation is integrated along the longitudinal direction, it yields the requisite length of water surface curve.

1. Basic assumptions

The following assumptions are made to analyse the gradually varied flow:

(1) The channel is prismatic. Channel section and alignment remain the same.

(2) The bed slope is small. The depths of flow section d (normal to bed) and depth of flow y (vertical depth) are nearly equal.

(3) The energy loss at a section having the same velocity and hydraulic radius is the same as for a uniform flow.

(4) The energy correction factor α is nearly unity.

(5) The pressure distribution is hydrostatic.

(6) The roughness coefficient is independent of depth of flow and constant throughout the channel reach under consideration.

2. Dynamic equation of gradually varied flow

Consider the profile of a gradually varied flow, of length dx, Fig.12.19. Let water be flowing with mean velocity U and the depth of flow at section 1 be d. The total head H above the datum at this section is given by

$$H = d \cos \theta + z + \alpha\, U^2/2g \qquad \qquad ...(12.87)$$

where z is the datum head and α is the energy correction factor. The longitudinal slope of the bed of channel is θ. Conventionally, the X-axis is assumed along the channel bed and Y-axis normal to its bed.

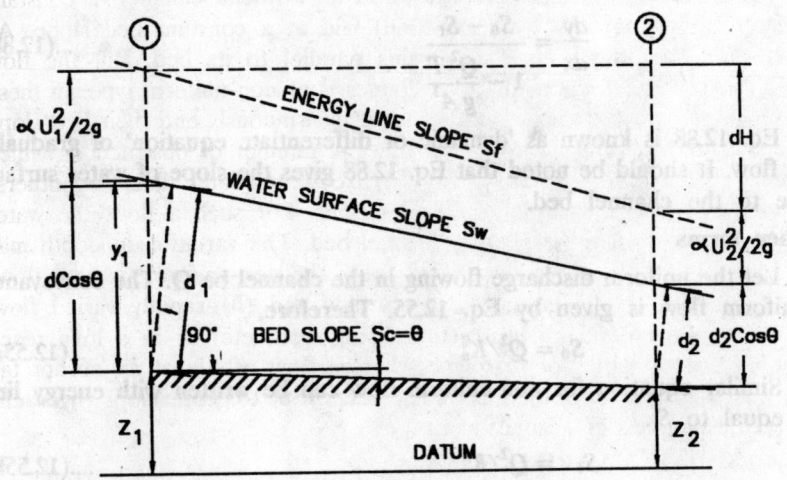

FIG. 12.19. DERIVATION OF GRADUALLY VARIED FLOW EQUATION

Differentiate Eq. 12.87 with respect to y,

$$\frac{dH}{dx} = \frac{dz}{dx} + \cos \theta\, \frac{d\,(d)}{dx} + \alpha\, \frac{d}{dx} (U^2/2g) \qquad ...(i)$$

The slope θ and energy correction factor $\propto$ are assumed constant along X-axis. The bed slope is assumed positive if it ascends and negative if it descends in the direction of flow. Hence,

$$S_o = - \frac{dx}{dx} \quad \text{and} \quad S_f = - \frac{dH}{dx} \qquad ....(ii)$$

Substituting these values in Eq. (i)

$$- S_f = - S_0 + \cos\theta \times \frac{d\,(d)}{dx} + \propto \times \frac{d}{d\,(d)} (U^2/2g) \times \frac{d\,(d)}{dx}$$

Rearranging the terms,

$$\frac{d\,(d)}{dx} = \frac{S_o - S_f}{1 + \propto [d\,(U^2/2g)/d\,(d)]}$$

Since slope angle θ is small and so $y \approx d$. Also, $\propto$ is assumed to be unity.

$$\frac{dy}{dx} = \frac{S_0 - S_f}{1 + d\,(U^2/2g)/dy}$$

$$\frac{dy}{dx} = \frac{S_0 - S_f}{1 + d\,(Q^2/2gA^2)/dy}$$

$$\frac{dy}{dx} = \frac{S_0 - S_f}{1 + \dfrac{Q^2}{2g} \times \dfrac{(-2)}{A^3} \times \dfrac{dA}{dy}}$$

From Eq. 12.61, $dA/dy = T$

$$\frac{dy}{dx} = \frac{S_0 - S_f}{1 - \dfrac{Q^2 T}{g A^3}} \qquad ...(12.88)$$

Eq. 12.88 is known as 'dynamic or differentiate equation' of gradually varied flow. It should be noted that Eq. 12.88 gives the slope of water surface relative to the channel bed.

3. Other forms

Let the uniform discharge flowing in the channel be Q. The conveyance for uniform flow is given by Eq. 12.55. Therefore,

$$S_0 = Q^2/K_n^2 \qquad ...(12.55a)$$

Similar equation for non-uniform flow can be written with energy line slope equal to S_f.

$$S_f = Q^2/K^2 \qquad ....(12.55b)$$

Dividing Eq. 12.55a by 12.55b

$$S_f/S_o = K_n^2/K^2 \qquad ...(12.89)$$

In Eq. 12.4. the symbol Z simply represents the numerical value of $\sqrt{A^3/T}$, whereas in Eq. 12.62a, Z_c represents the section factor for critical flow.

$$Z^2 = A^3/T \qquad \text{....(12.4)}$$

$$Z_c^2 = Q^2/g \qquad \text{...(12.62a)}$$

Dividing Eq. 12.62a by Eq. 12.4,

$$\frac{Z_c^2}{Z^2} = \frac{Q^2}{g} \times \frac{T}{A^3} \qquad \text{...(12.90)}$$

Substituting Eqs. 12.89 and 12.90 in Eq. 12.88,

$$\frac{dy}{dx} = \frac{S_0 \left[1 - S_t/S_0\right]}{\left[1 - Q^2 T/gA^3\right]}$$

$$= \frac{S_0 \left[1 - K_n^2/K^2\right]}{\left[1 - Z_c^2/Z^2\right]} \qquad \text{...(12.91)}$$

It is applicable to any shape of channel section. The conveyance K is a function of y and is equal to

$$K_n = \frac{A R^{2/3}}{n}$$

For a wide rectangular channel, $R \approx y$

$$K_n = B y_n^{5/3}/n$$

and

$$K = B y^{5/3}/n$$

Thus

$$K_n^2/K^2 = (y_n/y)^{10/3} \qquad \text{...(12.92)}$$

The section factor Z is also expressed in terms of y.

$$Z^2 = A^3/T = B^2 y^3$$

and

$$Z_c^2 = \frac{Q^2}{g} = \frac{B^2 q^2}{g} = B^2 y_c^2$$

Since $y_c^3 = q^2/g$ for critical flow in a rectangle channel.

Hence

$$\frac{Z_c^2}{Z^2} = (y_c/y)^3 \qquad \text{....(12.93)}$$

Substituting the values of $(Kn/K)^2$ and $(Z_c/Z)^2$ in Eq. 12.91

$$\frac{dy}{dx} = \frac{S_0 \left[1 - (y_n/y)^{10/3}\right]}{\left[1 - (y_c/y)^3\right]} \qquad \text{...(12.94)}$$

This equation is used to plot the surface profiles on various slopes. It is to be noted that if Chezy's equation is used instead of Manning's equation in Eq. 12.92, then

$$K_n = C B y_n^{3/2}$$

and

$$K = C B y^{3/2}$$

Hence

$$K_n^2/K^2 = (y_n/y)^3$$

The dynamic equation then becomes

$$\frac{dy}{dx} = \frac{S_0 \left[1 - (y_n/y)^3\right]}{\left[1 - (y_c/y)^3\right]} \qquad \qquad ...(12.95)$$

12.20 WATER SURFACE SLOPE WITH RESPECT TO HORIZONTAL

Consider a channel reach between two sections 1 and 2 whose bed is inclined at slope S_0 to the horizontal (Fig. 12.20). The water surface shown by AC is inclined at a slope S_w to the horizontal line AD. The line AB is drawn parallel to channel bed.

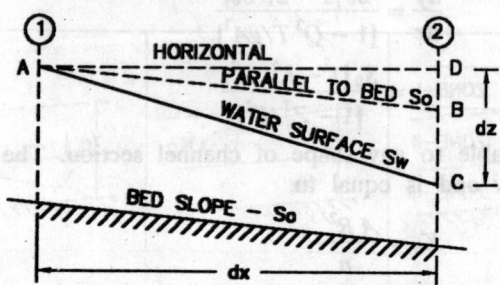

FIG. 12.10. DERIVATION OF GRADIENT OF WATER SURFACE

Thus BC is the distance by which the water depth is reduced between sections 1 and 2, dx distance apart. The change in datum head of water surface (relative to a horizontal line AD) is $z_1 - z_2$, or Δz in a distance dx. The slope of water surface with respect to bed is indicated by dy/dx, whereas relative to horizontal it is given as S_w.

$$S_w = dz/dx = CD/AC$$

$$= \frac{BD + BC}{AC} = \frac{BD}{AC} + \frac{BC}{AC}$$

But $BD/AC =$ bed slope S_0, and $BC/AC = - dy/dx$. Therefore,

$$S_w = S_0 - dy/dx \qquad \qquad ...(12.96a)$$

If water surface rises in the direction of flow, dy/dx is positive.

Therefore, $S_w = S_0 + dy/dx$ ...(12.96b)

12.21 CLASSIFICATION OF SURFACE CURVES

1. Various slopes

The bed slope of channel is compared to the critical slope (for given discharge and other flow conditions) and are classified accordingly.

(1) Mild slope: If bed slope $S_0 < S_c$, it is termed as mild slope which means $y_n > y_c$ as is evident from Eq. 12.40 for given discharge Q.

(2) Steep slope: If bed slope $S_0 > S_c$, it is termed as steep slope; which means $y_n < y_c$.

(3) Critical slope: If bed slop $S_0 = S_c$, it is critical slope and $y_n = y_c$.

(4) Horizontal slope: If bed slope $S_0 = 0$, $y_n = \infty$, it is horizontal slope.

(5) **Adverse slope:** If bed slope $S_o < 0$, it means the channel is rising in the direction of flow. It is known as adverse slope. The normal depth y_n cannot be determined as the roots of quadratic equation (Manning's equation) are imaginary.

Out of these, first three bed slopes are known as 'sustaining slopes' and last two slopes are known as 'non-sustaining slopes.

2. Various zones

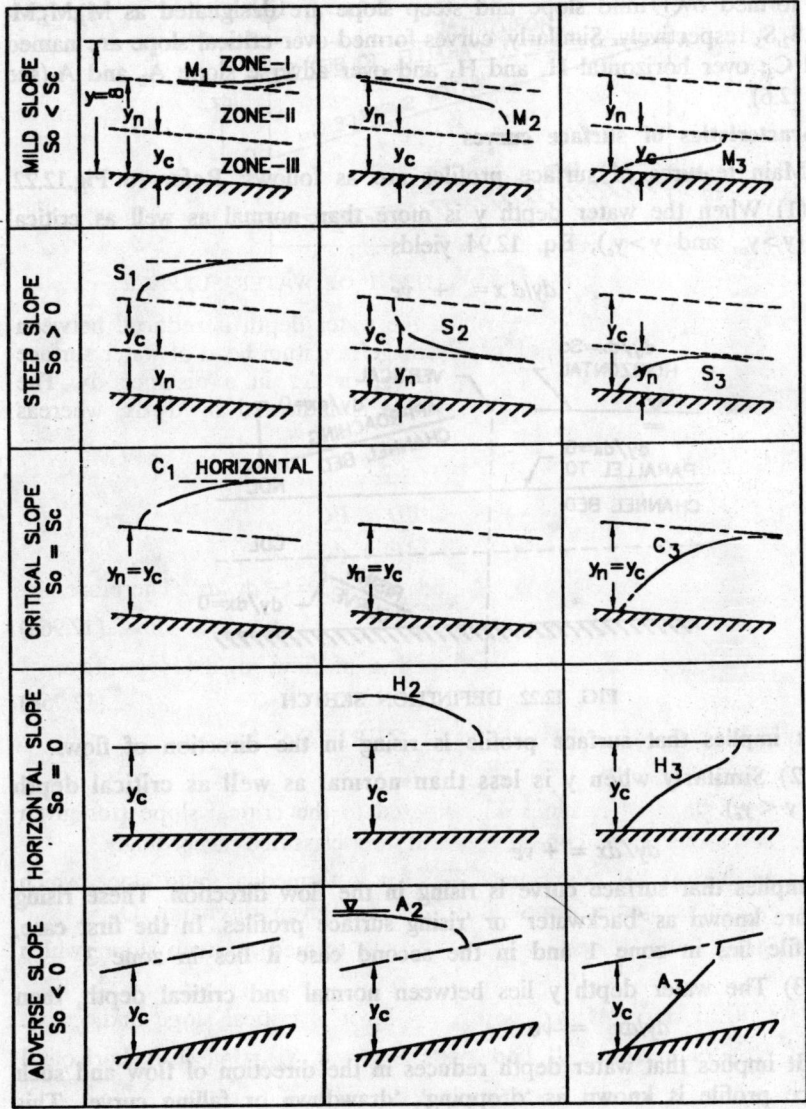

FIG. 12.21. VARIOUS TYPES OF CURVES

There are four governing lines between which a surface profile may lie. These are (i) channel bed (ii) normal depth line or NDL (iii) critical depth line or CDL and (iv) a line at large distance from channel bed; it is expressed as $y = \infty$. These four lines form three zones. The region between top two lines is known as zone 1, between middle two lines as zone 2 and between last two lines as zone 3. In this way, there should be fifteen types of surface curves. In practice, there are in all twelve possible types of curves: three types of curves form over each of mild and steep slopes and two curves form over each of critical, horizontal and adverse slopes, see Fig. 12.21. The curves formed over mild slope and steep slope are designated as M_1, M_2, M_3 and S_1, S_2, S_3 respectively. Similarly, curves formed over critical slope are named C_1 and C_3; over horizontal H_2 and H_3 and over adverse slope A_2 and A_3 (see Table 12.6)

3. Characteristics of surface curves

Main features of surface profiles are as follows: Refer to Fig.12.22.

(1) When the water depth y is more than normal as well as critical depth ($y > y_n$, and $y > y_c$), Eq. 12.94 yields

$$dy/dx = + ve$$

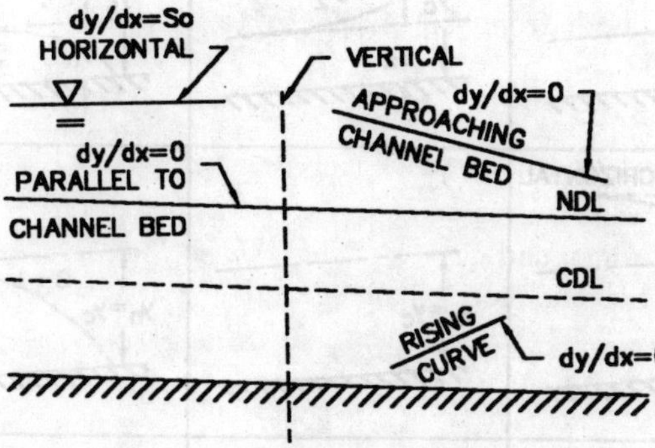

FIG. 12.22. DEFINITION SKETCH

It implies that surface profile is rising in the direction of flow.

(2) Similarly when y is less than normal as well as critical depth ($y < y_n, y < y_c$).

$$dy/dx = + ve$$

Implies that surface curve is rising in the flow direction. These rising curves are known as 'backwater' or 'rising surface profiles. In the first case, the profile lies in zone 1 and in the second case it lies in zone 3

(3) The water depth y lies between normal and critical depth, then

$$dy/dx = -ve$$

It implies that water depth reduces in the direction of flow and such a surface profile is known as 'dropping', 'drawdown or falling curve'. This means that the profiles in zone 2 are always drawdown curves.

(4) When $y \to y_n$, $\dfrac{dy}{dx} \to 0$, or water surface becomes parallel to channel bed. It means that water surface approaches normal depth line asymptotically.

(5) When $y \to y_c$, $\dfrac{dy}{dx} \to \infty$ or water surface cuts critical depth line at right angle. In other words, water surface becomes asymptotic to a vertical line at some point on the critical depth line, $y = y_c$.

(6) When $y \to \infty$, $\dfrac{dy}{dx} \to S_0$ or water surface becomes horizontal.

(7) When $y \to 0$, $\dfrac{dy}{dx} \to \dfrac{\infty}{\infty}$ or indeterminate. Near the bed the curvature of water surface becomes too large and assumption of small slope becomes invalid.

12.22 SURFACE PROFILES

Keeping these characteristics in mind, the surface profiles on any slope can be sketched easily.

1. Mild slope $(S_0 < S_c)$

The normal depth y_n can be computed from Manning's formula Eq. 12.40 and critical depth from Eq. 12.62a. Since $y_n > y_c$, $S_0 < S_c$, the NDL lies above CDL Fig. 12.23.

Zone 1 : $y > y_n > y_c$

$dy/dx = +ve$ or M_1 curve is backwater curve. In this zone the flow is subcritical $(y > y_c)$.

At right extreme end, $y \to \infty$ $dy/dx \to S_0$, that means water surface should eventually become horizontal.

At left extreme end, $y \to y_n$ $dy/dx = 0$ that means water surface should become parallel to bed at this end.

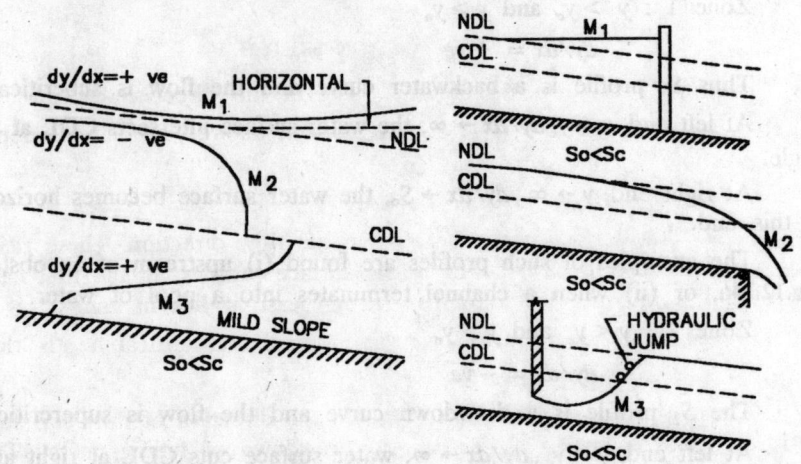

FIG. 12.23 SURFACE PROFILE - MILD SLOPE OF BED

Such a profile may form (i) behind a dam (Fig.12.23a), (ii) at change of slope from mild to milder one and (iii) in a small channel connecting two reservoirs with higher water level in the downstream reservoir.

Zone 2 : $y < y_n$ but $y > y_c$

$dy/dx = -$ ve or M_2 curve is drawdown curve and the flow in zone 2 is subcritical.

At left side end $y \to y_n$, $\dfrac{dy}{dx} = 0$, water surface should be horizontal.

At right side end $y \to y_c$, $dy/dx = \infty$, water surface cuts the CDL line at right angle.

Examples of such profile are seen at (i) free fall at the end of mild slope channel, Fig. 12.23b, (ii) at the junction of change of slope from milder to mild one; (iii) flow taking place from small section to enlarged section of the same channel.

Zone 3: $y < y_n$, also $y < y_c$

$dy/dx = +$ ve ; M_3 curve is backwater curve and the flow is supercritical:

At right end, $y \to y_c$; $\dfrac{dy}{dx} = \infty$ or water surface cuts the CDL line normally,

At left end, $y \to \infty$, $\dfrac{dy}{dx} = \dfrac{\infty}{\infty}$ or indeterminae. This type of profile is unknown near the bed level.

Flow occurring below sluice gate (Fig.12.23c) at the foot of a spillway or (ii) at the junction of steep to mild slope are examples of M_3 curves.

2. Steep slope $(S_o > S_e)$

The normal depth y_n lies below critical depth line over a steep slope, $y_n < y_c$; Fig. 12.24. Generally, a hydraulic jump preceds the S_1 profile.

Zone 1 : $y > y_c$ and $y > y_n$

$$dy/dx = + ve$$

Thus S_1 proflie is a backwater curve and the flow is subcritical

At left end, $y \to y_c$ $dy/dx \to \infty$, the water sutface intersects CDL at right angle.

At right end, $y \to \infty$, $dy/dx \to S_o$, the water surface becomes horizontal at this end.

The examples of such profiles are found (i) upstream of an obstacle, Fig.12.24a, or (ii) when a channel terminates into a pool of water.

Zone 2 : $y < y_c$ and $y > y_n$

$$dy/dx = - ve$$

The S_2 profile is a drawdown curve and the flow is supercritical.

At left end, $y \to y_c$, $dy/dx \to \infty$, water surface cuts CDL at right angle.

At right end, $y \to y_n$, $dy/dx \to 0$, the water surface becomes parallel or asymptotic to normal depth line.

The practical examples are found (i) at the change of mild to steep slope, Fig. 12.24b, and (ii) at junction of steep to steeper slope.

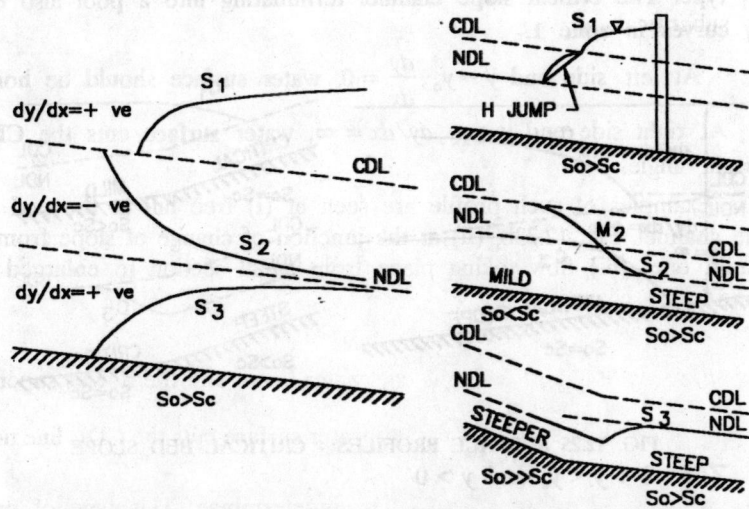

FIG. 12.24. SURFACE PROFILE - STEEP SLOPE OF BED

Zone 3 : $y < y_c$, also $y < y_n$

$$dy/dx = + ve$$

The S_3 profile is a backwater curve and flow is supercritical

At left end, $y \to 0$, dy/dx =indetermindate. At right end, $y \to y_n$, $\dfrac{dy}{dx} \to 0$, the water surface is asymtotic to NDL line.

Some of the examples are found (i) at the junction of steeper to steep slope, Fig. 12.24c, or (ii) the flow taking place below a sluice gate (sluice gate opening less than critical depth)

3. Critical slope: $S_o = S_c$

Since the normal depth and critical depth are the same, $y_n = y_c$, hence there is no zone 2 and C_2 curve does not exist. One may, otherwise, call C_2 profile as uniform critical flow. Fig. 12.25.

Zone 1: $y > y_c$ and $y_c = y_n$

$$dy/dx = + ve$$

Thus C_1 is a backwater curve and flow is subcritical.

At left end, $y \to y_n$, $dy/dx = 0$, that means it is asymptotic to a horizontal line.

At right end, $y \to \infty$, $dy/dx = S_0$, that means it tends to becomes horizontal.

If Chezy's equation is used, Eq. 12.95 is obtained, For critcal flow $(y_n = y_c)$ it reduces to $dy/dx = S_o$. Thus both C_1 and C_3 curves are straight lines parallel to horizontal line.

The profile at the break of slope from critical to mild slope, Fig. 12.25a is C_1 type. The critical slope channel terminating into a pool also creates a C_1 curves in zone 1.

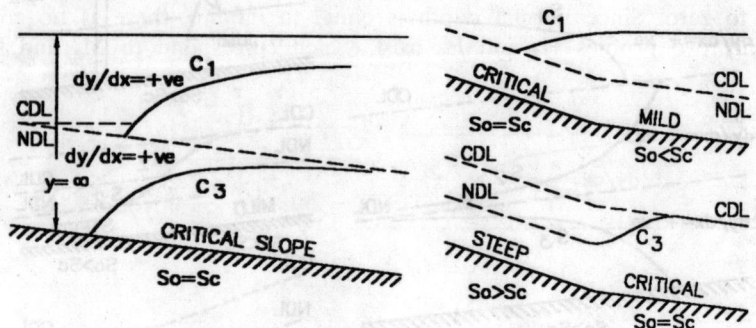

FIG. 12.25 SURFACE PROFILES - CRITICAL BED SLOPE

Zone 3 : $y < y_e$ and $y > 0$

$$dy/dx = + ve$$

The C_3 is again a rising profile or a backwater curve and the flow is supercritical.

At left end, $y \to 0$, $dy/dx \to \infty/\infty$, indeterminate ; hence the profile cannot be sketched at this end.

At right end $y \to y_e$, $dy/dx \to \infty$, hence profile meets CDL normally.

Some of this type of profiles are found (i) below sluice gate fitted in a channel and (ii) at the junction of steep to critical slopes.

4. Horizontal slope, $S_o = 0$ and $y_n = \infty$

These profiles could not be plotted with the help of Eq. 12.94 because of zero bed slope. Fig. 12.26.

From Eq.12.88,

$$\frac{dy}{dx} = -\frac{-S_f}{1 - \dfrac{Q^2 T}{g A^3}} \qquad \text{...(12.88)}$$

But From Eq. 12.40,

$$S_f = n \, U^2 / R^{4/3}$$

For a wide channel, $R \approx y$, therefore it reduces to

$$S_f = \frac{nQ^2}{A^2 y^{4/3}}$$

$$= \frac{n \, Q^2}{B^2 y^{10/3}}$$

Substituting it in Eq. 12.88

$$\frac{dy}{dx} = \frac{- n \, Q^2/B^2 y^{10/3}}{1 - (y_c/y)^3} \qquad \qquad ...(12.97)$$

These are limiting cases of M-profiles when the channel bed slope is reduced to zero. Since normal depth is equal to infinite, there is no zone 1 and only two profiles H_2 and H_3 exist, which correspond to M_2 and M_3 profiles.

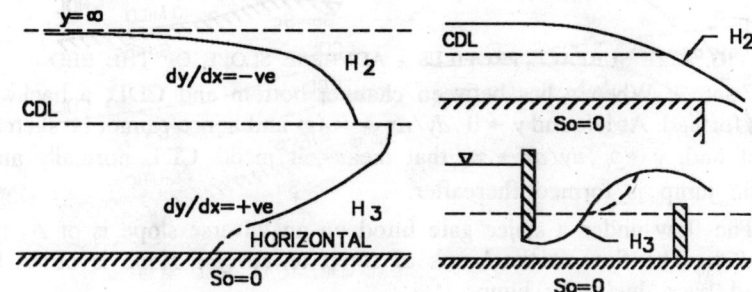

FIG. 12.26. SURFACE PROFILES - HORIZONTAL SLOPE OF BED

Zone 2 : $y < \infty$ but $y > y_c$

$$dy/dx = - ve$$

It means H_2 profiles is a drawdown curve

At left end, $y \to \infty$, $dy/dx \to S_o$ So that it becomes horizontal

At right end, $y \to y_c$, $dy/dx \to \infty$ so that it meets CDL normally.

Examples of this class occurs at the free fall from a horizontal channel. Fig. 12.26a.

Zone 3: $y > 0$ but $y < y_c$

$$dy/dx = + ve$$

At left end, $y \to 0$, $dy/dx = \infty/\infty$ i.e., indeterminate and so the profile cannot be drawn at this end.

At right end $y \to y_c$ so that, $dy/dx \to \infty$, which means that profile meets CDL normally. Thus, H_3 is a backwater profile.

The flow below a sluice gate and fitted on a horizontal channel is the example of this type, Fig. 12.26b.

5. Adverse slope: $S_o < 0$

Since the normal depth y_n is not real the A_1 proflile is impossible.

Zone 2 : y lie between $y = \infty$ and $y = y_c$, the A_2 profile lying in this zone is a drawdown curve. At left end $y \to \infty$ so $dy/dx \to S_o$ and the profile eventually becomes horizontal. At right end, $y \to y_n$, so $dy/dx \to \infty$ and the profile meets CDL normally. Fig 12.27a

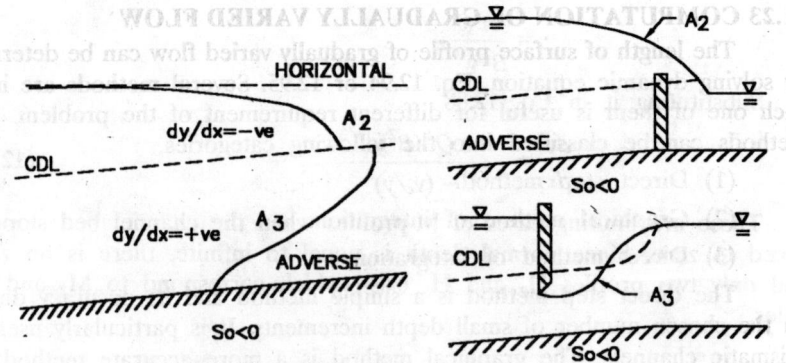

FIG. 12.27. SURFACE PROFILES - ADVERSE SLOPE OF THE BED

Zone 3: When y lies between channel bottom and CDL, a backwater curve is formed. At left end $y \to 0$, $dy/dx \to \infty/\infty$ and hence cannot be sketched. At right end, $y \to y_c$, $dy/dx \to \infty$, that means, it meets CDL normally and a hydraulic jump is formed thereafter.

The flow under a sluice gate fitted on an adverse slope is of A_3 type, Fig. 12.27b. The flow at the breek of steep to adverse slope is of A_3 type preceded by a hydraulic jump.

TABLE 12.6 TYPES OF FLOW PROFILES IN PRISMATIC CHANNELS.

Channel Slope	Symbol			Depth $\dfrac{dy}{dx}$ Relations	Types of curves	Type of flows
	Zone I	Zone II	Zone III			
Horizontal $S_o = 0$	None			$y>y_b>y_c$	None	None
		H_2		$y_n>y>y_c$	Draw down	Subsritical
			H_3	$y_n>y_c>y+$	Backwater	supercritical
Mild $0<S_o<S_c$	M_1			$y_n>y_c>y+$	Backwater	Subsritical
		M_2		$y>y_n>y_c-$	Drawdown	
			M_3	$y_n>y_c>y+$	Backwater	supercritical
Critical $S_o=S_c>0$	C_1			$y>y_n=y_c$	Backwater	Subsritical
		C_2		$y_c=y=y_n$	None	Critical
			C_3	$y_c=y_n>y+$	Backwater	Supercritical
Steep $S_o>S_c>0$	S_1			$y_c>y>y_n-$	Drawdown	Subcritical
		S_2		$y_c>y_n>y+$	Backwater	Supercritical
			S_3			Supercritical
Adverse $S_o<0$	None				None	None
		A_2		$y>y_n-$	Drawdown	Subsritical
			A_3	$y_c>y+$	Backwaer	Supercritical

11.23 COMPUTATION OF GRADUALLY VARIED FLOW

The length of surface profile of gradually varied flow can be determined by solving dynamic equation, Eq. 12.94 or 12.95. Several methods are in use; each one of them is useful for different requirement of the problem. These methods can be classified into the following categories.

(1) Direct step method.

(2) Graphical method of integration.

(3) Direct method of integration.

The direct step method is a simple method and its accuracy depends on the chosen number of small depth increments. It is particularly useful for prismatic channels. The graphical method is a more accurate method and can also be used for non-prismatic channels. There are several methods of direct integration e.g. Bresse's method, Chow's mehthod and Bakhmeteff method which are in use with different flow situations. Only first two methods and Chow's method are discussed in this text. The remaining integration methods can be referred to elsewhere.

1. Direct step method

The computation is made in steps and hence it is known as direct step method. The surface profile is subdivided into a number of small segments of pre-determined depths. Then the length of each segment is determined and finally summed up to get the length of profile.

Consider such a small segment of length Δx between sections 1 and 2. The depth of flow at these sections are y_1 and y_2 respectively. The bed slope of channel is S_0, hence $\Delta z = S_0 \times \Delta x$, Fig 12.28. The energy equation between these two sections can then be written as

$$S_0 \times \Delta x + y_1 + U_1^2/2g = y_2 + U_2^2/2g + S_r \times \Delta x$$

$$\Delta x (S_o - S_f) = E_2 - E_1$$

$$\Delta x = \frac{(E_2 - E_1)}{(S_o - S_f)} \qquad \qquad ...(12.98)$$

For the known discharge Q, the specific energy of the two section 1 and 2 can be determined. The energy line slope at section 1 and 2 is computed from Manning's formula, Eq. 12.40. The average* of these two values $\overline{S}_f (= (S_{f_1} + S_{f_2})/2)$ is then substituted in Eq. 12.98 and Δx is determined.

The method is repeated for different sugments. and the length of these segments is then added up to determine the total length of the surface profile,

The method is useful for prismatic channels only.

---

* Alternatively the values of area, and hydraulic radius are computed separately corresponding to y_1 and y_2 and then the average values of area and hydraulic radius are used to determine S_f.

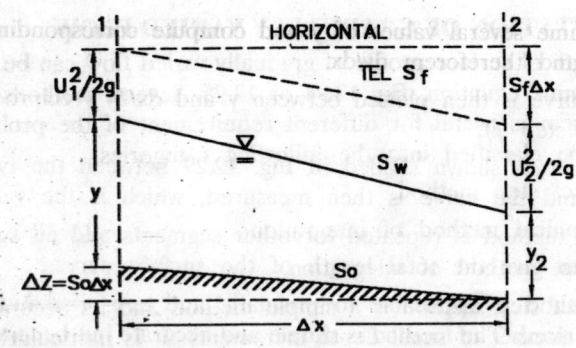

FIG. 12.28. DIRECT STEP METHOD

2. Graphical method of integration

Consider two channel sections 1 and 2 at a distance x_1 and x_2 respectively from a control section. Let the corresponding depths of flow at these sections be y_1 and y_2. The dynamic equation, Eq. 12.89 is

$$\frac{dy}{dx} = \frac{S_o - S_f}{1 - Q^2 T/gA^3} \qquad \text{...(12.88)}$$

The parameters T, A and S_f are all functions of y as discussed earlier. Therefore the above equation can be integrated with respect to y (between the two values of, y, i.e. y_1 and y_2).

$$\int_{x_1}^{x_2} dx = \int_{y_1}^{y_2} \frac{\left(1 - \dfrac{Q^2 T}{gA^3}\right)}{(S_o - S_f)} \cdot dy$$

or

$$x = \int_{y_1}^{y_2} f(y)\, dy \qquad \text{...(12.99)}$$

The method involves the following steps.

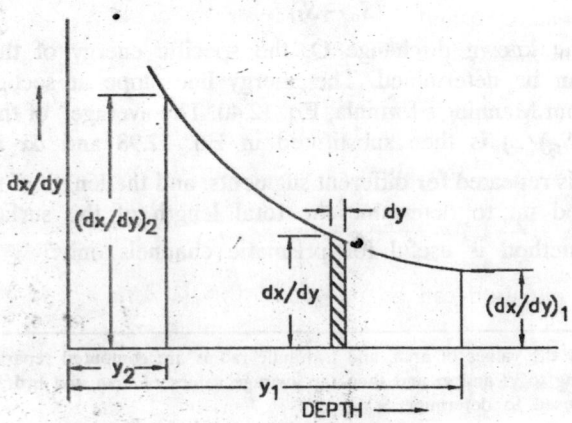

FIG. 12.29. GRAPHICAL INTEGRATION METHOD

(1) Assume several values of y and compute corresponding values of A, T and S_f and thereforem dy/dx.

(2) A curve is then plotted between y and dx/dy (reciprocal of dy/dx determined in step 1).

(3) The area shown shaded in Fig. 12.29 between the two limits of y, the x-axis and the curve is then measured, which is the value of x.

(4) The method is repeated for other segments and all such value of x are added to give the total length of the surface curve.

The method is applicable to prismatic and non-prismatic channel of any shape and slope. The method is simple and accurate but becomes laborious when applied to typical problems.

3. The numerical integration method

The differential equation, Eq. 12.91 for gradually varied flow may be inverted and then integrated between known water depths y_1 and y_2 to determine the length of surface profile.

$$x = \int_{y_1}^{y_2} \frac{dx}{dy} = \int_{y_1}^{y_2} \frac{[1 - (Z_c/Z)^2]}{S_0 [1 - (K_n/K)^2]} \qquad ...(12.100)$$

Since the equation cannot be expressed explicitly as a function of y and hence the direct integration of this equation is not possible. The channel reach is subdivided into small segments and the value of Z_c, K_n, K, etc., are determined at the edge of these segments and average value of these are then determined. These values are substituted in the above equation and the length of the segment is determined. Similar procedure is followed for all the segments. For illustration, Chow's method is given here which seems to be better than many methods suggested earlier. Recently Gill has suggested a method which gives more accurate results.

Chow's method. The conveyance and section factor are function of depth of flow and can be written as $K_n^2 = C_1 y_n^N$, $K^2 = C_1 y^N$, $Z_c^2 = C_2 y_c^M$ and $Z^2 = C_2 y^M$, where C_1 and C_2 are coefficients ; M and N are exponents. These values are substituted in Eq. 12.100.

$$\frac{dy}{dx} = \frac{S_0 [1 - (y_n/y)^N]}{[1 - (y_c/y)^M]} \qquad ...(12.101)$$

If $u = y/y_n$; the above equation may be expressed for dx as

$$dx = \frac{y_n}{S_0} \left[1 - \frac{1}{1 - u^N} + (y_c/y_n)^M \frac{u^{N-M}}{1 - u^N} \right] du \qquad ...(12.102)$$

This euqation can be integrated for the length x of the flow profile. Thus,

$$x = \frac{y_n}{S_0} \left[u - \int_0^u \frac{du}{1 - u^N} + (y_c/y_n)^M \int_0^n \frac{u^{N-M}}{1 - u^N} du \right] + C_2$$

$$...(12.103a)$$

Let $\qquad J = N/(N - M + 1), v = u^{N/J}$

Then $\qquad \displaystyle\int_0^u \frac{u^{N-M}}{1 - u^N} = \frac{J}{N} \int_0^u \frac{dv}{1 - v^J}$

Writing $\qquad \displaystyle\int_0^u \frac{du}{1 - u^N} = F(u, N)$

and $\qquad \displaystyle\int_0^u \frac{dv}{1 - v^J} = F(v, J)$

The Eq. 12.103a becomes

$$x = (y_n/S_0)[u - F(u, N) + (y_c/y_n)^M F(v, J) + C_2] \qquad ...(12.103b)$$

Solution of this equation between section 1 and 2 yields.

$$L = (x_2 - x_1)$$
$$= y_n/S_0 [(u_2 - u_1) - [F(u_2, N) - F_1(u_1, N)$$
$$+ \left(\frac{y_c}{y_n}\right)^M [F(v_2, J) - F(v_1 J)] \qquad ....(12.104)$$

The values of 'varied flow function'$F(u,N)$ were tabulated by Chow. Same table can also be used for $F(v,J)$ for known values of v and J. The values of M and N for different shape of channel are given in Table 12.7

TABLE 12.7
EXPONENT M AND N VALUES

Channel shape	M	N
Wide rectangular	3.0	3.33
Narrow and deep rectangular	3.0	2.00
Triangular	5.0	5.33
Trapezoidal	3.0 to 5.0	3.33 to 5.25

12.24 RAPIDLY VARIED FLOW

When the flow along a channel increases or decreases in a short reach, the flow is said to be rapidly varied flow. Flow downstream of overflow structures (spillways and weirs), flow through underflow structures (sluice gate) and flow from steep slope to mild slope channels are some of the examples of rapidly varied flow. While the flow takes place over the structures, the velocities remain high and depth remains less than critical flow. The downstrem channel is not able to sustain such a high velocity (due to mild slope) and hence there is corresponding rise in water level in a short reach accompanied by high turoulence. Similarly, when the supereritical flow meets a subcritical flow, there is an abrupt rise of water level. This rise of water level is known as 'hydraulic jump'. It is usually associated with a surface roller starting from the beginning of hydralic jump to nearly end of it. It casues violent mixing and air entrainment.

A hydraulic jump may be made use of (i) in the dissipation of energy at the foot of steep channels (chutes) as an energy dissipation device, (ii) for aeration of raw water, (iii) for mixing of chemicals in the industries, and (iv) for raising the water level on the downstrem side of measuring flume to maintain irrigation and similar other applications.

The flow in a hydraulic jump (rapidly varied flow) is quite complex. The hyraulic jump formed in a rectangular channel is only analysed here due to the limitation of space.

12.25 CLASSIFICATION OF HYDRAULIC JUMP

The United States Bureau of Reclaimation (USBR) has made extensive studies on the types of jump. The hydraulic jump formed over a horizontal floor has been classifed according to Froude's number of approaching flow.

(1) Critical flow : $N_{F1} = 1$.

(2) Undular jump : Between $N_{F1} = 1.0$ to 1.7, small disturbances are created on the water surface.

(3) Weak jump : Between $N_{F1} = 1.7$ to 2.5, the disturbances develope into small rollers and there is an abrupt rise in water level.

(4) Oscillating jump : Between $N_{F1} = 2.5$ to 4.5, the oncoming jet oscillates between the bed and surface and stronger rollers are noticed.

(5) Steady jump : In the range of $N_{F1} = 4.5$ to 9.0, a steady jump is formed in the channel. Its performance is best at this state of flow (energy dissipation efficiency varies from 45% to 70%). The jump remains standing at a point where the oncoming jet leves the bottom.

(6) Strong jump : At $N_{F1} = 9.0$ or greater, the water surface is quite rough due to high turbulence and fast moving surface rollers. The energy dissipation efficiency is about 85%.

12.26 ANALYSIS OF FLOW IN HYDRAULIC JUMP

The flow in a hydraulic jump can be analysed by the use of continuity equation and momentum equation.

Consider a control volume of the fluid, comprising a hydraulic jump, in a rectangular channel between sections 1 and 2. The notations are as shown in Fig. 12.30. The depth of flow at these sections are y_1' and y_2' respectively.

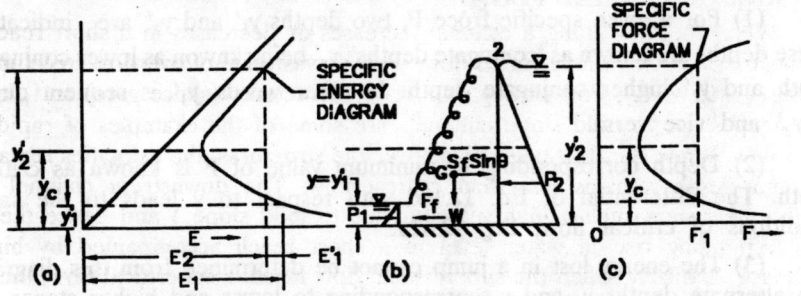

FIG. 12.30. HYDRAULIC JUMP IN A RECTANGULAR CHANNEL
(A) SPECIFIC ENERGY DIAGRAM (B) FORCE ACTING ON FLUID PRISM
(C) SPECIFIC FORCE DIAGRAM

The following assumptions are made :

(1) The flow is assumed to be uniform before and after the jump so that the pressure distribution is hydrostatic.

(2) The energy coefficient α and momentum coefficient β are assumed to be unity.

(3) The channel reach is of small length and hence the fricutional forces acting on the control volume can be neglected.

(4) The bed slope is small, therefore, the weight component of the fluid in the direction of flow $W \sin \theta$ can be neglected.

Applying momentum theorem to the control volume,

Σ External forces = Rate of change of momentum.

The |force| acting on the fluid prism are hydrostatic presssure forces, weight components of fluid and the boundary frictional forces. The pressure forces are given by $P_1 = w A_1 \overline{h_1}$ and $P_2 = w A_2 \overline{h_2}$. Thus

$$P_1 - P_2 + W \sin \theta - F_t = wQ/g \, (U_2 - U_1) \qquad ...(12.105a)$$

Substitute the values of P_1 and P_2 in Eq. 12.105a and neglect the weight component (θ being small) and boundary friction (length of jumps is small).

$$w A_1 \overline{h_1} - w A_2 \overline{h_2} = w \, Q/g \, (U_2 - U_1) \qquad ...(12.105b)$$

where $\overline{h_1}$ and $\overline{h_2}$ are the centroids of areas A_1 and A_2 respectively.

Using the continuity equation $A_1 U_1 = A_2 U_2 = Q$, and rearranging the various terms,

$$\frac{Q^2}{g A_1} + A_1 \overline{h_1} = \frac{Q^2}{g A_2} + A_2 \overline{h_2} = F \qquad ...(12.106)$$

The sum of momentum force Q^2/gA and pressure force $A \overline{h}$ is known as 'specifice force' F. Eq. 12.106 indicates that for given discharage Q, the specific force F remains constant at both sections 1 and 2. The specific force is found to be function of y (depth of flow) and can be plotted as shown in Fig. 12.30c. The plot between F and y is known as specific force diagram. The following observations can be made from Fig. 12.30c.

(1) For a given specific froce F, two depths y_1' and y_2' are indicated. These depths are known as 'conjugate depths'. y_1' being knwon as lower conjugate depth and y_2' higher conjugate depth. In other words, y_1' is sequent depth to y_2' and vice versa.

(2) Depth corresponding to minimum value of F is known as critical depth. The differential of Eq. 12.106 with respect to y leads to the same conditions of critical flow, Eq, 12.62a.

(3) The energy lost in a jump cannot be determined from this diagram. The alternate depths y_1 and y_2 corresponding to lower and higher stages are read from specifice energy diagram 12.30a. The difference of specific energy at these stages is the loss of energy in the jump.

11.27 CHARACTERISTICS OF HYDRAULIC JUMP

1. Relation between conjugate depths

For a hydraulic jump formed over a horizontal apron, Eq. 12.105b

$$w A_1 \bar{h}_1 - w_2 A_2 \bar{h}_2 = w Q/g \, (U_2 - U_1) \qquad ...(12.105b)$$

$$A_1 \bar{h}_1 - A_2 \bar{h}_2 = Q^2/g \, (1/A_1 - 1/A_2)$$

For a rectangular channel of width B,

$$A_1 = B y_1', A_2 = B y_2', h_1' = y_1'/2 \text{ and } \bar{h}_2 = y_2'/2$$

Substituting these values in Eq. 12.105b,

$$B y_1' y_1'/2 - B y_2' y_2'/2 = Q^2/g \, (1/B y_2' - 1/B y_1')$$

which simplifies to

$$y_1' y_2' (y_1' + y_2') = 2 q^2/g \qquad ...(12.107a)$$

where q is the discharge per unit width, Eq. 12.107a relates conjugate depths y_1' and y_2' in terms of q. Solving the quadratic equation in terms of y_2'

$$\frac{y_2'}{y_1'} = \frac{1}{2} \left[-1 \pm \sqrt{1 + \frac{8 q^2}{g y_1'^3}} \right]$$

Substituting $N_{F_1} = q/\sqrt{g y_1'^3}$,

$$y_2'/y_1' = \tfrac{1}{2}[-1 \pm \sqrt{1 + 8 N_{F_1}^2}] \qquad ...(12.107b)$$

It is known 'Belanger momentum equation'. Conversely the relationship between y_1' and y_2' can be derived from Eq. 12.107a.

$$y_1'/y_2' = \frac{1}{2}[-1 \pm \sqrt{1 + 8 N_{F_2}^2}] \qquad ...(12.108)$$

and

$$N_{F_2} = \frac{8 N_{F_1}}{\sqrt{(1 + 8 N_{F_1}^3 - 1)^3}} \qquad ...(12.109)$$

A dimensionless plot between y_2'/y_1' and N_{F_1} is shown in Fig. 12.31a.

2. Height of jump

The difference between the depths after and before the jump $(y_2' - y_1')$. is defined as the 'height of jump'. If it is divided by initial specific energy, 'relative height' is obtained.

$$h_j/E_1 = (y_2'/E_1 - y_1'/E_1) \qquad ...(12.110)$$

The height of jump varies with initial Froude's number, N_{F_1} and is given as

$$\frac{h_j}{E_1} = \frac{\sqrt{1 + 8 N_{F_1}^2} - 3}{N_{F_1}^2 + 2} \qquad ...(12.111)$$

The maximum height of jump equal to $0.507 \, E_1$ occurs at $N_{F_1} = 2.77$, Fig. 12.31b

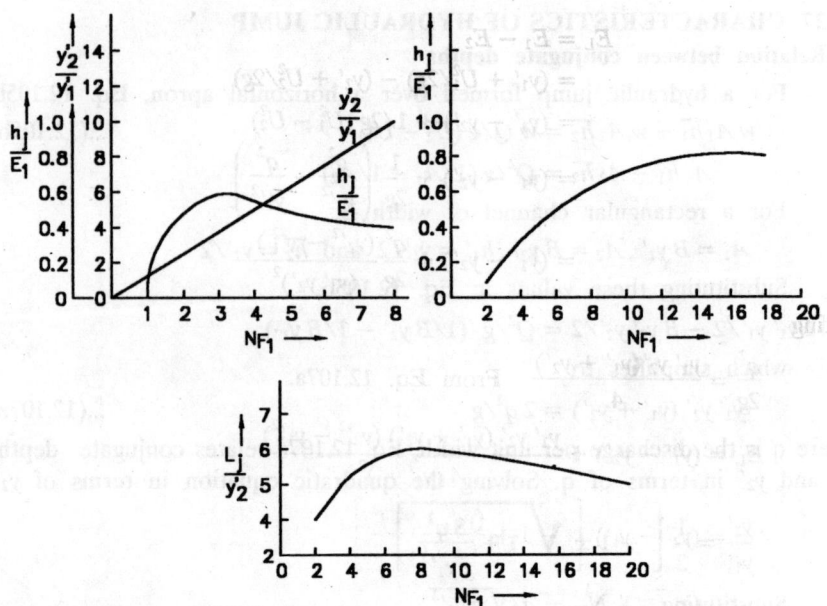

FIG. 12.31. CHARACTERISTICS OF A HYDRAULIC JUMP

3. Length of jump

It may be defined as the distance measured from the front face of the jumps, which is distinctly located, to a point on the surface of the water immediately downstream of the surface roller, where the surface becomes essentially horizontal. The length of jump cannot be determined by theory. As the downstream end of the jump cannot be ascertained with sufficient degree of accuracy, some scatter is found in the experimentsal data collected by many investigatiors. The dimensionless length parameter has been found to be a function of initial Froude's number N_{F_1} (Fig. 12.31c). The proposed relationship is of the form

$$L_j/y_2' = A (y_2' - y_1') \qquad ...(12.112a)$$

Here A is a contant and varies from 5 to 7. USBR uses the value of constant, A, as 6.9.

$$L_j/y_2' = 6.9 (y_2' - y_1') \qquad ....(12.112b)$$

It is intersting to note that length of surface roller is smaller than the length of the jump.

4. Energy loss in the jump

The specifie energy at sections 1 and 2 is written as

$$E_1 = y_1' + U_1^2/2g \qquad ...(12.113)$$

$$E_2 = y_2' + U_2^2/2g \qquad ...(12.114)$$

The difference of E_1 and E_2 is the energy lost in the jump.

$$E_L = E_1 - E_2$$

$$= (y_1' + U_1^2/2g) - (y_2' + U_2^2/2g)$$

$$= (y_1' - y_2') + 1/2g \, (U_1^2 - U_2^2)$$

$$= (y_1' - y_2') + \frac{1}{2g} \left(\frac{q^2}{y_1'^2} - \frac{q^2}{y_2'^2} \right)$$

$$= (y_1' - y_2') + \frac{q^2}{2g} \frac{(y_2'^2 - y_1'^2)}{(y_1' y_2')^2}$$

Writing

$$\frac{q^2}{2g} = \frac{y_1' y_2' (y_1' + y_2')}{4} \quad \text{From Eq. 12.107a.}$$

$$E_L = (y_1' - y_2') + \frac{y_1' y_2' (y_1' + y_2') (y_2'^2 - y_1'^2)}{4 (y_1' y_2')^2}$$

$$= (y_2' - y_1') \left[-1 + \frac{(y_1' + y_2')^2}{4 y_1' y_2'} \right]$$

$$= \frac{(y_2' - y_1')^3}{4 y_1' y_2'} \qquad \qquad ...(12.115)$$

$$\frac{E_L}{y_1'} = \frac{(y_2'/y_1' - 1)^3}{4 y_2'/y_1'}$$

and $E_1/y_1' = \left(1 + \dfrac{U_1^2}{2 g y_1'} \right) = \left(1 + \dfrac{N_{F_1}^2}{2} \right)$

Using Eq. 12.115 in association with Eqs. 12.113 and 12.107a and after simplification, the following expression for dimensionless energy loss E_L/E_1 is obtained.

$$\frac{E_L}{E_1} = \frac{8 N_{F_1}^4 + 20 N_{F_1}^2 - (8 N_{F_1}^2 + 1)^{3/2} - 1}{8 N_{F_1}^2 (2 + N_{F_1}^2)} \qquad ...(12.116)$$

The Eq. 12.116 is shown plotted in Fig. 12.31 b.

5. Efficiency of hydraulic jumps

The ratio of specific energy after the jump to that before the jump is defined as the efficiency of the jump. The dimensionless function E_2/E_1 depends on the Froude's number of approaching flow.

$$E_2/E_1 = \frac{(8 N_{F_1}^2 + 1)^{3/2} - 4 N_{F_1}^2 + 1}{8 N_{F_1}^2 (2 + N_{F_1}^2)} \qquad ...(12.117)$$

6. Surface profile of the jump

Knowledge of the surface profile is desirable for determining the pressure acting on the surface of hydraulic structure where the jump is formed, e.g., at downstream of weirs, etc. The pressure acting upon the structure is equal to the difference between vertical water load due to hydraulic jump and uplift pressure acting on the structure from below it. The free board required for many structure also needs prior knowledge about surface profile. Rajaratnam and Subramanya suggested a unique relationship between $y/0.75\,h_1$ and $x/\bar{x}$ (Fig. 12.32). The scaling parameter $\bar{x}$ is the distance from the beginning of the jump to a point on the X-axis where the depth of flow is 0.75 h_j. It is given by

$$\bar{x}/y_1' = 5.08\,N_{F_1} - 7.82 \qquad \qquad ...(12.118)$$

Eqs. 12.107b and 12.118 alongwith Fig. 12.32 enable the determination of surface profile for known values of y_1' and U_1.

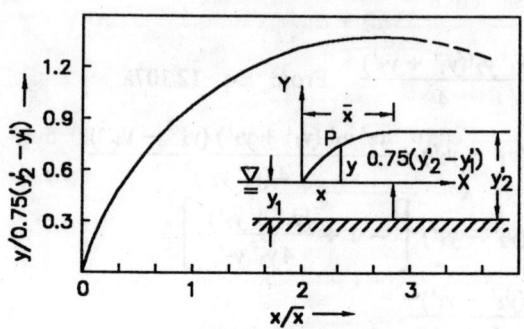

FIG. 12.32. SURFACE PROFILE OF A HYDRAULIC JUMPIC JUMP

12.28 HYDRAULIC JUMP IN NON-RECTAGULAR CHANNEL

For the channels of other shapes like triangular or trapezoidal, the method of section 12.27 cannot be used to find the relation between y_1', y_2' and Q. However, the pressure-momentum equation (Eq. 12.106) hold good for any shape of channel and hence the specific force remains constant for any section of the rapidly varied flow. The specific force diagram can be draum for non-rectangular channel for given discharge. The conjugate depth y_1' and y_2' can then be determined for known specific force F from this diagram and, thereafter all the characteristics of the hydraulic jump can be computed.

12.29 HYDRAULICY JUMP ON A SLOPING CHANNEL

There are many flow situations in which the hydraulic jump forms on a sloping bed. Supercritical flow occurring over the steep down-stream face of a spillway terminates into a jump at its foot, the flow occurring at the junction of mild to steep channel or adverse slope channel creates jump on the steep or adverse slope (in some cases). Such flows can be analysed, using momentum equation between sections 1 and 2. In this case weight component is of sufficient magnitude and cannot be left out. Again, writing the momentum equation between sections 1 and 2 per unit width of channel, (Refer to Fig. 12.30)

$$P_1 - P_2 + W\sin\theta - F_t = w\,Q/g\,(U_2 - U_1) \qquad ....(12.105a)$$

where $Q = U_1\,d_1$, $P_1 = 0.5\,w\,d_1^2\cos\theta$, $P_2 = 0.5\,w\,d_2^2\cos\theta$ and F_t is negligible. Since the profile of the jump is curved instead of straight line hence the weight of the fluid prism between sections 1 and 2 is

$$W = k \, w \, L_j \frac{(y_1' + y_2')}{2} \qquad \qquad ...(12.119)$$

k is a factor to take into account the effect of slope and the discrepancy caused by assuming the straight line profile of jump. Substituting these values in Eq. 12.105a,

$$(d_2/d_1)^3 - (2 \, G^2 + 1) \, d_2/d_1 + 2 \, G^2 = 0 \qquad ...(12.120)$$

where $\qquad G = \sqrt{\dfrac{N_{F1}}{\cos\theta - \dfrac{k \, L_j \sin\theta}{d_2 - d_1}}} \qquad ...(12.121)$

and $\qquad N_{F1} = \dfrac{U_1}{\sqrt{g \, d_1 \cos\theta}} \qquad ...(12.122)$

Since $d_1 = y_1' \cos\theta$ and $d_2 = y_2' \cos\theta$, Eq. 12.120 may then be written as

$$(y_2'/y_1')^3 - 2 \, (G^2 + 1) \, y_2'/y_1' + 2 \, G^2 = 0 \qquad ...(12.123)$$

The solution of above equation is

$$y_2'/y_1' = \tfrac{1}{2} \left[-1 \pm \sqrt{1 + 8 \, G^2} \right] \qquad ...(12.124)$$

Since k and L_j/h_j are expected to be functions of N_{F1} and θ, hence G can be written as $f(N_{F1}, \theta)$. The ratio y_2'/y_1' then ought to be function of N_{F1} and θ. Experimental results have resulted into empirical relations. Some simpler empirical relations suggested by Rajarathaam are

$$G^2 = k_1^2 \, N_{F1}^2 \qquad ...(12.125)$$

and $\qquad k_1 = 10^{0.027} \, \theta \qquad ...(12.126)$

where θ is in degrees

12.30 LOCATION OF JUMP

Theoretically speaking the jump will occur in a horizontal rectangular channel if the initial and sequent depths and the Froude's number of approaching flow satisfy Eq. 12.107b. For accurate location of jump, the length of jumps is also used. The location of jump in three typical cases is illustrated here.

Case1: Flow under a sluice gate. The flow is occurring under a sluice gate fitted on a mild slope channel. The water is headed up by a barrier fitted at downstream end, Fig.12.33. The method involves the following steps:

(1) Draw the surface profiles which are M_3 and M_2 type.

(2) Compute and plot the curve A'B which represents the sequent depth (SDL) corresponding to M_3 profile.

(3) Extend b.ck water's the profile M_2, i.e. CF which intersects $A'B$ at F'

(4) Compute initial sequent depth y_1' corresponding to the depth y_2' from Eq. 12.107b. And therefrom, determine the length of the jump.

(5) By trial and error, the intercept EF equal to the length of jump is fitted, as shown in Fig. 12.33. Thus F is located which is the downstream end of the jump.

(6) Draw a vertical from E which meets AB at G which is the starting point of the hydraulic jump.

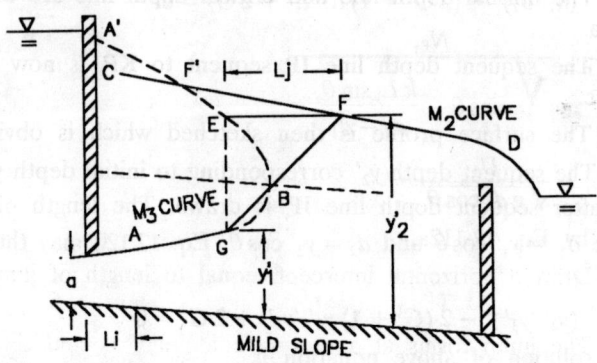

FIG. 12.33. CASE -1 : FLOW UNDER A SLUIC GATE

Case 2: Flow from steep to mild slope channel. While the flow takes place in a channel whose slope changes from steep to mild, the jump may either form on the steep channel or on the mild channel, Fig. 12.34. If the

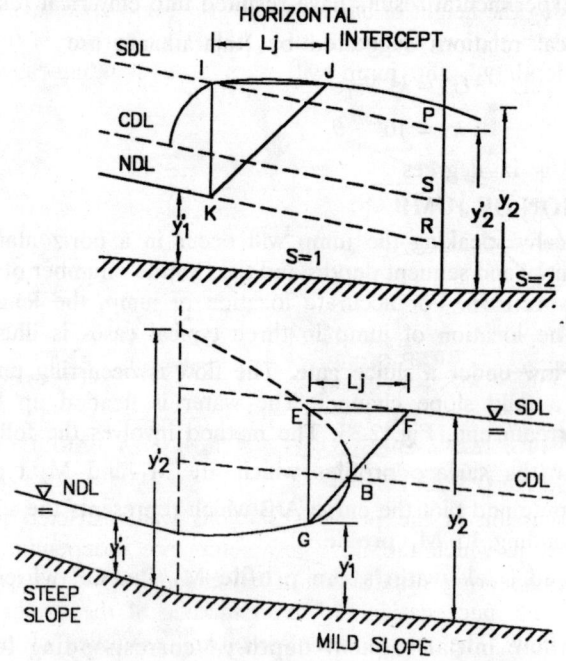

FIG. 12.34. CASE -2 : FLOW AT THE BREAK OF SLOPE

depth y_2 on mild channel is less than the depth y_2' sequent to initial depth y_1, the jump forms on the steep channel. If $y_2 > y_2'$ the jump will form on the mild channel. In the second alternate flow situation, the jump can be located by the method of case 1. For first alternate flow situation, the method given below is to be used.

(1) The normal depth line and critical depth line are drawn as usual, Fig. 12.34a.

(2) The sequent depth line IP sequent to KR is now drawn on the steep slope.

(3) The surface profile is then sketched which is obviously S_1 type.

(4) The sequent depth y_2' corresponding to initial depth y_1 is computed and thereafter sequent depth line IP is drawn. The length of jump is also computed by Eq. 12.112a.

(5) Draw a horizontal intercept, equal to length of jump, between IJ and IP.

(6) The jump forms at a section containing IJ and thus the position of jump is located.

Case 3: Flow upstream of barrier. Fig. 12.35 depicts the flow situation occurring in a steep channel upstream of a barrier. The initial depth of flow is y_1 and its sequent depth is y_2'. If the height of barrier is more than y_2', the jump will form upstream of it and it can be located by the method of case 2. Increasing the height of barrier moves the jump upstream while lowering the height moves it downstream. If the height of barrier becomes less than the sequent depth y_2', the jump will pass as a standing wave.

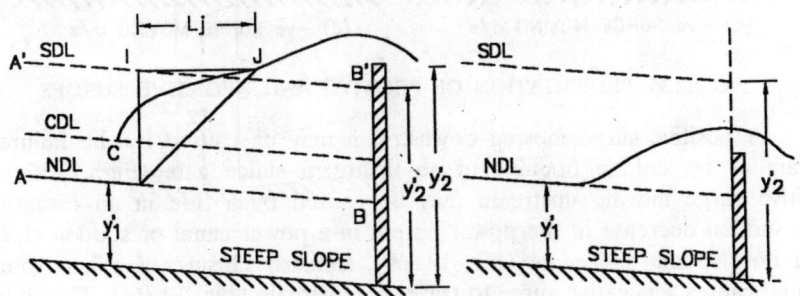

FIG. 12.35 - CASE -3 : FLOW BEHIND A BARRIER

12.31 SURGES AND WAVES

The discussion in the previous sections was restricted to the case of steady flow, i.e. in which the flow parameters are independent of the time. But in many engineering situations in open channel flow, the flow parameters do vary with time, necessiating an understanding of the principles governing the unsteady flow. The surges and waves are examples of unsteady flow.

12.32 SURGES

A surge is defined as a moving wave front which brings about an abrupt change in the depth of flow in the channel. It may move either upstream or downstream at velocity Uw (absolute velocity). The moving hydraulic jump is an example of a surge. Surges may be caused by the sudden opening or closing of sluice gates in the channel or by blockage of channel (partially or fully) by a landslide, etc.

A surge is known as positive or an elevation wave when it causes an increase in depth in the direction of its travel. A negative surge is the one which causes the decrease in the depth. Fig. 12.36 shows the propagation of positive and negative surges. It is to be noted that the flow becomes unsteady in the neighbourhood of surges.

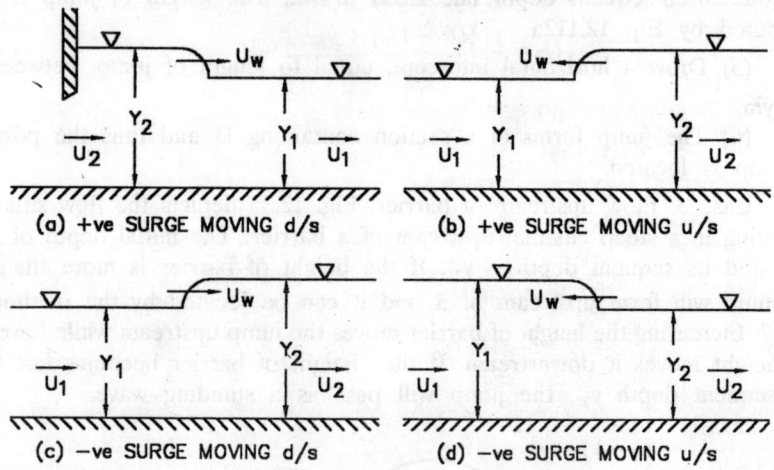

(a) +ve SURGE MOVING d/s

(b) +ve SURGE MOVING u/s

(c) −ve SURGE MOVING d/s

(d) −ve SURGE MOVING u/s

FIG. 12.36. PROPAGATION OF POSITIVE AND NEGATIVE SURGES

A positive surge moving downstream may be caused by the failure of a dam or by sudden opening of an upstream sluice gate (Fig. 12.36a). A positive surge moving upstream may be caused by a tide in an estuary or by a sudden decrease in the power output in a power canal or sudden closure of a downstream sluicegate (Fig. 12.26b). similarly closure of a headgate of a canal causes a negative surge to travel derenstream (Fig. 12.36c). The sudden opening of the gate at power house to increase power generation results in a negative surge moving upstream (Fig. 12.36d).

A surge is a rapidly varied unsteady flow phenomenon. However, when the surge is moving with a constant velocity Uw, the problem can be converted into one of the steady flow problem. It can be done by adding a velocity equal in magnitude and opposite in direction to the surge as well as to the fluid.

Consider a positive surge moving downstream which has been created due to sudden opening of a sluice gate, Fig. 12.37. Let the velocity of surge be Uw and that of fluid at section 1 and 2 be U_1 and U_2 respectively. Further let the depths at these sections be y_1 and y_2 respectively. In order to convert this problem into a steady flow case, superimpose a velocity Uw in the opposite direction to the surge as well as to the fluid. Thus, the velocity at section 1 and 2 becomes (U_1-U_w) and (U_2-U_w) respectively. The velocity of surge now becomes (U_w-U_w), that is zero or stationary.

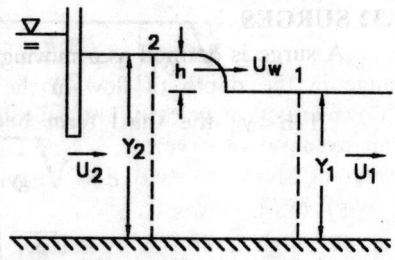

FIG. 12.37. ANALYSIS OF A SURGE

From continuity equation,

$$y_1 (U_1 - U_w) = y_2 (U_2 - U_w)$$

$$U_2 = \frac{y_1 (U_1 - U_w) + y_2 U_w}{y_2} \qquad ....(12.127)$$

Applying momentum equation to the fluid bounded by sections 1 and 2,

$$\frac{w (y_1^2 - y_2^2)}{2} = \frac{w}{g} y_2 (U_2 - U_w) [(U_1 - U_w) - (U_2 - U_w)]$$

$$= \frac{w y_2}{g} (U_2 - U_w) (U_1 - U_2) \qquad ...(12.128)$$

Substituting the value of U_2 from Eq. 12.128, and simplifying,

$$(U_1 - U_w)^2 = \frac{g y^2}{2 y_1} (y_1 + y_2) \qquad ...(12.129a)$$

Solving,

$$U_w = U_1 + \sqrt{\frac{g y_2}{2 y_1} (y_1 + y_2)} \qquad ...(12.129b)$$

In non-dimentional form, it can be written as

$$\frac{(U_w - U_1)^2}{g y_1} = \frac{1}{2} \frac{y_2}{y_1} \left(1 + \frac{y_2}{y_1}\right) \qquad ...(12.129c)$$

Eq. 12.129b gives the absolute velocity of the surge. The surge moves with a velocity relative to the velocity of flow at section 1 and is designated as the celerity of the surge.

$$\therefore \qquad c = (U_w - U_1)$$

$$= \sqrt{\frac{g y_2}{2 y_1} (y_1 + y_2)} \qquad ...(12.130)$$

The height of the surge h is defined as (y_2-y_1)

$$\therefore \qquad h = (y_2 - y_1) \qquad ...(12.131)$$

From Eqns. 12.130 and 12.131,

$$c = \sqrt{\frac{g (y_1 + h)}{2 y_1} (2y_1 + h)}$$

$$= \sqrt{gy_1 \left[1 + \frac{3}{2}\frac{h}{y_1} + \left(\frac{h}{y_1} \right)^2 \right]} \qquad \text{...(12.132)}$$

If $h < y_1$, the third term becomes too small and can be left out.

$$\therefore \qquad c = \sqrt{gy_1 \left(1 + \frac{3}{2} h/y_1 \right)}$$

$$= \sqrt{gy_1} \left(1 + \frac{3}{4} h/y_1 \right) \qquad \text{....(12.133)}$$

When the ratio h/y_1 is very small, the last term can also be left out,

$$c = \sqrt{gy_1} \qquad \text{...(12.134)}$$

The simplification was suggested by Lagrange and hence, Eq. 12.134 is known as 'Lagrange's celerity equation. In case of stasionary hydraulic jump, $U_w = 0$ and Eq. 12.130 reduces to

$$U_1 = \sqrt{\frac{gy_2}{2y_1} (y_1 + y_2)} \qquad \text{...(12.135)}$$

$$q = U_1 y_1 = \sqrt{\frac{gy_1 y_2}{2} (y_1 + y_2)} \qquad \text{...(12.136)}$$

which is the same equation as Eq.12.107a. Hence, the hydraulic jump is a special case of a surge.

The above equation is derived for a rectangular channel. For a prismatic channel of other shape, the general equation for celerity can be derived by applying the continuity and momentum equations.

$$c = (U_w - U_1) = \sqrt{\frac{g (A_2 \overline{h_2} - A_1 \overline{h_1})}{A_1 (1 - A_1/A_2)}} \qquad \text{...(12.137)}$$

where $\overline{h_1}$ and $\overline{h_2}$ are the depths of the centre of gravity of the areas A_1 and A_2 below water surface. In the above analysis, the effect of viscosity has been neglected which are not important for short channels otherwise the surge profile will change.

For a positive surge moving upstream in a rectangular channel, the corresponding equations are

$$y_1 (U_1 + U_w) = y_2 (U_2 + U_w) \qquad \text{...(12.138)}$$

$$\frac{(U_w + U_1)^2}{gy_1} = \frac{1}{2}\frac{y_2}{y_1} \left(1 + \frac{y_2}{y_1} \right) \qquad \text{...(12.139)}$$

Eqs. 12.129c and 12.139 may be written in alternate form as

$$\frac{(U_w - U_1)^2}{gy_2} = \frac{1}{2}\frac{y_1}{y_2} \left(1 + \frac{y_1}{y_2} \right) \qquad \text{...(12.140)}$$

$$\frac{(U_w + U_1)^2}{gy_2} = \frac{1}{2}\frac{y_1}{y_2} \left(1 + \frac{y_1}{y_2} \right) \qquad \text{...(12.141)}$$

12.33 WAVES

A wave is defined as a variation of velocity with time which travels through the fluid mdeium. The celerity of wave is the speed of propagation of such a change or disturbance relative to the fluid. These can be generated by the action of strong wind, motion of ships or by geophysical activities such as earthquake or tides.

Waves are characterised by their wave length λ, amplitude 'a' or height h(equal to 2a) and velocity c. The term λ/c gives the time required for one wave to pass a particular section and is known as the time period T, whereas $c/\lambda (= 1/T)$ is the number of waves passing a fixed section per unit time and is known as frequency of wave.

Waves may be of different types e.g. gravity waves formed over the water surface in which the gravity force is important, capillary waves influenced primarily by the surface tension and elastic waves governed essentially by fluid compressibility.

Thus if h/λ is much smaller than 0.5, the waves are called as shallow water waves or long waves. It is observed that fluid particles follow elliptical orbits in the plane of waves.

But if $h/\lambda > 0.5$, $\tan \dfrac{2\pi h}{\lambda} = 1.0$

$$c = \sqrt{\dfrac{g\lambda}{2\pi}} \qquad \qquad ...(12.142)$$

Such wave are known as deep water waves. In this case, the particles are found to follow circular orbits.

The deep water waves are those in which only the surface layers of the flow are disturbed by the movement of the waves. In contrast to it, the shallow water waves are those in which the entire depth of water is disturbed by the waves.

From the physical point of view, waves may be classified into two kinds.viz. oscillating waves and translatory waves. Oscillatory wave is periodic in character which imparts to the liquid an undulating motion having both components horizontal as well as vertical. The average mass transport is zero in oscillatory waves while there is net mass transport of fluid in the direction of motion in case of the translatory waves. Sea waves are oscillatory in nature whereas the moving hydraulic jump and tidal bore are examples of translatory waves.

The translatory wave can further be classified as solitary wave and train of waves. The solitary wave has a rising limb, a single peak and a recession limit, all is followed and preceded by speeding flow. A wave train is produced by the sequence of waves.

An oscillating wave can be either progressive or standing. A progressive wave has a sine profile and its amplitude is a function of time.

$$\eta = a \sin \dfrac{2\pi}{y} (x - c . t) \qquad \qquad ...(12.143)$$

Two progressive waves of the same amplitude and same period but travelling in opposite direction can be superimposed so as to result in a stationary wave. The amplitude of a stationary wave is given by

$$\eta = \eta_1 + \eta_2$$

$$= a \sin \frac{2\pi}{\lambda} (x - c_t) + a \sin \frac{2\pi}{\lambda} (x + c_t)$$

$$= 2a \cos \frac{2\pi t}{T} \cdot Sin \frac{2\pi x}{\lambda} \qquad ...(12.144)$$

The celerity c of an oscillatory wave is given by

$$c = \sqrt{\frac{g\lambda}{2\pi} \tan \left(\frac{2\pi h}{\lambda} \right)}$$

If $\qquad h/\lambda < 0.5 , \tan \dfrac{2\pi h}{\lambda} = \dfrac{2\pi h}{\lambda}$

$$\therefore \qquad c = \sqrt{gh} \qquad ...(12.145)$$

EXAMPLES 12.1-12.44

12.1 Derive an expression for discharge in terms of depth y in a channel with Manning's $n = 0.0125$ and bed slope $= 0.0025$ for (a) rectangular channel with bed width equal to 2.5 times its depth and (b) a parabolic channel with its profile following $T^2 = 16$ y, where T is the top width at water surface and y is the depth of water.

Solution

(a) Ractangular section,

From Eq. 12.40

$$U = (1/n) R^{2/3} S_1^{1/2}$$

$$Q = AU = (B y \times 1/n) R^{2/3} S_0^{1/2}$$

Here $\qquad B = 2.5 y$

$$A = By = 2.5 y^2$$

$$P = B + 2y = (2.5y + 2y) = 4.5 y$$

$$R = A/P = 2.5 y^2 / 4.5 y = (5/9) y$$

Hence $\qquad Q = 2.5 y^2 \times \dfrac{1}{0.0125} \times \left(\dfrac{5}{9} y \right)^{2/3} (0.0025)^{1/2}$

$$Q = 6.758 y^{8/3}$$

(b) Parabolic section,

$$A = \frac{2}{3} Ty = \frac{2}{3} \sqrt{16 y} \cdot y = (8/3) y^{3/2}$$

$$P = \left[T + \frac{8 y^2}{3 T} \right] = \left[\sqrt{16 y} + \frac{8}{3} \frac{y^2}{\sqrt{16 y}} \right]$$

$$P = [4 \sqrt{y} + \frac{2}{3} y^{3/2}] = \frac{2}{3} \sqrt{y} (6 + y)$$

$$R = \frac{A}{P} = \frac{(8/3\,y^{3/2})}{\frac{2}{3}\sqrt{y}\ (6+y)}$$

$$= \left(\frac{4y}{6+y}\right)$$

From Eq. 12.40

$$Q = AU = A\,(1/n)\,R^{2/3}\,S_0^{1/2}$$

$$Q = \frac{8}{3}\,y^{3/2} \times \frac{1}{0.0125}\left(\frac{4y}{6+y}\right)^{2/3}(0.0025)^{1/2}.$$

$$Q = 26.88\,y^{3/2}\,[y/(6+y)]^{2/3}$$

12.2 A circular conduit, 1 m diameter 4000 m long, is laid at a uniform slope of 1 in 1500 and connects two reservoirs. When the level in the reservoir is low the conduit runs partly full and it is found that normal depth of 0.6 m in the conduits gives discharge of 0.35 m^3/s. The Chezy's C = K R^n where K is constant and n is 1/6. Obtain the value of K and also the discharge when the conduit runs full; the difference in elevation of water surface being maintained at 5 m Neglect entrance and exit losses.

Solution

From Fig. 12.38, $\sin\theta = 0.1/0.5 = 0.2$

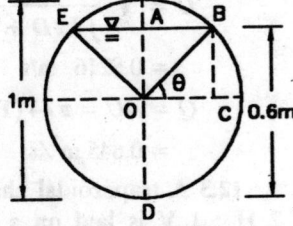

FIG. 12.38. EXAMPLE 12.2

$$\theta = 11.5°$$

So that $2\theta = 23°$

Area BDEB = Area of segment BDE + Area of traingle BOE

$$A = \frac{(180+23)}{360} \times \pi\,(0.5)^2 + 0.1 \times 0.49$$

$$A = 0.443 + 0.049 = 0.4917\ \text{m}^2$$

$$P = (203/360)\,\pi\,(1) = 1.77\ \text{m}$$

$$R = A/P = 0.4917/1.77 = 0.277\ \text{m}$$

The discharge is given by

$$Q = AU = AC\sqrt{RS}$$

$$= A\,(K R^{1/6})\sqrt{RS}$$

or

$$K = \frac{Q}{A R^{2/3} S^{1/2}}$$

$$= \frac{0.35}{0.4917\,(0.277)^{2/3}\,(1/1500)^{1/2}}$$

$$= 64.87 \approx 64.9$$

(b) When flowing full,

$$R = D/4 = 1/4 \text{ m}$$

$$C = K R^{1/6} = 64.9 \left(\frac{1}{4}\right)^{1/6}$$

$$= 51.51$$

The head loss due to friction is given by Darcy's formula, Eq. 10.51

$$h_f = f \frac{L}{D} \frac{U^2}{2g}$$

Substituting the value of U and bed slope S $= h_f/L$ in Eq. 12.36b

$$U^2 = C^2 RS = C^2 S D/4$$

$$\therefore \qquad f = 2g/C^2 = 2g/(51.51)^2 = 0.0296$$

Applying Bernoulli's equation between two reservoirs,

$$S = h_f + U^2/2g$$

$$= \frac{fL}{D} \cdot \frac{U^2}{2g} + \frac{U^2}{2g} = \frac{U^2}{2g}\left(f \cdot \frac{L}{D} + 1\right)$$

$$U = \sqrt{\frac{10g}{fL/D + 1}} = \sqrt{\frac{9.81 \times 10}{(0.0296 \times 4000/1) + 1}}$$

$$= 0.8216 \text{ m/s}$$

$$Q = AU = \pi/4 \, (1)^2 \times 0.8216$$

$$= 0.645 \,\text{m}^3/\text{s}$$

12.3 A trapezoidal channel having bottom width of 6 m and side slopes of 2 H : 1 V is laid on a bottom slope of 0.0016. If the discharge flowing in the channel is 10 m³/s calculate the normal depth and normal velocity. Assume n = 0.025.

Solution

$$A = (B + zy)y$$

$$= (6 + 2y)y \qquad\qquad ...(i)$$

$$P = (B + 2\sqrt{5}y) \qquad\qquad ...(ii)$$

$$P = (6 + 2\sqrt{5}\,y)$$

$$R = \frac{A}{P} = \frac{(6 + 2y)y}{(6 + 2\sqrt{5}\,y)} \qquad\qquad ...(iii)$$

Using Eq. 12.40,

$$U = 1/n \, R^{2/3} S^{1/2} = Q/A$$

$$\frac{10}{(6+2y)y} = \frac{1}{0.025}\left[\frac{(6+2y)y}{(6+2\sqrt{5}y)}\right]^{2/3}\left[\frac{1}{0.0016}\right]^{1/2}$$

$$[(3+y)y]^{5/2} = 12.35y + 16.57 \qquad\qquad ...(iv)$$

Method 1: Eq.(iv) is solved by trial,

$y_n = 0.962$ m = normal depth

$$A = [6 + 2 \times 0.962] \, 0.962 = 7.62 \text{ m}^2$$

$$U_0 = 10/7.62 = 1.31 \text{ m/s}$$

Method 2: Eq. 12.40 alongwith continuity equation yields

$$Q = AU = A \times 1/n \, R^{2/3} \, S^{1/2}$$

or

$$A R^{2/3} = \frac{n \, Q}{\sqrt{S}} = \frac{0.025 \times 10}{\sqrt{0.0016}} = 6.25$$

Thus, the normal depth should be such that it yields the product $AR^{2/3}$ equal to 6.25

y	A	R	$R^{2/3}$	$AR^{2/3}$
1.5	13.5	1.06	1.04	14.04
0.75	5.63	0.60	0.73	4.11
1.0	8.00	0.76	0.84	6.72
0.96	7.60	0.74	0.82	6.23
0.962	7.62	0.74	0.82	6.25

The required normal depth $y_n = 0.962$ m

Method 3: A graph is plotted between y and $AR^{2/3}$. The value of y corresponding to $AR^{2/3}$ equal to 6.25 then gives the required normal depth.

y	A	R	$R^{2/3}$	$AR^{2/3}$
0.25	1.63	0.23	0.38	0.62
0.50	3.50	0.43	0.57	2.0
0.75	5.63	0.60	0.73	4.11
1.0	8.0	0.76	0.84	6.72
1.25	10.63	0.92	0.95	10.10

$y_n = 0.962$ m.

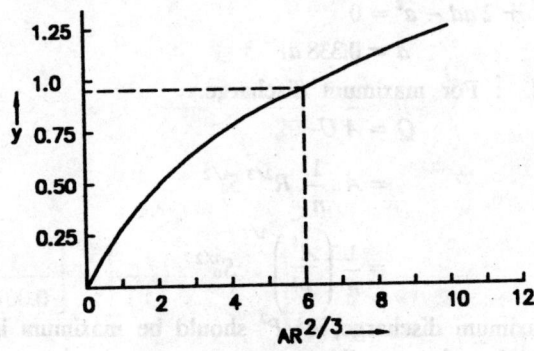

FIG. 12.39. EXAMPLE 12.3

12.4. Water flows in a channel of the shape of isocales triangle of bed width a and sides making an angle of 45° with the bed. Determine the relation between depth of flow 'd' and bed width 'a' for maximum velocity condition and maximum discharge condition. Use Manning's formula and d should be less than 0.5 a.

Solution

Case I : For maximum velocity.

$$A = \left(ad - 2 \times \frac{d \times d}{2} \right)$$

$$= ad - d^2$$

$$P = (a + 2 \times \sqrt{2}\, d)$$

$$\frac{dA}{dd} = a - 2d$$

$$\frac{dP}{dd} = 2\sqrt{2}$$

From Eq. 12.40,

$$U = \frac{1}{n} . R^{3/2} S_0^{1/2}$$

$$= \frac{1}{n} \left(\frac{A}{P} \right)^{2/3} S_0^{1/2}$$

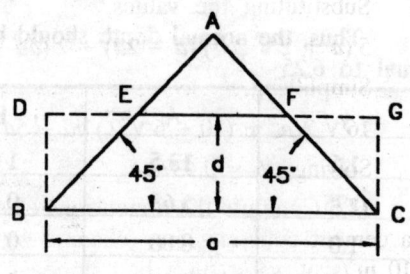

FIG. 12.40. EXAMPLE 12.4

For maximum velocity (A/P) should be maximum i.e. A/P should be differentiated and resulting expression should be equated to zero.

Differentiating A/P w.r. to d,

$$\frac{d}{dd}(A/P) = \frac{P\,dA/dd - A\,dP/dd}{P^2} = 0$$

Substituting the values.

$$(a + 2\sqrt{2}\, d)(a - 2d) - (ad - d^2) 2\sqrt{2} = 0$$

Simplifying.

$$2\sqrt{2}\, d^2 + 2ad - a^2 = 0$$

Solving $d = 0.338\, a.$

Case 2 : For maximum discharge.

$$Q = A U$$

$$= A . \frac{1}{n} . R^{2/3} S_0^{1/2}$$

$$= \frac{1}{n} \left(\frac{A^5}{P^2} \right)^{1/3} S_0^{1/2}$$

For maximum discharge, A^5/P^2 should be maximum i.e. A^5/P^2 should be differentiated and equated to zero.

$$\frac{d}{dd}(A^5/P^2) = \frac{P^2 .5A^4 \frac{dA}{dd} - A^5 .2P \frac{dP}{dd}}{P^4} = 0$$

$$A^4 P \left[5P \frac{dA}{dd} - 2A \frac{dP}{dd} \right] = 0$$

$$5P \frac{dA}{dd} - 2A \frac{dP}{dd} = 0$$

Substituting the values,

$$5(a + 2\sqrt{2}\,d)(a - 2d) - 2(ad - d^2)2\sqrt{2} = 0$$

Simplifying,

$$16\sqrt{2}\,d^2 + (10 - 6\sqrt{2})ad - 5a^2 = 0$$

Solving, $d = 0.4378\,a$

12.5 Compute the dimensions of the most economical trapezoidal section of a cement concrete lined channel with side slope 1 :1 to carry a discharge of 10 m³/s of water on a bed slope of 1 in 1600. Assume Manning's rugosity n as 0.015.

Solution

$$A = (B + zy)y \qquad ...(i)$$

$$P = (B + 2y\sqrt{1 + z^2}) \qquad ...(ii)$$

$$R = \frac{A}{P} = \frac{(B + zy)y}{(B + 2y\sqrt{1 + z^2})} \qquad ...(iii)$$

For most economical section,

$$R = y/2 \qquad ...(iv)$$

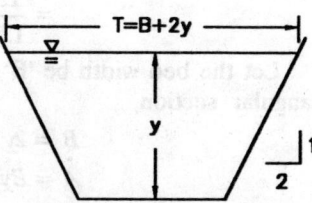

FIG. 12.41. EXAMPLE 12.5

From Eqs. (i) and (ii)

$$\frac{y}{2} = \frac{(B + zy)y}{B + 2y\sqrt{1 + z^2}} \qquad ...(v)$$

Also T/2 = length of sloping side

or $\qquad (B + 2zy)/2 = y\sqrt{1 + z^2}$

or $\qquad B = (2\sqrt{2}\,y - 2y) = 0.83\,y \qquad ...(vi)$

From Eq. 12.40

$$Q = AU = (B + y)y \times 1/n\,(y/2)^{2/3}\,(1/1600)^{1/2}$$

$$10 = \frac{(0.83\,y + y)\,y^{5/3}}{0.015 \times (2)^{2/3}\,(1600)^{1/2}}$$

$$1.83\,y^{8/3} = 10 \times 0.015 \times (2)^{2/3} \times 400$$

Solving, $y = 1.86$ m

$$B = 0.83\,y = 0.83 \times 1.86$$

$$= 1.54 \text{ m}$$

12.6 A channel of least penimater is to be designed and of rectangular, triangular, trapezoidal or circular section to supply 12 m³/s of water of flowing at velocity of 1.5 m/s. Assume Maning's $n = 0.015$. Compare the perineter of these sections and determine the section of maximum perimeter.

Solution

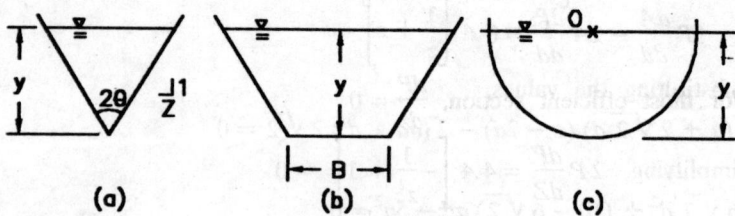

(a)   (b)   (c)

FIG. 12.42. EXAMPLE 12.6

(a) Rectangular :

Given $Q = 12$ m³/s, $U = 1.5$ m/s

$$A = \frac{Q}{U}$$

$$= \frac{12}{1.5} = 8\, m^2 \qquad \text{...(i)}$$

Let the bed width be 'B' and depth of flowy be y. For most economical rectangular section,

$$B = 2y$$
$$A = By = 2y \cdot y$$
$$= 2y^2 \qquad \text{...(ii)}$$

From Eqs. (i) and (ii)

$$2y^2 = 8$$
$$y = \sqrt{4} = 2m$$
$$B = 2y = 2 \times 2 = 4\ m$$
$$P_1 = B + 2y$$
$$= 4 + 2 \times 2 = 8\ m$$

(b) Triangular section :

Consider a triangular section of vertex angle 20°

$$\tan \theta = z$$

$$A = 2\left[\frac{y \times yz}{2}\right] = y^2 z \qquad \text{...(iii)}$$

$$P = 2\left[\sqrt{y^2 + y^2 z^2}\right] \qquad \text{...(iv)}$$

$$= 2y\sqrt{1 + z^2}$$

From Eqs (iii), $y = \sqrt{A/z}$

From. Eq. (iv) $P = \dfrac{2\sqrt{A}}{\sqrt{z}}\,(\sqrt{1+z^2})$

$$P = 2\sqrt{A}\left[\sqrt{\dfrac{1}{z}+z}\,\right]$$

$$P^2 = 4A\left[\dfrac{1}{z}+z\right]$$

For most efficient section, $\dfrac{dP}{dz} = 0$

$$2P\dfrac{dP}{dZ} = 4A\left[-\dfrac{1}{z^2}+1\right] = 0$$

$$z^2 = 1$$

$$z = 1$$

$$\tan\theta = \tan 45° = 1$$

Hence vertex angle $= 2\theta = 90°$

$$A = y^2 Z$$

$$8 = y^2 \tan 45°$$

$$y = \sqrt{8} = 2.828 \text{ m}$$

Perimeter $P_2 = 2y\sqrt{1+z^2}$

$$= 2y\sqrt{1+(1)^2} = 2\sqrt{2}\,y$$

$$= 2\sqrt{2} \times 2.828 = 8 \text{ m}$$

(c) Trapezoidal section:

For most efficient section

side slope $= 1$ vertical to z horizontal

$$= 1V:\sqrt{3}\,H$$

$$z = \sqrt{3} \qquad\qquad\qquad\qquad ...(v)$$

From Eq. 12.45a,

$$\dfrac{B+2zy}{2} = y\sqrt{1+z^2}$$

$$B = (2y\sqrt{1+z^2} - 2zy)$$

$$= \left[2y\sqrt{1+\left(\dfrac{1}{\sqrt{3}}\right)^2} - 2\times\dfrac{1}{\sqrt{3}}y\right]$$

$$= \dfrac{2}{\sqrt{3}}y \qquad\qquad\qquad\qquad ...(vi)$$

$$A = [By + zy^2]$$

$$= [(2y\sqrt{1+z^2} - 2zy)y + zy^2]$$

$$= [2y^2\sqrt{1+z^2} - zy^2]$$

$$= \left[2y^2 \sqrt{1 + \left(\frac{1}{\sqrt{3}} \right)^2} - \frac{1}{\sqrt{3}} \times y^2 \right]$$

$$= \left(\frac{4}{\sqrt{3}} y^2 - \frac{y^2}{\sqrt{3}} \right)$$

$$= \sqrt{3} \, y^2 \qquad \qquad ...(vii)$$

Substituting the value of A from Eq. (i)

$$\sqrt{3} \, y^2 = 8$$

$$y = \left(\frac{8}{\sqrt{3}} \right)^{1/2} = 2.149 \text{ m}$$

$$P_3 = [B + 2y \sqrt{1 + z^2})$$

Substituting from Eq. (vi) for B.

$$P_3 = [2y \sqrt{1 + z^2} - 2zy + 2y \sqrt{1 + z^2}]$$

$$= [4y \sqrt{1 + z^2} - 2zy]$$

$$= \left[4y \sqrt{1 + \left(\frac{1}{\sqrt{3}} \right)^2} - 2 \times \frac{1}{\sqrt{3}} y \right]$$

$$= \left(\frac{4}{\sqrt{3}} y - \frac{2}{\sqrt{3}} y \right)$$

$$= \frac{2}{\sqrt{3}} y \qquad \qquad ...(viii)$$

$$P_3 = \frac{2}{\sqrt{3}} \times 2.149 = 7.445$$

(d) Circular section

For a semi circular section,

$$A = \frac{1}{2} [\pi R^2]$$

Assuming

$$R = y$$

$$8 = \frac{1}{2} \pi y^2$$

$$y = \sqrt{\frac{16}{\pi}} = 2.257 \text{ m}$$

$$P_4 = \frac{1}{2} [2 \pi R]$$

$$= \pi \times 2.257 = 7.093 \text{ m}$$

The perimeter of various shaped channels is shown below

(a) Rectangular $P_1 = 8$ m

(b) Triangular $P_2 = 8$ m

(c) Trapezoidal $P_3 = 7.445$ m

(d) Circular $P_4 = 7.093$ m

Thus, least perimeter : Circular section and Maximum perimeter : Rectangular and Triangular section,

12.7 Compute the discharge carried by a rectangular channel 3 m wide, depth of water 1 m and laid at a bed slope of 1 m 1500. use Manning 's rugosity coefficient n = 0.015. Also determine the increase in discharge carried by a rectangular channel of most efficient section keeping same area of lining.

Solution

(a)
$$A = 3 \times 1 \doteq 3 \text{ m}^2$$
$$P = (3 + 2 \times 1) = 5\text{m}$$
$$R = \left(\frac{A}{P}\right)$$
$$= \frac{3}{5} = 0.6 \text{ m}$$
$$Q_1 = A U$$
$$= A . \frac{1}{n} . R^{2/3} S_0^{1/2}$$
$$= 3 \times \frac{1}{0.015} (0.6)^{2/3} \left(\frac{1}{1500}\right)^{1/2}$$
$$= 3.673 \text{ m}^3/\text{s}$$

(b) For most economical section,
$$B = 2y$$
$$P = (B + 2y)$$
$$= (2y + 2y) = 4y$$

Area of lining/m. length $= 4y = 5$
$$4y = 5$$
$$y = 1.25 \text{ m}$$
$$B = 2y$$
$$= 2 \times 1.25 = 2.5 \text{ m}$$
$$A = By$$
$$= 2.5 \times 1.25$$
$$= 3.125 \text{ m}^2$$
$$R = \frac{y}{2}$$
$$= \frac{1.25}{2} = 0.6125 \text{ m}$$
$$Q_2 = A U = A . \frac{1}{n} . R^{2/3} S_0^{1/2}$$

$$= 3.125 \times \frac{1}{0.015} \times (0.6125)^{2/3} \left(\frac{1}{1500}\right)^{1/2}$$

$$= 3.879 \text{ m}^3/\text{s}$$

Increase in discharge $= Q_2 - Q_1$

$$= 3.879 - 3.673$$

$$= 0.206 \text{ m}^3/\text{s}$$

$$\% \text{ increase} = \frac{Q_2 - Q_1}{Q_1} \times 100$$

$$= \frac{3.879 - 3.673}{3.673} \times 100$$

$$= 5.62 \%$$

12.8 A river has a cross section, shown in Fig. 12.43 during the high flood. It has an average bed slope of 0.001. The channel has water to a depth of 2 m in the shallow section and 5 m in the deep section. The value of n for shallow section is given as 0.038 whereas for deep section as 0.028. Compute the discharge through this section.

Solution

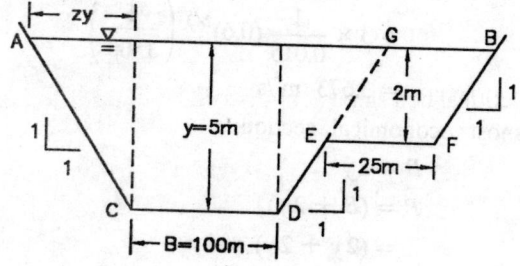

FIG. 12.43. EXAMPLE 12.8

Section ACDEG,

$$A_1 = \left[By + 2\left(y \times \frac{yz}{2}\right)\right]$$

$$A_1 = [B + zy]y$$

$$= (100 + 1 \times 5) \times 5$$

$$= 525 \text{ m}^2$$

$$P_1 = [B + \sqrt{2}\,y + \sqrt{2}\,(y - 2)]$$

$$= [100 + \sqrt{2}\,(5 + 3) = 111.31 \text{ m}^2$$

$$R_1 = \frac{525}{111.31} = 4.72$$

$$Q_1 = A_1 \frac{1}{n_1} R^{2/3} S_0^{1/2}$$

$$= 525 \times \frac{1}{0.028} \times (4.72)^{2/3} (0.001)^{1/2}$$

$$= 1668 \text{ m}^3/\text{s}$$

Section GEBF,

$$A_2 = 25 \times 2 = 50 \text{ m}^2.$$

$$P_2 = (25 + 2\sqrt{2}) = 27.83 \text{ m}$$

$$R_2 = A_2/P_2 = 50/27.83 = 1.8 \text{ m}$$

$$Q_2 = A_2 \times 1/n_2 R_2^{2/3} S_0^{1/2}$$

$$= \frac{50 \times (1.8)^{2/3} \times (0.001)^{1/2}}{0.038} = 61.57 \text{ m}^3/\text{s}$$

Total discharge $Q = Q_1 + Q_2$

$$= 1668 + 61.57$$

$$= 1729.57 \text{ m}^3/\text{s}$$

12.9 A trapezoidal channel has bed width 6 m, side slopes of 2 H: 1 V and n = 0.025; determine

(a) normal bed slope at normal depth of 0.962 m when it carries a discharge of 10 m³/s

(b) Critical bed slope and corresponding normal depth when it carries 10 m³/s,

(c) normal critical bed slope at normal depth of 0.962 m and corresponding discharge.

Solution

$$A = (B + zy) y$$

$$= (6 + 2 \times 0.962) \times 0.962$$

$$= 7.62 \text{ m}^2$$

$$P = (B + 2y\sqrt{1 + z^2})$$

$$= (6 + 2 \times 0.962 \sqrt{1 + (2)^2}$$

$$= 10.31$$

$$R = A/P = \frac{7.62}{10.31} = 0.74 \text{ m}$$

$$U = Q/A = \frac{10}{7.62} = 1.31 \text{ m/s}$$

(a) From Eq. 12.40

$$U = \frac{1}{n} R^{2/3} S_0^{1/2}$$

$$1.31 = \frac{1}{0.025} (0.74)^{2/3} (S_0)^{1/2}$$

$$S_0 = \frac{(1.31 \times 0.025)^2}{(0.74)^{4/3}}$$

$$= 0.0016 \text{ at } y_n \text{ equal to } 0.962 \text{ m}$$

(b) For given $Q = 10 \text{ m}^3/\text{s}$, the critical depth is y_c (say) From Eq. 12.62 c

$$\frac{A^3}{T} = \frac{Q^2}{g} = \frac{(10)^2}{9.81}$$

$$\frac{A^3}{T} = 10.19$$

where $\qquad A = (6 + 2y_c)\,y_c$

$$T = (6 + 4y_c)$$

Therefore, $\qquad \dfrac{(6y_c + 2y_c^2)^3}{(6 + 4y_c)} = 10.19$

Solving it by trial, $y_c = 0.61$ m

$$A = (6 + 2 \times 0.61) \times 0.61 = 7.83 \text{ m}^2$$

$$P = (6 + 2\sqrt{5} \times 0.61) = 8.728 \text{ m}$$

$$R = A/P = 7.83/8.728 = 0.897$$

$$U = 1/n\, R^{2/3}\, S_c^{1/2}$$

$$S_c = 0.001178$$

which will maintain uniform and critical flow at a depth of 0.61 m

(c) For given $y_n = 0.962$ m,

$$A = 7.62 \text{ m}^2$$

$$P = 10.31 \text{ m}$$

$$T = (6 + 4 \times 0.962) = 9.85 \text{ m}$$

$$D = A/T = 7.62/9.85 = 0.773 \text{ m}$$

Now from Eq. 12.62 a

$$Q^2/g A^2 = A/T$$

$$U_c = \sqrt{g D} = \sqrt{9.81 \times 0.773}$$

$$= 2.74 \text{ m/s}$$

Hence from Eq. 12.40

$$2.74 = \frac{1}{0.025} (7.62/10.31)^{2/3} (S_{cn})^{1/2}$$

$S_{cn} = 0.007$, that will maintain critical flow at normal depth of 0.962 m.

$$Q = AU$$

$$= 7.62 \times 2.74 = 20.88 \text{ m}^3/\text{s}$$

12.10 A channel is to be designed to give a constant velocity of flow of 1.8 m/s at all depths of flow. The lower portion of the channel is rectangular and is to carry minimum discharge. The rectangular section is to be designed with best proportions, the bottom width being 1.5m. Determine the depth of flow when the width at the water surface be 10m. Assuming Manning's $n = 0.015$, determine the bed slope of the channel.

Solution

For lower portion, the section is rectangular and for its best proportions,

$$B = 2y$$

$$y = B/2 = \frac{1.5}{2}$$

$$y = 0.75 \text{ m}$$

Also $R = y/2 = 0.375$ m

Using Manning's formula

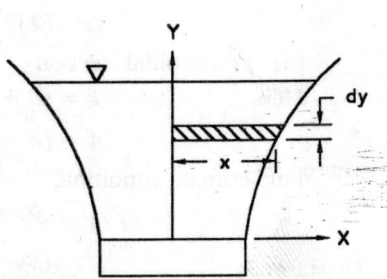

FIG. 12.44. EXAMPLE 12.10

$$U = \frac{1}{n} . R^{2/3} S^{1/2}$$

$$1.8 = \frac{1}{0.015} (0.375)^{2/3} S^{1/2}$$

Solving $S = 0.0027$

Now, for upper portion, the section is defined by Eq. 12.54a.

$$y = R \log_e [x + \sqrt{x^2 - R^2}] + C_1$$

Given conditions are; $x = 1.5/2 = 0.75$m; $y = 0$

∴ $0 = R \log_e [x + \sqrt{x^2 - R^2}] + C_1$

Solving $C_1 = - R \log [0.75 + \sqrt{(0.75)^2 - (0.375)^2}$

Hence, $y = R \log_e [x + \sqrt{x^2 - R^2}] / [0.75 + \sqrt{(0.75)^2 - (0.375)^2}]$

For $x = 5$ m.

$y = 0.375 \log_e [5 + \sqrt{(5)^2 - (0.375)^2}] / [0.75 + \sqrt{(0.75)^2 - (0.375)^2}]$

$$= 0.375 \log_e \left(\frac{9.986}{1.3995} \right) = 0.737 \text{ m}$$

∴ Total depth of flow $= (0.75 + 0.737)$

$$= 1.487 \text{ m}$$

12.11 Obtain the expressions for critical depth in (i) a triangular channel section with central angle 2θ, (ii) in a trapezoidal section with bottom width B and side slope 1:z.

Solution

(i) Triangular section

$$\frac{Q^2}{g} = \frac{A^3}{T}$$

Here $A = y^2 \tan \theta$

$T = 2 y_c \tan \theta$

$$\therefore \qquad Q^2/g = \frac{(y_c^2 \tan \theta)^3}{(2\, y_c \tan \theta)}$$

$$= \frac{y_c^5 \tan^2 \theta}{2}$$

$$y_c = (2\, Q^2/g \tan^2 \theta)^{1/5}$$

(ii) Trapezoidal section

Here
$$T = (B + 2\, y_c\, z)$$

$$A = (B\, y_c + y_c^2\, z)$$

For critical condition,

$$Q^2/g = A^3/T$$

$$= \frac{(B y_c + z y_c^2)^3}{(B + 2z\, y_c)}$$

$$RHS = \frac{[z y_c^2\,(B/z y_c + 1)]^3}{[z y_c\,(B/z y_c + 2)]} = \frac{z^3 y_c^6\,(B/z y_c + 1)^3}{[z y_c\,(B/z y_c + 2)]}.$$

$$\therefore \qquad \frac{Q^2}{g} = \frac{z^2 y_c^5\,(B/z y_c + 1)^3}{(B/z y_c + 2)}$$

Multiplying by $z^3\,/\,B^5$ on both sides.

$$\frac{Q^2 z^3}{g\, B^5} = \frac{z^5 y_c^5}{B^5}\,\frac{(B/z y_c + 1)^3}{(B/z y_c + 2)}$$

$$\frac{Q^2 z^3}{g\, B^5} = \frac{(B/z y_c + 1)^3}{(B/z y_c)^5\,(B/z y_c + 2)}$$

Similarly,

$$\frac{E_c}{B} = \frac{[3B/z y + 5]}{2\left(\dfrac{B}{z y_c}\right)[B/z y_c + 2]}$$

can be obtained for specific energy E.

12.12 Obtain an expression for critical depth for a parabolic channel section given by $x^2 = k\, y$. Therefrom determine y_e for a discharge of 1.5 m³/s. Assume k = 2 in the above equation.

Solution

$$x^2 = k\, y$$

$$x = \sqrt{k\, y}$$

$$T = 2x = 2\sqrt{k}\,\sqrt{y}$$

Also,
$$A = 2x\, dx$$

$$A = 2\int x\, dy$$

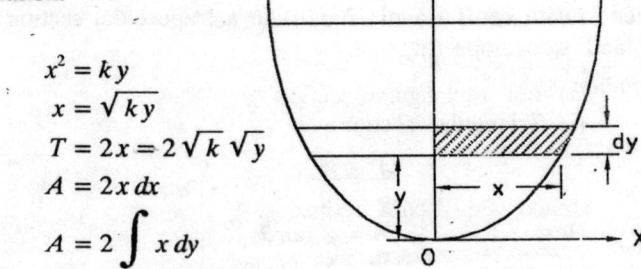

FIG. 12.45. EXAMPLE 12.12

$$= 2 \int_0^y \sqrt{k} \sqrt{y} \, dy$$

$$= 2\sqrt{k} \cdot \frac{y^{3/2}}{\frac{3}{2}}$$

$$A = \frac{4}{3}\sqrt{k} \, y^{3/2}$$

From Eq. 12.62 a,

$$\frac{A^3}{T} = \frac{Q^2}{g}$$

$$\frac{\left[\frac{4}{3}\sqrt{k} \cdot y_e^{3/2}\right]^3}{2\sqrt{k}\sqrt{y}} = \frac{Q^2}{g}$$

$$\frac{\frac{64}{27} \cdot k^{3/2} y_c^{9/2}}{2\sqrt{k}\sqrt{y_c}} = \frac{Q^2}{g}$$

$$y_e = \left[\frac{27}{32} \cdot \frac{Q^2}{gk}\right]^{1/4}$$

For $\qquad Q = 1.5 \text{ m}^3/\text{s}$

$$y_e = \left[\frac{27}{32} \cdot \frac{1.5^2}{9.81 \times 2}\right]^{1/4}$$

$$y_e = 0.558 \text{ m}.$$

12.13 An irrigation channel carries a discharge of 46 m³/s. Determine the critical depth of flow in each case.

(a) rectangular channel with bottom width 11.5 m,

(b) a triangular channel with each of the side slopes of 1.5 H : 1V, and (c) a trapezoidal channel with bottom width of 10 m and side slopes 1 H : 1 V on one side and 1/2H : 1 V on the other side.

Solution

The critical depth is determined from Eq. 12.62a.

$$Q^2 \, T/g \, A^3 = 1$$

(a) For rectangular section,

$$A = B y_e$$

$$T = B$$

Hence, Eq. 12.62a reduce to

$$y_c = (q^2/g)^{1/3}$$

$$= \left[\frac{\left(\frac{46}{11.5}\right)^2}{9.81}\right]^{1/3} = 1.117 \text{ m}$$

(b) For triangular section

$$A = \frac{1}{2}(y_c \times 3y_c)$$

$$= 1.5 y_c^2$$

$$T = 3 y_c$$

Hence

$$A^3/T = Q^2/g$$

$$\frac{(1.5 y_c^2)^3}{3 y_c} = \frac{(46)^2}{9.81}$$

$$y_c^5 = \frac{(46)^2}{9.81} \times \frac{3.0}{3.75}$$

$$y_c = 2.86 \text{ m}$$

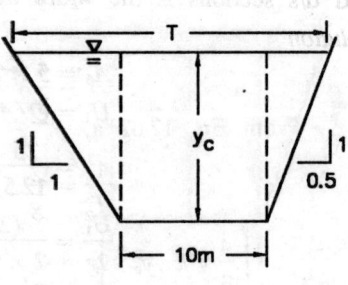

FIG. 12.46. EXAMPLE 12.13

(c) Trapezoidal section

$$A = [10 y_c + 0.5 y_c \times y_c/2 + y_c \times y_c/2]$$

$$= (10 y_c + 0.75 y_c^2)$$

$$T = (10 + 0.5 y_c + y_c)$$

$$= (10 + 1.5 y_c)$$

Substituting these values in Eq. 12.62a,

$$\frac{(10 y_c + 0.75 y_c^2)^3}{(10 + 1.5 y_c)} = \frac{Q^2}{g}$$

$$\frac{(10 y_c + 0.75 y_c^2)^3}{(10 + 1.5 y_c)} = \frac{(46)^2}{9.81} = 215.70 \qquad \text{...(i)}$$

Method 1 : Solve Eq. (i) by trial, $y_c = 1.25$ m

Method 2 : $A^3/T = Q^2/g$

Taking square root,

$$\frac{A\sqrt{A}}{\sqrt{T}} = \frac{Q}{\sqrt{g}}$$

$$A\sqrt{D} = Z_c = \text{section factor}$$

$$A\sqrt{D} = (46/\sqrt{9.81}) = 14.68$$

Computation is done in tabular form

y	A	T	$\sqrt{A/T} = \sqrt{D}$	$Z_c = A\sqrt{D}$
0.5	5.188	10.75	0.695	3.60
1.0	10.75	11.50	0.967	10.39
1.5	16.88	12.25	1.167	19.47
1.25	13.67	11.875	1.073	14.67

Required critical depth $= 1.25$ m.

12.14 A rectangular channel, 5 m wide, carries a discharge of 25 m³/s at a depth 2.5 m, (a) compute the width at section 2 downstream to obtain critical flow. (b) If the width at section 2 is reduced to 4 m, what should be the depth of flow at 2. (c) How are the depths of flow affected at u/s and d/s sections if the width at contracted section is reduced to 2.5 m.

Solution

$$A_1 = 5 \times 2.5 = 12.5 \text{ m}^2$$

$$U_1 = Q/A_1$$

$$= \frac{25}{12.5} = 2 \text{ m/s}$$

$$\frac{U_1^2}{2g} = \frac{(2)^2}{2 \times 9.81} = 0.204 \text{ m}$$

$$E_1 = (y_1 + U_1^2/2g)$$

$$= 2.5 + 0.204 = 2.704 \text{ m}$$

(a) For obtaining critical flow at 2,

$$E_1 = E_2 = E_c$$

Also

$$E_c = \frac{3}{2}y_c$$

$$= \frac{3}{2}\left[\frac{(Q/B_2)^2}{g}\right]^{1/3}$$

$$= \frac{3}{2}\left[\frac{(25/B_2)^2}{9.81}\right]^{1/3} \qquad \text{...(iii)}$$

Equating E_c to E_1

$$\frac{3}{2}\left[\frac{(25/B_2)^2}{9.81}\right]^{1/3} = 2.704$$

$$\left[\frac{(25/B_2)^2}{9.81}\right] = \left(2.704 \times \frac{2}{3}\right)^3$$

$$(25/B_2)^2 = 9.81 \times \left(\frac{2}{3} \times 2.704\right)^3$$

Solving, $\qquad B_2 = 3.298$ m.

With E_1 constant

$$y_c = (q^2/g)^{1/3}$$

$$= \left[\frac{(25/5)^2}{9.81}\right]^{1/3}$$

$$= 1.366 \text{ m.}$$

(b) Width of section 2 (downstream)

$$E_2 = E_1$$

$$\left[y_2 + \frac{U_2^2}{2g} \right] = 2.704$$

$$\left[y_2 + \left(\frac{25}{4y_2} \right)^2 \right] = 2.704$$

$$\left[y_2 + \frac{1.991}{y_2^2} \right] = 2.704$$

Solving by trial and error,

$$y_2 = 2.34 \text{ m} > 1.366 \text{ m}$$

The flow at section 2 is subentical $(y_2 > y_c)$

(c)
$$B_2 = 2.5 \text{ m}$$

$$q_2 = (Q/B_2)$$

$$= \frac{25}{2.5} = 10 \text{ m}^3/\text{s/m}$$

$$y_c = \left(q_2^2/g \right)^{1/3}$$

$$= \left(\frac{10^2}{9.81} \right)^{1/3} = 2.169 \text{ m}$$

$$E_c = \frac{3}{2} y_c$$

$$= \frac{3}{2} \times 2.169 = 3.253 \text{m}.$$

Since $E_1 = 2.704 < E_c$, the flow can not take place unless (i) water level on u/s rises and E_1 increases or (ii) discharge decreases so that E_c decreases and becomes equal to E_c.

Therefore, $E_1 = E_c = 3.253\text{m}$, let u/s depth be y_1'.

Then,
$$\left[y_1' + \frac{(Q/B y_1')^2}{2g} \right] = 3.253$$

$$\left[y_1' + \frac{\left(\frac{25}{2.5 y_1'} \right)^2}{2 \times 9.81} \right] = 3.253$$

$$y_1' + \frac{5.097}{(y_1')^2} = 3.253$$

Solving,
$$y_1' = 2.08 \text{ m}$$

$$y_2' = y_c = 2.169 \text{ m}$$

Since $y_1' < y_c$, the flow u/s is supercritical.

12.15 A rectangular channel 3.0 m wide carries a discharge of 10 m³/s at a depth of 1.5 m. If the channel width is reduced to 2.25 m and bed level is lowered by 0.75 m at the location of canal syphon, determine the difference in water levels between upstream and contracted sections, if any. The transition is smooth causing negligible energy loss.

Solution

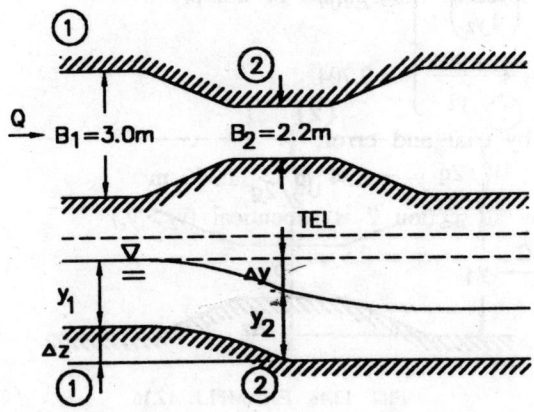

FIG. 12.47. EXAMPLE 12.15

$$A_1 = 3 \times 1.5 = 4.5 \text{ m}^2; \quad A_2 = 2.25 y_2 \text{ m}^2$$

$$U_1 = \frac{Q}{A_1}$$

$$= \frac{10}{4.5} = 2.22 \text{ m/s}$$

$$U_1^2/2g = \frac{(2.22)^2}{2 \times 9.81} = 0.25$$

Since there is no energy loss between sections 1 and 2,

$$E_2 = E_1 = \left(z_1 + y_1 + \frac{U_1^2}{2g} \right)$$

$$\left(y_2 + \frac{U_2^2}{2g} \right) = \left(0.75 + 1.5 + 0.25 \right)$$

$$y_2 + \left(\frac{10}{2.25 y_2} \right)^2 \times \frac{1}{2g} = 2.45$$

$$y_2 + \frac{1.006}{y_2^2} = 2.45$$

There are two possible values of y_2 Solving for subcritical flow

$$y_2 = 2.25 \text{ m}$$

As it is obvious if there is no energy loss, the water level will be horizontal and $y_1 = y_2 - \Delta z$

$$= 2.25 - 0.75 = 1.5 \text{ m (given)}$$

• It is to be noted that the assumptions of no energy loss in expanding flow is not correct.

12.16 A wide rectangular channel carries a discharge of 2.9 m³/s per meter width at a depth of 1.61 m. Compute the height of hump to be provided at the bed to produce critical flow over the hump. Also compute the corresponding drop in water level at the section of hump.

Solution

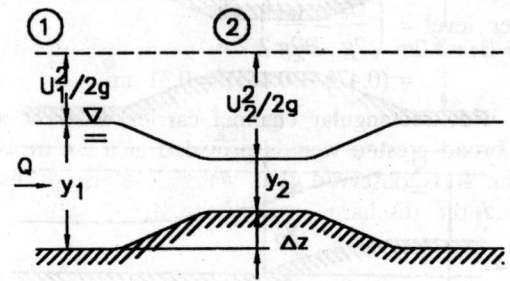

FIG. 12.48. EXAMPLE 12.16

$$U_1 = \frac{q}{y_1}$$

$$= \frac{2.9}{1.61} = 1.8 \text{ m/s}$$

$$\frac{U_1^2}{2g} = 0.165 \text{ m}$$

$$E_1 = \left(y_1 + \frac{U_1^2}{2g} \right)$$

$$= (1.61 + 0.165) = 1.775 \text{ m}$$

$$y_c = (q^2/g)^{1/3}$$

$$= \left[\frac{(2.9)^2}{9.81} \right]^{1/3} = 0.95 \text{m}$$

$$E_c = \frac{3}{2} y_c$$

$$= \frac{3}{2} \times 0.95 = 1.425 \text{m}$$

For critical flow $N_F = \dfrac{U_c}{\sqrt{g\,y_c}} = 1$

$$\frac{U_c^2}{2g} = \frac{y_c}{2}$$

$$= \frac{0.95}{2} = 0.475 \text{ m}$$

Let Δz be the height of hump and assuming no energy loss between sections 1 and 2,

$$E_1 = E_c + \Delta z$$

$$\Delta z = E_1 - E_c$$

$$= 1.775 - 1.425$$

$$= 0.35 \text{ m}$$

Drop in water level $= \left(\dfrac{U_c^2}{2g} - \dfrac{U_1^2}{2g} \right)$

$$= (0.475 - 0.165) = 0.31 \text{ m}.$$

12.17 A 4.2 wide rectangular channel carries water at a depth of 2.1 m. A 0.35 m high broad crested weir is provided at a 2.4 m wide contracted section downstream. It is observed that water level drops by 0.15 m over the hump. Compute the discharge carried by the channel.

Solution

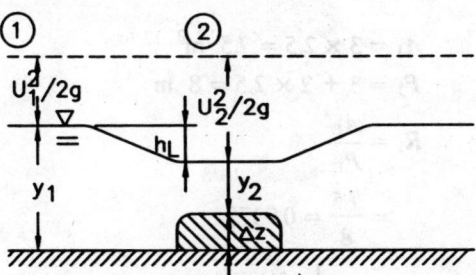

FIG. 12.49. EXAMPLE 12.17

Applying Bernoulli's theorem between sections 1 and 2,

$$\left(y_1 + \frac{U_1^2}{2g} \right) = \left(\Delta z + y_2 + \frac{U_2^2}{2g} \right) \qquad \text{...(i)}$$

Since there is no energy loss between 1 and 2, one can write,

$$\frac{U_2^2}{2g} = \frac{U_1^2}{2g} + h_L$$

$$= \frac{U_1^2}{2g} + h_L \qquad \text{...(ii)}$$

Substituting from Eq. (ii) into Eq. (i)

$$\left(y_1 + \frac{U_1^2}{2g} \right) = \left(\Delta z + y_2 + \frac{U_1^2}{2g} + h_L \right)$$

$$y_1 = \Delta z + y_2 + h_L$$

$$y_2 = y_1 - \Delta z - h_L$$

$$= (2.1 - 0.35 - 0.15) = 1.6,$$

From Eq. (ii)

$$\frac{U_2^2}{2g} = \frac{U_1^2}{2g} + 0.15$$

$$\frac{\left(\dfrac{Q}{B_2 y_2}\right)^2}{2g} - \frac{\left(\dfrac{Q}{B_1 y_1}\right)^2}{2g} = 0.15$$

$$\left(\frac{Q}{2.4 \times 1.6}\right)^2 - \left(\frac{Q}{4.2 \times 2.1}\right)^2 = 0.15 \times 2 \times 9.81$$

Solving, $\qquad Q = 7.317 \ \text{m}^3/\text{s}.$

12.18 Uniform flow occurs in a 3.0 m wide rectangular channel (bed slope 0.003) at a depth of 2.5 m. Due to sedimentation, the channel bed is raised at certain section Calculate the maximum height of hump without affecting the upstream depth. Use Manning's rugosity coefficient as 0.012. If the depth of water at upstream section is raised to 2.9 m, determine the height of hump.

Solution

$$A_1 = 3 \times 2.5 = 7.5 \ \text{m}^2$$

$$P_1 = 3 + 2 \times 2.5 = 8 \ \text{m}$$

$$R_1 = \frac{A_1}{P_1}$$

$$= \frac{7.5}{8} = 0.9375$$

$$Q = A \cdot \frac{1}{n} R^{2/3} S_0^{1/2}$$

$$= 7.5 \times \frac{1}{0.012} (0.9375)^{2/3} (0.003)^{1/2}$$

$$= 31.41 \ \text{m}^3/\text{s}$$

$$U_1 = \frac{Q}{A_1}$$

$$= \frac{31.41}{7.5} = 4.188 \ \text{m/s}$$

$$U_1^2/2g = 0.894 \ \text{m}$$

$$E_1 = (y_1 + U_1^2/2g)$$

$$= (2.5 + 0.894) = 3.394 \ \text{m}$$

(a) The maximum height of hump $= \Delta z$ m. It will correspond to critical flow at 2. i.e $y_2 = y_c$

$$q = \frac{Q}{B}$$

$$= \frac{31.41}{3} = 10.47 \text{ m}^3/\text{s/m}$$

$$y_c = (q^2/g)^{1/3} = 2.236$$

$$E_c = \frac{3}{2} y_c$$

$$= \frac{3}{2} \times 2.236 = 3.354 \text{ m}$$

Applying Bernoulli's theorem,

$$E_1 = E_c + \Delta z$$

$$\Delta z = (E_1 - E_c)$$

$$= 3.394 - 3.354$$

$$= 0.04\text{m}$$

(b) The depth of water at upstream is raised to 2.9 m due to hump, the flow at downstream section at hump will still be critical.

Let the height of hump be $= \Delta z$.

Then $E_1' = E_c + \Delta z$

$$\left(y_1' + \frac{U_1'^2}{2g} \right) = E_c + \Delta z \qquad \text{...(i)}$$

Since the discharge flowing in channel remains same, E_c remains same as in case (a).

Now $$U_1' = \frac{Q}{B y_1'}$$

$$= \frac{31.41}{3 \times 2.9} = 3.61 \text{ m/s}$$

$$\frac{(U_1')^2}{2g} = 0.664\text{m}$$

Hence from Eq. (i)

$$(2.9 + 0.664) = 3.354 + \Delta z$$

$$\Delta z = (2.9 + 0.664 - 3.354)$$

$$= 0.21 \text{ m}.$$

12.19 Uniform flow occurs at a depth of 2 m in a long rectangular channel, 3.5 m wide, and laid at a slope of 0.0064. If n = 0.02, compute

(a) maximum height of hump to produce the critical depth at downstream section,

(b) width of contraction which will produce critical depth without increasing upstream depth of flow.

Solution

(a) $$A_1 = 2 \times 3.5 = 7 \text{ m}^2$$

$$P_1 = (3.5 + 2 \times 2) = 7.5 \text{ m}^2$$

$$R_1 = A_1/P_1 = 7/7.5 = 0.933 \text{ m}$$

From Eq. 12,40,

$$U_1 = 1/n \, R_1^{2/3} \, S_c^{1/2}$$

$$= 1/0.02 \, (0.933)^{2/3} \, (0.0064)^{1/2}$$

$$= 3.82$$

$$U_1^2/2g = 0.744 \text{ m}$$

$$E_1 = (y_1 + U_1^2/2g) = (2 + 0.744).$$

$$= 2.744 \text{ m}$$

$$Q = A_1 U_1$$

$$= 7 \times 3.82 = 26.74 \text{ m}^3/\text{s}$$

$$y_c^2 = (q^2/g)$$

$$= [(26.74/3.5)^2/9.81]$$

$$= 5.95$$

$$y_c = 1.81 \text{ m}$$

$$E_c = (3/2) \, y_c = 3/2 \times 1.81 = 2.718 \text{ m}$$

Equating the specific energy at two sections

$$E_1 = E_2 + \Delta z = E_c + \Delta z$$

$$\Delta z = E_1 - E_c$$

$$= 2.744 - 2.718$$

$$= 0.026 \text{ m}$$

(b) Let the width of contracted section be B_2.

$$q = (Q/B_2) = (26.74/B_2)$$

$$(y_c)^3 = (26.74/B_2)^2/g$$

$$y_c = [(26.74/B_2)^2/g]^{1/3}$$

$$E_c = (3/2) \, y_c = 3/2 \, [(26.74)^2/B_2^2 g]^{1/3}$$

Equating the specific energy at sections 1 and 2

$$E_1 = E_c$$

$$2.744 = 3/2 \, [26.74)^2/B_2^2 g]^{1/3}$$

Solving, $B_2 = 3.46 \text{ m}$

12.20 In a rectangular channel, 5 m wide, the water flows at a depth of 2 m with a velocity 2.5 m/s. The channel width is reduced to 2.5 m and at the same time, the bottom is raised by 0.25 m to create a hump on the bed. By what extent is the water surface on the upstream affected by change of section?

Solution

$$Q = A U$$

$$= (5 \times 2) \times 2.5 = 25 \text{ m}^3/\text{s}$$

The discharge intensity at the contracted section,

$$q = Q/B_2 = 25/2.5 = 10 \text{ m}^2/\text{s/width}$$

Critical depth at contracted section,

$$y_c = (q^2/g)^{1/3}$$
$$= [(10)^2/9.81]^{1/3} = 2.165 \text{ m}$$

Specific energy at contracted section,

$$E_c = (3/2) y_c = 3/2 \times 2.165$$
$$= 3.25 \text{ m}$$

Specific energy at upstream section,

$$E_1 = (y_1 + U_1^2/2g)$$
$$= \left[2 + \frac{(2.5)^2}{2 \times 9.81} \right]$$
$$= (2 + 0.319) = 2.319 \text{ m}$$

Since $E_1 < E_c$, no flow can take place unless (i) the water level on upstream rises and E_1 increases or (ii) the discharge reduces so that E_c decreases.

Let the water level on upstream become y_1 metre

$$E_1 = (y_1 + U_1^2/2g)$$

Thus, the specific energy at upstream section should, at least, be equal to specific energy at downstream section.

$$E_1 = E_2 + \Delta z = E_c + \Delta z$$
$$(y_1 + U_1^2/2g) = (3.25 + 0.25)$$
$$\left[y_1 + \frac{(25/5 y_1)^2}{2 \times 9.81} \right] = 3.5$$
$$y_1 + \frac{1.285}{y_1^2} = 3.5$$

Solving it by trial, $y_1 = 3.42 \text{ m}$

Rise in water level $= 3.42 - 2.0$
$$= 1.42 \text{ m}$$

12.21 A 24 m wide rectangular channel carries water at a depth of 2.5 m and is laid at bed slope of 0.0008. Two piers, 2.25 m wide and 4.5 m long, are constructed in the water way to facilitate the construction of foot bridge. The nose of piers are made rounded so as to cause negligible energy loss to the flow between them. Determine the water depth upstream of piers. Take Mannings n = 0.02.

Solution

Under normal condition,

$$A_n = 24 \times 2.5 = 60 \text{ m}^2$$
$$P_n = 24 + 2 \times 2.5 = 2.9 \text{ m}$$

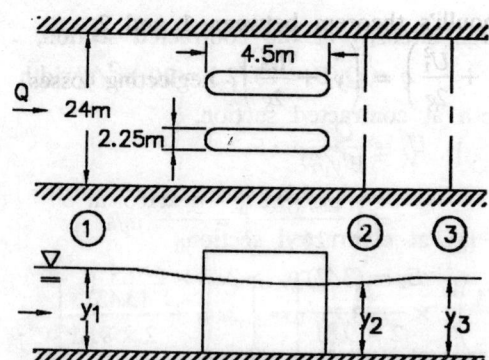

FIG. 12.50 EXAMPLE 12.21

$$R_n = 60/29 = 2.07$$

$$Q = A\,U = A\,\frac{1}{n}.R^{2/3}\,S_0^{1/2}$$

$$= 60 \times \frac{1}{0.02}\,(2.07)^{2/3}\,(0.0008)^{1/2}$$

$$= 137.823 \ \text{m}^3/\text{s}$$

$$U_3 = \frac{Q}{A_3}$$

$$= \frac{137.823}{60} \qquad (A_n = A_3)$$

$$= 2.297 \ \text{m/s} \qquad\qquad\qquad ...(i)$$

When piers are constructed, the water way is constricted at section 2,

$$B_2\,y_2\,U_2 = Q$$

$$U_2 = \frac{137.823}{(24 - 2 \times 0.25)\,y_2}$$

$$= \frac{7.068}{y_2} \qquad\qquad\qquad ...(ii)$$

Now apply momentum equation between 2 and 3.

$$w\,\frac{B}{2}\,(y_2^2 - y_3^2) = \frac{w\,Q}{g}\,(U_3 - U_2)$$

$$y_2^2 - (2.5)^2 = \frac{137.823 \times 2}{9.81 \times 24}\left(2.297 - \frac{7.068}{y_2}\right)$$

Simplifying,

$$y_2^3 - 8.94\,y_2 + 9.69 = 0$$

Solving, $\qquad\qquad y_2 = 2.06\text{m}$

From Eq. (i) $\quad U_2 = \dfrac{7.068}{2.06} = 3.43 \ \text{m/s}$

Apply Bernoulli's theorem between 1 and 2,

$$\left(y_1 + \frac{U_1^2}{2g}\right) = \left(y_2 + \frac{U_2^2}{2g}\right), \text{ neglecting losses.}$$

where

$$U_1 = \frac{Q}{B y_1}$$

$$= \left(\frac{137.823}{24 y_1}\right) = \frac{5.74}{y_1} \text{ m/s}$$

$$\left[y_1 + \left(\frac{5.74}{y_1}\right)^2 \times \frac{1}{2 \times 9.81}\right] = \left[2.06 + \frac{(3.43)^2}{2 \times 9.81}\right]$$

Simplifying, $y_1^3 - 2.66 y_1^2 + 1.681 = 0$

Solving, $\quad\quad y_1 = 2.37 \text{m}$

$$U_1 = \frac{137.823}{24 \times 2.37} = 2.423 \text{ m/s}$$

$$N_{F1} = \frac{U_1}{\sqrt{g y_1}}$$

$$= \frac{2.423}{\sqrt{9.81 \times 2.37}} = 0.5$$

Therefore, the flow u/s of piers is subcritical and depths of flow is 2.37 m.

12.22 A trapezoidal channel of base width 6 m and side slopes 2H:IV carries a flow of 60 m³/s at a depth of 2.5 m. There is a gradual transition to a rectangular section 6 m wide accompanies by a gradual lowering of channel bed by 0.6 m. Find (a) the depth of water in rectangular section and change in water surface level (b) In case, the drop in W.S. is to be restricted to 0.3 m, what is the amount by which the bed must be lowered (assume no losses).

Solution

(a) At section 1, (Trapezoidal section)

$$A_1 = \left(6 \times 2.5 + 2 \times \frac{2.5 \times 5}{2}\right) = 27.5 \text{ m}^2$$

$$U_1 = \frac{60}{27.5} = 2.182 \text{ m/s}$$

$$U_1^2/2g = 0.243 \text{ m}$$

$$E_1 = (2.5 + 0.243) = 2.743 \text{ m}$$

At section 2, (Rectangular section)

$$A_2 = 6 \times y_2$$

$$U_2 = \frac{60}{6 y_2} = \frac{10}{y_2}$$

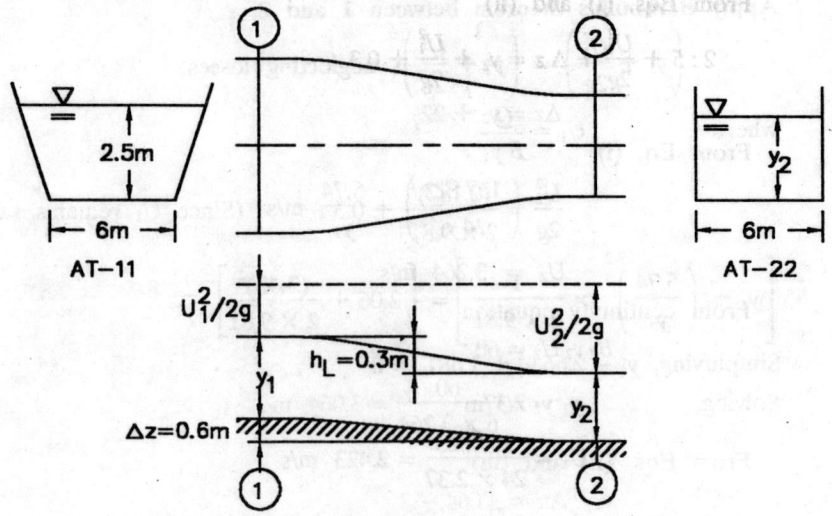

FIG. 12.51 EXAMPLE 12.22

$$U_2^2/2g = \frac{(10/y_2)^2}{2 \times 9.81} = \frac{5.1}{y_2^2}$$

$$E_2 = (y_2 + 5.1/y_2^2)$$

Apply Bernoulli's equation between 1 and 2,
(no energy loss)

$$E_1 + \Delta z = E_2$$

$$2.743 + 0.6 = y_2 + \frac{5.1}{y_2^2}$$

Simplifying,

$$y_2^3 - 3.343 y_2 + 5.1 = 0$$

Solving, $y_2 = 1.85$ m

Depth in rectangular channel $= 1.85$

Change or drop in W.L. $= 2.5 - 1.85 = 0.65$ m.

(b) In this case, drop in W.L. $= 0.3$ m.

$$\frac{U_2^2}{2g} = \frac{U_1^2}{2g} + 0.3 \qquad \qquad ...(i)$$

Again applying Bernoulli's equation between 1 and 2,

$$E_1 + \Delta z = E_2$$

where Δz is drop in bed level of rectangular channel,

$$y_1 + \frac{U_1^2}{2g} + \Delta z = y_2 + \frac{U_2^2}{2g} \qquad \qquad ...(ii)$$

From Eqs. (i) and (ii)

$$2:5 + \frac{U_1^2}{2g} + \Delta z = y_2 + \frac{U_1^2}{2g} + 0.3$$

$$\Delta z = y_2 + 22 \quad ;$$

From Eq. (i):

$$\frac{U_2^2}{2g} = \frac{(2.182)^2}{2 \times 9.81} + 0.3 \qquad \text{(Since } U_1 \text{ remains same)}$$

$$U_2 = 3.264 \text{ m/s}$$

From continuity equation

$$B_2 y_2 U_2 = 60$$

$$y_2 = \frac{60}{6 \times 3.264} = 3.064 \text{ m} \qquad \qquad \text{...(iii)}$$

From Eqs. (ii) and (iii)

$$\Delta z = 3.064 - 2.2$$

$$= 0.864$$

Drop in bed level = 0.864 m.

12.23 The bed of a river, 20 m wide, has a slope of 1 in 15000 and Chezy's C = 60. A dam across the river has a spillway with its top in the form of a broad creasted weir, 18 m wide; the height of sill being 4 m above the river bed.

Assuming that the whole of the river flow passes over the spillway, find the afflux at the dam when the depth of water at a upstream section is 1.5 m. Neglect the effect of ends of the spillway and assume the banks vertical and of the same material as the bed.

Assume coefficient of discharge for the spillway as 0.9.

Solution

Neglecting the velocity of approach and taking the top of weir as datum,

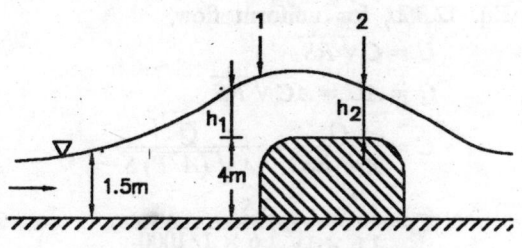

FIG. 12.52 EXAMPLE 12.23

$$E_1 = E_2$$

$$H = h_1 = h_2 + U_2^2/2g$$

$$U_2 = \sqrt{2g(h_1 - h_2)}$$

and
$$Q = C_d \, (b_2 \, h_2) \times \sqrt{2g \, (h_1 - h_2)}$$

Fox maximum discharge, $h_2 = \frac{2}{3} E_c = \frac{2}{3} h_1$

$$= \frac{2}{3} H = \frac{2}{3} \text{ (total head)}$$

Also
$$U_2 = \sqrt{2g \, (H - \frac{2}{3} H)} = \sqrt{\frac{2}{3} gH}$$

and
$$Q = 0.9 \times (18 \times \frac{2}{3} H) \sqrt{\frac{2}{3} gH}$$

$$= 27.7 \, H^{3/2}$$

From Eq. 12.36b,

$$U = C\sqrt{RS}$$

$$Q = A_1 U_1$$

$$= (20 \times 1.5) \left[60 \sqrt{\frac{20 \times 1.5}{(20 + 2 \times 1.5)} \times \frac{1}{15000}} \right]$$

$$= 16.85 \, \text{m}^3/\text{s}$$

Hence, $27.7 \, H^{3/2} = 16.85$

$$H = (0.61)^{2/3} = 0.72 \text{ m}$$

Therefore, afflux $= (h_1 - h_2)$

$$= (0.72 - \frac{2}{3} \times 0.72)$$

$$= 0.24 \text{ m}$$

12.24 A wide channel laid to a slope of 1 in 1000 carries a discharge of 3.5 m³/s per metre width at a depth of 1.6m. (a) Find out the value of C, assuming the flow to be uniform. (b) If the depth varies gradually from 1.5 m to 1.7 m at a location 300 m downstream, what will be the value of C ?

Solution

(a) From Eq. 12.36b, for uniform flow,

$$U = C\sqrt{RS}$$

$$Q = AU = AC\sqrt{RS}$$

or
$$C = \frac{Q}{A\sqrt{RS}} = \frac{Q}{A\sqrt{(A/P)\,S}}$$

or
$$C = \frac{3.5}{1.6 \times 1\sqrt{1.6 \times 1/1000}}$$

(since $R \approx y$ for wide channel)

$$= 54.69$$

(b) For gradually varried flow,

$$E_1 = y_1 + U_1^2/2g = (1.5 + U_1^2/2g)$$

$$E_2 = y_2 + U_2^2/2g = (1.7 + U_2^2/2g)$$

From Eq. 12.98

$$\Delta x = \frac{E_1 - E_2}{S_o - S_f}$$

$$(S_o - \overline{S}_f) = \frac{\Delta E}{\Delta x} = \frac{(1.5 + U_1^2/2g) - (1.7 + U_2^2/2g)}{300}$$

From continuity equation, $A_1 U_1 = A_2 U_2$

$$U_2 = \frac{A_1 U_1}{A_2} = \frac{1.5 \times 1 \times U_1}{1.7 \times 1}$$

$$U_2 = 0.882 U_1$$

$$\therefore \qquad (S_o - \overline{S}_f) = \frac{U_1^2/2g - (0.882 U_1)^2/2g - 0.2}{300}$$

$$= \frac{(0.0113 U_1^2 - 0.2)}{300}$$

The velocity of the upstream section is

$$U_1 = \frac{Q}{A_1} = \frac{3.5}{(1.5 \times 1)} = 2.33 \text{ m/s}$$

$$\therefore \qquad \dot{S} - \overline{S}_f = \frac{0.0113 (2.33)^2 - 0.2}{300} = -0.00046$$

$$\overline{S}_f = (1/1000 + 0.00046) = 0.00146 \qquad \qquad ...(i)$$

From Eq. 12.36 b

$$S_{f_1} = \frac{U_1^2}{C^2 R_1} \approx \frac{U_1^2}{C^2 y_1} = \frac{U^2}{C^2 \times 1.5}$$

$$= 0.666 U_1^2/C^2$$

$$S_{f_2} = \frac{U_2^2}{c^2 R_2} \approx \frac{U_2^2}{C^2 y_2} \approx \frac{10.882 U_1^2}{C^2 \times 17}$$

$$= 0.458 U_1^2/C^2$$

$$S_{\overline{f}} = \frac{S_{f_1} + S_{f_2}}{2} = \frac{(0.666 + 0.458)}{2} \frac{U_1^2}{C^2}$$

$$= 3.06/C^2 \qquad \qquad ...(ii)$$

From Eqs (i) and (iii),

$$3.06/C^2 = 0.00146$$

$$C = \sqrt{\frac{3.06}{0.00146}} = 45.78$$

12.25 A river, 90 m wide and 3 m deep, has a stable bed and vertical banks with a surface slope of 1 in 2500. Estimate the length of back water curve produced by an afflux of 2 m. Take n = 0.035.

Solution

$$A_1 = 90 \times 3 = 270 \text{ m}^2$$

$$P_1 = 90 + 2 \times 3 = 96 \text{ m}$$

$$R_1 = A_1/P_1 = 270/96 = 2.81 \text{ m}$$

$$Q = A_1 \left(\frac{1}{n}\right) R_1^{2/3} S^{1/2}$$

$$= 270 \times 1/0.035 \times (2.81)^{2/3} (1/2500)^{1/2}$$

$$= 307.23 \text{ m}^3/\text{s}$$

$$E_1 = y_1 + \frac{(Q/A_1)^2}{2g}$$

$$= 3 + \frac{(307.23/270)^2}{2 \times 9.81} = 3.066 \text{ m}$$

E_2 at section 2 where $y_2 = 3 + 2 = 5$ m

$$= \left[5 + \frac{(307.23/90 \times 5)^2}{2 \times 9.81}\right] = 5.0238 \text{ m}$$

$\overline{S_f}$ is computed at the middle of two section

$$y \text{ mean} = \frac{3+5}{2} = 4 \text{ m}$$

$$A_m = 90 \times 4 = 360 \text{ m}^2$$

$$P_m = (90 + 2 \times 2) = 98 \text{ m}$$

$$R_{m1} = A_m/P_m = 360/98 = 3.673 \text{ m}$$

From Eq. 12.40,

$$U_m = 1/n \, R_m^{2/3} S_t^{1/2}$$

$$S_f = \frac{n^2 U_m^2}{R_m^{4/3}}$$

$$= \frac{(0.035)^2 (307.23/360)^2}{(3.673)^{4/3}}$$

$$= 0.0001574$$

From Eq. 12.98,

$$\Delta x = \frac{E_2 - E_1}{S_o - \overline{S_f}}$$

$$= \frac{5.0238 - 3.066}{1/2500 - 0.0001574}$$

$$= 8070 \text{ m}$$

12.26 A wide canal conveys water at a normal depth of 1 m and is laid at a bed slope of 1 m in 1000. A weir is constructed to divert the water into a canal. The depth of water required behind the weir is 2m. Determine the distance upstream of the weir where the depth will be 1.5m. Use Chezy's formula and take C = 55.

Solution

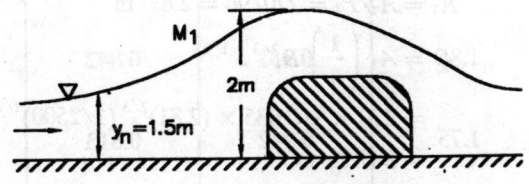

FIG. 12.53 EXAMPLE 12.26

From Eq. 12.95,

$$\frac{dy}{dx} = \frac{S_o\left[1 - (y_n/y)^3\right]}{\left[1 - (y_c/y)^3\right]}$$

when Chezy's equation is used.

or

$$dx = \frac{dy}{S_o} \frac{\left[1 - (y_c/y)^3\right]}{\left[1 - (y_n/y)^3\right]}$$

From Eq. 12.36b, $U = C\sqrt{RS}$ ...(i)

$$Q = AC\sqrt{RS}$$

$$q = Q/B = A C \sqrt{RS}/B$$

For wide channel, $R \approx y_n$

$$q = AC\sqrt{y_n S_o}/B = y_n C \sqrt{y_n S_o}$$

$$= C y_n^{3/2} \sqrt{S_o}$$

$$= 55 (1)^{3/2} \times \sqrt{1/1000} = 1.74 \text{ m}^3/\text{s/m}$$

$$y_c = (q^2/g)^{1/3}$$

$$= \left[\frac{(1.74)^2}{9.81}\right]^{1/3}$$

$$= 0.676 \text{ m}$$

Since $y_n > y_c$ it, is mild slope Moreover, $y > y_n > y_c$, M_1 curve will be formed upstream of wair.

The depth of water changes from 2 m at the weir to 1.5 m at upstream section. Taking each step of rise of water level as 0.1 m, the computation is made in tabular form.

From Eq.(i)

$$dx = \frac{0.1}{1/1000} \frac{\left[(1 - 0.676/y)^3\right]}{\left[1 - (1/y)^3\right]} = \frac{100\left[1 - 0.676/y)^3\right]}{\left[1 - (1/y)^3\right]}$$

Depth	Mean depth	$1 - (0.676/y)^3$	$[1 - 1]/y^3$	Δx
2.0				
	1.95	0.958	0.865	110.72
1.9				
	1.85	0.951	0.842	112.94
1.8				
	1.75	0.942	0.813	115.91
1.7				
	1.65	0.931	0.777	119.84
1.6				
	1.55	0.917	0.731	125.44
1.5				

Total $= 584.83$ m

Thus, the required distance from weir $= 585$ m.

12.27. A trapezoidal channel (Bed width 4 m, side slope 1 H : 1 V) s laid at a bed slope of 0.0016 and carries a discharge of 2.5 m³. The depth of flow decreases in the direction of flow and is found 0.5 m at certain section. Name the surface profile formed and determine its length by directs stop method.

Solution :

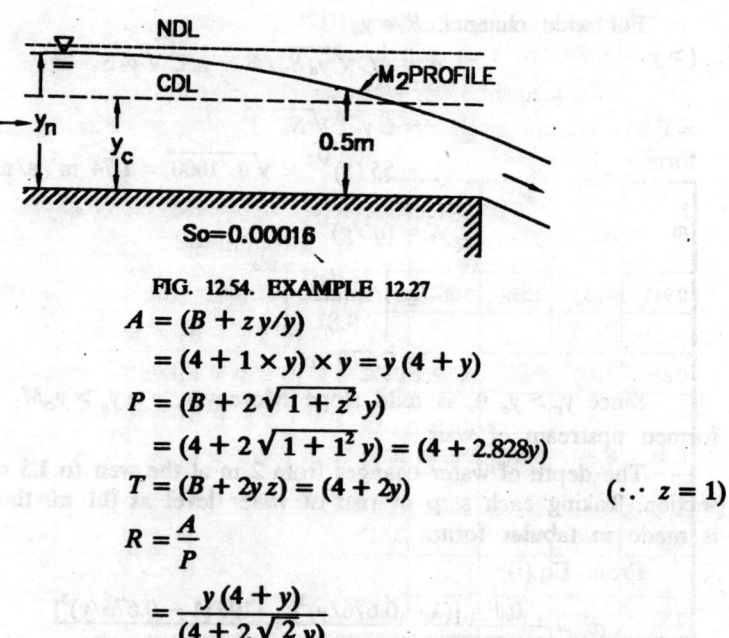

FIG. 12.54. EXAMPLE 12.27

$$A = (B + zy/y)$$
$$= (4 + 1 \times y) \times y = y(4 + y)$$
$$P = (B + 2\sqrt{1 + z^2}\, y)$$
$$= (4 + 2\sqrt{1 + 1^2}\, y) = (4 + 2.828y)$$
$$T = (B + 2yz) = (4 + 2y) \qquad (\because z = 1)$$
$$R = \frac{A}{P}$$
$$= \frac{y(4 + y)}{(4 + 2\sqrt{2}\, y)}$$

Using Equation 12.40

$$Q = AU$$

$$2.5 = Ay(4+y) \times \frac{1}{0.02} \left(\frac{y(4+y)}{4 + 2\sqrt{2}\,y} \right)^{2/3} (0.00016)^{1/2}$$

$$\frac{y^{5/3}(4+y)^{5/3}}{(4 + 2\sqrt{2}\,y)^{2/3}} = \frac{0.02 \times 2.5}{\sqrt{0.00016}}$$

$$\frac{y^{5/3}(4+y)^{5/3}}{4 + 2\sqrt{2}\,y)^{2/3}} = 3.953$$

Solving by trial and error,

$$y_n = 0.952 \text{ m}$$

(2) Calculate y_c

$$\frac{Q^2}{g} = \frac{A^3}{T}$$

$$\frac{(2.5)^2}{9.81} = \frac{[y(4+y)]^3}{[4 + 2y]}$$

$$\frac{y^3(4+y)^3}{(4 + 2y)} = 0.637$$

Solving by trial and error

$$y_c = 0.332 \text{ m}$$

Since $y_n > y_c$, $S_0 < S_c$ or bed slope is mild and water surface profile will be of M-family.

The surface curve will lie between 0.962 m (y_n) and 0.5 m ($> y_c = 0.332$ m), it will be M_2 cure.

The length of drawdown curve M_2 is computed between 0.99 y_n = 0.943 m and given depth 0.5 m. The computations are made in tabular form.

y m	A m²	U m/s	$\frac{U^2}{2g}$ m	E m	ΔE m	R m	S_f ×10⁻⁴	$\overline{S_f}$ ×10⁻⁴	$(S-\overline{S_f})$ ×10⁻⁴	Δx m	ΣΔx m
0.943	4.661	0.536	0.0147	0.957		0.699	1.852		-0.950	1421.05	
					0.135			2.550			1421.05
0.80	3.840	0.651	0.0216	0.822		0.613	3.249		2.582	360.20	
					0.093			4.182			1781.25
0.70	3.290	0.760	0.0294	0.729		0.550	5.114		5.271	165.08	
					0.087			6.871			1946.33
0.60	2.760	0.906	0.0418	0.642		0.484	8.628		10.634	74.29	
					0.079			12.234			
0.50	2.250	1.100	0.0630	0.563		0.416	5.840				2020.62

12.28 Water flows from under a sluice into a very wide rectangular channel. The bed slope is 1/1000. The sluice is regulated to discharge 5 m^3/s/metre width of channel so that the depth at the venacontracta becomes 0.5 m. Will a hydraulic jump form in the channel or not? If so, find the location of the jump. Take n = 0.02.

Solution

$$y_c = (q^2/g)^{1/3}$$

$$y_c = (5^2/9.81)^{1/3} = 1.366 \text{ m}$$

Since the depth at vena contracta is less than y_e, the jump is likely to form in the channel.

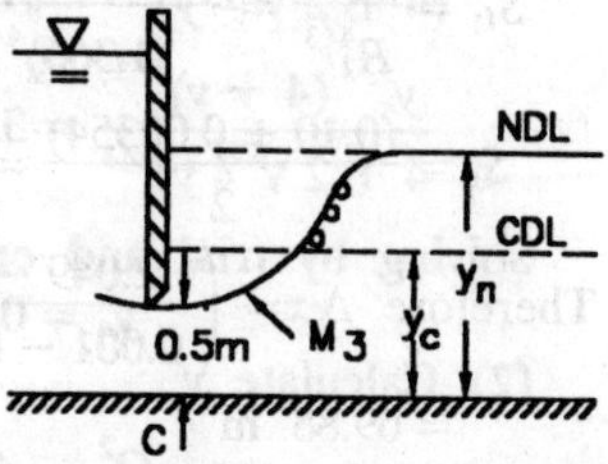

Using Eq. 12.40,

$$U = 1/n \, R^{2/3} \, S_o^{1/2}$$

Since the channel is very wide $R \approx y_n$,

FIG. 12.55 EXAMPLE 12.28

$$U = q/y_n = (1/0.02) \times y^{2/3} \times (1/1000)^{1/2}$$

$$y_r^{5/3} = 5 \times 0.02 \times (1000)^{1/2} = 6.324$$

$$y_n = 2.0 \text{ m}$$

Since $y_n > y_e$, the channel slope is mild. Also y_1 (depth at vena contracta) $< y_e$, the surface curve will lie in zone 3 or M3 curve will form.

From Eq. 12.107b,

$$\frac{y_2'}{y_1'} = \frac{1}{2} \left[-1 \pm \sqrt{1 + \frac{8 \, q^2}{g \, y_1'^3}} \right]$$

where y_1' and y_2' are conjugate depths. For $y_1' = 1.366$ m, sequent depth y_2' is determined,

$$\left(\frac{y_2'}{1.366} \right) = \frac{1}{2} \left[-1 \pm \sqrt{1 + \frac{8 \times 5 \times 5}{9.81 \times (1.366)^3}} \right]$$

$$= \frac{1}{2} \left[-1 \pm \sqrt{1 + 8} \right] = 1$$

$$y_2' = 1.366 \text{ m}$$

Let the jump form x distance from the section of vena contracta, in which depth varies from 0.5 m to 1.366 m.

$$\Delta x = \frac{E_2 - E_1}{S_o - S_t}$$

$$E_1 = \left(y_1 + \frac{U_1^2}{2g} \right) = \left[0.5 + \frac{(5/0.5)^2}{2 \times 9.81} \right] = 5.597 \text{ N m/N}$$

$$E_2 = \left(y_2 + \frac{U_2^2}{2g} \right) = \left[1.366 + \frac{(5/1.366)^2}{2 \times 9.81} \right] = 2.049 \text{ N m/N}$$

$$S_o = 1/1000 \, ; U_1 = 10 \text{ m/s}$$

$$\overline{S_t} = \frac{S_{f_1} + S_{f_2}}{2} \, ; \, U_2 = 3.66 \text{ m/s}$$

$$S_{f_1} = \frac{n^2 U_2^2}{R_2^{4/3}} \approx \frac{(0.02)^2 (10)^2}{(0.5)^{4/3}} = 0.10$$

$$S_{f_1} = \frac{n^2 U_2^2}{R_2^{4/3}} = \frac{(0.02)^2 (3.66)^2}{(1.366)^{4/3}} = 0.00354$$

$$\overline{S_t} = \frac{(0.10 + 0.00354)}{2} = 0.05177$$

Therefore $\Delta x = \left(\dfrac{2.049 - 5.597}{0.001 - 0.05177} \right)$

$$= 69.88 \text{ m}$$

Thus the jump will form nearly 70 m from the vena contract.

12.29 A wide rectangular channel carries a discharge of 5.1 m³/s/metre width of channel. (a) If the channel bed slope changes suddenly from 0.0009 to 0.0050, sketch the possible flow profiles (b). If the channel bed slope is reversed, (0.0050 to 0.0009), sketch the possible surface profiles, Assume Chezy's $C = 50$.

Solution

For a wide rectangular channel, $R \approx y$

$$q = y_n \cdot C \sqrt{y_n S_a}$$

$$y_n = \left(\frac{q}{C \sqrt{S_0}} \right)^{2/3}$$

(a) Normal depth for S_{01} and S_{02}

$$y_{n1} = \left[\frac{5.1}{50 \sqrt{0.0009}} \right]^{2/3} = 2.261 \text{ m}$$

$$y_{n2} = \left[\frac{5.1}{50 \sqrt{0.0050}} \right]^{2/3} = 1.276 \text{ m}$$

Critical depth,

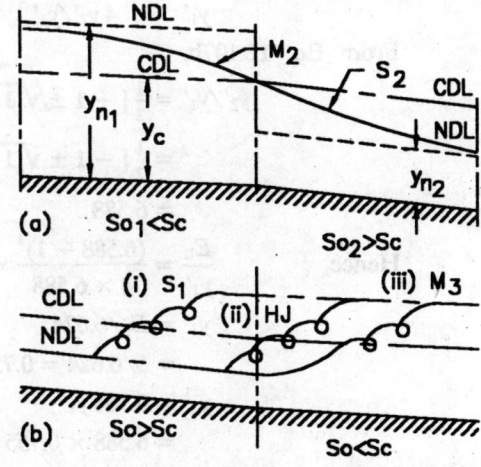

FIG. 12.56. EXAMPLE 12.29

$$y_c = \left(\frac{q^2}{q} \right)^{1/3}$$

$$= \left(\frac{5.1^2}{9.81} \right)^{1/3} = 1.384 \text{ m}$$

Since $y_{n1} > y_c$, S_{01} is mile slope and $y_{n2} < y_c$, S_{02} is steep slope. Thus the channel is a combination of mild to steep slope.

The resulting curve on mild slope will lie between y_n and y_e i.e. M_2 type and an steep slope, it will lie between CDL and NDL i.e. it will be S_2 type (See Fig. 12.56a)

(b) When the channel bed slopes are reversed, it will be a combinations of steep to mild slope.

In this case, there are three possibilities depending upon sequent depth downstream and anyone surface profile can form.

(i) Hydraulic jump on steep slope and then S_1 curve.

(ii) Hydraulic jump at junction.

(iii) M_3 curve on mild slope and then hydraulic jump.

12.30 If the energy loss in a jump formed in a rectangular channel is 5 m when $N_{F_1} = 5$, determine y_1', y_2'.

Solution

From Eq. 12.115,

$$E_L = \frac{(y_2' - y_1')^3}{4 y_1' y_2'}$$

Dividing by y_1' on both sides,

$$\frac{E_L}{y_1'} = \frac{(y_2'/y_1' - 1)^3}{4 y_2'/y_1'} \qquad \text{...(i)}$$

From Eq. 12.107b,

$$y_2'/y_1' = \frac{1}{2}[-1 \pm \sqrt{1 + 8 N_{F_1}^2}]$$

$$= \frac{1}{2}[-1 \pm \sqrt{1 + 8 \times (5)^2}]$$

$$= 6.588 \qquad \text{...(ii)}$$

Hence,

$$\frac{E_L}{y_1'} = \frac{(6.588 - 1)^3}{4 \times 6.588} = 6.624$$

$$y_1' = E_L/6.624$$

$$= 5/6.624 = 0.755 \text{ m}$$

$$y_2' = 6.588 y_1'$$

$$= 6.588 \times 0.755$$

$$= 4.972 \text{ m}$$

12.31 A horizontal bed channel, 20 m wide, has a hydraulic jump on it, which has resulted in a change of depth of flow from 1 m to 3 m. Find the discharge flowing in the channel.

Solution

From Eq. 12.107b

$$y_2'/y_1' = \frac{1}{2}[-1 \pm \sqrt{1 + 8 q^2/g y_1'^3}]$$

or	$3/1 = \frac{1}{2}[-1 \pm \sqrt{1 + 8\,q^2/(9.81 \times 1^3)}\,]$
or	$\sqrt{1 + 0.815\,q^2} = 7$
or	$q = 7.674 \text{ m}^3/\text{s/m width}$
	$Q = B\,q = 153.48 \text{ m}^3/\text{s}$

12.32 At the foot of a 30 m wide spillway from a dam when the discharging velocity is 28.2 m/s and the depth of flow is 0.96 m, a hydraulic jump is formed on a horizontal apron. Calculate the height and energy dissipated in the jump.

Solution

$$Q = A_1 U_1$$
$$= 0.96 \times 30 \times 28.2 = 812.16 \text{ m}^3/\text{s}$$

$$N_{F1} = \frac{U_1}{\sqrt{g\,y_1}}$$

$$N_{F1} = \frac{28.2}{\sqrt{9.81 \times 0.96}} = 9.19$$

From Eq. 12.107b,

$$y_2'/y_1' = \frac{1}{2}[-1 \pm \sqrt{1 + 8\,N_{F1}^2}\,]$$

$$= \frac{1}{2}[-1 \pm \sqrt{1 + 8 \times (9.19)^2}\,]$$

$$y_2'/y_1' = 12.506$$
$$y_2' = 12.506 \times 0.96$$
$$= 12.0 \text{ m}$$

Height of the jump $= y_2' - y_1'$
$$= (12.0 - 0.96)$$
$$= 11.04 \text{ m}$$

From Eq. 12.115,

$$E_L = \frac{(y_2' - y_1')^3}{4\,y_1'\,y_2'}$$

$$= \frac{(12.0 - 0.96)^3}{4 \times 12.0 \times 0.96}$$

$$= 29.2 \text{ N m/N}$$

12.33 A rectangular channel, 3 m wide, carries water. The initial Froude's number of the flow upstream of hydraulic jump is 2.0 and the height of the jump is 2 m. Determine the Froude's number at a section downstream of the jump and the associated energy loss in the jump.

Solution

From Eq. 12:107b

$$y_2'/y_1' = \frac{1}{2}[-1 \pm \sqrt{1 + 8N_{F1}^2}]$$

$$= \frac{1}{2}[-1 \pm \sqrt{1 + 8 \times (2)^2}] \qquad \text{...(i)}$$

$$= 2.372$$

Also   height of jump $= y_2' - y_1'$ ...(ii)

$$2 = (y_2' - y_1')$$

Solving Eqs. (i) and (iii)

$$2.372 y_1' - y_1' = 2$$

$$y_1' = 1.457 \text{ m}$$

$$y_2' = 3.457 \text{ m}$$

Now $$\frac{NF_2}{NF_1} = \frac{U_2}{\sqrt{gy_2'}} \times \frac{\sqrt{gy_1'}}{U_1}$$

Also $$U_1 y_1 = U_2 y_2$$

From Eqs. (iii) and (iv)

$$\therefore \qquad NF_2 = NF_1 \, (y_1'/y_2')^{3/2}$$

$$= 2 \times (1.457/3.457)^{3/2} = 0.547 \text{ m}$$

From Eq. 12.115,

$$E_L = \frac{(y_2' - y_1')^3}{4y_1' y_2'}$$

$$= \frac{(3.457 - 1.457)^3}{4 \times 1.457 \times 3.457} = 0.397 \text{ N m/N}$$

12.34 A 4 m wide rectangular channel carries a discharge of 6.2 m³/s. A hydraulic jump is formed in the channel and the depth after the jump is formed is known to be 2.0 m (a) What should be the depth of flow before the jump, (b) the energy loss and (c) power lost in the jump.

Solution

$$U_2 = \frac{6.2}{4 \times 2} = 0.775 \text{ m/s}$$

$$NF_2 = \frac{U_2}{\sqrt{g y_2}}$$

$$= \frac{0.775}{\sqrt{9.81 \times 2.0}} = 0.175$$

From Eq. 12.98,

$$\frac{y_1'}{y_2'} = \frac{1}{2} \left[-1 \pm \sqrt{1 + 8N_{F2}^2} \right]$$

$$=$$

$$= 0.0579$$

$$y_1' = 0.1158 \text{ m}$$

From Eq. 12.103,

Energy loss, $\quad E_1 = \dfrac{(y_2' - y_1')^3}{4\,y_1\,y_2}$

$$= \dfrac{(2 - 0.1158)^3}{4 \times 2 \times 0.1158} = 7.221 \text{ m}$$

Power dissipated, $P = w\,Q\,E_L$

$$= 9.81 \times 6.2 \times 7.221\ W$$

$$= 439.18 \text{ kW}$$

12.35 Water flows over a spillway of a dam at a depth of 2.75 m over its crest. The crest is located at 29.25m above the downstream bed level of the stream Calculate the tail water depth required to form the jump on the horizontal flow, length of jump and energy lost in the jump.

Solution

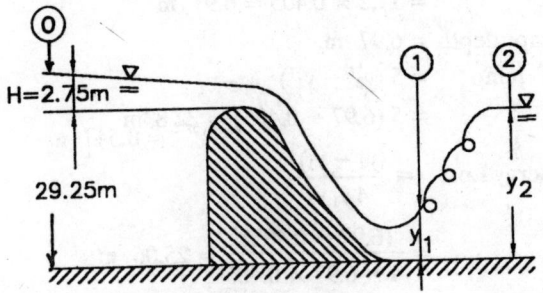

FIG. 12.57. EXAMPLE 12.35

Discharge per unit width q is given by

$$q = \dfrac{2}{3}\,Cd\,\sqrt{2g}\,H^{3/2}$$

$$= \dfrac{2}{3} \times 0.75\,\sqrt{2 \times 9.81}\,(2.75)^{3/2}$$

$$= 10.10\ \text{m}^3/\text{s/m}$$

Apply Bernoulli's Equation to 0 and 1,

$$(2.75 + 29.25) + 0 + 0 = y_1' + 0 + \dfrac{(10.10/y_1')^2}{2g}$$

$$32 = y_1' + \dfrac{5.199}{y_1^{2'}}$$

Solving by trial and error,

$$y_1' = 0.405 \text{ m},$$

$$U_1 = \dfrac{q}{y_1}$$

$$= \frac{10.10}{0.405} = 24.94 \text{ m/s}$$

$$NF_1' = \frac{U_1}{\sqrt{9.81 \times 0.405}} = 12.51$$

Since the flow at the toe is supercritical it is assumed that jump may form on horizontal apron,

From Eq. 12.97 b,

$$\frac{y_2'}{y_1'} = \frac{1}{2}[-1-+\sqrt{1 + 8NF_1^2}]$$

$$= \frac{1}{2}[-1 \pm \sqrt{1 + 8 \times (12.51)^2}]$$

$$= 17.2 y_1'$$

$$= 17.2 \times 0.405 = 6.97 \text{ m}$$

Post jump depth = 6.97 m.

Length of jump $\quad = 5\,(y_2' - y_1')$

$$\doteq 5\,(6.97 - 0.405) = 32.83\text{m}$$

Energy Loss $\quad = \dfrac{(y_2 - y_1)^3}{4 y_1 y_2}$

$$= \frac{(6.97 - 0.405)^3}{4 \times 6.97 \times 0.405} = 25.06 \text{ m}$$

12.36 A spillway is designed to discharge 5 m³/s per metre length. After flowing over the spillway, water flows on to a horizontal concrete apron (n = 0.015). The velocity of flow at the toe is observed to be 15 m/s and tail water depth is limited to 3 m. Calculate the minimum length of apron to contain the jump on the apron and consequent energy lost.

Solution

Given $\quad\quad q = 5 \text{ m}^3/\text{s/m}$

$$y_2' = 3 \text{ m}$$

From Eq. 12.98,

$$\frac{y_1'}{y_2'} = \frac{1}{2}[-1 \pm \sqrt{1 + 8NF_2^2}]$$

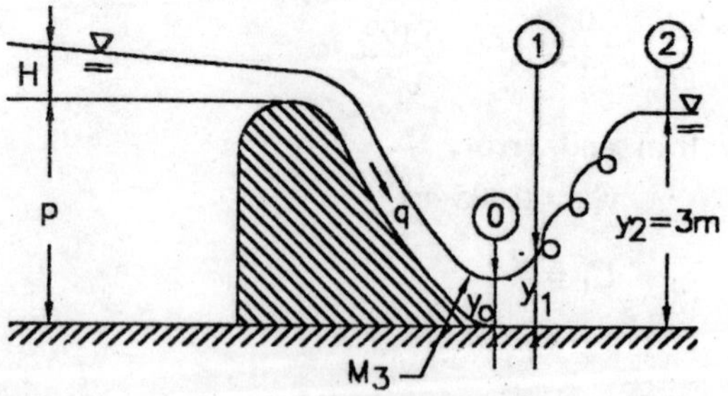

FIG. 12.58. EXAMPLE 12.36

where
$$N.F_2^2 = \frac{q^2}{g y_2'^3}$$

$$\frac{y_1'}{y_2'} = \frac{1}{2}\left[-1 \pm \sqrt{1 + 8 \cdot \frac{q^2}{g y_2'^3}}\,\right]$$

$$= \frac{1}{2}\left[-1 \pm \sqrt{1 + \frac{8\,(5)^2}{9.81 \times (3)^3}}\,\right]$$

$$\frac{y_1'}{y_2'} = 0.162$$

$$y_1' = 0.162 \times 3 = 0.487 \text{ m}$$

Also, depth of flow at the toe of spillway,

$$y_0 = \frac{q}{U_0}$$

$$= \frac{5}{15} = 0.333$$

Since $y_0 < y_1'$ i.e. conjugate depth required to form the jump with $y_2' = 3$ m, a backward curve H_3 will be formed on the horizontal apron.

Length of jump:

The H_3 curve will be formed between $y = 0.333$ m to 0.487 m.

$$E_0 = y_0 + \frac{U_0^2}{2g}$$

$$= 0.333 + \frac{(1.5)^2}{2 \times 9.81} = 11.80 \text{ m}$$

$$E_1 = y_1 + \frac{U_1^2}{2g}$$

$$= 0.487 + \frac{(10.267)^2}{2 \times 9.81} = 5.86 \text{ m}$$

where
$$U_1 = \frac{q_1}{y_1}$$

$$= \frac{5}{0.487} = 10.267 \text{ m/s}$$

$$U_0 = \frac{1}{n} \cdot R_0^{2/3} S_f^{1/2} \approx \frac{1}{n} \cdot y_0^{2/3} S_{f0}^{1/2}$$

$$15 = \frac{1}{0.015}(0.333)^{2/3} S_{f0}^{1/2}$$

$$S_{f0} = \left[\frac{0.015 \times 15}{(0.333)^{2/3}}\right]^2 = 0.2194$$

Similarly,
$$U_1 = \frac{1}{n} y^{2/3} S_{f1}^{1/2}$$

$$10.267 = \frac{1}{0.015} \times (0.487)^{2/3} S_{f1}^{1/2}$$

$$S_{f1} = \left[\frac{10.267 \times 0.015}{(0.487)^{2/3}} \right]^2 = 0.0619$$

$$\overline{S_f} = \frac{S_{f0} + S_{f1}}{2}$$

$$= \frac{0.2194 + 0.0619}{2} = 0.4407$$

Hence length of H_3 curve,

$$\Delta x = \left[\frac{E_0 - E_1}{S_0 - S_f} \right]$$

$$= \frac{11.80 - 5.86}{0 - 0.1407} = 29.85 \text{ m}$$

Length of hydraulic gump $= 5(y_2' - y_1')$

$$= 5(3 - 0.487) = 12.565 \text{ m}$$

Length of apron $= 29.85 + 12.565$

$$= 42.415 \text{ m}$$

Energy lost $= \dfrac{(y_2' - y_1')^3}{4 y_1' y_2'}$

$$= \frac{(3 - 0.487)^3}{4 \times 0487 \times 3} = 2.72 \text{ m}$$

Alternatively,

$$E_2 = \left(y_2 + \frac{U_2^2}{2g} \right)$$

$$= \left(\frac{3 + (5/3)^2}{2 \times 9.81} \right) = 3.1415 \text{ m}$$

$$\Delta E = (E_2 - E_1)$$

$$= 5.86 - 3.1415 = 2.712 \text{ m.}$$

12.37 A wide channel of rectangular section, 8 m wide, is laid to a bed slope of 1 in 64 and carries a discharge of 40 cumec (m³/s).

A barrier across the channel raises the water surface to 3 m just upstream of the barrier. Find the length of the water surface profile upto the hydraulic jump upstream. Assume Manning's n = 0.025.

Solution

From Eq. 12.64

$$y_c^3 = (q^2/g) = (Q/B)^2/g$$

$$y_c = (40/8)^2/9.81 = 1.37 \text{ m}$$

From Eq. 12.40

$$U = (1/n) R^{2/3} S^{1/2}$$

$$Q = AU = A \times 1/n \, R^{2/3} S_0^{1/2}$$

$$40 = 1/0.025 \, (8 y_n) \, (y_n)^{2/3} \, (1/64)^{1/2}$$

Since $R \approx y_n$

$$y_n^{5/3} = 1$$

$$y_n = 1 \text{ m}$$

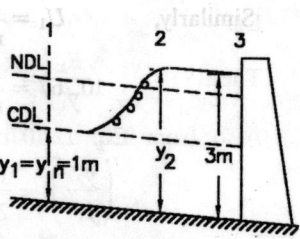

FIG. 12.59. EXAMPLE 12.37

Since $y_n < y_c$, the bed slope is steep. As the water level should change from 1.0 m ($< y_c$) to 3 m ($> y_n$) behind the barrier, S_1 curve is formed.

From Eq. 12.107b

$$y_2'/y_1' = 1/2 \left[-1 \pm \sqrt{1 + 8 N_{F1}^2} \right]$$

where

$$N_{F1} = \frac{Q/B \, y_1'}{\sqrt{g \, y_1'}} = \frac{40/(8 \times 1)}{\sqrt{9.81 \times 1}} = 1.60$$

$$y_2'/y_1' = 1/2 \left[-1 \pm \sqrt{1 + 8 \times (1.6)^2} \right].$$

$$y_2' = 1/2 \left[-1 \pm 4.634 \right] = 1.817 \text{ m}$$

The length of the surface profile between sections 2 and 3 is computed using step method.

y	U	$U^2/2g$	E	ΔE	S_f	$S_{\bar{f}}$	$S_o - S_{\bar{f}}$
3	1.67	0.143	3.143		4×10^{-4}		
1.8	2.3	0.4	2.20	0.943	22.5×10^{-4}	13.25×10^{-4}	142.8×10^{-4}

From Eq. 12.98,

$$\Delta x = \frac{E_2 - E_1}{S_o - S_f}$$

$$= \frac{0.943}{142.8 \times 10^{-4}} = 66 \text{ m}$$

12.38 For a discharge of 10 m³/s per meter width flowing in a channel, a hydraulic jump is formed. The head loss in the hydraulic jump is 20 m. Determine the pre-jump and post-jump depths.

Solution

The loss of energy in the hydraulic jump is given by,

$$E_L = \frac{(y_2' - y_1')^3}{4 y_1' y_2'}$$

or

$$\frac{E_L}{y_1'} = \frac{(y_2'/y_1' - 1)^3}{4 (y_2'/y_1')}$$

Let $\qquad y_2'/y_1' = r$

Then $\qquad \dfrac{E_{L'}}{y_1} = \dfrac{(r-1)^3}{4r}$

Also from Eq. 12.107b,

$$\left(\dfrac{y_2'}{y_1'}\right) = \dfrac{1}{2}[-1 + \sqrt{1 + 8q^2/gy_1'^3}]$$

$$r = \dfrac{1}{2}\left[-1 \pm \sqrt{1 + 8\,(10^2/9.81 \times y_1'^3}\,\right]$$

$$r = \dfrac{1}{2}[-1 \pm \sqrt{1 + 81.55/y_1'^3}]$$

Solving Equations (i) and (ii) by trial and error, the values of r and y_1' can be obtained.

$$r = 14.98$$
$$y_1' = 0.44$$
$$y_2' = 6.591\text{m}$$

Alternatively, the solution can be obtained by tabular computations. The method is as follows

(1) Assume y_1'

(2) Determine $N_{F_1} = q^2/gy_1'^3$

(3) Compute $y_2'/y_1' = \dfrac{1}{2}[-1 \pm \sqrt{1 + 8\,NF_1^2}]$

(4) Compute $= E_L = [y_2' - y_1')^3/4\,y_1'\,y_2']$

(5) If computed E_L is smaller, decrease y_1' so that y_2' will increase and will yield large E_1; and vice versa.

Thus $\qquad y_1' = 0.44$ m (see Table below)

$\qquad\qquad\qquad y_2' = 6.59$ m

y_1'	NF_1^2	y_2'/y_1'	y_2'	E_L
1	10.20	4.044	4.004	1.74
0.5	81.58	12.28	6.140	14.63
0.4	159.27	17.35	6.94	25.21
0.45	111.86	14.46	6.51	18.98
0.44	119.66	14.98	6.59	20.06

12.39 Water flows in a rectangular channel at a depth of 2.0 m and a velocity of 1.0 m/s. The discharge of water is suddenly trebled. Find the increase in depth of flow.

Solution

$$U_2 y_2 = 3\,U_1 y_1 = 3 \times 1 \times 2 = 6\,m^3/s/m \qquad\qquad ...(i)$$

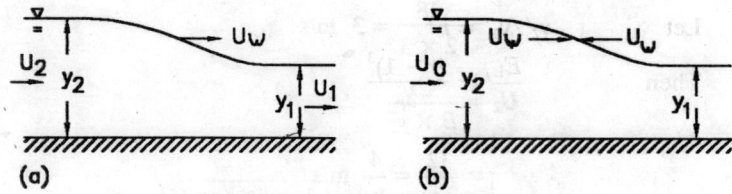

FIG. 12.60. EXAMPLE 12.39

By applying a velocity U_w in the upstream direction to the surge as well as fluids, the problem reduces to a steady flow.

The continuity equation yields,

$$(U_2 - U_w) y_2 = (U_1 - U_w) y_1$$
$$(U_2 - U_w) y_2 = (1 - U_w) \times 2 \qquad \qquad ...\text{(ii)}$$

The momentum equation yields,

$$\frac{w}{2} (y_2^2 - y_1^2) = \frac{w}{g} \cdot (U_1 - U_w) y_1 (U_1 - U_2)$$

Substituting the values of U_1 and y_1,

$$\frac{1}{2} (y_2^2 - 4) = \frac{1}{g} (1 - U_w) \times 2 \times (1 - U_2) \qquad \qquad ...\text{(iii)}$$

Solving, Eqs. (i) to (iii) by trial and error,

$$y_2 = 2.45 \text{ m}.$$

12.40 A horizontal rectangular channel 3 m wide and 2 m depth conveys water at 18 m³/s. If the flow rate is suddenly reduced to 2/3ʳᵈ of its original volume, compute the magnitude and speed of u/s surge.

Solution

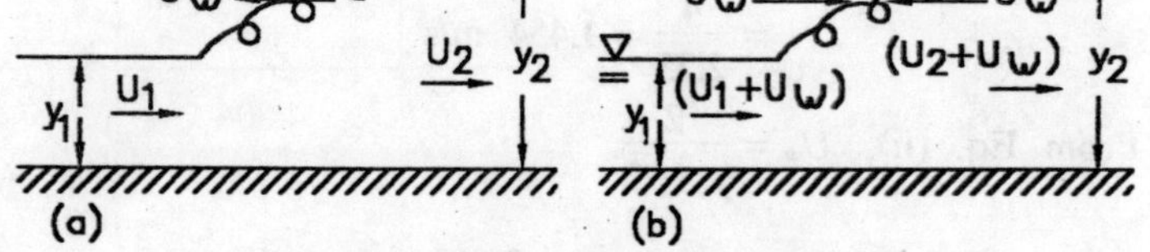

FIG. 12.61. EXAMPLE 12.40

Superimpose U_w in the downstream direction to simulate it to steady flow.

Given $y_1 = 2$ m, $B_1 = 3$ m, $Q_1 = 18$ m³/s, $Q_2 = \dfrac{2}{3} \times 18 = 12$ m³/s.

$$U_1 = \frac{Q_1}{B_1 y_1}$$

$$= \frac{18}{2 \times 3} = 3 \text{ m/s}$$

$$U_2 = \frac{Q_2}{B \times y_2}$$

$$= \frac{12}{3 y_1} = \frac{4}{y_2} \text{ m/s} \qquad \qquad ...(i)$$

From continuity equation,

$$y_1 (U_1 + U_w) = y_2 (U_2 + U_w)$$

$$2 (3 + U_w) = y_2 \left(\frac{4}{y_2} + U_w \right)$$

$$U_w (2 - y_2) = -2$$

$$U_w = \frac{2}{y_2 - 2}$$

From Eq. 12.139 c,

$$\frac{(U_1 + U_w)^2}{g y_1} = \frac{1}{2} \cdot \frac{y_2}{y_1} \left(1 + \frac{y_2}{y_1} \right)$$

$$\frac{\left(3 + \dfrac{2}{y_2 - 2} \right)^2}{9.81 \times 2} = \frac{1}{2} \cdot \frac{y_2}{2} \left(1 + \frac{y_2}{2} \right)$$

$$\left(3 + \frac{2}{y_2 - 2} \right)^2 = 2.4525 \, y_2 \, (2 + y_2)$$

Solving by trial and error,

$$y_2 = 2.75 \text{ m}$$

From Eq.(i), $\qquad U_2 = \dfrac{4}{y_2}$

$$= \frac{4}{2.75} = 1.454 \text{ m/s}$$

From Eq. (ii), $\quad U_w = \dfrac{2}{y_2 - 2}$

$$= \frac{2}{2.75 - 2} = 2.667 \text{ m/s}.$$

The surge will move upstream with $U_w = 2.667$ m/s

Height of surge $\quad = y_2 - y_1$

$$= 2.75 - 2.0 = 0.75 \text{ m}.$$

12.41 A tidal estuary is flowing at the rate of 1.8 m/s and the depth of flow is 2 m. Owing to the tide in the sea, the level of water rose rapidly and the resulting surge or tidal bore took one hour to reach 19.8 km. upstream.

Compute the height of the bore above the initial depth of bore. Also determine the speed and direction of the flow after the bore has passed

Solution

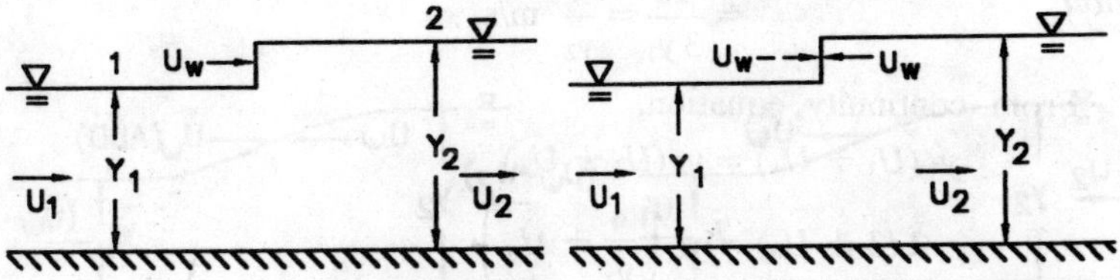

FIG. 12.62. EXAMPLE 12.41

$$U_1 = 1.8 \text{ m/s}, y_1 = 2 \text{ m}$$

$$U_w = \frac{19.8 \times 1000}{60} = 5.5 \text{ m/s}$$

Adding U_w in the downstream direction to the surge and flow, the surge becomes stationary and the velocity of flow becomes $(U_1 + U_w) = c$.

$$(U_1 + U_2) = c = \sqrt{\frac{gy_2(y_1 + y_2)}{2y_1}}$$

$$(1.8 + 5.5) = \sqrt{\frac{9.81 \times y_2(2 + y_2)}{2 \times 2}}$$

Simplifying, $y_2^2 + 2y_2 - 21.72 = 0$

From which, $y_2 = 3.76 \text{ m}$

Height of the bore, $h = (y_2 - y_1)$

$$= (3.76 - 2) = 1.76 \text{ m}$$

Normal flow in the river $= U_1 y_1$

$$= 1.8 \times 2 = 3.6 \text{ m}^3/\text{s/m}$$

Flow taken by the bore $= (y_2 - y_1) U_w$

$$= (3.76 - 2) \times 5.5$$

$$= 9.68 \text{ m}^3/\text{s/m}$$

Net flow in the direction of bore

$$= (9.68 - 3.6) = 6.06 \text{ m}^3/\text{s/m}$$

Speed of flow after the bore has passed

$$= \frac{6.06}{y_2}$$

$$= \frac{6.06}{3.76} = 1.61 \text{ m/s}$$

The direction of flow is opposite to the initial direction of flow.

12.42 A rectangular channel has a positive surge moving with a velocity of 10 m/s in the downstream direction. If the velocity of flow after the surge has passed is found to be 6 m/s and its depth of water is raised to 3.0 m, determine the depth and velocity of flow before the passage of surge.

Solution

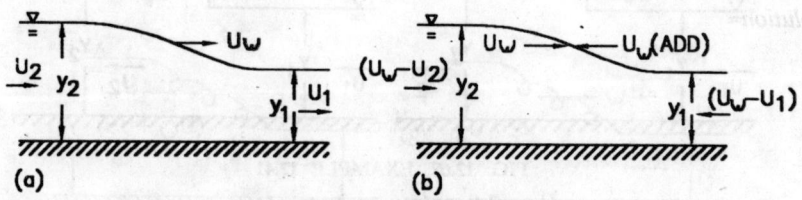

FIG. 12.63. EXAMPLE 12.42

Superimposing U_w to the surge and flow in the upstream direction, a simulated stredy flow is obtained.

Given $U_w = 10$ m/s, $U_2 = 6$ m/s, $y_2 = 3.0$ m

From Fig. 12.63 (b), using continuity equation,

$$y_1 (U_w - U_1) = y_2 (U_w - U_2)$$
$$y_1 (10 - U_1) = 3 (10 - 6)$$
$$y_1 (10 - U_1) = 12$$

Solving, $U_1 = \left(10 - \dfrac{12}{y_1} \right)$ ...(i)

From Eq. 12.129 c,

$$\frac{(U_w - U_1)^2}{g y_1} = \frac{1}{2} \frac{y_2}{y_1} \left(1 + \frac{y_2}{y_1} \right)$$

$$\frac{(10 - U_1)^2}{g y_1} = \frac{1}{2} \times \frac{3}{y_1} \left(1 + \frac{3}{y_1} \right)$$ ...(ii)

From Eqs. (i) and (ii)

$$\frac{\left[10 - \left(10 - \dfrac{12}{y_1} \right) \right]^2}{g y_1} = \frac{1}{2} \frac{3}{y_1} \left(1 + \frac{3}{y_1} \right)$$

$$\frac{14.679}{y_1^3} = \frac{1.5}{y_1} \left(1 + \frac{3}{y_1} \right)$$

$$\frac{14.679}{1.5 y_1^2} = 1 + \frac{3}{y_1}$$

$$y_1^2 + 3 y_1 - 9.786 = 0$$

Solving, $y_1 = 1.269$ m

From Eq. (i), $U_1 = \left(10 - \dfrac{12}{y_1} \right)$

$$= \left(10 - \frac{12}{1.696}\right) = 3.91 \text{ m/s}$$

12.43 Water is flowing in a wide river at normal depth of 2.0 m. A tidal bore is observed the river to move upstream at a velocity of 6.5 m/s and depth of flow become 4.5 m. Calculate the velocities of water before and after the bore.

Solution

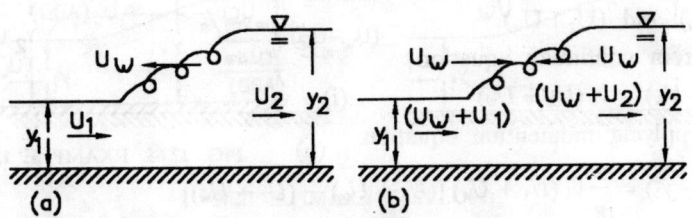

FIG. 12.64. EXAMPLE 12.43

To make of flow relatively stredy, superimpose U_w in the downstream direction.

Given $\qquad y_1 = 2$ m, $y_2 = 4.5$, $U_w = 6.5$ m/s

From continuity equation,

$$y_1 (U_w + U_1) = y_2 (U_w + U_r)$$

$$2 (6.5 + U_1) = 4.5 (6.5 + U_2)$$

$$U_1 = \frac{4.5}{2} (6.5 + U_2) - 6.5$$

$$= 8.125 + 2.25 \, U_2 \qquad \qquad \text{...(i)}$$

Also from Eq. 12.139c,

$$\frac{(U_w + U_1)^2}{g y_1} = \frac{1}{2} \frac{y_2}{y_1} \left(1 + \frac{y_2}{y_1}\right)$$

$$\frac{(6.5 + U_1)^2}{9.81 \times 2} = \frac{1}{2} \times \frac{4.5}{2} \times \left(1 + \frac{4.5}{2}\right)$$

$$\frac{(6.5 + U_1)^2}{19.62} = 3.656$$

$$U_1 = 1.969 \text{ m/s}$$

From Eq. (i) $1.969 = 8.125 + 2.25 \, U_2$

$$U_2 = -1.64 \text{ m/s}$$

This means, the water will flow in the upstream direction after the bore has passed.

12.44 A steady flow occurs in a rectangular channel at a depth of 1.5 m and velocity 2 m/s. The sides of the channel are 3 m high and the channel is 1 km. long. Due to the sudden closure of the sluice gate at the downstream end, the surge is generated which travels upstream. Determine whether the water spills over the sides and how much time the surge will take to reach the upstream end of the channel?

Solution :

The problem is made of steady flow by adding U_w in the downstream direction to the surge as well as to the fluids. The velocities, at sections 1 and 2 become $(U_1 + U_w)$ and $(U_2 + U_w)$.

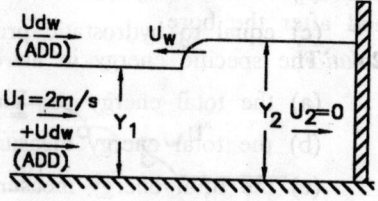

From continuity equation

$$y_1 (U_1 + U_w) = y_2 (U_2 + U_w) \qquad \text{...(i)}$$

Applying momentum equation,

FIG. 12.65. EXAMPLE 12.44

$$\frac{w}{2} (y_2^2 - y_1^2) = \frac{w}{g} y_1 (U_1 + U_w) [(U_1 + U_w) - (U_2 + U_w)] \qquad \text{...(ii)}$$

Since the water at the downstream end is completely stopped, $U_2 = 0$. Substituting the values and simplifying,

$$1.5 (2 + U_w) = y_2 (U_w) \qquad \text{...(i)}$$

$$\frac{(y_2^2 - 1.5)^2}{2} = \frac{1.5}{g} (2 + U_w) (2) \qquad \text{...(ii)}$$

Solving by trial and error,

$$y_2 = 2.31 \text{ m}$$

From Eq. (i)

$$U_w (y_2 - 1.5) = U_1 y_1 = 2 \times 1.5$$

$$U_w = 3.7 \text{ m/s}$$

Since the depth after the surge has passed, i.e. y_2 is 2.31 m and the sides of the channel are 3 m high, the water will not spill out.

Time required to reach the upstream end,

$$= \frac{1000}{3.70}$$

$$= 270 \text{ s or } 4.50 \text{ minutes.}$$

Objective questions

12.1 The turbulent flow occurs in an open channel when Reynolds number is equal to

(a) 500   (b) 2000   (c) 4000

(d) 1000   (e) none of these answers

12.2 Mark the correct statement

(a) uniform flow can occur in a horizontal channel

(b) ideal fluid can flow at normal depth in an open channel

(c) the specific energy diagram should always be tangential to a 45° line

12.3 The water flows in a channel whose bed is convex upward. The pressure at any point on the bed will be

(a) more than hydrostatic pressure

(b) less than hydrostatic pressure

(c) equal to hydrostatic pressure

12.4 The specific energy in an open channel is

(a) the total energy per unit mass

(b) the total energy measured above a horizontal datum

(c) the total energy measured above the channel bed

(d) total energy measured above the water surface

(e) none of these ansseres

12.5 The critical depth is the depth of flow at which

(a) the discharge is minimum

(b) the discharge is maximum

(c) the specific energy is maximum

(d) the Froude's number is more than unity

12.6 The critical depth in a non-prismatic channel is expressed by

(a) $QT^2/g \ A^3 = 1$

(b) $Q^2 \ T/g \ A^3 = 1$

(c) $Q^2 \ A^3/g \ T^3 = 1$

(d) $Q^2/g \ A^3 = 1$

(e) none of these answers

12.7 The maximum rate of discharge per unit width q of a rectangular channel is

(a) $g \, y_c^3$ (b) y_c^3/g (c) $\sqrt{g/y_c^3}$

(d) $\sqrt{g y_c^3}$ (e) none of these answers

12.8 Alternate depth of flow in a channel are

(a) the depths at which the specific force is the same

(b) the depths at which the specific energy is the same

(c) at which the total energy remains same

(d) at which the discharge per unit width remains the same

(e) none of these answers

12.9 Tranquil flow always occurs at depth

(a) above normal depth   (b) below normal depth

(c) above critical depth   (d) below critical depth

(e) none of these answers

12.10 The minimum possible specific energy in a rectangular channel 3 m wide and carrying a discharge of 12 m³/s in Nm/N is

(a) 2.12   (b) 1.717   (c) 1.632

(d) 14.425   (e) none of these answers⁻

12.11 The best hydraulic section is defined as

(a) the section that has a maximum area

(b) the section that has minimum area

(c) the section that has minimum roughness coefficient

(d) the least expensive canal cross section

(e) none of these answers

12.12 The most efficient rectangular section is the one which has

(a) $y = B$ (b) $y = 2 B$ (c) $B = 2 y$

(d) $B = y/3$ (e) none of thses answers

12.13 A channel carries water at subcritical depth. The channel width is reduced gradually at a point downstream so as to obtain the desired width. The depth of flow in the contracted section will be

(a) less than upstream depth

(b) more than upstream depth

(c) less than critical depth

(d) is always equal to the critical depth

(e) none of these answers

12.14 The supercritical flow takes place in a channel and a hump is provided at a section on downstream side so that the critical flow occurs at the contracted section. If the height of hump increases further,

(a) the upstream depth is reduced

(b) the upstream depth is increased

(c) the critical flow occurs at the contracted section

(d) no flow takes place

(e) none of these answers

12.15 The dynamic equation of gradually varied flow is

(a) $\dfrac{dy}{dx} = \dfrac{(S_o - S_f)}{(1 - N_F^2)}$ (b) $\dfrac{dy}{dx} = \dfrac{S_o + S_f}{1 - N_F^2}$

(c) $\dfrac{dy}{dx} = \dfrac{S_o - S_f}{1 + N_F^2}$ (d) $\dfrac{dy}{dx} = \dfrac{S_o + S_f}{1 + N_F^2}$

(e) none of these answers

12.16 The critical depth meter

(a) measures the depth at the critical section

(b) must have tranquil flow immediatly upstream

(c) always requires the formation of hydraulic jump

(d) is always preceded by a hydraulic jump

(e) none of these answers

12.17 The specific force is written as

(a) $\dfrac{Q^2}{A} + w\bar{h}$

(b) $\dfrac{Q^2}{gA} + A\bar{h}$

(c) $\dfrac{Q^2 T}{gA^3} + w\bar{h}$

(d) $\dfrac{Q^2 T}{gA^3} + wA\bar{h}$

(e) none of these answers

12.18 A hydraulic jump occurs when

(a) supercritical flow meets critical flow

(b) supercritical flow meets subcritical flow

(c) subcritical flow meets supercritical flow on downstream side

(d) none of these answers

12.19 Specify the name of possible curve formed at the junction of

(a) mild to steep slope   (b) mild to critical slope

(c) mild to adverse slope   (d) horizontal to mild slope

(e) steep to steeper slope

12.20 The pre jump and post jump depth are related as

(a) $y_2'/y_1' = \frac{1}{2}\left[-1 \pm \sqrt{1 + N_{F1}^2}\right]$

(b) $y_1'/y_2' = \frac{1}{2}\left[-1 \pm \sqrt{1 + 8N_{F1}^2}\right]$

(c) $y_2'/y_1' = \frac{1}{2}\left[-1 \pm \sqrt{1 + 8N_{F1}^2}\right]$

(d) $y_2'/y_1' = \left[-\frac{1}{2} \pm \sqrt{1 + 8N_{F1}^2}\right]$

(e) none of these answers

Problems

12.1 Drive an expression for discharge in terms of depth y in a channel with Manning's n = 0.0125 and bed slope 0.0025 for (a) a tringular channel with two sides sloping at 1:1 and 1.5:1 respectively. (b) a trapezoidal channel with bed width equal to three times depth and side slopes 2 H : 1 V.

12.2 A concrete lined trapezoidal channel has bed width of 1.5 m and bed slope of 1 in 1800. If the depth of flow is 1.5 m and side slopes are 1.5 H : 1 V, determine the discharge carried by the channel by (a) Manning's formula and (b) Kutter's formula. Assume Manning's n = 0.015.

12.3 A trapezoidal channel has to be designed to carry 10 m³/s at a velocity of 2 m/s, so that the concrete lining for the bed and sides is minimum. Calculate (i) the area of lining required per metre length of canal and (ii) the bed slope of the canal. Assume Manning's n = 0.015 side stope 1 : 1.

12.4 Prove that the section of a channel in which the flow is critical at any section takes the form expressed by

$$x^2 \, h^3 = Q^2/32 \, g$$

where x is the half the top width and h is the distance of the water surface below energy line.

12.5 A flow of 100 lit/s flows down in a rectangular channel (flume) of width 0.6 m and having adjustable slope of bottom. If Chezy's C = 56, find the bottom slope necessary for uniform flow with a depth of flow of 0.30 m. Also find the conveyance of the flume.

12.6 A wide channel carries a flow of 2.75 m³/s per metre width, the depth of flow being 1.5 m. Calculate the rise in floor level required to produce a critical flow condition. What is the corresponding fall in the surface level?

12.7 For the purpose of measurement, the width of rectangular channel is reduced from 3 m to 2 m and the floor level is raised by 0.3 m in elevation at the given section when the depth of approaching flow is 2 m. What rate of flow would be indicated by 0.15 m drop in surface elevation at the contracted section?

12.8 A stream, 45 m wide, has an average depth of 3 m. The surface slope is 1 in 12000. Find out the length of backwater curve caused by an afflux of 2.4 m. Use Manning's n = 0.03.

12.9 A quantity of 90 m³/s of water is flowing in a rectangular channel, 6 m wide. If the depth of flow is 2 m and a jump is established, what would be the depth downstream of the jump? Also calculate loss of energy and relative energy loss.

12.10 A hydraulic jump forming below a sluice gate produces a change in depth from 0.6 m to 1.6 m (a) what are the heads on the gate (b) the discharge flowing per meter width and (c) the change in the total head within the jump?

12.11 In a rectangular channel, the discharge flowing per unit width is 1.6 m³/s and height of jump is 2.0 m. Determine the conjugate depths.

12.12 Draw the, surface profile for the rectangular channel, 7 m wide and carrying a discharge of 15 ³/s. Take Manning's n = 0.015.

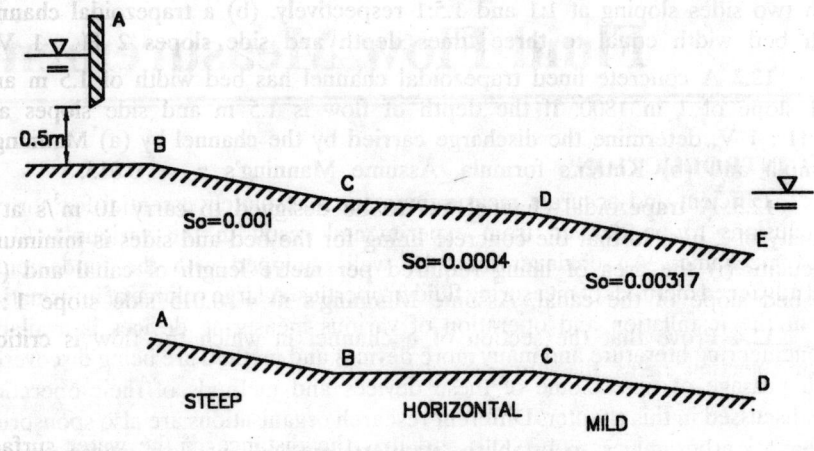

FIG. 12.66. PROBLEM 11.12

Fluid Flow Measurement

13.1 INTRODUCTION

Efficient and accurate measurements are absolutely essential for correct conclusions to be derived from experimental result in the various field of fluid mechanics. An engineer must be well equipped with the fundamental and advanced methods of measuring fluid properties. A large volume of information about the installation and operation of various measuring devices is available in engineering literature and many more devices and method are being discovered with passage of time. Some of these devices and methods of their operation are discussed in this chapter. Different research organisations are also sponsoring extensive programmes to establish 'standard methods of flow measurement'. The latest standards or codes are published inthe current literature.. These standard instructions about the methods/devices form part of activity of many national/international/societies/association, e.g. American standards, British standards. In India, B.I.S. (Bureau of Indian Standards, previously known as Indian Stadnards Institution) publishes the various 'standards or codes' and are arranged alphabetically in the index book. Some of these codes are mentioned at the ends of the chapter, Table 13.2.

For the analsysis of a fluid problem, four basic equations are available for use. These are (1) the equation of State,(2) the continuity equation, (3) the energy equation and (4) the dynamic or momentum equation. The equations can also be used for the specific problem of fluid flow measurement. In analysing the action of flow meters, it is customary to set-up a relation assuming certain ideal conditions and then use experimentally determined calibration coefficients to take into account the deviations from the ideal conditions.

13.2. MEASUREMENT OF FLUID PROPERTIES

1. Density

Of the various fluid properties the important ones are fluid density and visconsity. The density of liquids can be measured by (a) weighing a known volume of liquid, (b) hydrostatic weighing, (c) hydrometer and (d) U-tube.

(a) *Pycnometer.* The pycnometer is used to measure the density. It is a glass vessel of known weight W_1 and volume V. If the weight of vessel filled with liquid be W_2 at temperature t, the specific weight or weight density is given by

$$w_s = \frac{W_2 - W_1}{V} \qquad \qquad ...(13.1)$$

(b) *Hydrostatic weighing.* A plummet of known volume V is first weighed in air (W_a) It is then immersed in the liquid of unknown specific weight and weiged (W_1). The specific weight of the liquid (w_s) is given by

$$w_s = \frac{W_a - W_1}{V} \qquad \qquad ...(13.2)$$

(c) *Hydrometer.* The most common method of determining specific weight of liquid is by means of hydrometer, Fig. 13.1a. It consists of cylinderical vessel containing heavy material at its bottom and a small diameter graduated tube on its upper end. While the hydrometer is immersed in the liquid, the reading of hydrometer at the surface of the liquid directly indicates specific weight of the liquid.

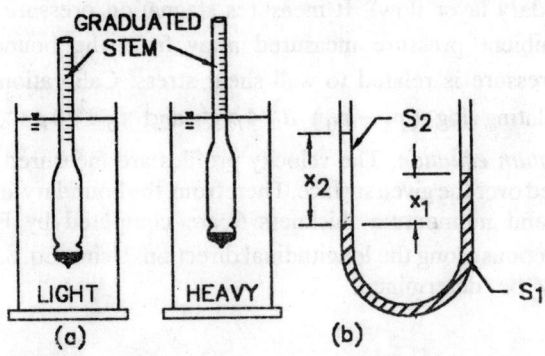

FIG. 13.1. DETERMINATION OF SPECIFIC WEIGHT OF LIQUID

(d) *U-tube method.* Another method which sometimes can be used is by means of a U-tube. The U-tube is filled up with the liquid of unknown specific density, Fig. 13.1b. A liquid of known density is then poured in it. Let us assume that the column of liquid in one arm is x_1 and its unknown density is w_1 When it supports a column x_2 of a liquid of known density, w_2, Then

$$w_1 = \frac{w_2 \times x_2}{x_1} \qquad \qquad ...(13.2)$$

2. Viscosity

Another important fluid property is its viscosity, which is used for the study of problems of real fluid. The devices used for measurement of viscosity are known as 'viscosimeter or viscometer.' These are (a) concentric cylinder viscometer (b) Falling sphere viscometer (c) Tube type and (d) Industrial viscometer, e.g. Saybolt viscometer or Redwood viscometer. These have been discussed in chapter 7 (Refer section 7.12)

13.3 MEASUREMENT OF SHEAR

The motion of real fluid is resisted by frictional forces or shear stress along its boundaries. Fluid mechanics researchers also need to know the shear stress exerted by one layer on its adjoining layer. There is no device which directly measures the shear stress present between fluid layers. It can only be deduced from fluid mechanics equations. The wall shear stress τ_0 can be measured by the following methods.

(a) Preston tube (b) Momentum integral equation(c) Empirical formulas, e.g. Ludwig-Tillman formula (d) Standard charts, e.g. Clauser's chart, Cole's chart, etc.

(a) *Preston tube method.* Preston tube is a small diameter tube 'd' (say) which is placed at the boundary and faces against the flow Fig. 13.2a. The tube is so placed that it is immersed in the buffer zone of turbulent boundary layer. (A similar device developed earlier by Stanton, was used for laminar boundary layer flow). It measures stagnation pressure p_s. Let the free stream or ambient pressure measured away from the boundary be p_0 The differential pressure is related to wall shear stress. Calibration curve has been developed relating log $(p_s - p_0)$ $d^2/4\rho v^2$ and $\tau_0 d^2/4\rho v^2$, (Fig. 13.2.b).

Momentum equation. The velocity profiles are measured in the boundary layer developed over the given surface. Therefrom, the boundary layer displacement thickness δ_x and momentum thickness θ are computed by Eqs. 8.2 and 8.3 at different sections along the longitudinal direction. Using Eq. 8.10, the boundary shear τ_0 may be determined.

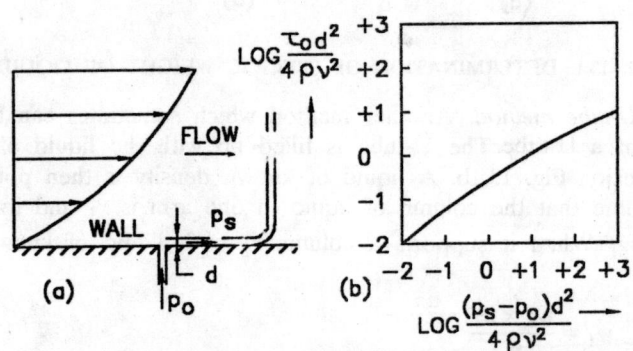

FIG. 13.2. CALIBRATION CURVE FOR PRESTON TUBE

(a) *Ludwieg Tillmann's formula.* The wall shear may also be determined by

$$\tau_0/\rho\, U_0^2 = 0.123 \times 10^{-0.678H} \, (U\theta/v)^{-0.268} \tag{13.3}$$

where H is the ratio of δ_* and θ is known as shape factor.

(b) *Standard charts.* The velocity distribution Eq. 9.19b is applicable in the vicinity of the wall. This equation is plotted in the form of charts (with slight modification) relating $c_f = \dfrac{2 U_x^2}{U_0^2}$ and R_e. Knowing R_e, the local drag coefficient c_f or wall shear stress can be read from these chars.

13.4 THEORY OF ORIFICES

An orifice is an opening in the side or bottom of a tank or in a plate which is placed normal to the axis of the pipe. The fluid from the tank is discharged into atmosphere in the form of a jet. It is known as 'free orifice'. If the jet emerges out into the fluid mass which stands above the level of the orifice, it is termed as 'submerged orifice', If the water level stands below the top level of orifice, it is known as partially submerted orifice'. Similarly, if the water stands above the top of orifice, it is termed as 'fully submerged orifice.'

An orifice is known as 'sharp edged', if the thickness of the plate containing the orifice is small as compared to the diameter of the opening, or its upstream edge has been bevelled as shown in (first from left) Fig. 13.3d. The orifice at (middle) in Fig. 13.3d is blunt edge and at (right end) is bell mouthed. The diameter 'd' of the orifice is too small as compared to the head acting at its centre (d < H) and is known as 'small orifice'.

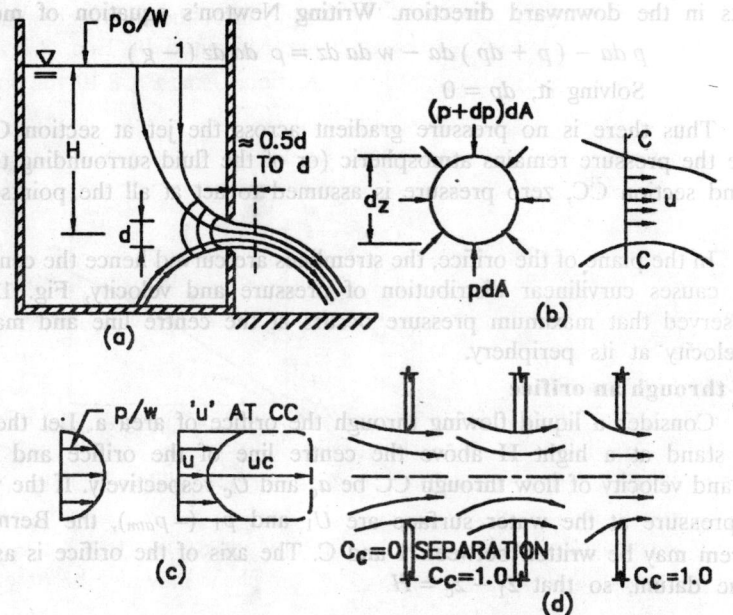

FIG. 13.3. FLOW THROUGH AN ORIFICE

An standard orifice is the one with sharp edge or an absolutely square shoulder so that there is only a line contact with the fluid stream.

Consider the flow of liquid taking place through an orifice of diamter d Fig. 13.3a. Let the head of water above the centre line of orifice be H.

As the stream lines approach the opening, they are converged theoretically. The convergence should continue for infinite distance from the plane of orifice. But owing to the friction between the jet and surrounding fluid, the stream lines converge upto section CC, known as section of "vena contracta". This section lies nearly at a distance of 0.5 d from the upstream face of the orifice. Beyond CC, the jet starts diverging, its direction becomes downward and flowtakes place under gravity. Thus, it is seen that the curvature of streamlines is changed from concave upwards to convex upwards. Hence there exists a point of inflextion at CC on the sreamlines, Fig. 13.3b.

Characteristics of section CC. The streamlines become horizontal and parallel to each other. The area of cross section of the jet is minimum and the velocity of flow is U_c. The velocity in each stream tube remains invariant and hence the pressure remains constant in each stream tubeFig. 13.3. (b). As the jet comes out into atmosphere (or into another liquid) the pressure remains the same at all the points of the section CC, equal to atmospheric pressure (or pressure of outside liquid as the case may be).

Consider a fluid element of area da located at CC which is acted upon by pressures p and p + dp on its lower and upper edges, dz apart. (Fig 13.3b). The fluid mass of the elements is $\rho da\,dz$ on which the verticial acceleration g acts in the downward direction. Writing Newton's equation of motion,

$$p\,da - (p + dp)\,da - w\,da\,dz = \rho\,da\,dz\,(-g)$$

Solving it, $dp = 0$ ...(13.4)

Thus there is no pressure gradient across the jet at section CC and hence the pressure remains atmospheric (or of the fluid surrounding the jet). Beyond section CC, zero pressure is assumed to act at all the points of the jet.

In the plane of the orifice, the stremlines are curved hence the centrifugal force causes curvilinear distribution of pressure and velocity, Fig. 13.3c. It is observed that maximum pressure occurs at the centre line and maximum jet velocity at its periphery.

Flow through an orifice

Consider a liquid flowing through the orifice of area a. Let the liquid level stand at a hight H above the centre line of the orifice and let the area and velocity of flow through CC be a_c and U_c respectively. If the velocity and pressure at the water surface are U_1 and p_1 ($= p_{atm}$), the Bernoulli's theorem may be written between 1 and C. The axis of the orifice is assumed as the datum, so that $z_1 - z_c = H$.

$$\frac{p_1}{w} + z_1 + \frac{U_1^2}{2g} = \frac{p_c}{w} + z_c + \frac{U_c^2}{2g} + losses$$

The losses between sections 1 and 3 are assumed to be zero. Therefore,

$$p_a / w + (z_1 - z_c) + U_1^2 / 2g = p_c / w + U_c^2 / 2g$$

$$p_a / w + H + U_1^2 / 2g = p_c / w + U_c^2 / 2g$$

$$U_c = \sqrt{2g \left(\frac{p_a - p_c}{w} + H - \frac{U_1^2}{2g} \right)} \qquad \qquad ...(13.5)$$

If the jet emerges out into the atmosphere, $p_c = p_1 = p_a$. Moreover, the velocity of fluid particles U_1, known as velocity of approach, with which it approaches the orifice is quite small (area of tank $>>$ area of orifice) and hence can be left out. Therefore, the velocity of flow U_c is given as

$$U_c = \sqrt{2gH} \qquad \qquad ...(13.6)$$

It is well known theorem of 'Torricelli', who first discovered it. It gives the theoretical velocity of flow.

2. Jet coefficients

(a) *Coefficient of velocity C_v.* For the flow of real fluid the actual velocity U (say), of jet which is attained at CC is found to be less than theoretical velocity U_c owing to the friction losses taking place between 1 and C. These losses are taken into account with the use of a coefficient, C_v, known as a *coefficient of velocity*. It is the ratio of actual velocity of the jet to the theoretical velocity. Thus,

$$C_v = \frac{U}{U_{th}} = \frac{U}{\sqrt{2gH}} \qquad \qquad ...(13.7)$$

Coefficient of contraction. The jet of liquid while passing through the orifice of area 'a' gets contracted to the area a_c at the section of vena contracta CC. The ratio of area 'a_c' to 'a' is defined as the *coefficient of contraction* C_c. Its varies from 0.5 to 1.0, depending on the shape of the entrance and type of orifice. For the ideal flow through a rectangular sharp edged orifice and also for standard orifice, the value of C_c is given by

$$C_c = \pi / (\pi + 2) = 0.611 \qquad \qquad ...(13.8)$$

The coefficient merely determises the size of jet that issues out through a certain area.

(c) *Coefficient of discharge.* The discharge flowing through an orifice can be known from the continuity equation. As such, the theoretical discharge Q_{th} flowing out of an orifice (without consideration of friction losses).

$$Q_{th} = a \sqrt{2gH} \qquad \qquad ...(13.9)$$

The actual discharge is the product of the area of jet at section of vena contracta, CC, and its velocity at the same section.

$$Q_{ac} = a_c U = C_c a C_v \sqrt{2gH} = C_c C_v a\sqrt{2gH} \qquad \qquad ..(13.10)$$

The actual discharge can also be computed by multiplying Q_{th} with a coefficient of discharge, C_d. Thus

$$Q_{ac} = C_d a \sqrt{2gH} \qquad \qquad ..(13.11)$$

Here the coefficient of discharge is defined as the ratio of actual discharge to the theoretical discharge flowing through the orifice.

The head H is the difference of pressure acting on the upstream and downstream faces of the orifice. Let the pressure acting on upstream face be H_1 and on downstream face H_2, so that

$$H = H_1 - H_2$$

and $\quad Q = C_d a \sqrt{2g(H_1 - H_2)}$ ...(13.12)

Comparing Eq. 13.10 and 13.11

$$C_d = C_c \, C_v \qquad \qquad ...(13.13)$$

The value of C_d varies in the range of 0.59 to 0.68. For the standard orifice, its value is 0.62×0.98 or 0.61. The coefficient of discharge decreases with increase in its size and also with increase in head acting on it.

3. Determination of coefficients

(a) *Coefficient of velocity.* Various methods for its determination are discussed below.

(i) The simplest method is to measure the velocity of jet at the section of vena contracta (at its centre) by means of a small pitot tube (section 13.10) and then taking the ratio of U to $\sqrt{2gH}$. It gives approximate result.

(2) Another method is the 'jet trajectory methods, Fig. 13.4. Consider the flow taking place through an orifice under head H. Let the section CC be located at a distances x_1 and y_1 with reference to tank wall. Referring to the section CC as the origin, the co-ordinates of any point P on the underside of the jet are measured by means of a pair of horizontal and vertical scales. Let these be x_2 and y_2. From the statics, the horizontal and vertical distance traversed by a fluid particle P in time t can be written. Thus

$$x = (x_2 - x_1) = U \times t$$

$$y = (y_2 - y_1) = \frac{1}{2} g t^2$$

Eliminatng t between these two equations,'

$$U = \frac{x}{\sqrt{2y/g}}$$

The coefficient of velocity C_v. is the ratio of U to theoretical velocity. Therefore,

$$C_v = \frac{U}{\sqrt{2gH}} \qquad ...(13.14a)$$

$$= \frac{x}{\sqrt{2y \cdot g} \times \sqrt{2gH}}$$

$$= \sqrt{\frac{x^2}{4y\,H}} \qquad ...(13.14b)$$

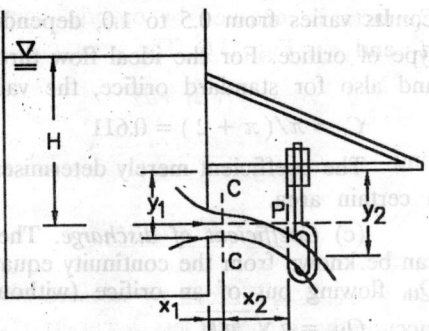

FIG. 13.4. TRAJECTORY METHOD OF DETERMINING C_v

(3) By use of momentum equation. In Fig. 13.5 is shown a tank suspended on a knife edge which is in the balanced condition. It contains liquid upto a height H above the centre line of orifice which is choked. While the flow takes place through the orifice the change in momentum of the jet causes

an equal and opposite unbalanced force F on the opposite wall. The tank is levelled again by adding weight W on it. Taking moment about knife edge,

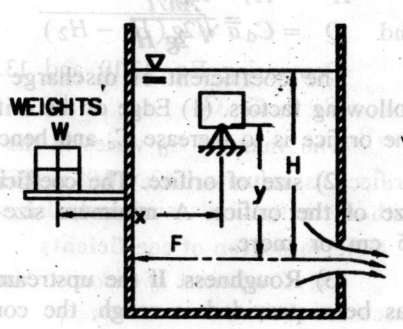

$$F = \frac{Wx}{y}$$

Applying moemntum theorem to the fluid in the tank

$$\Sigma F_x = \frac{wQ}{g}(U_{2x} - U_{1x})$$

The force is equal to ΣF_x, U_{x1} is initial velocity which is zero and U_{x2} is the actual velocity U of jet, which is unknown. The discharge Q is measured by volumetric method.

FIG. 13.5. DETERMINATION OF Cv BY MOMENTUM THEOREM

$$F = (wQ/g)(U)$$

Thus the actual velocity is determined and then the ratio of the velocity U to $\sqrt{2gH}$ results in the coefficient of velocity.

$$C_v = \frac{gF}{wQ\sqrt{2gH}} \qquad (13.15)$$

(b) *Coefficient of contraction.* The actual area at the section of vena conracta is measued by outside calipers in the two normal directions, say, d_1 and d_2, Fig 13.6. The area of jet at CC is

$$a_c = \pi/4\left\{(d_1+d_2)/2\right\}^2$$

and $\quad C_c = \dfrac{area\ of\ jet}{area\ of\ opening\ or\ orifice}$

$$= \frac{\pi/4\left\{(d_1+d_2)/2\right\}^2}{a} \qquad ...(13.16)$$

As it is difficult to measure the jet diameters accurently, it yields less accurate result.

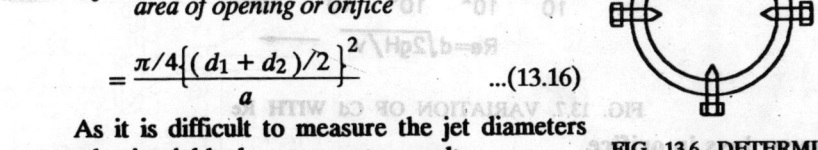

FIG. 13.6. DETERMINA-TION OF Cc

(c) *Coefficient of discharge.* The actual discharge can either be measured by gravitational or volumetric method. In the first method the water flowing through the orifice in time t is collected in a tank and weighed. The rate of flow is the ratio of the weight of fluid to the product of the time and its specific weight.

In the volumetric method the water is collected in a tank of area A (in plan) for t seconds. If the rise in liquid is h $(= h_2 - h_1)$, the actual discharge is A h/t. The coefficient of discharge is then determined as

$$C_d = \frac{Q_{ac}}{Q_{th}}$$

$$= \frac{Ah/t}{\sqrt{2g\ H}} \qquad \qquad ...(13.17)$$

The coefficient of discharge for a circular orifice depends on the following factors. (1) Edge of the orifice. The effect of rounding the edges of the orifice is to increase C_c and hence C_d.

(2) size of orifice. The coefficient reduces slightly with increase in the size of the orifice. A minimum size of orifice is 7.5 cm when the head is 35 cm or more.

(3) Roughness. If the upstream face of the surface in which the orfice has been provided is rough, the contraction is reduced, thereby increasing C_c and C_d.

(4) Velocity of approach. With higher velocity of approach the C_d is increased.

(5) Viscosity. The effect of viscosity is studied by means of Reynolds number. The variation of C_d with R_e ($= d \ \sqrt{2g\ H}/v$)is shown in Fig. 13.7. At lower head, the effect of viscosity is pronounced causing lesser contraction and higher value of C_r and C_d.

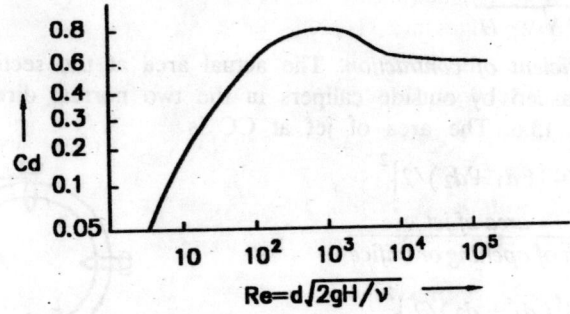

FIG. 13.7. VARIATION OF Cd WITH Re

4. Energy loss in orifice

The energy loss (due to friction, at the entrance to the orifice, etc) in an orifice can be determined by equating the total head on the upstream and downstream faces of the orifice (Fig. 13.3a).

$$\frac{p1}{w} + \frac{U_1^2}{2g} + H = \frac{pa}{w} + \frac{U^2}{2g} + h_L$$

As the jet emerges out in the atmosphere with a velocity U and the velocity of approach U_1 is neglected, hence

$$h_L = (H - U^2/2g)$$

The velocity of jet $U = C_v \sqrt{2g\ H}$, therefore,

$$h_L = (1 - C_v^2) H$$
$$= (1/C_v^2 - 1) U^2/2g \qquad \qquad ...(13.18c)$$

13.5 THEORY OF LARGE ORIFICE

When the size of orifice is large (say $d \approx H$) the head acting on the lower and upper edge is substantially different. This causes sufficient variation in pressure along the vertical dimension of the orifice and hence, the use of head acting at the centre line does not give true velocity of flow through the orifice.

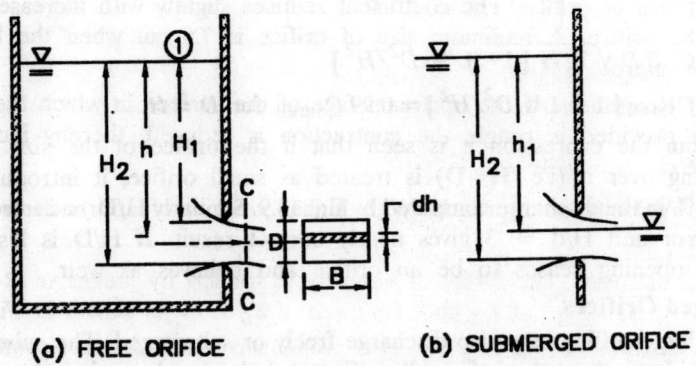

(a) FREE ORIFICE   **(b) SUBMERGED ORIFICE**

FIG. 13.8. FLOW THROUGH A LARGE ORIFICE

Consider a rectangular orifice of width B and height D. The head on its upper and lower edges are H_1 and H_2 respectively. Take an elementary strip of width B and thickness dh at a depth h below free water surface (Fig. 13.8). The discharge through this elementary strip is dQ.

From continuity equation,

$$dQ = C_d \, B \, dh \, \sqrt{2gh} \qquad \qquad ...(13.19a)$$

Integrating, with head varying from H_1 to H_2,

$$\therefore Q = \int dQ$$

$$= C_d \, B \, \sqrt{2g} \int_{H_i}^{H_2} \sqrt{h} \; dh$$

$$= \frac{2}{3} C_d \, B \, \sqrt{2g} \, [H_2^{3/2} - H_1^{3/2}] \qquad \qquad ...(13.19b)$$

The liquid approaches the orifice with a velocity U_1. If it is also to be considered, the limit of integration in Eq. 13.19b should be taken as. $H_1 + U_1^2/2g$ and $H_2 + U_1^2/2g$ Then,

$$Q = \frac{2}{3} C_d \, \sqrt{2g} \, B \, [\, (H_2 + U_1^2/2g)^{3/2} - (H_1 + U_1^2/2g)^{3/2} \,] \qquad ...(13.20a)$$

If the orifice is supposed to be small, the head acting on it at its centre would be $H = (H_1 + H_2)/2$. From Fig. 13.8 $H_1 = H + D/2$ and $H_2 = H - D/2$ and hence Eq. 13.19b can be written as

$$Q = \frac{2}{3} C_d \sqrt{2g} \left[(H + D/2)^{3/2} - (H - D/2)^{3/2} \right]$$

This equation can be expanded by binomial theorem, and the terms of higher order may be dropped. Therefore,

$$Q_{large} = \frac{2}{3} C_d B \sqrt{2g} \left[\frac{3}{2} \sqrt{H} D - \frac{1}{64} \frac{1}{H^{3/2}} D^3 \right]$$

$$= C_d B D \sqrt{2gH} \left[1 - 1/96 \, D^2/H^2 \right]$$

$$= Q_{small} \left[1 - 1/96 \, D^2/H^2 \right] = 0.99 \, Q_{small} \text{ for } D = H.$$

From the expression it is seen that if the orifice of the size of the head acting over it (i.e. H = D) is treated as small orifice, it introduces an error of 1% in the discharge computed by Eq. 13.9. Similarly H/D = 2 introduces 0.26% error and H/d = 3 gives nearly correct result. If H/D is less than 0.68, the opening ceases to be an orifice and behaves as weir,

Submerged Orifices

A large orifice may also discharge freely or submerged. The submerged orifice is identical to that of small orifice and the head causing the flow is the differene between the pressures on the upstream and downstream of the orifice. In case the orifice discharges partially submerged, that is, the liquid level on the downstream side is below its top edge but above the lower edge, as shown in Fig. 13.8b, the discharge is determined by assuming the upper portion of orifice running free and lower portion running (the portion of the orifice between downstream liquid level and its lower edge) as submerged orifice. Thus

$$Q = Q_{free} + Q_{submeged}$$

$$= \frac{2}{3} C_d B \sqrt{2g} \left[h_1^{3/2} - H_1^{3/2} \right] + C_d B (H_2 - h_1) \sqrt{2g} \, h_1$$

$$\text{...(13.20b)}$$

assuming the same coefficient of discharge.

13.6 THEORY OF MOUTHPIECES

If a short length of pipe, 1 to 3 times the diameter of pipe, is fixed to the opening, the discharge flowing out is increased. Such a short pipe is called a mouthpiece or short tube. The mouthpiece may be cylinderical, convergent or divergent in shape and are accordingly named. The mouthpiece projecting outside from the tank wall is called as 'external mouthpiece whereas projecting inward from the tank wall (at the orifice) is called an 'internal or re-entrant mouthpiece'.

A standard mouthpiece has a length of 2.5 times diameter and a square edged entrance.

1. External mouthpiece

Consider an external mouthpiece of diameter d, fitted to a tank containing liquid to a height H above the centre line of the mouthpiece. As discussed earlier, the streamlines approaching the opening get converged upto a section of vena contracta (which now lies inside the mouthpiece) and thereafter expands and fills the mouthpiece completely. The mouthpiece is then said to be running full. While the flow takes place through the mouthpiece, the losses taking place in it are (i) due to friction from 1 to C and (ii) due to sudden expansion C to 2.

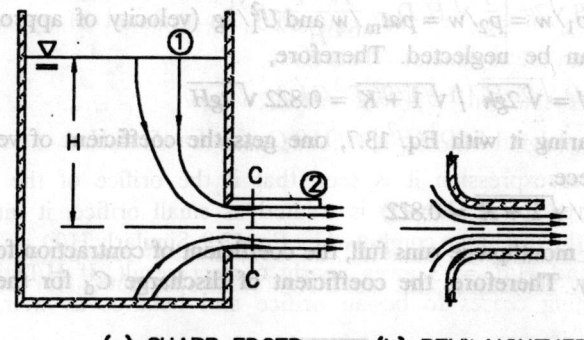

(a) SHARP EDGED   (b) BELL MOUTHED
MOUTH PIECE   MOUTH PIECE

FIG. 13.9 FLOW THROUGH AN EXTERNAL MOUTHPIECE

(a) *Discharge.* If the velocity of flow at vena contracta is U_c and at section 2 is U, then from Eq. 13.18c.

$$h_{L1} = (1/C_v^2 - 1) U_c^2/2g \qquad ...(13.18c)$$

Substituting $U_c = U/C_c$, where C_c and C_v are the coefficient of contraction and coefficient of velocity for the given opening (behaving as an orifice),

$$h_{L1} = (1/C_v^2 - 1) \frac{1}{2g} \times \frac{U^2}{C_c^2} \qquad ...(13.21a)$$

Assuming $C_v = 0.98$ and $C_c = 0.62$ for the given orifice,

$$h_{L1} = 0.104 \, U^2/2g \qquad ...(13.21b)$$

The head loss due to sudden expansion is computed from Eq. 5.62b.

$$h_{L2} = \frac{(U_c - U)^2}{2g}$$

$$= \frac{(U/C_c - U)^2}{2g} = \frac{U^2}{2g} (1/C_c - 1)^2 \qquad ...(13.22a)$$

$$= 0.375 \, U^2/2g \text{ , assuming } C_c = 0.62 \qquad ...(13.22b)$$

Therefore, total head loss in the mouthpiece is

$$h_L = [(1/C_v^2 - 1) 1/C_c^2 + (1/C_c - 1)^2] \frac{U^2}{2g} = 0.479 \frac{U^2}{2g}$$

$$= K \frac{U^2}{2g} \text{ (say)} \qquad ...(13.23)$$

Applying the Bernoulli's theorem between 1 and 2.

$$\frac{p_1}{w} + H + \frac{U_1^2}{2g} = \frac{p_2}{w} + \frac{U_2^2}{2g} + h_L$$

$$\frac{p_1}{w} + H + \frac{U_1^2}{2g} = \frac{p_2}{w} + \frac{U_2^2}{2g} + \frac{KU^2}{2g} \qquad \ldots(13.24a)$$

Here $p_1/w = p_2/w = pat_m/w$ and $U_1^2/2g$ (velocity of approach head) is small and can be neglected. Therefore,

$$U_2 = U = \sqrt{2gh} \ / \sqrt{1 + K} = 0.822 \sqrt{2gH} \qquad \ldots(13.24b)$$

Comparing it with Eq. 13.7, one gets the coefficient of velocity C_v for the mouthpiece.

$$C_v = 1/\sqrt{1 + K} = 0.822$$

As the mouthpiece runs full, the coefficient of contraction for the mouthpiece is unity. Therefore, the coefficient of discharge C_d for the mouthpiece is

$$C_d = C_c \, C_v = 1 \times 1/\sqrt{1 + K}$$
$$= 1/\sqrt{1 + K} = 0.822$$

Neglecting h_{L1} in Eq. 13.23 to find K,

$$C_d = C_v = \frac{1}{\sqrt{(1/C_c - 1)^2 + 1}} = 0.853 \qquad \ldots(13.25)$$

The discharge through the mouthpiece can be computed as

$$Q = C_d \, a \sqrt{2gH} \ ; \ \text{where} \ a = (\pi/4) \, d^2 \qquad \ldots(13.26)$$

The value of C_v and hence C_d for water is nearly 0.82 and slightly varies with head and diameter of the mouthpiece.

(b) *Pressure head at C:* The pressure head at CC is different than atmospheric pressure. Applying Bernoulli's theorem between 1 and C;

$$p_a/w + H + U_1^2/2g = pc/w + U_c^2/2g$$

$$p_c/w = H_a + H + U_1^2/2g - U_c^2/2g$$

Nelgect $U_1^2/2g$ being small. Substitute $U_c = U/C_c$

and $\qquad U = C_v \sqrt{2gH} = 0.853 \sqrt{2gH}$

$$p_c/w = H_a + H - (C_v^2/C_c^2) H \qquad \ldots(13.27a)$$

$$= H_a + H - (0.853^2/0.62^2) H$$

$$= H_a - 0.893 \, H \qquad \ldots(13.27b)$$

The pressure at vena contracta is less than atmospheric pressue by an amount equal to 0.893 H. It also implies theoretically that if the head of the liquid is $H_a/0.893$ metre, zero pressure will be acting at the section CC. But it is not practical because when the pressure at any section falls down to vapour pressure of fluid, the cavitation may start and the flow may separate from the boundary.

Using actual value of $C_v = 0.822$

$$p_c/w = H_a - 0.757 H \qquad ...(13.27c)$$

(c) *Maximum discharge* : Applying Bernoulli's theorem between sections 1 and 2 and neglecting h_{L1}

$$H = \left[\frac{U^2}{2g} + \frac{(U_c - U)^2}{2g} \right]$$

$$= [U^2/2g + (1/C_c - 1)^2 U^2/2g]$$

$$= U^2/2g [1 + (1/C_c - 1)^2]$$

$$U = \sqrt{ 2gH/[2 - 2/C_c + 1/C_c^2] }$$

Then, discharge $Q = AU = (\pi d^2/4) \sqrt{ 2gH/[2 - 2/C_c + 1/C_c^2] }$

where $C_c = a_c/a = dc^2/d^2$

$$Q = \frac{\pi}{4} \sqrt{2gH} \, d^2 / \sqrt{2 - 2 d^2/d_c^2 + d^4/d_c^4}$$

$$\equiv K_1 d^2 d_c^2 / \sqrt{2d_c^4 - 2 d^2 d_c^2 + d^4}$$

For maximum discharge $dQ/dd = 0$, therefore,

$$\frac{dQ}{dd} = K_1 d_c^2 \left[\frac{2d}{\sqrt{2d_c^4 - 2d^2 d_c^2 + d^4}} + \frac{d^2 (-1/2) (0 - 4d \, d_c^2 + 4d^3)}{(2d_c^4 - 2d^2 d_c^2 + d^4)^{3/2}} \right] = 0$$

Solution of this equation yields, $d = \sqrt{2} \, d_c$

$$d/dc = \sqrt{2} \qquad ...(13.28)$$

$$Q_{max} = (\pi d^2/4) \sqrt{2gH} \left[\frac{1}{\sqrt{2 - 2(\sqrt{2})^2 + (\sqrt{2})^4}} \right]$$

$$= \sqrt{2} \left(\pi \frac{d^2}{4} \sqrt{2gH} \right)$$

Discharge through an orifice of equal diameter d is

$$Q = (\pi d^2/4) \times \sqrt{2gH}$$

Percentage increase in discharge

$$= \frac{Q_{mouthpiece} - Q_{orifice}}{Q} \times 100$$

$$= \frac{C_{dm} \times a \sqrt{2gH} - C_{do} \times a \sqrt{2gH}}{C_{do} \, a \sqrt{2gH}} \times 100$$

$$= \left(\frac{C_{dm} - C_{do}}{C_{do}} \right) \times 100 \qquad ...(13.30)$$

In this case, percentage increase in discharge

$$= \left(\frac{Q_{max} - Q}{Q} \right) \times 100 \qquad ...(13.31a)$$

Percentage increase $= (\sqrt{2} - 1) \times 100$

$$= 41.4 \% \qquad ...(13.31b)$$

2. Internal or Re-entrant Mouthpiece

A short cylindrical tube 2d to 3d projecting inside the tank is called "Re-entrant or Borda's mouthpieice". It is named after Borda who showed mathematically and experimentally that C_c for such an mouthpiece is equal to 0.5. While the flow takes place for such a mouthpiece, the streamlines have to turn by 180°. causing large contraction of the jet. Thus, there are two possible cases of flow patterns through Borda's mothpiece; (a) mouthpiece running free and (b) mouthpiece running full. Fig. 13.10.

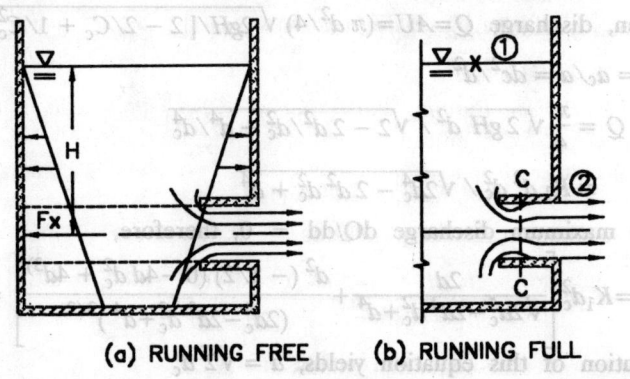

(a) RUNNING FREE   **(b) RUNNING FULL**

[FIG. 13.10. FLOW THROUGH A RE-ENTRANT MOUTHPIECE

(a) *Mouthpiece running free :* Consider an internal mouthpiece of diameter d (area a) fitted to the tank (Fig. 13.10a) while the flow takes place through the mouthpiece, the jet contracts upto the section CC and comes out of it free, i.e. without touching the walls of mouthpiece. The pressure distribution on the opposite walls of the tank are hydrostatic except in the region near the opening, where actual pressure distribution is shown by dotted lines. Thus an unbalanced force equal to (w aH) is assumed to be imposed on the tank walls as a result of change of momentum of the fluid coming out of the mouthpiece. Applying momentum theorem to the fluid body in the tank.

$$F_x = (w \, Q/g) \, U_{2x} - U_{1x})$$

$$w \, a \, H = (wQ/g) \, U_c \qquad (\because \; U_{1x} = 0) \qquad ...(13.32a)$$

Using continuity equation.

$$Q = a_c \, U_c \quad \text{and} \quad U_c = C_v \sqrt{2gH}$$

Eq. 13.32a becomes.

$$aH = a_c \, U_c^2/g$$

$$= a_c \times C_v^2 \times 2H$$

$$a = 2\, C_v^2\, a_c$$

Therefore, coefficient of contraction for re-entrant mouthpiece becomes

$$C_c = a_c/a$$

$$= 1/2\, C_v^2 \qquad\qquad\qquad ...(13.32c)$$

For water to flow through a mouthpiece with sharp entrance, C_v is 0.98 hence,

$$C_c = 0.52 \qquad\qquad\qquad ...(13.32d)$$

The value of C_c will be 0.5, if C_v is assumed to be 1.0. Thus discharge through mouthpiece running free is given by

$$Q_{free} = a_c\, U_c$$

$$= C_c\, a \times C_v\, \sqrt{2gH}$$

$$= 0.52 \times 0.98\, a\, \sqrt{2gH}$$

$$= 0.51\, a\, \sqrt{2gH} \qquad\qquad\qquad ...(13.33)$$

(b) *Mouthpiece Running Full* : Referring to Fig. 13.10b, it is seen that the jet converges from entrance section to the section CC; beyond section CC it expands and fills the mouthpiece. To analyse the flow, apply Bernoulli's Theorem between section 1 and 2.

$$\frac{p_a}{w} + H = \frac{p_a}{w} + \frac{U^2}{2g} + h_L$$

where

$$h_L = (U_c - U)^2/2g = (U^2/2g)(1/C_c - 1)^2$$

Putting

$$C_c = 0.5 \, ; h_L = U^2/2g$$

$$\therefore \qquad H = U^2/2g + U^2/2g$$

$$H = \frac{U^2}{g}$$

Hence

$$U = \sqrt{gH} \qquad\qquad\qquad ...(13.34)$$

Comparing it with Eq. 13.7,

$$C_v = 1/\sqrt{2} = 0.707 \qquad\qquad\qquad ...(13.35)$$

The discharge flowing through re-entrant mouthpiece running full,

$$Q_{full} = aU$$

$$Q_{full} = a\, \sqrt{gH} \qquad\qquad\qquad ...(13.36)$$

Comparing it with Eq. 13.26.

$$C_d = 1/\sqrt{2}$$

Alternatively, $C_d = C_c \times C_v = 1.0 \times 1/\sqrt{2} = 1/\sqrt{2} \qquad ...(13.37)$

Since coefficient of contraction for outlet section of mouthpiece running full is. 1.0

Pressure at CC: Apply Bernoulli's theorem between sections 'CC' and outlet section 2.

$$\frac{p_c}{w} + \frac{U_c^2}{2g} = \frac{p_a}{w} + \frac{U^2}{2g} + \frac{U^2}{2g}$$

$$\frac{p_c}{w} = \frac{p_a}{w} + \frac{U^2}{g} - \frac{U_c^2}{2g}$$

But $\dfrac{U_c^2}{2g} = \left(\dfrac{U}{C_c}\right)^2 / 2g = 4\dfrac{(U^2)}{2g}$ (Putting $C_c = 0.5$)

$$\therefore \frac{p_c}{w} = \frac{p_a}{w} + \frac{U^2}{g} - 2\frac{U^2}{g}$$

$$= \left(\frac{p_a}{w} - \frac{U^2}{g}\right)$$

$$= \left(\frac{p_a}{w} - H\right) \qquad \qquad ...(13.38)$$

Theoretically, the pressure at venta contracta lowers down by head of liquid behind it.

13.7 UNSTEADY FLOW THROUGH ORIFICE

1. Flow from a Tank into Atmosphere[*]

Consider a tank of plan area A, to which an orifice or mouthpiece is fitted. Let the liquid stand to a height H_1 above the centre line of opening. When the liquid flows out of the tank, the liquid level lowers down to a height H_2 above the centre line in time t (say). Let us assume that the liquid in the tank stands to the height h at any instant t and the correspondng discharge is Q. In the time interval dt, the liquid level falls by dh, Fig. 13.11.

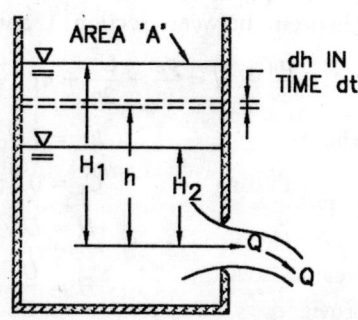

FIG. 13.11. UNSTEADY FLOW THROUGH AN ORIFICE

Therefore, $Q\,dt = -A\,dh$ ...(13.39a)

The negative sign is used to indicate the reducton in head h with increase in time t. Eq. 13.39a is the fundamental equation of unsteady flow.

Integrating Eq. 13.39a in the range of head from H_1 and H_2.

$$\int_T dt = -\int_{H_1}^{H_2} \frac{A\,dh}{Q} \qquad \qquad ...(13.39b)$$

The expression for discharge Q is to be substituted for the type of device used, whether it is an orifice, or a mouthpiece or even a weir. Moreover, the area of the tank, in plan A may either be consant or may vary with

---

[*] See Examples 13.7 to 13.10.

head (as in case of triangular or circular cylinder lying horizontally). In such a case, A is expressed in terms of head and substituted in Eq. 13.39b.

Case 1. for constant area;

$$T = -A \int_{H_1}^{H_2} \frac{dh}{Q}$$

From Eq. 13.11, $Q = C_d \, a \, \sqrt{2g \, h}$

$$T = A \int_{H_2}^{H_1} \frac{dh}{C_d \, a \, \sqrt{2gh}} = \frac{A}{C_d \, a \, \sqrt{2g}} \int_{H_2}^{H_1} \frac{dh}{\sqrt{h}}$$

$$= \frac{2A}{C_d \, a \, \sqrt{2gh}} \left[\sqrt{H_1} - \sqrt{H_2} \right] \qquad \qquad ...(13.40)$$

Case 2. When the discharge Q_1 also enters the tank simultaneously to the outflow Q, the Eq. 13.39a modifies to

$$A \, dh = (Q_1 - Q) \, dt$$

or

$$dt = A \, dh/(Q_1 - Q) \qquad \qquad ...(13.41a)$$

The inflow and outflow are now substituted in tems of head h.

Let $\qquad\qquad Q_1 = K \sqrt{h}$, then

$$dt = \frac{A \, dh}{K\sqrt{h} - C_d \, a \, \sqrt{2g \, h}}$$

Integrating,

$$T = \left[\int_{H_1}^{H_2} \frac{A \, dh}{K\sqrt{h} - C_d \, a \, \sqrt{2g \, h}} \right] \qquad ...(13.41b)$$

(see solved Examples 13.7 to 13.10)

2. Time of flow from one tank to another

Fig 13.12 shows a tank which is divided into two compartments, of area A_1 on the left side and of area A_2 on the right side. An orifice is provided in the partition wall so that the liquid may flow from one side to other. Suppose the liquid stands to a height H_1' in the left tank and to a height H_2' in the right tank. Let the difference in liquid levels be H_1 at the beginning. It is required to find the time taken for the difference of level to become H_2.

At a certain instant of time, let the difference in liquid beween two tanks be h and let the discharge dQ flow through the orifice in time dt. This will cause the liquid level to fall in the left tank by dH (say) and, therefore, the liquid will rise by dH A_1/A_2 in the right tank.

The new difference in liquid level becomes

$$= (h - dH - dH \, A_1/A_2)$$

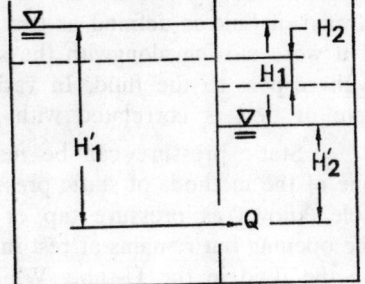

FIG. 13.12 FLOW FROM ONE TANK TO ANOTHER TANK

$$= h - dH \ (1 + A_1/A_2) \qquad \qquad ...(13.42)$$

The change of head causing the flow

$$dh = [\text{initial difference} - \text{final difference}]$$

$$dh = h - [\,h - dH \ (1 + A_1/A_2)\,]$$

$$dh = dH \ (1 + A_1/A_2)$$

or $\qquad dH = \dfrac{dh}{(1 + A_1/A_2)} \qquad \qquad ...(13.43)$

From Eq. 13.39 a

$$Q \, dt = - A_1 \, dH$$

Substituting the value of dH from Eq. 13.43

$$dt = \frac{- A_1 \, dH}{C_d \, a \sqrt{2gh}} = \frac{- A_1}{C_d \, a \sqrt{2g} \sqrt{h}} \ \frac{dh}{(1 + A_1/A_2)} \qquad ...(13.44)$$

Integrating for head varying from H_1 to H_2

$$\int_0^T dt = \frac{-A_1}{C_d \, a \sqrt{2g} \ (1 + A_1/A_2)} \int_{H_1}^{H_2} \frac{dh}{\sqrt{h}}$$

$$T = \frac{A_1}{C_d \, a \sqrt{2g} \ (1 + A_1/A_2)} \left[\frac{h^{1/2}}{1/2}\right]_{H_2}^{H_1}$$

$$= \frac{2 A_1 (\sqrt{H_1} - \sqrt{H_2})}{C_d \, a \sqrt{2g} (1 + A_1/A_2)} \qquad \qquad ...(13.45a)$$

If both the tanks were of the same size, $A_1 = A_2$

$$= \frac{A_1 (\sqrt{H_1} - \sqrt{H_2})}{C_d \, a \sqrt{2g}} \qquad \qquad ...(13.45b)$$

It is immaterial, whether the flow takes place from left to right or right to left, the time of flow will be the same; provided the reduction in level is same in both the cases.

13.8 MEASUREMENT OF STATIC PRESSURE

The accurate measurement of pressure (force per unit area) in a fluid at rest is comparatively easy, whereas an accurate measurement of pressure within a moving stream of fluid is quite difficult. The static pressure in a stream of fluid is defined as the pressure that would act on a pressure gauge if it were moving alongwith the stream so as to be at rest or relatively static with respect to the fluid. In various flow measurements, the velocity or the rate of flow is correlated with the static pressure.

Static pressure can be measured in various ways. Fig. 13.13a, shows one of the methods of static pressue measurement by means of static pressure hole, known as pressure tap or piezometric opening. The fluid flows past the opening but remains at rest in the opening and hence exerts static pressure on the fluid in the U-tube. While drilling the pressure tap, care should be taken that the hole is of sufficient size (minimum 3 mm diameter); it is at right angle to the flow and the surface has got no projections or burrs (i.e., the pressure tap is flush with internal surface). A variety of manometers, or gauges hae been developed for such measurement, (refer to section 2.4).

The static pressures on the smooth surface of a pipe wall, an airfoil or any other object can be measured by these piezometric tappings. These tappings measure the pressures at their locations only. If the stream lines are straight and have no curvature, the pressure throughout the cross section remains the same. Frequently, in pipeline a number of pressure tappings are drilled along the pipe periphery and a piezometric ring is fitted at this cross section. The average of these measured pressures yield an accurate static pressure in the cross section.

The static pressue variation along a cross section (where the flow direction is known with fair accuracy) can be measured by means of a static tube. Such a tube is merely a small smooth cylinder with rounded or pointed upstream end. In the side of this cylinder, the piezometric holes or circumferential slot are provided, through which the pressure is transmitted to gauge or manometer. Assuming perfect alignment with the flow, the flow past the tube will be symmetrical -and of mean velocity U_0. Hence the pressue at the piezometric hole is slightly less than p_0, but this error can be minimised by making the tube diameter as small as possile.

Transducers

For rapidly fluctuating pressures, however, these manometers or gauges are not suitable. In such case, pressure sensitive devices are used, which employ a diaphragm and electronic means to indicate the pressure variation on a dial. These are broadly classified into four groups : (a) Electrostatic devices (b) Electromagnetic devices (c) Photo electronic devices and (d) Resistance devices.

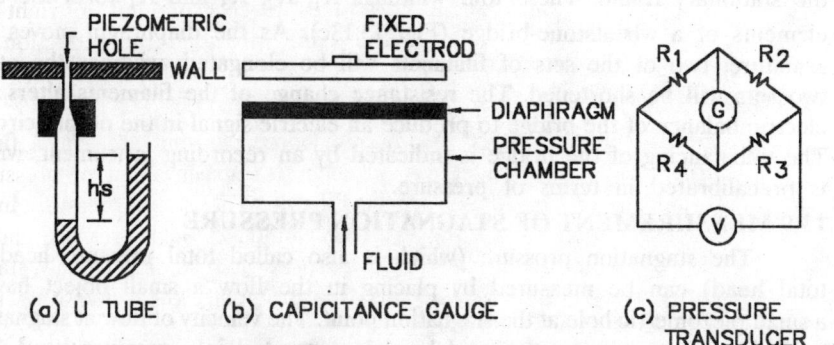

FIG. 13.13. STATIC PRESSURE MEASUREMENT BY PRESSURE TRANSDUCER

(a) Electrostatic devices make use of the piezoelectric properties of certain crystalline substance and the variation of the capacitance of a capacitor, e.g., rochelle salt and quartz. Fig. 13.13b illustrates schematically a gauge (useful in water) described by Ippen and Raichlen. Liquid fills the pressure chamber and acts on the circular flexible diaphragm. The diaphragm is firmly clamped on the chamber wall around its periphery. A fixed electrode is held a small distance away from the diaphragm separated by a thin air gap. A change in the instantaneous pressure of the liquid causes a deflection of diaphragm. This deflection can be noted by electronically measuring the change in capacitance between the fixed electrode and the diaphragm. Such type of devices are also used in an acoustic microphones where the fluid is air.

(b) **Electromagnetic devices make use of industance changes in the magnetic** sysem to generate small voltage in a coil. A diaphragm of magnetic material can be held in close proximity to one pole face of a permanent magnet so that an air gap is formed in the magnetic circuit. A coil of wire composed of a large number of turns is wound on the magnet. The pressure applied to one side of a diaphragm will deflect it, change the air gap and thus cause a flux change. This fllux change is then converted into pressure indication.

(c) **Photoelectronic devices use photoelectric properties of certain material** to convert a pressure into an electric effect. A beam of light from an electric filament bulb is directed towards an emmission type of photo-cell. The centre of the diaphragm is attached to a vane that moves in front of a fixed vane and varies the area of the beam light. Thus pressure variation of the diaphragm vary the electric response of the photocell, which in turn can be indicated on some instrument as a cathode ray oscilloscope.

(d) Resistance devices make use of the variation of electrical resistance of a material with applied strain. This transducer is an electromechanical device that transmits minute changes of diaphragm displacement to sensible resistance changes. It consists of a stationary frame to which an armature is supported in such a way so as to allow free movement in the line of displacement. Four windings of strain sensitive resisance wires are wound by rigid pins in the stationary frame. These four windings R_1, R_2, R_3 and R_4 form the four elements of a wheatstone-bridge (Fig. 13.13c). As the diaphragm moves the armature, two of the sets of filaments will be elongated, whereas the other two sets will be shortened. The resistance change of the filaments alters the electric balance of the bridge to produce an electric signal in the output circuit. The unbalancing of the bridge is indicated by an recording instrument, which is precalibrated in terms of pressure.

13.9 MEASUREMENT OF STAGNATION PRESSURE

The stagnation prossure (which is also called total pressure head or total head) can be measured by placing in the flow a small object having a small piezometric hole at the stagnation point. The velocity of flow at stagnation point is zero and hence the total head is converted into pressure head. For this purpose any symmetrical object like cylinder, cone or hemisphere can be placed in the flow so that its axis is in the direction of the flow; in this way, the piezometric opening faces the flow. Henry Pitot (1723) measured accurately the stagnation pressure by means of a small cylindrical tube which is now known as Pitot tube ; (Pitot tube indeed means stagnation tube only). Fig. 13.14a.

For the measurement of stagnation pressure the direction of flow should be known in advance. There are many devices for determining the direction of flow such as a cylinder or direction finding tube as shown in Fig. 13.14b. The pressure distribution at the front face of the tube is shown in the Fig. 13.14b. It is obvious that if the tube faces exactly opposite the direction of flow the piezometric tube at B and C will show equal pressure. Theoretically the critical angle for B and C should be 30° each for ideal incompressible fluid but experimentally it has been determined as 39.25°. The device consists of a small diameter cylinder with a partition. Two small piezometric holes B and C are drilled in it which are then connected to two piezometers or twc limbs of a U-tube manometer. The device is placed in pipe or channel such that the piezometric holes face the flow. The tube is rotated until the pressure in the two limbs is equal (or the difference in the two limbs of the manometer is zero).

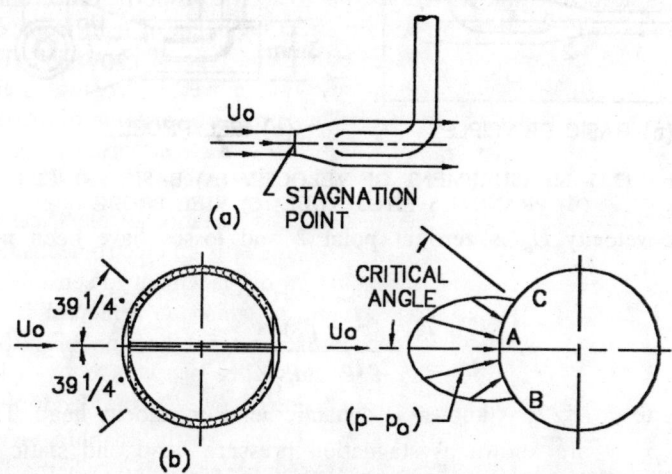

FIG. 13.14. STATIC PRESSURE MEASUREMENT

13.10 MEASUREMENT OF VELOCITY

1. Velocity measurement

The local velocity in a cross section can be measured by means of (a) Pitot static tube or by (b) Hot wire anemometer.

(a) *Pitot tube placed in an incompressile fluid.* Fig 13.15 shows the arranement of velocity measurement in a pipe at any point 1 (say). The static pressue at point 1 is p_0 which can be measured by means of a static tube or by a gauge connected through a piezometric opening. Let the velocity at this point be U_0. The stagnation pressure at the same level as 1 can be measured by means of a stagnation tube. Let the total pressure be p_s. Applying Bernoulli's theorem between 1 aɪ.d 2,

$$\frac{p_0}{w} + \frac{U_0^2}{2g} = \frac{p_s}{w} + \frac{U_s^2}{2g}$$

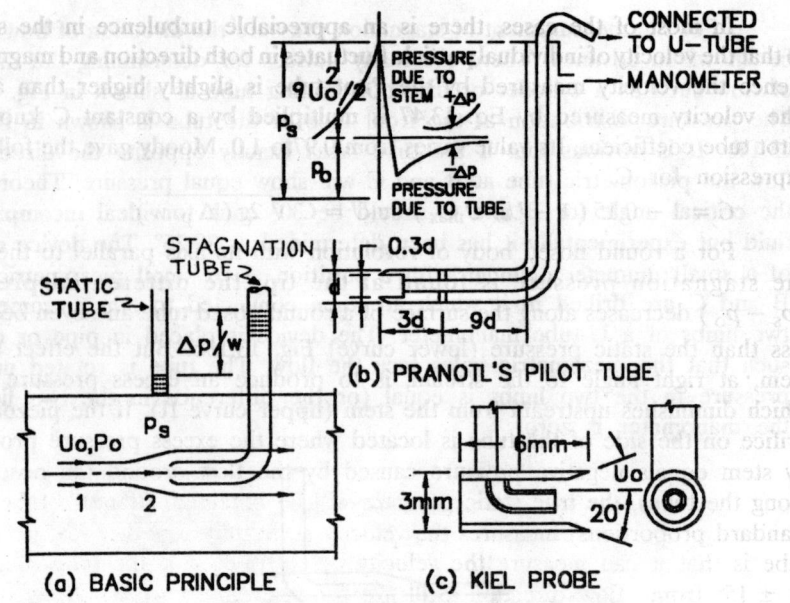

FIG. 13.15. MEASUREMENT OF VELOCITY (A) BASIC PRINCIPLE
(B) PRANDTL'S PITOT TUBE (C) KIEL PROBE

The velocity U_s is zero at point 2 and losses have been neglected. Therefore,

$$U_0^2/2g = (p_s - p_0)/w \qquad ...(13.46a)$$

$$U_0 = \sqrt{2g\,(p_s - p_0)/w} \qquad ...(13.46b)$$

The term $U_0^2/2g$ is known as dynamic head or velocity head. The terms p_s/w and p_0/w are known as stagnation pressure head and static pressure head. Thus velocity U_0 is computed by taking separate readings of p_s and p_0 and using Eq. 13.46b.

A typical Pitot static tube was designed by Prandtl and is sometimes known as 'Prandtl's Pitot tube'. It consists of a bell-mouthed small diameter tube with a piezometric hole at its tip. It is surrounded by another tube. Two piezometric holes are provided at the opposite ends of a horizontal diameter of the outer tube. The hole in the tip is connected to one leg of a manometer and the side holes to another leg of the same manometer. For accurate measurement, the manometer is mounted on a board inclined at an angle θ to the horizontal. The vertical difference of the pressures in the two limbs is then determined and used in Eq. 13.47.

$$U_0 = \sqrt{2g\,(p_s - p_0)/w}$$
$$= \sqrt{2g \times l\,(S_w/S - 1)\sin\theta} \qquad ...(13.47)$$

In most of the cases, there is an appreciable turbulence in the stream so that the velocity of individual particle fluctuates in both direction and magnitude. Hence the velocity measured by the Pitot tube is slightly higher than actual. The velocity measured by Eq. 13.47 is multiplied by a constant C known as Pitot tube coefficient. Its value varies from 0.97to 1.0. Moody gave the following expression for C.

$$C = 1 - 0.15 (1 - U_o/U_{max}) \quad ; \quad U = C \sqrt{ 2g (\Delta p/w)}$$

For a round nosed body of revolution with its axis parallel to the flow, the stagnation pressure is found at the tip; the differential pressure ($p_s - p_o$) decreases along the surface of a round nosed tube and even becomes less than the static pressure (lower curve) Fig. 13.15b. But the effect of the stem,· at right angle to the stream, is to produce an excess pressure head, which diminishes upstream from the stem (upper curve II). If the piezometric orifice on the side of the tube is located where the excess pressure produced by stem equals negative pressure caused by the flow around the nose (and along the tube), the true static pressure will be obtained. Prandtl's tube (with standard proportions) measures the velocity accurately. Another feature of this tube is that it can measure the velocity correctly even if the tube is aligned at ± 15° from flow direction. Still greater insensitivity to angularity of flow may be obtained by flow past the Pitot tube by providing a shroud or cover. Such an arrangement is called a Kiel's probe, Fig. 13.15c. In this instrument, a separate arrangement is made to measure the static pressure. Such a device is used exclusively in aeronautics (science of the study of air). It measures stagnation pressure within 1% accuracy. The instrument can be used for yaw angle upto ±54°.

The mean velocity through a pipe may be measued by dividing the cross section of pipe into segments of equal area and measuring the velocity at the centre of these segments at two points located at opposite ends of the diameter.

In case of open channels, the section is divided into segments and the velocity traverse is taken along the vertical section at the centre of each segment. The area of the velocity diagram yields the discharge per unit width (q) of the channel. Thus, the mean velocity is determined by dividing q by the depth of flow, i.e.,

$$U_o = \frac{\text{area of velocity diagram}}{\text{Depth of flow}}$$

$$= q/y$$

Alternatively, the velocity is measued at 0.6 times the depth of flow, which is assumed to be the mean velocity of flow. The other method is to measure the velocity at 0.2 and 0.8 time the depth of flow and the mean of these two velocities gives the mean velocity.

$$U_o = \frac{U_{0.2y} + U_{0.8y}}{2}$$

The same procedure may also be followed with a currentmetre (described later)

(b) *Pitot tube placed in compressible flow.* For velocity measuement in compressible flow separate measurment of static pressure, stagnation pressure and stagnation temperature are required; First two are measured by static tube and Pitot tube respectively and the temperature is measured by temperature probe. The temperature probe consists of a small thermocouple surrounded by a jacket with open upstream end and small holes at the rear. The temperature close to the stagnation temperature is measured by means of the thermocouple. The flow may be subsonic ($N_M < 1$) or supersonic ($N_M > 1$). In case of subsonic flow past the Pilot tube the, velocity U_0 is given by

$$U_0 = \sqrt{\frac{2k}{k-1}\frac{p_0}{\rho_0}[(p_s/p_0)^{(k-1)/k} - 1]}$$

Here k is the ratio of specific heats, c_p/c_v, c_p is the specific heat at constant pressure and c_v at the constant volume.

Next consider the steady flow around the Pitot tube mounted in a supuersonic stream (Fig. 13.16) in which $N_M > 1$. It is seen that there is a short region forward of the stagnation point of the Pitot in which there is a normal compression shock. Across this shock wave there is a pressure rise from the upstream static pressure p_0 to p_1 (just behine the shock) while N_{M0}. changes from N_{M0} (>1) to subsonic value N_{M1} (<1). The pressure p_1 and N_{M1} for subsonic flow behind shock wave are given by

NORMAL SHOCK WAVE

$\dfrac{U_0}{P_0}$ N_{Mo}

P_s PILOT

13.16. MEASUREMENT OF VELOCITY IN COMPRESSIBLE FLOW

$$\frac{p_1}{p_0} = \frac{1 + kN_{Mo}^2}{1 + kN_{M1}^2} \qquad \qquad ...(13.49)$$

$$N_{M1}^2 = \frac{N_{Mo}^2(k-1) + 2}{2k\,N_{Mo}^2 - k + 1} \qquad \qquad ...(13.50)$$

The stagnation pressue p_s at point C is given by

$$\frac{p_s}{p_1} = \left[1 + \frac{k-1}{2}N_{M1}^2\right]^{k/(k-1)} \qquad \qquad ...(13.51)$$

Combining Eq. 13.49 and 13.51

$$\frac{p_s}{p_1} = N_{Mo}^2 \left(\frac{k+1}{2}\right)^{k/(k-1)}$$

$$\times \left[\frac{2k\,N_{Mo} - k + 1}{N_{Mo}^2(k+1)}\right]^{[1 - k/(k+1)]} \qquad ...(13.52)$$

The Mach number or the approaching velocity U_0 can be computed from Eq. 13.52.

(c) *Hot wire anemometer.* This device can be used to measure the velocity of flow at any point, even in the region where Pitot tube cannot be used such as in boundary layer, corners of duct, etc. The fluctuating component of velocities (or related quantities like turbulent shear, etc.) can also be measured by this instrument as it has a very quick response to changes of velocity.

The device (Fig 13.17) consiss of a short length of fine platinum or tungston wire (d = 0.01 mm or so) mounted in a probe. This probe forms an arm of a wheatstone-bridge. The wire is heated by electric current and placed in the flow at desired point. As the fluid flows past the wire, it cools down the wire and changes its resisance. This will simultanously changes the current/voltage across the wire. In one method, a constant current is allowed through the wire and hence the change in voltage is a direct measure of the velocity of flow, Fig. 13.17b. In the second method, a constant voltage is applied across the wire and hence the corresponding, variation in current will indicate the fluid velocity, Fig. 13.17c. The instrument is precalibrated in the known velocity of same fluid by means of Pitot tube (as the density of fluid also varies with the temperature).

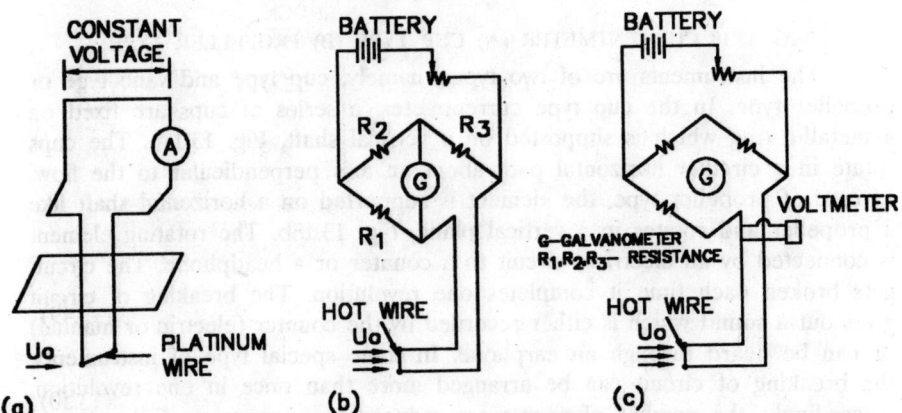

FIG. 13.17. HOT WIRE ANEMOMETER (A) BASIC PRINCIPLE (B) CONSTANT VOLTAGE (C) CONSTANT CURRENT HOT WIRE ANEMOMETER

The instrument cannot be used with much success in liquid as the gas bubbles and solid particles stick to the wire and disturbs its calibration. Hence in liquids, instead of this instrument another instrument known as hot film anemometer is used for measuring turbulent velocity fluctuations; the film acting as a continuous media. For its details refer else-where.

2. Velocity measurement in channels

There are various methods of velocity measurement in an open channel; only two methods, namely anemometer or currentmeter and salt velocity method, are disscussed here.

(a) *Anemometer.* The instruments used for air velocity is known as anemometer and that used for water is known as currentmeter, Fig. 13.18. These instruments consist of a rotating element, supported over a shaft and a counter or head phone to count the rotation of the element. The instrument works on the principle that the drag force exerted by the fluid on the rotating element depends on the density of the fluid as well as on its velocity. The anemometer must be made to operate with minimum friction.

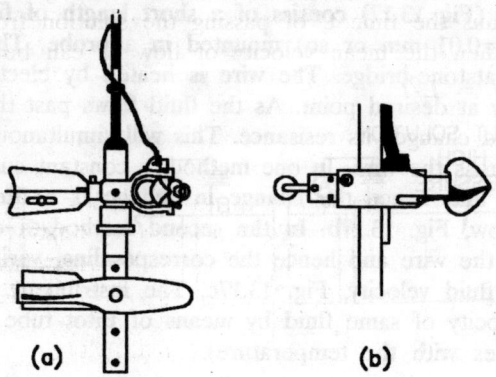

(a)   (b)

FIG. 13.18 CURRENTMETER (A) CUP TYPE ,(B) PROPELLER TYPE

The instruments are of two types, namely, cup type and vane type or propeller type. In the cup type currentmeter, a series of cups are fixed on a metallic ring which is supported on a vertical shaft, Fig. 13.18a. The cups rotate in a circular horizontal path about an axis perpendicular to the flow. In case of propeller type, the element is supported on a horizontal shaft like a propeller and rotates in a vertical plane, Fig. 13.18b. The rotating element is connected by an electrical circuit to a counter or a headphone. The circuit gets broken each time it completes one revolution. The breaking of circuit gives out a sound which is either recorded by the counter (electric or manual) or can be heard through an earphone. In some special type of instruments, the breaking of circuit can be arranged more than once in one revolution. Accordingly, the number of counts are reduced by appropriate factor (equal to the number of counts the circuit breaks in one revolution). The instrument is calibrated before hand in the stream of known velocity or in a laboratory flume and its calibration coefficient C is determined. While using the meter, only the number of counts are observed and multiplied by the coefficient, C.

$$U = CN \qquad \text{...(13.53)}$$

The calibration curve is prepared which a plot between N (r.p.m.) and the velocity of flow U (in metre per second).

The cup type instrument has an advantage that the cups rotate in the same direction and at the same rate regardless of the direction of velocity whether positive or negative. Therefore, this is not suitable where there are eddies. The propeller type registers the component of the velocity along its axis. It will rotate in opposie direction for negative flow and is thus more dependable type of meter.

(b) *Salt velocity method.* In this method, two electrodes with an electrical circuit containing a battery and an ammeter are placed at some distance apart, say L. The ammeter indicates a null point in the beginning. A concentrated dose of salt solution is now suddenly introduced in the flow from an upsream point. As soon as the salt solution crosses the electrodes, the ammeter shows the deflection. Thus the time t, of passing the solution from A to B can be noticed and then the mean velocity of flow U can be determined.

$$U = L/t$$

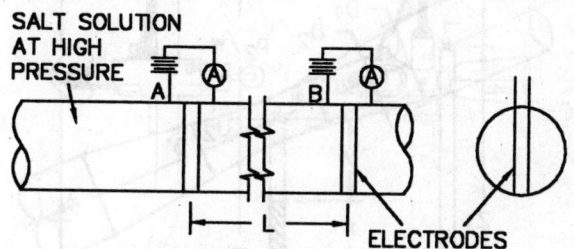

FIG. 13.19. SALT VELOCITY METHOD

13.11 MEASUREMENT OF DISCHARGE

The discharge through a pipe can be measured either by direct volumetric or weight measurements or by means of the various discharge measuring devices. Some of these devices are (i) Venturimeter (ii) Flow nozzle (iii) Orificemeter and (iv) Elbowmeter. Each one of them are described in this section.

The discharge flowing in a channel can be measured by means of weirs and notches which are described in the next section.

1. Venturimeter.

The instrument is named after Venturi, an Italian who investigated its principle. It functions on the principle that the local reduction in pressure is produced with contraction of flow. Clemens Hershel (1842-1930) developed this instrument to measure the discharge.

It consists of an **upstream** section of the same size as the pipe, and which has a bronze liner and contains a piezometric ring for the measurement of static pressure, a converging conical section, a cylindrical throat with a bronze liner containing a piezometric ring, and a gradually diverging conical section leading to the cylindrical section of the size of pipe (Fig. 13.20). A differential gauge or pressure gauges are attached to the pressure tappings at 1 and 2. The size of the venturimeter is specified by the diameter of pipe and diameter of throat, e.g. 10 cm × 5 cm, etc. The ratio of throat diameter D_2, to entrance section diameter D_1 i.e. D_2/D_1 gives larger difference of pressure between these two sections. However, the low pressure of the throat may cause cavitation and hence D_2 can only be reduced to a finite value.

The angle of convergence is 20° whereas the angle of divergence may be from 5° to 7°. The smaller angle of divergence is needed so that the decelerating flow in the diverging cone is not separated from the walls.

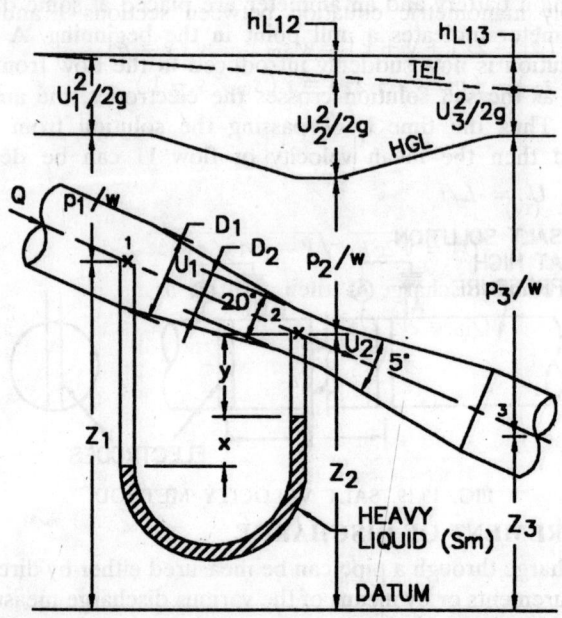

FIG. 13.20. FLOW THROUGH AN VENTURIMENTER

To ensure accurate measurements, the meter should be installed downstream of a straight and uniform pipe; the length should be free from fittings, misalignment and any other source that may cause large scale turbulence in the flow. The length of straight pipe should be at least 30 times diameter and preferably 50 times its diameter. Straightening vanes may also be provided upstream of the meter to further reduce rotational motion in the flow.

Consider a liquid of specific gravity s flowing through a venturimeter inclined at an anle θ to the horizontal. Let the discharge flowing through it be Q and the diameters at inlet and throat be D_1 and D_2 respectively (Fig. 13.20). The difference of pressue between 1 and 2 is measured by means of a U-tube manometer conaining a heavy liquid of specific density s_m. (In case of inverted U-tube, a lighter liquid is used). The inlet and throat sections are situated a height of z_1 and z_2 from an arbitrary datum.

Applying Bernoulli's theorem between 1 and 2.

$$\frac{p_1}{ws} + z_1 + \alpha \frac{U_1^2}{2g} = \frac{p_2}{ws} + z_2 + \alpha_2 \frac{U_2^2}{2g} + losses. \qquad ...(i)$$

Neglecting losses and assuming $\alpha_1 = \alpha_2 \approx 1.0$,

$$(U_2^2 - U_1^2)/2g = (p_1/ws + z_1) - (p_2/ws + z_2) \qquad ...(ii)$$

From continuity equation, $U_1 A_1 = U_2 A_2$ ...(iii)

From Eqs. (ii) and (iii),

$$U_2^2/2g \, (1 - A_2^2/A_1^2) = (p_1/ws + z_1) - (p_2/ws + z_2) = h \quad \text{(say)} \quad \text{...(iv)}$$

Now apply manometric equation between sections 1 and 2,

$$p_1 + w s \left[(z_1 - z_2) + y + x \right] = w s_m x - w s y = p_2$$

or

$$(p_1/ws + z_1) - (p_2/ws + z_2) = x(s_m/s - 1)$$

or

$$h = x\left(\frac{S_m}{s} - 1\right) \qquad \text{...(v)}$$

From Eq. (iv)

$$U_2 = \sqrt{2gh}/\sqrt{1 - (A_2/A_1)^2}$$

The theoretical discharge is then written as

$$Q_{th} = A_2 \, U_2$$

$$= \frac{A_1 A_2 \sqrt{2g \, h}}{\sqrt{A_1^2 - A_2^2}} \qquad \text{...(13.54a)}$$

Substituting the value of h from Eq. (v)

$$Q_{th} = A_1 A_2 \frac{\sqrt{2g \times x \, (s_m/s - 1)}}{\sqrt{A_1^2 - A_2^2}} \qquad \text{...(13.54b)}$$

The actual discharge flowing through the venturimeter will be slightly less than given by Eq. 13.54b, since the energy losses have not been considered. Using C_v as the coefficient of velocity, and C_c as the coefficient of contraction at section 2 (which is unity),

$$Q = \frac{C_d A_1 A_2 \sqrt{2g \, h}}{\sqrt{A_1^2 - A_2^2}} \qquad \text{...(13.55a)}$$

where coefficient of discharge $C_d = C_c \cdot C_v = C_v$

It can also be written as

$$Q = C_d \, C \sqrt{h} \qquad \text{...(13.55b)}$$

Here $C = A_1 A_2 \sqrt{2g}/\sqrt{A_1^2 - A_2^2}$ is known as 'meter constant' and it depends only on the, geometric dimensions of the meter.

Considering the energy loss, h_L, through the meter, Eq. 13.55b can be written as

$$Q = C \sqrt{h - h_L} \qquad \text{...(13.56)}$$

Equating Eq. 13.55b and 13.56

$$Q = C_d \, C \sqrt{h} = C \sqrt{h - h_L}$$

$$C_d = \sqrt{1 - h_L/h} \qquad \text{...(13.57a)}$$

Alternatively,

$$h_L = h(1 - C_d^2) = h(1 - C_v^2) \qquad \text{...(13.57b)}$$

The ratio of h_L/h is the fraction of energy lost in the meter and hence C_d can be computed if h_L/h is known. This loss is ordinarily 0.1 to 0.2 times h and mostly occurs in the diverging cone.

The value of C_d varies in the range of 0.95 to 0.99. Dimensional analysis shows that C_d is a function of Reynolds number at throat, inside surface roughness of venturimeter and the ratio D_2/D_1. The variation of C_d with R_e for various D_2/D_1 for turbulent flow is shown in Fig. 13.21. With increase in smoothness of the internal surface of the meter, the value of C_d also increases. The value of C_d may be more than unity for venturimeters that are unusually smoth inside. It does not mean that there are no energy loses through the venturimeter. The reason for $C_d > 1$ is that α_1 and α_2 have been assumed to be unity whereas $\alpha_1 > \alpha_2$. The velocity distribution at section 2 is nearly uniform and at section 1 it is not so. This causes a higher velocity at section 1 than what has been assumed at 1.

From Eqs. (i) and (iii)

$$U_1' = A_2 \sqrt{2gh} \; / \; \sqrt{A_1^2 - \alpha_2 A_2^2} \qquad \qquad ...(vi)$$

It is obvious that U_1' given by Eq. (vi) is larger than given by Eq. (ii)

$$U_1 > U_1' \qquad \qquad ...(13.58)$$

Usually the meter is pre-calibrated (i.e., its Cd is determined)

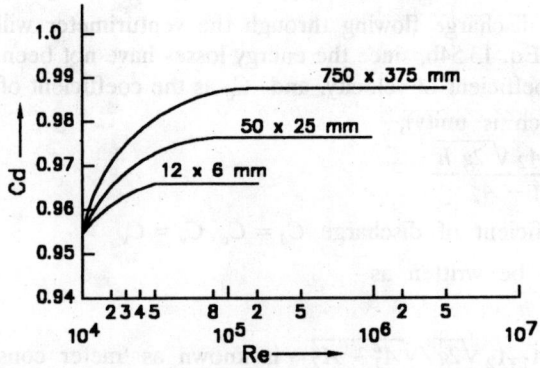

FIG. 13.21 VARIATION OF Cd WITH Re

2. Flow Nozzles

Nozzles are used for the creation of jets in engineering practice and when these are placed in the pipe line or at its ends to measure the discharge,these are known as flow nozzles. As illustrated in Fig. 13.22a, the flow nozzle may be regarded as a venturimeter without gradually tappering diffuser on the outlet side. Hence, the jet of water coming out of short cylindrical tip remains unguided and this entails greater energy loss in the nozzle as compared to venturimeter. The differential pressures between 1 and 2 is measured by means of different arranement of pressure gauges in the nozzles of different shapes. In the flow nozzles of different shapes, different arrangement of piezometric openings are made. There are various designs of flow nozzles that are in use, e.g. VDI (Varein Deutscher Ingenieure) nozzles, ISA nozzles (International Standards Association nozzles), etc. Eq. 13.55a for the venturimeter can also be used for the flow nozzles, namely,'

$$Q = \frac{C_d A_1 A_2}{\sqrt{A_1^2 - A_2^2}} \sqrt{2gh} \qquad \qquad ...(13.55a)$$

In a few cases, some of the terms are regrouped and the equation is written as

$$Q = K A_2 \sqrt{2g\ h} \qquad \qquad ...(13.59)$$

where $K = C_d / \sqrt{1 - (A_2 / A_1)^2}$ \qquad \qquad ...(13.60)

is known as flow coefficient. The dimensionless term $1/\sqrt{1-(A_2/A_1)^2}$ is commonly called the velocity of approach factor. The dimensional analysis and dynamic similarity show that K is function of Reynolds number of approach flow ($U_1 D_1/\nu$), nozzle dimensions (i.e. D_2/D_1), nozzle shape and the head under which the flow takes place. A typical variation is shown in Fig. 13.22b.

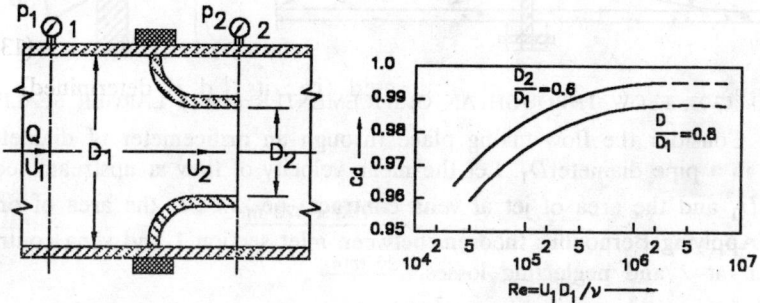

FIG. 13.22. FLOW NOZZLE AND VARIATION OF Cd WITH $U_1 D_1/\nu$

3. Orificemeter

It is the most simple device frequently used for measuring the discharge of liquid. A thin plate with a concentric circular hole cut in it, is clamped between the flanges of the pipeline as shown in Fig. 13.23. The edges of the orifice are bevelled or squared so as to minimise friction losses. As discussed in case of orifices (section 13.4) the stream-lines curve or converge as they approach the orifice opening, bend around the edge of the hole, and continue to curve and converge beyond the orifice. At some distance from the plane of the orifice, the jet has minimum area which is the section of vena contracta. Usually, it lies at 0.5 times the pipe diameter from the upstream face of the plate. The distance to the venacontracta is not a constant but decreases as D_2/D_1 increases. The static pressure connections are made on both sides of the plate. The inlet or upstream tap is located at a point between 0.5 times the pipe diameter and 2 times the pipe diameter from upstream face of the plate; commonly a distance of one pipe diameter is employed. The centre of downstream pressue tap is placed at the minimum pressure location, which is assumed to be at vena contracta. In some arrangements, the pressure connections are casted as an integral part of orifice plate and are located at 2.5 cm from upstream and downstream faces of the plate.

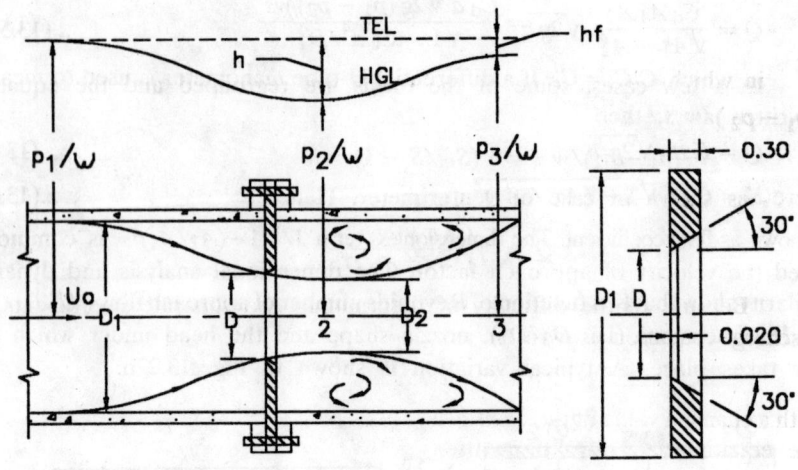

FIG. 13.23. FLOW THROUGH AN ORIFICEMENTER (TO A LARGER SCALE)

Consider the flow taking place through an orificemeter of diameter d fitted in a pipe diameter D_1. Let the mean velocity of flow at upstream section 1 be U_1 and the area of jet at vena contracta be A_2. Let the area of orifice be a. Applying Bernoulli's theorem between inlet section 1 and vena contracta section at 2 and neglecting losses,

$$p_1/ws + U_1^2/2g = p_2/ws + U_2^2/2g \qquad \text{...(i)}$$

From continuity equation

$$U_1 \pi D_1^2/4 = U_2 \, \pi D_2^2/4 \qquad \text{...(ii)}$$

The coefficient of contraction $C_c = A_2/a \, (D_2/d)^2$ and therefore, the continuity equation yields

$$U_1 = C_c \, (d^2/D_1^2) \, U_2 \qquad \text{(iii)}$$

Eleminating U_1 from Eqs. (i) and (iii)

$$U_2^2/2g \, [\, 1 - C_c^2 \, (d/D_1)^4 \,] = (p_1 - p_2)/ws$$

$$U_2 = \frac{\sqrt{2g \, (p_1 - p_2)/ws}}{\sqrt{1 - C_c^2 \, d^4/D_1^4}} \qquad \text{...(13.61)}$$

The actual velocity at vena contracta is $U_{2a} = C_v \, U_2$

$$U_2 = C_v \, \frac{\sqrt{2g \, (p_1 - p_2)/ws}}{\sqrt{1 - C_c^2 \, d^4/D_1^4}} \qquad \text{...(13.62)}$$

The discharge is then determined from continuity equation.

$$Q = a_2 \, U_{2a}$$

$$Q = C_c \, a \, U_{2a}$$

$$= \frac{C_c \, a \, C_v \sqrt{2g \, (p_1 - p_2)/ws}}{\sqrt{1 - C_c^2 \, d^4/D_1^4}}$$

$$= \frac{C_d \, a \, \sqrt{2g \, (p_1 - p_2)/ws}}{\sqrt{1 - C_c^2 \, d^4/D_1^4}} \qquad \ldots(13.63a)$$

in which $C_c C_v = C_d$. If a differential U-tube manometer is used to measure $(p_1 - p_2)/w \; s$, then

$$(p_1 - p_2)/w \; s = x \, (S_m/S - 1) = h \qquad \ldots(13.64)$$

as shown in case of venturimeter. Hence,

$$Q = \frac{C_d \, a \, \sqrt{2g \, h}}{\sqrt{1 - C_c^2 \, d^4/D_1^4}}$$

Because of the difficulty of determining two separate coefficients, the discharge equation is written as

$$Q = C_{d1} \, a \, \sqrt{2g \, h/ \, [1 - d^4/D_1^4]} \qquad \ldots(13.64)$$

with a changed value of the coefficients of discharge. For the ease of computation, the equation may also be written as

$$Q = K_1 \, a \, \sqrt{2gh}$$

where $\qquad K_1 = C_{d1} \, / \, \sqrt{1 - d^4/D_1^4} \qquad \ldots(13.66)$

Any of the form of discharge formula can be used for the determination of discharge. The discharge coefficient (C_{d_1} or K_1) may be known by fitting the plate in place and calibrating it as usual.

The coefficient of discharge depends on Reynolds number $U_1 D_1/\nu_1$, the ratio d/D_1 and finish of the plate and surface of the plate, for Re in the rane of 10^3 to 10^4. At higher Reynolds number, the viscous effects are damped out and C_d is influenced only by d/D_1 and shape of the orifice and at low Reynolds number the inertia forces are less predominant and hence C_d is effected only by Reynolds number. A typical variation of C_d with R_e and d/D_1 is shown in Fig. 13.24. As in case of venturimeter, for

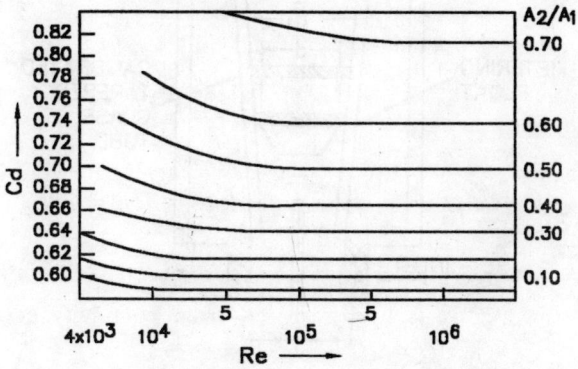

FIG. 13.24. VARIATION OF COEFFICIENT OF DISCHARGE
WITH REYNOLDS NUMBERS

accurate measurements the orifice plate should be preceded by a straight length of pipe (nearly 50 pipe diameters).

4. Elbowmeter

An elbow fitted in a pipe can also be used as a flow measuring device. Sometimes, the elbowmeter can be quite convenient and economical. Two pressure connections are made on the inner and outer curves of the elbow and are connected to a differential gauge. The centrifugal or dynamical action of the fluid on flowing in a curved path causes a difference of pressure between inner and outer curves of the elbow; being higher static pressure at the outer curve. The elbow should be preceded by sufficient length of straight pipe. Lansford has done sufficient amount of experimental work on various type of 90° bends. The basic equation proposed by him is

$$C_1 (U^2/2g) = (p_1 w + z_1) - (p_2/w + z_2) = h \qquad ...(13.67)$$

The coefficient C_1 varies from 1.3 to 3.2, the magnitude depending on the size and shape of the elbow. The discharge may, then, be computed from continuity equaton.

$$Q = A U$$
$$= A \sqrt{2g h} / \sqrt{C_1}$$
$$= C A \sqrt{2g h} \qquad ...(13.68)$$

The value C is determined by calibrating the elbowmeter in advance.

5. Rotameter

It consists of a transparent tapered tube which is held vertical with larger opening at the top and a rotating free 'float' (actually heavier than the liquid). Notches are made in the float which causes it to rotate and thus

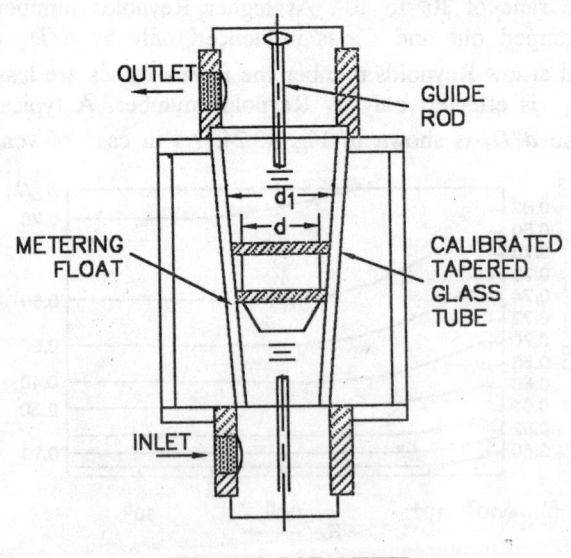

FIG. 13.25 ROTAMETER

maintain its central position in the tube, Fig. 13.25. The fluid passes vertically upwards through the tube. With no flow, the float rests on a stop on the lower end. With flow taking place in the pipe, the float rises towards the upper, larger diameter of the tube. There is a corresponding position for each flow which is obtained by its pre-calibration. This meter is sometimes known as area type of meter, because the variable annular space is provided between float and tube.

13.12. WEIRS AND NOTCHES

A weir or notch may be used for measurement of the flow of liquid in an open channel. The weir, in effect, is 'any regular obstruction over which the liquid is made to flow'. An opening made in a thin sheet of metal, masonry or any other material through which liquid flows in such a way that the jet springs free of its upstream face (actually there is a line contact between the jet over the opening) is known as notch. The jet of water flowing over the weir or (notch) is known as nappe and top surface of a weir is known as 'crest'. If the wall thickness of obstruction is sufficiently large to support the nappe, it is known as weir. The overflow section of a dam is 'a special type of weir known as spillway which can also be used as flow measuring device.

The flow over weir is caused due to the difference of water level on its upstream and downstream sides. If the water level on downstream is below the crest, the nappe springs 'free on to the downsream side. Such a weir is called a freely flowing weir or free weir. If the water level on downstream side is above the crest of weir so that the nappe is partially submerged the weir is known as 'submerged weir'. The other classification is made on the basis of the shape of opening or notch, e.g. rectangular weir, triangular notch (or V-notch), trapezoidal weir, etc. Generally, the crest of the notches are made sharp and are known as sharp edged notches.

While analysing the weir flow, the following assumptions need to be made; (i) the velocity distribution on the upstream side of the weir is uniform, (ii) the pressure in the nappe is zero, (iii) the fluid particles move horizontally as they flow over the weir crest and (iv) the effect of viscosity, surface tension, turbulence and secondary flows may be neglected.

'Consider the flow taking over a sharp edged weir as shown in Fig. 13.26. The upstream face of the weir plate should be smooth and the plate should be strictly vertical. The crest should have a square upstream edge, a top width of 1.5 mm to 3.0 mm and a bavel on the downsream side so that the nappe springs clear, making a line contact for all heads. While the flow approaches the weir, it is contracted and the water surface is lowered by 0.15 H. The head causing the flow is measured above the weir crest at least at a distance of 4 H from upstream face. The approach channel should be long enough so that velocity distribution above the crest is as shown in Fig. 13.26. Let the the height of weir be P. Various other dimensions of the nappe are also depicted in Fig. 13.26. It is also observed that periodic spirals are formed just upstream of the crest and near the base of the weir. The periodic spiral also influences the flow over the weir in an uppredictable manner. Thus, it is evident that the discharge over the weir depends on the form of crest and sides of weir, height of weir, width of approach channel, length of weir and head over the crest.

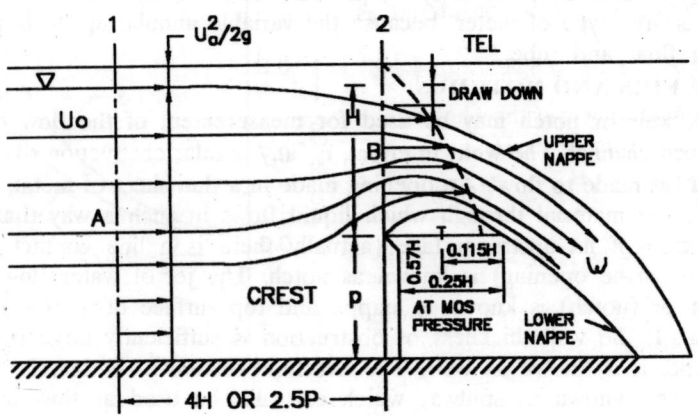

FIG. 13.26 VELOCITY AND PRESSURE DISTRIBUTION OVER A SHARPE CRESTED WEIR

1. Rectangular weir

Consider a sharp edged rectangular weir of length 'L' and height 'P' installed in a channel of width L_1. Let the head over the crest be H measured at some distance upstream, i.e. at section A. When the flow takes place, the nappe is contracted sideways as shown in Fig. 13.27. Take a small strip of thickness dh at a depth h below free water surface. It is assumed that the water level is not lowered at the nappe. The discharge passing through this elementry strip is δQ. Applying Bernoulli's equation between 1 and 2,

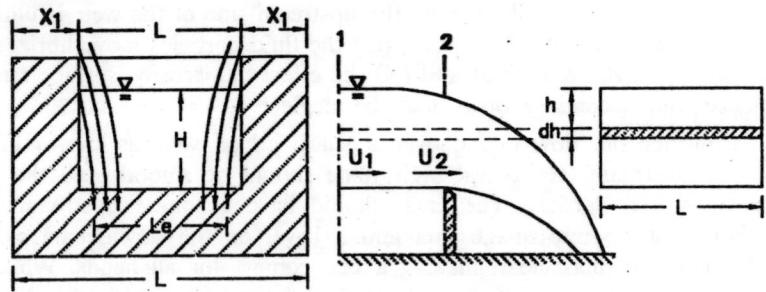

FIG. 13.27. FLOW OVER A RECTANGULAR WEIR

$$H + \frac{U_1^2}{2g} = (H - h) + \frac{U_2^2}{2g} + \text{losses(neglected)}$$

$$U_2 = \sqrt{2g(h - U_1^2/2g)} \qquad \qquad ...(13.69)$$

Application of continuity equation yields,

$$\delta Q = a_2 U_2$$

$$= L\, dh\, \sqrt{2g\, (h - U_1^2/2g)}$$

When the velocity of approach with which water approaches the weir from section 1 to 2 is considered as small,

$$\delta Q = L\, dh\, \sqrt{2gh} \quad ...(13.70)$$

Integrating over the whole range of H, i.e., from 0 to H,

$$\int \delta Q = \int_0^H L\, dh\, \sqrt{2g\, h}$$

$$Q = \frac{2}{3}\sqrt{2g}\, L\, H^{3/2} \quad ...(13.71)$$

Some of the energy of flowing liquid is always lost in traversing from 1 to 2, hence it is accounted for by using C_v. At the same time, the nappe is contracted and area at nappe becomes less than normal area. Using coefficient of contraction C_c.

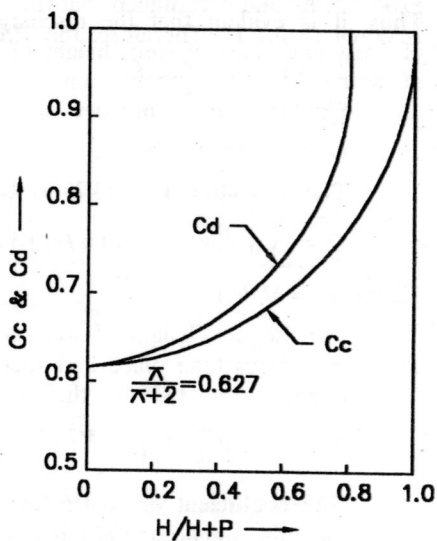

FIG. 13.28 VARIATION OF C_c AND C_d WITH $H/(H+P)$ FOR SHARP CRESTED WEIR

$$Q = \frac{2}{3}C_c\, C_v\, \sqrt{2g}\, L\, H^{3/2}$$

or $\quad Q = \frac{2}{3}C_d\, \sqrt{2g}\, L\, H^{3/2}$ $\qquad\qquad$ ...(13.72)

If the velocity of approach is appreciable and cannot be neglected, the integration of Eq. 13.70 is done from h_a to $H + h_a$. The velocity of approach head,

$$h_a = U_1^2/2g \qquad\qquad ...(13.73)$$

and $\qquad\qquad U_1 = Q/[L_1(P + H)] \qquad\qquad$ (13.74)

Therefore $\displaystyle\int \delta Q = \int_{h_a}^{H+h_a} C_d\, \sqrt{2g}\, L\, h^{1/2}\, dh$

$$Q = \frac{2}{3}C_d\, \sqrt{2g}\, [(H + h_a)^{3/2} - h_a^{3/2}] \qquad ...(13.75)$$

The velocity of approach correction is made by trial. Initially the head h_a is omitted and discharge Q is determined. Then the velocity of approach is calculated by Eq. 13.74 and hence $h_a\ (= \propto U_1^2/2g)$. Now the discharge is recalculated. The procedue is repeated till previous Q is same as calculated in the next step. The energy correction factor α varies from 1.01 to 1.15. Usually, it is assumed to be unity.

Francis Formula

As explained earlier, the jet is contracted sideways due to the presence of the side of the weir and a correction is applied. Francies (1815-1892) conducted experiments and determined that the contraction by each end of an obstruction is equal to 0.1 H. Therefore, the effective length of flow of a weir becomes

$$L_e = L - 2 \times 0.1\,H \qquad \qquad ...(13.76a)$$

Similarly, for n number of end contractions,

$$L_e = (L - 0.1\,n\,H)$$

The discharge Eq. 13.75 is then modified as

$$Q = \frac{2}{3}C_d\sqrt{2g}\,(L - 0.1\,n\,H_1)\,[\,(H + h_a)^{3/2} - h_a^{3/2}\,] \qquad ...(13.77)$$

Here $H_1 = H + h_a$

In case, the length of weir is equal to the width of the channel, no end contractions take place and such weirs are known as 'suppressed weirs.' The discharge Eq. 13.77 is then written as

$$Q = \frac{2}{3}C_d\sqrt{2g}\,L\,[\,H_1^{3/2} - ha^{3/2}\,] \qquad ...(13.78)$$

The coefficient of contraction C_c and coefficient of discharge C_d are shown plotted against $H/(H + P)$ in Fig. 13.28.

The C_d is given by

$$C_d = 0.611 + 0.075\,H/P \qquad ...(13.79)$$

At low heads, the discharge is also affected by the viscosity and surface tension. Ranga Raju and Asawa have found from their experimental investigations that the correction K (to account for these forces) is related to $R_e^{0.2}\,N_w^{0.6}$; Reynolds number R_e being given by $g^{1/2}\,H^{3/2}/v$ and Weber number by $N_w = \rho\,gH^2/\sigma$.

hence $\qquad\qquad Q_1 = K\,Q \qquad\qquad\qquad ...(13.79)$

Some of the values of K for rectangular and triangular weirs are given in Table 13.1

Table 13.1. Correction factor K

$R_e^{0.2}\,N_w^{0.6}$	30	60	100	200	400	600	1000
K	1.27	1.20	1.16	1.09	1.04	1.01	1.0

Calibration. A weir to be used needs calibration before it is installed. The discharge Q is then expressed as a function H.

$$Q = K\,H^n$$

Take log on both sides

$$\log\,Q = n\,\log H + \log K \qquad ...(13.81)$$

where K and n are unknown. The discharge is measured by volumetric or any other device and head H is measured by means of gauges (point gaguge or hook gauge). For various sets of head H, the corresponding Q is determined. A plot of Q versus H on log- log graph then gives a straight line. The slope of this line gives the value of n and the intercept on the Q scale gives the value of K.

Ventilation. For the discharge over the rectangular weir, in the above theory, it is assumed that the pressure remains atmospheric on the upper and lower sides of the nappe. In case of contracted weir, the air enters the underside of the nappe from its sides. In case of suppressed weir, the air present below nappe is entrapped in the flowing jet of water and hence the pressure on the underside of it becomes less than atmospheric. The nappe starts fluctuating and finally clings to the downstream face of weir. The reduced pressue below nappe causes increased effective head on the jet of water and hence the discharge flowing over the crest is increased. Proper ventilation holes are, therefore, provided on the side of channel to supply the air below the nappe. The maximum amount of air required is

$$q_a = 0.1 \, q / (H_p / H)^{1.5} \qquad \qquad \text{...(13.82)}$$

in which q_a and q are rates of flow of air and waer in $m^3/$ sec per mere of weir length, H is the head on the weir and H_p is the depth of water on the downstream side of weir. Hickox (1944) has made experimenal investigation on this aspect of the flow.

Other formulae. Various investigators have modified Eq. 13.77 for the discharge. Some of them are given here.

(a) Francis formula : Francis assumed a constant value of 0.623 for C_d in Eq. 13.77 and combined $2/3 \, C_d \sqrt{2g}$ to obtain one constant. The discharge equation is then written as

$$Q = 1.84 \, (L - 0.1 \, n \, H_1) \, (H_1^{3/2} - ha^{3/2}) \qquad \text{...(13.83)}$$

It is known as **Francis formula** for the contracted weir and is sometimes used for ready calculation.

(b) **Bazin's formula**

$$Q = (0.405 + 0.003/H_1) \sqrt{2g} \, L \, H_1^{3/2} \qquad \text{...(13.84)}$$

where $H_1 = H + \propto U_1^2/2g$ ...(13.85)

and $\propto = 1.6$ ...(13.86)

(c) Rehbock formula :

$$Q = (1.782 + 0.24 \, H_e/\rho) \, L \, [H_e^{3/2}] \qquad \text{...(13.87)}$$

without velocity of approach.

$H_e = (H + 0.0011) \; metre$ ...(13.88)

3. Triangular weir

A triaangular weir is V-shaped weir, cut from a thin metallic plate and is symmetrical about its apex. Its edges are made sharp on the inner side. This type of weir is useful for measuring discharge even at low head. Since the width of flow is small, ventilation of nappe is not necessary.

Consider the flow occurring over a triangular weir, of apex angle 2θ, under head H. Take an elementry strip of width 2 x and height dh at a depth h below free water surface, Fig. 13.29.

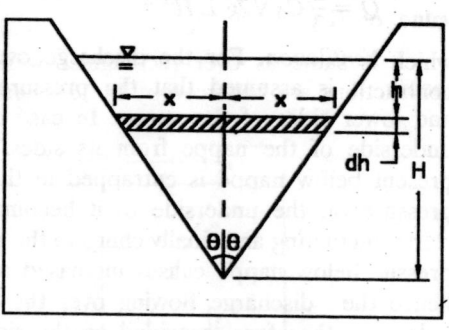

The discharge through the elementry strip is δQ.

$$\delta Q = (2 x d h)(\sqrt{2gh})$$

The width of strip is given as

$$x = (H - h)\tan\theta$$

Therefore,

$$\delta Q = 2(H - h)\tan\theta\sqrt{2g}\sqrt{h}\ dh$$

FIG. 13.29. FLOW OVER TRIANGULAR WEIR

Integrating the equation between limits 0 and H

$$\int dQ = 2\sqrt{2g}\tan\theta\int_0^H (H - h)\sqrt{h}\ dh$$

$$Q = (8/15)\sqrt{2g}\tan\theta\,[H^{5/2}]$$

Using the coefficient of discharge C_d

$$Q = 8/15\ C_d\sqrt{2g}\tan\theta\ H^{5/2} \qquad\qquad ...(13.89)$$

For a right angled V-notch,

$$Q = 8/15\ C_d\sqrt{2g}\ H^{5/2} \qquad\qquad ...(13.90)$$

The coefficient of discharge C_d for V- notch is generally smaller than for rectangular notch. C_d for rectangular notch is nearly 0.62 whereas for traingular notch it is 0.6 or so. The effect of velocity of approach is usually neglected for the flow over V-notch, since the cross sectional area of nappe is small.

4. Trapezoidal weir

A trapezoidal weir of base width B and side slope θ is shown in Fig. 13.30. The discharge through it can be considered as occurring through a rectangular weir of width B and a triangular weir of apex angle 2θ.

$$Q_{trap} = Q_{rect} + Q_{triangular}$$

$$= \frac{2}{3}C_{d1}\sqrt{2g}(L - 0.1\ n\ H)H^{3/2} +$$

$$8/15\ C_{d2}\sqrt{2g}\tan\theta\ H^{5/2} \qquad\qquad ...(13.91a)$$

Assuming $C_{d1} = C_{d2}$ and $n = 2$,

$$Q = \frac{2}{3}C_{d1}\sqrt{2g}\ H^{3/2}[(L - 0.2H) + 4/5\tan\theta\ H] \qquad\qquad ...(13.91b)$$

Weir of side slope 1 H : 4 V' (or $\tan\theta = \frac{1}{4}$) is known as 'Cipolleti weir'. The discharge over it is given by,

$$Q = \frac{2}{3} C_d \sqrt{2g} \, L \, H^{3/2} \qquad \qquad ...(13.91c)$$

which is same as over rectangular weir. This means that the effect of end contractions are balanced by the discharge over the triangular portion of weir.

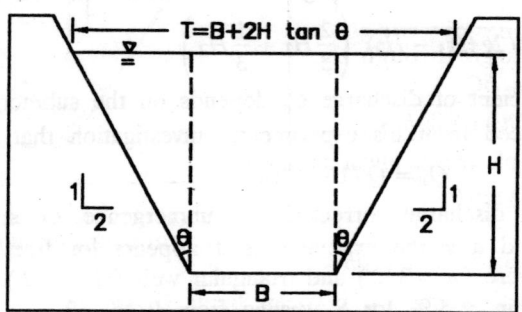

FIG. 13.30. FLOW OVER TRAPEZOIDAL WEIR

5. Submerged weir

If the water surface on the downstream side is higher than the crest of the weir (Fig. 13.31), the weir is said to be submerged weir. The ratio of head on the upstream side H_1 to water depth H_2 on the downstream side is known as 'submergence ratio $S = H_2/H_1'$. Two kinds of submergence are recongnisable, (i) the plunging nappe, in which the weir nappe is similar to the free flow but plunges to the bed of the channel which occurs at low submergence and (ii) surface nappe, in which the nappe remains on or near the surface. The water remains more or less undisturbed. It occurs at high submergence.

Consider the flow occurring over a weir with upstream and downstream heads as H_1 and H_2 respectively, Fig. 13.31. The flow over the weir may be divided into two portion, i.e. (i) discharge Q_1 occurring between head H_1 and H_2 as free weir flow and (ii) discharge Q_2 between H_2 to crest as submerged orifice flow working under a head $(H_1 - H_2)$.

Thus total $Q = Q_1 + Q_2$

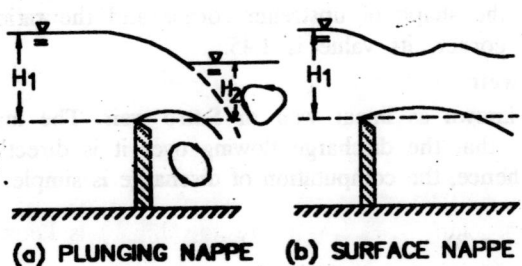

(a) PLUNGING NAPPE   (b) SURFACE NAPPE

FIG. 13.31. FLOW OVER A SUBMERGED WEIR

$$= \frac{2}{3} C_{d1} \sqrt{2g} \, L \, (H_1 - H_2)^{3/2} + C_{d2} L \, H_2 \sqrt{2g \, (H_1 - H_2)} \qquad ...(13.92)$$

If $C_d = C_{d1} = C_{d2}$, the discharge formula then becomes

$$Q = C_d L \sqrt{2g \, (H_1 - H_2)} \left[\frac{2}{3} (H_1 - H_2) + H_2 \right]$$

$$= C_d L \sqrt{2g \, (H_1 - H_2)} \left(\frac{2}{3} H_1 + \frac{1}{3} H_2 \right)$$

The coefficient of discharge C_d depends on the submergence ratio S. Villemonte deduced from his experimental investigation that

$$Q_1 = Q \, (1 - S^n)^{0.385}$$

where Q_1 is the discharge corrected for submergence, Q is the free flow over the weir and n is the exponent as it appears for free flow equation for rectangular were ($n = 3/2$) and triangular weir ($n = 5/2$). The equation yields result within ± 5 % for S varying from 0 to 0.9.

6. Broad crested weir

The weir whose crest is a flat surface in contrast to a line contact of sharp crested weir are known as broad crested weir. If the width of crest is less than 0.5 H, the nappe springs clear of it and weir functions as a sharp crested weir. In case crest width is between 0.5 H to 0.66 H, the flow conditions become unstable but if crest width is more than 0.66 H, the weir behaves as a broad crested weir. The flow approaching the weir from upstream section drops down to a minimum depth (indeed it is critical depth of flow, refer to section 12.17.) on the crest and becomes a parallel flow thereafter, see Fig. 13.32. Thus it is a critical flow meter. The discharge is given by

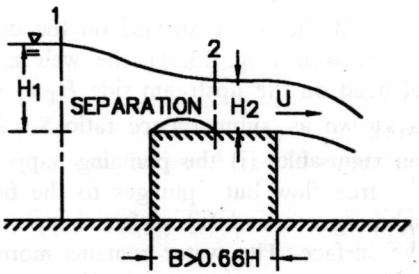

FIG. 13.32. FLOW OVER A BROAD CRESTED WEIR

$$Q = C L H^{3/2} \qquad ...(13.95)$$

The value of coefficient C is found to be 1.703 for theoretical discharge and depends on the shape of upstream corner and the ratio of L/H. For upstream square corner, its value is 1.45.

7. Proportional weir

It is also known as linear weir or Sutro weir. The major advantage of such a weir is that the discharge flowing over it is directly proportional to the head and hence, the computation of discharge is simple. The discharge equation is

$$Q = K \, (H - a/3) \qquad ...(13.96)$$

where $K = 2 \, C \, W$

The profile of the weir is defined by the Eq. 13.97.

$$(x/2W) = \left[1 - \left(\frac{2}{\pi} \right) \tan^{-1} (\sqrt{y/a}) \right] \qquad ...(13.97)$$

The value of k varies from 0.6 to 0.65. The major restriction of the weir is that head should not be lower than a/3.

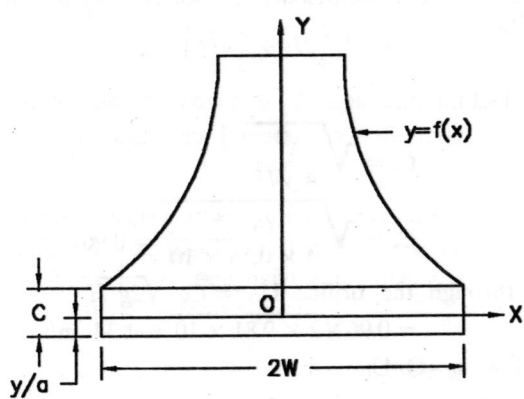

FIG. 13.33. FLOW THROUGH A PROPORTIONAL WEIR

There are many other similar proportional notches. In logarithmic notch, Q varies directly with the logarithm of head. A great amount of research work has been done at Indian Institute of Science and Technology, Banglore on the different types of weirs.

TABLE 13.2

ISI Code	Description
3818-1966	Code of practice for use of currentmeter (cup meter) for water flow
9163-1979 (Part I)	Constant rate injection method for the measurment of steady flow by dilution method
1915-1979	Estimation of incompressible fluid flow in closed conduits by bend meters
4467-1967	Methods of measurement of fluid flow by means of venturimeter
6059-1971	Liquid flow measurement in open chennels by weirs and flumes – (weirs of finite crest width for free discharge)
9108-1979	Liquid flow measurement in open channels using thin plate weir.
9117-1979	End depth method for the estimation of liquid flow measurement in open channels by weirs and flumes.
6063-1971	Method of measurement of flow in open channels using standing wave flume.
2959-1964 Part I)	Method of measurement of fluid flow by means of orifice plates and nozzles
1918-1979	Method for measurement of fluid pressure by means of manometers.

Examples : 13.1 – 13.36

13.1 Water discharges at the rate of 100 lit/s through a 12 cm diameter vertical sharp edged orifice placed under a constant head of 10 m. A point on the jet, measured from the vena-contracta, has co-ordinates 4.5 m horizontal and 0.55 m vertical. Find the coefficients of velocity, contraction and discharge for the given orifice.

Solution

From Eq. 13.14.

$$C_v = \sqrt{\frac{x^2}{4\,y\,H}}$$

$$C_v = \sqrt{\frac{(4.5)^2}{4 \times 0.55 \times 10}} = 0.96$$

Velocity of flow through the orifice $U_o = C_v \sqrt{2g\,H}$

$$= 0.96 \sqrt{2 \times 9.81 \times 10} = 1.34 \text{ m/s}$$

Actual area of flow $a_c = Q/U_o$

$$= \frac{100 \times 10^{-3}}{13.45} = 0.00743 \text{ m}^2$$

Area of the orifice $= \pi\,(0.12)^2/4 = 0.00113 \text{ m}^2$

Coefficient of contraction $C_c \quad = \dfrac{\text{area of jet}}{\text{area of opening}}$

$$= \frac{0.00743}{0.0113} = 0.657$$

Coefficient of discharge $C_d = C_v \times C_c$

$$= 0.96 \times 0.657 = 0.63$$

13.2 A 10 cm diameter orifice discharges 45 lit/s water under a head of 2.8 m. A flat plate held normal to the jet just downstream from the vena-contracta requires a force of 0.32 kN to resist the impact of the jet. Find the coefficients of discharge, velocity and contraction.

Solution

Applying momentum theorem to the jet of water,

$$F_x = w\,Q/g\,(U_{2x} - U_{1x})$$
$$= w\,Q/g\,(0 - U_o) = -(w\,Q\,U_o/g)$$

But $\qquad F_1 = -F_x = (w\,Q\,U_o/g)$

$$0.32 = \frac{9.81 \times 45 \times 10^{-3}\,U_o}{9.81} \qquad (w = 9.81 \text{ kN/m}^3)$$

$$U_0 = 7.11 \text{ m/s}$$

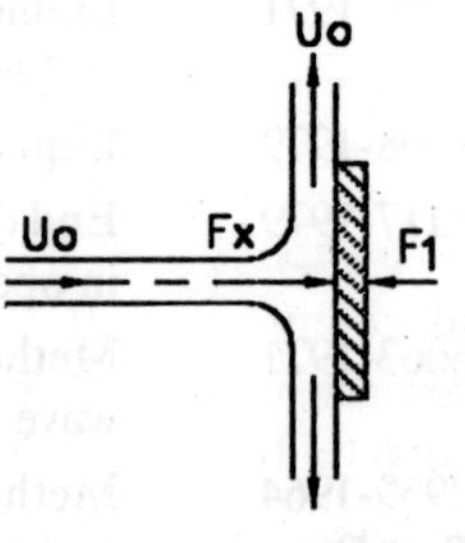

Theoretical velocity

$$U_{th} = \sqrt{2g\,H}$$

$$U_{th} = \sqrt{2 \times 9.81 \times 2.8} = 7.41 \text{ m/s}$$

FIG. 13.34. EXAMPLE 13.2

Hence $\qquad C_v = \dfrac{\text{Actual velocity}}{\text{theoretical velocity}}$

$$= \dfrac{7.11}{7.41} = 0.96$$

Theoretical discharge $\quad Q_{th} = \pi\,(0.1)^2 \times 7.41/4$

$$= 0.0581\ \text{m}^3/\text{s}$$

Hence $\qquad C_d = \dfrac{\text{Actual discharge}}{\text{theoretical velocity}}$

$$= \dfrac{0.045}{0.0581} = 0.775$$

$$C_c = C_d/C_v$$

$$= 0.775/0.96 = 0.807$$

13.3 Oil flows through a standard 25 mm diameter orifice under a 5.5 m head at the rate of 0.003 m³/s. The jet strikes a wall 1.5 m away and 0.12 m vertically below center line of the contracted section of the jet. Compute coefficients of contraction, velocity and discharge.

Solution

Given $\qquad d = 0.025$ m, $H = 5.5$ m, $Q = 0.003$ m³/s

$$x = 1.5\ \text{m},\ y = 0.12\ \text{m},$$

$$C_v = \sqrt{\dfrac{x^2}{4\,y\,H}}$$

$$= \sqrt{\dfrac{(1.5)^2}{4 \times 0.12 \times 5.5}} = 0.923$$

$$C_d = \dfrac{Q}{a\,\sqrt{2\,g\,H}}$$

$$= \dfrac{0.003}{\dfrac{\pi}{4}\,(0.025)^2 \times \sqrt{2 \times 9.81 \times 5.5}} = 0.588$$

$$C_c = \dfrac{C_d}{C_v}$$

$$= \dfrac{0.588}{0.923} = 0.637$$

13.4 A tank 3.5 m high contains oil (s = 0.9) to a height of 2.67 m and compressed air under a pressure of 25 k P_a over it. An orifice, 7.5 cm diameter fitted 5 cm above the bottom of tank discharges the oil into atmosphere. Estimate the rate volume of oil discharged per minute. Assume $C_d = 0.62$

Solution

Total head over the orifice

$$= (2.67 - 0.05) + \frac{25 \times 1000}{9810 \times 0.9}$$

$$= 5.45 \text{ m}$$

$$Q = C_d . a . \sqrt{2gH}$$

$$= 0.62 \times \frac{\pi}{4} (0.05)^2 \sqrt{2 \times 9.81 \times 5.45}$$

$$= 0.62 \times 1.9625 \times 10^{-3} \times 10.34$$

$$= 0.01258 \text{ m}^3/\text{s}$$

Discharge/min$= 0.01258 \times 60 = 0.755 \text{ m}^3/\text{min}$

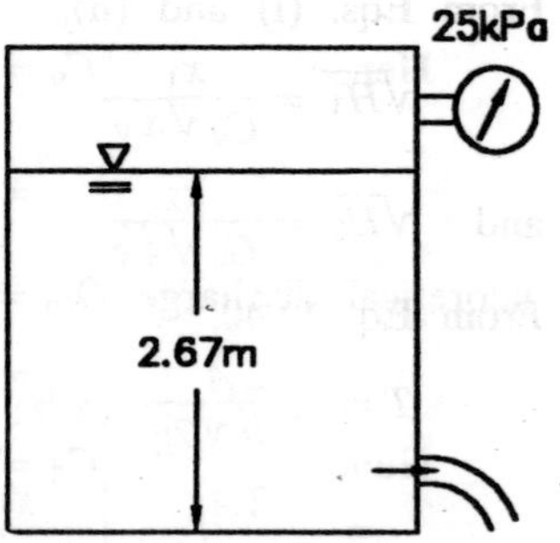

FIG. 13.35. EXAMPLE 13.4

13.5 A jet H metres below the water surface meets a horizontal plane at a point whose co-ordinates with respect to the centre of the orifice are $(a, - h)$. Show that the loss of head due to friction is $(H - a^2/4h)$.

solution

The water flows under a head H and produces a jet of velocity U. Therefore,

Loss of head due to friction $= (H - U^2/2g)$.

From Eq. 13.14a, $\quad C_v = U / \sqrt{2g H}$ ...(i)

or $\qquad U^2 /2g = C_v^2 H$ ...(ii)

From Eq. 13.14b, $\quad C_v = \sqrt{\dfrac{x^2}{4y H}} = \sqrt{\dfrac{a^2}{4Hh}}$ ...(iii)

Hence, $U^2/2g = (a^2/4 H h) H = a^2/4h$ ...(iv)

From Eqs. (i) and (iv)

$$h_L = (H - a^2/4h)$$

13.6 A cylindrical tank, 1 m in diameter, is filled with water and is provided with an orifice, $(C_d = 0.64 , C_v = 0.98)$, 5 cm in diamtar in its vertical side. Jet of water issuing out óf the orifice strikes a horizontal floor 20 cm below the centre of orifice. As the head in the tank falls, the striking jet on the floor approaches the tank. Determine the rate of approach of the tank.

Solution

Let the water stand initiatly to a height H_1 and after an interval of time T, it falls to H_2. The jet of water correspondingly shifts from x_1 (at the beginning) to x_2 at the end of T.

From Eq. 13.14b,

$$C_v = \frac{x_1}{\sqrt{4y H_1}}$$ ...(i)

also $\quad C_v = \dfrac{x_2}{\sqrt{4y H_2}}$ ...(ii)

From Eqs. (i) and (ii),

$$\sqrt{H_1} = \frac{x_1}{C_v \sqrt{4y}} \qquad \qquad ...(iii)$$

and

$$\sqrt{H_2} = \frac{x_2}{C_v \sqrt{4y}} \qquad \qquad ...(iv)$$

From Eq. 13.40,

$$T = \frac{2A}{C_d \, a \sqrt{2g}} (\sqrt{H_1} - \sqrt{H_2}) \qquad \qquad ...(13.40)$$

$$= \frac{2A}{C_d \, a \sqrt{2g}} \left[\frac{x_1}{C_v \sqrt{4y}} - \frac{x_2}{C_v \sqrt{4y}} \right]$$

Therefore, rate of approach of jet, dx/dt is given by

$$\frac{(x_1 - x_2)}{T} = \frac{C_d \, a \sqrt{2g} \, C_v \sqrt{4y}}{2A}$$

$$= \frac{0.64 \times 0.98 \times \pi/4 \, (0.05)^2 \times \sqrt{19.62} \, \sqrt{4 \times 0.2}}{2 \times \pi/4 \times (1)^2}$$

$$= 0.031 \text{ m/s or } 0.31 \text{ cm/s}$$

13.7 Two orifices were placed in the side of a tank at depths H_1 and H_2 from the water surface and at height h_1 and h_2 from the base of the tank repsectively. If the two jets from orifices intersect at a height k from a plane through the base of the tank, prove that

$$k = (H_1 h_1 - H_2 h_2)/(H_1 - H_2)$$

Solution

Let the two jet interest at P at a height k from the datum plane passing through the base of the tank. Let the point P lie at a distance x from the tank.

From Eq. 13,14b, for orifice 1,

$$C_v = \sqrt{\frac{x^2}{4 y_1 H_1}} \qquad \qquad ...(i)$$

Similarly, for orifice 2,

$$C_v = \sqrt{\frac{x^2}{4 y_2 H_2}} \qquad \qquad ...(ii)$$

Equating Eqs. (i) and (ii)

$$\sqrt{x^2/4 y_1 H_1} = \sqrt{x^2/4 y_2 H_2}$$

$$y_1 H_1 = y_2 H_2$$

But $y_1 = (h_1 - k)$ and $y_2 = (h_2 - k)$,

therefore, $(h_1 - k) H_1 = (h_2 - k) H_2$

Solving $k = \dfrac{(H_1 h_1 - H_2 h_2)}{(H_1 - H_2)}$

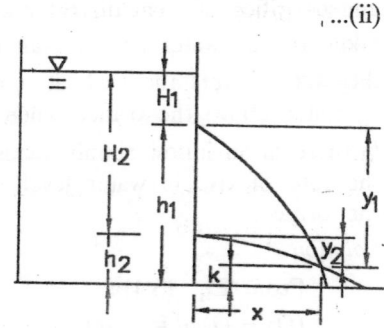

FIG. 13.36. EXAMPLE 13.7

13.8 A rectangular opening, 1 m wide and 3 m deep, is discharging water from a tank. If the water level in the tank is 1 m above the top edge of the orifice, determine the discharge through the opening considering it to be a large orifice. What percentage of error in the calculated value will be introduced, if it is considered to be a small orifice? Assume $C_d = 0.625$.

Solution

Considering the orifice as large, Eq. 13.19.b,

$$Q = \frac{2}{3} C_d \, B \sqrt{2g} \, [H_2^{3/2} - H_1^{3/2}]$$

$$= \frac{2}{3} \times 0.625 \times 1 \times \sqrt{2g} \, [H_2^{3/2} - H_1^{3/2}]$$

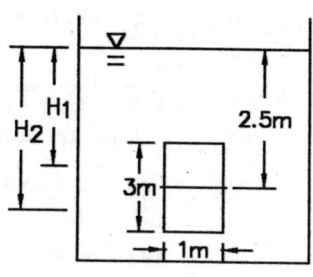

Since the water level is 1 m above the top edge of the orifice,

$$H_1 = 1 \text{ m and } H_2 = 3 + 1 = 4 \text{ m}$$

$$Q_1 = \frac{2}{3} \times 0.625 \times 1 \times \sqrt{2g} \, [(4)^{3/2} - (1)^{3/2}]$$

FIG. 13.37. EXAMPLE 13.8

$$= 12.92 \text{ m}^3/\text{s}$$

Considering the orifice as small, head at the centre of the orifice

$$= \left(1 + \frac{3}{2}\right) = 2.5 \text{ m}$$

From Eq. 13.17,

$$Q_2 = C_d \, a \sqrt{2g \, H}$$

$$= 0.625(3 \times 1) \sqrt{2 \times 9.81 \times 2.5}$$

$$= 13.13 \text{ m}^3/\text{s}$$

Percentage error

$$= \frac{Q_2 - Q_1}{Q_1} \times 100$$

$$= \frac{13.13 - 12.92}{12.92} \times 100$$

$$= 1.6 \%$$

13.9. A vertical cylindrical tank, 2 m diameter, is provided with a sharp edged orifice of 5 cm diameter at its bottom ($C_d = 0.6$). Find (a) the time taken by the water level to fall from 3 m to 1 m above the orifice. (b) If the water enters the tank at a constant rate of 0.01 m³/s, find the depth of water above the orifice when the level in the tank becomes steady. (c) If there is an inflow simultaneously to the tank at a rate of 0.02 m³/s, find the rate of rise in water level when the water level reaches 1.5 m above the orifice.

Solution

From Eq. 13.41a,

$$(Q_1 - Q) \, dt = A \, dh$$

(a) When there is no inflow $Q_1 = 0$

$$dt = \frac{-A \ dh}{Q} = \frac{+A \ dh}{C_d \ a \ \sqrt{2g} \ \sqrt{h}}$$

Integrating for h varying from H_1 to H_2

$$T = \frac{-A}{C_d \ a \ \sqrt{2g}} \left[\int_{H_1}^{H_2} \frac{dh}{\sqrt{h}} \right] = \frac{2A \ (\sqrt{H_1} - \sqrt{H_2})}{C_d \ a\sqrt{2g}}$$

$$= \frac{2 \times \frac{\pi}{4} \ (2)^2}{0.6 \times \pi/4 \ (0.05)^2 \ \sqrt{2 \times 9.81}} \ (\sqrt{3} - \sqrt{1})$$

$$= 881.3 \ \text{seconds}$$

(b) When dh = 0,

$$Q_1 = Q = C_d \ a \ \sqrt{2g \ h}$$

$$\sqrt{h} = \left[\frac{0.01}{0.6 \times \pi/4 \ (0.05)^2 \ \sqrt{2 \times 9.81}} \right] = 1.917$$

$$h = 3.675 \ \text{m}$$

(c) When $Q_1 = 0.02 \ \text{m}^3/\text{s}$

$$\frac{dh}{dt} = \frac{Q_1 - Q}{A}$$

$$\frac{dh}{dt} = \left[\frac{0.02 - 0.6 \times \pi/4 \ (0.05)^2 \ \sqrt{2 \times 9.81 \times 1.5}}{\pi/4 \ (2)^2} \right]$$

$$= \left[\frac{0.02 - 0.0064}{\pi} \right] = 0.014 \ \text{m/s}$$

13.10 A tank of square cross section, area 0.1 m^2, is placed in the upright position. An orifice of 1 cm diameter is situated in one of the vertical sides near the bottom. Water flows to the tank at the top at a constant rate of 0.3 m^3/h. The jet of water at a certain moment strikes the floor at a point P which lies 0.6 m horizontally away from the vena contracta and 0.5 m vertically below it. Determine the rate of change of water level at the instant under consideration and also the head above the centre of the orifice. Assume $C_d = 0.65$ and $C_v = 0.95$.

Solution

Let the jet strike a point P (x,y) at a certain moment. Let its actual velocity of water through the orifice be U_a. Therefore, the fluid particle moves a distance x and y in time t.

$$x = U_a t \qquad \qquad ...(i)$$

$$t = x/U_a = 0.6/U_a$$

and

$$y = \frac{1}{2} g t^2$$

$$t^2 = \frac{2y}{g} = \frac{2 \times 0.5}{g} \qquad \qquad ...(ii)$$

$$t = \sqrt{1/g}$$

From Eqs. (i) and (ii)

$$U_a = 0.6 \sqrt{g} = 1.88 \text{ m/s}$$

Also $C_v = \dfrac{U_a}{\sqrt{2g\,H}}$

$$H = \frac{U_a^2}{2g\,C_v^2} = \frac{(1.88)^2}{2 \times 9.81 \times (0.95)^2} = 0.2 \text{ m}$$

Hence, the outflow

$$Q = C_d\,a\sqrt{2g\,H}$$

$$= 0.65 \times \pi/4\,(0.01)^2\,\sqrt{2 \times 9.81 \times 0.2}$$

$$= 0.0001 \text{ m}^3/\text{s}$$

$$= 0.3636 \text{ m}^3/h$$

Since inflow is less than outflow, the water level in the tank is falling at the given moment

From Eq. 13.41a,

$$(Q_1 - Q)\,dt = A\,dh$$

$$\frac{dh}{dt} = -\left[\frac{Q - Q_1}{A}\right] = -\left[\frac{0.3636 - 0.30}{0.1}\right]$$

$$= -0.936 \text{ m/h}$$

13.11. A cylindrical tank, 1 m diameter and 2 m long, is filled with water and placed with its axis horizontal. Find the time required to lower the depth of water by 0.6 m through an orifice, 5 cm diameter, placed at the bottom of the tank. Take $C_d = 0.62$.

Solution

Let the water level stand at a height h above the orifice at particular instant of time. The water level falls by a depth dh in the time interval dt. Therefore,

$$A\,dh = -Q\,dt = -C_d\,a\,\sqrt{2g\,h}\,dt \qquad \text{...(i)}$$

The area A of the tank also varies with h. At any moment t,

$$A = AB \times L = 2\,(BC) \times L$$

In $\triangle$ OBC, BC

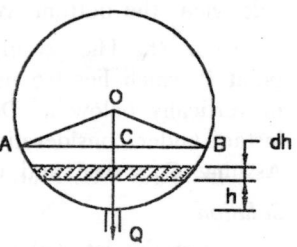

FIG. 13.38. EXAMPLE 13.11

$$= \sqrt{(OB)^2 - (OC)^2} = \sqrt{(R)^2 - (R - h)^2}$$

$$= \sqrt{2Rh - h^2}$$

$$\therefore \quad A = 2L\sqrt{2Rh - h^2} \qquad \text{...(ii)}$$

Substituting the values in Eq. (i)

$$2L\sqrt{2Rh - h^2}\,dh = -C_d\,a\,\sqrt{2g}\,\sqrt{h}\,dt$$

$$dt = -\frac{2L\sqrt{2Rh - h^2}\,dh}{C_d\,a\,\sqrt{2g}\,\sqrt{h}}$$

Integrating for h varying from H_1 to H_2

$$T = \int_o^T dt = -\int_{H_1}^{H_2}\frac{2L\sqrt{2R - h}}{C_d\,a\sqrt{2g}}$$

$$T = \frac{2 \times 2}{0.60 \times \dfrac{\pi}{4} \times (0.05)^2 \times \sqrt{2 \times 9.81}}\int\limits_{H_1}^{H_1}\sqrt{2 \times 0.5 - h}\,dh$$

$$= 742\left[\frac{(1 - h)^{3/2}}{3/2} \times (-1)\right]_{0.4}^{1}$$

$$= -742 \times \frac{2}{3}[0 - (0.6)^{3/2}] = 229.9 \text{ seconds.}$$

13.12. A hopper in the form of a truncated cone is used to discharge water. It is 1 m in diameter at its top and 0.3 m at the bottom. The height of the hopper is 1 m. An orifice of 4 cm diameter is fitted at the bottom of the hopper. Determine the time required to empty the tank by 0.5 m, assuming the tank to be full in the beginning.

Solution

From Eq. 13.39b,

$$T = \int dt = -\int\frac{A\,dh}{Q}$$

$$T = \int_{H_2}^{H_1} A\,dh/C_d\,a\sqrt{2gh} \quad ...(i)$$

From $\triangle$ AGO and $\triangle$ EKO

$$\frac{1/2}{x + 1} = \frac{0.3/2}{x}$$

$$x = 3/7$$

From $\triangle$ MLO and $\triangle$ EKO

$$\frac{D/2}{h + x} = \frac{0.3/2}{x}.$$

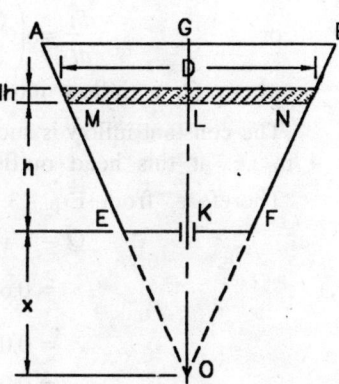

FIG. 13.39. EXAMPLE 13.12

$$D = \left(0.3 + \frac{7}{10}h\right)$$

Area
$$A = \frac{\pi}{4}D^2 = \frac{\pi}{4}\left(0.3 + \frac{7h}{10}\right)^2 \quad ...(ii)$$

From Eqs. (i) and (ii)

$$T = \int_{H_2}^{H_1}\frac{\pi}{4}\left(0.3 + \frac{7h}{10}\right)^2 \times \frac{dh}{0.6 \times \pi/4\,(0.04)^2\sqrt{2g}\,\sqrt{h}}$$

$$= \int_{0.5}^{1} \frac{235.14\,(0.09 + 4.2\,h + 0.49\,h^2)}{\sqrt{h}}\,dh$$

$$T = \int_{0.5}^{1} \left[\frac{21.16}{\sqrt{h}} + 98.76\sqrt{h} + 115.2\,h^{3/2} \right]\,dh$$

$$= \left(21.16\,\frac{h^{1/2}}{1/2} + 98.76\,\frac{h^{3/2}}{3/2} + 115.2\,\frac{h^{5/2}}{5/2} \right]_{0.5}^{1}$$

$$= [42.32\,(\sqrt{1} - \sqrt{0.5}) + 65.84\,[(1)^{3/2} - (0.5)^{3/2}]$$
$$+ 46.08\,[(1)^{5/2} - (0.5)^{5/2}]]$$

$$= 92.88 \ \text{seconds}$$

13.13 A 1 m × 1 m tank is 5 m deep. It contains a 100 mm diameter orifice ($C_d = 0.65$) at its base. The tank receives a constant supply of water (from its top) that would maintain water level 4 m above the orifice. Calculate the rate of rise of water level in the tank (a) when the tank is empty and when supply just enters the tank and (b) when the head over the crifice is 2 m.

Solution

From Eq. 13.41,

$$A\,dh = (Q_1 - Q)\,dt$$

$$\text{or} \qquad \frac{dh}{dt} = \left(\frac{Q_1 - Q}{A} \right)$$

where Q_1 is inflow into the tank where and Q is outflow.

The constant inflow is such that the water level in the tank is maintained at 4 m i.e. at this head outflow is same as inflow.

Therefore, from Eq. 13.11,

$$Q = C_d\,a\,\sqrt{2g}\,\sqrt{h}$$

$$= 0.65 \times \frac{\pi}{4} \times (0.1)^2\,\sqrt{2g}\,\sqrt{4}$$

$$= 0.022604\,\sqrt{4}$$

$$= 0.0452 \ \text{m}^3/\text{s}$$

When tank is empty and supply just enters the tank,

$$\frac{dh}{dt} = \frac{(0.0452 - 0.022604\,\sqrt{H})}{1 \times 1}$$

when $\qquad H = 0, \quad \dfrac{dh}{dt} = \dfrac{0.0452}{1} = 0.0452 \ \text{m/s}$

(b) when the head over orifice is 2 m,

$$\frac{dh}{dt} = \frac{(0.0452 - 0.022604\,\sqrt{2})}{1 \times 1} = 0.0320 \ \text{m/s}$$

13.14 Water is discharged through an external mouthpiece, of 5 cm diameter, under a head of 3 m. Find the discharge and pressure at the vena contracta. Assume coefficient of contraction as 0.64.

Solution

Applying Bernoulli's equation between points 1 at the water surface and 3 at the outlet of the mouthpiece,

$$0 + 3 + 0 = \frac{U^2}{2g} + \frac{(U_c - U)^2}{2g} \quad \text{(Refer Fig. 13.9)}$$

But $\quad a_c U_c = a U$

or $\quad U_c = \frac{a}{a_c} U = \left(\frac{U}{0.64}\right)$

Therefore, $\quad 3 = U^2/2g \, [1 + (U_c/U - 1)^2]$

$$= U^2/2g \, [1 + (1/0.64 - 1)^2]$$

$$U = \frac{\sqrt{2g \times 3}}{\sqrt{1 + \left(\frac{1}{0.64} - 1\right)^2}} = 6.686 \text{ m/s}$$

$$C_v = \frac{1}{\sqrt{1 + \left(\frac{1}{0.64} - 1\right)^2}} = 0.78$$

$C_c = 1.0$ for the outlet section of mouthpiece running full

$$C_d = 0.78 \times 1 = 0.78$$

Discharge $\quad Q = a \times U$

$$= \pi/4 \, (0.05)^2 \times 6.686 = 0.0131 \text{ m}^3/\text{s}$$

$$U_c = U/0.64 = 6.686/0.64 = 10.45 \text{ m/s}$$

Applying Bernoulli's equation to water surface and vena contracta.

$$10.3 + 3 + 0 = p_c/w + 0 + U_c^2/2g.$$

$$p_c/w = 13.3 - (10.45)^2/(2 \times 9.81)$$

$$= 7.734 \text{ m absolute}$$

$$p_c = 75.87 \text{ kPa absolute}$$

13.15 An internal mouthpiece has a diameter of 4 cm and is fitted to a tank. If the head above the centre line of mouthpiece is 1.6 m and coefficient of velocity C_v is 0.96, determine C_e, C_d and discharge when the mouthpiece is running free. Also compare the discharge through a Borda's mouthpiece (internal mouthpiece) with that from an external mouthpiece of the same diameter. Assume coefficient of contraction for the orifice as 0.64.

Solution

(a) From Eq. 13.32a,

$$C_c = 1/2\, C_v^2$$

$$= \frac{1}{2 \times (0.96)^2} = 0.543$$

$$C_d = C_c \times C_v$$

$$= 0.543 \times 0.96 = 0.52$$

$$Q = C_d\, a\, \sqrt{2gH}$$

$$= 0.52 \times (\pi/4)\,(0.04)^2 \sqrt{2 \times 9.81 \times 1.6}$$

$$= 0.00366 \text{ m}^3/\text{s}$$

(b) From Eq. 13.25,

$$C_d = \frac{1}{\sqrt{1 + (1/C_c - 1)^2}}$$

$$= \frac{1}{\sqrt{1 + (1/0.64 - 1)^2}} = 0.871$$

$$Q = C_d\, a\, \sqrt{2gH}$$

$$= 0.871 \times \pi/4\,(0.04)^2 \sqrt{2 \times 9.81 \times 1.6}$$

$$= 0.00613 \text{ m}^3/\text{s}$$

Percentage increase $= \dfrac{0.00613 - 0.00366}{0.00613} \times 100 = 40.28\%$

13.16. A venturimeter is fitted to a 15 cm diameter pipeline carrying water which is inclined at 60° to the horizontal plane. The throat diameter of the venturimeter is 5 cm and is placed higher than the inlet side. The difference in pressure head between the throat and the inlet which are 0.9 m apart is equivalent of 7.5 cm of mercury. Calculate the rate of flow of water. Assume $C_d = 0.98$.

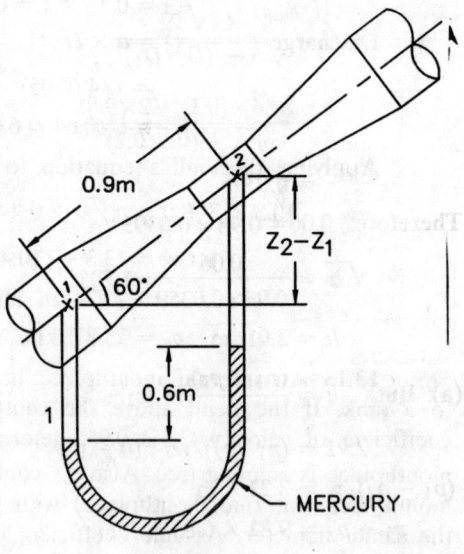

FIG. 13.40. EXAMPLE 13.16

Solution

From Eq. 13.55b,

$$Q = C_d\, C\, \sqrt{h}$$

where

$$C = \frac{A_1 A_2 \sqrt{2g}}{\sqrt{A_1^2 - A_2^2}}$$

$$= \frac{A_2 \sqrt{2g}}{\sqrt{1 - (A_2/A_1)^2}}$$

$$= \frac{\pi/4 \, (0.05)^2 \times \sqrt{2 \times 9.81}}{\sqrt{1 - (0.05/0.15)^4}} = 0.875 \times 10^{-2}$$

$$h = (p_1/w + z_1) - (p_2/w + z_2) = (p_1 - p_2)/w + (z_1 - z_2)$$

$$= (13.6 \times 0.075) + (0 - 0.78) = 0.24 \text{ m}$$

$$(\because \quad z_1 - z_2 = 0.9 \sin 60° = 0.78 \text{ m})$$

$$Q = C_d C \sqrt{h}$$

$$= 0.98 \times 0.875 \times 10^{-2} \sqrt{0.24}$$

$$= 4.2 \times 10^{-3} \text{ m}^3/\text{s}$$

$$= 4.2 \text{ lit/s}$$

13.17 Crude oil of specific gravity 0.85 flows upwards at volume rate of flow of 0.06 m³/s through a vertical venturimeter which has an inlet diameter of 200 mm and a throat diameter of 100 mm. The vertical distance between the pressure tappings is 300 mm and they are connected to two pressure gauges. Determine the difference of pressure between two sections. If the two limbs of a manometer are connected to these pressure tappings, determine the difference in mercury column in the manometer. Take $C_d = 0.98$

Solution

From Eq. 13.55b,

$$Q = C_d C \sqrt{h}$$

$$C = \frac{A_2 \sqrt{2g}}{\sqrt{1 - (D_2/D_1)^4}}$$

$$= \frac{\pi/4 \times (0.1)^2 \sqrt{2 \times 9.81}}{\sqrt{1 - (0.1/0.2)^4}}$$

$$= 0.0395$$

Therefore, $0.06 = 0.98 \times 0.0395 \sqrt{h}$

$$\sqrt{h} = \frac{0.06}{0.98 \times 0.0359} = 1.705$$

$$h = 2.91 \text{ m}$$

(a) But $h = \frac{(p_1 - p_2)}{ws} + (z_1 - z_2)$

$$2.91 = (p_1 - p_2)/ws + (0 - 0.3)$$

$$(p_1 - p_2)/w = 3.21 \text{ m}$$

$$p_1 - p_2 = 9.81 \times 0.85 \times 3.21$$

$$= 26.766 \text{ kPa}$$

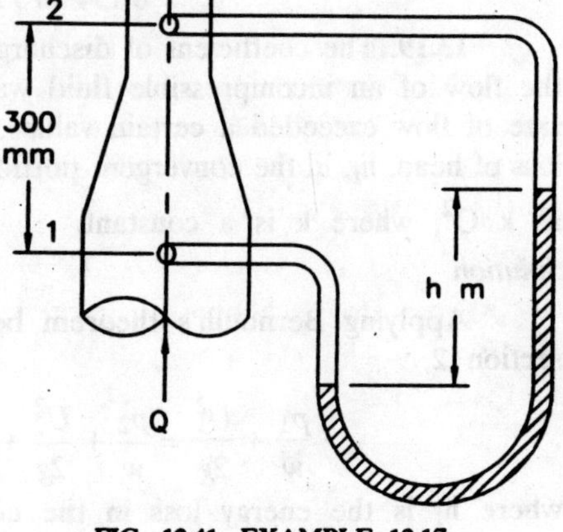

FIG. 13.41. EXAMPLE 13.17

(b) When the differential pressure is measured by means of U-tube manometer,

$$h = x (S_m/S - 1)$$
$$2.91 = x (13.6/0.85 - 1)$$
$$x = 2.91/15.0 = 0.194 \text{ cm of mercury}$$

13.18 The intet and outlet diameters of a horizontal venturimeter are 0.30 m and 0.10 m respectively. The liquid flowing through the meter is water. The pressure intensity at the inlet is 150 kPa while the vacuum pressure head at the throat is 37 cm of mercury. Calculate the discharge flowing through the venturimeter. Assume that the 4% of the differential head is lost between the inlet and the throat. Find also coefficient of discharge.

Solution

From Eq. 13.57a;

$$C_d = \sqrt{1 - h_L/h} = \sqrt{1 - 0.04} = 0.98$$

Let the pressure at inlet be p_1 and at throat p_2

$$p_1/w = 150/9.81 = 15.29 \text{ m}$$
$$p_2/w = -37 \text{ cm of mercury}$$
$$= -0.37 \times 13.6 = -5.032 \text{m}$$
$$(p_1 - p_2) w = [15.29 - (-5.032)] = 20.32 \text{ m}$$

Now
$$C = \frac{A_1 A_2 \sqrt{2g}}{\sqrt{A_1^2 - A_2^2}} = \frac{A_2 \sqrt{2g}}{\sqrt{1 - (D_2/D_1)^4}}$$

$$= \frac{\pi/4 (0.1)^2 \sqrt{2 \times 9.81}}{\sqrt{1 - (0.1/0.3)^4}} = 0.035$$

From Eq. 13.55b,

$$Q = C_d C \sqrt{h}$$
$$= 0.98 \times 0.035 \sqrt{20.322}$$
$$= 0.154 \text{ m}^3/\text{s}$$

13.19. The coefficient of discharge for venturimeter used for measuring the flow of an incompressible fluid was found to be constant, provided the rate of flow exceeded a certain value. Show that under these conditions, the loss of head, h_f, in the convergent portion of the venturimeter can be expressed as $k Q^2$, where k is a constant.

Solution

Applying Bernoulli's theorem between entrance section 1 and throat section 2,

$$\frac{p_1}{w} + \frac{U_1^2}{2g} = \frac{p_2}{w} + \frac{U_2^2}{2g} + h_f$$

where h_f is the energy loss in the convergent cone

$$\therefore \quad \frac{p_1 - p_2}{w} = h = \frac{U_2^2 - U_1^2}{2g} + h_f$$

or
$$h - h_f = U_1^2 / 2g \, (U_2^2 / U_1^2 - 1)$$

But
$$A_1 U_1 = A_2 U_2, \text{ therefore } U_2 / U_1 = A_1 / A_2$$

$$\therefore \quad (h - h_f) = U_1^2 / 2g \, (A_1^2 / A_2^2 - 1) \qquad \qquad \text{...(ii)}$$

Hence
$$U_1 = \frac{\sqrt{2g \, (h - h_f)}}{\sqrt{(A_1^2 / A_2^2 - 1)}}$$

and
$$Q_{ac} = A_1 U_1$$

$$= \frac{A_1 \sqrt{2g \, (h - h_f)}}{\sqrt{(A_1^2 / A_2^2 - 1)}} \qquad \qquad \text{...(iii)}$$

Let the theoretical discharge be Q_{th} and coefficient of discharge be C_d, hence,

$$Q_{ac} = C_d Q_{th}$$

$$= \frac{C_d A_1 \sqrt{2gh}}{\sqrt{(A_1^2 / A_2^2 - 1)}} \qquad \qquad \text{...(iv)}$$

From Eqs. (iii) and (iv)

$$h - h_f = C_d^2 h$$

$$h = h_f / (1 - C_d^2) \qquad \qquad \text{...(v)}$$

From Eqs. (iii) and (v)

$$Q_{ac} = \frac{A_1 \sqrt{2g}}{\sqrt{A_1^2 / A_2^2 - 1}} \sqrt{h_f \, (h/h_f - 1)}$$

$$= \frac{A_1 \sqrt{2g}}{\sqrt{A_1^2 / A_2^2 - 1}} \sqrt{h_f \left\{ \frac{1}{1 - C_d^2} - 1 \right\}}$$

$$= \frac{C_d A_1 \sqrt{2g} \sqrt{h_f}}{\sqrt{(A_1^2 / A_2^2 - 1)(1 - C_d^2)}}$$

Since C_d is a constant,

$$h_f = k Q^2$$

where
$$k = \frac{(A_1^2 / A_2^2 - 1)(1 - C_d^2)}{2g A_1^2 C_d^2}$$

13.20 Determine the maximum discharge that can be carried without covitation by a horizontal venturimeter 200 mm × 100 mm. The pressure at inlet is 12 kP_a (gauge). Take vapour pressure of water as $4 kp_a$ (absolute) and C_d as 0.96.

Solution

The discharge will be maximum when the differential head between inlet and throat is maximum. Since inlet pressure is given, Δh will be maximum when $p_2 = pv = 4\,kp_a$ (abs.)

Pressure at inlet in absolute system is,

$$p_1 \text{ (abs.)} = p_a + p_1 \text{ (gauge)}$$
$$= 100 + 12 = 112\,h\,p_a$$

(assuming $p_a = 100\,kp_a$)

For horizontal venturimeter, $(z_1 = z_2)$

$$\frac{(p_1 - p_2)}{w} = \frac{(112 - 4) \times 1000}{9810} = 11.009 \text{ m}$$

$$\Delta h = 11.009 \text{ m}$$

Given, $C_d = 095$

$$C = \frac{A_1 A_2 \sqrt{2g}}{\sqrt{A_1^2 - A_2^2}}$$

$$= \frac{A_2 \sqrt{2g}}{\sqrt{1 - (A_2/A_1)^2}}$$

$$= \frac{\frac{\pi}{4}(0.1)^2 \sqrt{2 \times 9.81}}{\sqrt{1 - (100/200)^4}} = 0.0359$$

From Eq. 13.55h,

$$Q = C_d . C . \sqrt{h}$$
$$= 0.96 \times 0.0359 \times \sqrt{11.009}$$
$$= 0.1144 \text{ m}^3/\text{s}$$

13.21 A horizontal venturimeter is used to measure the discharge through a 300 mm diameter pipeline. The ratio of inlet to throat diameter is 2 : 1. The difference in pressures between inlet and throat is measured as 3 m of water and loss of head through the meter is found to be one-eighth of throat velocity head. Calculate the discharge in pipeline.

Solution

Applying Bernoulli's equation between inlet and throat,

$$\frac{p_1}{w} + z_1 + \frac{U_1^2}{2g} = \frac{p_2}{w} + z_2 + \frac{U_2^2}{2g} + h_L$$

For horizontal venturimeter, $z_1 = z_2$,

$$h_L = \frac{1}{8} . \frac{U_2^2}{2g} \quad \text{(Given)}$$

$$\left(\frac{p_1}{w} + z_1\right) - \left(\frac{p_2}{w} + z_2\right) = \frac{U_2^2 - U_1^2}{2g} + \frac{1}{8} . \frac{U_2^2}{2g}$$

$$h = \frac{1}{2g}\left(\frac{9}{8} \cdot U_2^2 - U_1^2\right)$$

From continuity equation,

$$A_1 U_1 = A_2 U_2$$

$$U_2 = \frac{A_1 U_1}{A_2} = \left(\frac{D_1}{D_2}\right)^2 \cdot U_1$$

$$= \left(\frac{2}{1}\right)^2 \cdot U_1 = 4\, U_1$$

Hence

$$h = \frac{1}{2g}\left[\frac{9}{8} \cdot (4\, U_1)^2 - U_1^2\right]$$

$$= \frac{1}{2g}[17\, U_1^2] = 17 \cdot \frac{U_1^2}{2g}$$

$$U_1 = \sqrt{\frac{2gh}{17}}$$

∴

$$Q = A_1 U_1$$

$$= \frac{\pi}{4}(0.3)^2 \times \sqrt{\frac{2gh}{17}}$$

$$= \frac{\pi}{4} \times (0.3)^2 \sqrt{\frac{2 \times 9.81 \times 3}{17}} = 0.13146 \text{ m}^3/\text{s}.$$

13.22 Find the discharge of water flowing through a pipe 30 cm diameter placed is an inclined position where a venturimeter is inserted having a throat diameter as 15 cm. The difference of pressure measured by a liquid of sp. 0.6 in an inverted U-tube manometer and is equal to 30 cm. The loss of head between the main and the throat is 0.2 times the kinetic head of the pipeline.

Solution

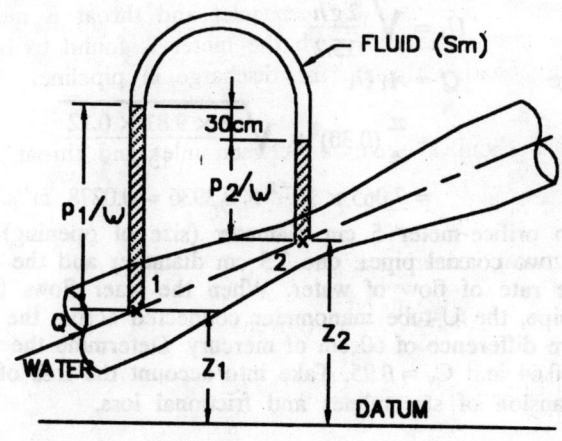

FIG. 13.42. EXAMPLE 13.22

Given $\qquad D_1 = 0.30$ m, $D_2 = 0.15$ m, $S_m = 0.6, h = 0.3$ m,

$$h_L = 0.2 \, U_1^2/2g$$

Applying Bernoulli's equation between 1 and 2,

$$\left(\frac{p_1}{ws} + z_1 + \frac{U_1^2}{2g} \right) = \left(\frac{p_2}{ws} + z_2 + \frac{U_2^2}{2g} \right) + h_L$$

$$\left(\frac{p_1}{ws} + z_1 \right) - \left(\frac{p_2}{ws} + z_2 \right) = \left(\frac{U_2^2 - U_1^2}{2g} \right) + 0.2 \frac{U_1^2}{2g}$$

$$h = \left(\frac{U_2^2}{2g} - 0.8 \frac{U_1^2}{2g} \right) \qquad \qquad \text{...(i)}$$

Also from manometric equation,

$$h = x \left(1 - \frac{S_m}{S} \right)$$

$$= 0.30 \left(1 - \frac{0.6}{1} \right) = 0.12 \text{ m}$$

From continuity equation,

$$A_1 U_1 = A_2 U_2$$

$$U_2 = \frac{A_1}{A_2} \cdot U_1 = \left(\frac{D_1}{D_2} \right)^2 \cdot U_1$$

$$= \left(\frac{0.30}{0.15} \right)^2 \cdot U_1 = 4 \, U_1 \qquad \qquad \text{...(ii)}$$

From Eqs. (i) and (ii)

$$h = \left(\frac{(4 \, U_1)^2}{2g} - 0.8 \frac{U_1^2}{2g} \right)$$

$$= (16 - 0.8) \frac{U_1^2}{2g}$$

$$U_1 = \sqrt{\frac{2gh}{15.2}}$$

Discharge $\qquad Q = A_1 U_1$

$$= \frac{\pi}{4} (0.30)^2 \times \sqrt{\frac{2 \times 9.81 \times 0.12}{15.2}}$$

$$= 7.065 \times 10^{-2} \times 0.3936 = 0.0278 \text{ m}^3/\text{s}.$$

13.23 An orifice-meter 5 cm diameter (size of opening) is fitted at the junction of two coaxial pipes, one 7.5 cm diameter and the other 10 cm to measure the rate of flow of water. When the waer flows from smaller pipe to large pipe, the U-tube manometer connected across the orificemeter reads a pressure difference of 60 cm of mercury. Determine the rate of flow, assuming $C_c = 0.64$ and $C_v = 0.95$. Take into account the loss of energy due to sudden expansion of streamlines and frictional loss.

Solution

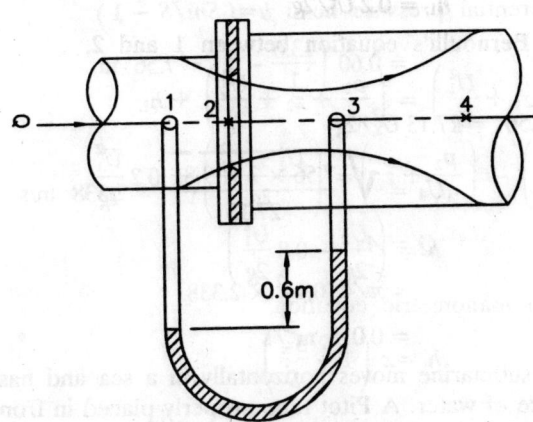

FIG. 13.43. EXAMPLE 13.23

Let the velocity through the orifice be U_2 and at vena contracta be U_3.

The frictional loss in an orifice

$$= (1/C_v^2 - 1)\, U_2^2/2g$$

The head loss due to sudden expansion

$$= \frac{(U_3 - U_4)^2}{2g}$$

Applying Bernoulli's theorem between 1 and 4

$$\frac{p_1}{w} + \frac{U_1^2}{2g} = \frac{p_4}{2} + \frac{U_4^2}{2g} + (1/C_v^2 - 1)\, U_2^2/2g + (U_3 - U_4)^2/2g$$

From continuity equation,

$$A_1 U_1 = A_2 U_2 = A_3 U_3 = A_4 U_4$$

Therefore,

$$(p_1 - p_4)/w = U_4^2/2g\, [1 + (1/C_v^2 - 1)\, U_2^2/U_4^2$$
$$+ (U_3/U_4 - 1)^2 - U_1^2/U_4^2]$$
$$= U_4^2/2g\, [1 + (1/C_v^2 - 1)\, A_4^2/A_2^2 + (A_4/A_3 - 1)^2 - A_4^2/A_1^2]$$

But $\qquad A_4/A_2 = (0.1)^2/(0.05)^2 = 4$

$$A_4/A_3 = (0.1)^2/(0.05)^2\, C_c = 4/0.64 = 6.25$$

$$A_4/A_1 = (0.1)^2/(0.075)^2 = 1.777$$

Substituting these values,

$$(p_1 - p_4)/w = U_4^2/2g\, [1 + (1/0.95^2 - 1)\, 4^2$$
$$+ (6.25 - 1)^2 - (1.777)^2]$$

$$= 27.13 \, U_4^2/2g$$

But differential pressure head $h = (Sm/S - 1)$

$$= 0.60 \left(\frac{13.6}{1} - 1 \right) = 7.56 \text{ m}$$

Hence $7.56 = 27.13 \, U_4^2/2g$

$$U_4 = \sqrt{\frac{7.56 \times 2 \times 9.81}{27.13}} = 2.338 \text{ m/s}$$

$$Q = A_4 \, U_4$$

$$= \pi/4 \, (0.1)^2 \times 2.338$$

$$= 0.018 \text{ m}^3/\text{s}$$

13.24. A submarine moves horizontally in a sea and has its axis much below the surface of water. A Pitot tube properly placed in front of submarine and along its axis is connected to the two limbs of a U-tube containing mercury. The difference in mercury level is found to be 17 cm. Find the speed of the submarine knowing that the specific weight of sea water is 10.25 kN/m³.

Solution

From Eq. (13.46b)

$$U = C \sqrt{2g h}$$

where

$$h = x \, (S_m/S - 1)$$

$$= 0.17 \, (13.6/1.025 - 1)$$

$$= 2.085 \text{ m}$$

Assuming constant of Pitot tube $= 1.0$

$$U = \sqrt{2 \times 9.81 \times 2.085}$$

$$= 6.397 \text{ m/s}$$

Since the Pitot tube is placed in front of the submarine, Pitot tube measures the velocity of fluid relative to the submarine.

Hence speed of submarine $= 6.397$ m/s

13.25 A Pitot static tube is mounted on an aeroplane to indicate the relative speed of the plane. What differential pressure intensity will the instrument register when the plane is travelling at a speed of 200 km/hr in a wind flowing at 60 km/hr. against the direction of wind ? Take sp. wt. of air as 12.65 N/m³.

Solution

Wind speed relative to the plane

$$= 60 - (- 200)$$

$$= 260 \text{ km/hr}$$

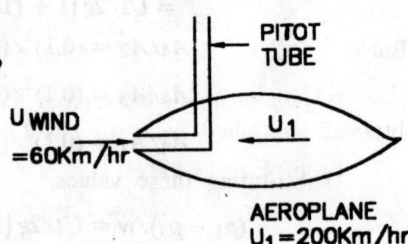

PITOT TUBE

U WIND =60Km/hr

U₁

AEROPLANE U₁=200Km/hr

FIG. 13.44. EXAMPLE 13.25

$$= \frac{260 \times 1000}{3600} = 72.22 \ \text{m/s}$$

Also $\qquad U = C \sqrt{2 g \left(\Delta p / w\right)}$

Assuming $\qquad C = 1$

$$72.22 = \sqrt{2 \times 9.81 \times \Delta p / 12.65}$$

$$\Delta p = \frac{(72.22)^2 \times 12.65}{2 \times 9.8} = 3362.84 \ \text{N/m}^2$$

$$= 3.363 \ kP_a$$

13.26 A Pitot static tube is used to measure the velocity of water in a pipe. The stagnation pressure is $59 \ k P_a$ and static pressure head is $49 \ kP_a$. Calculate the velocity of flow assuming $C_v = 0.98$.

Solution

$$U = C \sqrt{2 g \left(p_{\text{stagnation}} - p_{\text{static}} / w\right)}$$

$$= 0.98 \sqrt{2 \times 9.81 \times \frac{(59 - 49) \times 1000}{9810}}$$

$$= 4.38 \ \text{m/s}$$

13.27. A Pitot static tube is placed at various points along a diameter of a 50 cm pipe in which water is flowing. The pressure difference is measured by a U-tube manometer containing mercury and water. Compute the discharge flowing through the pipe. The following readings were obtained.

Distance from centre line, cm	0	5	10	15	20	22.5	24
Manometer reading, cm	15	14.5	14.1	12.6	10.3	8.0	6.2

Solution

Consider a small elementary area of thickness dr at a radius r, so that

$$dQ = u \pi d \left(r^2\right)$$

Integrating, $\qquad Q = \int dQ = \int_0^{R^2} u \pi d \left(r^2\right)$

$$= \pi \int_0^{R^2} u \ d \left(r^2\right)$$

A plot is made between u and d (r^2) and the area of the curve so obtained multiplied by π to give the discharge Q.

From Eq. 13.46b,

$$U_0 = C \sqrt{2g h}$$

Distance m	0	0.05	0.10	0.15	0.20	0.225	0.24
Manometer reading m	0.15	0.145	0.141	0.126	0.103	0.08	0.062
Velocity (m/s)	2.36	2.28	2.216	1.98	1.62	1.25	0.975
$(\text{Rad})^2 \times 10^{-4}$	0	25.0	100.0	225.0	400.0	506.3	576.0

Assuming the constant of the meter C as unity, and substituting the differential head h as

$$h = x\,(S_m/S - 1) = 12.6\,x$$

and

$$U_0 = 15.72\,\sqrt{x}\quad \text{m/s}$$

The plot is made with the following scale

$$U : 1\,\text{cm} = 0.5\,\text{m/s}\ ,\ r^2\ ;\ 1\,\text{cm} = 1/150\,\text{m}^2$$

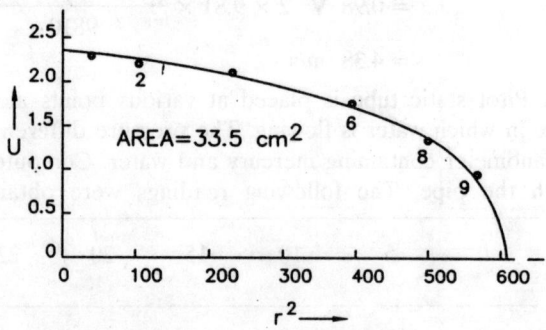

FIG. 13.45. EXAMPLE 13.27

Area of the U versus r^2 curve $= 33.5 \times 0.5 \times 1/150\ \text{m}^3/\text{s}$

Therefore, $Q = \pi\,[33.5 \times 0.5 \times 1/150]$

$$= 0.3506\ \text{m}^3/\text{s}$$

13.28 The following data were taken by a currentmeter across a river cross section 20 m wide at the water surface. Assuming the calibration equation for currentmeter as

$$U = C N = 0.0125\ N$$

Compute the rate of volume flowing in the river.

Station from one bank	0	1	2	3	4	5	6	7	8
Depth, m	0	1	1.16	1.23	1.33	1.46	14	1.17	0
R.P.M. at 0.2y	0	50	58	67	55	53	51	45	0
R.P.M. at 0.8 y	0	40	50	60	50	40	41	32	0

Solution

Let the depths at various section be y_0, y_1, y_2, etc. The discharge through each segment is determined by continuity equation.

$$Q_{01} = B \frac{(U_0 + U_1)}{2} \frac{(y_0 + y_1)}{2}$$

$$Q_{12} = B \frac{(U_1 + U_2)}{2} \frac{(y_1 + y_2)}{2} \quad \text{and so on.}$$

Station	Depth	Average depth	$U_{0.2x}$	$U_{0.8y}$	Average Velocity	$Q = B\, y_{av}\, U_{av}$
0	0		. 0		0	
		0.5			0.2813	0.3516
1	1		0.625	0.500		
		1.08			0.619	1.6713
2	1.16		0.725	0.625		
		1.20			0.7345	2.2035
3	1.23		0.838	0.75		
		1.28			0.7253	2.321
·4	1.33		0.688	0.625		
		1.40			0.619	2.1665
5	1.46		0.663	0.500		
		1.43			0.5785	2.068
6	1.40		0.638 ·	0.513		
		1.28			0.5285	1.6912
7	1.17		0.563	0.40		
		0.585			0.2408	0.352
8	0		0	0		

$$Q_T = 12.825 \text{ m}^3/\text{s}$$

$U_0\, 2y$ and $U_0\, zy$ are computed at given section by above equation

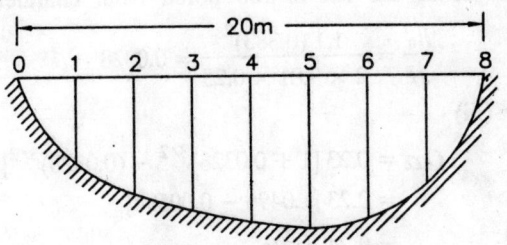

FIG. 13.46. EXAMPLE 13.28

The total discharge Q_T is the sum of all these discharges flowing through the segments.

$$Q_\tau = \Sigma (Q_1 + Q_2 + \ldots\ldots)$$

The width of each segment $B = 20/8 = 2.5$ m

$\therefore \qquad Q_T = \Sigma (2.5 \, y_{av} \, U_{av})$

13.29. A rectangular notch, 1.0 m wide and 0.25 m high, is provided in a long rectangular channel, 1.2 m wide. The water flows over the notch under a head of 0.25 m. Calculate the discharge (a) neglecting the velocity of approach (b) considering the velocity of approach. Assume the kinetic energy correction factor $\alpha \approx 1.1$ and use Francies formula, $Q = 1.84 \, LH^{3/2}$.

Solution

(a) Neglecting velocity of approach.

$$Q_1 = 1.84 \, LH^{3/2}$$

$$= 1.84 \times 1 \times (0.25)^{3/2}$$

$$= 0.23 \text{ m}^3/\text{s}$$

(b) Considering the velocity of approach,

$$Q_2 = 1.84 \, L \, H^{3/2} [(1 + h_a/H)^{3/2} - (h_a/H)^{3/2}]$$

where $\qquad h_a/H = \alpha \, U_a^2/(2gH)$ \hfill ...(i)

and $\qquad U_a = Q/B \, (P + H)$ \hfill ...(ii)

$$Q_2 = 1.84 \times 1 \times (0.25)^{3/2} [(1 + h_a H)^{3/2} - (h_a/H)^{3/2}]$$

$$= 0.23 [(1 + h_a/H)^{3/2} - (h_a/H)^{3/2}] \qquad \text{...(iii)}$$

Since the computation of velocity of approach needs the value discharge which is unknown, the problem is solved by successive approximation.

First trial : Initially assume, $U_a = 0$

$$Q_{21} = 0.23 \text{ m}^3/\text{s}$$

From Eqs. (i) and (ii)

$$U_a = \frac{Q}{B \, (P + H)} = \frac{0.23}{1.2 \, (0.25 + 0.25)} = 0.383 \text{ m/s}$$

where $\qquad P$ = height of the sill of the notch from channel bottom.

$$\frac{h_a}{H} = \frac{1.1 \, (0.383)^2}{2 \times 9.81 \times 0.25} = 0.0328$$

From Eq. (iii)

$$Q_{22} = 0.23 [1 + 0.0328)^{3/2} - (0.0328)^{3/2}]$$

$$= 0.23 [1.0496 - 0.00594]$$

$$= 0.24 \text{ m}^3/\text{s}$$

Second trial :

$$U_a = \frac{0.24}{1.2\,(0.25 + 0.25)} = 0.4 \text{ m/s}$$

$$\frac{ha}{H} = \frac{1.1\,(0.4)^2}{2 \times 9.81 \times 0.25} = 0.0358$$

Hence

$$Q_{23} = 0.23\,[1 + 0.0358)^{3/2} - (0.0358)^{3/2}]$$

$$= 0.23\,[1.0542 - 0.00677]$$

$$= 0.251 \text{ m}^3/\text{s}$$

Third trial :

$$U_a = 0.251/1.2 \times 0.5 = 0.418 \text{ m/s}$$

$$ha/H = 1.1\,(0.418)^2/(2 \times 9.81 \times 0.25) = 0.0392 \text{ m/s}$$

Hence

$$Q_{24} = 0.251\,[(1 + 0.0392)^{3/2} - (0.0392)^{3/2}]$$

$$= 0.251\,[1.0594 - 0.00766]$$

$$= 0.264 \text{ m}^3/\text{s}$$

This way, the computation is continued till the desired accuracy is obtained.

13.30 Water flows over a rectangular weir, 1 m wide under a head of 15 cm and afterwards passes over a V-notch. The coefficiencts of discharge for rectangular and V-notch are 0.62 and 0.69 respectively. Find the depth of water over the triangular weir.

Solution

For rectangular notch,

$$Q = \frac{2}{3}\,C_{d1}\,\sqrt{2g}\,L\,H^{3/2}$$

$$= \frac{2}{3} \times 0.62 \times \sqrt{2 \times 9.81} \times 1 \times (0.15)^{3/2}$$

$$= 0.1064 \text{ m}^3/\text{s}$$

For triangular notch,

$$Q = (8/15)\,C_{d2}\,\sqrt{2g}\,\tan\theta \times (H)^{5/2}$$

The same discharge passes over the V-notch and assuming it to be right angled V-notch,

$$Q = \frac{8}{15} \times 0.69\,\sqrt{2 \times 9.81}\,\tan\frac{90°}{2} \times (H)^{5/2}$$

$$H^{5/2} = \frac{15}{8} \times 0.1064 \times \frac{1}{0.69\,\sqrt{2 \times 9.81}} = 0.0653$$

$$H = 0.3356 \text{ m}$$

13.31 A rectangular channel, 1.7 m wide, carries a maximum flow of 0.15 m³/s and minimum 0.08 m³/s. It discharges over a right angled V-notch. At what level should the notch be placed so that the depth of water in the channel does not exceed 1 m ? What is the minimum depth of water ? Assume $C_d = 0.6$ and neglect velocity of approach.

Solution

Let the notch be placed z m above the channel bottom so that

$$H = (1 - z) \text{ m}$$

From Eq. 13.90

$$Q = (8/15) \, C_d \sqrt{2g} \, H^{5/2}$$

$$0.15 = 8/15 \times 0.6 \times \sqrt{2 \times 9.81} \, H_1^{5/2}$$

$$H_1^{5/2} = \frac{0.15 \times 15}{8 \times 0.6 \times \sqrt{2 \times 9.81}} = 0.1058$$

$$H_1 = 0.407 \text{ m} = (1 - z)$$

$$z = 0.593 \text{ m}$$

Thus the notch should be placed 0.593 m above the channel bottom. When the minimum discharge flows through the notch,

$$0.08 = 8/15 \times 0.6 \sqrt{2 \times 9.81} \, H_2^{5/2}$$

$$H_2 = \left(\frac{0.08 \times 15}{8 \times 0.6 \times \sqrt{2 \times 9.81}} \right)^{2/5} = 0.316 \text{ m}$$

Hence mimimum depth of water $= (0.593 + 0.316)$

$$= 0.91 \text{ m}$$

13.32. A weir, 36 m long, is divided into 12 equal bays by vertical posts, each 0.6 m wide. Determine the discharge over the weir if the head over the crest is 1.2 m and velocity of approach is given as 2 m/s.

Solution

Since there are 12 bays, there will be 11 vertical posts, each of 0.6 m width.

Length of clear water bay $= 36 - 11 \times 0.6 = 29.4$ m

Since there are 12 bays, there will be $2n = 2 \times 12$ or 24 end contractions.

Using Francis formula,

$$Q = 1.84 \, [L - 0.1 \, n \, H_1] \, [H_1^{3/2} - h_a^{3/2}]$$

where $\qquad H_1 = H + h_a$

and $\qquad h_a = U_a^2/2g$

$$= (2)^2/2 \times 9.81 = 0.204 \text{ m}$$

Hence $\qquad H_1 = 1.2 + 0.204 = 1.404$ m

Substituting the values,

$$Q = 1.84 \, [29.4 - 0.1 \times 24 \times 1.404] \, [1.404)^{3/2} - (0.204)^{3/2}]$$

$$= 75.26 \text{ m}^3/\text{s}$$

13.33 A canal carries a discharge varing from 0.1 m^3/s to 0.65 m^3/s. A sharp crested weir user is to be used to measure the discharge with an accuracy of 1 % in this entire range. The head over the weir can be measured with an accuracy of 0.5 mm. Find out the maximum length of weir required to satisfy above condition. Take $C_d = 0.62$ and neglect velocity of approach.

Solution

From Eq. 13.71,

$$Q = \frac{2}{3} C_d \sqrt{2g} \, L_e \, H^{3/2} = kH^{3/2} \qquad \text{...(i)}$$

where L_e = effective length of weir

$$= (L - 2H) \qquad \text{...(ii)}$$

Differentating Eq. (ii) w.r. to H,

$$dQ = 1.5 \, k \, H^{1/2} \, dH \qquad \text{...(iii)}$$

From Eqs. (ii) and (iii)

$$\frac{dQ}{Q} = 1.5 \frac{dH}{H}$$

Let minimum head be H_{min} and $dH = 0.5 \times 10^{-3}$ m (Given)

$$0.01 = 1.5 \times \frac{0.5 \times 10^{-3}}{H_{min}}$$

$$H_{min} = \frac{1.5 \times 0.5 \times 10^{-3}}{0.01} = 0.075 \text{m}$$

Thus, the head over weir H' should be more than 0.075 m for all the discharge,

From Eq. (i)

$$Q = \frac{2}{3} \times 0.62 \times \sqrt{2 \times 9.81} \, L_e \, (0.075)^{3/2}$$

$$0.1 = 0.0376 \, L_e$$

$$L_e = \frac{0.1}{0.0376} = 2.66 \text{ m}$$

$$(L - 0.1 \, n \, H) = 2.66$$

$$L = 2.66 + 0.1 \times 2 \times (0.075)$$

$$= 2.66 + 0.015 = 2.675 \text{m}$$

13.34 A triangular notch is used to measure flow in a channel under a head of 20 cm If the discharge is to be measured with 3% accuracy. What is the maximum velocity of approach that can be neglected ?

Solution

For a triangular notch,

$$Q = \frac{8}{15} C_d \sqrt{2g} \, \tan \frac{\theta}{2} \, H^{5/2} \qquad \text{...(i)}$$

$$= K H^{5/2} \qquad \text{...(ii)}$$

Differentiating Eq. (ii) w.r. to H,

$$dQ = \frac{5}{2} K H^{3/2} dH \qquad \text{...(iii)}$$

From Eqs. (ii) and (iii)

$$\frac{dQ}{Q} = 2.5 \frac{dH}{H}$$

Given

$$\frac{dQ}{Q} = 0.03, H = 0.2 \text{ m,}$$

$$0.03 = 2.5 \frac{dH}{0.2}$$

$$dH = \frac{0.03 \times 0.2}{2.5} = 2.4 \times 10^{-3} \text{m}$$

If velocity of approach is U_a

$$\frac{U_a^2}{2g} = dH = 2.4 \times 10^{-3}$$

$$U_a = \sqrt{2 \times 9.81 \times 2.4 \times 10^{-3}} = 0.217 \text{ m/s.}$$

13.35A triangular slot is cut in a metallic plate with base width of 1.5 m and apex angle of 60°. It is used as a notch and placed at the end of the channel. The base is horizontal and one of the vertex remains above the water surface. If the head above base is 0.4 m, what is the discharge, assume $C_d = 0.6$.

Solution

The given notch is trapezoidal and discharge over it is equal to the difference of discharge over a rectangular notch of crest length L and a triangular notch of vertex angle θ

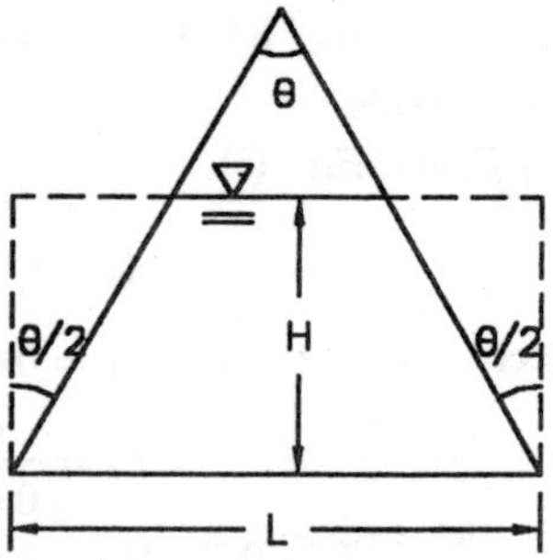

$$Q = Q_{\text{rect}} - Q_{\text{Triangular notch}}$$

$$= \frac{2}{3} C_d \sqrt{2g} \, L \, H^{3/2} - \frac{8}{15} C_d \sqrt{2g} \tan\frac{\theta}{2} H^{5/2}$$

$$Q = \frac{2}{3} C_d \sqrt{2g} \, H^{3/2} \left(L - \frac{4}{5} \tan\frac{\theta}{2} \right)$$

Substituting the values,

$$Q = \frac{2}{3} \times 0.6 \times \sqrt{2 \times 9.81} \times (0.4)^{3/2} \left[1.5 - \frac{4}{5} \times 0.4 \times \tan\frac{60}{2} \right]$$

$$= 0.4483 \, [1.5 - 0.1848]$$

$$= 0.589 \text{ m}^3/\text{s.}$$

FIG. 13.47. EXAMPLE 13.35

13.36 A weir has been so designed that its end contractions are suppressed and it lowers the water surface in the reservoir from a head of 2 m over the horizontal crest to 1 m in a time of 40 minutes. Determine the length of the weir. Use Francis formula. The area of the water surface A, in square metres varies by the expression

$$A = 10^4 (75 + 0.5 H^2)$$

where H is the head over the crest.

Solution

The fundamental equation is

$$Q \, dt = -A \, dH$$

or

$$dt = -A \, dH/Q$$

For rectangular weir,

$$Q = 1.84 \, L \, H^{3/2}$$

Sobstituting the value of Q

$$dt = \frac{-A \, dH}{1.84 \, L \, H^{3/2}} = \frac{10^4 (75 + 0.5 H^2) \, dH}{1.84 \times L \, H^{3/2}}$$

$$dt = (10^4/1.84 \, L) \, (75 \, H^{-3/2} + 0.5 \, H^{1/2}) \, dH$$

Integrating for h varying from 2 m to 1 m,

$$T = \int dt = \frac{-10^4}{1.84 \times L} \left[\int_2^1 75 \, H^{-3/2} + 0.5 \, H^{1/2} \right] dH$$

$$40 \times 60 = \frac{10^4}{1.84 \times L} \left[75 \frac{H^{-1/2}}{-1/2} + 0.5 \frac{H^{3/2}}{3/2} \right]_1^2$$

$$L = \frac{10^4}{1.84 \times 40 \times 60} \left[-150 \left(\frac{1}{\sqrt{2}} - 1 \right) + \frac{1}{3} \left(2^{3/2} - 1^{3/2} \right) \right]$$

$$L = 100.87 \text{ m}$$

Objective Questions

13.1 The pressure distribution at the upstream face of the orifice is

(a) hydrostatic   (b) parabolic

(c) atmospheric   (d) none of these answers

13.2 An orifice of 2 cm diameter is fitted to a tank containing water to a depth of 4 m above the centre of orifice. The pressure at the vena contracta will be, in metre,

(a) 10.3   (b) 9   (c) 1.3

(d) 8.86   (e) none of these answers

13.3 A pipe of 6 cm length is fitted outside an opening in the vertical side of tank. The pressure at the vena contracta will be, in metres,

(a) 10.3   (b) 4.7   (c) 5.6

(d) 4   (e) none of these answers

The coefficients of velocity and contraction may be assumed to be 0.98 and 0.62 respectively

13.4 The energy loss in the orifice is

(a) $H (1 - C_v^2)$

(b) $(H - U_a^2/2g)$

(c) $U_a^2/2g - U_c^2/2g$

(d) $(1/C_v^2 - 1) H$

(e) none of these answers

13.5 The coefficient of contraction for an orifice is 0.62. If an external mouthpiece is fitted to this opening, its coefficient of discharge will be

(a) 0.62   (b) 0.98   (c) 0.852

(d) 0.75   (e) non of these answer

13.6 The stagnation pressure at a point is measured by

(a) static tube

(b) piezometric tube

(c) Pitot static tube

(d) total head tube

(e) none of these answers

13.7 The Pitot static tube measures

(a) mean velocity   (b) static pressure

(c) dynamic pressure   (d) difference in total and static pressure

(e) none of these answers

13.8 The hot wire anemometer is used to measuer

(a) velocity of water   (b) velocity of air

(c) pressure intensities in gases

(d) stagnation pressure in gases

(e) none of these answers

13.9 A 5 cm Borda's mouthpiece discharges 0.008 m³/s under a head of 3 m. The coefficient of velocity is

(a) 0.97   (b) 0.94   (c) 0.98

(d) 1.0   (e) none of these answers

13.10 Mark the correct statement. The coefficient of discharge for venturimeter

(a) increases with increase in Reynolds number

(b) decreases with increase in Reynolds number

(c) does not depend on Reynolds number

(d) increases upto certain values of Reynolds number and then becomes constant

(e) none of these answers

13.11 A venturimeter is preferable to an orificemeter because

(a) it measures the discharge accurately

(b) it is cheaper

(c) the energy loss is less

(d) the coefficient of discharge remains constant

(e) none of these answers

13.12 The discharge through a horizontal pipe is measured by means of a venturimeter. If the pipe is made vertical and carries same discharge, the difference in the levels of mercury in the two legs of the U-tube manometer will

(a) increase   (b) decrease

(c) remain the same (d) none of these answers

13.13 In laboratory the right angled notch measures the discharge of 1 m^3/s under a head of 0.1 ± 0.001 m. The percentage error in the discharge measurement will be

(a) 1.5   (b) 2.5   (c) 1.0

(d) 0.1   (e) none of these answers

13.14 A weir will behave as broad crested weir when

(a) the flow over it becomes critical

(b) the thickness of the crest is more than 0.66H

(c) the thickness of the crest is at least equal to the head H

(d) the flow over it becomes supercritical

(e) none of these answers

13.15 The coefficient of discharge for a weir depends on

(a) R_e and N_M (b) R_e, N_w (c) R_e, N_F

(d) R_e alone   (e) none of these answers

Problems

13.1 A sharp edged orifice, 10 cm in diameter, is provided in the side of a closed tank. If the tank contains a liquid of specific gravity 1.5 to a height of 4 m above the orifice, calculate the actual discharge and head lost. Assume $C_d = 0.61$ and $C_v = 0.98$. If it is required to increase the discharge by 50%, what should be the pressure in the tank?

13.2 The head loss in the flow through a 5 cm diameter orifice under a certain head is 0.2 m and velocity of jet is 7.5 m/s. Determine head H, coefficient of velocity C_v and diameter of jet. Also determine the discharge flowing out of the orifice. Take $C_d = 0.62$.

13.3 The velocity of jet flowing through an orifice can be determined from the determination of the positions of three points A,B and C in the path of the jet. If the points B and C lie at a horizontal distance of x_1 and x_2 from A and at a vertical distance of y_1 and y_2 below A respectively, prove that the velocity of jet U is given by

$$U = \sqrt{g\, x_1\, x_2\, (x_2 - x_1)/2\, (x_1\, y_2 - y_1\, x_2)}$$

13.4 A tank of constant cross sectional area consists of an orifice of 5 cm diameter in its vertical side near its bottom. The jet of water coming out from the orifice strikes at a point on a horizontal plane, 1.5 m vertically below the centre of orifice. After an interval of 15 seconds, it was observed that the jet of water strikes at a point 75 cm behind the previous point. Determine the cross sectional area of the tank. Use $C_d = 0.61$ and $C_v = 0.98$.

13.5 A mouthpiece is fitted at the bottom of a boiler drum which is 2 m in diameter and 10 m long. The drum is laid horizontally and is half full of water. Determine the time required to empty the boiler; the diameter of mouthpiece is 10 cm. Assume coefficient of discharge for the mouthpiece as 0.8.

13.6 A hemi spherical vessal of 2 m radius with base horizontal is filled with water upto the top. Find the time required to empty it through an orifice of 7.5 cm diameter located at its lowest point. Take $C_d = 0.60$.

13.7. A cylindrical tank of internal diameter 0.6 m, length 1.5 m and axis vertical, has a 5 cm diameter sharp edged orifice ($C_d = 0.6$) at the bottom. The orifice discharge freely in the atmosphere. The tank is open at the top and intially, it is empty. If the water was admitted into the tank from the top of the tank at a constant rate of 0.015 m³/s, in how much time will the tank be filled up ? And how much water will escape during this period through the orifice ?

13.8. A tank is suspended over a knife edge which is 0.9 m above the orifice. The head above the orifice, 12 cm in diameter, is 1.2 m. A weight of 0.25 kN placed at 0.6 m from the knife edge balances the tank while the water discharges from the tank at the rate of 0.35 m³/s. Determine the coefficients of velocity, contraction and discharge.

13.9 A cylindrical mouthpiece, 10 cm in diameter, is attached to the opening of the same size at the bottom of the tank. The total depth of water in tank is maintained at 7.5 m. Determine the discharge flowing through the mouthpiece, if $C_d = 0.8$. Also determine the total energy loss in the mouthpiece. If the vapour pressure is 20 kPa and coefficient of contraction for the section of vena contracta is 0.62, determine the minimum pressure anywhere in the mouthpiece. Determine the maximum permissible head and maximum permissile discharge flowing though the mouthpiece.

13.10. Water flows through a 5 cm diameter external cylindrical mouthpiece under a head of 4 m. If 90% of the head loss takes place between the contracted section and the outlet and $C_v = 0.90$ for the mouthpiece, calculate the discharge.

A small hole is provided in the contracted section to connect a piezometer tube, the lower end of which dips below in a mercury sump. Determine, to what height the mercury will rise in the piezometric tube and what is the minimum pressure at the contracted section?

13.11 A venturimeter with a 7.5 cm diameter throat is installed in a 15 cm pipeline. The pressure at the entrance to the meter is 70 kPa gauge and it is undersirable that the pressure should, at any point, fall below 2.5 m absolute. Determine the maximum rate of flow passing through the meter. Assume C_d as 0.96 and specific weight of liquid flowing through the meter as 9 kN/m³. Take $p_{atm} = 100$ kPa

13.12 Show that for incompressible fluid flowing through a venturimeter, the energy lost per unit weight of fluid in the convergent cone is given by

$$h_1 = (1/C_v^2 - 1)(1 - D_2^4/D_1^4) U_2^2/2g$$

13.13 A venturimeter, 30 cm × 15 cm, is provided in a vertical pipeline carrying oil, of specific gravity 0.8, the throat being higher than entrance section by 30 cm. A differential U-tube mercury manometer is used to measure the difference of pressure which recorded the difference as 20 cm. Determine the rate of flow of oil. Assume the coefficient of discharge for the venturimeter as 0.96.

13.14 A pitot static tube is used to measure the velocity of water in a pipe. The tube registers the stagnation pressure of 10 cm and static pressure as 8 cm of water. Determine the velocity of flow in the pipe. Take C_v for the Pitot satic tube as 0.99.

13.15 A Pitot tube is mounted on an aeroplane to indicate the speed of plane relative to the wind blowing past it. If the plane is moving at a speed of 200 km/h through a wind of 60 km/h (in the opposite direction), what difference of pressure will be recorded by the instrument? Specific weight of air = 1.2 kg/m³

13.16 In order to measure the discharge through a rectangular channel, 1.4 m wide and 1.2 m deep, a sharp edged rectangular weir is used. The length of the weir is 1 m and coefficient of discharge is 0.6. Determine the rate of flow in the channel when head over the weir is 0.6 m. Take into account the end contractions and velocity of approach in the computation.

13.17 Show that the flow Q over a rectangular weir of crest length H can be expressed by

$$Q = A(L - CH)H^{3/2}$$

where H is the head of water over the weir and A and C are constants

A rectangular weir, crest length 1.5 m, carries a discharge of 0.17 m³/s under a head of 0.15 m and a discharge of 0.43 m³/s under a head of 0.30 m. What will be the discharge when the head is 0.25 m?

13.18 Water flows in a channel of trapezoidal shape (bed width = 9 m and side slope 1:1) and then passes over a Cipoletti weir. Determine the discharge flowing in the channel when the depth of water in the channel is 3.2 m. The sill of weir is located at 1.2 m above the channel bed. The length of crest at the base is 2 m. Use Francis formula and make corrections for end contractions and velocity of approach.

13.19 The catchment area of a reservoir is 25 sq. km. The maximum rainfall in the catchment is 10 mm /per hour and 10 percent of it reaches the reservoir. A waste weir is required to be constructed in the area to the measure the discharge. The waste weir has to carry piers of 0.6 m width over a span of 2.5 m. Determine the length of the waste weir so that the depth of water does not exceed 0.75 m.

13.20 Water is flowing over a sharp edged weir from a reservoir; the water surface area is 0.85 km^2 and the depth of water over weir crest is 2 m. The length of the crest is 12 m. Find the time required to lower the water level to 0.5 m above the weir crest. Assume the reservoir side to be vertical and $C_d = 0.62$.

14

Dynamic Action of Fluids

14.1 INTRODUCTION

Whenever the velocity of a stream of fluid is changed either in magnitude or direction, external forces are required to be applied on the stream. The deflection of the stream may be accomplished by a moving vane (plane or curved). When a jet of fluid strikes a moving vane, it deflects the jet and changes its momentum; the forces are exerted between vane and jet and the work is done by the displacement of vane. Fluid machines make use of this principle.

A fluid machine is a device which either converts the fluid energy into mechanical energy or vice versa. The various types of turbines fall in the first category whereas the centrifugal pump, blowers and compressors fall in the second category of machines. All these machines are known as rotodynamic machines, also known as turbomachines. These machines have a rotating element which causes the conversion of one form of energy into another. There is another class of machines which is known as positive displacement machines, in which the fluid is displaced by the movement of mechanical element such as a moving plunger (reciprocating pump), or a gear system (gear pump) etc.

14.2 DYNAMIC FORCE

14.2.1 Free Jet

A free jet is a stream of liquid which issues from a nozzle into atmospheric air. Water flowing under pressure in a pipe may be converted into a free jet by fitting a nozzle at the end of the pipe. The nozzle provides a smooth and gradually reducing area of flow and converts the pressure energy into velocity energy.

If the total energy at the end of pipe (section 1) is H, the velocity at the exit end of nozzle is

$$U = k_v \sqrt{2gH}$$

Here k_v is the coefficient of the velocity for the nozzle and takes into account the frictional losses in the nozzle. The value of k_v is very nearly unity (really it varies from 0.95 to 1.0).

14.2.2 Dynamic Force of the Stream

Whenever the velocity of a stream of fluid (i.e.,a free jet) is changed either in direction or in magnitude, a force is required. By the Newton's third law of motion, an equal and opposite force is exerted by the fluid upon the body producing the change. This is called a 'dynamic force' to distinguish it from the forces due to hydrostatic pressure.

As discussed in Chapter 5, the force exerted by the fluid upon the body (or vice versa) can be determined by the use of impulse momentum equation. It states that the rate of change of momentum brought in any direction of a fluid mass in a control volume is equal to the summation of all the external forces acting in the same direction.

$$F_x = \frac{W}{g}(\Delta U_x) = \rho Q (\Delta U_x) \qquad (14.1)$$

Referring to Fig. 14.1, let a jet of water discharge Q, strike a plate (vane); U_1 and U_2 are the mean velocities at sections 1 and 2, F_x is the force acting on the fluid mass (jet of water) and ΔU_x is the change in velocity (in x-direction) brought in by the presence of plate in the path of the jet. Hence,

Summation of all the external forces

= Mass of fluid striking the plate/sec × change in velocity of jet

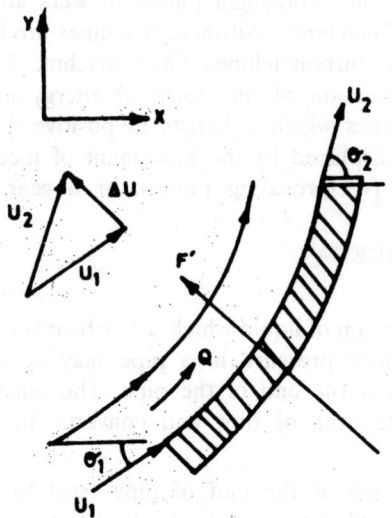

FIG. 14.1. DEFINITION SKETCH

$$F_x' = \frac{W}{g}(\Delta U_x) = \rho Q (\Delta U_x) \qquad (14.1)$$

$$F_x' = \rho Q (U_2 \cos \theta_2 - U_1 \cos \theta_1) \qquad (14.2)$$

Similarly $\qquad F_y' = \rho Q (\Delta U_y) = \rho Q (U_2 \sin \theta_2 - U_1 \sin \theta_1) \qquad (14.3)$

The resultant dynamic force F exerted by the body on the fluid is

$$F' = \frac{W}{g}(\Delta U) \qquad (14.4)$$

where $F' = \sqrt{(F_x')^2 + (F_y')^2}$ and $\Delta U = \sqrt{(\Delta U_x)^2 + (\Delta U_y)^2} \qquad (14.5)$

The direction of F' will be the same as that of $\Delta\,U$ (see inset to Fig. 14.1). The force F exerted by the fluid on the body will be equal in magnitude and opposite in direction to that of F'

Thus $$F = -F' = \frac{W}{g}(-\Delta U) \tag{14.6}$$

Alternatively from Eqs. 14.2 and 14.3,

$$F_x = \frac{W}{g}(U_1\cos\theta_1 - U_2\cos\theta_2) \tag{14.7}$$

and $$F_y = \frac{W}{g}(U_1\sin\theta_1 - U_2\sin\theta_2) \tag{14.8}$$

14.2.3 Relation Between Absolute and Relative Velocity

In the analysis of fluid problem, it will be necessary to deal with both the absolute and relative veclocities. The absolute velocity of a body is its velocity relative to the earth.

The relative velocity of a body is its velocity relative to a second body which may be stationery or in motion relative to the earth. The absolute velocity of the first body is the vectorial sum of its velocity relative to the second body and the absolute body of the second body. See Fig. 1.2.

In Fig. 14.2, u is the absolute velocity of the plate (vane), U is the absolute velocity of the jet of water and U_r is the relative velocity of the jet of water relative to the moving vane.

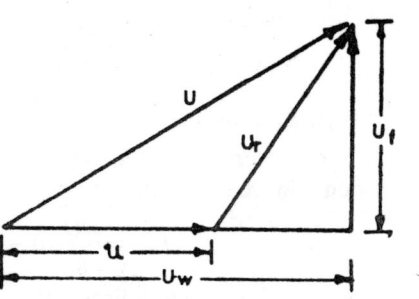

FIG. 14.2. RELATIVE AND ABSOLUTE VELOCITIES

$$\overline{U_r} = \overline{u} + \overline{U} \tag{14.9}$$

The absolute velocity U can be resolved into two component U_w and U_f, i.e. in the direction of u and normal to it respectively.

$$\overline{U} = \overline{U_w} + \overline{U_r} \tag{14.10}$$

14.3 DYNAMIC THRUST EXERTED BY A FLUID JET

Let a free jet of water strike against a flat plate; the plate may be held either normally or at an angle to the direction of jet, the jet of water issuing out of a nozzle (of area of cross section a) with the mean velocity U strikes the plate. A force F is exerted on the plate and vice versa. The mass of fluid issuing out of the nozzle per second is Q = (=a U). The magnitude and direction of this force can be determined by the use of impulse momentum equation, Eq. 14.1.

The following assumptions are made in the analysis of flow.

(i) The plate is assumed to be smooth and so no frictional loss occurs as the jet of water glides along the plate.

(ii) No loss of energy occurs due to the impact of jet on the plate and hence the absolute velocity of jet remains unchanged before and after striking the plate.

(iii) The pressure remains atmospheric all round the jet.

(iv) The plate is of finite size and so no change in the velocity occurs between any two sections of the jet due to the difference in their elevations.

14.4 FLAT PLATE OF FINITE SIZE

14.4.1 Stationary Flat Plate Held Normal to the Jet

Let a jet of water of area a and mean velocity U strike a stationary flat plate held normal to it. The jet is deflected by 90° after impact and then glides along the plate. Thus it will have no component of velocity in the direction of jet after impact. (Fig. 14.3).

The mass of water striking/sec $= \dfrac{W}{g} = \dfrac{wQ}{g}$

The change in velocity of jet in X-direction

$$= (U_{2x} - U_{1x})$$
$$= (0 - U)$$

Hence from Eq. 14.1

Force exerted on the fluid = mass striking the plate/sec × change of velocity in X-direction

$$F_x' = \frac{wQ}{g}(0 - U) = -\frac{wQU}{g} \tag{14.11}$$

The negative sign indicates that F_x' should act in the opposite direction.

The force acting on the flat plate by the jet is

$$F_x = -F_x'$$

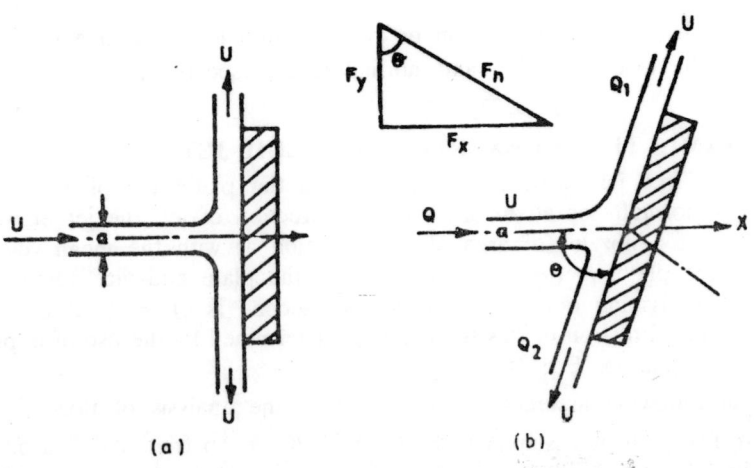

(a) (b)

FIG. 14.3. (A) STATIONARY FLAT PLATE HELD NORMALLY (B) STATIONARY FLAT PLATE HELD AT AN ANGLE TO THE DIRECTION OF JET

or $\qquad F_x = \dfrac{wQU}{g} = \dfrac{waU^2}{g}$ $\qquad\qquad$ (14.12)

14.4.2 Stationary Flat Plate Inclined to the Jet

When the jet strikes the plate, the discharge Q is divided into two unequal parts; discharge Q_1 flowing upward and discharge Q_2 flowing downwards, Fig. 14.3(b). Initially, these two components are unknown, hence first the force, normal to the plate, F_N is determined.

The force along the plate, F_T, will be zero; since there is no impact of jet on the plate in the tangential direction and water simply glides over it. The plate is assumed smooth and pressure remains unaltered all round the jet and therefore the velocity is assumed to remain unchanged.

The velocity of jet U can be resolved into two components; U cos θ along the plate and U sin θ normal to the plate. Therefore,

F_N = Mass striking the plate/ sec $\times$ change in velocity in the normal direction.

$$F_N = \frac{wQ}{g}(U \sin \theta - 0) = \frac{wa\, U^2 \sin \theta}{g} \qquad (14.13)$$

The force F_N can now be resolved into two components, in X (in the direction of jet) and Y directions.

$$F_X = F_N \sin \theta = \left(\frac{w\,a\,U^2 \sin \theta}{g}\right) \sin \theta = \frac{w\,a\,U^2}{g} \sin^2 \theta \qquad (14.14)$$

$$F_Y = F_N \cos \theta = \left(\frac{w\,a\,U^2}{g} \sin \theta\right) \cos \theta = \frac{w\,a\,U^2}{g} \sin \theta \cos \theta \qquad (14.15)$$

Similarly, the force F_T along the plate is given by

F_T = change: in momentum of the fluid/sec

$$0 = \frac{w}{g}[(Q_1 U - Q_2 U) - (Q U \cos \theta)] \qquad ...(14.16a)$$

Solving, $\qquad Q \cos \theta = Q_1 - Q_2$ $\qquad\qquad$ ...(14.16b)

From continuity equation, $Q = Q_1 + Q_2$ $\qquad\qquad$ ...(14.17)

Simplifying Eqs. 14.16b and 14.17,

$$Q_1 = Q\,(1 + \cos \theta)/2 \qquad ...(14.18a)$$

$$Q_2 = Q\,(1 - \cos \theta)/2 \qquad ...(14.18b)$$

14.4.3 Jet striking a moving inclined flat plate

Consider a smooth flat plate moving with velocity u in the direction of jet. Let the area and mean velocity of jet be 'a' and U respectively. Thus by the principle of relative velocity, the plate may be assumed to be stationary, if a velocity - u is superimposed on the velocity of jet U, i.e. the relative velocity of the jet is (U - u) with respect to plate.

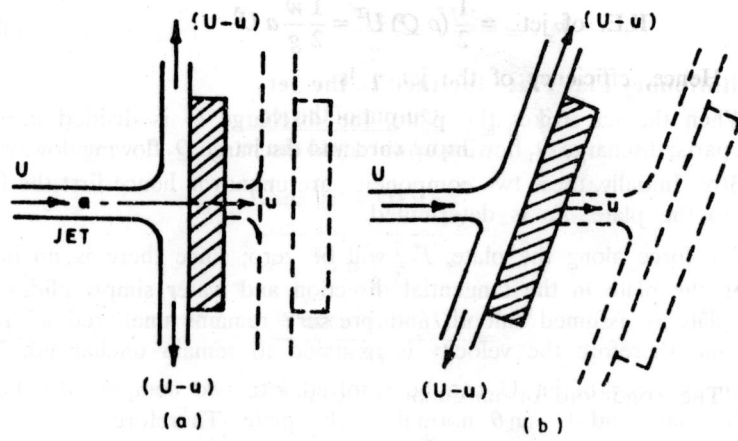

FIG. 14.4. INCLINED PLATE IN TRANSLATION

Mass of fluid striking the plate/sec $= \dfrac{w}{g} a (U - u)$

Therefore, $F_N =$ mass striking/sec $\times$ change in velocity in the normal direction

$$F_N = \frac{w}{g} a (U - u) [(U - u) \sin \theta - 0]$$

$$= \frac{w a (U - u)^2}{g} \sin \theta \qquad (14.20)$$

and $\qquad F_T = 0$

since the mass of the fluid striking the plate is zero and water simply glides over the plate.

The normal force F_N can be now resolved in the direction of jet and normal to it.

$$F_x = F_N \sin \theta = \frac{w a}{g} (U - u)^2 \sin^2 \theta \qquad (14.21)$$

$$F_y = F_N \cos \theta = \frac{w a}{g} (U - u)^2 \sin \theta \cos \theta \qquad (14.22)$$

Since the plate is moving in the direction of jet, this force F_x will do work on the plate which is given by Eq. 14.23.

Work done by the force in the direction of jet

$$= F_x u$$

$$= \left[\frac{w}{g} a (U - u)^2 \sin^2 \theta \right] \times u$$

$$= [\text{Output of the jet}] \qquad (14.23)$$

The input energy supplied to the jet is given by its kinetic energy.

$$\text{K.E. of jet} = \frac{1}{2}(\rho\, Q)\, U^2 = \frac{1}{2}\frac{w}{g}\, a\, U^3 \qquad (14.24)$$

Hence, efficiency of the jet η is ,

$$\eta = \frac{\text{Output of the jet}}{\text{Input energy to the jet}}$$

$$= \frac{\dfrac{w}{g}\, a\, u\, (U - u)^2 \sin^2\theta}{\dfrac{1}{2}\dfrac{w}{g}\, a\, U^3}$$

$$= \frac{2\,(U - u)^2\, u \sin^2\theta}{U^3} \qquad \ldots(14.25)$$

The condition for maximum efficiency is

$$\frac{d\eta}{du} = 0$$

$$= \frac{2\sin^2\theta}{U^3}\,[u \times 2\,(U - u)\,(-1) + (U - u)^2 \times (1)]$$

Simplifying, $(U - u)\,(U - 3\,u) = 0$

so that $\qquad\qquad U = u \text{ or } U = 3\,u \qquad\qquad \ldots(14.26)$

The second result is useful to determine the maximum efficiency.

$$\eta_{max} = \frac{2\sin^2\theta\,(3u - u)^2}{27\, U^3} = \frac{8}{27}\sin^2\theta \qquad \ldots(14.27)$$

If $\theta = 90°$, the jet will be striking the plate in the normal direction. This case is not practical as it requires continuous lengthening of jet.

14.4.4 Series of flat plates

Consider a series of flat plates which are mounted on the periphery of a wheel as shown in Fig. 14.5. As soon as the jet, area a and mean velocity U, strikes one of the flat plate, it moves forward and another plate comes in front of the jet and intercepts the jet. Likewise, the jet is continuously intercepted. Thus it may be considered that the whole mass of the fluid issuing out of the jet, i.e. ρ a U, is fully intercepted by a plate which may be in motion with tangential velocity u (= angular velocity of wheel × radius of wheel = ωr)

Mass striking per second $= \rho$ a U

Relative velocity of jet w.r. to the plate $= (U - u)$

$$\therefore \qquad F_x = \rho\, a\, U\,[(U - u) - 0] = \frac{w}{g}\, a\, U\,(U - u) \qquad \ldots(14.28)$$

Work done per second $= F_x \times u$

$$= \frac{w}{g}\, a\, U \times (U - u)\, u = \text{output of the jet} \qquad \ldots(14.29)$$

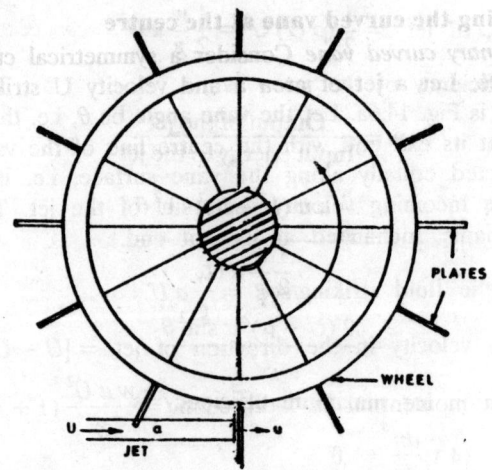

FIG. 14.5. SERIES OF FLAT PLATES MOUNTED ON A WHEEL

Input energy supplied to the jet/sec $= \dfrac{1}{2}\dfrac{w}{g}\,a\,U^3$

$\therefore$ Efficiency $\eta = \dfrac{Output\ of\ the\ jet}{Input\ of\ the\ jet}$

$$= \left[\dfrac{\dfrac{w}{g}\,a\,U\,(U-u)\times u}{\dfrac{w\,a\,U^3}{2g}}\right]$$

$$= \left[\dfrac{2u\,(U-u)}{U^2}\right] \qquad\qquad ...(14.30)$$

For maximum efficiency,

$$\dfrac{d\eta}{du} = 0$$

$$= \dfrac{2}{U^2}[(1)\,(U-u)+u\,(-1)]$$

Simplifying, $u = U/2$

Hence, $\eta_{max} = \dfrac{2\,(U/2)\,(U-U/2)}{U^2} = 0.5$ or 50% ...(14.31)

The maximum efficiency obtained is 50% when a series of plates are mounted on the periphery of a wheel and the wheel moves with a periphery velocity equal to half the jet velocity.

14.5 DYNAMIC FORCE EXERTED BY A JET ON CURVED SURFACE

Instead of the plate being flat, it may be made curved in shape and the jet may either strike the curved plate (or vane) at it centre and may come out at its ends (Fig. 14.6) or it may enter at one of its ends and may be discharged at the other end. (Fig. 14.8).

14.5.1 Jet striking the curved vane at the centre

(a) *Stationary curved vane* Consider a symmetrical curved vane having a smooth surface. Let a jet of area a and velocity U strike the vane at its centre as shown is Fig. 14.6a. Let the vane angle be θ, i.e. the angle subtended by the tangent at its exit end with the centre line of the vane. After impact, the jet is deflected equally along the vane surface, i.e. it makes an angle $(\pi - \theta)$ with the incoming velocity vector U of the jet. The magnitude of the velocity remains unchanged at its exit end.

Mass of the fluid striking/sec $= \dfrac{w}{g} a U$

Change is velocity in the direction of jet $= [U - U \cos (\pi - \theta)]$

Change in momentum in x-direction $= \dfrac{w a U^2}{g} (1 + \cos \theta)$

From Eq. 14.1,

$$F_x = \frac{w a U^2}{g} (1 + \cos \theta) \qquad \qquad ...(14.32)$$

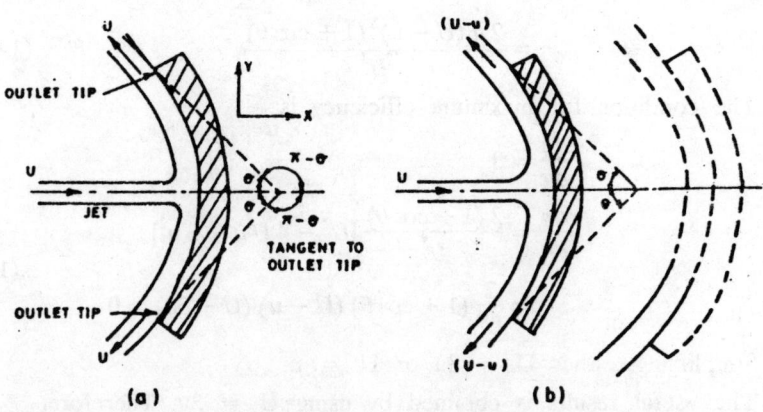

FIG. 14.6. (A) STATIONARY CURVED VANE (B) CURVED VANE IN TRANSLATION

(b) *Curved vane in translation* Let the curved vane move with velocity u in the direction of jet. Therefore, the relative velocity of the jet with respect to the curved vane will be (U - u), Fig. 14.6b.

∴ Mass striking the vane/sec $= \dfrac{w}{g} a (U - u)$

Change in velocity in X-direction

$$= [(U - u) - (U - u) \cos (\pi - \theta)]$$

From Eq. 14.1,

$$F_x = \text{mass striking/sec} \times \text{change in velocity in x-direction}$$

$$= \frac{w}{g} a (U - u) \left[(U - u) (1 - \cos (\pi - \theta) \right]$$

$$= \frac{w}{g} a \, (U - u)^2 \, (1 + \cos \theta) \qquad (14.33)$$

When the vane is in translation, work is done on the vane by the jet and vice versa.

Work done/sec $= F_x . u$

$$= \frac{w \, a \, (U - u)^2}{g} (1 + \cos \theta) \times u \qquad (14.34)$$

= Output of the jet

Input energy to the jet $= \frac{1}{2} mass \times U^2 = \frac{1}{2} \left(\frac{w}{g} a \, U \right) U^2$

$$= \frac{1}{2} \frac{w \, a \, U^3}{g}$$

$\therefore \qquad \eta = \dfrac{\text{Output of the jet}}{\text{Input to the jet}}$

$$= \frac{w \, a \, u \, (U - u)^2 \, (1 + \cos \theta)/g}{w \, a \, U^3/2g}$$

$$= \frac{2 \, u \, (U - u)^2 \, (1 + \cos \theta)}{U^3} \qquad (14.35)$$

The condition for maximum efficiency is

$$\frac{d\eta}{du} = 0$$

$$\frac{d\eta}{du} = \frac{2 \, (1 + \cos \theta)}{U^3} [U^2 - 4 \, U u + 3 \, u^2]$$

$$= \frac{2}{U^3} (1 + \cos \theta) \, (U - u) \, (U - 3u) = 0$$

Simplifying, either U = 3u or U = u

The useful results is obtained by using U = 3u, Therefore,

$$\eta_{max} = \frac{2 \, (1 + \cos \theta) \, u \, (3 \, u - u)^2}{(3 \, u)^3}$$

$$= \frac{8}{27} (1 + \cos \theta)$$

(i) When $\theta = 90°$, the curved vane becomes a flat plate, and

$$\eta_{max} = \frac{8}{27} \qquad (14.36b)$$

(ii) When $\theta = 0°$, the curved vane becomes a semi-circular surface, and

$$\eta_{max} = \frac{16}{27} \qquad (14.36c)$$

(c) *Series of curved vanes* The case of a single moving vane is not a practical proposition for performing useful work as the distance between jet and vane goes on increasing. After sometime, the vane moves much further away from the jet, and no portion of the jet impinges on the vane. Alternatively, a series of curved vanes may be mounted on the periphery of a wheel and a jet, area a and mean velocity U, strikes at the centre of the vane. As soon as one vane moves forward, another vane comes in front of the jet. In this manner, the jet is being intercepted continuously. Let the rotational speed of the wheel be ω (or its tangential velocity be u) and let inlet blade angle be θ.

$\therefore$ Mass of the fluid striking the vanes/sec. $= \rho\, a\, U = \dfrac{w}{g} a\, U$

Relative velocity of the jet with respect to the vane moving with a peripheral velocity u, i.e., $U_r = (U - u)$.

From Eq. 14.1

$$F_x = \text{mass striking/sec} \times \text{change in velocity in x} - \text{direction}$$

$$= \frac{w\,a\,U}{g} [(U - u) - (U - u) \cos(\pi - \theta)]$$

$$= \frac{w\,a\,U}{g} (U - u)(1 + \cos\theta) \qquad\qquad ...(14.37)$$

The work done by the jet on the vane/sec $= F_x . u$

$$= \frac{w\,a\,U}{g} (U - u)(1 + \cos\theta) \times u$$

$$= \text{Output of the jet} \qquad\qquad ...(14.38)$$

The input energy to the jet

$$= \frac{1}{2} \frac{w\,a\,U}{g} (U^2) = \frac{1}{2} \frac{w}{g} a\, U^3 \qquad\qquad ...(14.39)$$

From Eqs. 14.38 and 14.39,

Efficiency $\eta = \dfrac{w\,a\,U\,(U - u)\,u\,(1 + \cos\theta)/g}{w\,a\,U^3/2g}$

$$= \frac{2(1 + \cos\theta)(U u - u^2)}{U^2}$$

For obtaining maximum efficiency, $\dfrac{d\eta}{du} = 0$

$$\frac{2(1 + \cos\theta)}{U^2}(U - 2u) = 0$$

Hence $\eta_{max} = \dfrac{2(1 + \cos\theta)(2u \times u - u^2)}{4u^2}$

$$= \frac{(1 + \cos\theta)}{2} \qquad\qquad ...(14.40)$$

(i) When $\theta = 90°$, the curved vane behaves as a series of flat plates and Eq. 14.40 yields the same result as Eq. 14.31.

(ii) When $\theta = 0°$, the curved vanes becomes a semi-circular and $\eta_{max} = 100$ %.

Thus theoretically one can obtain 100% efficiency from series of smooth semi-circular vanes. Pelton wheel uses a modified form of these curved vanes.

14.5.2 Jet Striking the Curved Vane at one end

(a) *Stationary curved vane* Consider a stationary curved vane AB of Fig. 14.7. Let OX be the normal at the centre of the vane and tangents at A and B make an angle θ and φ respectively with the centre line OX. These are known as inlet blade angle θ and outlet blade angle φ respectively. Let the jet strike the vane tangentially at inlet tip A and come out tangentially at outlet tip B. Thus the jet makes an angle θ at inlet and φ at outlet to the centre line OX. In other words, the jet is deflected by an angle $\pi - (\theta + \varphi)$ from its initial position. Taking positive X and Y directions as shown in Fig. 14.7, the jet will have a velocity component in the positive X-direction ($= U \cos \theta$) at its inlet and a velocity component in the negative X-direction ($= - U \cos \varphi$) at its outlet tip. This fact can also be described as the jet

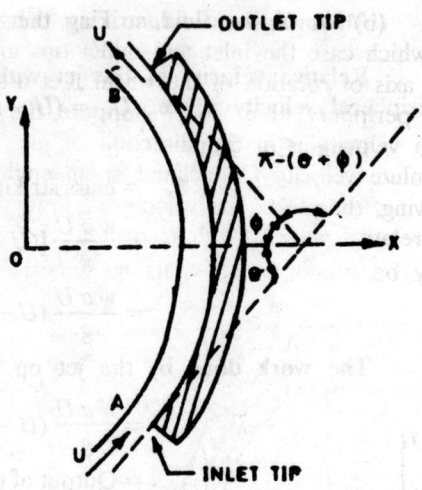

FIG. 14.7. JET STRIKING AT ONE OF THE TRIPS

is deflected by $(\pi - \varphi)$ from its + ve X-axis and hence the velocity component in the direction of OX at the outlet will be $U \cos (\pi - \varphi)$.

Mass of fluid striking the vane/sec at A $= \dfrac{w}{g} A U$

Change of momentum per second in the direction of OX

$$= [U \cos \theta - U \cos (\pi - \varphi)]$$

From Eq. 14.1, the force exerted by the jet in the normal direction or X-direction is given by

$$F_x = \frac{w}{g} a U [U \cos \theta - U \cos (\pi - \varphi)]$$

$$= \frac{w a U^2}{g} (\cos \theta + \cos \varphi) \tag{14.41a}$$

If the vane is semi circular, $\theta = \varphi = 0$

$$F_x = 2 \left(\frac{w a U^2}{g} \right) \tag{14.41b}$$

The force exerted by the jet on a semi circular vane is thus twice as great as that on a flat plate. This is due to the fact that with a semi circular vane, use is made of the reaction of the leaving fluid which exerts the same force on the vane in leaving as in entering.

In the same way, the force exerted on a vane in the tangential direction or Y-direction can be computed.

$$F_y = \frac{w}{g} a U [U \sin \theta - U \sin \varphi]$$

$$= \frac{w}{g} a U^2 [\sin \theta - \sin \varphi] \tag{14.42}$$

(b) *Moving curved vane* First consider the case of axial flow machines in which case the inlet and outlet tips are located at the same distance from the axis of rotation of the wheel. Let a series of vanes be located all around the periphery of a wheel. Suppose the curved vane of Fig, 14.8 is moving with velocity u in the direction of jet. The jet enters the inlet tip with an absolute velocity U, inclined at an angle α with ab. Since the vane itself is moving, therefore, the velocity of fluid with which it enters the vane will be its relative velocity with respect to the vane. The relative velocity U_r at inlet may be found by substracting vectorially u from U.

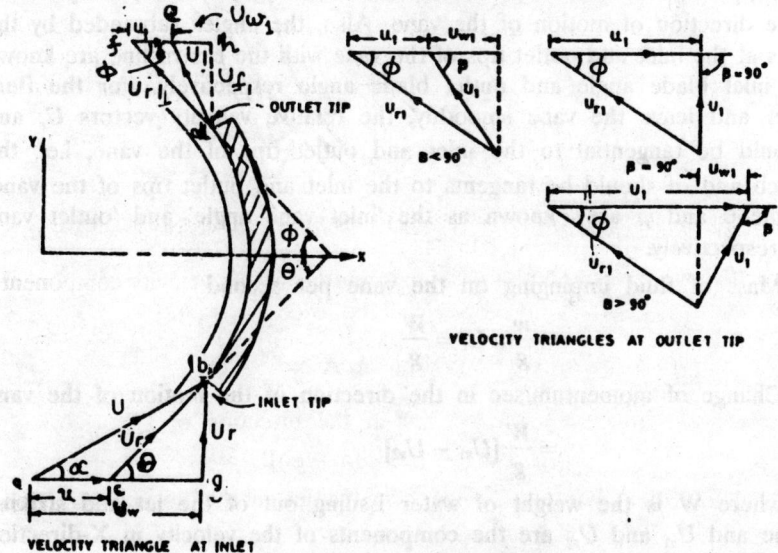

VELOCITY TRIANGLES AT OUTLET TIP

INLET TIP

VELOCITY TRIANGLE AT INLET

FIG. 14.8. JET STRIKING TANGENTIALLY AT ONE OF THE TIPS OF A MOVING CURVED VANE

Referring to Fig. 14.8, draw ab to represent absolute velocity U at the entrance and ac to represent velocity of vane u in magnitude and direction. Then cb represents the relative velocity of the jet. If the fluid is to enter the vane smoothly (without shock) at its entrance, the relative velocity should be parallel to cb, and it should be tangent to the vane at its inlet tip.

The fluid will glide over the vane and will leave at exit with relative velocity U_{r1} (say). The absolute velocity of the leaving jet of fluid may now be determined by drawing the velocity triangle at the outlet. Draw df to represent U_{r1} and fe to represent velocity of vane u_1 ($= u$ for axial flow machine) in magnitude and direction at exit. If the jet is to leave the vane smoothly, U_{r1} should be parallel to df and tangential at the outlet tip. Then de gives the absolute velocity in magnitude and direction of the fluid leaving the vane. Let it make an angle β with the direction of motion of the vane.

The absolute velocity of fluid U with which it enters the vane may be resolved into two components; one in the direction of motion of the vane and is known as velocity of whirl U_w and another normal to the direction to motion of the vane and is known as the velocity of flow U_f. These two components are represented by cg, and bg in Fig. 14.8. Thus, the triangle abg is known as the 'velocity triangle at inlet'.

Similarly, the absolute velocity U_1 at exit may be resolved into velocity of whirl U_{w1} in the direction of motion and velocity of flow U_{f1} in the normal direction. These are shown plotted as eh and dh respectively in Fig. 14.8. Thus, the triangle dfh is known as 'velocity triangle at outlet'.

Suppose the vectors U_r and U_{r1} make an angle θ and φ respectively with the direction of motion of the vane. Also, the angles subtended by the tangents at the inlet and outlet tips of the vane with the centre line are known as the inlet blade angle and outlet blade angle respectively. For the fluid to enter and leave the vane smoothly, the relative velocity vectors U_r and U_{r1} should be tangential to the inlet and outlet tips of the vane, i.e., the vector cb and df should be tangents to the inlet and outlet tips of the vane, the angle θ and φ are known as the 'inlet vane angle' and 'outlet vane angle' respectively.

Mass of fluid impinging on the vane per second

$$= \frac{w}{g} a U_r = \frac{W}{g}$$

Change of momentum/sec in the direction of the motion of the vane

$$= \frac{W}{g}[U_{x1} - U_{x2}]$$

where W is the weight of water issuing out of the jet and striking the vane and U_{x1} and U_{x2} are the components of the velocity in X-direction at its inlet tip and outlet tip.

From Δ b c g

$$U_{x1} = U_r \cos \theta = (U_w - u)$$

and from Δ d f h

$$U_{x2} = U_{r1} \cos (\pi - \varphi) = - U_{r1} \cos \varphi$$

The value of $U_{r1} \cos \varphi$ will depend on the actual value of β; for axial flow machines $u_1 = u$. (See Fig. 14.8)

From Δ d f h

(i) when $\beta < 90°$, $U_{x2} = -U_{r1}\cos\varphi = -[u + U_w]$

(ii) when $\beta = 90°$, $U_{x2} = -U_{r1}\cos\varphi = -(u)$

(iii) when $\beta < 90°$, $U_{x2} = -U_{r1}\cos\varphi = -(u - U_w)$

Thus the force acting on the vane in the direction of motion of the vane is given by

(i) when $\beta < 90°$,

$$F_x = \frac{W}{g}[(U_w - u) - \{-(u + U_{w1})\}]$$

$$= \frac{W}{g}(U_w + U_{w1}) \qquad ...(14.43a)$$

(ii) when $\beta = 90°$,

$$F_x = \frac{W}{g}[(U_w - u) - (-u)] = \frac{W}{g}(U_w) \qquad ...(14.43b)$$

(iii) when $\beta > 90°$,

$$F_x = \frac{W}{g}[(U_w - u) - \{-(u - U_{w1})\}]$$

$$= \frac{W}{g}(U_w - U_{w1}) \qquad ...(14.43c)$$

In general,

$$F_x = \frac{W}{g}[U_w \pm U_{w1}] \qquad ...(14.43)$$

Work done/sec $= F_x . u$

$$F_x = \frac{W}{g}[U_w u \pm U_{w1} u] \qquad ...(14.44)$$

The work done by the jet on the vane is also equal to the rate of change of kinetic energy of the jet per second.

Work done/sec $= \left[\dfrac{WU^2}{2g} - \dfrac{WU_1^2}{2g}\right] = \dfrac{W}{2g}(U^2 - U_1^2) \qquad ...(14.45)$

The efficiency η of the jet can now be determined

$$= \frac{Output\ of\ the\ jet}{Input\ to\ the\ jet}$$

$$= \frac{\dfrac{W}{g}[U_w u \pm U_{w1} u_1]}{\dfrac{1}{2}\dfrac{WU^2}{g}} = \frac{2(U_w u \pm U_{w1} u_1)}{U^2} \qquad ...(14.46)$$

Also $\qquad \eta = \dfrac{\dfrac{W}{2g}[U^2 - U_1^2]}{\dfrac{W}{g}\dfrac{U^2}{2}} = \left[\dfrac{U^2 - U_1^2}{U^2}\right]$

$$= [1 - U_1^2/U^2]$$ ...(14.47)

It follows from this equation that for a given value of α the efficiency will be maximum when U_1 is minimum. The velocity U_1 can not be zero otherwise the jet can not move out of the vane, i.e., it should have some finite value. Alternatively U_1 will be minimum when β is small (when β is acute U_{w1} will add to U_w and increase the efficiency). In the extreme case, β may be zero, this means U_{r1}, u and U_{w1} are co-linear. Assuming no friction loss over the vaves.

$$U_{r1} = U_r$$
$$U_1 = U_{W1} = (U_{r1} - u) = (U_r - u) \qquad \text{(i)}$$

If α is also zero, i.e. the U, u and U_r are co-linear

$$U_r = (U - u) \qquad \text{(ii)}$$

From Eqs (i) and (ii)

$$U_1 = U - 2u$$

Theoretically,

$$U_1 = 0 ; u = U/2 \qquad \text{(14.48)}$$

This means the efficiency will be 100% for semi-circular vanes moving at half the jet velocity. Slightly modified semi circular (or bowl type) vanes are used in the axial flow impulse turbines (e.g., Pelton Wheel).

14.5.3 Flow Over a Radial Vane

In axial flow machines, the distance of the water molecules from the axis of rotation remains same, therefore, the action of the stream can be determined by computing the force exerted by moving fluid (by the application of linear momentum theorem) and thereafter the torque exerted on the vanes can be computed. In case of radial flow machines, the radial distance of the water molecules (from the axis or rotation) varies along the path of the flow from inlet tip to outlet tip (See Fig. 14.9). Hence, the reaction of the jet on the vanes is determined by evaluating the rate of change in the moment of momentum (or angular momentum) which is also the torque imparted on the vanes by the fluid and vice versa. (Ref. sec. 5.13)

Angular momentum theorem. The sum of all the externally applied torquc on a given control volume of fluid is equal to the time rate of change in the angular momentum of the control volume about an axis of rotation, which is normal to the plane of rotation. The torque is the moment of the force and angular momentum is the moment of momentum about the axis of rotation.

Consider the vane of Fig. 14.9 to be one of a series of vanes fixed radially to the rim of a rotating wheel. Let the water enter at radius R at the outer periphery with velocity U. Since the wheel is also revolving with angular velocity ω rad/sec., the water enters the wheel smoothly with a relative velocity U_r. The inlet velocity triangle a b g is shown in the Fig. 14.9. Similarly the water jet comes out at the inner periphery at a radius R_1. The outlet velocity triangled d f h is also shown in the same figure.

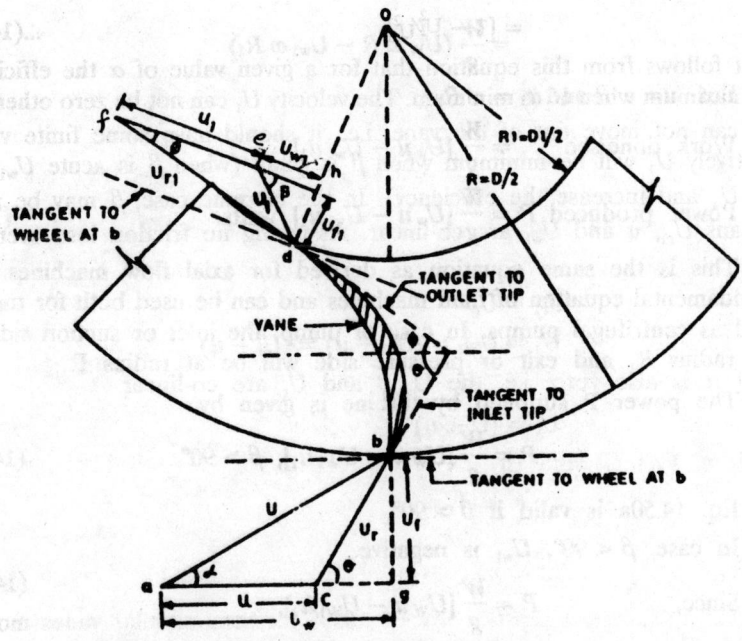

FIG. 14.9. CURVED VANES MOUNTED RADIALLY ON
THE PERIPHERY OF A WHEEL

The mass of the fluid striking the vane/sec

$$= \frac{w}{g} Q = \frac{w a_r U_r}{g} = \frac{W}{g}$$

The tangential momentum of the fluid entering the vane at its entrance

$$= \frac{W}{g} (U_w)$$

Moment of momentum of the fluid at the entrance

$$= \frac{W}{g} (U_w R)$$

Similarly moment of momentum of the fluid at exit

$$= \frac{W}{g} (U_{w1} R_1)$$

From angular momentum theorem,

Torque applied on the wheel = Rate of change of moment of momentum

$$T = \frac{W}{g} (U_w R - U_{w1} R_1) \tag{14.49}$$

Work done/second

$$= T \times \omega$$

$$= \frac{W}{g} (U_W \omega R - U_{w1} \omega R_1)$$

But $u = \omega R$ and $u_1 = \omega R_1$

$\therefore$ Work done/sec $= \frac{W}{g} [U_W u - U_{w1} u_1]$

Power produced $P = \frac{W}{g} [U_w u - U_{w1} u_1]$ watts. $\hspace{1cm}$ (14.50)

This is the same equation as derived for axial flow machines. It is the fundamental equation of fluid machines and can be used both for turbines as well as centrifugal pumps. In case of pump, the inlet or suction side will be at radius R_1 and exit or pressure side will be at radius R.

The power P supplied by turbine is given by

$$P = \frac{W}{g} [U_w u - U_{w1} u_1], \beta > 90° \hspace{1cm} (14.50a)$$

Eq. 14.50a is valid if $\beta > 90°$.

In case, $\beta < 90°$, U_{w1} is negative.

Since, $\hspace{1cm} P = \frac{W}{g} [U_w u - U_{w1} u_1],$

$$= \frac{W}{g} [U_w u + U_{w1} u_1] \hspace{1cm} (14.50b)$$

When $\beta = 90°$, $U_{w1} = 0$;

$$P = \frac{W}{g} [U_w u] \hspace{1cm} (14.50c)$$

The power input to the jet = K.E. of the jet

$$= \frac{1}{2} \cdot \frac{W}{g} \cdot U^2$$

Efficiency $\hspace{1cm} \eta = \dfrac{\dfrac{W}{g} [U_w u \pm U_{w1} u_1]}{\dfrac{1}{2} \left[\dfrac{W}{g} \cdot U^2 \right]}$

$$\eta = \frac{2 (U_w u \pm U_{w1} u_1)}{U^2} \hspace{1cm} (14.46)$$

If the head transmitted between the wheel and fluid is Hr, then from Eq. 14.50 a to c.

$$P = W \times H_r$$

or $\hspace{1cm} H_r = \left[\frac{U_w u \pm U_{w1} u_1}{g} \right] \hspace{1cm} (14.51)$

This is Euler's equation of fluid machines which gives the total head that would be developed (or absorbed) by a runner without loss.

The actual head under which the machine operates equals the runner head minus all the internal hydraulic losses h_L between the inlet and discharge flanges of the machine. Thus, for pumps,

$$H = \eta_H H_r = (H_r - h_L) \qquad (14.52)$$

For turbines,

$$H = \frac{H_r}{\eta_H} = (H_r + h_L) \qquad (14.53)$$

where η_H is the hydraulic efficiency which is always less than unity.

Example 14.1 to 14.10

14.1. A jet of water 8 cm in diameter, delivering a flow of 105 lit/sec, strikes normally a flat smooth plate. Determine (a) the thrust on the plate if it is at rest, (b) the thrust, and work done on the plate and its efficiency if the plate is moving in the same direction as the jet with a velocity of 12 m/s, (c) the thrust, and work done on the plate and efficiency if the single plate in case (b) is replaced by a series of plates moving with a velocity of 12 m/s.

Solution.

(a) The normal thrust on the plate at rest is given by Eq, 14.12,

$$F_N = \frac{w \, a \, U^2}{g}$$

Area of the jet $= \frac{\pi}{4} \times (0.08)^2 = 0.00502$

Velocity of jet $U = \frac{Q}{a} = \frac{105}{1000 \times 0.00502} = 20.9 \text{ m/s}$

$$F_N = \frac{9810 \times 0.00502 \times (20.9)^2}{9.81}$$

$$= 2192.78 \text{ N}$$

Since the plate is at rest, u = 0

Work done $= F \times u = 0.$

(b) The normal thrust on the moving plate is given by Eq. 14.19

$$F_N = \frac{w \, a \, (U - u)^2}{g} \sin \theta$$

Here $\sin \theta = 1.0$ since $\theta = 90°$

$$F_N = \frac{9810 \times 0.00502 \times (20.9 - 12)^2}{9.81}$$

$$= 397.63 \text{ N}$$

Work done per second by the jet on the plate

$$= F \times u$$

$$= 397.63 \times 12$$

$$= 4771.56 \text{ Nm}$$

Output power $= 4771.56\,\text{Nm}$

Input power $=$ kinetic energy of the jet

$$= \frac{1}{2}\left(\frac{w\,a\,U}{g}\right)U^2$$

$$= \frac{1}{2} \times \frac{(9810 \times 0.00502 \times 20.9)}{9.81}(20.9)^2$$

$$= 22914.62\ \text{N-m/s}$$

Efficiency of jet $\eta = \dfrac{Output}{Input} \times 100$

$$= \frac{4771.56}{22914.62} \times 100$$

$$= 20.82\%$$

(c) When the single plate is replaced by a series of flat plates, the mass of fluid striking the plates is given by

Mass of fluid striking/sec $= \dfrac{w\,a\,U}{g}$

$$\therefore \qquad F_N = \frac{w\,a\,U}{g}(U-u)$$

$$= \frac{9810 \times 0.00502 \times 20.9}{9.81} \times (20.9 - 12)$$

$$= 933.77\ \text{N}$$

Work done by the jet per second the plates

$$= 933.77 \times 12$$

$$= 11205.24\ \text{N-m}$$

Output power $= 11205.24\ \text{N-m/s}$

Input power $= 22914.62\ \text{N-m/s}$

$$\%\,\eta = \frac{11205.24}{22914.62} \times 100$$

$$= 48.89\ \%$$

14.2 A rectangular plate, waghing 60 N, is suspended vertically by a hinge on the top horizontal edge. The centre of gravity of the plate is 10 cm from the hinge. A horizontal jet of water 2 cm diameter, whose axis is 15 cm below the hinge impinges normally on the plate with a velocity of 5 m/s. Find the horizontal force applied at the centre of gravity to maintain the plate in its vertical position. Find the corresponding velocity of the jet, if the plate is deflected through 30° and the same force continues to act at the centre of gravity of the plate.

Solution.

Area of jet $\qquad = \dfrac{\pi}{4}\left(\dfrac{2}{100}\right)^2 = 0.000314\ \text{m}^2$

Weight of the plate = 60 N.

Velocity of the jet = 5 m/s

Let the force F acts at the centre of gravity of the plate as shown in Fig. 14.10.

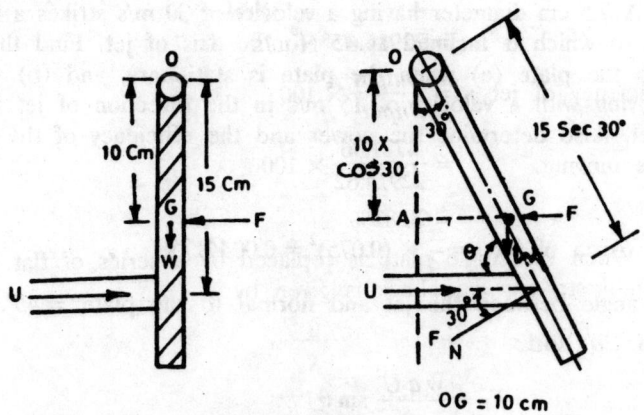

FIG. 14.10. EXAMPLE 14.2

The force exerted by the jet in the normal direction to the vertical plate

$$= \frac{w\,a\,U^2}{g}$$

$$F_N = \frac{9810 \times 0.000314 \times (5)^2}{9.81}$$

$$= 7.85\ \text{N}$$

Take moment about the hinge O,.

$$F_N \times 0.15 = F \times 0.10$$

$$F = \frac{7.85 \times 0.15}{0.10}$$

$$= 11.78\ \text{N}$$

(b) The plate is deflected as shown in Fig. 14.10 (b). The angle between the jet and the plate is 60°. The force acting normal to the plate is given by Eq. 14.13

$$F_N = \frac{w\,a\,U^2}{g}\sin\theta$$

$$F = \frac{9810 \times 0.000314 \times (U)^2}{9.81}\times\sin 60°$$

$$= 0.272\,U^2$$

Taking moment about the hinge O,

$$F_N \times 0.15 \sec 30° = 60 \times (AG) + F \times OA$$

$$0.272\, U^2 \times 0.15 \times 1.155 = 60 \times 0.10 \times 0.5 + 11.78 \times 0.10 \times 0.866$$

(Since $AG = 0.10 \sin 30°$
and $OA = 0.10 \cos 30°$)

$$\therefore \qquad U = 9.23 \text{ m/s.}$$

14.3 A 7.5 cm diameter having a velocity of 30 m/s strikes a flat plate, the normal to which is inclined at 45° to the axis of jet. Find the normal pressure on the plate (a) when the plate is stationary, and (b) when the plate is moving with a velocity of 15 m/s in the direction of jet and away from the jet. Also determine the power and the efficiency of the jet when the plate is moving.

Solution.

(a) Area of jet $= \dfrac{\pi}{4} \times (0.075)^2 = 0.004417 \text{ m}^2$

The angle between the jet and normal to the plate $= 45°$.

From Eq. 14.13,

$$F_N = \frac{w\, a\, U^2}{g} \sin \theta$$

$$F_N = \frac{9810 \times 0.004417 \times (30)^2}{9.81} \sin 45°$$

$$F_N = 2811.4 \text{ N}$$

(b) When the plate is moving with a velocity of 15 m/s, the normal

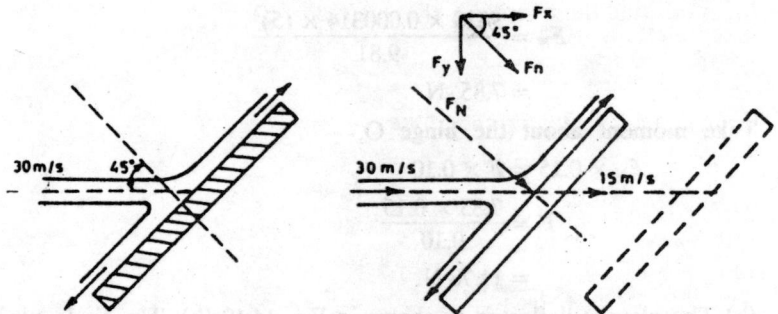

FIG. 14.11. EXAMPLE 14.3

force F_N is given Eqn. 14.19.

$$F_N = \frac{w\, a\, (U - u)^2}{g} \cdot \sin \theta$$

$$= \frac{9810 \times 0.004417 \times (30 - 15)^2}{9.81} \sin 45°$$

$$= 702.85 \text{ N}$$

Work done per second by the jet in the direction of jet

$$= F_x \times u$$
$$= F_N \sin \theta \times u$$
$$= 702.85 \times \sin 45° \times 15$$
$$= 7455.98 \text{ N–m}$$

Output of the jet $= 7455.98$ N–m/s
$$= 7455.98 \text{ W}$$

Input of the jet $= \left(\dfrac{w}{g} a U\right) \dfrac{U^2}{2}$

$$= \left(\dfrac{9810 \times 0.004417 \times 30}{9.81}\right) \dfrac{(30)^2}{2}$$

$$= 59629.5 \text{ W}$$

$$= \% \, \eta = \dfrac{7455.98}{59629.5} \times 100$$

$$= 12.5 \ \%$$

14.4 A jet of water from a nozzle is deflected through 60° from its original direction by a curved plate which it enters without shock with a velocity of 30 m/s and leaves with a velocity 25 m/sec. If the weight of fluid discharged from the nozzle is 8 N/s, calculate the magnitude and direction of the resultant force on the vane, taking the vane as stationary.

Solution.

Let the force F act on vane at an angle α to the horizontal.

Mass of the fluid striking the plate
$$= \dfrac{8}{9.81} = 0.815 \text{ kg/s}$$

Change in velocity in the direction of jet
$$= 30 - 25 \cos 60°$$

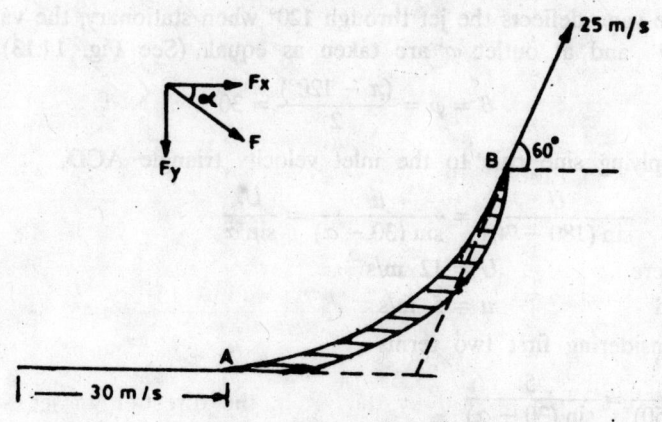

FIG. 14.12   EXAMPLE 14.4

∴   Force acting in the direction of jet F_x

$$= 0.815 \left(30 - 25 \times \frac{1}{2} \right) = 14.26 \text{ N}$$

Similarly, the force acting in the Y-direction

$$= 0.815 \times \text{ change in vel. in Y-direction}$$
$$= 0.815 \times [0 - 25 \sin 60°]$$
$$= - 17.64 \text{ N}$$

ve sign indicate that F_y acts vertically downward.

∴   Resultant force $F = \sqrt{F_x^2 + F_y^2}$

$$= \sqrt{(14.26)^2 + (- 17.64)^2}$$
$$= 22.68 \text{ N}$$

The direction of resultant F with reference to X axis is   given   by tan α

$$\tan \alpha = \frac{F_y}{F_x}$$
$$= - \frac{17.64}{14.26} = - 1.237$$

- ve sign indicates that the α is measured in clockwise direction.

$$= \tan^{-1} (- 1.237)$$
$$= 51.05°.$$

14.5 A jet of water moving at 12 m/s impinges on a concave shaped vane to deflect the jet through 120° when stationary. If the vane is moving at 5 m/s, find the angle of the jet so that there is no shock at inlet. Also determine the absolute velocity at exit in magnitude and direction and work done per unit weight of water. Assume the vane to be smooth.

Solution

The vane deflects the jet through 120° when stationary, the vane angles at inlet θ and at outlet φ are taken as equal. (See Fig. 14.13)

$$\theta = \varphi = \frac{(\pi - 120°)}{2} = 30°$$

Applying sine rule to the inlet velocity triangle ACD,

$$\frac{U}{\sin (180 - 30)} = \frac{u}{\sin (30 - \alpha)} = \frac{U_r}{\sin \alpha}$$

where $U = 12$ m/s

and $u = 5$ m/s

Considering first two terms

$$\frac{12}{\sin (150)} = \frac{5}{\sin (30 - \alpha)}$$

∴ $\sin (30 - \alpha) = 0.2083$

$$\alpha = 17.98°$$

Now considering first and third term.

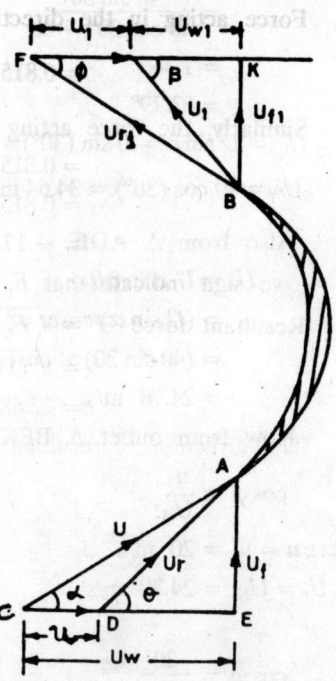

$$\frac{12}{\sin (150)} = \frac{U_r}{\sin 17.98}$$

$$U_r = \frac{12 \sin (17.98)}{\sin (150)}$$

$$= 7.41 \text{ m/s}$$

$$U_r = U_{r1} = 7.41 \text{ m/s}$$

Now consider outlet velocity triangle. Applying consine rule,

$$U_1^2 = u_1^2 + U_{r1}^2 - 2 u_1 U_{r1} \cos 30$$

$$(\text{since } \varphi = 30)$$

Since $u = u_1 = 5$ m/s

$$U_1^2 = (5)^2 + (7.41)^2 - 2 \times 5 \times 7.41 \cos 30$$

$$U_1 = 3.96 \text{ m/s.}$$

From outlet velocity triangle,

$$\tan \beta = \frac{U_{f1}}{U_{w1}}$$

$$= \frac{U_{r1} \sin 30°}{U_{r1} \cos 30° - u_1}$$

FIG. 14.13 EXAMPLE 14.5

$$= \frac{7.41 \times 0.5}{(7.41 \times \sqrt{3/2} - 5)} = 2.61$$

$$\beta = 69°$$

14.6 A jet of water having velocity of 40 m/s strikes a curved vane which is moving with a velocity of 20 m/s. The jet makes an angle of 30° with the direction of the vane at inlet and leaves at an angle of 90° to the direction of motion of vane at outlet. Draw velocity triangles at inlet and outlet so that water enters the vane at inlet and leaves the vane without shock.

Solution

The velocity triangles at inlet and outlet are drawn in Fig. 14.14 where $\alpha = 30°$ and $\beta = 90$.

Also $U = 40$ m/s, $u = 20$ m/s.

From $\triangle$ ADE,

$$\tan \theta = \frac{U_f}{(U_w - u)} = \frac{U \sin \alpha}{(U \cos \alpha - u)}$$

$$= \frac{40 \sin 30°}{40 \cos 30° - 20},$$

$$= 1.366$$

$$= 53.79°$$

$$\left[\because \quad U_f = U \sin \alpha = 40 \sin (30°) = 20 \text{ m/s} \right.$$

$$\left. U_w = 40 \cos (30°) = 34.64 \text{ m/s} \right]$$

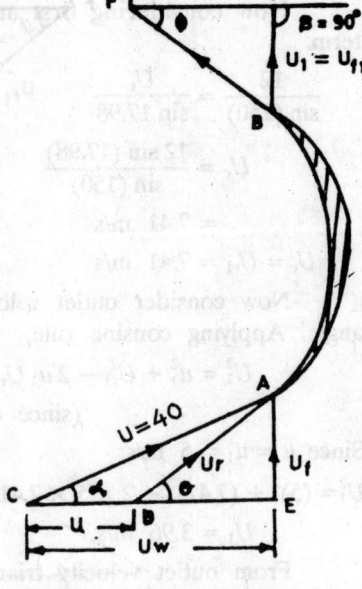

FIG. 14.14 EXAMPLE 14.6

Also from $\triangle$ ADE,

$$U_r = U_f \, cosec \, \theta$$

$$= (U \sin \alpha) \, cosec \, \theta$$

$$= (40 \sin 30) \times cosec \, (53.79)$$

$$= 24.78 \text{ m/s}.$$

Now from outlet $\triangle$ BFK

$$\cos \varphi = \frac{u_1}{U_{r1}}$$

where $u = u_1 = 20$ m/s

$\quad U_r = U_{r1} = 24.78$ m/s

$\therefore \qquad \cos \varphi = \dfrac{20}{24.78}$

$$= 0.8071$$

$$\varphi = 36.18°.$$

14.7 A jet of water having a velocity of 35 m/s impinges on a series of vanes moving with a velocity of 20 m/s. The jet makes an angle of 30° to the direction of motion of vanes when entering and leaving at an angle of 120°. Draw the velocity triangles and find (a) the angle of vane tips so that water enters and leaves without shock, (b) the 'work done per newton of water entering the turbine, and (c) efficiency of the turbine.

Solution.

Given $\qquad U = 35$ m/s, $\qquad u = 20$ m/s

$\qquad\qquad\qquad \alpha = 30°, \qquad \beta = (180 - 120°) = 60°$

From inlet $\triangle$ ACE

$$U_f = U \sin \alpha$$

$$= 35 \sin (30) = 17.5 \text{ m/s}$$

$$U_w = U \cos \alpha$$

$$= 35 \cos (30°)$$

$$= 30.3 \text{ m/s}$$

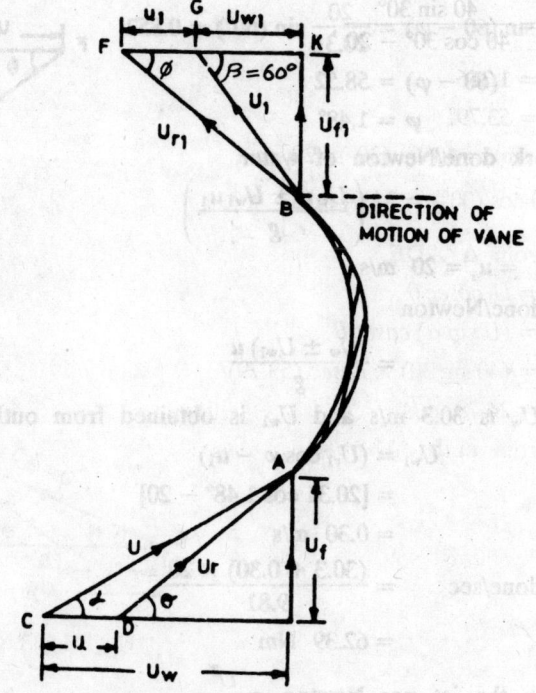

FIG. 14.15 EXAMPLE 14.7

From Δ ADE,

$$\tan \theta = \frac{U_f}{(U_w - u)}$$

$$= \frac{17.5}{(30.3 - 20)} = 1.697$$

$$\theta = 59.5°$$

Also

$$U_r = \frac{U_f}{\sin \theta}$$

$$= \frac{17.5}{\sin (59.5)} = 20.31 \text{ m/s}$$

Assume the vanes to be smooth,

$$U_r = U_{r1} = 20.31 \text{ m/s}$$

Apply sine rule to outlet Δ BFG,

$$\frac{U_{r1}}{\sin (180 - \beta)} = \frac{u_1}{\sin (60 - \varphi)}$$

$$\frac{20.31}{\sin (60)} = \frac{20}{\sin (60 - \varphi)}$$

$$\sin(60 - \varphi) = \frac{20}{20.31} \sin(60°) = 0.852$$

$$(60 - \varphi) = 58.52$$

$$\varphi = 1.48°$$

(b) Work done/Newton of water

$$= \left(\frac{U_w u \pm U_{w1} u_1}{g} \right)$$

Since $u = u_1 = 20$ m/s

Work done/Newton

$$= \frac{(U_w \pm U_{w1}) u}{g}$$

where U_w is 30.3 m/s and U_{w1} is obtained from outlet Δ BFK

$$U_{w1} = (U_{r1} \cos \varphi - u_1)$$
$$= [20.31 \cos 1.48° - 20]$$
$$= 0.30 \text{ m/s}$$

∴ Work done/sec $= \dfrac{(30.3 + 0.30) \times 20}{9.81}$

$$= 62.39 \text{ Nm}$$

Input to the jet per Newton $= \dfrac{U^2}{2g}$

$$= \frac{(35)^2}{2 \times 9.81} = 62.43 \text{ Nm}$$

$$\% \eta = \frac{62.39}{62.43} \times 100$$

$$= 99.9 \%$$

14.8 A jet of water having a velocity of 45 m/s, impinges without shock on a series of vanes moving at 15 m/s, the direction of motion of the vanes being inclined at 20° to that of jet. The relative velocity at outlet is 0.9 times of that at inlet, and the absolute velocity of water at exit is to be normal to the motion of the vanes.

Find (a) vane angles at entrance and exit, (b) Work done on vanes per newton of water supplied by the jet, and (c) hydraulic efficiency.

Solution

Applying cosine rule to inlet Δ ACD; Refer Fig. 14.16

$$U_r^2 = (U^2 + u^2 - 2U \cdot u \cos \alpha)$$
$$U_r^2 = [(45)^2 + (15)^2 - 2 \times 45 \times 15 \, (cos \, 20°)]$$
$$U_r = 31.32 \text{ m/s}$$

∴ $U_{r1} = 0.9 \, U_r$

$$= 28.19 \text{ m/s}$$

From inlet Δ ACE

$U_f = U \sin \alpha$ and $U_w = U \cos \alpha$

From inlet Δ ADE

$$\tan \theta = \frac{U_f}{(U_w - u)}$$

$$= \frac{45 \sin (20°)}{45 \cos (20) - 15}$$

$\theta = 29°.26'$

From outlet Δ BFK, $u = u_1$

$$\cos \varphi = \frac{u_1}{U_{r1}}$$

$$= \frac{15.0}{28.19}$$

$\varphi = 57° 51'$

(b) Work done/sec/Newton

$$= \frac{(U_w u \pm U_{w1} u_1)}{g}$$

(Since $\beta = 90°$, $U_{w1} = 0$),

$\therefore$ Work done/sec/Newton, $= \dfrac{U_w u}{g}$

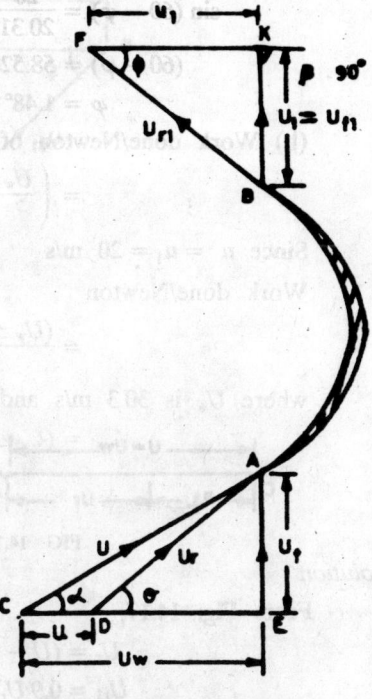

FIG. 14.16 EXAMPLE 14.8

$$= \frac{45 \cos 20° \times 15}{9.81}$$

$$= 64.66 \text{ N-m/N}$$

(c) Input to the jet per Newton

$$= \frac{U^2}{2g}$$

$$= \frac{(45)^2}{2 \times 9.81} = 103.2 \text{ N-m/N}$$

$$\% \eta = \frac{64.66}{103.2} \times 100$$

$$= 62.65 \%$$

14.9 A 2.5 cm diameter jet having a velocity of 70 m/s impinges without shock on a series of vanes which move in the same direction as the jet. The shape of each vane is such that, if stationary, it would deflect the jet through and angle of 150°. Friction reduces the relative velocity by 10% as water flows across the vanes and there is further windage loss given by $0.4\, u^2/2g$ N m/N of water. Find (a) the velocity of vanes corresponding to maximum efficiency and the value of this efficiency, (b) the corresponding force on the vanes, in and at right angles to the direction of their motion.

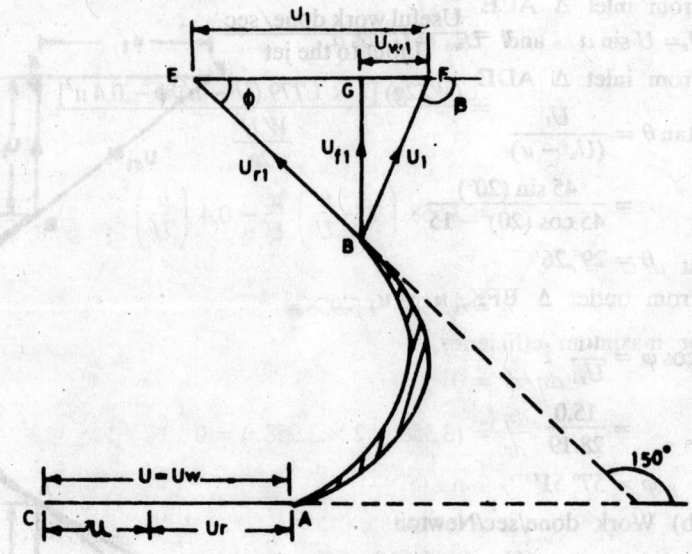

FIG. 14.17 EXAMPLE 14.9

Solution

From Fig. 14.17,

$$U_r = (U - u) = (70 - u)$$
$$U_{r1} = 0.9 \, U_r = 0.9 \, (70 - u)$$
$$U_w = U = 70 \text{ m/s}$$

and $\qquad U_{w1} = (u_1 - U_{r1} \cos \varphi)$

But $\quad u = u_1$ and $\varphi = (180 - 150) = 30°$

$\therefore \qquad U_{w1} = [u - 0.9 \, (U - u) \cos 30°]$

$$= \left[u - 0.9 \, (U - u) \frac{\sqrt{3}}{2} \right]$$

Work done/sec $\quad = \dfrac{W}{g} \left[U_w u - U_{w1} u \right]$

$$= \frac{W}{g} \left[U - \left\{ u - 0.9 \, (U - u) \frac{\sqrt{3}}{2} \right\} \right] u$$

$$= \frac{W}{g} \left[1.779 \, (U - u) \right] u$$

$\therefore \quad$ Useful work done/sec $= \dfrac{W}{g} \left[1.779 \, (U - u) \, u \right] - 0.4 \, W \dfrac{u^2}{2g}$

Input to the jet $\quad =$ kinetic energy of the jet

$$= \frac{W U^2}{2g}$$

Efficiency is given by

$$\eta = \frac{\text{Useful work done/sec}}{\text{Input to the jet}}$$

$$= \frac{(W/2g)\,[2 \times 1.779\,(U - u)\,u - 0.4\,u^2]}{\dfrac{W U^2}{2g}}$$

$$= 3.558 \left(1 - \frac{u}{U}\right) \frac{u}{U} - 0.4 \left(\frac{u}{U}\right)^2$$

Put $u/U = r$

$\therefore$ $\qquad\qquad \eta = 3.558\,r - 3.958\,r^2$

For maximum efficiency,

$$\frac{d\eta/dr = 0}$$

$\therefore$ $\qquad\qquad \dfrac{d\eta}{dr} = (3.558 - 2 \times 3.958\,r) = 0$

$$r = 0.449$$

i.e. $\qquad\qquad u = 0.449\,U = 0.449 \times 70 = 31.43 \text{ m/s}$

Maximum efficiency $= (3.558 - 3.958 \times 0.449) \times 0.449$

$$= 0.799 \text{ or } 79.9\%$$

Force acting on the vane in the direction of jet

$$= \frac{W}{g}[U_w - U_{w1}]$$

Weight of water impinging the vane/sec

$$= 9810 \times \frac{\pi}{4} \times (0.025)^2 \times 70$$

$$= 1347.65 \text{ N}$$

and $\qquad\qquad U_{w1} = 31.43 - 0.9\,(70 - 31.43)\dfrac{\sqrt{3}}{2}$

$$= 1.368 \text{ m/s}$$

$$F_x = \frac{1347.65}{9.81}[70 - 1.368]$$

$$= 9428.25 \text{ N}$$

Force acting on the vane at right angles to the direction of the motion of the vane is F_y

$$F_y = \frac{W}{g}[U_{f1} - U_f] \qquad\qquad\qquad [\because U_f = 0]$$

$$= \frac{1347.65}{9.81}[U_{r1}\sin\varphi]$$

$$= 137.37\,[0.9\,(70 - 31.43)\sin 30]$$

$$= 2384.35 \text{ N}$$

14.10 A jet of water having a velocity of 30 m/s strikes a series of curved vanes radially mounted on a wheel, with outer and inner radius as

0.5 m and 0.25 m respectively. The wheel rotates at 200 rpm. The jet makes an angle of 20° with the tangent at inlet and leaves with velocity 5 m/s at an angle of 130° to the tangent to the wheel at outlet. Determine (a) vane angles at inlet and outlet, (b) work done per second per newton of water (c) efficiency of the wheel. Water enters the wheel radially inward.

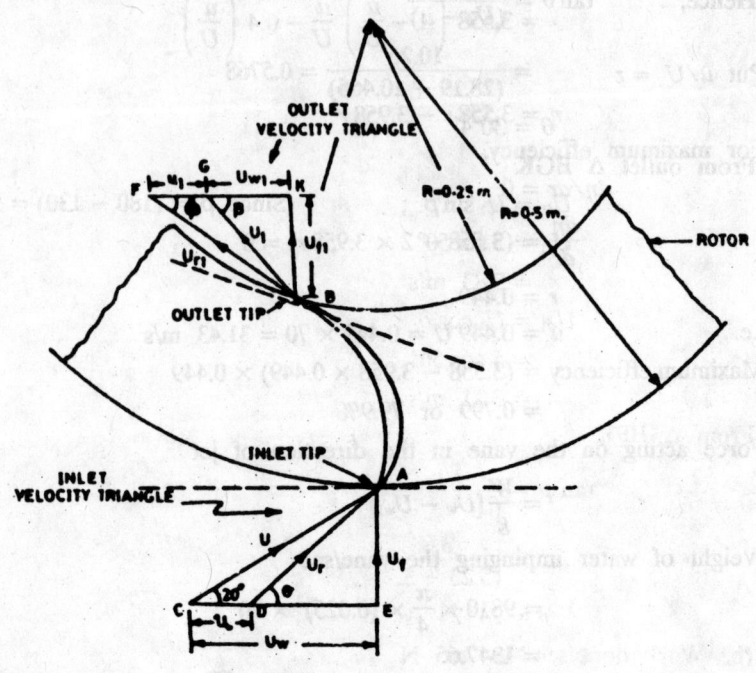

FIG. 14.18 EXAMPLE 4.10

Solution

The following data are given :

$$\alpha = 20°, R = 0.5\,m, R_1 = 0.25\,m, U = 30 \text{ m/s}$$

$$\beta = 130°, N = 200\,rpm, U_1 = 5 \text{ m/s}$$

$$u = \frac{2\pi R N}{60}$$

$$= \frac{2 \times \pi \times 0.5 \times 200}{60} = 10.466 \text{ m/s}$$

$$u_1 = \frac{2\pi R_1 N}{60}$$

$$= \frac{2 \times \pi \times 0.25 \times 200}{60} = 5.23 \text{ m/s}$$

Apply cosine rule to Δ ACD,

$$U_r^2 = (U^2 + u^2 - 2U \times u \times \cos\alpha)$$

$$U_r^2 = [(30)^2 + (5.23)^2) - 2 \times 30 \times 5.23 \times \cos 20°]$$

$$U_r = 25.15 \text{ m/s}$$

Then

$$U_t = U \sin (20°) = 10.26 \text{ m/s}$$

$$U_w = U \cos (20°) = 28.19 \text{ m/s}$$

Hence,

$$\tan \theta = \frac{U_t}{(U_w - u)}$$

$$= \frac{10.26}{(28.19 - 10.466)} = 0.5768$$

$$\theta = 30°4'$$

From outlet Δ BGK

$$U_{f1} = U_1 \sin \beta \; ; \qquad \text{(Since } \beta' = (180 - 130) = 50°)$$

$$U_{f1} = 5 \sin 50°$$

$$= 3.83 \text{ m/s}$$

$$U_{w1} = U_1 \cos \beta$$

$$= 5 \cos 50°$$

$$= 3.21 \text{ m/s}$$

From Δ BFK

$$\tan \varphi = \frac{U_{f1}}{(u_1 + U_{w1})}$$

$$= \frac{3.83}{(5.23 + 3.21)} = 0.453$$

$$\varphi = 24° 24'$$

(b) Work done/sec/Newton

$$= \frac{(U_w u + U_{w1} u_1)}{g}$$

$$= \left(\frac{28.19 \times 10.466 + 3.21 \times 5.23}{9.81} \right)$$

$$= 31.78 \text{ N–m/N}$$

Input to the jet/Newton = Kinetic energy of water

$$= \frac{U^2}{2g}$$

$$= \frac{(30)^2}{2 \times 9.81}$$

$$= 45.87 \text{ N–m/N}$$

Efficiency

$$= \frac{Work\ done/sec/Newton}{Input/Newton}$$

$$= \frac{31.78}{45.87} \times 100$$

$$= 69.28 \%$$

Objective Question

14.1 Select from the following list the correct assumptions made for analysing the flow of a jet that is intercepted by a fixed or moving vane.

(1) The momentum of the jet is unchanged

(2) The absolute speed does not change along the vane

(3) The fluid flows on to the vane without shock

(4) The flow from the nozzle is steady

(5) The jet leaves without any velocity

(6) Friction between jet and vane is neglected

(7) The velocity remains uniform over the cross-sectional areas of the jet before and after impinging on the vanes

(8) The cross sectional area of jet is unchanged

(a) 1, 3, 4, 6   (b) 2, 3, 6, 7

(c) 3, 4, 5, 6   (d) 1, 2, 3, 4

(e) 3, 4, 6, 7

14.2 A jet of cross sectional area 'a' and velocity U strikes a flat plate moving with a velocity u. The fluid mass striking the plate per second is

(a) $\rho\, a\, U$ (b) $\rho\, a\, (U - u)$

(c) $\rho\, a\, (U + u)$ (d) $\rho\, a\, U u$

14.3 A jet of water, area 'a' and velocity U, strikes a series of flat plate. The force acting on the plate is

(a) $\rho\, a\, U\, (U - u)$ (b) $\rho\, a\, (U - u)^2$

(c) $\rho\, a\, U u$ (d) $\rho\, a\, U\, (U + u)$

(e) None.

14.4 A plate is inclined at an angle θ to the axis of a jet (area a and velocity U). If the plate is also moving in the direction of jet the force acting in the normal direction is

(a) $\rho\, a\, (U - u)\sin\theta$ (b) $\rho\, a\, (U - u)^2\cos\theta$

(c) $\rho\, a\, (U - u)^2$ (d) $\rho\, a\, (U + u)^2\sin\theta$

(e) None.

14.5 A fluid jet strikes a curved moving vane. The velocity triangles at inlet and outlet represent the flow conditions. The force acting on the vane in the direction of motion is

(a) $\dfrac{W}{g}(U_w - U_{w1})$ (b) $\dfrac{W}{g}(U_t - U_{t1})$

(c) $\dfrac{W}{g}(U_r - U_{r1})$ (d) $\dfrac{W}{g}(U - U_1)$

(e) None.

14.6 A oil jet of specific gravity 0.8 discharges 5 kg/sec onto a fixed vane which deflect the jet through 90°. The jet leaves the vane at a velocity of 30 m/s. The force acting in the direction of approach velocity is, in newton.

   (a) 15.29   (b) 120   (c) 150   (d) 1471.5   (e) None.

14.7 A water jet having a velocity of 40 m/s and cross sectional area 0.005 m^2 strikes onto a vane moving at 14 m/s in the same direction as the jet. The mass of fluid having its momentum changes per unit time in kg/sec, is

   (a) 70   (b) 130   (c) 200   (d) 3380   (e) None.

14.8 A jet having a velocity of 30 m/s flows onto a vane (angle $\theta = 150°$ having a velocity of 15 m/s in the same direction as the jet. The velocity of whirl and velocity of flow at the outlet is given by

   (a) $U_{w1} = 2$, $U_{f1} = 7.5$ (b) 12.99, 7.5

   (c) $-$ 12.99, 8.66   (d) 15, 7.5

   (e) None.

14.9 A jet of water strikes at the centre of a symmetrical curved vane with a absolute velocity U. A series of such vanes are mounted on the periphery of a wheel. The maximum efficiency obtained from such a system is

   (a) 8/27   (b) 16/27   (c) 50 %   (d) 100 %   (e) None.

14.10 The jet of water from a nozzle flows onto a curved vane at its entrance tip at an angle α and flows out at its other tip or exit at an angle β. The vane moves with a velocity u in the direction of the axis of the vane. The expression for work done is

   (a) $\dfrac{W}{g}(U_w u - U_{w1} u_1)$ (b) $\dfrac{W}{g}(U_f u - U_{f1} u_1)$

   (c) $\dfrac{W}{g}(U_w + U_{w1}) u$ (d) $\dfrac{W}{g}(U_f + U_{f1}) u$

   (e) $\dfrac{W}{g}(U_w u \pm U_{w1} u_1)$

Problems 14.1-14.2

   14.1 State the angular momentum theorem. Derive an expression to determine the power developed (or consumed) by a hydraulic machine.

   14.2 What is the fundamental equation of fluid machine. How is it affected if the angle β is acute, right angle or obtuse.

14.3 A jet having a velocity U strikes a single curved vane moving in the same direction as the jet with velocity u, so that the velocity of jet relative to vane is (U – u). The vane causes the jet to be reversed in direction. In flowing over the vane the relative velocity head of water is reduced by 23%. Show that the maximum efficiency is obtained when U = 3u, and that the maximum efficiency is 55.62%.

14.4 If the single vane of Problem 14.3 is replaced by series of similar vanes, show that the maximum efficiency is obtained when U = 2 u and it is equal to 93.87%.

14.5 A jet of water 5 cm in diameter is moving at 15 m/s. It strikes a flat plate which is inclined at 30° to the jet. Find the force on the plate in the direction of jet when (a) the plate is stationary (b) the plate is moving at 3 m/s in the direction of jet.

14.6 A water jet issues from a nozzle 5 cm diameter, strikes a plate with a velocity of 30 m/s. The plate makes an angle of 60° to the horizontal. If frictional losses reduce the velocity of stream leaving the plate to 25 m/s, find (a) the component force in the direction of jet, (b) the component of force normal to the jet, (c) the magnitude and direction of resultant of force exerted by the jet on the plate.

14.7 A square plate of uniform thickness is hinged about its horizontal upper edge. Each side of the plate is 0.4 m long and its weight is 125 N. A horizontal jet of water 2 cm in diameter impinges on the plate at a point 0.2 m below the upper edge. The velocity of the jet is m/s. Determine (a) the force which must be applied at the lower edge in order to keep the plate vertical ? (b) If the plate is allowed to swing freely, find the inclination to the vertical which the plate assumes under the action of the jet.

14.8 A 7.5 cm diameter jet of water discharging at a rate of 196 lit/s strikes on a series of curved vanes tangentially. The vanes when stationary, will deflect the jet through an angle of 120°. Calculate the magnitude and direction of action of resultant force when vanes are stationary. Also determine the magnitude of the resultant force, work done/per second on the vanes, and the hydraulic efficiency of the vanes if the latter move in the direction of jet at a speed of 12.5 m/s.

14.9 A jet of water issues from a nozzle 0.5 cm diameter and implinges axially on a hemispherical cup which is observed to turn it through a total angle of 160°. It is found that 100 N of water is discharged in 40 seconds and force exerted on the vane is 5 N. Determine the ratio of the velocity of water as it leaves the vane to the velocity of water as it enters the vane.

14.10 A series of curved vanes (entrance angle 30° and exit angle 15°) deflect a jet of water 10 cm² in area, moving at 4.5 m/s and inclined at 15° to the line of motion of the vane. Find (a) the velocity of vane so that the water enters and leaves the vane without shock (b) the magnitude and direction of resultant force acting on the vane (c) and the velocity of water at exit, in magnitude and direction.

14.11 An inward flow radial turbine has its inner and outer radial of 0.3 m and 0.5 m respectively. Water enters the blades of the runner with a velocity of 45 m/s making an angle of 40° with the tangent to the wheel at its inlet tip. Water leaves the runner with a velocity of 8 m/s. If the blade angle at the inner and outer tipes are 30° and 25° respectively, determine (a) the speed of the turbine wheel at its inlet and outlet tip (b) work done per newton of water and (c) efficiency of the hydraulic machine.

14.12 A 40 m/s velocity jet of water strikes a series of vanes moving at m/s. A jet is inclined at an angle of 20° to the direction of motion of the vanes. The relative velocity of jet at outlet is 0.9 times of the value at inlet, and the absolute velocity of water at exit is to e normal to the motion of vanes. Determine (a) the vane angles at entrance and exit (b) work done per second per unit weight of water and (c) hydraulic efficiency.

15

Fluid Machines —Turbines

15.1 INTRODUCTION

Fluid machine is a mechanical contrivance which serves to interchange energy between moving parts of the machine and the liquid flowing through it. The fluid machine is in essence an energy convertor. The energy may exist in various forms, e.g. hydraulic energy, mechanical energy, thermal energy, etc. The hydraulic energy possessed by a flowing fluid may be either in the form of kinetic energy or pressure energy or in both these forms. The mechanical energy is the one which is associated with the moving or rotating parts of a fluid machine usually, transmitting power.

The fluid machines can be classified on the basis of direction of energy transfer. Thus, all machines in which hydraulic energy is transferred into mechanical energy (in the form of a rotating shaft, or in some other moving parts) are known as 'Turbines' or hydraulic motors. In contrast to it, all those machines in which the mechanical energy is transferred into hydraulic energy are known as 'Pumps'. Thus, in the first category of machines, the work is done by the fluid on the machine and in this process, the energy is extracted from the flowing fluid. Whereas, in the second category of machines, the work is done by the moving parts of the machine on the fluid and energy is added to it.

The fluid machines can further be classified as 'Positive displacement or fluid static machines' and 'Rotodynamic or fluid kinematic machines'. In positive displacement machines, the fluid is drawn or forced into a finite space bounded by mechanical parts and is sealed in it by mechanical means (like plunger cylinder arrangement alongwith inlet and outlet valves). The fluid is then forced out of the space by means of mechanical thrust. Thus, the flow rate is governed by the dimensions of the space and the frequency of filling/emptying of the space. Some of the machines of this category are reciprocating pump, hydraulic press and hydraulic accumulator (See chapter 16 and 18).

In rotodynamics machines, there is no such sealing of fluid. All the rotodynamic machines have got a rotating part known as runner (turbine), impeller (pump) or rotor (compressor) which rotate continuously and freely in the fluid. This rotation changes the angular momentum of the fluid contained between the inlet and outlet of the machines and thus causes the transfer of the energy. The hydraulic turbines (Chapter 15), Centrifugal pumps (Chapter 17), hydraulic torque transmitter (Chapter 18) are some of the examples of this class of machines.

15.2 HYDRAULIC TURBINES

A turbine is a machine which transfers hydraulic energy of flowing water into mechanical energy of the rotating shaft. The hydraulic turbines are, sometimes, called prime movers or hydraulic motors since they utilise hydraulic energy and convert it into mechanical energy similar to an electric prime mover which utilises electric energy and converts it into mechanical energy.

Hydraulic turbines are designed for service of hydro-electric power plants (HEPP) where they drive electric generators. Water stored in a reservoir upstream of a dam (water level in the upstream reservoir is known as head water HW or head race) is directed by means of pressure pipes, known as penstocks, to the turbine and is, finally, discharged into tail race/tail water TW (Water level in the downstream reservoir). The complete unit of turbine coupled with an electric generator is called hydro- electric unit (Fig. 15.1). In this way, a hydroelectric unit transforms the hydraulic energy of the flowing water into mechanical energy and then into electric energy.

15.3 CLASSIFICATION OF TURBINES

15.3.1 Classification Based on Energy

The hydraulic turbines are broadly classified into two categories, depending on the form of hydraulic energy they utilise, viz., (a) Impulse turbine and (2) Reaction turbine.

Impulse turbine: In the impulse turbine unit, all the hydraulic energy of water is converted into kinetic energy before it enters the impulse turbine. This is accomplished by means of one or more number of contracting nozzles. The jet or jets of water from the nozzles strike against a number of buckets fixed on the periphery of a wheel, called runner, and do work over it. Thereafter, the flowing water falls into a river or downstream reservoir (tailrace). Since whole of the hydraulic energy of water is converted into velocity energy, and the turbine runner runs freely in air, the pressure remains atmospheric everywhere in the turbine. Hence, the casing of impulse turbine has no hydraulic function to perform. It is only necessary to prevent splashing of water and to lead it to tailrace and further, to serve as a safe guard against accident.

Reaction turbine: Reaction turbine are those in which water entering the turbine has got pressure as well as kinetic energy. This means that only a part of available hydraulic energy is transformed into kinetic energy before it enters the turbine under pressure. The pressure drops in the runner and the water may be discharged at exit at a pressure below atmospheric pressure (if a draft tube is provided at its exit) or at atmospheric pressure (no draft tube is provided at the exit). Thus nowhere in the turbine runner the pressure is atmospheric, therefore, the runner should always run full. And an airtight casing is absolutely necessary for a reaction turbine.

The turbines can further be classified according to

(a) the direction of flow

(b) the head of water available

(c) the specific speed of the turbine.

15.3.2 Classification According to the Direction of Flow

The turbines can be classified according to the direction of flow through them (i.e., over the runner), namely, radial flow, axial flow and mixed flow turbines.

(i)*Radial flow turbines* In radial flow turbines, the water enters the turbine in the radial direction and comes out of it also radially. This means, throughout the passage, the water flows in radial direction over the runner vanes. The radial flow turbines may be inward flow radial turbines or ourward flow radial turbines depending on whether water flows inwardly or outwardly through the runner. One of the turbine of this category is old designed Francis turbine.

(ii) *Axial flow turbines* In axial flow machines, the water flows parallel to the axis of the turbine. Propeller turbine is one of the example of this class.

(iii) *Mixed flow turbines* In mixed flow turbines, the water enters the turbine radially at the outer circumference and come out axially at the exit. Thus, water changes its direction (of flow) while flowing over the runner vanes from radial to axial direction. Modern design of Francis turbine is an example of this class.

15.3.3 Classification According to the Head

The head of water under which a turbine can function efficiently can also be the one of the criteria for clssifying the turbine, e.g., (i) low head turbines, (ii) medium head turbines and (iii) high head turbines.

(i) *Low head turbines* Turbines working under a head of 3 to 50 meters are called low head turbine. Examples of this type are propeller turbine, Kaplan turbine, etc.

The tubular type turbine, known as bulb turbine, is the latest development for very low head plants. It consists of axial flow (fixed blades) propeller turbine coupled with a generator. The assembly is housed in a bulb casing and hence the name. This turbine has been very useful to harness tidal power.

(ii) *Medium head turbine* These turbines work between a head of 30 m to 500 meters. Francis turbine is the example of this class.

(iii) *High head turbines* These turbines operate at or above 100 m head. Impulse turbine, which uses exclusively the kinetic energy of the flowing water, and especially Pelton wheel is the common example of this type.

As the given value of heads are overlapping each other, it is difficult to classify the turbines according to the heads alone.

15.3.4 Classification Based on Specific Speed

The specific speed of a turbine is defined as the speed of a geometrically similar turbine which would produce one unit of power while working under unit head. The turbine can also be classified according to the specific speed.

The turbines are classified as (i) low specific speed turbine, (ii) medium specific speed turbine and, (iii) high specific speed turbine.

The Pelton wheel is a low specific speed turbine. If it uses single nozzle, its specific speed ranges from 20 to 35 r.p.m.

Reaction turbines have got higher range of specific speed. Francis turbine is a medium specific speed turbine and its value varies from 60 to 300 r.p.m.

The axial flow turbines like propeller and kaplan turbines are high specific speed turbines with speeds ranging from 300 to 1000 r.p.m.

15.3.5 Classification According to the Disposition of Turbine Shaft

Sometimes turbines are classified according to the disposition of the turbine shaft. For example, vertical shaft turbine and horizontal shaft turbine.

15.4 ELEMENTS OF A HYDROELECTRIC POWER PLANT

A hydro-electric power plant is constructed downstream of a suitable selected site for a dam or a reservoir, i.e. where sufficient amount of runoff may be made available at sufficient head throughout the year for the production of power. Water from this source is led down by means of a big size tunnel or a pipe- line which is known as penstock to the site of turbine (or power house). A forebay may be provided at the head of penstock when the power house is located away from the upstream reservoir (main storage of water); otherwise it is not provided. A forebay is a small size reservoir which stores water temporarily whenever not required by the turbine and draws from it when the demand exceeds the normal supply. The water is then fed to the turbine through canals. A generator or an electric alternator is coupled with the turbine which produces electric power. This power is then transmitted to the industries, domestic suppliers, etc. by means of transmission lines.

Turbines used at the power house may be impulse type or reaction type. In case of impulse turbine, a nozzle is fitted at the end of penstock which transforms all the available hydraulic energy into kinetic energy in the form of jet. The jet of water then strikes over the buckets mounted all round the periphery of a wheel which is coupled with an electric alternator or an electric generator to produce electric power. This power is then transmitted through various electric installations.

In case of reaction turbine, the penstock supplies the water at one end of the spiral casing. The water under pressure flows over the runner vanes and does work over it and runs the wheel. The water is then, discharged through the eye or exit of the turbine, generally into a diverging pipe. This pipe is known as draft tube which discharges into the downstream channel.

The level of water surface in the upstream reservoir before it is diverted for power development is known as 'Head race or Head water HW'. The water level in the downstrem channel is known as 'Tail race or Tail water TW'.

15.5 DEFINITIONS

Some of the definitions of basic terms used in the following text are described below.

(1) *Specific Energy* : The amount of energy contained in one r   of flowing water (1 N) is called its specific energy.

$$e = \frac{p}{w} + Z + \frac{\alpha U^2}{2g} \tag{15.1}$$

where p and Z refer to the pressure and datum energy above an arbitrary chosen datum respectively and U is the mean velocity of flow and α is the kinetic energy correction factor.

(2) *Gross Head or Static Head* (H_1) It is defined as the difference between the elevations of head race and tail race when no water is flowing through the penstoke and is denoted by H_1 (See Fig. 15.1)

$$H_1 = H_{HW} - Z_{TW} \tag{15.2}$$

It is also called 'total head or static head'.

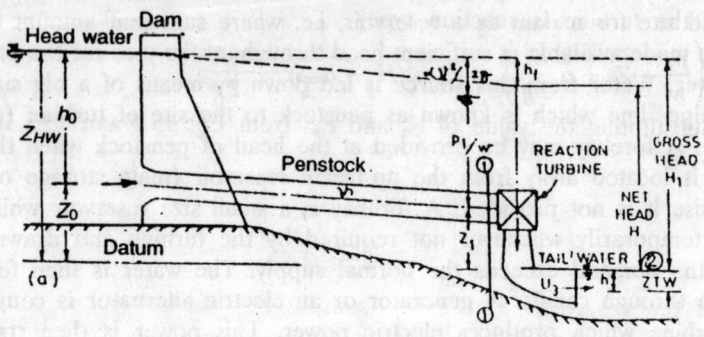

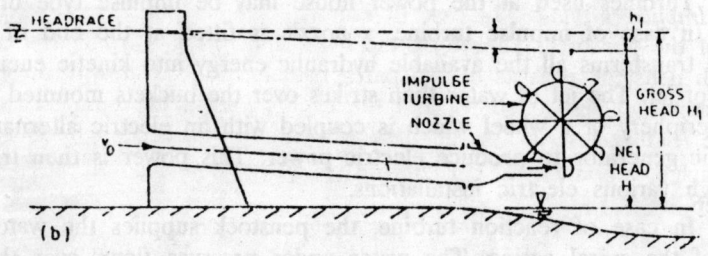

FIG. 15.1 SCHEMATIC DIAGRAM OF HYDRO-ELECTRIC PLANT

(3) *Net Head or Available Head* (H) It is defined as the difference between the specific energies e_{in} and e_{out} at the turbine inlet and turbine exit respectively.

$$H = e_{in} - e_{out} \tag{15.3}$$

It is approximately equal to the difference of gross head H_1 and frictional and other losses occurring in the penstock.

The energy at the inlet e_{in} and at the exit e_{out} of the turbine is given by Eq. 15.4 and 15.5 (Fig. 15.1)

$$e_{in} = p_1/w + Z_1 + \alpha_1 U_1^2/2g \tag{15.4}$$

$$e_{out} = p_2/w + Z_2 + \alpha_2 U_2^2/2g = \alpha_2 U_2^2/2g \tag{15.5}$$

Since pressure at point 2 at downstream water surface, p_2 is atmospheric and Z_2 is zero, being the chosen datum.

The pressure at the inlet, p_1, can be determined by applying Bernoulli's equation to a point 'O' at the water level in the forebay (or reservoir) and '1' at inlet to the turbine.

$$\frac{p_0}{w} + Z_0 + \alpha_0 \frac{U_0^2}{2g} = \frac{p_1}{w} + Z_1 + \alpha_1 \frac{U_1^2}{2g} + h_{loss} \qquad (15.6)$$

where $\left(\dfrac{p_0}{w} + Z_0\right) = H_1$ (Fig. 15.1), U_0 is the velocity in the forebay and h_{loss} is the sum of the losses in the penstock (including loss in the draft tube, if the turbine is reaction type)

$$\therefore \quad \left(\frac{p_1}{w} + Z_1 + \alpha \frac{U_1^2}{2g}\right) = e_{in} = (H_1 - h_{loss}) + \frac{\alpha_0 U_0^2}{2g} \qquad (15.7)$$

Substituting the value of e_{in} and e_{out} from Eq. 15.7 and 15.5 into Eq. 15.3,

$$H = e_{in} - e_{out}$$

$$= \left[H_1 - h_{loss} + \alpha_0 \frac{U_0^2}{2g}\right] - \alpha_2 \left(\frac{U_2^2}{2g}\right) \qquad (15.8)$$

If the difference in velocity energies at the forebay and at the exit to the turbine is small, it can be neglected.

$$\therefore \qquad H = (H_1 - h_{loss}) \qquad (15.9)$$

Impulse turbines In case of impulse turbine, a nozzle is fitted at the base of the penstock. Therefore, the head loss in the transmission of power through penstock consists of two parts, namely frictional loss in the penstock of diameter D and length L, and the energy loss in the nozzle of diameter d. The friction loss, h_{ft}, in the penstock can be determined by using Darcy Weisbach equation, Eq. 9.51. Therefore, the available head at the end of penstock is given by

$$H = [H_1 - h_f]$$

$$= \left[H_1 - \frac{fL Q^2}{12.1 D^5}\right] \qquad (15.10)$$

For obtaining optimum power from a hydro-electric power plant h_f should be as small and diameter of penstock as great as possible.

The available head H at the end of penstock is further reduced by nozzle loss. If the velocity of jet through the nozzle is U, the frictional loss through it can be computed by introducing a coefficient of velocity k_v for the nozzle.

$$\therefore \qquad U = k_v \sqrt{2gH} \qquad (15.11)$$

The value of this coefficient k_v varies from 0.97 to 1.0.

Reaction Turbine In case of reaction turbine, the available head H can be computed by Eqn. 15.10. Since the water under pressure flows into airtight casing, its velocity varies from point to point.

(4) *Work done* The analysis of flow of water over the vanes of the runner has already been described in chapter 14. The velocity triangles shown in Fig. 14.8 are applicable to axial flow machines whereas those in Fig. 14.9 are applicable to radial flow machines. The water flowing over the vanes does work on the runner and in turn, energy is extracted by the runner. The work done by W newton of water is given by Eq. 14.44,

$$\text{Work done} = \frac{W}{g}(U_w u \pm U_{w1} u_1)$$

In this equation (Eq. 14.50), the +ve sign is used if the outlet blade angle $\beta < 90°$ and -ve sign is used if the outlet blade angle $\beta > 90°$; U_W and U_{w1} are the velocity of whirl and u and u_1 are peripheral speed of wheel at the turbine inlet and outlet respectively.

15.6 LOSSES AND EFFICIENCIES

All the hydraulic machines convert energy from one form into another and in this process of conversion of energy, a fraction of input energy is lost. Thus, if these losses are small, the machine is said to be 'good or efficient' and vice-versa. The efficiency of a machine, in a way, represent how good is the machine in conversion of energies. The hydraulic machine consists of many parts and the flow through them is too complex. Hence, it is always convenient for analytical and design purposes to consider the component losses as well as their sum total and to express each component losses in the efficiency form.

The actual energy transfer in a turbine occurs in its runner. Firstly the water enters the casing of the turbine and friction losses take place in it. Thereafter, fluid passes through the blade passages and imparts energy to them. Two major losses take place in the runner. The inevitable contact between the fluid moving over the solid surfaces gives rise to boundary layer development and hence to frictional losses. Whereas the need for the fluid to change direction results in separation or shock losses. But these losses may be augmented by secondary flows which may occur within the runner due to pressure distribution across it (pressure drag) and are prominent at off design points of separation.

Thus, if h_r is the head loss in the runner and $Q_r (= Q - Q_v)$ is the volumetric flow through the runner, the energy loss in the runner is then given by

$$P_r = w\, Q_r\, h_r \tag{15.12}$$

But it is found that the flow rate through the runner is usually less than that entering the casing of the turbine simply because some fluid passes through the clearance between the runner and the casing. Thus, if we denote the volumetric flow rate by Q_v, leaking past the runner and if H_r is the 'total head' across the runner, the power loss due to leakage may be expressed as

$$P_v = w\, Q_v\, H_r \tag{15.13}$$

In most machines, the runner is surrounded by a stationary casing so that the fluid passes through the parts of the casing before it enters the runner and also after leaving it. Thus, losses due to friction (and possibly due to separation) occur in casing also. If the flow rate through the casing is Q and the loss of head in the casing is h_c, then the power lost in the casing is given by

$$P_c = w Q h_c \qquad (15.14)$$

The internal losses of the machines, i.e. those occurring in the runner and casing, due to friction and separation are called hydraulic losses. It also includes the losses occurring in the draft tube of a reaction turbine.

Finally, there are mechanical losses of energy such as in the bearings and sealing glands which must be taken into account. It is normal practice to include within this category losses due to disc friction (sometimes referred as windage loss). The disc friction is the power required to spin the bladeless runner at the required speed. Thus the windage loss accounts for the friction between the outer surfaces of the runner rotating in the fluid and the casing. It is now possible to consider the energy balance for the whole machine.

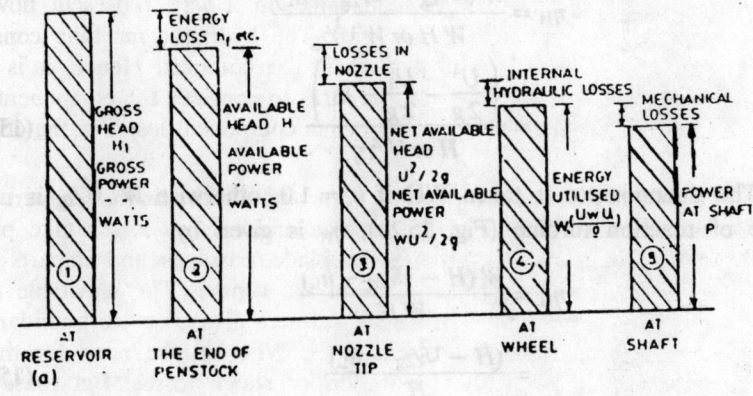

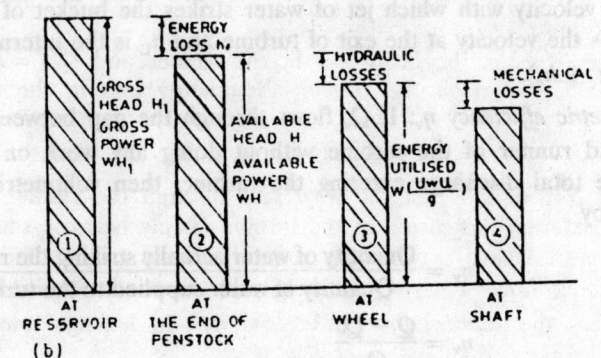

FIG. 15.2 DISTRIBUTION OF ENERGY AT DIFFERENT STAGES OF TURBINE

$$\text{Input power} = (\text{Runner loss} + \text{casing loss}) + \text{leakage loss}$$
$$+ \text{mechanical loss} + \text{shaft power output.}$$
$$w\,Q\,H = w\,(Q_r\,h_r + Q\,h_c + Q_v\,H_r) + P_m + P \tag{15.15}$$

The distribution of energy available and that lost at different stages for impulse turbines and reaction turbines are shown in Fig. 15.2.

Efficiencies For a turbine of any type, the efficiencies at different stages are computed as follows:

Hydraulic efficiency η_H The hydraulic efficiency is defined as the ratio of the power delivered to the shaft to the available power of the fluid flowing through the runner

$$\eta_H = \frac{W\,(U_w\,u \pm U_{w1}\,u_1)/g}{WH}$$

$$= \frac{(U_w\,u \pm U_{w1}\,u_1)}{gH} \tag{15.16}$$

Alternatively, for impulse turbine (Fig. 15.2a), η_H is also given by

$$\eta_H = \frac{W\,(U^2/2g - U_1^2/2g - h_L)}{WH \text{ or } W\,U^2/2g}$$

$$= \frac{\left(\dfrac{U^2}{2g} - \dfrac{U_1^2}{2g} - h_L\right)}{H \text{ or } U^2/2g} \tag{15.17}$$

The denominator is taken WH if $k_v = 1.0$, otherwise $W \cdot U^2/2g$ is used. In case of reaction turbine (Fig. 15.2b), η_H is given by

$$\eta_H = \frac{W\,(H - U_1^2/2g - h_L)}{WH}$$

$$= \frac{(H - U_1^2/2g - h_L)}{H} \tag{15.18}$$

In the above expressions, Eqns. 15.16 to 15.18, U is the inlet velocity of water (or velocity with which jet of water strikes the bucket of an impulse turbine), U_1 is the velocity at the exit of turbine and h_L is the internal hydraulic losses (i.e. $h_r + h_c$).

Volumetric efficiency η_v: If Q_v flows through the gap between the guide apparatus and runner of the turbine without doing any work on the runner and Q is the total discharge entering the turbine, then volumetric efficiency η_v is given by

$$\eta_v = \frac{\text{Quantity of water actually striking the runner}}{\text{Quantity of water supplied to the turbine}}$$

$$\eta_v = \frac{Q - Q_v}{Q} \tag{15.19}$$

Ordinarily, this leakage is a very small percentage and for some machines (impulse turbine) does not exist but under unfavourable conditions, it is occassionally an important item.

Mechanical efficiency η_M : It is the ratio of the power P delivered by the turbine to that delivered by the fluid at the shaft

$$\eta_M = \frac{P}{WH''} = \frac{P}{W(U_w u \pm U_{w1} u_1)/g} \qquad (15.20)$$

where $H'' = (U_w u \pm U_{w1} u_1)/g$ watts is often known as the power delivered to the shaft/unit weight of water or head utilised.

Overall or total efficiency η_0: It is the ratio of the power available at the turbine shaft to that power input to the turbine.

$$\eta_0 = \left(\frac{P}{WH}\right) \qquad (15.21)$$

It is commonly designated as efficiency and is also given by

$$\eta_0 = \eta_H \, \eta_v \, \eta_M \qquad (15.22a)$$

as can be shown from Eqns. 15.16 to 15.22. In M.K.S. system of units WH/75 is normally known as 'Water Horse Power' or W.H.P.

When η_v is unity or it is not to be considered,

$$\eta_0 = \eta_H \, \eta_M \qquad (15.22b)$$

15.7 IMPULSE TURBINES

Impulse turbines are high head turbines, head ranging from 600 m to 2000 m. In the impulse turbine the total energy of flowing water is first converted into kinetic energy of the following water before the jet strikes the vanes and the pressure remains atmospheric throughout the turbine periphery.

Several types of impulse turbines have been proposed in the past, which may be categorised as radial flow turbines and axial flow turbines. Out of these, the only one that has survived is 'Pelton Wheel', named in honour of Laster Pelton (1829-1903) who contributed much in the development of this turbine.

(i)*Radial Flow Turbine* This type of turbine is not much in use. In these turbine, the water enters the wheel through fixed guide blades. As the water flows over the moving vanes a centrifugal head is impressed on it by the revolving wheel. It slightly increases the relative velocity of water in an inward flow turbine. Thus

$$\frac{U_r^2}{2g} = \frac{U_{r1}^2}{2g} + \left(\frac{u^2}{2g} - \frac{u_1^2}{2g}\right) - h_L \qquad (15.23)$$

where U_r and U_{r1} are the relative velocities at the inlet and outlet to the wheel, u and u_1 denote peripheral velocities at these ends respectively, and h_L is loss of head in the turbine.

Axial Flow Turbines: In this type of turbines, water enters and leaves the wheel at equal distance from the axis of the wheel, i.e. $R = R_1$ and so

$u = u_1$. Hence, no centrifugal force (or head) acts on the water as it flow from inlet to exit side. Therefore, the relative velocity at the exit U_{r1} is slightly different than the relative velocity U_r at the inlet side by the blade frictional loss h_L, i.e.

$$\frac{U_{r1}^2}{2g} = \frac{U_r^2}{2g} - h_L \tag{15.24a}$$

In case, the loss h_L is small,

$$U_{r1} = U_r \tag{15.24b}$$

Pelton wheel belongs to this category of the turbine.

15.8 Pelton Wheel

It is an axial flow impulse turbine and consists of vanes, commonly known as buckets of elliptical shape. These buckets are attached to the periphery of a rotating wheel as shown in Fig. 15.3. One or two (or more) number of nozzles project a jet of water tangentially to the bucket's pitch circle. Hence, Pelton wheel is sometimes also known as tangential flow impulse turbine. The buckets are of double hemispherical cup type as shown in Fig. 15.3. Thus each cup has got a partition between them. The jet of water strikes at the centre of each bucket.

As the water flows axially in both directions over the buckets, equal and oppositely directed axial thrust, $\dfrac{W}{g}(U_f - U_{f1})$, acts on the shaft of the turbine. In this way (due to the special shape of buckets) the axial thrust is eliminated and the turbine is saved of unnecessary stresses in its various component parts.

The basis of design of nozzle and the buckets of a Pelton wheel are as follows:

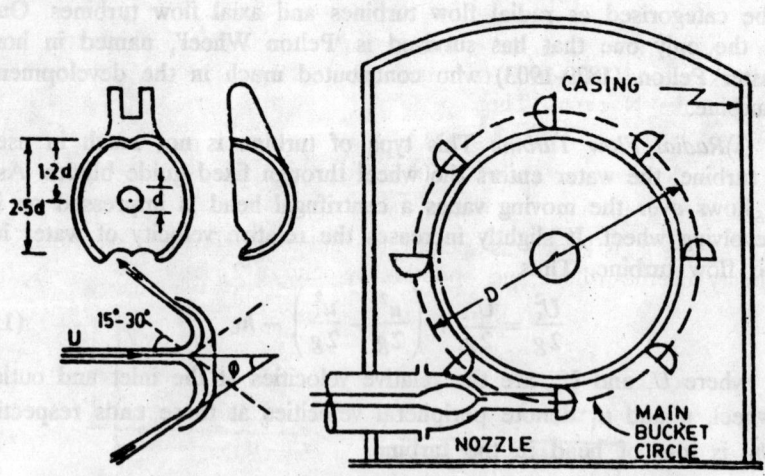

FIG. 15.3. PELTON WHEEL—DIAGRAMMATIC ARRANGEMENT.

Nozzle: The issuing jet of water should be solid, uniform and free from surface sprays under varying rates of discharge.

Buckets: (1) The bucket pitch should be such that all the jet's fluid is intercepted and deflected.

(2) The jet enters the buckets smoothly and without shock losses from the time bucket first cuts the jet until last water is deflected.

(3) Every particle of water flows over the bucket surface without sudden change in direction.

(4) The relative deflection is as nearly 180° as possible allowing for the necessary lateral velocity to carry the fluid away from the wheel.

(5) The discharging (absolute) velocity U_1 is as low as possible.

Fig. 15.3 is the diagram of the bucket of a Pelton wheel satisfying the above requirements.

Let H be the available head at the entrance of the nozzle supplying water to the wheel which produces the velocity U of the jet coming out of the nozzle.

$$U = k_v \sqrt{2gH} \tag{15.11}$$

where k_v is the coefficient of the velocity of the nozzle and takes into account the frictional losses in the nozzle. The jet is directed towards the direction of motion of blades (buckets) at inlet (each half bucket serves as a blade).

Referring to velocity triangle at inlet, Fig. 15.4, inlet blade angle $\theta = \alpha = 0°$.

This being an axial flow turbine the peripherial velocity of the wheel at inlet, u, is same as that outlet, u_1,

∴ $u = u_1 =$ peripherial velocity of mean bucket circle.

Mean bucket circle is an imaginary circle passing through the centre of buckets and tangential to nozzle axis. Let its diameter be D and let the wheel make N r.p.m. Then

$$u = \frac{\pi D N}{60} = u_1 \tag{15.25a}$$

Also $$u = k_u \sqrt{2gH} \tag{15.25b}$$

Here k_u is known as speed ratio and it is defined as ratio of peripherial velocity of the wheel and spouting velocity $\sqrt{2gH}$.

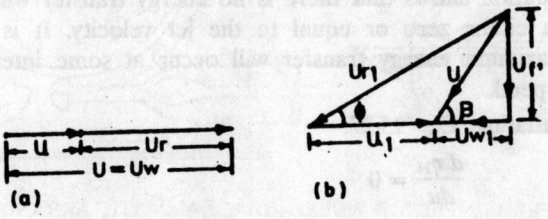

(a)   (b)

FIG. 15.4 VELOCITY TRIANGLES FOR A PELTON WHEEL

Now referring to inlet velocity triangle of Pelton wheel, Fig. 15.4

$$U = U_w \tag{i}$$

$$U_r = (U - u) \tag{ii}$$

The relative velocity U_r reduces slightly while the water flows over the bucket due to blade surface friction. Hence, the relative velocity at outlet U_{r1} is given by

$$U_{r1} = k\, U_r = k\, (U - u) \tag{iii}$$

The multiplying factor k takes into account the blade surface friction. Referring to outlet velocity diagram,

$$U_{w1} = (U_{r1} \cos \varphi - u_1) = (k\, U_r \cos \varphi - u_1)$$

$$= [k\, (U - u) \cos \varphi - u] \tag{iv}$$

The sign of the U_{w1} will be negative as it is directed away from the bucket (see Fig. 15.4) and $u = u_1$.

The total energy (per unit weight) transferred to the wheel is given by Euler's equation, Eq. 14.44

$$E = \left(\frac{U_w u - U_{w1} u_1}{g} \right) \tag{14.44}$$

$$= \frac{u}{g} (U_w - U_{w1})$$

E or work done/unit weight of water

$$= \frac{u}{g} (U_w - U_{w1})$$

Substituting the values of U_w and U_{w1} from Eqs. (i) and (iv)

$$E = \frac{u}{g} [U + \{k\, (U - u) \cos \varphi - u\}]$$

$$= \frac{u}{g} [(U - u)(1 + k \cos \varphi)] \tag{15.26}$$

The hydraulic efficiency η_H is given by

$$\eta_H = \frac{\text{Work done/unit weight of water}}{\text{Energy (head) available at the outlet of nozzle}}$$

$$= \frac{[u\,(U - u)(1 + k \cos \varphi)]/g}{(U^2/2g)} \tag{15.27}$$

This equation shows that there is no energy transfer when the velocity of the vane is either zero or equal to the jet velocity. It is reasonable to expect that maximum energy transfer will occur at some intermediate value of the vane speed.

Differentiating Eq. 15.27.

$$\frac{d\,\eta_H}{du} = 0$$

Therefore, for a maximum efficiency

$$U - 2u = 0$$

or

$$u = U/2 \tag{15.28}$$

Substituting this value back into Eq. 15.27, the maximum efficiency is obtained

$$(\eta_H)_{max} = \frac{U}{2}\left(\frac{U}{2}\right)\frac{(1 + k\cos\varphi)}{(U^2/2)} = \frac{(1 + k\cos\varphi)}{2} \tag{15.29}$$

In an ideal case, assuming no blade friction, there is no reduction of the relative velocity over the vane and therefore, k = 1.0. Also, if outlet blade angle $\varphi = 0°$, and k_v for nozzle is unity, the hydraulic efficiency η_H will be 1.0 or 100%.

$$(\eta_H)_{max} = \frac{1}{2}(1 + \cos\varphi) = 1.0 \; or \; 100\% \tag{15.30}$$

Alternatively, sometimes the hydraulic efficiency may also be expressed as

$$\eta_H = 2k_u(k_v - k_u)(1 + k\cos\varphi) \tag{15.31}$$

Working proportions of Pelton Wheel : It has been shown above that for an ideal case, $k_u = 0.5$, $k_v = 1.0$ and $\varphi = 0°$, it is possible theoretically to obtain 100% hydraulic efficiency. In actual practice, it is not so.

(a) Velocity of jet : $U = k_v\sqrt{2gH}$

k_v account for frictional losses in the nozzle which is inevitable and its value, therefore, will never be unity. It ranges from 0.97 to 1.0; usually, its value being taken as 0.985.

(b) Peripheral velocity : $u = k_u\sqrt{2gH}$

k_u is known the speed ratio and it is found by testing Pelton Wheel that maximum efficiency is not attained at $k_u = 0.5$. Its value ranges from 0.44 to 0.46.

(c) Blade friction k: In practice, there is always frictional losses over he bucket surface and its value varies from 0.80 to 0.85.

(d) Finally, the vane outlet angle φ : If blade (vane) outlet angle is, ρ, the water flowing over the vane is deflected by $(\pi - \varphi)$. If φ is taken)°, water discharged from one bucket will strike the back of the preceeding ɔucket and thus reduce the wheel efficiency. Thus φ should have atleast such value that water falls clcar off the bucket. Usually, φ is taken as 15° to avoid the interference between oncoming and outgoing jets.

Due to above considerations, the hydraulic efficiency of the Pelton Wheel is found to be 85% to 90%. Further, in case of Pelton Wheel, the ratio of wheel diameter, D, to the jet diameter d known as jet ratio, ranges from 11 to 14. Usually, its value is taken as 12.

$$\text{Jet ratio, m} = \frac{D}{d}$$

Number of Buckets : The number of buckets to be mounted on the periphery of the Pelton Wheel is given by empirical formula.

$$\text{Number of buckets} = \left(\frac{m}{2} + 15\right) \qquad (15.32)$$

Alternatively, the number of buckets could be computed by

$$n = \frac{2\pi}{\theta} = \frac{2\pi}{\sqrt{1 - \left(\dfrac{R + d/2}{R_e}\right)^2}} \qquad (15.33)$$

Since $\qquad \sin\theta \approx \theta = \sqrt{1 - \{R + d/2\}^2/R_e^2}$

where R is the radius of pitch circle, d is the diameter of nozzle and R_e is the extreme (outer) radius of runner and θ is the angle between two consecutive buckets.

15.9 Multiple Jet Pelton Wheel

Usually, the power developed by a Pelton Wheel with single nozzle is quite low and insufficient. Therefore, to develop more power under constant head H, more discharge should strike the buckets, since

$$P = w\,Q\,H\,\eta_0$$
$$P \propto Q\,H$$

But the discharge Q, flowing out of a nozzle is given by

$$Q = k_v\,a\,\sqrt{2gH} \;;$$

k_v being unaltered hence more discharge means more area of cross section of the nozzle. Now, if the diameter of the nozzle is increased, the diameter D of the wheel shall have to be increased to keep the constant value of jet ratio m. But it is not desirable to increase the wheel diameter. Therefore, more area of the cross section of the jet can be provided by increasing the number of nozzles to 2, 4 or at the maximum 6. If the number of nozzles is increased beyond 6, the water from one nozzle will interfere with that of other nozzle. Moreover, the manufacturing and operations become too much tedius.

15.10 DESIGN OF PELTON WHEEL

A Pelton wheel is required to be designed to develop power P while working under head H and running at speed N rpm. The suitable value of overall efficiency η_0, coefficient of velocity k_v, speed ratio k_u and jet ratio m are assumed.

1. Determine the discharge Q required to develop power P watts

$$Q = P/WH\eta_0 \ \text{m}^3/\text{s} \qquad (i)$$

2. Calculate the jet velocity U,

$$U = k_v\sqrt{2gH} \qquad (ii)$$

3. Compute the total area of jet required,

$$A = \frac{Q}{U} \; m^2 \tag{iii}$$

4. Now, obtain the speed of the wheel u,

$$u = k_u \sqrt{2gH} \tag{iv}$$

5. The wheel diameter D, can now be obtained

$$D = 60 \, u / \pi \, N \tag{v}$$

6. Assuming a suitable value of jet ratio m, the diameter of the nozzle can be computed.

$$d = \frac{D}{m} \tag{vi}$$

7. Required number of nozzles can now be found out,

$$\text{Required number } n_1 = \frac{A}{\pi/4 \, d^2} \tag{vii}$$

8. If the value of n_1 is fractional, it is rounded up to next higher number and keeping the value of m more or less same.

9. Total number of buckets n can be determined from Eq. 15.32 or 15.33

$$n = (m/2 + 15) \tag{15.34}$$

10. The standard dimensions of the bucket are adopted as shown in Fig. 15.3.

15.11 REACTION TURBINES

Because of the rigid relationships between the head H and peripheral speed u; and also between the diameter of the wheel D and nozzle diameter d, it is readily seen that as the head diminishes, the diameter of the wheel (to develop a given output P) increases progressively greater and the speed of revolution N progressively decreases. If the head falls below 150 m, Pelton wheel becomes so slow and unwieldy that they are unsuitable for ordinary use. In such situations, relatively fast moving reaction turbines come to one's rescue. There are many design of reaction turbines, out of which only Francis Turbine, Propeller turbine and Kaplan turbine are in much use and are described hence after.

In reaction turbine, a part of the total head H acting on the turbine is transformed into kinetic energy and the rest remains as pressure head. The water first enters a set of movable blades (guide blades) and, thereafter, passes over a set of fixed runner vanes. There exists a difference of pressure between these two sets of blades which is called 'reaction pressure' and is responsible for the motion of the runner vanes. The parameter which describes the reaction turbine is known as degree of reaction R.

$$R = \frac{\text{Static pressure drop}}{\text{Total energy transferred}} \tag{15.35a}$$

By the application of Bernoulli's equation to the inlet and outlet sections of a runner vane, one can write,

$$\frac{p - p_1}{w} = E - \frac{(U^2 - U_1^2)}{2g} \tag{15.36}$$

where E is the total energy available at the turbine runner = H meter per newton of water. Thus, if the pressure is constant at the inlet and outlet sections then such a turbine behaves purely as a impulse turbine. If on the other hand, $U = U_1$, then $E = (p - p_1)/w$ and this represents purely reaction turbine. The intermediate type of turbine is described by the degree of reaction R.

$$\therefore \qquad R = \left[E - \frac{U^2 - U_1^2}{2g} \right] \Big/ E = \left[1 - \frac{U^2 - U_1^2}{2gE} \right] \tag{15.35 b}$$

But from Euler's equation, Eq. 14.44

$$E = \frac{U_w u}{g} \qquad (\text{ for } \beta = 90°)$$

Hence, $$R = \left[1 - \frac{U^2 - U_1^2}{2 U_w u} \right] \tag{15.35 c}$$

15.12 FRANCIS TURBINE

It is radial flow reaction turbine which works under medium head. It was designed by a French engineer James B. Francis in 1829. A lot of improvements have been made in its design in course of time and modern Francis turbine is a mixed flow type in which water enters at the outer periphery of the turbine radially and leaves the runner axially at its centre. Its overall efficiency varies from 80% to 90%.

15.12.1 Various Components

The essential components of a Francis turbine are : (a) scroll casing, (b) guide vanes or wicket gates, (c) runner and runner vanes and (d) exit and draft tube.

(a) *Scroll casing* : The big size pipe, known as penstock, carrying water from the head race ends into a casing which feeds the water to the turbine. The water is to be fed under pressure all over the periphery of the turbine and its velocity should remain constant. The turbine runner is, therefore, enclosed by an airtight casing. As the water flows along the casing, it also enters over the periphery of the guide vanes and thus flow at subsequent sections gradually decreases. To maintain the velocity of flow in the casing constant, the area of flow of the casing should also decrease gradually at subsequent sections. Therefore, the casing is a passage of gradually decreasing area of flow and it is called 'spiral casing'.

As the water flows under pressure (sometimes very high), the design of casing should be such that the stresses developed in the material of the casing are within permissible limit. Therefore, the spiral casing is made up of R.C.C. for medium head, and for high head it is made up of cast steel, welded or rivetted plates of steel or even of cast iron.

(b) *Guide mechanism* : The water from the casing passes through the gradually contracting passages formed by a series of guide vanes or wicket gates spaced evenly around the periphery of the runner. These are made up of cast steel or brass and are of aerofoil shape. Their main function is to guide the water to enter over the runner vane at designed velocity and designed angle (as per the inlet velocity triangle). Each guide blade is capable of rotation around its pivot and all these blades are connected by a regulating guide ring. By regulating this ring, the passages between the guide blades can be fully closed and thus the flow through them can be regulated. This rotating system is known as guide mechanism and is required for governing of turbine (See section 15.17).

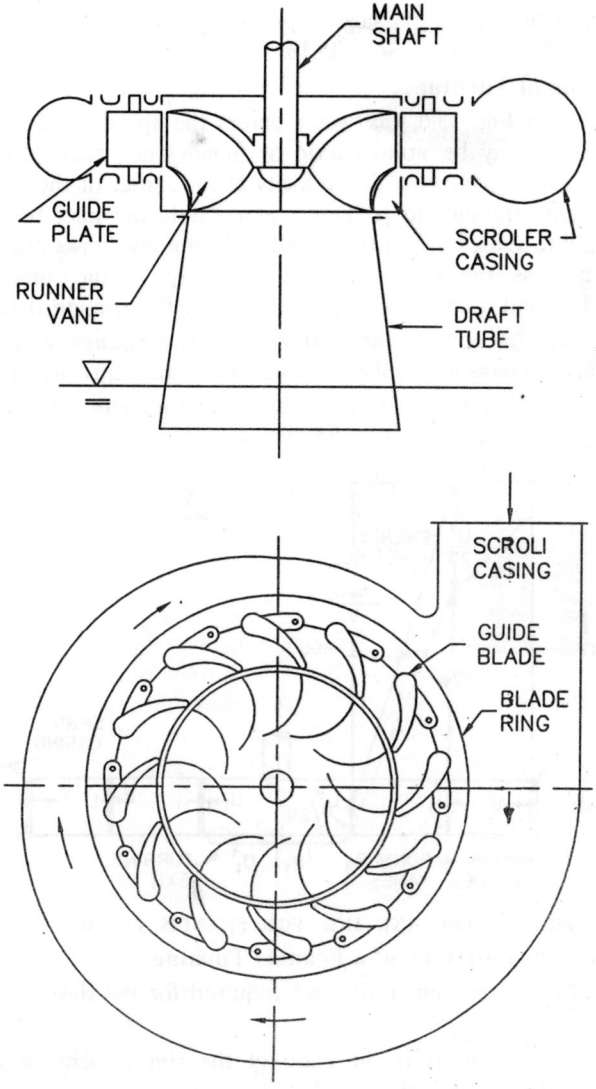

FIG. 15.5 FRANCIS TURBINE

(c) *Turbine runner* : The water from the guide blades enters the runner which consists of a number of curved vanes (about 12 or 16 or more) evenly arranged around its periphery. The proper shape and its various angles (α, θ, φ and β) are designed with the data given Sec. 15.12.2. Usually these are so designed that the flow at the exit is radial or $\beta = 90°$. This way, the whirling component of the velocity U_{w1} is eliminated. The water enters the runner radially at its outer periphery and comes out of it axially at its outer periphery. The runner is keyed to a shaft and transfers the torque to the generator through it.

(d) *Exit* : The water from the runner is discharged to the tail race through an air tight pipe or passage of gradually increasing area, called 'draft tube', which is described in Sec. 15.13.

15.12.2 Working of Turbine

As shown in Fig. 15.6, the water enters the spiral casing with velocity 'v' (pressure in it may be atmospheric or higher) and then passes through the contracting guide passages. The velocity at the outlet of the guide passage changes to U and pressure to p. Thus water enters the inlet tip of the vane at desired absolute velocity U in the radial direction and flows over the runner vane. In the process, the water transfers the energy to the runner (given by Euler's equation) and a small amount h_L is lost in the friction over the vanes. The water is discharged to the exit end of the runner with a velocity U_1 ; the pressure remains atmospheric (if no draft tube is provided) or becomes -ve (if draft tube is provided at its exit). Thus the total energy line and hydraulic gradient line may be drawn (Fig. 15.6).

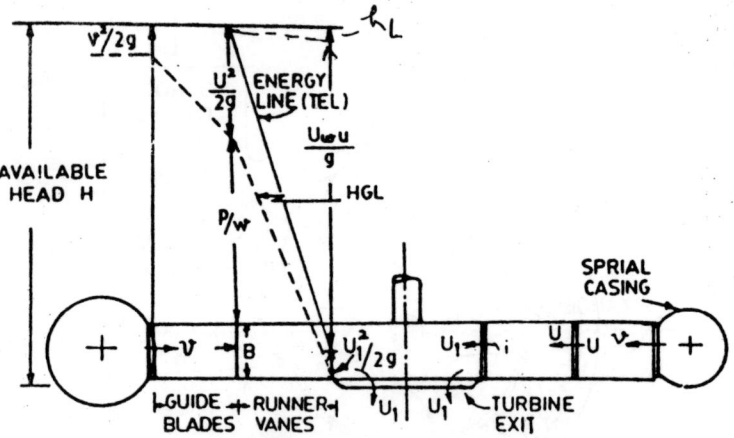

FIG. 15.6 TEL AND HGL FOR FRANCIS TURBINE

15.12.3 Working Proportions of a Francis Turbine

The following important ratios are required for the design of a Francis Turbine.

(a) Speed ratio Φ. It is the ratio of the rim velocity at inlet, u, to the theoretical velocity, $\sqrt{2gH}$

$$\Phi = \frac{u}{\sqrt{2gH}} \qquad (15.37)$$

Its value varies within wide range, i.e. from 0.6 to 0.9.

(b) Flow ratio ψ ; It is the ratio of the velocity of flow at inlet to theoretical velocity $\sqrt{2gH}$

$$\psi = \frac{U_f}{\sqrt{2gH}} \qquad (15.38)$$

Its value ranges from 0.15 to 0.30.

(c) Breadth ratio n. It is the ratio of the width of the wheel B to the diameter D (at inlet) of the wheel.

$$\therefore \qquad n = \frac{B}{D} \qquad (15.39)$$

Its value ranges from 0.2 to 0.4.

15.12.4 Design of Francis Turbine

Design calculation includes the determination of the size of runner and its various angles α, β, θ and φ to develop power P while working under head H and running at N r.p.m. The appropriate values of η_H, η_0, flow ratio ψ, speed ratio Φ and breadth ratio n are assumed for the design of proper runner. It is to be noted that the turbine runners (prototype) are manufactured after proper model testing and modification (if any) incorporated in its design. The design is given in steps.

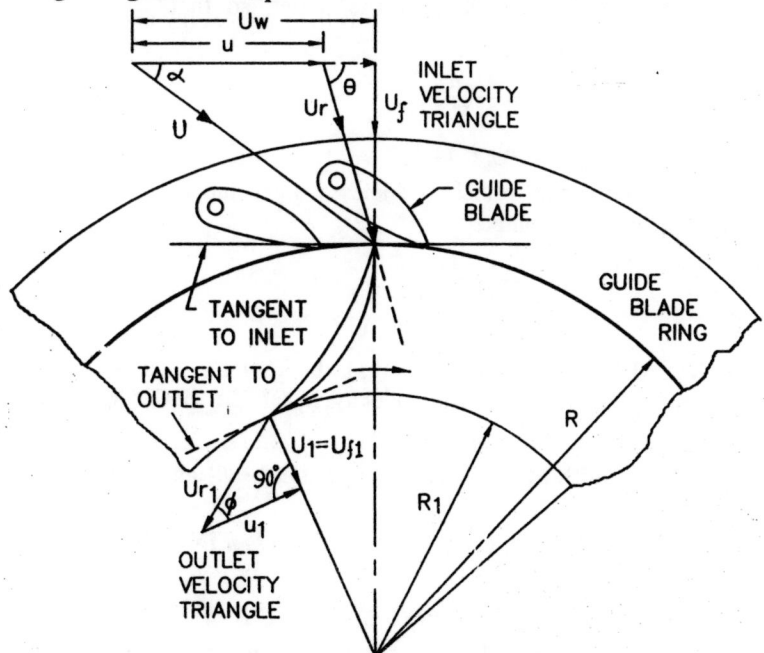

FIG. 15.7 VELOCITY TRIANGLES FOR FRANCIS TURBINE (U IS RIM
VELOCITY AND U_w IS WHIRL VELOCITY AT INLET)

(a) Compute the discharge Q required to produce power P watts.

$$\therefore \qquad Q = \frac{P}{w\, H\, \eta_0}\, m^3/s \qquad\qquad\qquad \text{(i)}$$

(b) Obtain the velocity of flow U_f

$$U_f = \psi\, \sqrt{2gH}\ \ m/s \qquad\qquad\qquad \text{(ii)}$$

(c) The discharge Q flowing through the runner for Francis Turbine is given

$$Q = (\pi D - z\, t)\, B\, U_f \qquad\qquad\qquad \text{(15.40 a)}$$

where z is the number of runner blades and t is the thickness of each blade. Sometimes, the clear passage of flow is expressed as certain fraction "k" of total circumferential area. B and D are the breadth and diameter of the wheel at its inlet end.

$$\therefore \qquad Q = k\, \pi\, D\, B\, U_f \qquad\qquad\qquad \text{(15.40 b)}$$

Using breadth ratio n, diameter D at inlet is determined

$$D = \sqrt{\frac{Q}{k\, \pi\, n\, U_f}} \qquad\qquad\qquad \text{(iii)}$$

(d) Compute peripheral velocity u,

$$u = \Phi\, \sqrt{2gH} \qquad\qquad\qquad \text{(iv)}$$

(e) The whirling velocity U_w at the inlet is now computed. It is assumed that the water discharges radially at the outlet, so that

$$U_{w1} = 0$$

$$\therefore \qquad \eta_H = \frac{U_w\, u}{g\, H}$$

$$U_w = g\, H\, \eta_H / u \qquad\qquad\qquad \text{(v)}$$

(f) Referring to the velocity trangles at inlet and outlet, the inlet blade angle θ and α are computed.

$$\tan\theta = \frac{U_f}{(U_w - u)} \qquad\qquad\qquad \text{(vi)}$$

$$\tan\alpha = U_f / U_w \qquad\qquad\qquad \text{(vii)}$$

(g) The diameter of the runner at the outlet D_1 varies from D/3 to 2D/3. Assuming $D_1 = D/2$, the rim velocity u_1 at the outlet is obtained.

$$u_1 = \pi\, D_1\, N / 60 \qquad\qquad\qquad \text{(viii)}$$

(h) Let the width of the wheel at the outlet be B_1 and its blade thickness be t_1.

$$Q = (\pi D_1 - z\, t_1)\, B_1\, U_{f1} = k_1\, \pi\, D_1\, B_1\, U_{f1} \qquad\qquad \text{(15.40c)}$$

Also at inlet

$$Q = (\pi\, \bar{D}\, z\, t)\, B\, U_f = k\, \pi\, D\, B\, U_f \qquad\qquad \text{(15.40d)}$$

Usually, the velocity of flow is assumed constant at the runner inlet and outlet and k is taken equal to k_1

Therefore, $B_1 = 2B$. \qquad\qquad\qquad (ix)

(i) The outlet blade angle is now determined, since $U_1 = U_{f1}$,

$$\tan \varphi = (U_{f1}/u_1) \tag{x}$$

(j) The number of runner vanes should either be one more or one less than the number of guide vanes to avoid periodic impulses.

15.13 THEORY OF DRAFT TUBE

The draft tube is an integral part of a reaction turbine. It is a gradually expanded closed passage provided at the exit of the turbine. It enables the turbine to be set above tail race water level without losing any head thereby. Also, it reduces the velocity of water finally discharging into the tailrace. Thus, the draft tube has two main functions to perform.

(1) It permits a negative or suction head to be established at runner exit (as can be seen by the use of Bernoulli's theorem), thus making it possible to set the turbine above the tail race water level.

(2) It acts a recuperator of energy, converting a large proportions of energy rejected from the runner into useful pressure energy.

Let U_1 be the absolute velocity of water leaving the runner blade and it is the same with which it enters the draft tube (U_1). The pressure at the entrance to the draft tube is p_2 (say). Let the quantities at the exit of draft tube be U_3 and p_3. the turbine be set H_s metre (say) above the tail race level. Usually, the draft tube discharges below water level. Let it be immersed by h_3 metre and h_L be the loss of head in the draft tube, Fig. 15.8.

Applying Bernoulli's theorem between the entrance and exit section of draft tube

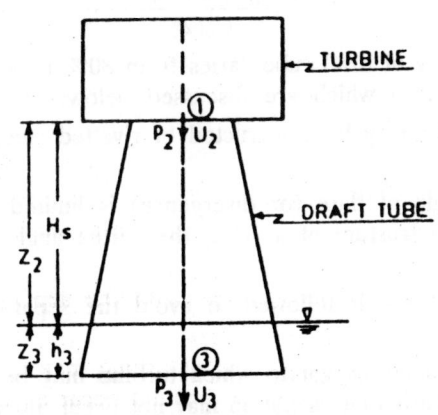

FIG. 15.8 A DRAFT TUBE

$$\frac{p_2}{w} + z_2 + \frac{U_2^2}{2g} = \frac{p_3}{w} + z_3 + \frac{U_3^2}{2g} + h_L$$

But

$$\frac{p_3}{w} = \frac{p_a}{w} + h_3$$

$$z_2 = H_s = \text{datum head at entrance section}$$

$$z_3 = -h_3 = \text{datum head at exit section}$$

Substituting these values,

$$\frac{p_2}{w} = \left(\frac{p_a}{w} + h_3\right) + (z_3 - z_2) + \frac{U_3^2}{2g} - \frac{U_2^2}{2g} + h_L$$

$$= \left(\frac{p_a}{w} + h_3\right) + (-h_3 - H_s) - \frac{U_2^2 - U_3^2}{2g} + h_L$$

$$= \left[\frac{p_a}{w} - \left\{H_s + \frac{U_2^2 - U_3^2}{2g} - h_L\right\}\right]$$

Generally, the energy loss in the draft tube h_L is expressed as

$$h_L = k\,(U_2^2 - U_3^2)/2g$$

Therefore,

$$\frac{p_2}{w} = \left[\frac{p_a}{w} - \left\{H_s + (1 - k)\left(\frac{U_2^2 - U_3^2}{2g}\right)\right\}\right] \quad \text{...(15.41)}$$

The quantity under last bracket is +ve, this means, that the pressure at the entrance to the draft tube is -ve or below atmospheric pressure. Further, if a draft tube is not fitted, the loss of velocity energy would be $U_2^2/2g$. By fitting the flared draft tube, the kinetic energy lost is only ($U_3^2/2g + h_L$). Thus, the head equal to the difference of these two quantities have been recuped.

The efficiency of the draft tube η_{DT} is thus defined as

$$\eta_{DT} = \frac{\text{Actual recuped pressure head}}{\text{Velocity energy at the entrance to draft tube}}$$

$$= \frac{(U_2^2/2g - U_3^2/2g - h_L)}{U_2^2/2g} = \frac{(1 - k)\,(U_2^2 - U_3^2)}{U_2^2} \text{...(15.42)}$$

The efficiency of draft tube varies from 80% to 90%. There are other points of interest also which are discussed below:

(1) The draft may be constructed of rivetted steel plates or moulded in concrete.

(2) The angle of flare (or divergence) is limited in such a way that the draft tube is a frustum of a cone, the vertex angle of which is limited to 8°

This requirement is followed to avoid the separation of flow in the tube.

(3) The optimum height to which turbine may be set above tail race is decided on the basis that cavitation may not occur anywhere in the turbine, particularly at the entrance to the draft tube. The optimum height $(H_s)_{max}$ can be determined from Eq. 15.41. The pressure at the exit of turbine runner and also at the draft tube entrance should not be less than vapour pressure of water p_v.

From Eq. 15.41,

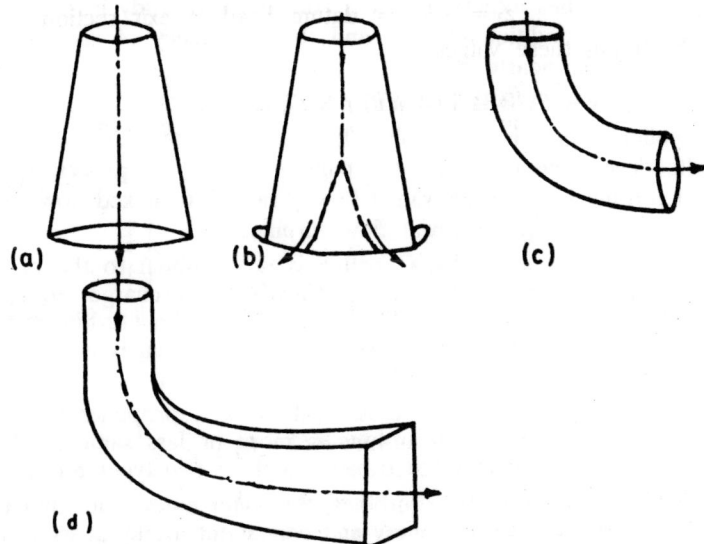

FIG. 15.9 DIFFERENT TYPES OF DRAFT TUBES.

$$\left[H_s + \frac{U_2^2 - U_3^2}{2g} - h_L \right] = \frac{(p_a - p_2)}{w}$$

$$\therefore \quad \left[(H_s)_{\text{max}} + \frac{(U_2^2 - U_3^2)}{2g} - h_L \right] \not> \frac{(p_a - p_v)}{w} \quad \text{absolute} \qquad (15.43)$$

If $p_a/w = 10.3$ m and $p_v/w = 2.5$ m is assumed,

$$\left[(H_s)_{\text{max}} + \frac{(U_2^2 - U_3^2)}{2g} - h_L \right] \not> 7.8 \text{ m.}$$

(4) There are various types of draft tube which are used with different type of reaction turbines and at different site, Fig. 15.9. The axial flow turbine work under low head and hence straight flaring type draft tube are unsuitable. In such cases, a draft tube with circular inlet and rectangular exit with a right angled bend in between (type d) is used. The water although enters in it vertically but leaves in horizontal direction. Such a draft tube can be accommodated in a lesser vertical distance and gives good recupation of pressure energy. But its efficiency is slightly lower than straight flared type draft tube, i.e., nearly 80%.

(5) There are different designs of draft tube which have been developed to turn the water through 90° with the least loss of energy. Among these, Moody spreading draft tube is shown in Fig. 15.9 (b) which has got a solid core at its centre (In some design, the central core is extended upto the runner). In case of reaction turbine, water leaves the runner with little rotation at full load condition. But at part load, usually it leaves with a large component of whirling velocity and the flow approaches a free vortex flow. It has been shown earlier that, as the radius of a free vortex approaches zero, the whirl

component approaches infinity; which is conductive to eddy loss. The central core avoids such condition of flow and thus efficiency of such draft tube remains quite high; nearly 90%.

15.14 PROPELLER TURBINE/KAPLAN TURBINE

Propeller turbine is essentially a low head turbine which produces high outputs. Its development results as a culmination of the process of finding a modified turbine from purely radial flow (Francis) to mixed flow (modified Francis) and then to purely axial flow turbine.

The power developed by a turbine is proportional to the product of total head (net), H and the flow rate Q. Clearly the discharge required must increase as the available head falls. Thus, a purely axial flow turbine is obtained as maximum flow rate may be passed through the passages between runner vanes i.e., when the flow is parallel to the axis.

Fig. 15.10 shows a typical cross section of a propeller turbine. The details of setting of a propeller turbine is more or less same as that of a Francis turbine. The main difference between these two types are as follows:

(1) In case of mixed flow turbines, the water enters the runner in the radial direction at its outer periphery and comes out axially at its inner ring. Thus it has got a finite component of radial velocity. But in case of axial flow turbines, the water looses all its components of radial velocity and flow becomes purely axial by the time it reaches the runner vane.

(2) The number of runner vanes is reduced from 12 or more in Francis turbine to 3,4 or 5 only.

15.14.1 Various Components

The main components of a Propeller turbine are spiral casing, stay vanes (rings) or speed ring, guide vanes and draft tube.

The spiral casing is of sufficiently large size to accommodate the large flow rate of water and distribute it uniformly all over the periphery of the turbine with small velocity. From strength point of view as well as to guide the water, the guide vanes are supplemented by additional vanes known as stay vanes or speed ring outside the guide assembly. The stay vanes behave as a column and are so shaped as to conform to the natural streams which are spiral in character. The water entering from the casing first passes past the stay vanes then past the guide ring in the radial direction and thereafter takes a right angle turn into axial direction and flows over the runner vanes. These runner vanes may be either stationary (Propeller turbine) or movable (Kaplan turbine). The purpose of the guide blades is to impart whirling motion to the fluid so that when it reaches the runner, it is essentially a free vortex motion $U \propto 1/R$.

In the simplest form of axial flow runner, the vanes are cast integrally with the shaft, also called hub or boss, as in case of Propeller turbine or may be pivoted and fitted with adjusting gear as in case of Kaplan turbine. By means of this gear, the runner vane angles can be adjusted at part load condition. It is the main difference between a Propeller turbine and Kaplan turbine. Runner vanes are made up of stainless steel. They must be long enough to accommodate the larger flow rate and consequently the consideration of strength required to transmit tremendous torque involved impose the necessity for large blade chords. Thus the pitch to chord ratio of 1.0 to 1.5 are used and hence the number of blades is small, usually 3 to 5. Finally, the water from the runner is discharged to tailrace through elbow type draft tube.

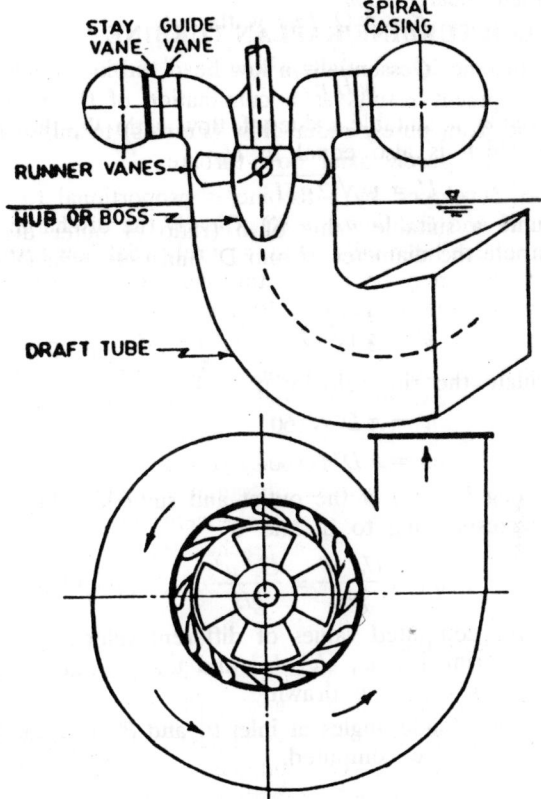

FIG. 15.10 A KAPLAN TURBINE

Being an axial flow type, the inlet and outlet are at same radial distance from the central axis but the diameter of inlet and outlet varies from the diameter of the boss to the diameter of outer periphery of the runner (Fig. 15.10). Thus the rim velocity u to u_1 varies from near the boss to outer periphery and so the corresponding velocity diagrams and hence the required runner inlet and outlet vane angles also vary. Therefore the shape of the runner vanes is warped i.e., it gradually changes over its radial width.

15.14.2 Design of Propeller (or Kaplan) Turbine

Let a Kaplan turbine be required to be designed to develop P watts of power while working under a head H metre and running at N r.p.m. The appropriate values of η_0, Φ, ψ and n are assumed for the purpose of design.

Being an axial flow turbine, the area of flow remain same at its inlet and outlet and therefore, the velocity of flow remains constant throughout the runner i.e. $U_f = U_{f1}$. Let the quantities near the boss be indicated by single dash (') and that at outer rim by double dash (").

(1) Calculate the required discharge Q to produce power P from the expression

$$P = w Q H \eta_0 \text{ watts}$$

or

$$Q = \frac{P}{w H \eta_0} m^3/s \tag{i}$$

(2) Assuming a suitable value of flow ratio Φ, the velocity of flow U_f is obtained which is also equal to U_{f1}

$$U_f = \psi \sqrt{2gH} \tag{ii}$$

(3) Assume a suitable value of n (ratio of outer diameter to inner diameter). Compute the diameter of hub D' and outer rim D" from discharge relation.

$$Q = \frac{\pi}{4} [(D'')^2 - (D')^2] U_f \tag{15.44}$$

(4) Calculate the rim velocity u' and u"

$$u' = \pi D' N/60 \tag{iii}$$
$$u = \pi D'' N/60 \tag{iv}$$

(5) Assuming $U_{w1} = 0$ at the outlet and suitable values of η_H, compute U'_w and U_w'' corresponding to u' and u"

$$\eta_H = \frac{U_w' u'}{gH} = \frac{U_w'' u''}{gH} \tag{v}$$

(6) With the computed values of different velocities at the inner rim (hub) and at outer rim, i.e., u', U_w', U_f' and u", U_w'' and U_f'', the velocity triangles at these ends can be drawn.

(7) The runner blade angles at inlet θ' and θ'' near the hub and outer periphery, respectively are computed.

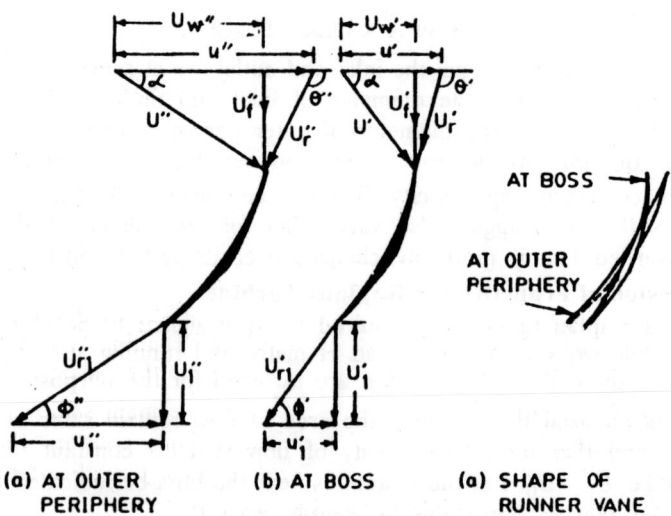

(a) AT OUTER   (b) AT BOSS   (a) SHAPE OF
     PERIPHERY   RUNNER VANE

FIG. 15.11 SHAPE OF RUNNER VANES AT DIFFERENT RADIAL DISTANCES.

$$\tan \theta' = \frac{U_f}{(u' - U_w')} \text{ and } \tan \theta'' = \frac{U_f}{(u'' - U_w'')} \qquad \text{(vi)}$$

(8) Similarly outlet blade angles φ' and φ'' are determined

$$\tan \varphi' = \frac{U_1'}{u'} = \frac{U_{f_1}}{u}, \text{ and } \tan \varphi'' = \frac{U_1''}{u''} \qquad \text{(vii)}$$

(9) By repeating the above procedure for various radial distances the complete shape of the blade for its full radial width may be obtained.

15.15 KAPLAN TURBINE

Although the propeller turbine stands almost unrivalled when large output must be produced under low-head but it has got one quite serious disadvantage, viz., its efficiency is quite low at part load. This drop in efficiency at part load is caused due to greater loss of energy due to shock (or formation of eddies) at the runner inlet and rejection of large amount of kinetic energy at the turbine exit. The Kaplan turbine (which was developed by Kaplan of Czechoslovakia in early 1920) is similar in construction to propeller turbine except that it has got variable pitch propeller. By this arrangement the angles of inclination of the runner vanes can be adjusted at part load (while the turbine is in motion) so as to obtain maximum possible efficiency.

At part load, lesser discharge Q will flow through the turbine runner than at designed full load. Therefore, the values of U_f and α decrease but the value of peripheral velocity u at the inlet remains same (even at part load as the turbine is coupled with a constant speed generator). Thus, the water enters at quite different angle θ' over the runner inlet and water suffers a shock at the entrance. Moreover, the whirling component of velocity at runner outlet U_{w1} does not remain zero (Refer Fig. 15.12). Both these causes of energy loss are eliminated in the Kaplan turbine by the adjustment of runner

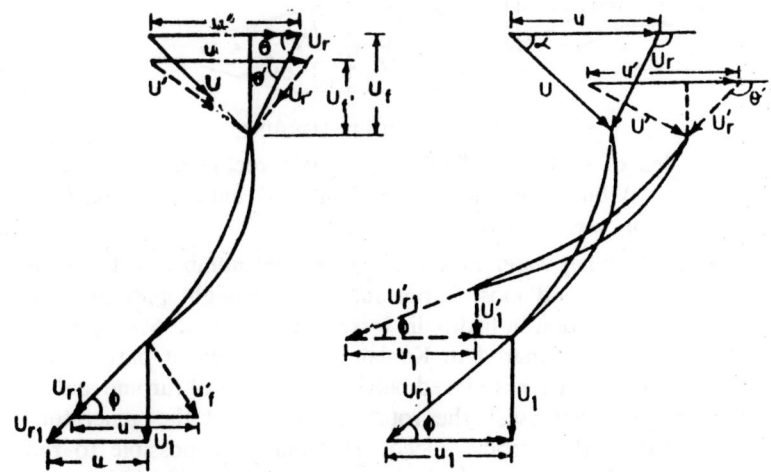

(a) PROPELLER TURBINE (b) KAPLAN TURBINE

FIG. 15.12 VELOCITY TRIANGLES FOR A KAPLAN TURBINE

vanes at appropriate angle and its efficiency remains as high as at full load (except at less than 20% of full load).

15.16 TUBULAR/BULB TURBINE

Kaplan turbine when employed for very low heads (5m to 15m) has to be installed below tail race level, thus requiring an excessive excavation. Therefore, cost of such installation is high. Further, the water has to pass through many bends and curved passages which causes the loss of energy and lower turbine efficiency.

In 1937, Arno Fischer (Germany) developed a modified axial flow turbine whose shaft could be set either vertically or inclined. It was named as 'tubular turbine'. The turbo-generator set using tubular turbine has an outer casing having the shape of a bulb. If the axis of the rotation of the turbine set is made horizontal, it is known as bulb set and the turbine used as bulb turbine. This turbine is quite useful to work at very low head (5m to 15m). The bulb unit is a water tight assembly of turbine and generator submerged below water level. The axis of rotation coincides with the axis of the straight passage of water.

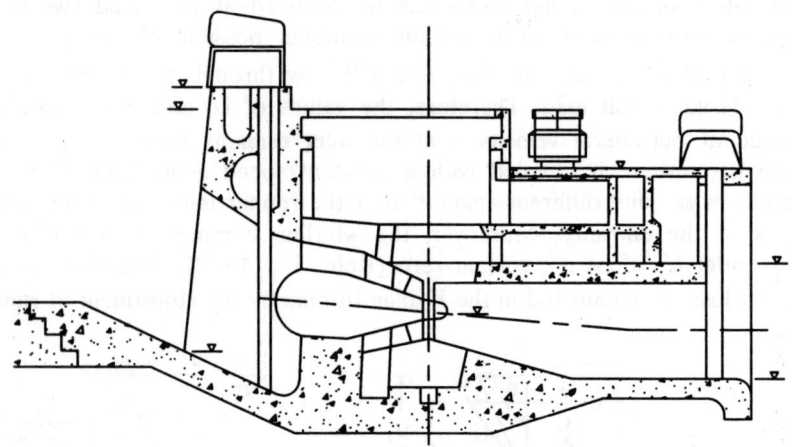

FIG. 15.13 BULB TURBINE

The idea of such axial flow turbine with rectilinear draft tube is quite old (1920 or so) but could not be implemented until a compact and water sealed alternator was developed.

In bulb turbine, water flow has a minimum number of turns and bends throughout the unit and most important is the straight passage through the draft tube. The reduction in hydraulic losses gives a 3% to 5% higher efficiency for bulb turbine as compared to Kaplan turbine, even at part load. In some bulb turbine a step up gear is placed between the shaft of turbine and generator. The step up gear increases the rotational speed of the generator 5 to 10 times over that of the turbine speed. This makes it possible to reduce the dimensions of both turbine and generator and thus requiring lesser space for installation. The step up gear is a concentric planetory gear drive which is rather intricate and costly item.

Another special type of the horizontal hydro-electric unit employing axial flow turbine is, so called, straight flow unit or straflow, the distinguishing feature of this type is that the generator rotor is set on the peripheral edge of the turbine runner. Such units are of great importance to tidal power plants.

The major demerit of bulb turbine is that, it is completely submerged under water so maintenance is difficult. Also generator chamber should be water tight. Even then high moisture remains in the chamber which is a major source of trouble. Another serious problem associated with it is to ensure reliable performance of bearings, especially of turbine bearings that take up a large radial load caused by the large overhang mounted runner. The practice is, therefore, to have a centre of gravity of the runner as close as possible to the bearing.

15.17 GOVERNING OF TURBINE

A turbine is designed to develope a 'rated output' (at maximum efficiency) which will maintain a full load (or torque) of the shaft at normal speed. Whenever the load on the turbine changes, say drops, the speed of the turbine shoots up, (since output α load $\times$ speed, i.e., $P \alpha T \omega$).

Usually, the turbines are coupled with alternators and hence must run at the same speed. But the speed of the alternator is governed by the number of poles 'p' in it and the frequency 'f' at which electric current is to be supplied, none of which can vary with the changes in the load.

$$\text{Synchronous speed}^1 \ N_{syn} = 60 f/p = \frac{3000}{p} \qquad (15.45)$$

This means that the turbine must also run at constant speed (i.e. N_{syn}) which is its normal speed, whatever may be the variation in the load on the turbine. The operation of maintaining the constant speed whenever there is a variation in the load is known as 'governing of turbines'.

15.17.1 Principal of Governing

Generally, the turbine work at maximum efficiency, produces output power P while running at speed N and supplies torque T to the shaft (i.e., load on the shaft is T).

The output power $= Torque \times angular\, velocity$

$$P = T \omega \qquad \qquad ...(15.46a)$$

also $\qquad P = w\, Q\, H\, \eta_0 \text{ watts} \qquad ...(15.46b)$

$\therefore \qquad P \alpha Q\, H \alpha T N \qquad ...(15.46c)$

---

1 In India, electricity is supplied at 50 cycles per second.

.1 is obvious from Eq. 15.46c, that to maintain the speed constant when the load on the turbine changes suddenly the output should change accordingly. But output is also proportional to the rate of flow Q and head H impressed on the turbine. The later is the difference of head race and tail race elevations and hence remain unchanged. This means that the flow rate Q must change suddenly as soon as the load on the turbine changes. This is known as 'principle of governing'.

15.17.2 Governing of Turbines

If the discharge Q is changed suddenly so as to maintain a constant speed the momentum of the flowing water in the penstock will be destroyed suddenly. This may result in the development of high inertia pressure in the penstock (water hammer). Thus as the load variation takes place almost instantaneously and a corresponding instantaneous regulation of discharge can only be done at heavy risk of damaging the pipe line due to water hammer. To avoid this situation to develop, the flow rate should be moderated down (or up) gradually so that the pressure rise remain within permissible limits. Thus the governing of turbines involves two stages:

1. *Speed Regulation* To maintain the speed of the turbine constant, the discharge should be regulated immediately and simultaneously with the changes in the load. This is known as 'speed regulation'.

2. *Pressure Regulation* At the same time. the pressure rise in the penstock should remain within permissible safe limits and therefore, the discharge Q should be moderated slowly. This is known as 'pressure regualation'.

It may be seen that these two requirements are contrary to each other and has to be followed by different means in different types of turbines.

15.17.3 Governing of Pelton Wheel

As discussed above, to maintain the speed constant, the discharge should vary simultaneously with the variation in the load. In case of Pelton Wheel, the water from the penstock flows through the nozzle of diameter 'd' and the discharge Q is given by

$$Q = aU = \left(\frac{\pi}{4}d^2\right)k_v\sqrt{2gH}$$

Since the head impressed on the turbine remains unchanged, therefore, $Q \propto d^2$. Thus, by regulating the diameter of the nozzle, the discharge can be regulated. Of course, this can be done by any ordinary throttle valve but it may cause large hydraulic losses, a streamlined body, called 'spear' connected with a spear rod is used. The spear moves axially within the penstock and the nozzle and thus regulates the cross sectional area of the flow (in the nozzle), thereby regulates the discharge. This process is known as 'speed regulation by spear'.

The serious objection to the use of spear is the development of high inertia pressure in the penstock following a rapid closure or opening of the nozzle. In case of Pelton Wheel this objection is overcome by moving spear slowly and in the mean time, the excess flow is disallowed to strike the buckets by means of a deflector. As soon as the load on the turbine falls, the deflector (which is also connected with the shaft) comes in front of the jet and excess water is diverted away from the wheel. In the course of time, the spear moves slowly, raduces the nozzle diameter corresponding to changed load condition and thus maintains the turbine speed constant. After the turbine speed is resorted to normal, and spear moves to appropriate location, the deflector comes back to OFF position.

In hydraulic turbines, these two operations are done with the help of an 'oil pressure governor', also known as 'centrifugal governor'. This operation (regulation of speed and pressure) is known as double regulation. The oil pressure governor is connected to the turbine shaft and take 3 seconds to resort the constant speed of the turbine.

15.17.4 Double Regulation by Oil Pressure Governor

Fig. 15.14(a) shows an automatic oil pressure governor used with Pelton Wheel. It consists of the following major components:

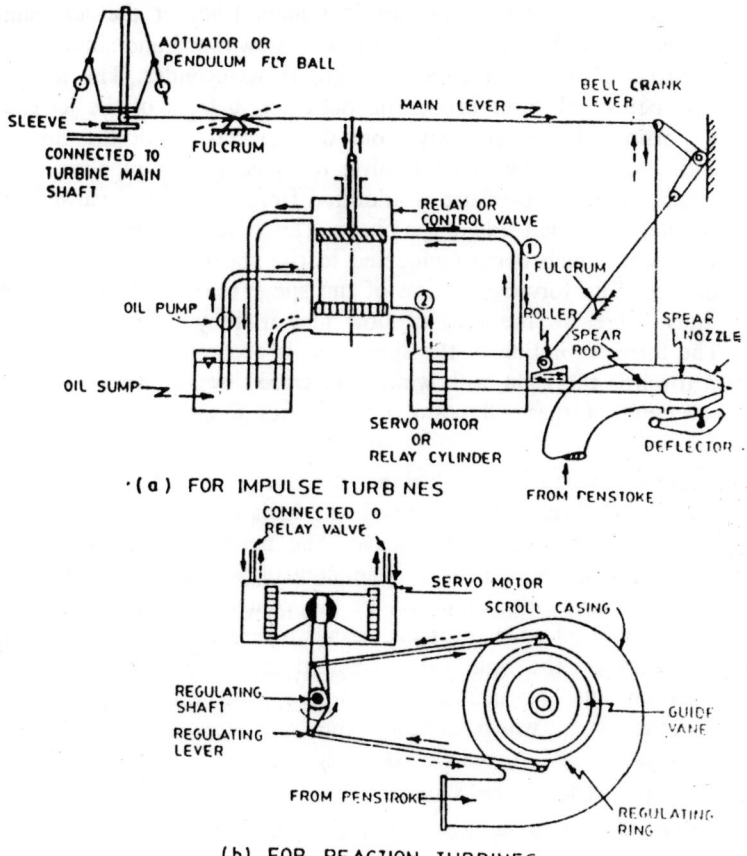

(b) FOR REACTION TURBINES

FIG. 15.14 AUTOMATIC OIL PRESSURE GOVERNOR (A) PELTON
WHEEL (B) FRANCIS AND KAPLAN TURBINE.

1. *Servomotor or relay cylinder* It consists of a cylinder and a piston moving inside it. It operates the turbine gates or the spear.

2. *Relay valve or distribution valve* It controls the flow of oil under pressure on either side of the servomoter cylinder.

3. *Actuator or pendulum* It functions by the action of centrifugal force and is driven by the turbine main shaft.

4. *Oil pump* It supplies the oil to the relay valve at about 15 atmospheric pressure or more and it is driven by the turbine shaft.

5. *Oil supply pipeline* It conveys oil between the oil sump and relay valve.

Let us consider a situation in which the load on the turbine decreases resulting in the increase in its speed. Now since the pendulum is connected to the turbine main shaft, the balls of the pendulum move outward (with increase in the speed of the turbine) and this results in an upward movement of the sleeve. As the sleeve moves up, the main lever at the left hand is raised which causes the bell crank lever to move downward and simultaneously pushes the piston of the control valve down in its cylinder. The downward motion of the bell crank lever brings the deflector in front of the jet thereby diverting a portion of the jet away from the buckets. With the downward position of the piston of the control valve, the passage for pipeline 2 opens (Fig. 15.14) and oil under pressure is admitted from the control valve cylinder to the servomoter on the left side of the piston. The servomotor piston, therefore, moves to the right, which being connected to the spear rod causes the spear to move forward. The forward motion of the spear reduces the nozzle outlet area and thus decreases the rate of flow and thereby its normal speed is resorted. The forward motion of the spear rod is accompanied by the motion of the cam towards the right with which the crank lever moves upward. The upward movement of the bell crank lever brings the deflector back to its normal position.

Whenever the load on the turbine increases, the speed of the turbine decreases. Due to this reduction in speed, the balls move downward resulting in the downward movement of the sleeve. The main lever at the left hand is lowered which pulls the piston of the control valve up in the cylinder. With the upward motion of the piston of the control valve, the passage for pipe line 1 opens and oil under pressure rushes from the control valve cylinder to the servo-motor on the right side of the piston. The servo-motor piston then moves to the left. This increases the nozzle outlet area by the backward movement of the spear, which occupies the normal position so that again the normal speed of the turbine is resorted.

15.17.5 Governing of Reaction Turbine

The rate of flow in the reaction turbine is controlled by varying the area of flow passage between the adjacent guide blades. As shown in Fig. 15.14(b), the guide vanes of a reaction turbine are pivoted and are connected by levers and links to the regulating ring. The regulating ring is then connected to the regulating lever by means of two regulating rods. Thereafter this regulating lever is connected to a regulating shaft which is operated by servometer piston of an oil pressure governor, Fig. 15.14(b). The motion of the servometer piston is transmitted to the regulating ring which causes all guide blades to turn simultaneously in one direction and thus the area of the flow passage between the adjacent guide blades is reduced or increased depending on the load on the turbine.

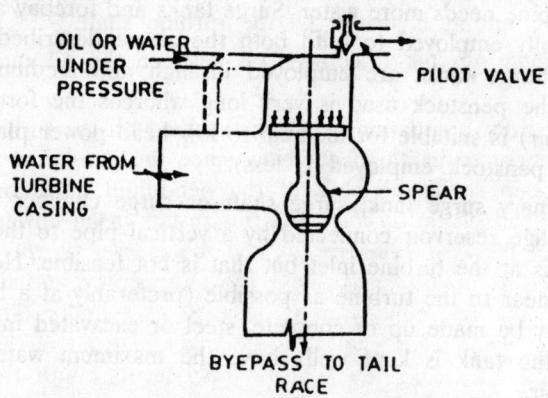

FIG. 15.15 RELIEF VALVE

A sudden drop in the load on a turbine would require a rapid closure of the guide vane. But it may create high inertia pressure in the penstock. In order to keep the pressure within permissible safe limits (pressure regulation) and at the same time to facilitate the rapid closure of the guide blades, a relief valve is usually provided (Fig. 15.15). The relief valve bye passes the excess flow of water directly to the tail race and thus help in maintaining safe pressure in the penstock (just like a deflector of a Pelton wheel).

In case of Kaplan turbine in addition to the guide blades, the runner vanes are also adjustable. As such, the governor is required to operate both sets of vanes simultaneously. The governor does not differ much from that for Francis turbine described above except that it is also provided with a control valve for the runner vanes servomoter. The servometer control valves for both runner vanes and guide vanes, are interconnected to ensure that for a given guide vane opening there shall be definite runner vane inclination. In this way, higher efficiency is obtained even at part load.

15.18 RUN AWAY SPEED

If the external load of a turbine while working under a maximum head and full gate opening is disconnected anyhow, i.e., the load drops to zero, the turbine will race up and will attain a maximum speed. This maximum or limiting speed is known as "runaway speed" and hence all the rotating parts must be designed to withstand the stresses developed due to high speed. For Pelton wheel the runaway speed varies from 1.8 to 1.9 times its normal speed; for Francis turbine it varies from 2 to 2.5 times its normal speed and for Kaplan turbine it varies from 2.5 to 3 times normal speed (Refer also to the characteristic curves for these turbines).

15.19 SURGE TANKS

Two methods, jet deflector and relief valve for Pelton wheel and Francis turbine respectively are used to avoid the creation of excessive pressure in the event of the turbine gates (guide vanes) are closed suddenly. But when the load on the turbine increases, neither of these devices can be of any help as the turbine needs more water. Surge tanks and forebay are the devices which are usually employed to fulfil both the above described requirements (see 15.17.2). Surge tanks are employed in high and medium head power plants where the penstock used is very long whereas the forebay (which is a small reservoir) is suitable for medium to low head power plants (for which the length of penstock employed is less).

An ordinary surge tank, surge shaft or surge chanber is a open top cylindrical storage reservoir connected by a vertical pipe to the penstock. Its ideal location is at the turbine inlet but that is not feasible. Hence, it should be located as near to the turbine as possible (preferably at a higher elevated section). It may be made up of concrete, steel or excavated in the rock. The upper lip of the tank is kept well above the maximum water level in the supply reservoir.

When the load on the turbine is steady and normal and there are no velocity variations in the pipeline, there will be a normal hydraulic gradient line o a a_1 (Fig. 15.16). The water level in the surge tank will be lower than the supply reservoir water level by an amount equal to the friction head loss in the pipe connecting the reservoir with the surge tank. When the load on the turbine is reduced, the turbine gates are partially or fully closed and water flowing towards the turbine is stored in the surge tank in he space between level 'a' and 'b' and a rising hydraulic gradient line o b b_1 is developed.

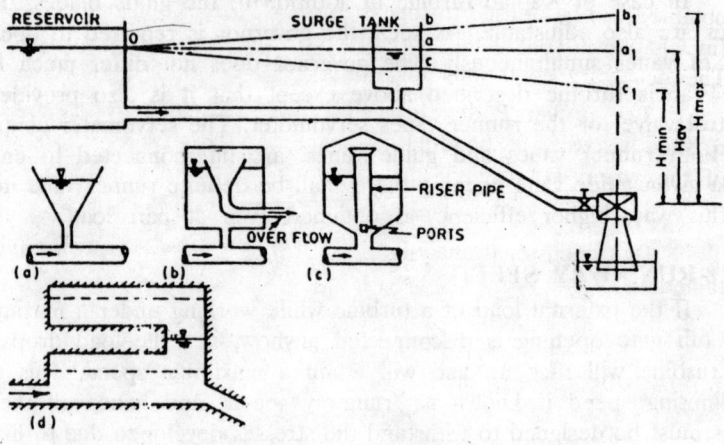

FIG. 15.16 SURGE TANK

The retarding head so built up in the surge tank reduces the velocity of flow in the pipeline to a value corresponding to the reduced discharge required by the turbine.

When the load on the turbine increases, the governer opens the turbine gates to increase the rate of flow entering the runner. The increased demand of water by the turbine is met by the water stored between levels 'a' and 'c' in the surge tank. As such, the water level in the surge tank falls and a falling hydraulic gradient line (HGL) o c c₁ is established. In other words, the surge tank develops an accelerating head which increases the velocity of flow in the penstock to a value corresponding to the increased discharge required by the turbine.

There are various types of surge tanks as shown in Fig. 15.16. The type (a) is conical, type (b) has an internal bellmouth spillway which permits the overflow to be disposed off easily and type (c) is known as differential surge tank. It has got a central riser pipe having small ports or orifices at its lower end. The main advantage of this type is that for the same stabilising effect, its capacity may be less than that for a simple cylindrical tank. This is because in this tank retarding and accelerating heads are developed more promptly. In a simple cylindrical tank, these heads builds up gradually. Moreover, no water is wasted as the water from the riser pipe spills over in the tank itself and can be utilised whenever it is required to be supplied to the turbine. The type (d) surge tank can be used at some suitable sites where the topography permits it to be excavated in the adjoining rocks itself.

15.20 SIMILARITY LAWS

Every machine is designed to meet a specific duty, usually referred to as design point. It should develop a designed power P while working under a head H and running at speed N. The design points is normally associated with maximum efficiency of the machine. To ensure that the turbine will behave the way it has been designed, its performance should be known before the critical turbine (prototype) is manufactured. Hence, a dynamical similar model is tested experimentally and its performance is determined. The results so obtained can be utilised to suggest the modification, if any. As discussed earlier (in Chapter 6) the model should be dynamically similar to that of prototype. The necessary conditions for this can be obtained by dimensional analysis.

The power P developed by the turbine depends on mass density ρ, fluid viscosity μ, head H, discharge Q, speed N and specific dimension of the wheel D.

$$P = f(\rho, D, Q, N, g, H, \mu) \qquad (15.47a)$$

By dimensional analysis the following dimensionless parameters are obtained

$$\left[\frac{P}{\rho N^3 D^5}\right] = f\left[\frac{Q}{N D^3}, \frac{gH}{N^2 D^2}, \frac{\rho N D^2}{\mu}\right] \qquad (15.47b)$$

Since most of the machines run at high speed and the flow in it is turbulent, the effect of viscosity will be insignificant. Therefore, the last term can be dropped out.

∴ $$K_p = f[K_Q, K_H] \qquad (15.48)$$

Thus for dynamically similar machines the above equation should be satisfied. The parameter K_p is known as power coefficient, K_Q as flow parameter and K_H as head coefficient. Therefore,

$$\left(\frac{P}{\rho N^3 D^5}\right)_m = \left(\frac{P}{\rho N^3 D^5}\right)_p \qquad (15.49)$$

$$\left(\frac{Q}{N D^3}\right)_m = \left(\frac{Q}{N D^3}\right)_p \qquad (15.50)$$

and $$\left(\frac{gH}{N^2 D^2}\right)_m = \left(\frac{gH}{N^2 D^2}\right)_p \qquad (15.51)$$

15.21 PERFORMANCE OF TURBINES

The turbines are required to work under varying conditions of head, speed, output and gate opening. It is, therefore, desirable to predict their behaviour under varying conditions of the above parameter. The variations in the working conditions of the turbine may be of the following nature :

(1) The head on the turbine may change and with it the output; the speed being correspondingly adjusted so that no sensible change in efficiency occurs; the gate opening remaining constant.

(2) The head and speed may remain steady, the output being varied by movements of the gates or the needle (spear). These are normal operating conditions for most of the turbines.

(3) Variations in the relationship between head and speed are common, particularly in low head units. Although the speed is permitted to fluctuate within very narrow limits, the head may vary through a range of 50% or more.

(4) With head and gate opening fixed, the speed may be allowed to vary by adjusting the load. These conditions are not often found outside the laboratory and the test plant.

15.22 PERFORMANCE UNDER UNIT HEAD

When comparing the performance of turbines of same type (e.g. Pelton or Francis etc.), it is often convenient to calculate their output while working head is reduced to unity, i.e. H = 1.0 metre such that their efficiency may remain unaffected. The primary condition for unchanged efficiency of a given turbine is that the velocity triangles under the working head H and under unit head should be geometrically similar. In Fig. 15.17 (a) ABC represents the inlet velocity triangles for a Francis turbine working under head H and abc represents the velocity triangle for the same turbine under unit head; the subscript 'u' being used consistently to represent unit conditions. The velocity

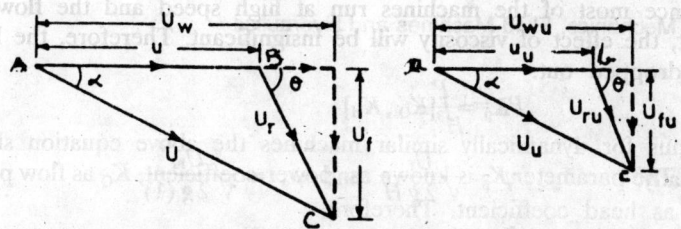

FIG. 15.17 VELOCITY TRIANGLES FOR FRANCIS TURBINE

triangles at exit need not be sketched since the turbines are assumed to discharge radially at outlet.

In both these triangles, the angles θ and α are assumed constant, therefore, 'ac' must be parallel to AC, because the direction of these vectors is fixed by the guide blade angle α. Also 'bc' must be parallel to BC because both these vectors must be along the tangent to the inlet tip of the blade to avoid shock at entry. Thus, the required condition of similarity is fulfilled. It follows that

$$\frac{u}{u_u} = \frac{U_w}{U_{wu}} = \frac{U_f}{U_{fu}} = \text{ constant } k \text{ (say)} \qquad (15.52)$$

Now, since the efficiency of the turbine should remain constant under head H and 1 metre.

$$\eta_H = \frac{U_w u}{gH} = \frac{U_{wu} U_u}{g\,(1)} \qquad (15.53)$$

Substituting the value of U_{wu} and u_u from Eq. 15.52,

$$\frac{U_w u}{gH} = \frac{U_w}{k} \times \frac{u}{k} \times \frac{1}{g}$$

Hence $\qquad k = \sqrt{H} \qquad (15.54)$

Thus, $\qquad u_u = \dfrac{u}{\sqrt{H}} \qquad (15.55a)$

$$U_{wu} = \frac{U_w}{\sqrt{H}} \qquad (15.55b)$$

$$U_{fu} = \frac{U_f}{\sqrt{H}} \qquad (15.55c)$$

Since $\qquad u_u = \dfrac{\pi D N_u}{60}$ and $u = \dfrac{\pi D N}{60}$

Hence $\qquad N_u = \dfrac{N}{\sqrt{H}} \qquad (15.56)$

Further, $\qquad Q = \pi D B U_f \qquad$ and $\qquad Q_u = \pi D B U_{fu}$

Hence $\qquad Q_u = \dfrac{Q}{\sqrt{H}} \qquad (15.57)$

and $\qquad P = w Q H \eta_0$ and $P_u = w Q_u (1) \eta_0$

$$\therefore \qquad P_u = \frac{P}{H^{3/2}} \qquad\qquad (15.58)$$

Finally, $\qquad \psi = \dfrac{U_f}{\sqrt{2gH}}$ and $\psi_u = \dfrac{U_{fu}}{\sqrt{2g(1)}} \qquad\qquad (15.59)$

$$\psi_u = \psi$$

and $\qquad \Phi = \dfrac{u}{\sqrt{2gH}}$ and $\Phi_u = \dfrac{u_u}{\sqrt{2g(1)}}$

$$\therefore \qquad \Phi_u = \Phi \qquad\qquad (15.60)$$

Although these identities have been deduced from the diagrams relating to Francis turbine, they are also applicable to all types of turbines. Therefore, in general, the various parameters can be determined as follows:

(1) All velocities under unit head will be obtained by reducing the corresponding velocities under head H by the factor $\sqrt{H}$ (see Eq. 15.55, etc).

(2) The unit speed N_u (in r.p.m) of the turbine is the working speed N divided by $\sqrt{H}$.

(3) Under unit conditions, a turbine has the same speed ratio Φ and the same flow ratio ψ as it has under its working head H.

(4) The unit power P_u of a turbine, that is, its output under unit head is found by dividing its normal power P by $H^{3/2}$.

The advantage of determining the performance of the turbine at unit head can be seen as follows. Let us assume that a given turbine runs at N r.p.m. under head H, develops power P and discharge Q flows through it. It is required to predict its performance under head H_1. Let us first compute various quantities under unit head in both cases. Since the same turbine is used in both these cases, therefore,

$$N_u = \frac{N}{\sqrt{H}} \text{ should be equal to } \frac{N_1}{\sqrt{H_1}}$$

$$N_1 = N \sqrt{\frac{H_1}{H}} \qquad\qquad (15.61)$$

Similarly, $\qquad Q_u = \dfrac{Q}{\sqrt{H}} = \dfrac{Q_1}{\sqrt{H_1}} \; ; \; Q_1 = Q \sqrt{\dfrac{H_1}{H}} \qquad\qquad (15.62)$

$$P_u = \frac{P}{\sqrt{H^{3/2}}} = \frac{P_1}{H_1^{3/2}} \; ; \; P_1 = P \left(\frac{H_1}{H} \right)^{3/2} \qquad\qquad (15.63)$$

The above treatment is based on the assumption that even at unit head, the hydraulic efficiency remain unaltered. This assumption is not strictly true since the hydraulic losses are proportionately higher at smaller head and therefore, the efficiency does fall slightly (Refer Sec. 15.24).

15.23 PERFORMANCE UNDER SPECIFIC CONDITIONS

The performance of the same type of turbines can be studies by the concept of unit quantities. But it does not provide an equitable basis to compare the turbines of different types (for example a Pelton Wheel and a Francis turbine, etc.). That is, to say, the reduction of turbine performance at a unit head is not a sufficient basis to compare turbines of various types, because each one of them behaves differently. For example, two runner of turbines, say one of them is Pelton wheel and other is Francis turbine, having same runner diameter, working under the same head will be found to run at different speeds, take up different discharges and develop outputs differently having no correlation between them. Hence, the next step (to that of unit quantities) forward is to use "specific quantities". Let us imagine a turbine identical in shape in all geometric proportions to the one to be compared and of such dimensions that it will develop one H.P. power under one meter of head. This imaginary turbine is called 'specific turbine' and its speed as specific speed. All the quantities associated with it are referred with a suffix 's', blade angles and the gate opening remaining the same.

Specific Speed : The specific speed N_s of any turbine is the speed in revolutions per minute of a turbine geometrically similar to the actual turbine, but of such a size that under corresponding conditions it will develop 1 h.p. under unit head.

It will be seen that the turbines exactly of same type, whatever their sizes, have same specific speed. To obtain a specific turbine, first assume the given turbine to be working under unit head and calculate velocities U_{wu}, U_{fu}, u_u, Q_u, N_u and P_u etc., (i.e. unit quantities); keeping it in mind that the turbine has same dimensions and geometric proportions. As a second step,

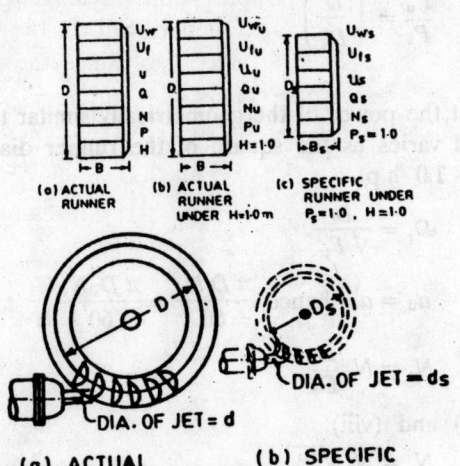

(a) ACTUAL RUNNER   (b) ACTUAL RUNNER UNDER H=1·0 m   (c) SPECIFIC RUNNER UNDER P_s=1·0 , H=1·0

DIA. OF JET = d

DIA. OF JET = ds

(a) ACTUAL   (b) SPECIFIC

FIG. 15.18 ACTUAL AND SPECIFIC RUNNER (A) ACTUAL TURBINE (B) ACTUAL TURBINE UNDER UNIT QUANTITIES (C) SPECIFIC TURBINE OF A REACTION TURBINE AND A PELTON WHEEL.

now reduce the dimensions of the turbine keeping all the geometric proportions the same (i.e. obtain a homologous turbine) such that it produces a unit power (i.e. 1 h.p.). Such a turbine runner is known as specific turbine. This turbine will discharge $Q = k \pi D B U_{fu} \alpha K D^2$, since B = n D and head still remaining 1 m (i.e. $H_u = H_s = 1$ m). This will correspondingly give U_{ws}, U_{fs}, u_s, N_s and P_s (1 h.p.) and its diameter will be D_s. Since the velocities and discharge are dependent upon head only which is 1 m in each case, therefore, $U_{ws} = U_{wu}, U_{fs} = U_{fu}$ etc.

The discharges through actual turbine under unit head Q_u and through specific turbine Q_s are given by

$$Q_u = \pi D B U_{fu} = \pi n D^2 U_{fu} \qquad \text{(i)}$$
$$Q_s = \pi D_s B_s U_{fs} = \pi n D_s U_{fs} \qquad \text{(ii)}$$

From Eqs. (i) and (ii)

$$\frac{Q_u}{Q_s} = \frac{\pi n D^2 U_{fu}}{\pi u D_s^2 U_{fs}} = \left(\frac{D}{D_s}\right)^2 \; ; \; \text{since } U_{fu} = U_{fs} \qquad \text{(iii)}$$

The powers developed by actual turbine and specific turbine are

$$P_u = w \, Q_u \, H_u \, \eta_0 / 75 \qquad \text{(iv)}$$

and
$$P_s = w \, Q_s \, H_s \, \eta_0 / 75 \qquad \text{(v)}$$

From Eqs. (iv) and (v)

$$\frac{P_u}{P_s} = \frac{w \, Q_u \, H_u \, \eta_0}{w \, Q_s \, H_s \, \eta_0} = \frac{Q_u}{Q_s} \; ; \; \text{since } H_u = H_s = 1.0 \text{ m} \qquad \text{(vi)}$$

From Eqs. (iii) and (vi),

$$\frac{P_u}{P_s} = \left(\frac{D}{D_s}\right)^2 \qquad (15.64)$$

This shows that the power of the geometrically similar turbines working under the same head varies as the square of the runner diameters. But for specific turbine, $P_s = 1.0$ h.p.

$$\therefore \qquad D_s = \frac{D}{\sqrt{P_u}} \qquad \text{(vii)}$$

Also $\qquad u_u = u_s$, hence $\dfrac{\pi D N_u}{60} = \dfrac{\pi D_s N_s}{60}$

Therefore, $\qquad N_s = N_u \dfrac{D}{D_s} \qquad \text{(viii)}$

From Eq. (vii) and (viii)

$$N_s = N_u \sqrt{P_u}$$
$$= \frac{N}{\sqrt{H}} \cdot \sqrt{\frac{P}{H^{3/2}}} \; ; \; N_s = \frac{N \sqrt{P}}{H^{5/4}} \qquad \text{...(15.65)}$$

This value of N_s which is the speed of specific runner is termed as 'specific speed'.

Similar to a Francis turbine, for a Pelton wheel the diameter of nozzle $d \propto$ diameter of wheel D. Therefore,

$$\frac{P_u}{P_s} = \frac{\pi/4\, d^2\, U_{fu}}{\pi/4\, d_s^2\, U_{fs}} = \frac{D^2}{D_s^2}$$

which is the same equation as Eq. 15.64 above.

(1) The significant aspect of the formula Eq. 15.65 is that it is independent of the size or dimensions of both, the actual turbine and specific turbine. That is to say, all the turbine of the same geometrical shape working under the same values of Φ and ψ and therefore, having the same efficiency, will have the 'same specific speed.'

(2) The specific speed refers to the performance of the turbine at the value of Φ giving maximum efficiency at normal full gate opening.

(3) Specific speed although is expressed in revolutions per minute is not a pure number but depends on the system of units used. Thus,

N_s (metric units) $= 4.44\, N_s$ (FPS units)

D_s (FPS units) $= 8.05\, D_s$ (metric units).

(4) The concept of specific speed is of utmost utility; the mere knowledge of numerical value of N_s for a given runner conveys quite a definite notion of the shape or proportions and type of the runner and its working performance to be predicted as explained henceafter.

15.23.1 Specific Speed of Pelton Wheel

Let us assume that the maximum efficiency of the single jet Pelton wheel is 85%. Further, assume $k_v = 0.98$ and $k_u = 0.46$. Therefore, the expressions for discharge and power are

$$Q = \frac{\pi}{4}\, d^2\, U = \frac{\pi}{4}\, d^2\, k_v\, \sqrt{2gH} \quad \text{m}^3/\text{s}$$

$$P = \frac{wQH}{75}\, \eta_0\, H.P. = \left(w\eta_0 \frac{\pi}{4}\, d^2\, k_v\, \sqrt{2g} \right) H^{3/2} \quad (15.66)$$

Then, $$u = \frac{\pi D N}{60} = 0.46 \sqrt{2gH}$$

or $$N = \frac{0.46 \times 60 \sqrt{2g}}{\pi D} \sqrt{H} \quad \text{r.p.m.} \quad (15.67)$$

Substituting these values in Eq. 15.65,

$$N_s = \frac{N\sqrt{P}}{H^{5/4}}$$

$$= \left(\frac{0.46 \times 60 \sqrt{2g} \sqrt{H}}{\pi D} \right) \frac{\left\{ 9810 \times \frac{\pi}{4}\, d^2\, k_v\, \sqrt{2g}\, \eta_0\, H^{3/2} \right\}^{1/2}}{H^{5/4}}$$

$$= \frac{242.1}{m} \qquad (15.68)$$

where $m = \dfrac{D}{d}$, Usually the value of D/d equal to 12 is used in the design of Pelton wheel. Only in the extreme case, its lowest value of 7 may be used. Thus N_s for single jet Pelton wheel ranges from 20 to 35, i.e. in a very narrow range.

Multiple jet Pelton Wheel : For a multiple jet Pelton wheel having n number of jets, so long as D, d, N and H remain constant, $Q_1 = n\, Q$ and $P_1 \alpha\, Q_1$; hence $P_1 = n\, P$. Since $N_s \alpha \sqrt{P}$, therefore, the value of N_s for multi jet Pelton wheel will be increased by $\sqrt{n}$ times. Thus, for a Pelton wheel with 4 jets and D/d = 12,

$$N_{s1} = N_s \sqrt{n} = \frac{242.1}{m} \sqrt{n} \qquad \qquad ...(15.69)$$

$$= 40.4 \text{ r.p.m.}$$

15.23.2 Specific Speed of Francis Turbine

The specific speed of Francis turbine can vary within wider range than that of Pelton wheel because it now depends on (i) the speed ratio Φ which itself depends on the inlet blade angle α, (ii) the flow ratio ψ and (iii) the breadth ratio B/D.

Let us again assume a constant value of Φ, ψ, n and η_0

Then, $$u = \Phi \sqrt{2gH} = \frac{\pi D N}{60} \; ; \; N = C_1 \Phi \sqrt{H}/D$$

$$Q = \pi B D U_f = \pi n D^2 \psi \sqrt{2g} \sqrt{H}$$

$$P = \frac{w Q H}{75} \eta_0 = \frac{w \pi n D^2 \psi \sqrt{2g}\; H^{3/2}}{75} \eta_0$$

$$= C_2 n D^2 \psi H^{3/2}$$

Substituting these values in Eq. 15.65

$$N_s = \frac{N \sqrt{P}}{H^{5/4}}$$

$$N_s = \frac{C_1 \Phi \sqrt{H}}{D} \times \frac{\sqrt{C_2 n D^2 H^{3/2} \psi}}{H^{5/4}}$$

$$= C \varphi \sqrt{n \psi} \qquad (15.70)$$

This shows that N_s of a Francis turbine depends upon Φ, ψ and n. Any alternation in any or all of these will alter the specific speed and hence a wide range of specific speed. For suitable performance of a Francis turbine, Φ ranges between 0.6 to 0.9, ψ ranges between 0.15 to 0.30 and the value of n varies from 0.15 to 0.30. Corresponding to these values of Φ, ψ and n, the specific speed varies between 60 to 300.

For developing same power P under same head, H, it is evident from Eq. 15.70 that a runner with smaller N_s runs slow (N is less), has a bigger specific runner diameter (D_s is large) and runs under high head (H is high) Similarly, a runner with higher N_s runs fast (N is comparatively more) has a smaller specific runner (D_s and so D is small and compact) and runs under low head. Thus a runner with $N_s = 300$ is quite fast works under medium head and of medium size (diameter of runner, etc.) as compared to a runner having $N_s = 20$, which will run slow, will work under high head and will be of bigger runner diameter. It is thus, obvious that first one is a reaction turbine

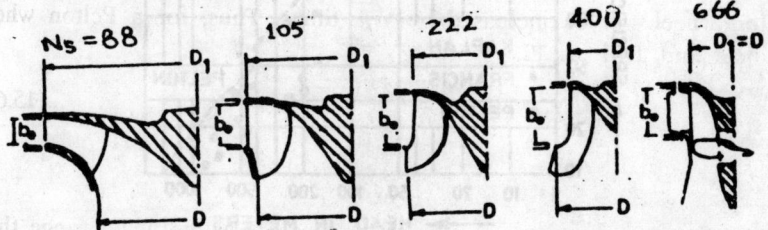

FIG. 15.19 VARIATION OF THE SHAPE OF THE RUNNER
WITH SPECIFIC SPEED

(possibly a Francis turbine) and second one is a Pelton wheel. With a change in the value of N_s, the shape of the runner also changes as is seen in Fig. 15.19, to accommodate different values of Φ, ψ and n.

15.23.3 Specific Speed of Propeller/Kaplan Turbine

These turbines have got highest value of N_s ranging from 300 to 1000 and are of great discharging capacities. The smaller the number of runner blades, the larger the discharging capacity. They work under low head and develop maximum power for each unit head of water. The expression for N_s can be determined as has been done for Francis turbine.

$$Q = \frac{\pi}{4} (D^2 - D_1^2) \, U_f = \frac{\pi}{4} (D^2 - D_1^2) \, \psi \, \sqrt{2gH}$$

where D and D_1 are the diameters of runner and the boss,

$$u = \frac{\pi D N}{60} = \Phi \sqrt{2gH}$$

$$\therefore \qquad N = \frac{60 \, \Phi \sqrt{2g} \sqrt{H}}{\pi D}$$

$$P = \frac{w Q N}{75} \eta_0 = \frac{w \eta_0}{75} \, \frac{\pi}{4} (D^2 - D_1^2) \, \psi \, \sqrt{2g} \, H^{3/2}$$

Substituting the values of N and P in Eq. 15.65,

$$N_s = \frac{60 \, \Phi \sqrt{2g} \sqrt{H}}{\pi D H^{5/4}} \left[\frac{w}{75} \eta_0 \frac{\pi}{4} (D^2 - D_1^2) \, \psi \, \sqrt{2g} \, H^{3/2} \right]^{1/2}$$

$$= 576.1 \, \Phi \sqrt{\eta_0 \psi \, (1 - D_1^2/D^2)} \qquad (15.71a)$$

For a Kaplan turbine, assuming $\eta_0 = 0.90$, $D_1/D = 0.35$ and $\psi = 0.70$.

$$N_s = 428.3 \, \Phi \qquad (15.71b)$$

Fig. 15.20 shows the range of specific speed for various types of turbines as well as the range of their working head, which has been obtained from the actual tests on the turbines of different designs.

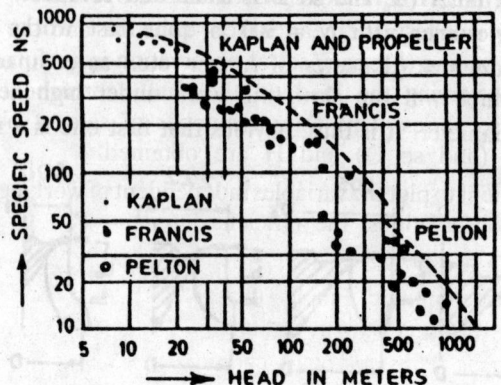

FIG. 15.20 RELATION BETWEEN HEAD AND SPECIFIC SPEED.

15.24 PERFORMANCE CHARACTERISTICS CURVES

The turbines are usually designed to work under a particular set of conditions (viz. at design point) of power, speed, discharge and head. But in practice ,they may be required to work under conditions different than those for which they have been designed. Exact behaviour of turbines under varies conditions of running producing power different than designed one, taking discharge Q ($Q \neq Q$ design) should be predetermined. This can be done either by means of field tests on actual machines or by model tests on small scale turbines of the actual one. (Refer to section 15.20). The results of these tests may be graphically plotted and these are known as 'characteristic curves' of that turbine. Such curves exhibit the behaviour of the turbine under all possible conditions of running and provide very useful informations to the designers and field engineers.

Turbines are usually tested under the following conditions and therefore, three types of characteristic curves are obtained.

(i) *Constant head characteristic curves* In this test the head and gate setting are maintained constant while the speed may be allowed to vary by adjusting the load on the shaft. Such conditions of running are of theoretical interest only and are not found outside the research laboratories.

(ii) *Constant speed characteristic curved* In this case the speed as well as head remain steady and the output power P is varied by the movement of turbine gate. These are normal conditions of working of a turbine; since usually a turbine is expected to work under constant head and is required to run at normal speed (equal to N_{syn} speed of the generator coupled with it). Therefore, such informations are of greatest use to a field engineer.

(iii) *Constant efficiency or Muschel curves* The primary purpose of plotting such curves is to find out a region of constant efficiency so that the turbine can be operated at maximum efficiency for the given load, head and discharge. It also helps in the selection of design conditions as explained henceafter.

15.25 CONSANT HEAD CHARACTERISTIC CURVES

For this type of test, the head is kept constant and the turbine is tested at different gate opening (i.e. each set of observation is performed at a different gate opening) by varying the load on the shaft; correspondingly the speed of the turbine also varies. This way, a number of sets of observations of P, N, gate opening (and so Q) and H are obtained.

It is convenient to plot the variables independent of working head. Therefore, from the above observations, the efficiency η_0 ($= P/w\, Q\, H$ in S.I. units), unit discharge Q_u ($= Q/\sqrt{H}$), unit power P_u ($= P/H^{3/2}$) and unit speed N_u ($= N/\sqrt{H}$) are computed. Finally, Q_u vs N_u, P_u vs N_u and η_0 vs N_u curves corresponding to different gate openings are plotted as shown in Fig. 15.21. These are known as 'constant head characteristic curves'. The major points of interest and importance for different types of turbines are discussed below:

15.25.1 Pelton Wheel

Fig. 15.21 shows constant head characteristic curves for Pelton wheel for gate opening 0.2, 0.5, 0.8 and 1.0 (curves 4, 3, 2 and 1).

(1) Since it is a purely axial flow turbine, no centrifugal force acts on the wheel and the discharge curves (Q_u vs N_u curves) are horizontal lines.

$$Q = area \times velocity$$

$$= \frac{\pi}{4} d^2 k_v \sqrt{2gH}$$

or

$$\frac{Q}{\sqrt{H}} = Q_u = \frac{\pi}{4} d^2 k_v \sqrt{2g} = c \times gate\ opening$$

Thus, for a fixed gate opening the unit discharge remains unaltered whatever may be the speed of the turbine.

(2) A glance on the efficiency curves reveal that these are parabola of nearly same shape for all gate settings. It is seen that peak efficiency has nearly the same magnitude and occurs at the same speed for all gate setting, curves 1, 2, 3 and 4. This speed corresponds to speed ratio k_u equal to 0.45 (since $u = k_u \sqrt{2gH} = \pi DN/60$ which means $k_u = (\pi D/60 \sqrt{2g})(N_u)$; or $k_u \alpha N_u$.

(3) The reason why the efficiency falls off at any other value of k_u is that the water leaves the bucket with an undue amount of unexpanded kinetic energy $U_1^2/2g$ which is wasted to the tailrace.

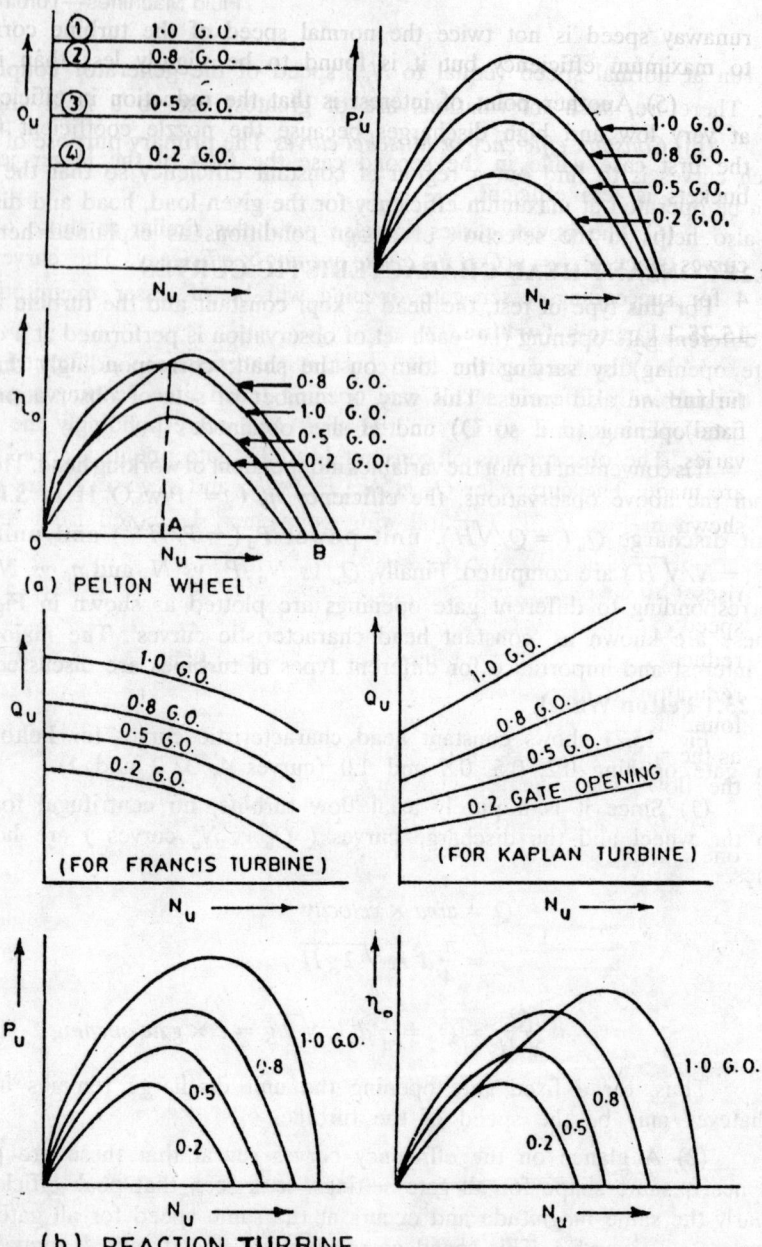

(a) PELTON WHEEL

(b) REACTION TURBINE

FIG. 15.21 CONSTANT HEAD CHARACTERISTIC CURVES (A) PELTON WHEEL TURBINE (B) FRANCIS AND KAPLAN TURBINE

(4) Under ideal conditions these efficiency curves should be true parabolas and runaway speed should be twice the normal speed (OB = 2 (OA)). But due to increased windage and friction losses at high speed the maximum or

runaway speed is not twice the normal speed of the turbine corresponding to maximum efficiency but it is found to be slightly less than it.

(5) Another point of interest is that the reduction in efficiency occurs at very low and high discharges because the nozzle coefficient falls off in the first case while in the second case the flow of the larger jet over the buckets is less efficient.

(6) The power curves are also parabolas similar to those of efficiency curves since P ($= w Q H \eta_0$) α *gate opening* $\times$ *efficiency*. The curves 2, 3 and 4 for succeeding lesser gate opening will be of lesser magnitude.

15.25.2 Francis Turbine

As discussed earlier, the constant head tests are performed on Francis turbine with different set of gate opening (each time keeping a gate opening fixed). The load is varied on the shaft and correspondingly the speed also varies. The observations of constant head H, gate opening, speed and power are made. The curves for Q_u vs N_u, P_u vs N_u and η_0 verses N_u are plotted and shown in Fig. 15.21. The following points may be noted from these curves.

(1) It is seen that discharge curves are falling curves, i.e. as the speed rises (Φ increases, the discharge diminishes). It is found that a rise in the speed N (or N_u) is accompanied by a rise in the runner speed u and a reduction in the value of U_f (refer velocity triangle Fig. 15.22) and so the reduction in discharge. The reduction in the discharge is more prominently found for radial flow type or mixed flow type turbine. The reason is that as the speed increases, the centrifugal head impressed on the flow and opposing the flow also increases and thus reduction in discharge.

(2) The power and efficiency curves are more or less parabolas; each one starting from zero, attaining a peak value and thereafter falling quickly.

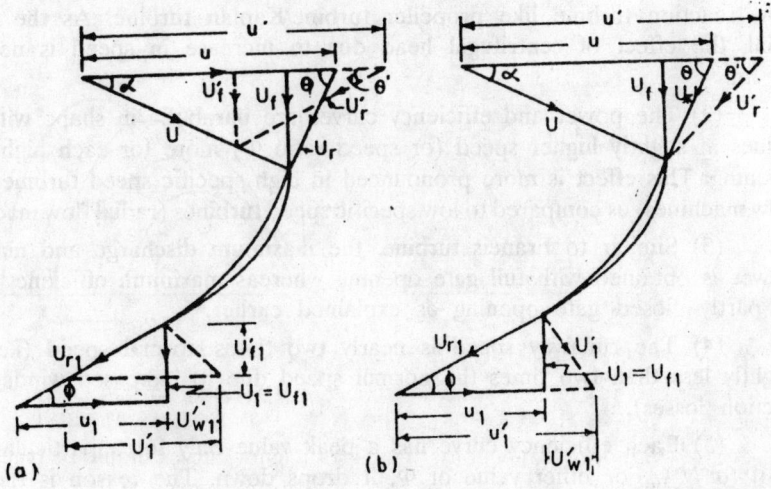

FIG. 15.22 EFFECT OF CHANGES IN SPEED ON VELOCITY TRIANGLES.

(3) The runaway speed is only about 50% more than the normal speed at the given gate opening. It is an obvious advantage of the inward flow turbine over an outward flow turbine in which case the runaway speed is 250% of the normal speed at peak efficiency.

(4) The peak efficiency (as well as peak power) for different gate openings do not occur at the same speed but it occurs at a slightly higher speed with each increase in gate opening.

(5) The maximum discharge and maximum power are obtained with wide open gate opening whereas maximum efficiency is obtained for a slightly closed gate opening. This is being done to provide an over load on the turbine but at a lesser efficient (say, at 0.9 gate opening). At full gate opening, the turbine develops greater power but with lesser efficiency.

(6) Each efficiency curve has a peak value for a particular value of unit speed N_u (and so also Φ) and for all other values of Φ, the efficiency falls off. This can be explained with the help of velocity triangles at inlet and at outlet. A turbine runner is designed for particular speed and corresponding velocity diagrams Fig. 15.22. But when the speed of the runner rises (for example) then centrifugal head impressed on the flow, which opposes the flow, also increases. This diminishes the discharge and thereby U_f reduces to U_f'. But rim velocity u has increased to u'. These changed velocities cause a modified velocity triangle at inlet (shown by dotted lines). Thus, water enters the runner with shock and eddying loss takes place at entry. Similarly, the outlet velocity triangle (shown by dotted lines) has also got changed, causing increased losses at exit. The combined effect of these losses is reduced efficiency.

15.25.3 Kaplan Turbine

(1) Fig. 15.21 shows the constant head characteristic curves for axial flow reaction turbine like propeller turbine/Kaplan turbine. As the flow is axial, the effect of centrifugal head due to increase in speed is negligible or nil.

(2) The power and efficiency curves are parabolic in shape with peak values at slightly higher speed (or speed ratio Φ) more for each higher gate opening. This effect is more pronounced in high specific speed turbines (axial flow machines) as compared to low specific speed turbines (radial flow machines).

(3) Similar to Francis turbine, the maximum discharge and maximum power is obtained with full gate opening whereas maximum efficiency occurs at partly closed gate opening as explained earlier.

(4) The runaway speed is nearly two times normal speed (i.e., it is slightly less than two times the normal speed due to increased windage and friction losses).

(5) Each efficiency curve has a peak value only for a particular value of Φ (or N_u). For other value of Φ, it drops down. The reason is the same as explained in case of Francis turbine (changed velocity triangles at changed speed). But in this case U_f does not change (see Fig. 15.22b).

15.25.4 Varying Head Characteristic Curves

Low head turbines are often required to work under conditions of constant speed and varying head. (The head may vary within a limit of 50% of the design head). Performance of a Francis turbine under these circumstances

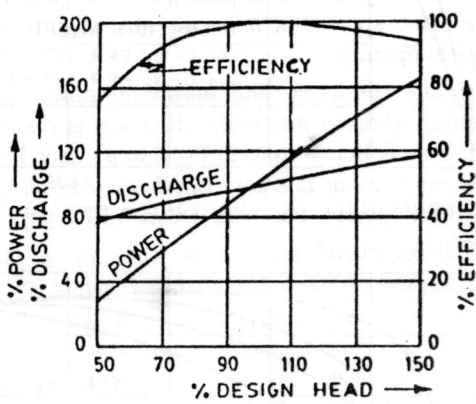

FIG. 15.23 PERFORMANCE CURVE UNDER VARYING HEAD.

at full gate opening is determined and plotted as shown in Fig. 15.23. It may be noticed from this figure that so long as the head does not vary more than 20% above or below the design value, the overall efficiency is not seriously impaired.

15.26 CONSTANT SPEED CHARACTERISTIC CURVES

Most turbines are required to run at constant speed so that the electrical generators to which they are coupled provide a fixed frequency and voltage. These characteristics, therefore, are of more practical use and are also known as operating characteristic curves.

In this case, the head and speed both, are kept constant and the load on the turbine shaft is allowed to vary which is adjusted by the change in gate opening (i.e. the quantity of water entering the turbine). After having a number of observations of P, Q, H and N (H and N are maintained constant), the load (i.e. torque) and efficiency of the turbine are calculated. Generally a graph is then plotted between fraction of full load (i.e. ratio of the load on the turbine to the design load) as abscissa and efficiency as ordinate. This curve is known as constant speed characteristic curve. Fig. 15.24

$$\text{Torque or load} = \frac{\text{Output power}}{\omega} = \frac{P \text{ watts}}{2\pi N/60}$$

and

$$\eta_0 = \frac{\text{Output power}}{\text{Input power}} = \frac{P \text{ watts}}{w Q H}$$

15.26.1 Pelton Wheel

(1) Fig. 15.24 (a) shows two curves for two different type of Pelton wheel, one for D/d = m = 12 and another for m = 7. Both the curves,

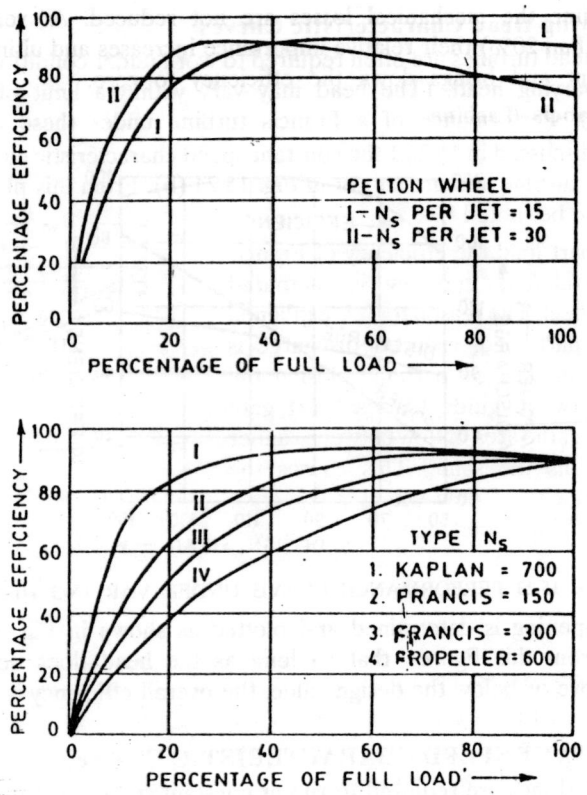

FIG. 15.24 CONSTANT SPEED CHARACTERISTIC CURVES
(a) PELTON WHEEL (b) FOR DIFFERENT TYPES OF TURBINES

in general, show a satisfactory performance at part load (a desirable aspect of Pelton wheel). But curve I for D/d = 12 is better as it gives nearly 80% efficiency even at 20% part load.

(2) Curve I shows an abrupt rise in efficiency from zero upto 20% of part load, then very gradual and continuous rise and finally approaches nearly 100% limit of efficiency. Curve II (for D/d = 7) shots up from 0 to 20% of load and at about 30% load, it attains the maximum efficiency (η_0 = 90%). Further rise in the load causes the curve to drop gradually and finally reaching a point of 78% of efficiency at 100% load. The reason for lower efficiency at higher discharge (and so higher power) for curve II is that the full nozzle opening provides a too big jet for the buckets and therefore full discharge may not be intercepted by the buckets. At part load the nozzle opening is so adjusted that the diameter of jet probably approaches to D/d = 12 and results in greater efficiency.

(3) Between 0% and 20% load a low efficiency (overall) is obtained. At this part load, of course, the output of wheel is reduced and so correspondingly the hydraulic losses are also reduced in much the same proportion. But in

the meantime the mechanical losses are not reduced. At very low outputs (load less than 20%) their relative importance increases and ultimately becomes predominant and brings down the efficiency to zero.

15.26.2 Francis Turbine

As discussed in 15.26.1 the constant speed characteristic curves are plotted for Francis turbine and are shown in Fig. 15.24 (b). From this plot the following points may be noted :

At part load the efficiency of Francis turbine is relatively too low as compared to Pelton wheel. The reason for it is explained below. At part load, reduced discharge is fed to the turbine by partially closing the passage between guide blades (part gate opening). But the area of flow between runner vanes remains the same. This causes the reduced velocity of flow which when combined with rim speed causes a distorted velocity triangles at inlet. This causes the shock losses at entry. Similarly the velocity triangle at the exit is distorted. Moreover, the velocity of whirl at the outlet U_{w1} also reappear (Fig. 15.25). Both these reasons cause lower efficiency at part load. Thus it is seen that the Francis turbine behaves very unsatisfactorily at part load.

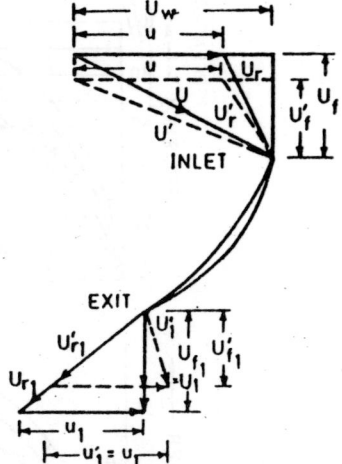

FIG. 15.25 VELOCITY TRIANGLE FOR FRANCIS TURBINE AT PART LOAD.

15.26.3 Kaplan Turbine

The constant speed characteristic curves for Propeller and Kaplan turbines are determined in the same way as discussed, in Sec. 15.26. The characteristics curves are of much the same shape as Francis turbine. Since propeller turbine has got higher specific speed and required larger discharge, its part load efficiency are lower than Francis turbine.

The Kaplan turbine has got adjustable runner blades besides movable guide blades. Therefore, the runner blades rotate and get adjusted at part load, resulting in higher efficiency even at part load. Kaplan turbine, as is seen from Fig. 15.24, gives best part load performance at constant speed.

15.27 CONSTANT EFFICIENCY CURVE (ISO-EFFICIENCY CURVE)

Fig. 15.26 shows the 'constant efficiency curve' (also known as Muschel's curves) which is a plot of unit power against unit speed for different gate opening and containing contour like efficiency curves plotted over it. These curves are not obtained by any separate test but from the constant head characteristic curves. The procedure of obtaining these curves is as follows:

Firstly horizontal lines are drawn at regular interval (say 10%, 20%, etc.) on a η_0 curve obtained from constant head tests. Now place P_u vs N_u curve just below the η_0 versus N_u curve. Project the line of intersections of 10% efficiency curve with 0.2 gate opening (say) on η_0 verses N_u curve to the, P_u verses N_u curve (corresponding to same gate opening), Likewise other points of intersection are transferred to P_u verses N_u curve corresponding to different gate opening. The procedure is repeated with $\eta_0 = 20\%, 30\%$, etc. Thereafter, the contours for different overall efficiency, η_0 (say 10%, 20%, 30%, etc.), are drawn on P_u verses N_u curves, Fig. 15.26. Thus iso-efficiency

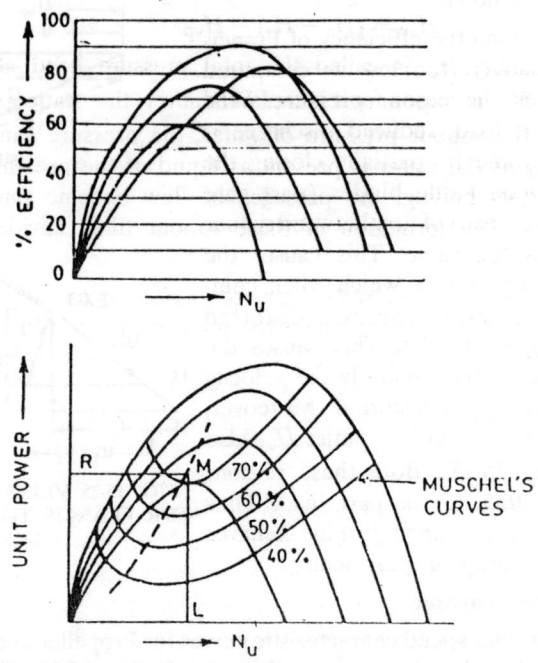

FIG. 15.26 ISO-EFFICIENCY CURVE (MUSCHEL'S CURVES)

curve corresponding to different gate openings are obtained which are applicable for different conditions of running. Join the points of peak values corresponding to different gate openings (shown by dotted lines in Fig. 15.26. This is 'the best efficiency curve'. The practical use of this curve can now be seen.

Let it be required to determine the best condition of running of a turbine which is to develop power P under head H. For this purpose first compute unit power P_u ($= P/H^{3/2}$) and draw a horizontal line RM (Fig. 15.26) to intersect the best efficiency curve at M. From this point M, drop a projection ML on the N_u axis (abscissa) and locate point L. Read the value of N_u (at point L) and so find N ($= N_u \sqrt{H}$). Also read the location of M, i.e., interpolate the gate opening and efficiency η_0 corresponding to point M. Thus for the best performance of the given turbine, it must run at speed N, at gate opening corresponding to point 'M' and at maximum η_0 (say 73% in the Fig. 15.26).

15.28 CAVITATION IN TURBINES

The hydraulic turbines are usually installed above the tailrace with draft tube. As a result the absolute pressure at some specific regions of the turbine is found to be below atmospheric pressure, From Eq. 15.41 it is found that

$$(H_a - H_s) = \left[\frac{p_2}{w} + \frac{(U_2^2 - U_3^2)}{2g} \right]$$

and
$$H_{SV} = (H_a - H_s) - H_{vp} \qquad (15.72)$$

The quantity H_{sv} is called the total pressure head above the vapour pressure and H_{vp} is vapour pressure. Whenever the static pressure at some point reaches the vapour pressure of water, the pressure can not be lowered than it, as long as the water is present as liquid. If the pressure lowers belows it the water stats boiling, the passages of flow become partly occupied by vapour cavities. The formation of these vapour filled cavities in the stream is called 'cavitation'.

The cavitation phenomenon can be explained as follows: Consider the flow through a turbine runner where the total draft (or suction pressure head) is excessive and where there is a failure of the vane contour to conform to the natural flow lines. At such a point (or region) in the runner, usually at the back of vanes near the disharging eye and near the outer periphery where relative velocity is high, the flowing stream parts from the vane surface and leves a void filled with eddies. And when absolute pressure is reduced to vapour pressure this void and cavities become filled with water vapour, air and other gases. As the flow continues downstream the static pressure rises again and then exceeds the vapour pressure. This way, when a particle of fluid reaches a place (where local pressure just attains vapour pressure limit at one instant and pressure rises above vapour pressure at another instant), the vapour will suddenly condense and return to liquid state producing a cavity. The bubbles burst and causes high impact along the surface. That is, there occurs explosion. This action is not limited to cavities so formed but extends into the pores of the metal also. The water rushes in to fill the collapsed cavities as well as vapour filled pores until stopped instantaneously by the bottom surface of the pores and water hammer action takes place here. This produces high intensity pressure; of the same order as the tensile strength of the metal. And under continual repetition of shock, the metal fails locally under fatigue and small particles are irregularly broken away, giving the surface a peculiar spongy appearance. This action is called 'cavitation or pitting'.

The resulting cavitation in the turbines, not only impairs the turbine performance, but it may damage the turbine itself. There may be several rattling, noise and vibration of machines and surrounding structures. The region of blade most susceptible of cavitation is near the discharging edge (on its back), which may become roughened, pitted and eventually destroyed. Of course, Pelton wheel are not that immune from cavitation, but the nozzles, needles and buckets are all liable to cavitation attack.

The incipient condition of cavitation is given by the use of Thoms's cavitation factor σ_c. It is defined as the ratio of H_{sv} (total pressure above the vapour pressure) and the net head absorbed by a turbine.

$$\therefore \qquad \sigma = \frac{H_{sv}}{H} = \frac{H_{atom} - H_s - H_{vp}}{H} \qquad (15.73)$$

where H_s is the suction head, i.e. the height of the turbine setting above the tailrace, H_{vp} is the vapour pressure head and H is the net head.

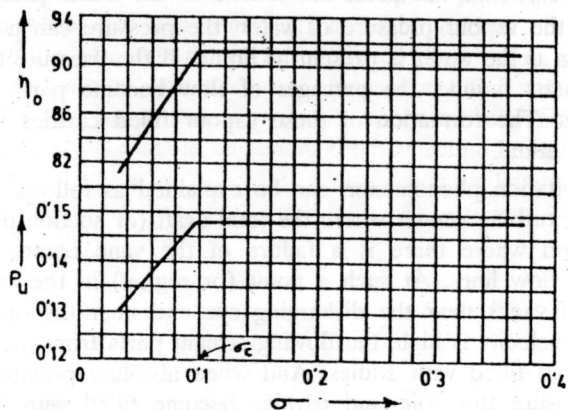

FIG. 15.27 PLOT BETWEEN σ AND η_0 AND P.

The turbine, in general, will be immune from cavitation if the value of σ becomes lower then the minimum value of σ ($= \sigma_c$). The minimum safe value of σ_c is known as critical value of Thoma's cavitation factor, There are several criteria to determine σ_c. One of the commonly used criteria establishes the σ_c as that value of σ at which there is drop in efficiency by 1% (arbitarily chosen value). But the reliable basis for determining σ_c and finding out the allowable value of H_s for the actual setting of turbine is obtained by conducting the cavitation tests on a homologous model under steady conditions of speed, gate opening and net head with increasing suction head H_s. If measured η_0 (or P in some cases) is plotted against σ, the point at which the efficiency (or power) begins to decline and is quite sharp, this point of break or inflextion is often known as sigma break.

The critical value of σ_c has been found to be related with specific speed for different turbines.

Francis turbine : $\sigma_c = 0.0317 \ (N_S/100)^2$ (15.74a)

Propeller turbine : $\sigma_c = 0.340 + .0024 \ (N_S/100)^{2.73}$ (15.74b)

Kablan turbine $\sigma_c = 1.1$ times for propeller turbine   (15.74c)

Remedial Measures :

(1) The surest way of preventing cavitation is to set the turbine sufficiently near the tail race level.

(2) If it becomes necessary to set the turbine at a higher suction head then the runner blades may be guarded against the effect of incipient cavitation by selecting special cavititation resistant metal, for example stainless steel, nickel steel and bronze.

(3) Alternatively stainless steel armoring may be welded on to the areas most likely to be attacked by cavitation.

15.29 SUCTION SPECIFIC SPEED

It is apparent that the magnitude of σ depends on the magnitude of H_{sv}, which is turn depends on the proportions and speed of the runner. In many instances a change in runner diameter or in vane angle does not affect the flow near the suction edges of the vanes and also does not influence actual cavitation behavior. From the principle of similarty a non-dimensional parameter may be found to account for cavitation in the turbines, This is known as suction specific speed (S). In parallel to the specific speed, the suction specific speed indicates the combination of suction operating conditions that will give similar flow and a similar degree of cavitation in machines which are geometrically similar in the suction passage- ways and in the low pressure portion of the runner. If cavitation is not present in the machine, the relationship between its performance variables will be independent of S.

It is defined as the speed of a geometrically similar turbine such that when it is developing 1 h.p., the total head H_{sv} is equal to 1 m (absolute units).

It is given by

$$S = \frac{N\sqrt{P}}{(H_{sv})^{5/4}} \qquad (15.75a)$$

But $\qquad H_{sv} = \sigma H,$

$$\therefore \qquad S = N\sqrt{P}/(\sigma H)^{5/4} \qquad (15.75b)$$

or $\qquad \sigma = \left(\frac{N_s}{S}\right)^{4/5} \qquad (15.75c)$

15.30 SELECTION OF TYPE OF TURBINE RUNNER

In a hydropower installation the engineer has to give a serious consideration to the choice or selection of the type of turbine runner so as to result economy and yield good performance under all expected conditions. The following are certain guiding factors:

(1) Head (H): under which the turbine is required to run is the first guide for a selection. Curves for different types of turbine runners between head and specific speed are given in Fig. 15.20. It is based on the data available regarding actual turbine installations working satisfactorily. From this diagram, by following the horizontal line corresponding to the given head, the type and specific speed of runner to be used can be read.

For example, for a head exceeding 1000 m, a single jet Pelton wheel is the only choise while for a head of 135 m or so either of Pelton or

Francis turbine can be used. Intersection of 135 m line also gives N_s of these turbines already in use under this head. Again should the head be 300 m, any one type of turbine out of Pelton wheel and Francis turbine may be adopted.

This indicates the flexibility of the head as a guide for final selection. So other factors should be given consideration before arriving at a final selection.

(2) Nature of the Load is the another very important guide in regard to final choice of the turbine runner. A efficiency-output curve's study (under constant design speed) for different turbines can be made. A Pelton wheel (N_s = 20) has fairly high and constant part load and overload efficiencies and so has a low specific speed Francies turbine (N_s = 100).

As the specific speed of Francis turbine becomes higher, its part load and overload efficiency declines while a Propeller turbine (N_s = 600) can be seen to have a very low efficiencies at part load and overloads. However, they possess high efficiency at rated loads. Kaplan turbine has highest efficiency at part, full or over load. Thus, Kaplan turbine is best choice to work at part load, then comes in succession Pelton wheel and finally Francis turbine is (see Fig. 15.24).

(3) Cost of turbine : Kaplan is the costliest and Francis turbine is the cheapest. If the turbines are required to operate for long times at part load or overload and a choice lies between 2 or more types of runners, the proceeding curves give a fair guidance-as a Pelton wheel should be preferred to a Francis turbine of low speed, a low N_s Francis turbine to a high N_s Francis turbine, a high N_s Francis turbine to a Propeller turbine and the Kaplan turbine is best choice to all. Thus cost should also be kept in view. If the turbines have to work nearly all the time at full loads then cost should be sole guiding factor.

(4) Highest possible specific speed of the turbine is a guide rule in the choice of runner type.

Examples 15.1-15.28

15.1 A Pelton wheel develops 4500 kW under a net head of 125 m while running at a speed of 200 r.p.m. Assuming k_v = 0.98, speed ratio k_u = 0.46, overall efficiency η_o = 88% and the ratio of nozzle diameter to pitch circle diameter, d/D = 1/9, determine (a) the discharge required, (b) the diameter of the wheel, (e) the diameter and number of jets required.

Solution

(a)
$$P = w\,Q\,H \text{ watts}$$

$$4500 \times 1000 = 9810 \times Q \times 125$$

$$Q = \frac{4500 \times 10^3}{9810 \times 125} = 3.67 \text{ m}^3\!/\text{s}$$

(b)
$$U = k_v \sqrt{2gH}$$

$$= 0.98 \sqrt{2 \times 9.81 \times 125} = 48.5 \text{ m/s}$$

Also
$$u = k_u \sqrt{2gH}$$
$$= 0.46 \sqrt{2 \times 9.81 \times 125} = 22.3 \text{ m/s}$$

The peripheral velocity u is also given by
$$u = \frac{\pi D N}{60} = 22.3$$
$$D = \frac{22.3 \times 60}{\pi \times 200} = 2.13 \text{ m}$$

(c) Since
$$d/D = \frac{1}{9}; d = \frac{2.13}{9} = 0.24 \text{ m}$$

Number of jets required
$$= \frac{Q}{\text{flow per jet}}$$
$$n = \frac{3.67}{\pi/4 \times (0.24)^2 \times 48.5} \approx 1.67$$
$$n \approx 2.0$$

15.2 A Pelton wheel driven by two similar jets transmits 3750 kW to the shaft when running at 375 rpm. The head from the reservoir level to the nozzle is 200 m and efficiency of power transmission through the pipelines and nozzles is 90%. The jets are tangential to a 1.45 m diameter circle. The relative velocity decreases by 10% as the water traverses the buckets which are so shaped that they would, if stationary, deflect the jet through 165°. Neglecting the windage losses, find (a) the efficiency of the wheel and (b) diameter of each jet.

Solution

(a) Since the efficiency of power transmission is 90%, the head at the base of the nozzle is
$$H = 0.9 \times 200 = 180 \text{ m.}$$

The jet velocity $U = \sqrt{2gH} = \sqrt{2 \times 9.81 \times 180}$
$$U = 59.5 \text{ m/s.}$$

The peripheral speed of the wheel is
$$u = \frac{\pi D N}{60}$$
$$= \frac{\pi \times 1.45 \times 375}{60} = 28.5 \text{ m/s}$$

The efficiency of Pelton wheel η_H is given Eq. 15.27.
$$\eta_H = \frac{u(U-u)(1 + k \cos \Phi)}{gH} = \frac{2u(U-u)(1 + k \cos \Phi)}{U^2}$$

Here
$$k = 0.9 \; ; \cos \Phi = \cos (\pi - 165°) = \cos 15°$$
$$\eta_H = \frac{2 \times 28.5 (59.5 - 28.5)(1 + 0.9 \times \cos 15°)}{(59.5)^2}$$
$$= 0.933 \text{ or } 93.3\%$$

(b) Since the efficiency of the runner is 93.3%, the total power to be developed by the jet

$$P_1 = \frac{3750}{0.933} = 4019.3 \text{ kW}$$

Thus, power per jet $P = \dfrac{4019.3}{2} = 2009.65$ kW

Hence, $2009.65 \times 10^3 = (w \, a \, U) \dfrac{U^2}{2g}$

$$= 9810 \left(\frac{\pi}{4} \times d^2 \right) \frac{U^3}{2 \times 9.81}$$

Solving, $d = \sqrt{\dfrac{2009.65 \times 19.62 \times 4 \times 1000}{9810 \times \pi \times (59.5)^3}}$

$$= 0.155 \text{ m.}$$

15.3 A Pelton wheel develops 1700 kW under a head of 500 m. The mean pitch circle diameter is 0.9 m and coefficient of velocity for the nozzle is 0.98. The buckets defect the jet by 170° and the relative velocity is reduced by 12% due to bucket friction. Take speed ratio $k_u = 0.47$ and actual efficiency of the wheel as 0.9 times the theoretical efficiency. Calculate (a) the hydraulic efficiency of the wheel (b) speed of the wheel and (c) the diameter of the nozzle.

Solution

(a) From Eq. 15.27

$$\eta_H = \frac{[u \, (U - u) \, (1 + k \cos \Phi)]/g}{(U^2/2g)}$$

$$\eta_H = \frac{2u \, (U - u) \, (1 + k \cos \Phi)}{U^2}$$

Here $u = k_u \sqrt{2gH} = 0.46 \sqrt{2 \times 9.81 \times 500} = 46.55$ m/s

$U = k_v \sqrt{2gH} = 0.98 \sqrt{2 \times 9.81 \times 500} = 97.06$ m/s

$k = 0.88 \, ; \Phi = (180° - 170°) = 10°$

$$\eta_H = \frac{2 \times 46.55 \, (97.06 - 46.55) \, (1 + 0.88 \cos 10°)}{(97.06)^2}$$

$$= 0.9318 \text{ or } 93.18\%$$

Since overall efficiency is 0.9 times the theoretical efficiency

$\eta_o = 0.9 \times 0.9318 = 0.8386.$

(b) The peripheral velocity $u = \dfrac{\pi D N}{60}$

$\therefore$ $N = \dfrac{60 \, u}{\pi D}$

$$= \frac{60 \times 46.55}{\pi \times 0.9} = 988.3 \text{ r.p.m.}$$

(c)

$$P = w \, Q \, H \, \eta_o \text{ watts}$$

$$Q = \frac{P}{w \, H \, \eta_0} = \frac{1700 \times 1000}{9810 \times 500 \times 0.8386}$$

$$= 0.4132 \text{ m}^3/\text{s}$$

Also,

$$Q = \left(\frac{\pi}{4} d^2 \right) U$$

∴

$$d = \sqrt{\frac{4 \, Q}{\pi \, U}} = \sqrt{\frac{4 \times 0.4132}{\pi \times 97.06}}$$

$$= 0.0736 \text{ m or } 7.36 \text{ cm.}$$

15.4 The water available for a Pelton wheel is $4 \text{ m}^3/\text{s}$ and the total head from reservoir to the nozzle is 250 m. The turbine has two runners with two jets per runner. All the four jets have the same diameters. The pipeline is 3000 m long. The efficiency of power transmission through the pipeline and nozzle is 91% and efficiency of each runner is 90%. The coefficient of velocity is 0.975 and coefficient of friction for pipe is 0.0045. Determine (a) the power developed by the turbine (b) the diameter of the jet and (c) the diameter of the pipeline.

Solution

Efficiency of power transmission $= \dfrac{H - h_f}{H}$

$$0.91 = \frac{250 - h_f}{250}$$

$$h_f = (250 - 250 \times 0.91) = 22.5 \text{ m}$$

Net head on the turbine $= (250 - 22.5)$

$$= 227.5 \text{ m.}$$

Velocity of jet $\quad U = k_v \sqrt{2 g H}$

$$= 0.975 \sqrt{2 \times 9.81 \times 227.5}$$

$$= 65.14 \text{ m/s}$$

Power available at the inlet to the turbine

$$= \text{ Kinetic energy of the jet}$$

$$= \frac{1}{2} \times \frac{9810}{9.81} \times 4.0 \times (65.14)^2 \text{ watts.}$$

$$= 8486.4 \text{ kW.}$$

But

$$\eta_H = \frac{\text{Power developed by turbine}}{\text{Input power to the turbine}}$$

Power developed by the turbine $= \eta_H \times Input \, power$

$$= 0.9 \times 8486.4$$

$$= 7637.76 \text{ kW.}$$

(b) Discharge per jet $= \dfrac{\text{total discharge}}{\text{number of jets}}$

$$= \dfrac{4.0}{4.0} = 1 \text{ cumec}$$

Also discharge per jet $= \dfrac{\pi}{4} d^2 \times U$

$\therefore$
$$d = \sqrt{\dfrac{4 \times 1}{\pi \times U}}$$

$$= \sqrt{\dfrac{4}{\pi \times 65.14}}$$

$$= 0.1398 \text{ m} \approx 14 \text{ cm}$$

(c) The head loss due to friction h_f is given by Darcy's formula.

$$h_f = \dfrac{f l Q^2}{12.1 D^5}$$

$$D = \left[\dfrac{f L Q^2}{12.1 \, h_f} \right]^{1/5} = \left[\dfrac{0.0045 \times 3000 \times 4^2}{12.1 \times 22.5} \right]^{1/5}$$

$$= 0.954 \text{ m}$$

15.5 The following data pertains to a single jet Pelton Wheel.

Head at the base of the nozzle $= 39.5$ m

Discharge from the nozzle $= 216$ lit/sec

Area of the jet $= 80 \text{ cm}^2$

Power at shaft $= 67.5$ kW

Hydraulic efficiency $= 92\%$

Calculate the power lost in (a) the nozzle (b) the runner (c) mechanical friction and (iv) overall efficiency.

Solution

(a) The discharge supplied by the jet $= a \times U$

$$\dfrac{216}{1000} = \dfrac{80}{(10)^4} \times U$$

$$U = \dfrac{2160}{80} = 27 \text{ m/s}$$

Power available at the base of the nozzle

$$= w Q H \text{ watts}$$

$$= 9810 \times \dfrac{216}{1000} \times 39.5 = 83.7 \text{ kW}$$

Power available at the exit of nozzle $= \dfrac{1}{2} \times \dfrac{w Q U^2}{g}$

$$= \frac{1}{2} \times \frac{9810}{9.81} \times \frac{216}{1000} \times (27)^2$$

$$= 78.73 \text{ kW}$$

Power lost in the nozzle = (Power at the base of nozzle - Power at the exit of nozzle)

$$(h_L)_{nozzle} = (83.7 - 78.73)$$

$$= 4.97 \text{ kW}$$

(b) From Eq. 15.16,

$$\eta_H = \frac{\text{Power developed by the wheel}}{\text{Power available at the exit of nozzle}}$$

$$0.92 = \frac{\text{Power developed by the wheel}}{78.73}$$

Power developed by the wheel $= 0.92 \times 78.73$

$$= 72.43 \text{ kW}$$

Power lost in mechanical friction

$$= \text{(Power developed by the wheel - Power available at shaft)}$$

$$= (72.43 - 67.5) = 4.93 \text{ kW}$$

Power lost in the runner $= (83.7 - 67.5) - (4.97 + 4.93)$

$$= 6.3 \text{ kW}$$

Overall efficiency $\eta_o = \dfrac{P}{w Q H}$

$$\eta_o = \frac{67.5}{78.73} \times 100$$

$$= 85.7\%$$

15.6 In an inward flow reaction turaine, the water enters readily and is also discharged radially. If the velocity of flow remains constant, show that the hydraulic efficiency is expressed by

$$\eta_H = \frac{2}{(2 + \tan^2 \alpha)}$$

where α is guide blade angle.

Solution

For a radial discharge

$$\eta_H = \frac{U_W u}{g H} \qquad \qquad (i)$$

Also, the net head

$$H = \left(\text{head utilised by the runner} + \frac{U_1^2}{2g} + \text{losses} \right)$$

Neglecting losses,

$$\overline{H} = \left(\frac{U_w u}{g} + \frac{U_1^2}{2g} \right)$$

Since the water is discharged radially and velocity of flow remains constant,

$$U_1 = U_{f1}$$

and

$$U_f = U_{f1}$$

$$\therefore \qquad H = \left(\frac{U_w u}{g} + \frac{U_{f1}^2}{2g} \right)$$

$$= \left(\frac{U_w u}{g} + \frac{U_f^2}{2g} \right)$$

From velocity triangle, $U_f = u \tan \alpha$

$$U_w = u$$

$$\therefore \qquad H = \left(\frac{u^2}{g} + \frac{u^2 \tan^2 \alpha}{2g} \right)$$

$$= \frac{u^2}{g} \left(\frac{2 + \tan^2 \alpha}{2} \right)$$

From Eqs. (i) and (ii)

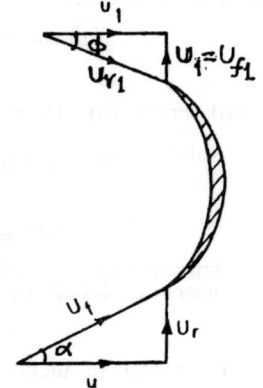

FIG. 15.28 EXAMPLE 15.6

$$\eta_H = \frac{U_w u}{gH}$$

$$\eta_H = \frac{u^2}{gH} \qquad (\because U_w = u)$$

$$\eta_H = \left(\frac{2}{2 + \tan^2 \alpha} \right)$$

15.7 An inward flow reaction turbine discharges radially and the velocity of flow is constant and equal to the velocity of discharge from the turbine. Show that the hydraulic efficiency is given by

$$\eta_H = \cfrac{1}{\left[1 + \cfrac{\frac{1}{2} \tan^2 \alpha}{\left(1 - \cfrac{\tan \alpha}{\tan \theta} \right)} \right]}$$

Solution

From the inlet velocity triangle,

$$U_f = U_w \tan \alpha$$

$$u = \left(U_w - \frac{U_f}{\tan \theta} \right) = \left(U_w - \frac{U_w \tan \alpha}{\tan \theta} \right)$$

$$= U_w \frac{(\tan \theta - \tan \alpha)}{\tan \theta} \qquad \qquad \text{...(i)}$$

For radial discharge at outlet, $U_{w_1} = 0$

Thus
$$-\frac{U_w u}{g} = \left(H - \frac{U_1^2}{2g} \right)$$

or
$$H = \left(\frac{U_w u}{g} + \frac{U_1^2}{2g} \right)$$
$$= \left(\frac{U_w u}{g} + \frac{U_{f_1}^2}{2g} \right)$$
$$= \left(\frac{U_w u}{g} + \frac{U_f^2}{2g} \right)$$

Substituting the value of U_f
$$H = \left(\frac{U_w u}{g} + \frac{U_w^2 \tan^2 \alpha}{2g} \right\}$$

Substituting the value of u
$$H = \left[\frac{U_w^2 (\tan \theta - \tan \alpha)}{g \times \tan \theta} + \frac{U_w^2 \tan^2 \alpha}{2g} \right]$$
$$= \frac{U_w^2}{g} \left[\frac{\tan \theta - \tan \alpha}{\tan \theta} + \frac{\tan^2 \alpha}{2} \right]$$
$$= \frac{U_w^2}{g} \left(1 - \frac{\tan \alpha}{\tan \theta} + \frac{\tan^2 \alpha}{2} \right) \qquad \ldots(i)$$

Now
$$\eta_H = \frac{U_w u}{g H}$$
$$= \frac{U_w \times U_w \left(1 - \dfrac{\tan \alpha}{\tan \theta} \right)}{g H} \qquad \ldots(ii)$$

Substituting the value of U_w^2 from Eq. (i) into Eq. (ii)
$$\eta_H = \frac{\left(1 - \dfrac{\tan \alpha}{\tan \theta} \right)}{\left[\left(1 - \dfrac{\tan \alpha}{\tan \theta} \right) + \dfrac{\tan^2 \alpha}{2} \right]}$$
$$= \frac{1}{\left[1 + \dfrac{\dfrac{1}{2} \tan^2 \alpha}{\left(1 - \dfrac{\tan \alpha}{\tan \theta} \right)} \right]}$$

15.8. Obtain an expression for work done per newton of water by a Pelton wheel in terms of mean bucket velocity u, jet velocity U and outlet blade angle θ, neglecting all frictional losses. If the loss due to bucket friction and shock can be expressed by $k_1 (U - u)^2/2g$ and that due to bearing friction by $k_2 u^2/2g$ where k_1 and k_2 are constants, show that maximum efficiency occurs when

$$n = \frac{u}{U} = \left(\frac{1 - \cos\theta + k_1}{2(1 - \cos\theta) + (k_1 + k_2)} \right)$$

Note : θ is equal to $(180 - \Phi)$

Solution

From Eq. 15.26, the energy transferred to the wheel per unit weight of water.

$$E = \frac{u}{g}(U - u)(1 + k\cos\Phi)$$

$$= \frac{u}{g}(U - u)(1 - \cos\theta) \quad \text{since} \quad \Phi = (180 - \theta)$$

$$\text{and} \quad k = 1.0$$

Considering the losses due to bucket friction and bearing friction

$$E = \frac{u}{g}(U - u)(1 - \cos\theta) - k_1 \frac{(U - u)^2}{2g} - k_2 \frac{u^2}{2g}$$

The input energy of the jet/weight of water

$$= \frac{U^2}{2g}$$

$\therefore$ Efficiency $\quad \eta_H = \dfrac{\dfrac{u}{g}(U - u)(1 - \cos\theta) - k_1 \dfrac{(U - u)^2}{2g} - k_2 \dfrac{u^2}{2g}}{\dfrac{U^2}{2g}}$

$$= \frac{2(Uu - u^2)(1 - \cos\theta) - k_1(U - u)^2 - k_2 u^2}{U^2}\}$$

$$= 2\left(\frac{u}{U} - \frac{u^2}{U^2}\right)(1 - \cos\theta) - k_1(1 - u/U)^2 - k_2 u^2/U^2$$

$$= 2(n - n^2)(1 - \cos\theta) - k_1(1 - n)^2 - k_2 n^2$$

For maximum efficiency $\dfrac{d\eta_H}{du} = 0$

But $\qquad n = u/U$

or $\qquad dn = \dfrac{1}{U} du$

Therefore, $\dfrac{1}{U} \cdot \dfrac{d\eta_H}{dn} = 0$

or $\qquad d\eta_H/dn = 0$

Diffierentation η_H w.r. to n and equating it to zero.

$$\frac{d\eta_H}{dn} = 2(1 - 2n)(1 - \cos\theta) - 2k_1(1 - n)(-1) - 2k_2 n = 0$$

or $\qquad (1 - 2n)(1 - \cos\theta) + k_1(1 - n) - k_2 n = 0$

or $$n\,[2\,(1-\cos\theta)+k_1+k_2=(1-\cos\theta)+k_1$$

or $$n=\frac{u}{U}=\left[\frac{1-\cos\theta+k_1}{2\,(1-\cos\theta)+k_1+k_2}\right]$$

15.9. Design a Francis turbine to develop 370 kW under a head of 70 m while running at 750 r.p.m. Assume ratio of width of the runner to diameter of runner as 0.1, flow ratio ψ as 0.15, hydraulic efficiency 95%, mechanical efficiency 84%. The water is discharged at exit, the velocity of flow remains constant and four percent of the flow area is blocked by the thickness of the vanes.

Solution

Given $P=370$ kW, $H=70$ m, $N=750$ r.p.m.

$$n=\frac{B}{D}=0.1\,,\psi=0.15\,,\eta_H=0.95\,,k=0.96$$

$\eta_M=0.84$ and $D_1=D/2$ (as usual)

(i) The overall efficiency η_0 is determined from Eq. 15.22 b

$$=0.95\times0.84=0.798$$

(ii) Also $$\eta_0=\frac{P\,watts}{w\,Q\,H}$$

$$0.798=\frac{370\times1000}{9810\times Q\times70}$$

$$Q=\frac{370\times1000}{9810\times70\times0.798}=0.675\text{ m}^3/\text{s}$$

(iii) $$U_{f_1}=U_f=\psi\,\sqrt{2gH}$$

$$U_f=0.15\,\sqrt{2\times9.81\times70}=5.559\text{ m/s}$$

(iv) $$Q=k\,\pi\,B\,D\,U_f$$

$$0.675=0.96\times3.14\times0.1D\times D\times5.559$$

$$D=\sqrt{\frac{0.675}{0.96\times3.14\times0.1\times5.559}}=0.635\text{ m}$$

$\therefore$ $$B=0.1\times D=0.0635\text{ m.}$$

(v) $$u=\frac{\pi\,D\,N}{60}$$

$$=\frac{\pi\times0.635\times750}{60}=24.92\text{ m/s}$$

(vi) $$\eta_H=\frac{U_w\,u}{g\,H}$$

$$0.95=\frac{U_w\times24.92}{9.81\times70}$$

$$U_w=\frac{0.95\times9.81\times70}{24.92}=26.17\text{ m/s}$$

(vii) From inlet velocity triangle.

$$\tan \alpha = \frac{U_f}{U_w}$$

$$= \frac{5.559}{26.17} = 0.2123$$

$$\alpha = 11° 59'$$

$$\tan \theta = \frac{U_f}{(U_w - u)}$$

$$= \frac{5.559}{(26.17 - 24.92)} = 4.4472$$

$$\theta = 77° 19'$$

(viii) Outlet diameter of the runner $= 0.5 \times$ inner diameter

$$D_1 = 0.5 \times 0.635 = 0.3175 \text{ m}$$

∴ $$B_1 = 0.1 \times 0.3175 = 0.031 \text{ m}$$

(ix) $$u_1 = \frac{\pi D_1 N}{60}$$

$$= \frac{\pi \times 0.3175 \times 750}{60} = 12.46 \text{ m/s}$$

(x) From outlet velocity triangle

$$\tan \Phi = \frac{U_{f_1}}{u_1}$$

$$= \frac{5.559}{12.46} = 0.4460$$

$$\Phi = 24° 02'$$

15.10. The guide blade angle of a Francis turbine is 8°, the runner vane angle at inlet and outlet are 110° and 20° respectively. The runner vanes reduce the flow area by 15%. The inner and outer diameters of the runner are 60 cm and 40 cm respectively. The widths at entrance and exit sections are 5 cm and 7.5 cm respectively. The pressure head at the entry to the guides is 29 m and kinetic energy there can be neglected. The pressure head at the discharge end is −2 m. If the losses in the guides and runner vanes is taken as 2.5 $U_f^2/2g$, determine (a) the speed of the runner for tangential flow to the runner vanes and (b) the power given to the runner by flowing water.

Solution

Given data :

$$\alpha = 8° , \theta = 110° , \Phi = 20° , k = 0.85,$$

$$D = 0.6 \text{ m}, D_1 = 0.4, \text{ m } B = 0.05 \text{ m}$$

$$B_1 = 0.075 \text{ m}, \text{ p/w} = 29 \text{ m}, h_1 = 2.5 \, U_1^2/2g$$

$$p_1/w = -2 \text{ m}, \quad h_L = 8 U_f^2/2g$$

(i) Area of flow at inlet $= A = k \pi DB$

$$A = 0.85 \times \pi \times 0.6 \times 0.05$$
$$= 0.0801 \text{ m}^2$$

Area of flow at outlet

$$A_1 = 0.85 \times \pi \times 0.4 \times 0.075$$
$$= 0.0801 \text{ m}^2$$

Since $A = A_1, U_f = U_{f_1} =$ velocity of flow.

(ii) From inlet velocity triangle, Fig. 15.29.

$$\tan(180 - 110) = \frac{U_f}{(u - U_w)} \qquad \ldots\text{(i)}$$

and

$$\tan 8° = \frac{U_f}{U_w} \qquad \ldots\text{(ii)}$$

From Eqs. (i) and (ii)

$$U_w = U_f \cot 8° = 7.11 U_f$$
$$u = 7.474 U_f \qquad \ldots\text{(iii)}$$
$$u_1 = \frac{u R_1}{R} = \frac{0.4}{0.6} \times 7.474 U_f \qquad \ldots\text{(iv)}$$
$$= 4.983 U_f$$

(iii) From outlet velocity triangle,

$$\tan 20° = \frac{U_{f_1}}{(u_1 - U_{w_1})}$$

$$0.364 = \frac{U_f}{(4.983 U_f - U_{w_1})}$$

$$U_{w_1} = 2.2355 U_f$$

(iv) Work done/newton

$$= \frac{U_w u - U_{w_1} u_1}{g}$$

$$= \frac{7.11 U_f \times 7.474 U_f - 2.2355 U_f \times 4.983 U_f}{g}$$

$$= 42.1 U_f^2/g \qquad \ldots\text{(v)}$$

(v) From outlet velocity triangle,

$$U_1^2 = (U_{f_1}^2 + U_{w_1}^2)$$

$$= (U_f^2 + (2.2355 U_f)^2) \qquad (\because U_{f_1} = U_f)$$

$$= (6 U_f^2)$$

Taking the tail race as the datum, the energy at the runner exit is given by

$$H_1 = \left(\frac{p_1}{w} + \frac{U_1^2}{2g}\right)$$

$$= \left(-2 + 6\frac{U_f^2}{2g}\right)$$

Similarly, the energy at the inlet $= H = 29$ m

$\therefore$ 29 = (Work done/newton losses in the guide and runner $+ H_1$)

$$= \left[42.1\frac{U_f^2}{g} + 2.5\frac{U_f^2}{2g}\right.$$

$$+ \left.\left(-2 + 6\frac{U_f^2}{2g}\right)\right]\frac{U_f^2}{g} = 0.628$$

$U_f = 2.48$ m

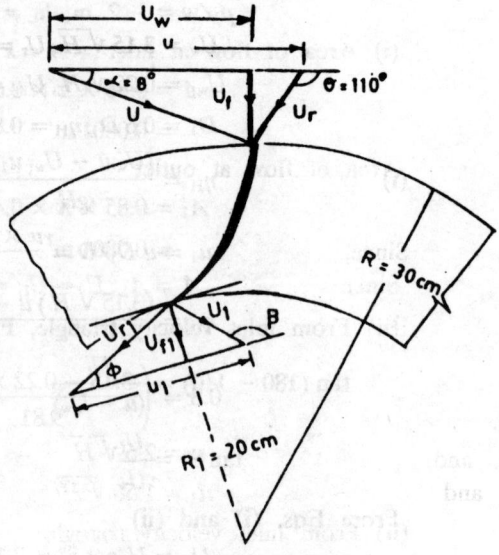

FIG. 15.29 EXAMPLE 15.10

(vi) From Eq. (iii),

$$u = 7.474 \times 2.48 = 18.55 \text{ m/s}$$

Also

$$u = \frac{\pi DN}{60}$$

$$N = \frac{18.55 \times 60}{\pi \times 0.6} = 590 \text{ r.p.m.}$$

From Eq. (v)

Work done/newton

$$= \frac{42.1 \times (2.48)^2}{9.81}$$

$$= 26.4 \text{ Nm/N}$$

Weight of water entering/sec $= wAU_f$

$$W = 9810 \times 0.0801 \times 2.48 = 1948.7 \text{ N}$$

$\therefore$ Power at runner $= 1948.7 \times 2.48$ N

$$= 51.44 \text{ kN}$$

15.11. The velocity of whirl at inlet to the runner of an inward flow reaction turbine is $3.15\sqrt{H}$ m/s and velocity of flow is $1.05\sqrt{H}$. The velocity of whirl at outlet is $0.22\sqrt{H}$ in the same direction as at inlet while velocity of flow at outlet is $0.83\sqrt{H}$. The outlet diameter of the runner is 0.6 times the inlet diameter and hydraulic efficiency of the turbine is 80%. Determine runner blade angles at inlet and outlet.

Solution

Given data :

$$U_w = 3.15 \sqrt{H},\ U_r = 1.05 \sqrt{H}$$
$$U_{w1} = 0.22 \sqrt{H},\ U_{r1} = 0.83 \sqrt{H}$$
$$D_1 = 0.6\, D\,,\, \eta_H = 0.8$$

(i)
$$\eta_H = \frac{(U_w u - U_{w1} u_1)}{gH}$$

Since,
$$u_1 = u\, D_1/D = \frac{u \times 0.6\, D}{D} = 0.6\, u$$

∴
$$\eta_H = \frac{(3.15 \sqrt{H})\, u - (0.22 \sqrt{H})\, 0.6\, u}{gH}$$

$$0.8 = \left(\frac{3.15 - 0.22 \times 0.6}{9.81} \right) \frac{\sqrt{H}\, u}{H}$$

$$u = 2.6 \sqrt{H}$$

and
$$u_1 = 1.56 \sqrt{H}$$

(ii) From inlet velocity triangle

$$\tan \theta = \frac{U_f}{(U_w - u)} = \frac{1.05 \sqrt{H}}{(3.15 - 2.6) \sqrt{H}}$$

$$= 1.910$$

$$\theta = 62° 22'$$

(iii) From outlet velocity triangle

$$\tan \Phi = \frac{U_f}{(u_1 - U_{w1})} = \frac{0.83 \sqrt{H}}{(1.56 - 0.22) \sqrt{H}}$$

$$= 0.6194$$

$$\Phi = 31° 46'$$

15.12. Two inward flow reaction turbines have the same diameters, viz. 0.6 m and the same efficiency. Both the runners work under the same head and they have the same velocity of flow, viz. 6 m/s. One of the runners, A, revolves at 520 rpm and has inlet blade angle 65°. If the other runner, B, has an inlet blade angle of 110°, at what speed should it run ?

Solution

Given data :

$$D_A = D_B = 0.6\, m\,,\, (\eta_H)_A = (\eta_H)_B$$

$$H_A = H_B\,;\, (U_f)_A = (U_f)_B = 6\ \text{m/s}$$

$$N_A = 520\ \text{rpm},\ \theta_A = 65°\ \text{and}\ \theta_B = 110°$$

(i)
$$u_A = \frac{\pi D N}{60} = \frac{\pi \times 0.6 \times 520}{60}$$

$$= 16.31\ \text{m/s}$$

(ii) From inlet velocity triangle,

$$\tan \theta = \tan 65° = \frac{U_f}{(U_w - u)}$$

$$2.144 = \frac{6}{(U_w - 16.31)}$$

$$U_w = 19.11 \ \text{m/s}$$

(iii) Since both runners have the same efficiency

$$\left(\frac{U_w u}{gH}\right)_A = \left(\frac{U_w u}{gH}\right)_B$$

or
$$\left(\frac{19.11 \times 16.31}{g \times H}\right) = \left(\frac{U_w u}{gH}\right)_B.$$

$$(U_w u)_B = 312 \qquad\qquad\qquad ...(\text{i})$$

(iv) From inlet velocity triangle for runner B,

$$\tan \theta_B = \frac{(U_f)_B}{(U_{wB} - u_B)}$$

or
$$\tan 110° = \frac{6}{(U_{wB} - u_B)}$$

or
$$(U_{wB} - u_B) = -2.18 \qquad\qquad\qquad ...(\text{ii})$$

Solving Eqs. (i) and (ii)

$$u_B = 18.8 \ \text{m/s}$$

Also
$$u_B = \frac{\pi D_B N_B}{60} = 18.8$$

$$N_B = \frac{18.8 \times 60}{\pi \times 0.6} = 600 \ \text{r.p.m.}$$

15.13 An inward flow reaction turbine having an efficiency of 75% is required to give 136 kW and works under a head of 9.15m. The velocity of the periphery of the wheel is $6\sqrt{H}$ m/s. The wheel is to make 120 r.p..m. The hydraulic losses in the turbine are 20% of the available energy. Determine (a) the guide blade angle at inlet, (b) the runner vane angle at inlet, (c) the diameter of the wheel at inlet, and (d) the width of the wheel at inlet. Assume radial discharge at exit.

Solution

Given data :

$$\eta_0 = 75\%, \ P = 136 \ \text{kW}, \ H = 9.15 \ \text{m},$$
$$u = 6\sqrt{H}, U_f = 2\sqrt{H}, N = 120 \ \text{r.p.m.}$$
$$\eta_H = (100 - 20) = 80\%$$

(i)
$$u = 6\sqrt{H}$$
$$= 6\sqrt{9.15} = 18.15 \ \text{m/s}$$

(ii)
$$U_f = 2\sqrt{H}$$

$$= 2 \sqrt{9.15} = 6.05 \text{ m/s}$$

(iii) $$\eta_H = \frac{U_w u}{gH}$$

$$0.8 = \frac{U_w \times 18.15}{9.18 \times 9.15} \text{ (for radial discharge)}$$

$$U_w = 3.956 \text{ m/s}$$

(iv) From inlet velocity triangle.

$$\tan \alpha = \frac{U_f}{U_w}$$

$$\tan \alpha = \frac{6.05}{3.956}$$

$$= 1.529$$

$$\alpha = 56° \ 49'$$

Also $$\tan \theta = \frac{U_f}{(u - U_w)}$$

$$= \frac{6.05}{(18.15 - 3.956)}$$

$$= 0.4622$$

$$\theta = 23° \ 5'$$

(v) $$u = \frac{\pi DN}{60}$$

$$18.15 = \frac{\pi \times D \times 120}{60}$$

$$D = \frac{60 \times 18.15}{\pi \times 120} = 2.89 \text{ m}$$

(vi) $$\eta_0 = \frac{P \, wats}{w \, Q \, H}$$

$$0.75 = \frac{136 \times 1000}{9810 \times Q \times 9.15}$$

$$Q = \frac{136 \times 1000}{9810 \times 9.15 \times 0.75} = 2.02 \text{ m}^3/\text{s}$$

(vii) Also $$Q = \pi DB U_f$$

$$2.02 = \pi \times 2.89 \times B \times 6.05$$

$$B = \frac{2.02}{\pi \times 2.89 \times 6.05} = 0.0367 \text{ m}$$

15.14 An inward flow reaction turbine working under a head of 8 m, has the guide angle of 25° and vane angle of 105°. Assuming the velocity for flow constant and radial discharge, determine hydraulic efficiency.

Solution

Given data :

$$H = 8 \text{ m}, \; \alpha = 25°, \theta = 105°$$
$$U_f = \text{constant}, \; B = 90° \; U_{w1} = 0$$

(i) From inlet velocity triangle

$$U_w = U \cos 25° = 0.9063 \, U$$
$$U_f = U \sin 25° = 0.4226 \, U$$

$$\tan 65° = \frac{U_f}{(u - U_w)}$$

$$u = (U_w + U_f \cot 75°)$$
$$= (0.9063 \, U + 0.4226 \, U \times \cot 75°)$$
$$= 1.0195 \, U$$

(ii) For radial discharge, $U_{w1} = 0$

$$\therefore \qquad \frac{U_w u}{g} = \left[H - \frac{U_1^2}{2g} \right]$$

$$= \left[H - \frac{U_{f_1}^2}{2g} \right]$$

$$= \left[H - \frac{U_f^2}{2g} \right] \quad \text{since } U_{f_1} = U_f = \text{ constant}$$

$$\left[\frac{0.9063 \, U \times 1.0195 \, U^2}{g} \right] = \left[H - \frac{(0.4226 \, U)^2}{2g} \right]$$

$$\frac{(0.924 \, U^2)}{9.81} = \left[8 - \frac{0.08929}{9.81} U^2 \right]$$

Solving, $\qquad U = 8.8 \text{ m/s}$

(iii) $\qquad \eta_H = \frac{U_w u}{gH}$

$$= \frac{(0.9063 \times 1.0195)(8.8)^2}{g \times 8}$$

$$= 0.911 \text{ or } 91.1 \, \%$$

15.15 A propeller turbine has outer diameter 4.5 m and diameter of central hub is 2 m. It develops 13250 kW under a head of 8 m with overall and hydraulic efficiencies as 88% and 94%. It runs at 115 rpm. Determine the vane angles at inlet and exit (a) at outer periphery and (ii) adjacent to central hub.

Solution

Given data,

$$D = 4.5 \, m, D_1 = 2 \, m$$

$$P = 13250 \ \text{kW}, \ H = 8 \ \text{m}$$
$$\eta_0 = 0.88, \ \eta_H = 0.94,$$
$$N = 115 \ \text{rpm.}$$

(i)
$$P = w \, QH \eta_0 \ \text{watts}$$
$$13250 \times 1000 = 9180 \times Q \times 8 \times 0.88$$
$$Q = \frac{13250 \times 1000}{9810 \times 8 \times 0.88} = 191.85 \ \text{m}^3/\text{s}$$

(ii)
$$Q = \frac{\pi}{4}(D^2 - D_1^2) \, U_t$$

$$U_t = \frac{4Q}{\pi \, (4.5^2 - 2^2)} = 15.04 \ \text{m/s}$$

(iii)
$$u = \frac{\pi \, DN}{60}$$

$$= \frac{\pi \times 4.5 \times 115}{60} = 27.08 \ \text{m/s}$$

$$u' = \frac{\pi \, D' \, N}{60}$$

$$= \frac{\pi \times 2 \times 115}{60} = 12.036 \ \text{m/s}$$

(iv)
$$\eta_H = \frac{U_w u}{gH}$$

$$0.94 = \frac{U_w \times 27.08}{9.81 \times 8}$$

$$U_w = \frac{0.94 \times 9.81 \times 8}{27.08} = 2.72 \ \text{m/s}$$

Also
$$\eta_H = \frac{U_w' \times u'}{gH}$$

$$0.94 = \frac{U_w' \times 12.036}{9.81 \times 8}$$

$$U_w' = \frac{0.94 \times 9.81 \times 8}{12.036} = 6.13 \ \text{m/s}$$

(v) From inlet velocity triangle (at outer radius)
$$\tan \alpha = \frac{U_t}{U_w}$$

$$= \frac{15.04}{2.72}$$

$$= 5.5294$$

$$\alpha = 79° \ 44'$$

$$\tan (\pi - \theta) = \frac{U_f}{(u - U_w)}$$

$$= \left(\frac{15.04}{27.08 - 2.72} \right) = 0.6174$$

$$\theta = 148° \, 18'$$

(vi) From outlet velocity triangle (at outer radius)

$$\tan \Phi = \frac{U_f}{u}$$

$$= \frac{15.04}{27.08} = 0.5554$$

$$\Phi = 29° \, 3'$$

(viii) Similarly at central hub,

$$\tan (\pi - \theta') = \frac{15.04}{(12.036 - 2.72)}$$

$$\tan (\pi - \theta') = 1.6144$$

$$\theta' = 121° \, 46'$$

$$\tan \Phi' = \frac{U_f}{u'}$$

$$= \frac{15.04}{12.036} = 1.2496$$

$$\Phi' = 51° \, 20'$$

15.16 A Kaplan turbine develops 1475 kW under a head of a 6 m with overall efficiency 85%. An elbow type draft tube with inlet diameter 3 m is provided at runner exit, set 2.5 m above the tail race level, gives a reading of 3 N/cm^2 on a vacuum gauge connected to the inlet. Determine the draft tube efficiency. If the output of the turbine is reduced to half, head and speed remaining unchanged, what would be the new reading of vacuum gauge after the governing.

Solution

Given data

$$P = 1475 \text{ kW}, \; H = 6 \text{ m},$$

$$\eta_0 = 85\%, D_1 = 3 \text{ m},$$

$$H_s = 2.5 \, m, p_2 = -3 \text{ N/cm}^2$$

(i) Neglecting the head losses in the draft, Eq. 15.41

$$\frac{p_2}{w} = - \left[H_s + \left(\frac{U_2^2 - U_3^2}{2g} \right) \right]$$

$$- \left[\frac{3 \times 10^4}{9810} \right] = - \left[2.5 + \left(\frac{U_2^2 - U_3^2}{2g} \right) \right]$$

$$\left(\frac{U_2^2 - U_3^2}{2g}\right] = 0.558$$

(iii)
$$\eta_0 = \frac{P}{w\,QH}$$

$$0.85 = \frac{1475 \times 1000}{9810 \times Q \times 6}$$

$$Q = \frac{1475 \times 1000}{0.85 \times 9810 \times 6} = 29.48 \text{ m}^3/\text{s}$$

$$a_2 = \frac{\pi}{4}\,(3)^2 = 7.065 \text{ m}^2$$

$$U_2 = \frac{29.48}{7.065} = 4.17 \text{ m/s}$$

$$\frac{U_2^2}{2g} = \frac{(4.17)^2}{2 \times 9.81} = 0.8874 \text{ m}$$

(iii) From Eq. 15.42

$$\eta_{DT} = \frac{(U_2^2 - U_3^2)/2g}{U_2^2/2g} \quad \left(\begin{array}{c}\text{no loss in the draft tube}\\ h_L = 0\end{array}\right)$$

$$= \frac{0.558}{0.8874}$$

$$= 0.6289 \text{ or } 62.89\%$$

(vi) If P is reduced to 1475/2 kW, discharge is also reduced by half

$$Q = \frac{29.48}{2} = 14.74 \text{ m}^3/\text{s}$$

∴
$$U_2 = \frac{14.74}{7.065} = 2.085 \text{ m/s}$$

$$\frac{U_2^2}{2g} = \frac{(2.085)^2}{2g} = 0.2215$$

$$\eta_{DT} = \frac{(U_2^2 - U_3^2)/2g}{0.2215}$$

or
$$\frac{U_2^2 - U_3^2}{2g} = 0.2215 \times 0.6289$$

$$= 0.1393$$

From Eq. 15.41,

$$\frac{p_2}{W} = \left[\frac{p_a}{w} - \left\{H_s + \frac{(U_2^2 - U_3^2)}{2g}\right\}\right]$$

$$= [10.3 - (2.5 + 0.1393) = 7.6607$$

$$p_2 = 7.6607 \times 9810 \text{ N/m}^2$$

$$= 7.51 \text{ N/cm}^2 \text{ absolute}$$

$$= - 2.79 \, \text{N/cm}^2 \text{ gauge}$$

15.17. The inlet area of a draft tube provided with a Francis turbine is X times the exit area of the tube. The head loss in the draft tube is kU^2 where U is the square root of the velocities at inlet and exit of the draft tube. Determine the efficiency of draft tube.

Solution

Given data $A_2 = X A_3, h_f = kU^2$

$$U = \sqrt{U_2 U_3}$$

(i) From continuity equations

$$U_3 = \frac{A_2}{A_3} U_2 = X U_2$$

$$\eta_{DT} = \frac{(U_2^2 - U_3^2)/2g - h_L}{U_2^2/2g}$$

$$= \left[\frac{(U_2^2 - X^2 U_2^2)}{2g} - kU^2 \right] / \left(\frac{U_2^2}{2g} \right)$$

$$= [1 - X^2 - 2gk]$$

15.18. A straight conical draft tube attached to a Francis turbine has an inlet diameter 3 m and its outlet area 20 m². The velocity of water at inlet is 5 m/s. The inlet is set 5 m above tail race level. Assuming the loss of head in the draft tube equals half the velocity head at its outlet, determine (a) the pressure head at the top of draft tube, (b) the total head at the top, taking tailrace level as datum, (c) power of water at outlet of runner, (d) power of water at the end of draft tube and (e) the power lost in the draft tube.

Solution

Given data $D_2 = 3 \, \text{m}, A_3 = 20 \, \text{m}^2, U_2 = 5$ m/s

$$H_s = 5 \text{ m}, \quad H_L = \frac{1}{2} (U_3^2/2g)$$

(i)
$$\frac{p_2}{w} = - \left[H_s + \frac{(U_2^2 - U_3^2)}{2g} \right] + h_L$$

$$= - \left[H_s + \frac{(U_2^2 - U_3^2)}{2g} \right] + \frac{1}{2} \left(\frac{U_3^2}{2g} \right)$$

From continuity equation,

$$U_3 = \frac{A_2}{A_3} U_2 = \frac{\pi/4 \times (3)^2}{20} \times 5$$

$$= 0.353 \, U_2 = 1.766 \text{ m/s}$$

∴
$$\frac{p_2}{w} = - \left[5 + \frac{(5^2 - 1.766^2)}{2 \times 9.81} \right] + \frac{1}{2} \cdot \frac{(1.766)^2}{2 \times 9.81}$$

$$= (- 6.115 + 0.0795)$$

$$= -6.07 \text{ m or } 6.07 \text{ m vacuum.}$$

(ii) Total head at the top of draft tube $= H$

$$H = \left(\frac{p_2}{w} + \frac{U_2^2}{2g} + z_2 \right)$$

$$= \left[-6.07 + \frac{(5)^2}{2 \times 9.81} + 5 \right]$$

$$= 0.2037 \text{ m.}$$

(iii) $\qquad Q = \dfrac{\pi}{4} \times (3)^2 \times 5 = 35.22 \text{ m}^3/\text{s}$

(iv) Power at the outlet of the runner $= w\,Q\,H$ watts

$$= 9810 \times 35.32 \times 0.2037 \text{ watts}$$

$$= 70.589 \text{ kW.}$$

(v) Powder at the end of draft tube

$$= w\,Q\,(U_3^2/2g)$$

$$= 9810 \times 35.32 \times \frac{1.766^2}{2 \times 9.81} \text{ watts}$$

$$= 55.077 \text{ kW}$$

(vi) Power lost in the draft tube

$$= (70.589 - 55.077)$$

$$= 15.51 \text{ kW}$$

15.19 An impulse turbine of 2.75 m diameter is rated at 11,000 kW at 300 rpm under a head of 490 m. It uses 2.7 m³/s discharge. If the turbine is operated under a head of 400 m, (a) what will be the speed, power and discharge ? (b) Determine the size of the wheel to develop 7000 kW power under a head of 300 m ? Also determine the speed and discharge,

Solution

Given data

$$D_1 = 2.75 \text{ m}, \; P_1 = 11000 \text{ kW,}$$

$$N_1 = 300 \text{ rpm}, \; H_1 = 490 \text{ m}$$

$$Q_1 = 2.7 \text{ m}^3/\text{s}, H_2 = 400 \text{ m.}$$

$$P_3 = 7000 \text{ kW}$$

(a) $\qquad \dfrac{P_2}{P_1} = \left(\dfrac{H_2}{H_1} \right)^{3/2} ; \; P_2 = P_1 \left(\dfrac{H_2}{H_1} \right)^{3/2}$

$$P_2 = \left(\frac{400}{490} \right)^{3/2} \times 11000 = 8113.13 \text{ kW}$$

$$\left(\frac{Q_2}{Q_1} \right) = \left(\frac{H_2}{H_1} \right)^{1/2} ; \; Q_2 = (H_2/H_1)^{1/2} \, Q_1$$

$$Q_2 = \left(\frac{400}{490}\right)^{1/2} \times 2.7 = 2.439 \text{ m}^3/\text{s}$$

$$\frac{N_2}{N_1} = \left(\frac{H_2}{H_1}\right)^{1/2} \; ; N_2 = \left(\frac{H_2}{H_1}\right)^{1/2} N_1$$

$$N_2 = \left(\frac{400}{490}\right)^{1/2} \times 300 = 271.05 \text{ rpm.}$$

(b) Since $D \propto \dfrac{1}{N}$

$$\frac{N_2}{N_1} = \frac{D_1}{D_2} = \left(\frac{H_2}{H_1}\right)^{1/2} = \left(\frac{300}{490}\right)^{1/2} = 0.7824$$

$$\therefore \qquad D_2 = \frac{D_1}{\left(\dfrac{H_2}{H_1}\right)^{1/2}}$$

$$= [2.75/0.7824] = 3.52 \text{ m}$$

$$\frac{Q_2}{Q_1} = \left(\frac{H_2}{H_1}\right)^{1/2}$$

$$Q_2 = Q_1 \times \left(\frac{H_2}{H_1}\right)^{1/2} = 27 \times 0.7824 = 2.11 \text{ m}$$

$$\frac{N_2}{N_1} = \left(\frac{H_2}{H_1}\right)^{1/2}$$

$$N_2 = N_1 \times \left(\frac{H_2}{H_1}\right)^{1/2} = 300 \times 0.7824$$

$$= 234.74 \text{ rpm.}$$

15.20. The reaction turbine at the Hoover dam installation have a rated capacity of 86000 kW at 180 rpm under a head of 148 m. The diameter of each turbine is 3.4 m and the discharge is 6.5 m³/s. Evaluate the speed coefficient (speed ratio), unit speed, unit power and specific speed.

Solution

Given data : ·

$$P = 86000 \text{ kW}, \; N = 180 \text{ rpm.}$$

$$H = 148 \text{ m}, \; D = 3.4 \text{ m} \; ; \qquad Q = 6.5 \text{ m}^2/\text{s.}$$

$$u = \frac{\pi DN}{60} = \Phi \sqrt{2gH}$$

$$\Phi = \frac{\pi DN}{60 \sqrt{2g} \sqrt{H}} = \frac{DN}{84.64 \sqrt{H}}$$

$$= \frac{3.4 \times 180}{84.64 \sqrt{148}} = 0.594$$

$$N_u = \frac{N}{\sqrt{H}} = \frac{180}{\sqrt{148}} = 14.\underline{79} \text{ r.p.m.}$$

$$P_u = \frac{P}{H^{3/2}} = \frac{86000}{(148)^{3/2}} = 47.76 \text{ kW}$$

$$N_s = \frac{N \sqrt{P}}{H^{5/4}} = N_u \sqrt{P_u}$$

$$= 14.79 \times \sqrt{47.76 \times 1.36} \quad (\because 1 \text{ kW} = 1.36 \text{ h.p.})$$

$$= 119.2 \text{ rpm.}$$

15.21. A reaction turbine, 0.5 m diameter, running at 600 rpm developed 195 kW when the flow was 0.74 m³/s. The pressure head at the entrance to the turbine was 28 m and the elevation of the turbine above the tailrace level was 1.90 m. The water entres the turbine with a velocity of 3.7 m/s. Calculate (a) the effective head, (b) the efficiency, (c) the speed expected under a head of 70 m, and (d) the power and discharge under the head of 70 m.

Solution

Given data

$$P = 195 \, kW \,, \quad Q_1 = 0.74 \text{ m}^3/\text{s}, \quad D = 0.5 \text{ m} , \frac{p_1}{w} = 28 \text{ m},$$

$$z_1 = 1.9 \text{ m} ; U_1 = 3.7 \text{ m/s} \quad H_2 = 70 \text{ m}$$

(a) Effective head

$$H_1 = \left(\frac{p_1}{w} + \frac{U_1^2}{2g} + z_1 \right)$$

$$H_1 = \left[28 + \frac{(3.7)^2}{2g} + 1.9 \right] = 30.6 \text{ m}$$

(b) Effective power

$$= w \, Q_1 \, H_1$$

$$P_1 = 9810 \times (0.74) \times (30.6) = 222 \text{ kW}$$

Efficiency $\qquad \eta = \dfrac{\text{Output Power}}{\text{Input power}}$

$$= \frac{195}{222} = 87.8\%$$

(c) For the same turbine,

$$\frac{N_1 D_1}{\sqrt{H_1}} = \frac{N_2 D_2}{\sqrt{H_2}}$$

$$\frac{600 \times 0.5}{\sqrt{30.6}} = \frac{N_2 \times 0.5}{\sqrt{70}}$$

$$N_2 = 907.5 \text{ r.p.m.}$$

(d) Similarly, $(k_p)_1 = (k_p)_2$

$$\frac{P_1}{D_1^2 H_1^{3/2}} = \frac{P_2}{D_2^2 H_2^{3/2}}$$

$$\frac{1.95}{(0.5)^2 (30.6)^{3/2}} = \frac{P_2}{(0.5)^2 (70)^{3/2}}$$

$$P_2 = 674.7 \text{ kW}$$

Also $\qquad (k_{Q1}) = (k_{Q2})$

$$\frac{Q_1}{D_1^2 \sqrt{H_1}} = \frac{Q_2}{D_2^2 \sqrt{H_2}}$$

$$\frac{0.74}{(0.5)^2 \sqrt{30.6}} = \frac{Q_2}{(0.5)^2 \sqrt{70}}$$

$$Q_2 = 1.119 \text{ m}^3/\text{s}$$

15.22 A Francis turbine working under a head of 30 m produces 13500 kW power when running at 120 rpm. If the local atmospheric pressure is 10.2 m of water and vapour pressure is 0.22 m of water. Calculate the safe height of the turbine above tail water level.

Solution

Given data

$$H = 30 \text{ m, } P = 13500 \text{ kW} \qquad N = 120 \text{ rpm,}$$

$$H_a = 12.2 \text{ m} \qquad\qquad H_{vp} = 0.22 \text{ m}$$

$$N_s = \frac{N \sqrt{P}}{H^{5/4}}$$

$$= \frac{120 \sqrt{13500 \times 1.36}}{(30)^{5/4}} \quad (\text{Since } 1 \text{ kW } = 1.36 \text{ hp})$$

$$= 231.41 \text{ rpm}$$

From Eq. 15.47 (a)

$$\sigma_c = 0.0317 \, (N_s/100)^2$$

$$= 0.0317 \left(\frac{231.41}{100}\right)^2 = 0.1697$$

But $\qquad\qquad \sigma_c = \dfrac{H_a - H_{wp} - H_s}{H}$

$$H_s = (H_a - H_{vp} - \sigma_c H)$$
$$= (10.2 - 0.22 - 0.1697 \times 30)$$
$$= 4.887 \text{ m.}$$

15.23 A Pelton wheel has a linear bucket speed $0.46 \sqrt{2gH}$ and a bucket circle diameter $D = 15$ times jet diameter. If $k_v = 0.97$ and η_0 is 82%, calculate specific speed and bucket circle diameter of the specific turbine.

Solution

Given data

$$u = 0.46 \sqrt{2gH}, \quad D/d = 15,$$
$$k_v = 0.97, \quad \eta_0 = 82\%$$

For Pelton wheel,

$$Q = \frac{\pi}{4} d^2 U$$
$$= \frac{\pi}{4} d^2 k_v \sqrt{2gH}$$
$$P = \frac{w\, QH}{75} \eta_0 \quad \text{h.p.}$$

Note : Power is found out in h.p. for use in N_s, formula.

$$P = \left(\frac{w}{75} \eta_0 \frac{\pi}{4} . k_v \sqrt{2g} \right) d^2 H^{3/2}$$

Also,

$$u = \frac{\pi DN}{60} = k_u \sqrt{2gH}$$
$$N = \frac{(60\, k_u \sqrt{2g}\, \sqrt{H}}{\pi D}$$

Substituting in Eq. 15.65

$$N_s = \frac{N \sqrt{P}}{H^{5/4}}$$

$$= \frac{60\, k_u \sqrt{2g}\, \sqrt{H}}{\pi D} \times \frac{\left(\dfrac{w}{75} \eta_0 \dfrac{\pi}{4} k_v \sqrt{2g} \right)^{1/2} d\, H^{3/4}}{H^{5/4}}$$

$$N_s = (60 \times 0.46 \sqrt{2 \times 9.81}) \times (w/75 \times 0.82 \times \pi/4 \times 0.98$$
$$\times \sqrt{2 \times 9.81})^{1/2} \left(\frac{d}{D} \right)$$

$$\therefore \qquad = \frac{247.75}{D/d}$$

For $\qquad D/d = 15,$

$$N_s = \frac{247.75}{15} = 16.5$$

Now $\qquad u_s = k_u \sqrt{2gH_s}$
$$= 0.46 \sqrt{2gH_s}$$

For specific turbine,

$$H_s = 1 \text{ m}$$
$$u_s = 0.46 \sqrt{2 \times 9.81 \times 1} = 2.038 \text{ m/s}$$

Also
$$u_s = \frac{\pi D_s N_s}{60}$$

$$D_s = \frac{60 \times 2.038}{\pi \times 16.5}.$$
$$= 2.36 \text{ m}$$

15.24 A turbine is to operate under a head of 25 m at 200 r.p.m. The discharge is 9 m³/s. If the efficiency is 90%, determine (a) specific speed of the turbine, (b) Power generated, and (c) the type of the turbine, (d) Performance under a head of 20 m.

Solution

Given data
$$H = 25 \text{ m}, \ N = 200 \text{ rpm}$$
$$Q = 9 \text{ m}^3/\text{s}, \eta_0 = 90\%$$

(a)
$$N_s = \frac{N \sqrt{P}}{H^{5/4}}$$

and
$$\eta_0 = \frac{P}{w QH}$$
$$P = w QH \eta_0 \text{ watts}$$
$$P = (9810 \times 9 \times 25 \times 0.9/1000) \text{ kW}$$
$$= 1986.525 \text{ kW}$$
$$= 2700 \text{ h.p.,}$$
$$N_s = \frac{200 \sqrt{2700}}{(25)^{5/4}}$$
$$= 185.89 \text{ r.p.m.}$$

(b)
$$P = 1986.525 \text{ kW}$$

(c) As the specific speed lies between 60 and 300, the Francis turbine is the choice.

(d) When the turbine works under a head of 20 m,
$$N_2 = N_1 \sqrt{H_2/H_1} = 200 \sqrt{20/25} = 1789 \text{ r.p.m.}$$
$$Q_2 = Q_1 \sqrt{H_2/H_1} = 9 \sqrt{20/25} = 8.05 \text{ m}^3/\text{s}$$
$$P_2 = P_1 (H_2/H_1)^{3/2} = 1986.25 (20/25)^{3/2} = 1421.44 \text{ kW}$$

15.25 A model of a Francis turbine build to a scale of 1:5 when tested at workshop was found to developed 3.0 kW at a speed of 360 r.p.m. under a head of 1.8 m. Estimate the equivalent speed and power of the full size turbine when working under a head of 5.8 m.

Solution

Given data :

$$L_m/L_p = 1/5, P_m = 3 \text{ kW}, N_m = 360 \text{ rpm}$$
$$H_m = 1.8 \text{ m} \quad H_p = 5.8 \text{ m}$$

(a) Speed of the motal under a head of 5.8 m

$$= 300 \sqrt{\frac{5.8}{1.8}} = 646 \text{ r.p.m.}$$

When model and prototype both works under a head of 5.8 m, their peripheral speed should be same.

$$u_m = u_p$$

$$\therefore \qquad D_m N_m = D_p N_p$$

or $$N_p = N_m \left(\frac{D_m}{D_p}\right) = 646 \times \frac{1}{5}$$

$$= 129 \text{ rpm}$$

(b) Power of model under 5.8 m head

$$= 3 \left(\frac{5.8}{1.8}\right)^{3/2} \qquad (\because P \propto H^{3/2})$$

$$= 17.35 \text{ kW}$$

Since $P \propto D^2$

$$\frac{P_p}{P_m} = \left(\frac{D_p}{D_m}\right)^2$$

or $$P_p = P_m (D_p/D_m)^2 = 17.35 (5)^2$$

$$= 433.8 \text{ kW}$$

As a check, the specific speed of the model and prototype may be computed and two values should agree.

$$(N_s)_m = \left(\frac{N\sqrt{P}}{H^{5/4}}\right)_m$$

$$= \left(\frac{360 \sqrt{4.076}}{(1.8)^{5/4}}\right)_m \qquad (\because P = 3 \text{ kW} = 4.076 \text{ h.p.})$$

$$= 348.6$$

$$(N_s)_p = \frac{129 \sqrt{433.8/0.736}}{(5.8)^{5/4}}$$

$$= 348.6$$

This simpliffced solution may now be corrected taking scale effect into account.

If the model efficiency on test had been found to be $(\eta_0)_m = 0.76$, then the prototype efficiency could be found out from

$$\frac{1 - (\eta_0)_m}{1 - (\eta_0)_p} = (n)^{1/4}$$

$$\frac{1 - 0.76}{1 - (\eta_0)_p} = (5)^{1/4}$$

Solving, $(\eta_0)_p = 0.84$

The corrected output of the prototype

$$= 433.8 \times \frac{0.84}{0.76}$$

$$= 479.46 \text{ kW}$$

15.26 Calculated the diameter, speed, and specific speed of a propeller turbine runner to develop 6182.4 kW under a head of 5 m. Given $\Phi = 2.1$ based on outer diameter, $\psi = 0.65$, diameter of boss $= 0.35$ times external diameter and overall efficiency $\eta_0 = 88\%$.

Solution

Given data :

$$P = 6182.4 \text{ kW}, \ H = 5 \text{ m}, \ \Phi = 2.1,$$

$$\psi = 0.65 \ , \quad D_1 = 0.35 \, D, \eta_0 = 0.88$$

(i)
$$\eta_0 = \frac{P}{w \, Q \, H}$$

$$Q = \frac{P}{w \, H \, \eta_0} = \frac{6182.4 \times 1000}{9810 \times 5 \times 0.88}$$

or
$$Q = 143.2 \text{ m}^3/\text{s}$$

(ii)
$$U_f = \psi \, \sqrt{2 \, g \, H}$$

$$= 0.65 \, \sqrt{2 \times 9.81 \times 5} = 6.438 \text{ m/s}$$

(iii)
$$Q = A_f \, U_f$$

$$A_f = \frac{143.2}{6.438} = 22.24 \text{ m}^2$$

But
$$A_f = \frac{\pi}{4} \, (D^2 - D_1^2) = \frac{\pi}{4} \, (D^2 - (0.35 \, D)^2)$$

∴
$$D = \sqrt{\frac{4 \times 22.24}{\pi \times (1 - 0.35^2)}} = 5.68 \text{ m}$$

(iv)
$$u = \Phi \, \sqrt{2 \, g H} = \frac{\pi \, D N}{60}$$

$$N = \frac{60 \, \Phi \, \sqrt{2 \, g H}}{\pi \, D}$$

$$= \frac{60 \times 21 \times \sqrt{2 \times 9.81 \times 5}}{\pi \times 5.68} = 69.95 \text{ r.p.m.}$$

(v)
$$N_s = \frac{N\sqrt{P}}{H^{5/4}}$$

$$= \frac{69.95\sqrt{6182.4/0.736}}{(5)^{5/4}}$$

$$= 857.46 \text{ r.p.m.}$$

15.27 Estimate the maximum height of a straight conical draft tube of a turbine producing 13616 kW while running at 120 r.p.m. and working at 26.6 m head. The draft tube exit dip at least 0.6 m below tail race level. Given

σ_c	0.05	0.10	0.16	0.23	0.31
N_s	138	178	220	266	310

Assume effective height of barometer as 9.8 m.

Solution

Given data :

$$P = 13616 \text{ kW}, \ N = 120 \text{ r.p.m.,}$$

$$H = 26.6 \text{ m} \ h_3 = 0.6 \text{ m}$$

(i)
$$N_s = \frac{N\sqrt{P}}{H^{5/4}}$$

$$= \frac{120\sqrt{13616/0.736}}{(26.6)^{5/4}}$$

$$= 278.18 \text{ r.p.m.}$$

From the given table, corresponding to N_s equal to 278.18 r.p.m.

$$\sigma_c = 0.2376$$

(ii)
$$\sigma_c = \left(\frac{H_a - H_s - H_v}{H}\right)$$

or
$$H_s = (H_a - H_v) - \sigma_c H$$

$$= (9.8 - 0.2376 \times 26.6)$$

$$= 3.48 \text{ m}$$

Maximum height of draft tube

$$= (3.48 + 0.6)$$

$$= 4.08 \text{ m}$$

15.28 Data below related to a laboratory test carried on a water turbine working under a design head of 8.5 m.

Unit speed	56	65	74	84	93	102
Unit power (kW)	8.83	9.2	9.5	9.5	9.35	8.98
Weight flow (kN/s)	39.6	38.9	38.1	37.25	36.3	35.2

Plot a curve of overall efficiency against N_u. Calculate the turbine speed N at maximum efficiency and hence determine the specific speed of the turbine. If the head is changed to 10 m, estimate the power developed and find from the graph overall efficiency at a speed of 250 r.p.m.

Solution

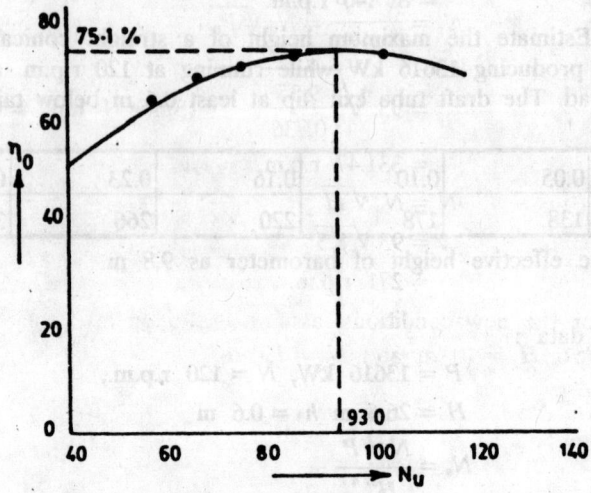

FIG. 15.30 EXAMPLE 15.28

Given data :

$H = 8.5$ m. Table of values of N_u, P_u and W.

From graph, (Fig. 15.30).

$(\eta_0)_{max} = 75.1\%$ at $N_u = 93$ r.p.m. and so $W = 36.3$

(i) From Eq. (i) $P_u = \dfrac{W \eta_0}{2.915}$

$= \dfrac{36.3 \times 0.751}{2.915}$

$= 9.35$ kW

Since $P_u = P/H^{3/2}$; or $P = P_u H^{3/2}$ ...(ii)

and $\eta_0 = \dfrac{P \, watts}{w \, Q \, H}$

$\therefore$ $\eta_0 = \dfrac{P_u H^{3/2}}{w \, Q \, H} = \dfrac{P_u \sqrt{H}}{W}$ where $W = w \, Q$ Newton

$= \dfrac{P_u \sqrt{8.5}}{W}$

$= 2.915 \dfrac{P_u}{W}$ ...(i)

Obtain N_u vs. η_0 values from above table.

N_u	56	65	74	84	93	102
$\%\eta$	65.0	68.95	72.7	74.4	75.1	74.7

From Eq. (ii), $\quad P = P_u H^{3/2} = 9.35 \,(8.5)^{3/2}$

$$= 231.7 \text{ kW}$$

$$N_s = \frac{N\sqrt{P}}{H^{5/4}} = N_u \sqrt{P_u}$$

$$= 93 \sqrt{\frac{9.35}{0.736}} \qquad \text{(Since 1 h.p. = 0.736 kW)}$$

$$= 331.47 \text{ r.p.m.}$$

$$N = N_u \sqrt{H}$$

$$= 93 \sqrt{8.5}$$

$$= 271 \text{ r.p.m.}$$

(ii) For the new conditions, assume maximum efficiency η_0 remaining same as 0.751, $H_2 = 10$ m and $N_2 = 250$ rpm.

Now $\qquad N_u = \dfrac{N_2}{\sqrt{H_2}} = \dfrac{250}{\sqrt{10}}$

$$= 79 \text{ r.p.m.}$$

Correspondingly, η_0 from graph is equal to $\eta_0 = 0.73$

$$N_s = N_u \sqrt{P_u}$$

or $\qquad P_u = (N_s/N_u)^2$

$$= \left(\frac{331.47}{79}\right)^2$$

$$= 17.60 \text{ hp. or } 12.957 \text{ kW}$$

$\therefore \qquad P = 12.957 \times (10)^{3/2}$

$$= 410.05 \text{ kW when } \eta_0 = 0.751$$

Therefore, actual power developed

$$P = 410.05 \times \frac{0.730}{0.751}$$

$$= 398.59 \text{ kW}$$

Objective Question :

15.1 The net head at the turbine is

(a) the sum of gross head and head loss in penstock,

(b) the sum of gross head, head loss in penstock and velocity head at the turbine exit.

(c) the difference between gross head and head loss in the penstock.

(d) the difference between gross head and the sum of head loss in the penstock and velocity head.

15.2 The difference between the power obtained from the turbine shaft and the power supplied by water at the entry to the turbine is equal to

(a) hydraulic losses,

(b) mechanical losses,

(c) sum of hydraulic, mechanical and volumetric losses,

(d) sum of mechanical and volumetric losses,

(d) sum of hydraulic and volumetric losses.

15.3 The hydraulic efficiency of a turbine is defined as

(a) $\eta_H = \dfrac{WH''}{WH}$

(b) $\eta_H = \dfrac{WH}{WH''}$

(c) $\dfrac{P}{WH''}$

(d) $\dfrac{WH''}{P}$

where $H'' = \dfrac{(U_w u \pm U_{w_1} u_1)}{g}$

15.4 The overall efficiency of a turbine is dependent on different losses occurring in the turbine. It is related to these by the following relation ship.

(a) $(\eta_v \eta_H \eta_M)^{1/3}$

(b) $\sqrt{\eta_v \eta_H \eta_M}$

(c) $\eta_v \eta_H \eta_M$

(d) $(\eta_v \eta_H \eta_M)/3$

(e) None

15.5 An impulse turbine

(a) is most suited to low head installation

(b) makes use of a draft tube

(c) converts pressure head into velocity head throughout the vanes.

(d) Operated by initial conversion to kinetic energy

(e) is high specific speed turbine.

15.6 A shaft transmits 147.2 kW at 600 r.p.m. The torque in kN m is

(a) 0.245

(b) 88320

(c) 2.34

(d) 2340

15.7 A reaction turbine discharge 35 m³/s under a head of 9 m and with an overall efficiency of 91%. The power developed in kW is

(a) 286.65

(b) 37.49

(c) 3.822

(d) 2812

(e) None

15.8 A draft tube is fitted to the exit of a reaction turbine, located at 1.82 m above tail race level. The efficiency of draft tube is 75% and velocity of flow at the entry to draft tube is 10 m/s. The pressure at the entrance section of draft tube is

(a) –5 m   (b) –3.82   (c) 10.2 m

(d) 1.82 m   (e) None

15.9 By fitting a draft tube at the exit of a reaction turbine, a portion of energy is recuped back. If this is given by

(a) $\dfrac{(U_2^2 - U_3^2)}{2g}$ (b) $\dfrac{(U_2 - U_3)^2}{2g}$

(c) $\left(H_s + \dfrac{U_2^2 - U_3^2}{2g} \right)$ (d) $\left(\dfrac{p_2}{w} + \dfrac{U_2^2}{2g} + H_s \right)$

where U_2 and U_3 are the velocities at entry and exit section of the draft tube, H_s is the datum head at entry and p_2 is the pressure at this section.

15.10 The specific speed of a turbine is expressed as

(a) $\dfrac{N \sqrt{P}}{H^{3/4}}$ (b) $\dfrac{N \sqrt{P}}{H^{5/4}}$

(c) $\dfrac{N H^{5/4}}{\sqrt{P}}$ (d) $\dfrac{N \sqrt{P}}{(gH)^{5/4}}$

15.11 Select the range of specific speed associated with each type

(a) Pelton wheel (single jet)   (i) 60–300

(b) Pelton wheel (multi jet)   (ii) 300–1000

(c) Francis turbine   (iii) 20–35

(d) Kaplan turbine   (iv) 35–60

15.12 The cavitation in a turbine would definitely occur if

(a) the pressure anywhere in the flow approaches the atmospheric value

(b) the pressure anywhere in the flow is lower than vapour pressure.

(c) the velocity of flow is too high

(d) the pressure in the flow falls to a value very close to the vapour pressure.

15.13 For cavitation free operation of a turbine, the critical value of Thoma's coefficient must satisfy the following condition

(a) $\sigma_c > \sigma_{inc}$ (b) $\sigma_c = \sigma_{inc}$

(c) $\sigma_c < \sigma_{inc}$ (d) none

where $\sigma_{inc} = \dfrac{(H_a - H_v - H_s)}{H}$

15.14 A $1:10$ model of a turbine develops 2 kW power while working under a head of 1.5 m. If the efficiency of the model is assumed be to the same as that of prototype, the power (kW) developed by the prototype while working under a head of 15 m is

(a) 20   (b) 63.24   (c) 6.32

(d) 10   (e) none

15.15 A turbine works under 50 m head. The peripheral speed of the turbine is 18.8 m/s. If is it required to work under 1 m head, the speed ratio is changed to

(a) 0.6   (b) 4.24

(c) 0.85   (d) none

Problems :

15.1 Differentiate between turbine and pump. How will you classify the turbines.

15.2 What do you understand by gross head, net head, and specific energy.

15.3 What are different losses occurring in a turbine. Define various efficiencies used with turbine.

15.4 Show that torque, T, delivered to the Pelton wheel per unit weight of water is given by

$$T = (U - u)(1 + k \cos \Phi) R/g$$

Hence derive the following expression for hydraulic efficiency.

$$\eta_H = 2 k_u (k_v - k_u)(1 + k \cos \Phi)$$

with usual notations.

15.5 Explain with the help of neat sketches why (a) Pelton wheel is shaped as a tangential flow impulse turbine though it works as an axial flow one. (b) The outlet tip of the buckets of Pelton wheel must have some angle even though maximum efficiency could be obtained with zero outlet angle.

15.6 Draw a sectional plan of a vertical shaft radial flow type reaction trubine and explain the purpose of providing a spiral casing and guide vanes.

15.7 What is a draft tube and what hydraulic functions are performed by it when connected to the exit of a reaction turbine. Derive an expression for draft tube efficiency. Sketch various types of draft tubes mentioning their merits.

15.8 Draw a neat sketch of a propeller turbine and how does it differ from that of a Kaplan turbine. What is the necessity of the stay vanes in a spiral casing.

15.9 What is a surge tank ? With the help of a illustrative sketch explain the working of the surge tank following a sudden change in load on turbine shaft.

15.10 What do you understand by characteristic curves of a turbine. Explain various types of characteristics curves of a turbine.

15.11 Explain with the help of velocity diagrams how the efficiency of a Kaplan turbine is maintained maximum in the event of load variation on the turbine shaft. How does this make Kaplan turbine superior to a propeller turbine in its performance at part load.

15.12 A Pelton wheel develops 8000 kW under a net head of 130 m at a speed of 200 rpm. Assuming $k_v = 0.98$, $\eta_H = 0.87$, $\Phi = 0.46$ and $d/D = 1/9$, determine (a) flow rate Q (b) mean diameter of wheel (c) diameter of nozzle (d) number of jets and (e) specific speed of the turbine. Assuming mechanical efficiency as 75%.

15.13 The buckets of a Pelton turbine deflect the jet through a total angle of 165° and owing to the surface friction the relative velocity of water leaving the buckets is 0.84 times that at entry. Draw velocity triangles and find the ratio of bucket velocity to jet velocity in order that the water shall leave the buckets without whirl. In such a turbine, the available head at the nozzle is 650 m, $k_v = 0.97$, the jet diameter 10 cm and mean bucket circle diameter 1.2 m. Determine (a) best running speed (rpm), (b) the impulsive force of the jet on the buckets at this speed, (c) power developed and (d) efficiency of buckets.

15.14 With the following data determine input power to the shaft and speed of the Pelton wheel.

Net head = 370 m, $k_v = 0.98$, speed ratio = 0.47, k = 0.9 and inlet blade angle $\Phi = 160°$. Also jet diameter = 18 cm.

15.15 An inward flow reaction turbine runner is required to operate under a head of 10 m at a speed of 176 rpm and to develop 1450 kW. Find the diameter of the runner inlet and outlet, the discharge, guide blade angle and runner vane angles at inlet and outlet. Assume following data : speed ratio $\Phi = 0.65$, flow ratio $\psi = 0.16$, velocity of flow constant, hydraulic efficiency = 0.86 and overall efficiency = 81%. Take the discharge as radial.

15.16 In an inward flow reaction turbine the supply head is 12 m and the maximum discharge is 0.25 m³/s. The external diameter is twice the internal diameter and the velocity of flow is constant and is equal to 0.15 $\sqrt{2gH}$. The runner vanes are radial at inlet and the runner rotates at 300 rpm. Determine (a) guide vane angle, (b) the vane angle at exit for radial discharge, (c) width of runner at inlet and exit. The vanes occupy 10% of the circumference and hydraulic efficiency is 80%.

15.17 An inward flow reaction turbine has radial tips at inlet (outer periphery) while at the exit (inner periphery) the blades make an angle of 30° with the forward tangent. The radius of the outer periphery is two times the radius of inner one and the turbine operates under a total head of 21 m. Assuming a constant radial velocity of flow and that the blade friction accounts for a dissipation of energy equivalent of 12% of k.E. at the outlet, determine the runner velocity at the rim, and hydraulic efficiency of the turbine, if the turbine discharges radially.

15.18 An inward flow reaction turbine (Francis type) has a runner 60 cm diameter and 5 cm width at the outer rim, the inner diameter being 39 cm. The wheel blade angles at the inlet and outlet are 95° (inside angle of the velocity triangle = 95°) and 14°, respectively. The velocity of flow is uniform throughout the wheel and 8% of the circumferential area of the runner is blocked by the blade thickness. The head on the turbine is 54 m, the hydraulic efficiency is 88%, overall efficiency is 81% and discharge at outlet is radial. Determine (a) the speed in r.p.m. and (b) power available at shaft.

15.19 An axial flow water turbine has a rotor of 8 m, overall diameter with a boss of 2 m diameter. The blade tips at the upper inlet side are inclined at $\tan^{-1}$ (2/5) to the tangential direction and at the lower outlet side at $\tan^{-1}$ (1/3). If the turbine is to work under a pressure difference of 8 m head at an efficiency of 85%, what will be its power output.

15.20 Water is supplied to an axial flow turbine under a gross head of 35 m. The mean diameter of runner is 2 m and it rotates at 145 r.p.m. Water leaves the guide vanes at 30° to the direction of runner rotation and at mean radius the angle of runner vane at outlet is 28°. If 7% of the gross head is lost in the casing and guide vanes and relative velocity is reduced by 8% due to friction in the runner determine the vane angle at inlet (at mean radius) and hydraulic efficiency of the turbine.

15.21 For a given inward reaction turbine, inlet blade angle θ speed ratio Φ, flow ratio ψ, the discharge is radial. Show that the hydraulic efficiency is given by

$$\eta_H = 2\,\Phi\,(\Phi + \psi \cot \theta)$$

15.22 A reaction turbine is equipped with a straight flaring draft tube having top and bottom diameters of 0.5 m and 0.75 m respectively. The water velocity at the top is 3 m/s where the elevation is 5 m above the level of the tail water. Assuming a loss in the draft tube equal to the half the velocity head at exit, compute the (i) pressure head at top (ii) the total head at top with reference to the tail race as a datum, (iii) total head at exit, (iv) power in water at top and at exit, (v) power lost in the draft tube due to friction and eddy formation.

15.23 A Kaplan turbine develops 1472 kW under a head of 6 m with efficiency of 85%. An elbow type draft tube with inlet diameter 3 m is provided at runner exit, set 2.5 m above tail race level gives a reading of 3.1 N/cm² on a vaccum gauge connected to tube inlet. Determine the draft tube efficiency. If the output of the turbine is reduced to 736 kW, head and speed remaining unchanged, what would be the reading of the vacum gauge after governing.

15.24 Derive an expression for N_s in terms of N, P and H with usual notations.

A quarter scale turbine model is tested under a head of 12 m. The full scale model is required to work under a head of 35 m and to run at

428 rpm. At what speed the model be run and if it develops 1000 kW and uses 1 m³/s at this speed, what power will be obtained from the full scale turbine assuming that its efficiency is 3% better than that of model. State the type of turbine used.

15.25 A model turbine constructed to a scale of 1 : 10. It is tested under a head of 8 m at 400 r.p.m. and gives 77% overall efficiency. Determine the speed of prototype and the ratio of the powers developed by the model and prototype. The prototype works under a head of 100 m. What will be the efficiency of the prototype if scale effect is considered.

15.26 A turbine develops 6624 kW when running at 100 r.p.m. the head on the turbine is 30 m. If the head on the turbine is reduced to 18 m, determine speed and power developed by it.

15.27 At hydro-electrical power house propeller turbines are rated at 36000 kW at 81.8 r.p.m. under a 13 m head. The exit diameter is 7.42 m. For a geometrically similar turbine to develop 27000 kW under an 11 m head, what speed and diameter should be used ? What percentage change in flow is probable?

15.28 The following data was obtained as a result of laboratory test on a prototype turbine under a working head of 10 m.

Speed (r.p.m)	168	195	222	252	279	306	325
Load at shaft (N)	4250	3840	3470	3060	2680	2300	2010
Discharge (m³/s)	3.96	3.90	3.81	3.72	3.65	3.52	3.43

Assuming the radius of brake drum as 3.26 m, compute and plot N_s vs Q_u, N_u vs P_u and N_u vs η_1 characteristic curves of turbine and therefrom determine the specific speed of the turbine.

16

Reciprocating Pump

16.1 INTRODUCTION

The pump is a mechanical device which when interposed in a pipeline transfers energy from external source to the liquid flowing through it. Thus, a pump may be defined as a machine which converts mechanical energy into hydraulic energy and then transfers it to the liquid flowing through it. Out of the hydraulic energy, mainly it it the pressure energy that is increased much more as compared to velocity energy or datum energy. This pressure energy is subsequently converted into potential energy and the liquid is lifted up from a lower level to a higher level.

There are wide diversity of types or design of pumps (See Fig. 16.1) but as regards their operating principles, all of them can be classified as:

1. Positive displacement pumps and

2. Rotodynamic pumps.

(1) *Positive Displacement Pumps* These are the pumps in which the liquid is sucked in or drawn into a finite space or a chamber and then this liquid is pushed out or lifted up due to the thrust of a moving part (piston or plunger) again and again. The chamber is filled up and emptied alternatively and thus the flow from such pump is fluctuating. The amount of liquid supplied per second mainly depends on the speed of the pump. The most common example of this category of pump is reciprocating pump.

(2) *Rotodynamic Pumps* All the Rotodynamic pumps have got a rotating part called impeller which is made to rotate freely in the liquid. The rotation of the impeller changes the angular momentum of the liquid flowing through it, thereby converting mechanical energy (of the rotating part) into the hydraulic energy of the flowing liquid through the impeller (in the form of increase of pressure energy). The well known example of this category is centrifugal pump.

16.2 CLASSIFICATION OF PUMPS

All the pumps can be classified on the basis of their operating principle, kind of action upon liquid, motion of working members and form of working members. The general classification of pumps is depicted in Fig. 16.1. Out of these pumps, the theory of reciprocating pump is given in the present chapter whereas centrifugal pump is described in the next chapter 17. For the description of other type of pumps one can refer elsewhere.

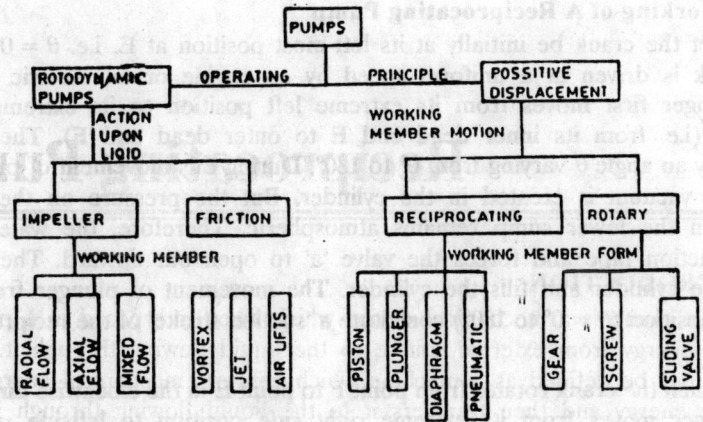

FIG. 16.1 GENERAL CLASSIFICATIONS OF PUMPS

16.3 RECIPROCATING PUMP

16.3.1 General Description

The diagrammatic view of a reciprocating pump is shown in Fig 16.2. It primarily consists of a piston or plunger P (or ram) which moves backward and forward inside a closed cylinder (or chamber). The plunger P is connected to a crank C by means of a connecting rod R. The crank is driven by power from an external source (or an electric motor or diesel engine). One way valves 'a' and 'b' are provided at the end of suction pipe S and at the entry to the delivery pipe D respectively. The pump is located at a height H_s above its centre line.

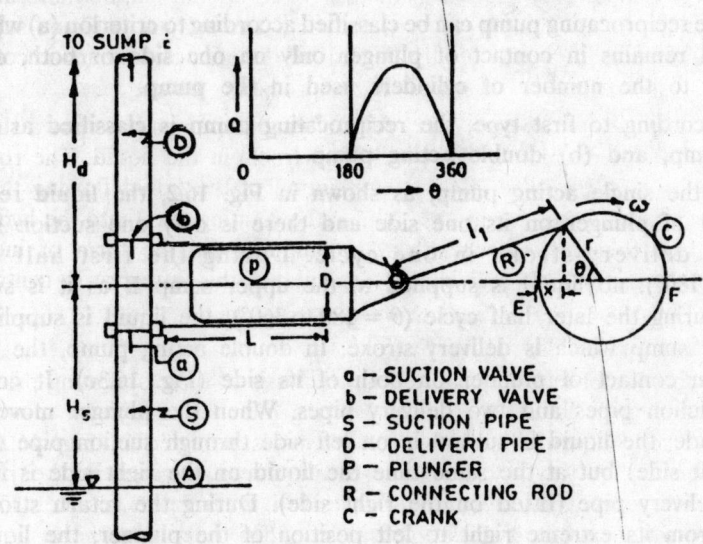

a — SUCTION VALVE
b — DELIVERY VALVE
S — SUCTION PIPE
D — DELIVERY PIPE
P — PLUNGER
R — CONNECTING ROD
C — CRANK

FIG. 16.2 DIAGRAMMATIC VIEW OF A RECIPROCATING PUMP

16.3.2 Working of A Reciprocating Pump

Let the crank be initially at its left-most position at E, i.e. $\theta = 0°$. Now the crank is driven at a uniform speed by an engine or an electric motor. The plunger first moves from its extreme left position to its extreme right position (i.e. from its inner dead end E to outer dead end F). The crank rotates by an angle θ varying from 0° to 180°. During this movement of plunger., a partial vacuum is created in the cylinder. But the pressure on the water surface in the lower sump remains atmospheric. Therefore, the water rises in the suction pipe and forces the valve 'a' to open out upward. The liquid enters the cylinder and fills the cylinder. The movement of plunger from left to right position ($\theta = 0°$ to 180°) constitute a 'suction stroke' of the reciprocating pump.

When the crank rotates from point F to point E in the clockwise direction, the plunger moves from its extreme right side position to leftside position (θ varies from 180° to 360°). This is what is known as 'delivery stroke'. The movement of the plunger from right to left side position forces the liquid (in the cylinder) to open the valve 'b' upward located in the delivery pipe. (At the same time, valve 'a' remains closed). The liquid rises in the delivery pipe and is supplied to upper sump B.

Thus the crank has rotated one full revolution ($\theta = 0°$ to 360°) and the plunger has moved from extreme left position to right (suction stroke) and then from extreme right position to left (delivery stroke). This is known as one cycle of the reciprocating pump. The same cycle is repeated again and again but the liquid is supplied only during delivery stroke, that is, the supply is intermittent.

16.4 CLASSIFICATION

The reciprocating pump can be classified according to criterion (a) whether the liquid remains in contact of plunger only on one side or both, or (b) according to the number of cylinders used in the pump.

According to first type, the reciprocating pump is classified as single acting pump, and (b) double acting pump.

In the single acting pump, as shown in Fig. 16.2, the liquid remains in contact of plunger on its one side and there is only one suction stroke and one delivery stroke in one cycle. During the first half cycle ($\theta = 0°$ to 180°), no liquid is supplied to the upper sump B as it is suction stroke. During the later half cycle ($\theta = 180$ to 360°), the liquid is supplied to the upper sump which is delivery stroke. In double acting pump, the liquid remains in contact of plunder on both of its side (Fig. 16.3c). It consists to two suction pipes and two delivery pipes. When the plunger moves left to right side, the liquid is sucked in on left side through suction pipe (fitted on the left side) but at the same time the liquid on the right side is forced up the delivery pipe (fitted on the right side). During the return stroke of plunger from its extreme right to left position of the plunger, the liquid is supplied through another delivery pipe (fitted on the left side) and the liquid is sucked in through suction pipe (fitted on the right side) from the lower sump. Thus it consists of two suction strokes and two delivery strokes in each cycle and hence the supply remains continuous.

According to the other criterion, the reciprocating pumps may be classified as : (i) Single cylinder pump, (ii) Double cylinder pump, (iii) Three cylinder pump, (iv) Duplex double cylinder pump, and (v) Quintuplex pump.

As the name indicates, single cylinder pump consists of one cylinder only and is shown in Fig. 16.3a; while double cylinder pump, also known as two throw pump consists of two cylinders with rams driven by cranks set at 180° as shown in Fig. 16.3b. The three cylinder pump consists of three cylinders with rams set at 120°.

Fig. 163c shows a double acting single cylinder pump. Fig. 16.3d shows a double acting pump with two cylinders in line and driven by a single crank. Although type shown in Fig. 15.3b, c and d, all yield the same gross discharge as type 'a' when driven at same speed. Out of type 'b', d and c, the former (type b and d) are more advantageous as the leakage past glands can at once be detected and remedied whereas the type 'c' must be dismantled before new packing rings can be inserted. Another two throw pump is shown in Fig. 16.3e which is known as 'outside end packed' pump and is better than type 'd'. In type 'e', the plunger/piston rod with glades is not required and it is sometimes used for high pressure hydraulic transmission systems.

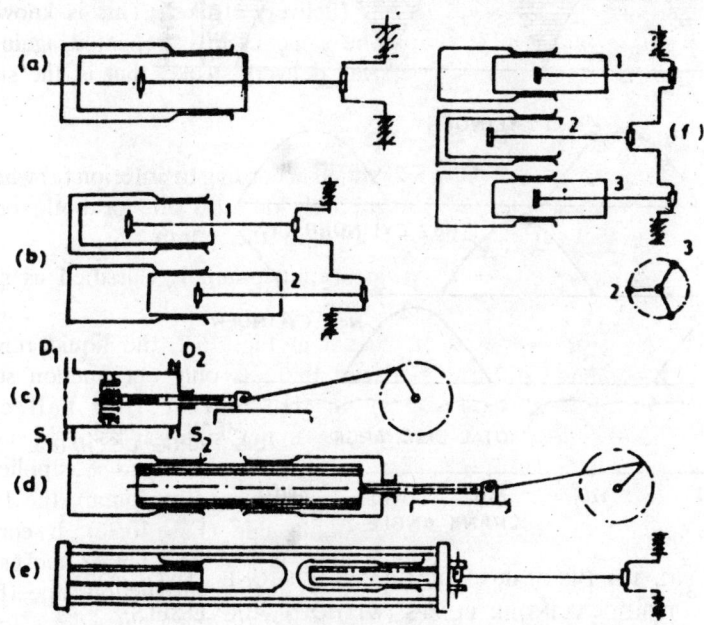

FIG. 16.3 MULTI CYLINDER PUMP.

The three throw pump having three cylinders and three cranks set at 120° is shown in Fig. 16.3f. It has the advantage that it provides the discharge more uniformly and creates inertia pressure as great as one sixth of that created by an equivalent single cylinder pump and thus its running is safer.

A duplex double acting pump is formed by combining two double acting single cylinder or two double acting double cylinder pump, each driven by a crank, the two cranks being set at 90°. This combination is equivalent to a four throw pump.

A quintuplex pump or five throw pump has five single acting cylinders driven from a shaft having cranks set at 72°. The discharge from such a pump is quite regular.

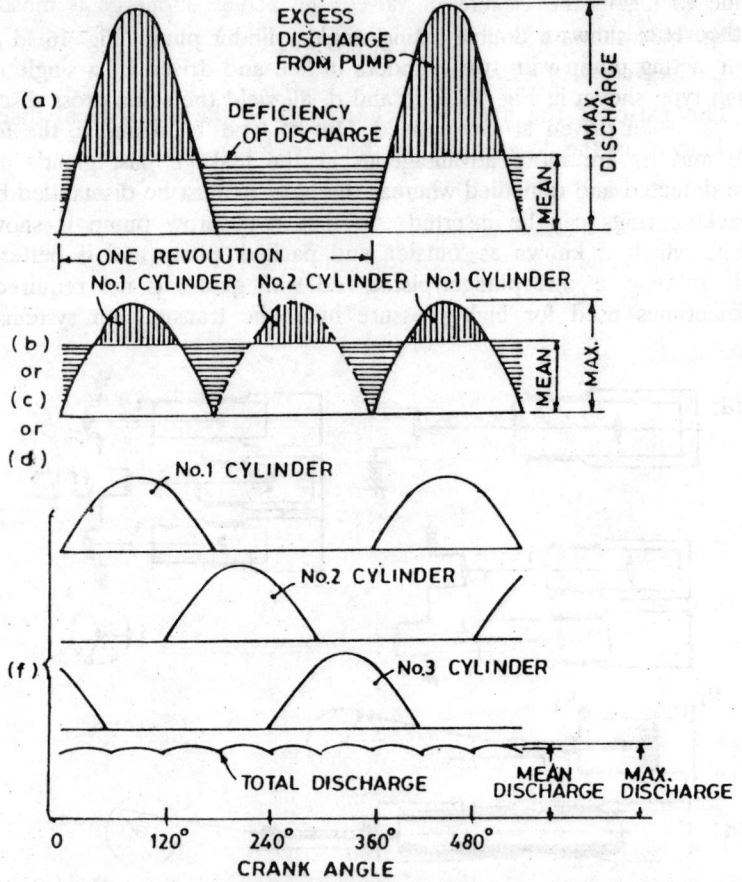

FIG. 16.4 DISCHARGE DIAGRAMS FOR ONE-, TWO-, AND THREE CYLINDER PUMPS (WITHOUT AIR-VESSELS)

16.5 SOME DEFINITIONS

Let us first consider a single acting pump. Referring to Fig. 16.2, let r be the radius of the crank and L be the length of the stroke, so that,

$$L = 2r$$

Let D be the diameter of the plunger so that its cross sectional area be A.

The volume swept per stroke $= A L$

$$= \frac{\pi}{4} D^2 \cdot L = \frac{\pi}{4} D^2 \cdot 2r$$

Theoretical discharge Q_{th} given out by pump,

$$Q_{th} = \frac{ALN}{60} = \frac{2ArN}{60} = \frac{\pi}{4} D^2 \cdot 2r \frac{N}{60} \qquad \qquad ...(16.1)$$

On account of leakage through valves and past piston or plunger and also due to lag in the closure of valves, the actual discharge is mostly less than theoretical discharge.

1. **Coefficient of discharge** C_d

The ratio of the actual discharge Q_a to the theoretical discharge Q_{th} is known as the 'coefficient of discharge 'C_d'

$$C_d = \frac{Q_a}{Q_{th}} \qquad \qquad ...(16.2)$$

and the value of C_d expressed in percentage is known as the volumetric efficiency of the pump

$$\text{Volumetric efficiency} = \frac{Q_a}{Q_{th}} \times 100 \qquad \qquad ...(16.3)$$

2. **Slip**

The difference between theoretical discharge and actual discharge is known as 'slip'.

$$\text{Slip} = (Q_{th} - Q_a) \qquad \qquad ...(16.4)$$

The ratio of the slip to the theoretical discharge is known as percentage slip

$$\% \ \text{Slip} = \frac{Q_{th} - Q_a}{Q_{th}} \times 100$$

$$= \left(1 - \frac{Q_a}{Q_{th}} \right) \times 100$$

$$= (1 - C_d) \times 100$$

$$= (100 - \text{Volumetric efficiency}) \qquad \qquad ...(16.5)$$

For the pumps maintained in good condition, the percentage slip is of the order of 2% or less. But when the delivery pressure is high (say 700 N/cm^2), the compressibility of liquid tends to increase the slip, especially when the clearance volume of the cylinder is excessive.

3. **Negative slip**

Generally the actual discharge supplied by a pump, Q_a, is less than theoretical discharge, Q_{th}. But in some cases, the theoretical discharge

Q_{th} is less than actual discharge Q_a. In that case, the slip defined as the difference of Q_{th} and Q_a is negative.

In a few cases, the pumps have to work under large suction head and small delivery head. If these pumps run at high speed, the inertia pressure built up in the suction side may be quite high in comparison to the pressure in the delivery pipe, outside the delivery valve. (Valve 'b' shown in Fig. 16.2). In such cases, some liquid may be pushed directly to delivery pipe before the end of suction stroke. In this way the actual discharge Q_a supplied to the upper sump will be larger than Q_{th}.

Now consider a double acting pump. In a double acting pump, there are two suction strokes and two delivery strokes in one cycle or in one revolution of the crank. Therefore, the theoretical discharge, Q_{th} supplied in each cycle is given by Eq. 16.6.

Theoretical discharge, Q_{th},

$$= \frac{ALN}{60} + \frac{(A - A_1)LN}{60}$$

$$= \frac{\pi}{4}D^2 \cdot \frac{LN}{60} + \frac{\pi(D^2 - d^2)}{4}\frac{LN}{60} \qquad ...(16.6)$$

where d is the diameter of the connecting rod. If diameter d is too small as compared to the diameter of the cylinder D, the theoretical discharge is given by

$$Q_{th} = \frac{2ALN}{60}$$

$$= 2\frac{\pi}{4}D^2 \cdot \frac{LN}{60} \qquad ...(16.7)$$

16.6 WORK DONE BY A PUMP

The expressions for work done by a reciprocating pump are now discussed and are given below:

16.6.1 Single Acting Pump

Let H_s be the suction head and H_d be the delivery head reckoned with the centre line of the pump. Then,

Theoretical work done/sec

$$= W Q_{th} (H_s + H_d) \frac{Nm}{s}$$

$$= w \frac{ALN}{60} (H_s + H_d) \qquad ...(16.8)$$

Theoretical power required to drive the pump

$$= w \frac{ALN}{60} (H_s + H_d) \text{ watts} \qquad ...(16.9)$$

However, the actual power required to derive the pump will be more than given by Eq. 16.9, to take into account the frictional and leakage losses in the pump.

Force acting on the plunger The expressions for the force acting on the plunger during both strokes are given below

Force acting on the plunger during suction stroke

$$= w A H_s$$

$$= w \frac{\pi}{4} D^2 H_s \qquad \qquad ...(16.10)$$

Force acting on the plunger during delivery stroke

$$= w A H_d$$

$$= w \frac{\pi}{4} D^2 . H_d \qquad \qquad ...(16.11)$$

16.6.2 Double Acting Pump

In case of double acting pump, the liquid is supplied in each half of the cycle, i.e. in each stroke and so the discharge supplied is double to that supplied by a single acting pump.

Theoretical work done/sec $= w \, Q_{th} \, (H_s + H_d)$

$$= w \, (H_s + H_d) \left[\frac{A L N}{60} + \frac{(A - A_1) L N}{60} \right] \quad ...(16.12a)$$

If the area of the plunger A_1 is too small as compared to the area of the cylinder A.

The theoretical work done/sec

$$= 2 w \, (H_s + H_d) \frac{A L N}{60} \qquad \qquad ...(16.12b)$$

In this case also, the actual power required to derive the pump will be more than theoretical power, given by Eq. 16.12 in watts, to account for the frictional and leakage losses past the plunger, etc.

Force acting on the plunger during suction stroke

$$= w A H_s + w \, (A - A_1) H_d \qquad \qquad ...(16.13)$$

Force acting on the plunger during delivery stroke

$$= w \, (A - A_1) H_s + w A H_d \qquad \qquad ...(16.14)$$

16.7 VARIATION OF VELOCITY AND PRESSURE DUE TO AC-CELERATION

16.7.1 Velocity and Pressure

During to and fro motion of the plunger, its speed does not remain uniform but it varies from its minimum value to maximum and then decreases to its minimum value as seen below. Since, the liquid in the cylinder remains in contact of plunger, its velocity also varies during a stroke. The variation in velocity causes the variation in pressure being exerted over the liquid. From the suction pipe, the liquid flows into the cylinder and thereafter flows out to the delivery pipe. Thus, the velocity of liquid in these pipes also varies during a stroke. This variation in velocity of liquid in the pipes causes non-uniform rate of flow and at the same time gives rise to the building up of inertia pressure. The magnitude of inertia pressure or acceleration head H_a created due to the acceleration of the plunder is now being computed.

In order to simplify the problem, it is usually assumed that the plunger moves in a simple harmonic motion. For this purpose, it is further assumed that the length of connecting rod l_1 is very long as compared to the radius of the crank.

Let the crank be rotating with an angular velocity ω rad/s. and the crank turn through an angle θ in the time t seconds.

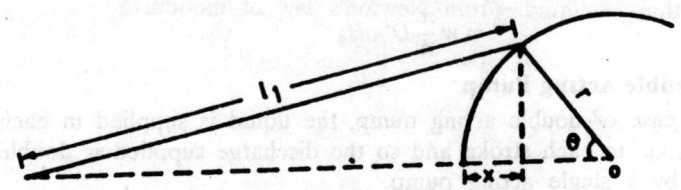

FIG. 16.5 MOTION OF A CRANK

From Fig. 16.5, $\theta = \omega t$

The displacement of plunger from its extreme right position, 'x' (i.e. $\theta = 0$) is given by

$$x = r - r \cos \theta$$
$$= r (1 - \cos \omega t) \qquad ...(16.15)$$

Velocity of plunger,

$$u = \frac{dx}{dt}$$
$$= \omega r \sin \omega t \qquad ...(16.16)$$

Acceleration of plunger.

$$f = \frac{d^2x}{dt^2} = \frac{du}{dt}$$
$$= \omega^2 r \cos \omega t \qquad ...(16.17)$$

Let 'A' be the cross sectional area of the cylinder and 'a' be the area of the pipe (either of the suction and delivery pipes). Then from continuity principle,

Velocity of liquid in the pipe $= u . \dfrac{A}{a}$

$$= \frac{A}{a} . \omega r \sin \omega t$$
$$= \frac{A}{a} \omega r \sin \theta \qquad ...(16.18)$$

Acceleration of liquid in the pipe

$$= f \cdot \frac{A}{a}$$

$$= \frac{A}{a} \omega^2 r \cos \omega t$$

$$= \frac{A}{a} \cdot \omega^2 r \cos \theta \qquad \ldots(16.19)$$

If l be the length of pipe (cross sectional area a) through which the liquid is flowing, the weight of water contained in it at any instant will be

$$= w a l$$

Let p_a represent the inertia pressure build up in the pipe due to the acceleration of liquid. From Newton's law of motion,

$$p_a \cdot a = \frac{wal}{g} \left(\frac{A}{a} \cdot \omega^2 r \cos \theta \right)$$

$$p_a = \frac{wl}{g} \frac{A}{a} \omega^2 r \cos \theta$$

$$H_a = \frac{p_a}{w} = \frac{l}{g} \frac{A}{a} \omega^2 r \cos \theta \qquad \ldots(16.20)$$

Eq. 16.20 shows that acceleration head H_a acting on the liquid in the pipe varies with crank angle θ.

At the beginning of stroke, when $\theta = 0°$, $\cos \theta = 1$, then

$$H_a = \frac{l}{g} \frac{A}{a} \omega^2 r \qquad \ldots(16.20a)$$

At the middle of stroke, when $\theta = 90°$, $\cos \theta = 0$, then

$$H_a = 0 \qquad \ldots(16.20b)$$

At the end of stroke, when $\theta = 180°$, $\cos \theta = -1$, then

$$H_a = -\frac{l}{g} \frac{A}{a} \omega^2 r \qquad \ldots(16.20c)$$

Thus, it is found that during the first half of the stroke ($\theta = 0°$ to $90°$), a positive acceleration head acts on the liquid in the pipe and during the later half of the stroke ($\theta = 90°$ to $180°$), a negative acceleration head acts on the liquid in the pipe. The above expressions are applicable to either the suction or delivery pipes; the length l and area a of the corresponding pipes, is being used.

If the motion of the plunger is not assumed as simple harmonic, the acceleration of the plunger f at the inner dead centre ($\theta = 0°$) is given by

$$f = \omega^2 r (1 + r/l_1) \qquad \ldots(16.21)$$

where l_1 is the length of the connecting rod.

The acceleration head H_a at the beginning of the stroke, $\theta = 0°$, is then given by

$$H_a = \frac{l}{g}\frac{A}{a}\omega^2 r\,(1 + r/l_1) \qquad ...(16.21a)$$

And at the end of stroke, $(\theta = 180°)$,

$$H_a = \frac{l}{g}\frac{A}{a}\omega^2 r\,(1 - r/l_1) \qquad ...(16.22b)$$

16.7.2 Instantaneous Rate of Discharge

The instantaneous velocity of water in the delivery pipe U_d is given by Eq. 16.18, using the area a_d as the area of delivery pipe,

$$U_d = \frac{A}{a_d}\cdot\omega r\sin\theta \qquad ...(16.23a)$$

$$= \left(\frac{D}{d_d}\right)^2 \omega r\sin\theta$$

$$= \left(\frac{D}{d_d}\right)^2 \cdot \frac{2\pi r N}{60}\sin\theta \qquad ...(16.23b)$$

The velocity U_d varies with the crank angle θ. The plot between U_d and θ is a sine curve.

Single Acting pump: The discharge supplied by a single acting can now be determined. Since there is only one delivery stroke in each cycle, the mean velocity of flow $(U_d)_{mean}$ can be obtained by integrating Eq. 16.23a and dividing by 2π

$$(U_d)_{mean} = \frac{1}{2\pi}\left[\int_0^\pi \left\{\frac{A}{a_d}\omega r\sin\theta\right\}d\theta\right]$$

$$= \frac{A}{a_d}\cdot\frac{\omega r}{\pi} \qquad ...(16.24)$$

Alternatively, $\qquad (U_d)_{mean} = \frac{Q_{th}}{a_d}$

$$= \frac{ALN}{60}\cdot\frac{1}{a_d} = \frac{A\,2rN}{60}\cdot\frac{1}{a_d}$$

$$= \frac{A}{a_d}\cdot\frac{\omega r}{\pi} \qquad ...(16.24)$$

From Eq. 16.23, the maximum velocity U_{max} is obtained for $\theta = 90°$.

$$(U_d)_{max} = \frac{A}{a_d}\cdot\omega r = \left(\frac{D}{d_d}\right)^2\omega r \qquad ...(16.25)$$

From Eqns 16.24 and 16.25, the ratio of mean velocity to maximum velocity in the delivery pipe is obtained

$$\frac{(U_d)_{mean}}{(U_d)_{max}} = \frac{1}{\pi} \qquad ...(16.26)$$

The instantaneous discharge Q supplied through a delivery pipe may be obtained by using continuity equation

$$Q = a_d U_d$$

Substituting the value of U_d from Eq. 16.23,

$$Q = a_d . \frac{A}{a_d} . \omega r \sin \theta$$

$$= A \omega r \sin \theta \qquad ...(16.27)$$

The discharge Q varies with crank angle θ. It is zero at the beginning of a delivery stroke ($\theta = 0$), maximum at the middle of the delivery stroke and becomes again zero at the end of stroke ($\theta = 180°$). The variation of discharge Q_{mean} is given by

$$Q_{mean} = a_d . U_{mean}$$

$$= a_d \left(\frac{A}{a_d} . \frac{\omega r}{\pi} \right)$$

$$= \frac{A \omega r}{\pi} \qquad ...(16.28)$$

The maximum discharge Q_{max} corresponding to $\theta = 90°$ is given by Eq. 16.27,

$$Q_{max} = a_d . \left(\frac{A}{a_d} . \omega r \right)$$

$$= A \omega r \qquad ...(16.29)$$

Dividing Eq. 16.28 by Eq. 16.29

$$\frac{Q_{mean}}{Q_{max}} = \frac{A \omega r / \pi}{A \omega r} = \frac{1}{\pi} \qquad ...(16.30)$$

Double Acting Pump: For a double acting pump, there are two delivery strokes in one cycle (i.e., in one revolution of the crank). The mean velocity is, therefore, given by Eq. 16.31.

$$(U_d)_{mean} = 2 . \frac{1}{2\pi} \left[\int_0^\pi \frac{A}{a_d} . \omega r \sin \theta \right]$$

$$= 2 \frac{A}{a_d} . \frac{\omega r}{\pi}$$

$$= 2 \left(\frac{D}{d_d} \right)^2 \frac{\omega r}{\pi} \qquad ...(16.31)$$

Again the ratio of mean velocity to maximum velocity can be obtained by dividing Eq. 16.31 by Eq. 16.25.

$$\frac{(U_d)_{mean}}{(U_d)_{max}} = \frac{2 (A/a_d) \frac{\omega r}{\pi}}{(A/a_d) \omega r} = \frac{2}{\pi} \qquad ...(16.32)$$

The instantaneous rate of discharge is again given by Eq. 16.27 and varies with crank angle θ, that is, it a sine curve. Since there are two delivery stroke in one cycle (or one complete revolution of the crank. i.e. one delivery stroke for $\theta = 0°$ to $180°$ and another for $\theta = 180°$ to $360°$, two sine curves are obtained with a phase difference of $180°$ (Fig. 16.4b). The mean discharge Q verses θ is a sine curve, Fig 16.4a. The mean discharge Q_{mean} is obtained as,

$$Q_{mean} = a_d\,(U_d)_{mean}$$

$$= a_d \times 2 \left(\frac{A}{a_d} \frac{\omega\,r}{\pi} \right)$$

$$= \left(\frac{2A\,\omega\,r}{\pi} \right) \qquad \qquad ...(16.33)$$

It is assumed that the area of the connecting rod is too small, otherwise

$$Q_{mean} = \left[\frac{A\,\omega\,r}{\pi} + \frac{(A - A_1)\,\omega\,r}{\pi} \right] \qquad ...(16.34)$$

Dividing Eq. 16.33 by Eq. 16.29

$$\frac{Q_{mean}}{Q_{max}} = \frac{2A\,\omega\,r/\pi}{A\,\omega\,r} = \frac{2}{\pi} \qquad \qquad ...(16.35)$$

16.8 INDICATOR DIAGRAM

16.8.1 Hypothetical Indicator Diagram

The work done by the plunger on the liquid during suction and delivery strokes (Eq. 16.8) can be represented diagrammetically, as shown in Fig. 16.6.

In this diagram, the line f e is drawn at a distance of atmospheric pressure, H_{atm} meter. above absolute zero pressure line on a suitably selected scale. The length of suction stroke, L is marked as 'd c' beginning at d and ending at c, and is drawn H_s meter below f e line, i.e. suction head H_s meter below atmospheric pressure line f e. In this way, the area of d c e f represents the work done by the plunger on the liquid during suction stroke on a suitable selected scale,

The delivery stroke begins at extreme right position of plunger and so it is marked as b and extends L distance from b and is marked as 'a'. Thus, the line a b represents the delivery stroke and it is drawn H_d meter above atmospheric pressure line f e. Thus, the area f e b a represents the work done by the plunger on the liquid during delivery stroke on the same scale. Thus, the total area a b c d is equal to L $(H_s + H_d)$ represents the theoretical work done by the plunger during one revolution of the crank of a single acting pump. This diagram can be obtained automatically by an indicator fitted on the cylinder of a pump. It is named as indicator diagram.

In case of double acting pumps, the volume of liquid supplied is twice that of the single acting pump and so the work done by it is also twice the area of the indicator diagram a b c d.

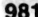

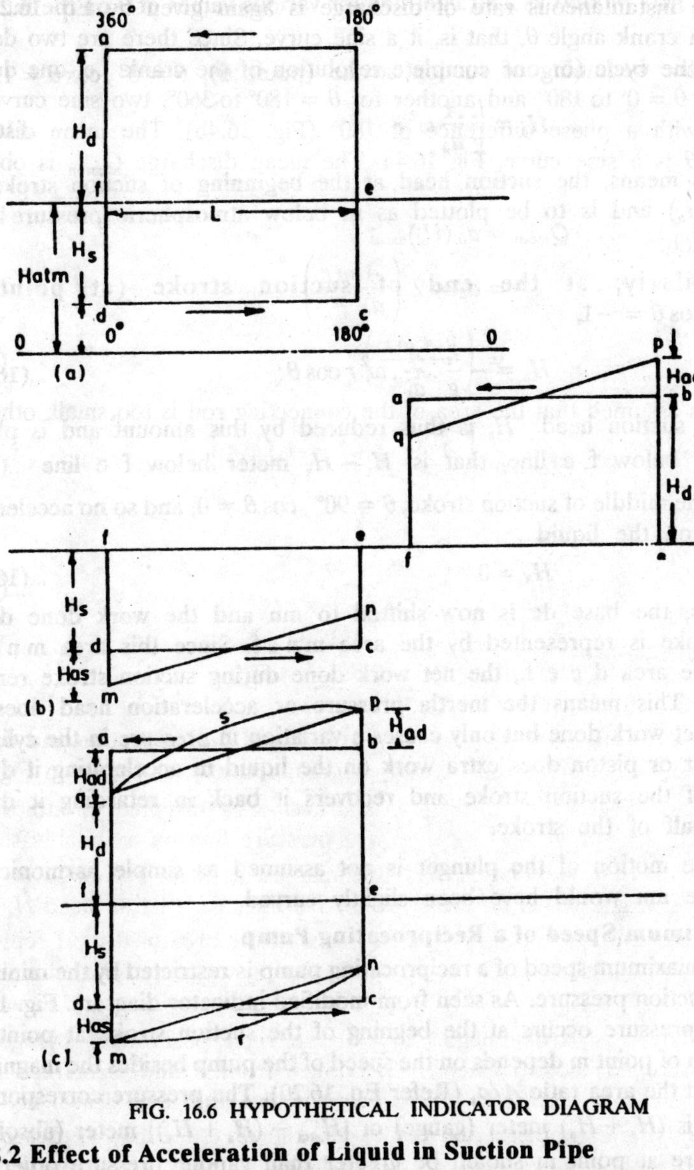

FIG. 16.6 HYPOTHETICAL INDICATOR DIAGRAM

16.8.2 Effect of Acceleration of Liquid in Suction Pipe

During the suction stroke, the acceleration head H_a acts on the liquid in the suction pipe. Therefore, the indicator diagram should be modified to take into account this acceleration head H_a, Let l_s and a_s be the length and area of the suction pipe respectively. The acceleration head H_a acting during the suction stroke is given by

$$H_a = \frac{l_s}{g}\frac{A}{a_s} \cdot \omega^2 r \cos\theta \qquad \text{...(16.20)}$$

This gets plotted as a straight line for various values of θ on the indicator diagram.

At the beginning of suction stroke (point d), $\theta = 0°$, $\cos \theta = 1$,

$$H_a = \frac{l_s}{g} \frac{A}{a_a} \omega^2 r \qquad \qquad ...(16.20a)$$

This means, the suction head at the beginning of suction stroke will be $(H_s + H_a)$ and is to be plotted as m below atmospheric pressure line fe in Fig. 16.6b.

Similarly, at the end of suction stroke (at point c), $\theta = 180°$, $\cos \theta = -1$,

$$H_a = -\frac{l_s}{g} \cdot \frac{A}{a_s} \cdot \omega^2 r \cos \theta \qquad \qquad ...(16.20b)$$

The suction head H_s is thus reduced by this amount and is plotted as point n below f. e line, that is, $H_s - H_a$ meter below f e line

At the middle of suction stroke, $\theta = 90°$, $\cos \theta = 0$, and so no acceleration head acts on the liquid

$$H_a = 0 \qquad \qquad ...(16.20c)$$

Thus, the base dc is now shifted to mn and the work done during suction stroke is represented by the area m n e f. Since this area m n e f is equal to the area d c e f., the net work done during suction stroke remains unaffected. This means the inertia pressure or acceleration head does not affect the net work done but only causes a variation in pressure in the cylinder. The plunger or piston does extra work on the liquid in accelerating it during first half of the suction stroke and recovers it back in retarding it during the later half of the stroke.

If the motion of the plunger is not assumed as simple harmonic, the straight line mn would have been slightly curved.

16.8.3 Maximum Speed of a Reciprocating Pump

The maximum speed of a reciprocating pump is restricted by the minimum allowable suction pressure. As seen from modified indicator diagram. Fig. 16.6b, the lowest pressure occurs at the begning of the suction stroke at point 'm'. The location of point m depends on the speed of the pump besides the magnitude of H_s, l_s and the area ratio A/a_s (Refer Eq. 16.20). The pressure corresponding to point m is $(H_s + H_a)$ meter (gauge) or $[H_{atm} - (H_s + H_a)]$ meter (absolute). This pressure at point m should be greater than vapour pressure otherwise, the separation of flow may take place in the pump cylinder and cavitation may start in the pump. If the atmospheric pressure and vapour pressure be assumed as 10.3 meter and 2.8 meter of water (absolute) respectively, then,

$$[H_{atm} - (H_s + H_a)] \; \not> \; (10.3 - 2.8)$$

$$\not> \; 7.5 \text{ metre (absolute) of water}$$

In the limiting case, the pressure at m may be allowed to occur equal to vapour pressure of liquid in absolute units.

$$H_{atm} - (H_s + H_a) = H_v$$

or $\quad (H_{atm} - H_v) = (H_s + H_a) = H_{sep}$

Substituting the value of H_a from Eq. 16.20,

$$H_s + \frac{l_s}{g} \frac{A}{a_s} . \omega^2 r = H_{sep} \qquad ...(16.36)$$

The maximum speed of the pump can be determined from Eq. 16.36. In designing of pump, the necessary condition is that the point m should not fall below separation pressure H_{sep} and this condition may be met by varying the values of $H_s, l_s,$ the area ratio A/a_s and the speed of the pump.

16.8.4 The Effect of Acceleration of Liquid in the Delivery Pipe

As discussed earlier, the liquid flowing in the delivery pipe is also accelerated due to the acceleration of plunger. The length delivery pipe is much more longer than the suction pipe and thus the acceleration head built up in the delivery pipe may be quite high. let l_d be the length and a_d be the area of delivery pipe then from Eq. 16.20.

$$H_{ad} = \frac{l_d}{g} \frac{A}{a_d} . \omega^2 r \cos \theta \qquad ...(16.20)$$

At the beginning of delivery stroke, $\theta = 0°$, $\cos \theta = 1$

$$H_{ad} = \frac{l_d}{g} \frac{A}{a_d} . \omega^2 r \qquad ...(16.20a)$$

At the middle of stroke, $\theta = 90°$, $\cos \theta = 0$,

$$H_{ad} = 0 \qquad ...(16.20b)$$

And, at the end of stroke, $\theta = 180°$, $\cos \theta = -1$,

$$H_{ad} = - \frac{l_d}{g} . \frac{A}{a_d} . \omega^2 r \qquad ...(16.20c)$$

Thus the plunger or piston is accelerated at the beginning of the delivery stroke and retarded at the end of delivery stroke and it is zero at the middle of stroke. The magnitude of pressure head acting on the plunger at the beginning of stroke is $(H_d + H_a)$ metre and at the end of stroke is $(H_d - H_a)$ metre above the atmospheric pressure.

Thus the acceleration head H_a is added at the beginning of stroke (i.e. at point b) and substracted at the end of delivery stroke (at point a) in Fig. 16.6b. This gets plotted as point p and q respectively in the indicator diagram. These are then joined by a straight line pq. Thus the base line a b is shifted to pq is Fig. 16.6b. And the modified indicator diagram f e p q is obtained. The area of f e p q represents the work done by the plunger during delivery stroke on some scale. Since this area f e p q is same as that of rectangle f e b a, the net work done during delivery stroke remains the same.

The pressure at the beginning of delivery stroke is $(H_d + H_a)$ metre above atmospheric pressure (corresponding point is p) whereas it is $(H_d - H_a)$ metre above atmospheric pressure at the end of delivery stroke (corresponding point is q is Fig. 16.6b). In absolute units the minimum pressure at the end of delivery stroke becomes $(H_{atm} + H_d - H_a)$ metre. For cavitation free performance of the pump, this pressure must not be less than 2.8 metre of water (vapour pressure of liquid). The limiting condition, therefore, occurs when

$$10.3 + H_d - H_a = 2.8$$
$$H_a = 7.5 + H_d \qquad \qquad ...(16.37)$$

The delivery pipe of a reciprocating pump can be arranged in either of the two ways as shown in Fig. 16.7. Let the length of delivery pipe l_d and delivery static lift H_d be same in both the cases shown in Fig. 16.7a and b. The condition as regards pressure, etc. at point Y and Y_1 will be same in both these cases because the magnitude of H_d and H_a are same at these points. But in the first arrangement (a), there is no delivery head remaining beyond Y, that is, H_d is zero. But still there is sufficient length of pipe in which acceleration head will be built up. Hence, the net pressure at Y in case 'a' may be negative at the end of delivery stroke. Hence, the separation of flow may take place at the bend Y. In the second arrangement, the pipe is first horizontal and then it is vertical so still there is sufficient height left beyong point Y_1 by which the liquid is to be lifted. Therefore, in this case there is no possibility of separation (since -ve value of H_a could be neutralised by +ve value of H_d).

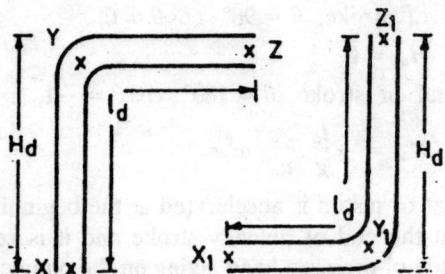

FIG. 16.7 VARIOUS ARRANGEMENTS OF DELIVERY PIPE.

16.8.5 Work Done Against Friction

As the water flows through suction and delivery pipe, it experiences the resistance due friction. The head loss due to friction can be computed using Darcy Weisbach equation, Eq. 7.51.

$$h_f = f \frac{l}{d} \frac{U^2}{2g}$$

where U is the velocity of flow in the pipe. But in this case the velocity U is found to vary with crank angle θ during both the strokes, Eq. 16.18.

$$U_s = \frac{A}{a_s} \omega r \sin \theta \qquad \qquad ...(16.18)$$

Thus the head lost in friction in suction pipe of length l_s and area a_s is given by

$$h_{fs} = \frac{f}{2g} \cdot \frac{l_s}{a_s} \left(\frac{A}{a_s} \cdot \omega r \sin \theta \right)^2 \qquad ...(16.38)$$

where f is the Darcy's coefficient of friction for suction pipe.

The head loss h_{fs} is found to vary with square of $\sin\theta$, that is, the relationship between h_{fs} and θ is parabolic and is shown plotted in Fig. 16.6c,

At the beginning of suction stroke, $\theta = 0$, $\sin\theta = 0$

$$h_{fs} = 0 \qquad ...(16.38a)$$

At the middle of suction stroke, $\theta = 90°$, $\sin\theta = 1$

$$h_{fs} = \frac{f}{2g} \frac{l_s}{d_s} \cdot \left(\frac{A}{a_s} \omega r \right)^2 \qquad ...(16.38b)$$

And at the end of suction stroke, $\theta = 180°$, $\sin\theta = 0$

$$h_{fs} = 0 \qquad ...(16.38c)$$

Similar expressions for head lost due to friction in the delivery pipe can be derived.

$$h_{fd} = \frac{f}{2g} \cdot \frac{l_d}{a_d} \left(\frac{A}{a_d} \omega r \sin \theta \right)^2 \qquad ...(16.39)$$

At the beginning of delivery stroke, $\theta = 0$, $\sin\theta = 0$

$$h_{fd} = 0 \qquad ...(16.39a)$$

At the middle of delivery stroke, $\theta = 90°$, $\sin\theta = 1$

$$h_{fd} = \frac{f}{2g} \cdot \frac{l_d}{d_d} \left(\frac{A}{a_d} \omega r \right)^2 \qquad ...(16.39b)$$

And, at the end of delivery stroke, $\theta = 180°$, $\sin\theta = 0$

$$h_{fd} = 0 \qquad ...(16.39c)$$

The work done against friction can now be added to the indicator diagram. In Fig. 16.6c, the parabola m r n represents the work done against friction during suction stroke.

Work done during suction stroke

$$= \text{area e f m r n}$$
$$= \text{area (e f d c + m r n)} \qquad ...(16.40a)$$

Similarly, the work done against friction during delivery stroke is represented by the parabola q p s and is added to the indicator diagram

Work done during delivery stroke

$$= \text{area f e p s q}$$
$$= \text{area (f e b a + p s q)} \qquad ...(16.40b)$$

Since the mean ordinate of a parabola is equal to two third of the maximum ordinate.

The mean ordinate of parabola (suction stroke)

$$= \frac{2}{3} h_{fs} = \frac{2}{3} \cdot \frac{f}{2g} \cdot \frac{l_s}{d_s} \left(\frac{A}{a_s} \omega r \right)^2 \qquad ...(16.41a)$$

Similarly, the mean ordinate of parabola (delivery stroke)

$$= \frac{2}{3} h_{fd} = \frac{2}{3} \cdot \frac{f}{2g} \cdot \frac{l_s}{d_d} \left(\frac{A}{a_d} \omega r \right)^2 \qquad ...(16.41b)$$

Let W be the weight of liquid pumped per second in one cycle of a single acting pump, then,

$$W = w \cdot \frac{A L N}{60} = w \cdot \frac{A 2r N}{60}$$

Total work done per second during suction stroke is given by,

$$= W. \text{ (area e f d c + area m r n)}$$

$$= W \left(H_s + \frac{2}{3} h_{fs} \right) \qquad (16.42a)$$

Similarly, the work done per second during delivery stroke

$$= W \text{ (area f e b a + area p s q)}$$

$$= W \left(H_d + \frac{2}{3} h_{fd} \right) \qquad ...(16.42b)$$

The total work done per second in one revolution of the crank of a single acting pump is given by

$$= w \frac{A L N}{60} \left(H_s + H_d'' + \frac{2}{3} h_{fs} + \frac{2}{3} h_{fd} \right) \qquad ...(16.43)$$

The absolute pressure acting on the plunger or piston during suction stroke for any crank angle θ is given by

$$= H_{atm} - (H_s + H_a + h_{fs})$$

$$= H_{atm} - \left[H_s + \frac{l_s}{g} \cdot \frac{A}{a_s} \omega^2 r \cos \theta \right.$$

$$\left. + \frac{f}{2g} \cdot \frac{l_s}{d_s} \left(\frac{A}{a_s} \omega r \sin \theta \right)^2 \right] \qquad ...(16.44a)$$

The absolute pressure acting on the piston during the delivery stroke for crank angle θ is given by

$$= H_{atm} + (H_d + H_a + h_{fd})$$

$$= H_{atm} + \left[H_d + \frac{l_d}{g} \frac{A}{a_d} \cdot \omega^2 r \cos \theta \right.$$

$$\left. + \frac{f}{2g} \cdot \frac{l_d}{d_d} \left(\frac{A}{a_d} \cdot \omega r \sin \theta \right)^2 \right] \qquad ...(16.44b)$$

It is noticed from above expressions, that the acceleration head is maximum at the end of stroke and zero at the middle of it while the head lost due to friction is zero at the end of stroke and maximum at the middle of stroke.

16.9 AIR VESSELS

The reciprocating pump supplies water at variable rate. It is zero during the suction stroke and gradually increases during delivery stroke and becomes maximum at the middle of delivery stroke. The flow rate then gradually reduces to zero at the end of delivery stroke. Thus, the liquid is supplied intermittently and at variable rate. Moreover, the suction pressure at the beginning of suction stroke H_s is reduced by acceleration head H_a, that is, it becomes $(H_s - H_a)$ which may cause the separation of flow and cavitation in the pump. To avoid such problems, air vessels are connected on the suction as well as delivery pipes at a point close to the pump.

The air vessel is a large cast iron chamber, which is closed at the top and has an opening at its base. The liquid may flow through this opening. The upper portion of the air vessel is charged with compressed air which helps in maintaining uniform rate of flow beyond the location of air vessel.

The air vessels serve the following objectives:

(a) maintain almost constant flow through suction and delivery pipes.

(b) reduction in the acceleration head and thereby the likelyhood of separation of flow is minimised.

(c) reduction of head loss due to friction, since the liquid flows at uniform rate in the most part of both the pipes.

(d) allows higher speed of running of the reciprocating pump, and

(e) it allows the setting of the pump at a sufficiently higher elevation. This is so, because the acceleration head generated is quite small (l_{sv} is small in Fig. 16.8) and thus $H_s - H_{as}$ remains within permissible limit even for higher H_s.

16.9.1 Air Vessel on Delivery Pipe

Let an air vessel be connected to the delivery pipe at 'X' and let the length of delivery pipe, upto the location of air vessel, be l_{dv} and beyond it to the supply sump B, be l_d (Fig. 16.8).

The liquid flows almost at uniform rate in the delivery pipe beyond the location of air vessel throughout the complete cycle. But the liquid is accelerated in the cylinder by the acceleration of the plunger and thereby in the pipe length l_{dv} during the first half of the delivery stroke and decelerated during the later half of the delivery stroke. Thus, the pump supplies the liquid at more than the mean flow rate during almost the first half of the delivery stroke. This excess water is stored in the air vessel at X and the air in it is compressed. In the later half of the delivery stroke, the liquid in the cylinder and in the delivery pipe length l_{dv} is decelerated. Thus, the pump supplies the liquid at a gradually decreasing rate. (Refer Fig. 16.8, Q versus L, length of stroke). During this portion of delivery stroke, the pressure of liquid in the pipe length l_{dv} remains less than the pressure of air in the upper portion of the air vessel. This causes the liquid to be pushed out of air vessel and thus the liquid flows at a uniform rate in the delivery pipe beyond air vessel.

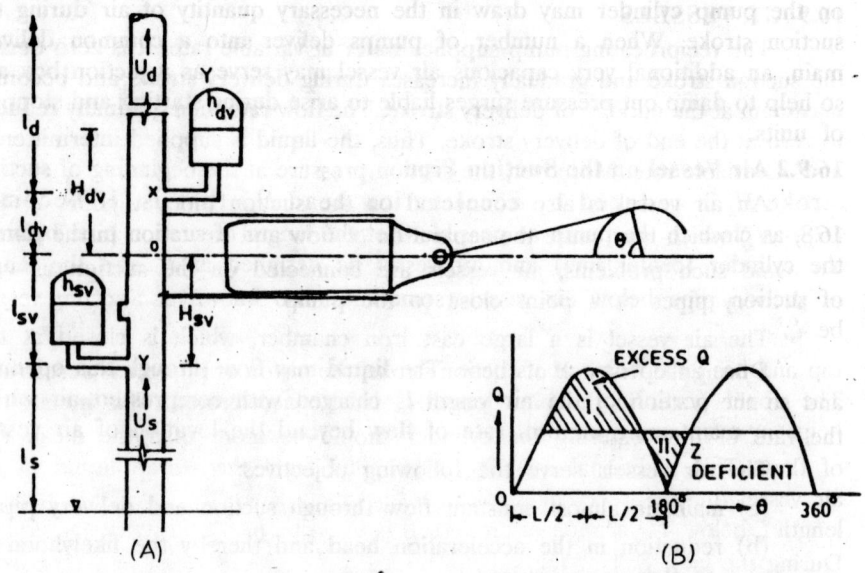

FIG. 16.8 (A) PUMP WITH AIR VESSEL (B) DISCHARGE CURVE.

Further, during suction stroke, no liquid is supplied by the pump. But the liquid from the air vessel continues to flow at uniform rate in the delivery pipe l_d beyond the location of air vessel during this suction stroke also. The flow from air vessel continues till the pressure of air in the air vessel and that of liquid on the pipe l_d becomes equal.

Thus, the water stored in the air vessel during delivery stroke volume 1 (shown shaded) is equal to the volume 2 (shown by hatched lines) in Fig. 16.8. In this way, almost uniform rate of flow is achieved in the delivery pipe (beyond point X) by fitting an air vessel on the delivery pipe. This also elimiates the creation of acceleration head H_a in the pipe length l_d (beyond the location of air vessel). In the pipe length l_{dv} (OX in the Fig. 16.8), the velocity of liquid fluctuates due to acceleration of plunger and correspondingly, the accelerating head H_{ad} is created in this length of pipe (which is quite small) and hence H_{ad} will also be too small.

As the liquid surface in the air vessel fluctuates the pressure of air may also fluctuate. This results in variation of pressure and velocity in the delivery pipe. These variation in pressure and velocity cause slight variation in the rate of flow of the liquid. The effect of the variation of air pressure in the air vessel may be reduced by making it large as compared to the area of the delivery pipe. Usually, it is sufficient to provide the volume of air vessel 6 to 9 times the capacity of the cylinder. Furthermore, some air contained in the upper portion of air vessel gets dissolved slowly into the liquid. Hence, the air in the air vessel must be renewed periodically. This is done in large pump by means of a special air compresser provided for the purpose; while in small pumps, an automatic air valve-a sniffing valv on the pump cylinder may draw in the necessary quantity of air during the suction stroke. When a number of pumps deliver into a common delivery main, an additional very capacious air vessel may serve as a juction box and so help to damp out pressure surges liable to arise during starting and stopping of units.

16.9.2 Air Vessel on the Suction Pipe

An air vessel is also connected on the suction pipe at point Y, Fig. 16.8, as close to the pump as possible. Let the length of suction pipe between the cylinder (center line) and air vessel be designed as l_{sv} and the length of suction pipe below air vessel (sometimes also known as vaccum vessel) be l_s.

During the first half of suction stroke, the piston or plunger is accelerated and so the water in the pipe length l_{sv} is also accelerated. This means that the rate of flow entering the cylinder should be more than the mean rate of flow. This additional quantity is supplied from the stored liquid in the air vessel during preceding stroke. At the same time, the liquid in the pipe length l_s below Y (location of air vessel) is assumed to flow at uniform velocity. During the later half of the suction stroke, the piston or plunger is retarded and so the liquid in the pipe length l_{sv}. This means, the liquid enters the cylinder at a lesser rate than mean rate of flow obtaining in the pipe length l_s below the location of air vessel. the excess liquid is stored in the air vessel to be utilised in the first half of the next cycle. Thus, throughout the suction stroke, the liquid flows at a uniform velocity, $(U_s)_{mean}$ in the pipe length l_s. It is only the small length of suction pipe l_{sv}, in which the liquid is accelerated or decelerated. Hence, the magnitude of $(H_a)_s$ developed during the suction stroke is too small and therefore, the pump running becomes free of separation and cavitation.

16.10 RATE OF FLOW INTO OR FROM AIR VESSEL

Single acting pump : Consider first the case of single acting pump. The liquid in the delivery pipe beyond air vessel will have a uniform mean velocity throughout the cycle, while the liquid is supplied by the pump at variable rate during the delivery stroke and no liquid is supplied during the suction stroke. Referring Eqns. 16.23 and 16.27.

Instantaneous velocity of flow issuing out of cylinder

$$= \left(\frac{A}{a_d} . \omega r \sin \theta \right) \text{ m/s} \qquad ...(16.23a)$$

Instantaneous rate of flow coming our of cylinder

$$= (A \omega r \sin \theta) \text{ m}^3/\text{s} \qquad ...(16.27)$$

Velocity of flow beyond air vessel = mean velocity of flow

$$= \left(\frac{A}{a_d} . \frac{\omega r}{\pi} \right) \text{ m/s} \qquad ...(16.24)$$

Rate of flow beyond air vessel = mean rate of flow

$$= \left(\frac{A \omega r}{\pi} \right) \text{ m}^3/\text{s} \qquad \text{...(16.28)}$$

∴ Rate of flow from air vessel into the delivery pipe

$$= \left(\frac{A \omega r}{\pi} - A \omega r \sin \theta \right) \qquad \text{...(16.45)}$$

If this equation is positive for crank angle θ, the liquid is supplied from the air vessel into the delivery pipe and if it is negative, the liquid flows into the air vessel from the cylinder.

In case of the air vessel connected on the suction pipe, the liquid flows at uniform rate in the suction pipe 'l_s' below air vessel and at fluctuating rate in the suction pipe l_{sv} beyond air vessel. This means the flow condition is reversed as compared to delivery pipe. Hence, the liquid will flow out from air vessel into the cylinder if above expression, Eq. 16.45 is a negative quantity. And it will flow into the air vessel from the suction pipe (length l_s) if the expression, Eq. 16.45, is a positive quantity.

In case, no liquid either enters or flows out of the air vessel, Eq. 16.45 should be equated to zero.

$$\therefore \qquad \sin \theta = \frac{1}{\pi} \qquad \text{...(16.46a)}$$

That is $\theta = 18°34'$ or $161°26'$ $\qquad \text{...(16.46b)}$

Thus for crank angle $\theta = 0°$ to $18°34'$ and $161°26'$ to $180°$, the instantaneous rate of flow is less than the mean rate of flow while for θ lying between $18°34'$ and $161°26'$, it is more than the mean rate of flow (inset Fig. 16.8)

Double acting pump : Now consider a double acting pump. In this case also, the instantaneous rate of flow is still given by Eq. 16.27.

$$Q_d = A \omega r \sin \theta \qquad \text{...(16.27)}$$

The liquid flows at uniform rate in the pipe length beyond air vessel on delivery side as well as in the pipe below air vessel on suction side.

The mean rate of flow is given by Eq. 16.33.

$$(Q_d)_{mean} = \frac{2 A \omega r}{\pi} \qquad \text{...(16.33)}$$

∴ The rate of flow from the air vessel

$$= \left(\frac{2 A \omega r}{\pi} - A \omega r \sin \theta \right) \qquad \text{...(16.47)}$$

If the expression, Eq. 16.47 is a positive quantity, the liquid will flow out from the air vessel in the delivery pipe and if it is a negative, the liquid will flow into the air vessel from the cylinder.

Since the condition of flow is reversed in case of an air vessel connected to a suction pipe, the liquid will flow out of air vessel if the Eq. 16.47 yields a negative quantity and liquid will flow into the air vessel from the suction pipe (length l_s) below it. if Eq. 16.47 yields a positive quantity.

When no flow takes place either into or out of the air vessel, Eq. 16.47 should be equated to zero.

$$\left(2\frac{A\omega r}{\pi} - A\omega r \sin\theta \right) = 0$$

$$\sin\theta = \frac{2}{\pi} \qquad \qquad ...(16.48a)$$

$$\theta = 34°32' \text{ or } 145° 28' \qquad ...(16.48b)$$

Thus, for a double acting pump, the instantaneous rate of flow remains less than mean rate of flow for the range of θ between 0° to 34°32′ and 140°28′ to 180°. While for crank angle varying between 34°32′ and 140°28′, the instantaneous rate of flow is more than the mean flow rate.

16.11 PRESSURE HEAD IN THE CYLINDER DURING DELIVERY STROKE (WITH AIR VESSEL)

The pressure head in the cylinder during delivery stroke consists of static head H_d, accelerating head H_{ad} in the delivery pipe length l_{dv} (from the cylinder to the air vessel), the head loss due to friction h_{f1} and h_{f2} in the pipe length l_{dv} and l_d respectively and the velocity head $U_d^2/2g$.

$$H_t = (H_d + H_{ad} + h_{f1} + h_{f2} + U_d^2/2g) \qquad ...(16.49)$$

The acceleration head H_{ad} is given by Eq. 16.20

$$H_{ad} = A/a_d \times l_{dv}/g \times \omega^2 r \cos\theta \qquad ...(16.20)$$

The frictional head loss h_{f1} in the pipe length l_{dv} is given by Eq. 16.39

$$(h_{f1})_d = \frac{f}{2g} \cdot \frac{l_{dv}}{d_d} \cdot \left(\frac{A}{a_d} \cdot \omega r \sin\theta \right)^2 \qquad ...(16.50)$$

The liquid flows at uniform velocity in the pipe length l_d and therefore, the head loss $(h_{f2})_d$ due to friction is given by

$$(h_{f2})_d = f\frac{l_d}{d_d} \cdot \frac{U_d^2}{2g} \qquad ...(16.51)$$

where mean velocity $U_d = \frac{A}{a_d}\left(\frac{\omega r}{\pi} \right) = \frac{ALN}{60\, a_d}$

$$= \frac{A\, 2\, r\, N}{60\, a_d} \qquad ...(16.24)$$

Substituting these values of various terms in Eq. 16.49, the total pressure H_{td} (gauge units) in the cylinder is given by

$$H_{td} = \left[H_d + \frac{A}{a_d} \cdot \frac{l_{dv}}{g} \omega^2 r \cos\theta + \frac{f}{2g} \cdot \frac{l_{dv}}{d_d} \right.$$

$$\left. \times \left(\frac{A}{a_d} \omega r \sin\theta \right)^2 + \frac{f}{2g} \cdot \frac{l_d}{d_d} (U_d)^2 + \frac{U_d^2}{2g} \right] \qquad ...(16.52)$$

This equation is shown plotted in Fig. 16.9 as the modified indicator diagram.

In absolute units, the total pressure $(H_{td})_{abs}$ is given by

$$(H_{td})_{abs} = H_{atm} + (H_t)_d \qquad ...(16.53)$$

Sometimes, it is found that the magnitude of H_{ad}, h_{fl} and $U_d^2/2g$ are too small and can be neglected. In that case, one can write.

$$(H_{td})_{abs} \approx H_{atm} + \left[H_d + \frac{f}{2g} \cdot \frac{l_d}{d_d} \cdot U_d^2 \right] \qquad ...(16.54)$$

Further, the pressure of air in the air vessel is assumed to be approximately the same as that of liquid in the delivery pipe reckoned above some datum (say, centre line of the cylinder). If h_{dv} be assumed as the pressure in the air vessel and the liquid may be standing at a height of H_{dv} in the air vessel above the centre line of cylinder Fig. 16.8, then

$$h_{dv} + H_{dv} = H_{atm} + (H_{td})_{abs} \qquad ...(16.55)$$

From this expression, the pressure of air in the air vessel can be computed.

16.10.2 Pressure Head in the Cylinder During Suction Stroke
(with Air Vessel)

In the suffix 'd' in the above expressions is replaced by suffix 's' the corresponding expressions for suction sides can be obtained. Thus,

$$(H_a)_s = \frac{A}{a_s} \cdot \frac{l_{sv}}{g} \omega^2 r \cos\theta \qquad ...(16.20)$$

$$(h_{f1})_s = \frac{f}{2g} \cdot \frac{l_{sv}}{d_s} \left(\frac{A}{a_s} \cdot \omega r \sin\theta \right)^2 \qquad ...(16.56)$$

$$(h_{f2})_s = f \frac{l_s}{d_s} \cdot \frac{U_s^2}{2g} \qquad ...(16.57)$$

where
$$U_s = \frac{A}{a_s} \cdot \frac{\omega r}{\pi} = \frac{ALN}{60\, a_s} = \frac{A\, 2rN}{60\, a_s} \qquad ...(16.24)$$

The pressure head in the cylinder during suction stroke (with air vessel) in gauge units is given by Eq. 16.58 and is shown plotted in Fig. 16.9.

$$(H_t)_s = [H_s + H_{as} + (h_{f1})_s + (h_{f2})_s + U_s^2/2g] \qquad ...(16.58)$$

$$= \left[H_s + \frac{A}{a_s} \cdot \frac{l_{sv}}{g} \cdot \omega^2 r \cos\theta + \frac{f}{2g} \cdot \frac{l_{sv}}{d_s} \right.$$

$$\left. \times \left(\frac{A}{a_s} \omega r \sin\theta \right)^2 + \frac{f}{2g} \cdot \frac{l_{sv}}{d_s} \cdot U_s^2 + \frac{U_s^2}{2g} \right] \qquad ...(16.59)$$

The total pressure in the cylinder in the absolute units is given by

$$(H_{ts})_{abs} = H_{atm} - (H_t)_s \qquad ...(16.60)$$

Sometimes, it is found that the magnitude of $H_{as}, (h_{f1})_s$ and $U_s^2/2g$ are small and can be neglected.

$$(H_t)_{abs} = \left[H_{atm} - \left(H_s + f \frac{l_s}{d_s} \cdot \frac{U_s^2}{2g} \right) \right] \qquad ...(16.61)$$

The pressure of air in the air vessel connected to the suction pipe remains sub-atmospheric. Let this pressure of air be h_{sv} and the liquid level in the air vessel stands at H_{sv} below the centre line of the cylinder. The pressure of air is assumed to be approximately equal to the total pressure of liquid in the suction pipe below same datum, say, the centre line of cylinder.

$$\therefore \quad (H_t)_{abs} = \left[H_{atm} - \left(H_s + f \frac{l_s}{d_s} \cdot \frac{U_s^2}{2g} \right) \right] \qquad ...(16.61)$$

The pressure of air in the air vessel connected to the suction pipe remains sub-atmospheric. Let this pressure of air be h_{sv} below the centre line of the cylinder. The pressure of air is assumed to be approximately equal to the total pressure of liquid in the suction pipe below same datum, say, the centre line of cylinder

$$\therefore \quad [h_{sv} + H_{sv}] = [H_{atm} - (H_{ts})_{abs}] \qquad ...(16.62)$$

Eq. 16.62 can be used to determine the pressure of air in the air vessel.

16.12 MODIFIED INDICATOR DIAGRAM

The indicator diagram is modified by connecting the air vessel on the delivery and suction pipes. The total pressure obtaining in the cylinder during delivery stroke is given by Eq. 16.52 and during suction stroke is given by Eq. 16.59. These are shown plotted for Fig. 16.9. The frictional head loss $(h_{f1})_d$ and $(h_{f1})_s$ are plotted as parabolas on the respective side whereas the frictional head loss $(h_{f2})_d$ and $(h_{f2})_s$ are plotted as rectangles in this figure.

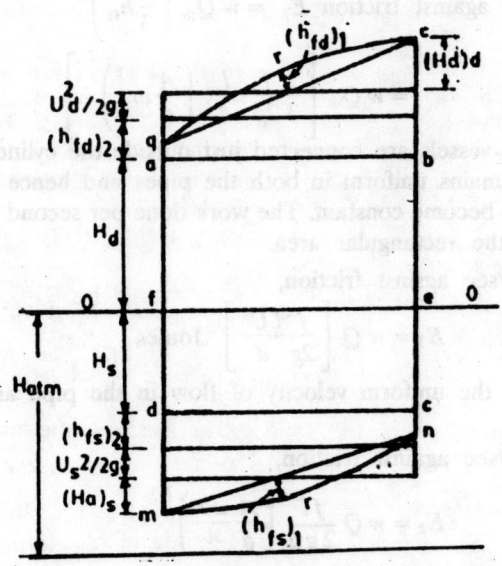

FIG. 16.9 MODIFIED INDICATOR DIAGRAM

16.13 WORK DONE BY A PUMP WITH AIR VESSEL

The theoretical work done per second by a reciprocting pump with air vessels fitted on both pipes suction as well as delivery one, is given by Eq. 16.63.

$$\text{Work done/sec} = w\,Q_{th}\left[H_s + H_d + \frac{2}{3}(h_{fl})_s + \frac{2}{3}(h_{fl})_d \right.$$

$$\left. + (h_{f2s} + h_{f2d}) + (U_s^2/2g + U_d^2/2g) \right] \qquad ...(16.63)$$

The acceleration heads H_{as} and H_{ad} do not affect the net work done and the frictional head loss $(h_{fl})_s$ and $(h_{fl})_d$ are used in Eq. 16.63 coresponding to crank angle $\theta = 90°$ (i.e. their maximum ordinate).

If the magnitude of $(h_{fl})_s$ and $(h_{fl})_d$ and velocity heads in these pipes be small, these can be neglected.

$$\therefore \text{Theoretical work done/sec} = W\,Q_{th}\,[(H_s + H_d) + (h_{f2})_s + (h_{f2})_d] \;...(16.64)$$

16.14 WORK SAVED BY FITTING AIR VESSEL

The following analysis applies equally to suction as well as delivery strokes.

Single acting pump : Firstly, consider the case of a single acting pump. If no air vessel is fitted with the pump, the pressure in the cylinder varies with crank angle θ and thereby the work done against friction h_{fl} also varies with crank angle θ. The work done against friction represented by a parabolic curve m r n, is given by E_1

$$\text{Work done against friction } E_1 = w\,Q_{th}\left(\frac{2}{3} h_{fl} \right)$$

$$= w\,Q_{th}\left[\frac{2}{3}\frac{f}{2g}\cdot\frac{l}{d}\cdot\left(\frac{A}{a}\omega r \right)^2 \right] \qquad ...(16.65)$$

Suppose air vessels are connected just outside the cylinder so that the velocity of flow remains uniform in both the pipes and hence the heads lost due to friction also become constant. The work done per second against friction is now given by the rectangular area.

Work done/sec agsinst friction,

$$E_2 = w\,Q\left[\frac{f}{2g}\frac{l\,U^2}{d} \right] \text{ Joules}$$

where U is the uniform velocity of flow in the pipe and is given by $(A/a)\,(\omega r/\pi)$.

$\therefore$ Work done/sec against friction,

$$E_2 = w\,Q\,\frac{fl}{2gd}\left(\frac{A}{a}\frac{\omega r}{\pi} \right)^2 \qquad ...(16.66)$$

Substracting Eq. 16.66 from Eq. 16.65.

Work saved/sec by fitting air vessel $= (E_1 - E_2)$

$$= w Q \frac{fl}{2gd} \left(\frac{A}{a} \omega r \right)^2 \left(\frac{2}{3} - \frac{1}{\pi^2} \right)$$

Percentage work saved/sec $= \dfrac{E_1 - E_2}{E_1}$

$$= \frac{2/3 - 1/\pi^2}{2/3} \times 100$$

$$= 84.8\% \qquad \qquad \dots(16.67)$$

Double acting pump: In this case also, the work done against friction E_1 remains same as for single acting pump Eq. 16.65 when no air vessel is connected to the pump.

When air vessels are connected on suction and delivery pipes, close to the pump cylinder, the velocity of flow in both the pipes remains uniform and is given by

$$(U)_{mean} = \frac{2A}{a} \frac{\omega r}{\pi}$$

∴ Work done per second against friction,

$$E_3 = w Q \frac{fl}{2gd} \left(2 \frac{A}{a} \frac{\omega r}{\pi} \right)^2 \text{ Joules} \qquad \dots(16.68)$$

Substracting Eq. 16.68 from Eq. 16.65,

Work saved by filtting air vessels $= (E_3 - E_1)$ Joules

$$= w Q \frac{fl}{2gd} \left(\frac{A}{a} \omega r \right)^2 \left(\frac{2}{3} - \frac{4}{\pi^2} \right) \qquad \dots(16.69)$$

Percentage work saved $\left(\dfrac{E_1 - E_3)}{E_3} \right) \times 100$

$$= \left(\frac{2/3 - 4/\pi^2}{2/3} \right) \times 100 = 39.2\% \qquad \dots(16.70)$$

16.14 MAXIMUM SPEED OF RECIPROCATING PUMP (WITH AIR VESSELS)

As discussed on section 16.8.3, the maximum speed of the pump is governed by the minimum pressure occuring in the cylinder during suction stroke. The minimum pressure in the cylinder should not fall below separation pressure at the beginning of suction stroke.

$$(H_s)_t = H_s + (H_a)_s + (h_{f2})_s + U_s^2/2g = H_{sep}$$

$$H_{sep} = \left[H_s + \frac{A}{a_s} \frac{l_{sv}}{g} \omega^2 r \cos \theta + f \frac{l_s}{d_s} \cdot \frac{U_s^2}{2g} + \frac{U_s^2}{2g} \right]$$

where velocity $U_s = \left(\dfrac{A}{a_s} \cdot \dfrac{\omega r}{\pi} \right)$

$$H_{sep} = \left[H_s + \frac{A}{a_s} \cdot \frac{l_{sv}}{g} \cdot \left(\frac{2\pi N}{60} \right)^2 r \cos\theta \right.$$

$$\left. + \frac{f l_s}{2 g d_s} \left(\frac{A}{a_s} \frac{\omega r}{\pi} \right)^2 + \frac{A}{a_s} \cdot \frac{\omega r}{\pi} \right] \qquad ...(16.71)$$

Using the limiting value of H_{sep} equal to 7.8 metre of water the maximum speed of hte reciprocating pump can be computed. Above equation gets slightly modified if small quantities are neglected.

$$H_{sep} = \left[H_s + \frac{f l_s}{2 g d_s} \cdot \left(\frac{A}{a_s} \cdot \frac{2\pi r N}{60} \right)^2 \right] \qquad ...(16.72)$$

16.15 PERFORMANCE OF RECIPROCATING PUMP

A reciprocating pump is required to work under different heads and to supply varying rates of discharge while running at speed N. The performance of a reciprocainting pump can be obtained by performing test on it. Mostly a reciprocating pump is expected to run at constant speed. Therefore, these test are performed at constant speed N by varying the pressure head H and recording the resultant discharge Q, the input power P and resultant efficiency η_0. Such curves are shown plotted in Fig. 16.10(a) and are known as 'operating characteristic curves'.

Under ideal conditions, the head discharge curve is a horizontal line meaning thereby that the discharge is independent of the head (Fig.16.10a). But in actual practice, some amount of the liquid leaks past the valves, plunger, etc in the pump. This results in a slightly. sloping straight line between H and Q.

The input power P verses head H curve for a reciprocating pump is also obtained as a straight line passing through origin while the pump runs at constant speed N. The output power from a pump can be obtained by substrating the losses from the input power P. These losses comprises of (1) mechanical losses(2) leakage losses and (3) hydraulic losses. When the pump runs at constant speed and supplies discharge at uniform rate under varying heads, the hydraulic losses remains substantially unchanged but the mechancial and leakage losses, both increase as the head on the pump increases. Hence, the ideal input power needed to be corrected and is shown plotted in Fig. 16.10 (b).

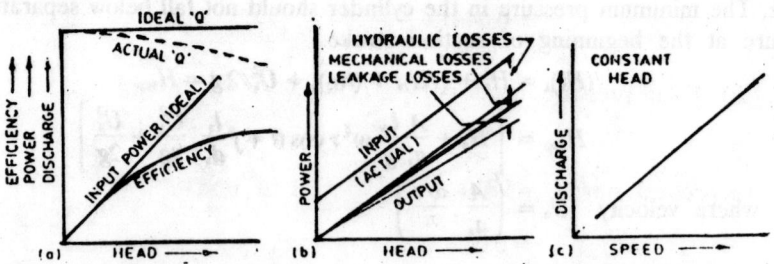

FIG. 16.10 CHARACTERISTIC CURVES FOR A RECIPROCATING PUMP

The ideal or theoretical efficiency verses head curve is also shown plotted in Fig. 16.10a. For a reciprocaitng pump, the maximum efficiency is as high as 0.95 or 95% or so is obtained.

Sometimes,. the reciprocaitng pumps are required to run at variable speed. The speed discharge curve for a reciprocating pump is shown plotted in Fig. 16.10 (c). It is observed that discharge veries lineraly with the speed as given by Eq. 16.1.

Example 16.1–16.12

16.1 A single acting reciprocating pump has a piston area of 0.15 m²
and a stroke of 30 cm. The cross sectional area of the delivery pipe is 0.03 m² and the water is lifted through a total height of 14 m. If the speed of the pump is 60 r.p.m. and the actual quantity of water lifted is 2650 lit/min, find the slip, the coefficient of discharge and the theoretical power required to derive the pump.

Solution

Given data: $A = 0.15$ m², $L = 0.3$ m, $a_d = 0.03$ m²,

$$H_s + H_d = 14 \text{ m}, \quad N = 60 \text{ rpm}, \quad Q_a = 2650 \text{ lit/min}$$

(i) Theoretical discharge of the pump

$$Q_{th} = \frac{A L N}{60}$$

$$= \frac{0.15 \times 0.3 \times 60}{60} = 0.045 \text{ m}^3/\text{s}$$

Actual discharge of the pump

$$Q_a = \frac{2650}{60 \times 1000} = 0.04416 \text{ m}^3/\text{s}$$

$$\text{Slip} = (Q_{th} - Q_a)$$

$$= (0.045 - 0.04416) = 0.00083$$

$$\% \text{ Slip} = \frac{0.00083}{0.045} \times 100 = 1.85\%$$

(ii) Coefficient of discharge

$$C_d = \frac{Q_a}{Q_{th}} \times 100$$

$$= \frac{0.04416}{0.045} \times 100 = 98.13\%$$

(iii) Total pressure head $= H_s + H_d$

$$= 14 \text{ m}$$

$$\text{Theoretical power} = 9810 \times \frac{2650}{1000 \times 60} \times 14 \text{ watts}$$

$$= 6.065 \text{ kW}$$

16.2 A single acting pump has a stroke of 0.3 m and a piston diameter of 15 cm. The centre of the pump is 5 m above water level in the sump and 3.5 m below delivery water level. The lengths of the suction and delivery pipes are 7 m and 40 m respectively and their diameters are 7.5 cm. The coefficient of friction for these pipes is 0.04. If the pump is working at 30 rpm, find the pressure head on the piston at the beginning, middle and end of both strokes and the power required to derive the pump. Neglect velocity head at the delivery end.

Solution

Given data $l_s = 7$ m, $l_d = 40$ m, $H_s = 5$ m,

$$H_d = 35 \text{ m}, \quad D = 0.15 \text{ m}, \quad d_s = d_d = 0.075 \text{ m},$$

$$N = 30 \text{ rpm}, \quad f = 0.04, \quad L = 2r = 0.3 \text{ m}.$$

At the two ends of the stroke, frictional head is zero whereas at the middle of stroke, the acceleration is zero.

(i) *Suction stroke*

At the beginning and end of stroke,

$$H_a = \frac{l_s}{g} \times \frac{A}{a_s} \times \omega^2 r$$

where

$$\omega = \frac{2\pi N}{60}$$

$$\omega = \frac{2\pi \times 30}{60}$$

$$= \pi \text{ rad/sec}$$

and

$$A/a = \left(\frac{0.15}{0.0075}\right)^2 = 4$$

∴

$$H_a = \frac{7}{9.81} \times \left(\frac{0.15}{0.075}\right)^2 \times (\pi)^2 \times \frac{0.3}{2}$$

$$= 4.22 \text{ m of water.}$$

At the middle of stroke,

$$h_{fs} = \frac{f l_s}{2 g d_s} \left(\frac{A}{a_s} \times \omega r\right)^2$$

$$= \frac{0.04 \times 7}{2 \times 9.81 \times 0.075} \times (4 \times \pi \times 0.15)^2$$

$$= 0.675 \text{ m}$$

Pressure at the beginning of stroke $= (H_s + H_a)$

$$= (5 + 4.22)$$

$$= 9.22 \text{ m of water (vacuum)}$$

Pressure at the end of stroke $= H_s - H_a$

$$= (5 - 4.22)$$

$$= 0.78 \text{ m of water (vaccum)}$$

Pressure at the middle of stroke $= (H_s + h_{fs})$

$$= (5 + 0.675)$$

$$= 5.675 \text{ m (vacuum)}$$

Delivery stroke

At the ends of stroke

$$H_a = \frac{l_d}{g} \times \frac{A}{a_d} \times \omega^2 r$$

$$= \frac{40}{9.81} \times \left(\frac{0.15}{0.075}\right)^2 \times \pi^2 \times 0.15 \quad (\because \omega = \pi \ rad/sec)$$

$$H_a = 24.12 \text{ m}$$

At the middle of stroke,

$$h_{fd} = \frac{f l_d}{2 g l_d} \times \left(\frac{A}{a_d} \times \omega r\right)^2$$

$$= \frac{0.04 \times 40}{2 \times 9.81 \times 0.075} (4 \times \pi \times 0.15)^2$$

$$= 3.86 \text{ m.}$$

Pressure at the beginning of stroke $= (H_d + H_a) = (35 + 24.12)$

$$= 59.12 \text{ m of water above atm. pressure}$$

Pressure at the end of stroke $= (H_d - H_a)$

$$= (35 - 24.12)$$

$$= 10.88 \text{ m of water above atm. pressure}$$

Pressure at the middle of stroke $= (H_d + h_{fd})$

$$= (35 + 3.86)$$

$$= 38.86 \text{ m of water above atm. pressure}$$

Work done/stroke $=$ Pressure $\times$ area $\times$ length

$$= w H \times \text{volume of cylinder}$$

$$= (\text{weight of water per stroke}) \times \text{head}$$

$$= WH$$

Weight W supplied per stroke

$$= 9810 \times \frac{\pi}{4} (0.15)^2 \times 0.3$$

$$= 51.98 \text{ N}$$

Work done during suction stroke $= W\left(H_s + \frac{2}{3} h_{fs}\right)$

$$= 51.98 \left(5 + \frac{2}{3} \times 0.675\right)$$

$$= 283.29 \text{ N-m}$$

Work done during delivery stroke

$$= W \left(H_d + \frac{2}{3} h_{fd} \right)$$

$$= 51.98 \left(35 + \frac{2}{3} \times 3.86 \right)$$

$$= 1953.0 \text{ N-m}$$

Total work done per revolution

$$= (283.29 + 1953) \text{ N-m}$$

$$= 2236.29 \text{ N-m}$$

$$\text{Power required} = \frac{2236.29 \times 30}{60} \text{ watts} \qquad (\text{Since } N = 30 \text{ rpm})$$

$$= 1118.15 \text{ watts.}$$

16.3 The following data pertains to a single acting reciprocating pump: Stroke L = 300 m, diameter of piston D = 125 mm, length of suction pipe l_s = 5 m, diameter of suction pipe d_s = 75 mm, suction head H_s = 3.0 m. Safe minimum pressure head = 2.0 m (absolute) and atmospheric pressure H_{atm} = 10.2 (absolute).

Determine the maximum speed at which it can be run without causing separation during suction stroke ?

Solution

Since the pressure head at the beginning of suction stroke will be minimum,

$$H_{sep} \leq [H_{atm} - (H_s + H_a)]$$

The acceleration head at the beginning of stroke,

$$(H_a)_s = \frac{l_s}{g} \times \left(\frac{A}{a_s} \right) \omega^2 r$$

$$= \frac{5}{9.81} \times \left(\frac{125}{75} \right)^2 \times \left(\frac{2 \times \pi \times N}{60} \right)^2 \times 0.15$$

$$= 0.00233 \text{ N}^2$$

Therefore, $\qquad 2 \leq [10.2 - (3 + 0.00233 \text{ N}^2)]$

or $\qquad 0.00233 \text{ N}^2 \leq 5.2$

or $\qquad\qquad N \leq 47.24 \text{ r.p.m.}$

Maximum speed of pump without causing secparation is 47.24 rpm.

16.4 A single acting reciprocating pump has a plunger 7.5 cm diameter and a stroke of 12.5 cm. It takes its supply from a pump 3.2 m below the pump through a pipe 5 m long and 3.1 cm diameter. It delivers to a tank 13.2 m above the pump through a 15 m long and 2.5 cm diameter. If separation occurs at 8.0 N/cm² below atmospheric pressure, find the maximum speed at which the pump may be operated without separation. Assume the SHM for the plunger of the pump.

Solution

Assuming the SHM, the maximum safe speed will correspond to the lowest point of the indictor diagram. Referring to Fig. 16.6.

Acceleration head at the beginning of suction stroke

$$H_a = \frac{l_s}{g} \times \frac{A}{a_s} \times \omega^2 r$$

$$= \left[\frac{5}{9.81} \times \left(\frac{0.075}{0.031} \right)^2 \times \left(\frac{0.125}{2} \right) \times \omega^2 \right]$$

(since $r = L/2$)

$$= 0.1865 \, \omega^2$$

Thus $\qquad H_{sep} = 8.0 \ \text{N/cm}^2$

$$= \frac{8.0 \times 10^4}{9810}$$

$$= 8.15 \ \text{m of water}$$

For limiting condition

$$H_{sep} = H_s + H_a$$

or $\qquad 8.15 = (3.2 + 0.1865 \, \omega^2)$

or $\qquad \omega = \sqrt{\dfrac{4.95}{0.1865}} = 5.152 \ \text{rad/sec}$

but $\qquad \omega = \dfrac{2\pi N}{60}$

$$N = \frac{60 \, \omega}{2\pi}$$

$$= \frac{60 \times 5.152}{2\pi}$$

$$= 49.22 \ \text{r.p.m.}$$

At the end of delivery stroke

$$H_{ad} = \frac{l_d}{d} \times \left(\frac{A}{a_d} \right) \times \omega^2 r$$

$$= \frac{15}{9.81} \times \left(\frac{0.075}{0.025} \right)^2 \times \left(\frac{0.125}{2} \right) \omega^2$$

$$= 0.86 \, \omega^2$$

For limiting condition,

$$H_{sep} = (H_{ad} - H_d)$$

$$8.15 = (0.86 \, \omega^2 - 13.0)$$

$$\omega = 4.96 \ \text{rad/sec.}$$

$$N = \frac{60 \, \omega}{2\pi}$$

$$= \frac{60 \times 4.96}{2 \times 3.14}$$

$$= 47.38 \ \text{r.p.m}$$

Thus the maximum speed of the pump for its safe running (no separation of flow) is 47.38 r.p.m.

16.5 A double acting reciprocating dump runs at 90 r.p.m. The diameter of the piston and stroke are 100 mm and 250 mm respectively. The suction pipe is 5 m long and 100 mm in diameter. Calculate the maximum permissible lift assuming no air vessel is fitted and separation occurs at 2 m of water absolute.

Solution

The acceleration head at the beginning of suction stroke is given by

$$(H_a)_s = \frac{l_s}{g} \times \frac{A}{a_s} \times \omega^2 r$$

where

$$\omega = \frac{2\pi N}{60}$$

$$= \frac{2\pi \times 90}{60} = 3$$

$$(H_a)_s = \frac{5}{9.81} \times \left(\frac{0.100}{0.100}\right)^2 \times (3\pi)^2 \times \left(\frac{0.250}{2}\right)$$

$$= 5.653 \ \text{m of water.}$$

The limiting condition, neglecting friction head loss in suction pipe is

$$H_{sep} \leq [H_a - (H_s + H_{as})]$$

$$2 \leq [10.3 - (H_s + 5.653)]$$

$$H_s \leq 2.643 \ \text{m.}$$

Maximum lift of the pump is 2.643 m.

16.6 A double acting recipocating pump has a cylinder 20 cm diameter and stroke of 40 cm. The pump delivers water to a height of 10 m through a pipe of 36 m long and 15 cm in diameter. A large air vessel is fitted in the delivery pipe at the level of pump but 2.5 m from the cylinder. If the pressure head in the cylinder at the beginning of delivery stroke is 12 m, find the speed of the pump in r.p.m. The head loss due to friction is given by the expression $h_f = \dfrac{0.03 \, l \, U^2}{2g \, d}$

Solution

The discharge through a double acting pump is given by

$$Q = \frac{2ALN}{60} \ \text{m}^3/\text{s}$$

But

$$\omega = 2\pi N/60$$

or
$$N = \frac{60\,\omega}{2\,\pi}$$

$$Q = 2\left(\frac{\pi D^2}{4} \times \frac{L}{60} \times \frac{60\,\omega}{2\,\pi}\right)$$

$$= \frac{D^2 L\,\omega}{4}$$

$$= \frac{(02)^2 \times 0.4 \times \omega}{4} = 0.004\,\omega \;\; \text{m}^3/\text{s}$$

Mean velocity

$$U = Q/a$$

$$= \frac{0.004\,\omega}{\pi\,(0.15)^2/4}$$

$$= 0.226\,\omega$$

The head loss due to frictioin in delivery pipe beyond air vessel

$$h_{\text{fd}} = 0.03 \times \frac{l_d}{d} \times \frac{U^2}{2g}$$

$$= 0.03 \times \frac{(36 - 2.5)}{0.15} \times \frac{(0.226\,\omega)^2}{2g}$$

$$= 0.01744\,\omega^2 \;\; \text{m. of water}$$

The acceleration head in this length 33.5 m is zero, i.e.

$$(H_a)_d = 0.0 \;\; \text{m.}$$

The acceleration head in 2.5 m of delivery pipe

$$(H_a)_d = \frac{l_{dv}}{g} \times \left(\frac{A}{a_d}\right) \times \omega^2 r$$

$$= \left[\frac{2.5}{9.81} \times \left(\frac{0.20}{0.15}\right)^2 \times (\omega^2) \times 0.20\right]$$

(since r = L/2)

$$= 0.09 \times \omega^2$$

Total pressure head in the cylinder during delivery stroke,

$$(H_t)_d = (H_d + h_{\text{fd}} + H_{ad} + \text{velocity head})$$

$$12 = (10 + 0.01744\,\omega^2 + \text{velocity head})$$

The velocity in delivery pipe $= \left(\dfrac{A}{a_d} \times \omega\,r\right)$

$$= \left(\frac{0.20}{0.15}\right)^2 \times \omega \times 0.2$$

$$= 0.355\,\omega$$

$$\therefore \qquad \frac{U_d^2}{2g} = \frac{(0.355\,\omega)^2}{2g} = 0.00644\,\omega^2$$

Hence
$$12 = 10 + (0.0174 + 0.9 + 0.00644)\,\omega^2$$

$$\omega^2 = 17.56$$

$$\omega = 4.19 \text{ rad/sec}$$

$$N = \frac{60\,\omega}{2\pi}$$

$$= \frac{60 \times 4.19}{2 \times \pi} = 40 \text{ r.p.m.}$$

16.7 A reciprocating pump draws water from a sump through a suction pipe 150 mm diameter and 12.5 m long, the water level being 3.2 m below the level of cylinder. The cylinder diameter is 225 mm, stroke 375 mm and the length of connecting rod is 1.5 m. The driving crank rotates at 20 r.p.m. Determine the pressure in the cylinder at the beginning of stroke (a) when no air vessel is fitted, (b) when air vessel is fitted at the cylinder level and distance 1.5 m from it. Assume $f = 0.04$

Solution

(1) No air vessel is fitted.

(a) Assuming simple harmonic motion,

$$(H_a)_s = \frac{l_s}{g} \times \left(\frac{A}{a_s}\right) \times \omega^2 r$$

$$= \frac{12.5}{9.81} \times \left(\frac{225}{150}\right)^2 \times \left(\frac{2\pi \times 20}{60}\right) \times \frac{0.375}{2}$$

$$H_{as} = 2.355 \text{ m of water}$$

Total pressure head in the cylinder
$$= (H_s + H_{as})$$
$$= (3.2 + 2.355)$$
$$= 5.555 \text{ m.}$$

(b) If simple harmonic motion is not assumed,

$$(H_a)_s = \frac{l_s}{g} \times \left(\frac{A}{a_s}\right) \times \omega^2 r \left(1 + \frac{r}{l_1}\right)$$

$$= 2.355 \left(1 + \frac{(0.375/2)}{1.5}\right)$$

$$= 2.649 \text{ m.}$$

Total pressure in the cylinder
$$= [H_s + (H_a)_s]$$
$$= [3.2 + 2.649]$$

(2) Air Vessel is fitted

Velocity of water in the suction pipe beyond air vessel,

$$U_s = \left(\frac{A}{a_s} \times \frac{\omega r}{\pi} \right)$$

$$= \frac{A}{a_s} \times \frac{2r \times N}{60} \qquad \left(\therefore \omega = \frac{2\pi N}{60} \right)$$

$$= \left(\frac{225}{150} \right)^2 \times 2 \times \frac{0.375}{2} \times \frac{20}{60}$$

$$= 0.281 \text{ m/s}$$

$$(h_{f1})_s = f \times \frac{l_s}{d_s} \times \frac{U_s^2}{2g}$$

$$= 0.04 \times \frac{(12.5 - 1.5)}{0.150} \times \frac{(0.281)^2}{2g}$$

$$= 0.0107 \text{ m of water}$$

(a) Assuming S.H. M.

$$(H_a)_s = \frac{l_s}{g} \times \left(\frac{A}{a_s} \right) \times \omega^2 r$$

$$= \left[\left(\frac{1.5}{9.81} \times \left(\frac{225}{150} \right)^2 \left(\frac{2\pi \times 20}{60} \right)^2 \times \frac{0.375}{2} \right) \right]$$

$$= 0.282 \text{ m of water.}$$

Total pressure head in the cylinder

$$= \left[H_s + (H_a)_s + (h_f)_s \right]$$

$$= \left[3.2 + 0.282 + 0.0107 \right]$$

$$= 3.4927 \text{ m of water below atmospheric pressure}$$

(b) If S.H.M. is not assumed

$$(H_a)_s = \frac{l_s}{g} \times \left(\frac{A}{a_s} \right) \times \omega^2 r \times (1 + r/l_1)$$

$$0.282 \times \left[1 + \frac{0.375/2}{1.5} \right]$$

$$= 0.3173 \text{ m}$$

Total pressure head in the cylinder.

$$= (H_s) + (H_a)_s + (h_f)_s$$

$$= (3.2 + 0.3173 + 0.0107)$$

$$= 3.528 \text{ m of water below atmospheric pressure}$$

16.8 In a reciprocating pump the velocity of water in the suction pipe varies from zero to U_s, the displacement being simple harmonic. Prove that the mean head loss due to friction, $(h_f)_s$ is given by

$$(h_f)_s = \frac{2}{3} \frac{fl_s \, U_s^2}{2g \, d_s}$$

where l_s and d_s are the length and diameter of the suction pipe respectively.

Solution

Referring to Fig. 16.5

$$x = r - r \cos\theta$$

$$\frac{dx}{dt} = \omega \, r \sin\theta ; \quad \text{where } \omega = d\theta/dt$$

∴ Velocity of water in suction pipe,

$$U_s = \frac{A}{a_s} \times \omega \, r \sin\theta \qquad \qquad ...(1)$$

Maximum velocity of water.

$$U_{max} = (U_s)_{max} = \frac{A}{a_s} \times \omega \, r \qquad \qquad ...(2)$$

From Eqs. (1) and (2)

$$U_s = U_{max} \sin\theta$$

$$U_s^2 = U_{max}^2 \, (1 - \cos^2\theta)$$

$$= U_{max}^2 \left[1 - \left(1 - \frac{x}{r} \right)^2 \right]$$

$$= U_{max}^2 \left(\frac{2x}{r} - \frac{x^2}{r^2} \right)$$

The head loss due to friction is given by

$$(h_f)_s = f \times \frac{l_s}{2g \, d_s} U_{max}^2 \left(\frac{2x}{r} - \frac{x^2}{r^2} \right)$$

The head loss due to friction $(h_f)_s$ varies with x^2, i.e. it is a parabolic with its maximum ordinate equal to $\dfrac{fl_s \, U_{max}^2}{2g \, d_s}$ at $x = r$.

Mean ordinate of the parabola $= \dfrac{2}{3} \times$ maximum ordinate

$$= \frac{2}{3} \left(f \frac{l_s}{d_s} \frac{U_s^2}{2g} \right)$$

16.9 A single acting reciprocating pumps has a piston 125 mm in diameter and 260 mm stroke and runs normally at 50 r.p.m. The axis of the barrel is horizontal and 4 m above the level of water in the sump. The suction pipe is 60 mm in diameter, 10 m long and has $f = 0.032$. An air vessel is fitted on the suction pipe close to the inlet valve to the cylinder. Calculate the work done during the suction stroke when (a) the pump runs at normal speed with air vessel functioning normally, (b) the air vessel is water logged and the pump runs at half the normal speed to avoid knocking.

Solution

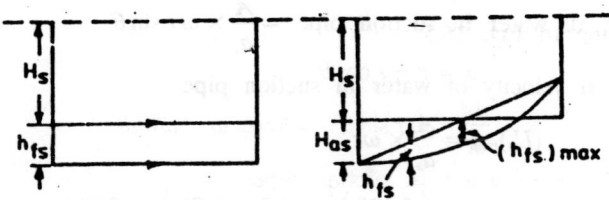

ZERO PRESSURE LINE

FIG. 16.11 EXAMPLE 16.9

(a) Air vessel functioning normally.

Discharge $\quad Q = \dfrac{2A\,rN}{60}$

The mean velocity of water in suction pipe.

$$U_s = \frac{Q}{a_s}$$

$$= 2r \times \left(\frac{A}{a_s}\right) \times \frac{N}{60}$$

$$= 0.260 \times \left(\frac{0.125}{0.060}\right)^2 \times \frac{50}{60}$$

$$= 0.94 \ \text{m/s}$$

The head loss due to friction

$$(h_f)_s = f\,\frac{l_s}{d_s}\frac{U_s^2}{2g}$$

$$= 0.032 \times \frac{10.0}{0.06} \times \frac{(0.94)^2}{2g}$$

$$= 0.24 \ \text{m,}$$

Net pressure on the piston $= w\,(H_s + h_{fs})$

$$= 9810\,(4 + 0.24) \ \text{N/m}^2$$

$$= 4.16 \ \text{N/cm}^2$$

Work done per stroke $= p \times A \times L$

$$= p \times A \times 2r$$

$$= (4.16 \times 10^4) \times \left(\frac{\pi}{4} \times 0.125^2\right) \times 0.260$$

$$= 132.665 \ \text{N-m}$$

(b) Air vessel is water logged : Refer to Fig. 16.11. In this case the water in the pipe will accelerate and will have maximum acceleration head H_{as}.

Velocity of water in suction pipe $= \dfrac{A}{a_s} \times \omega r \sin\theta$

Maximum velocity of water in suction pipe

$$(U_s)_{max} = \dfrac{A}{a_s} \times \omega r$$

$$(U_s)_{max} = \left(\dfrac{0.125}{0.060} \right)^2 \times \left(\dfrac{2\pi \times 25}{60} \right) \times \dfrac{0.260}{2}$$

$$(U_s)_{max} = 1.476 \text{ m/s}$$

Mean head loss due to friction

$$= \dfrac{2}{3} \times f \times \dfrac{l_s}{d_s} \times \dfrac{(U_s)^2_{max}}{2g}$$

$$= \dfrac{2}{3} \times 0.032 \times \dfrac{100}{0.06} \times \dfrac{(1.476)^2}{2 \times 9.81}$$

$$= 0.3948 \text{ m}$$

Mean pressure during suction stroke

$$= w (H_s + h_{f_s})$$

$$= 9810 (4 + 0.3948) \text{ N/m}^2$$

$$= 4.31 \text{ N/cm}^2$$

Work done per stroke

$$= \dfrac{4.31}{4.16} \times 132.665$$

$$= 137.45 \text{ N-m}$$

16.10 A double acting reciprocating pump has the following details. $D = 200$ mm. $L = 350$ mm, $N = 30$ r.p.m. If an air vessel in fitted on the suction side, determine the crank angle at which discharge to or from air vessel is zero. Also determine the discharge to or from the air vessel at an angle of $60°$.

Solution

Speed of the crank

$$\omega = \dfrac{2\pi N}{60}$$

$$\omega = \dfrac{2 \times 3.14 \times 30}{60} = 3.14 \text{ rad/sec.}$$

Instantaneous velocity of flow through suction pipe

$$= \frac{A}{a_s} \times \omega r \sin \theta$$

Instantaneous rate of flow going into cylinder

$$\doteq \left(\frac{A}{a_s} \times \omega r \sin \theta \right) \times a_s$$

$$= A \, \omega r \sin \theta \qquad \qquad ...(i)$$

Mean velocity of flow in the suction pipe before the location of air vessel

$$= \left(\frac{A}{a_s} \times \frac{\omega r}{\pi} \right)$$

Mean rate of flow in the suction pipe

$$= 2 \left(\frac{A}{a_s} \times \frac{\omega r}{\pi} \right) \times a_s$$

$$= 2 \left(\frac{A \, \omega r}{\pi} \right) \qquad \qquad ...(ii)$$

Rate of flow into or from the air vessel Q_a

$$= \left(\frac{2A \, \omega r}{\pi} - A \, \omega r \sin \theta \right) \qquad \qquad ...(iii)$$

The water will be supplied by the air vessel, if the sign of Q_s is –ve and it will be entering into the air vessel, if Q_a is +ve

Q_a will be zero when $\sin \theta = \dfrac{2}{\pi}$

At $\theta = 60°$, Discharge supplied by air vessel.

$$Q_a = \frac{\pi}{4} (0.2)^2 \times \left(\frac{0.350}{2} \right) \times \left(\frac{2\pi \times 30}{60} \right) \left[\frac{2}{\pi} - \sin 60° \right]$$

$$= 0.00395 \ \text{m}^3/\text{s}$$

16.11 A reciprocating pump has the following dimensions. Determine the power required to derive it, if the efficiency of the pump is 84%. Data given are

$D = 150$ mm, $L = 200$ mm, $N = 60$ r.p.m.

$d_s = 75$ mm, $l_s = 10$ m, $H_s = 3.0$ m.

$d_d = 50$ mm, $l_d = 40$ m, $H_d = 25$ m

Air vessels are fitted at 3 m and 5 m on the suction and delivery side respectively

Solution

Discharge $\qquad Q = \dfrac{A L N}{60}$

$$= \frac{\pi}{4} \times (0.15)^2 \times \frac{0.20 \times 60}{60}$$

$$= 0.00353 \ \text{m}^3/\text{s}$$

angular speed $\quad \omega = \dfrac{2 \pi N}{60}$

$$= \dfrac{2 \times 3.14 \times 60}{60} = 6.28 \ \text{rad/s}$$

Mean velocity on suction side

$$U_s = \left(\dfrac{Q}{a_s} \right)$$

$$= \dfrac{0.00353}{\pi/4 \times (0.075)^2} = 0.799 \ \text{m/s}$$

Mean velocity on delivery side

$$U_d = \left(\dfrac{Q}{a_d} \right)$$

$$= \dfrac{0.00353}{\pi/4 \times (0.05)^2} = 1.798 \ \text{m/s}$$

Instantaneous velocity in suction pipe

$$= \dfrac{A}{a_s} \times \omega \, r$$

$$= \left(\dfrac{0.150}{0.075} \right)^2 \times 6.28 \times \dfrac{0.2}{2} = 2.512 \ \text{m/s}$$

Instantaneous velocity in delivery pipe

$$= \dfrac{A}{a_d} \times \omega \, r$$

$$= \left(\dfrac{0.150}{0.050} \right)^2 \times 6.28 \times \dfrac{0.2}{2} = 5.65 \ \text{m/s}$$

Referring to Fig. 16.9,

Total pressure $(H_t)_s$ during suction stroke,

$$= \left[H_s + f \dfrac{(l_s - l_{sv})}{d_s} \times \dfrac{U_s^2}{2g} + \dfrac{2}{3} \times \dfrac{f}{2g} \times \dfrac{l_{sv}}{d} \times \left(\dfrac{A \omega r}{a_s} \right)^2 \right]$$

$$= \left[3.0 + \dfrac{0.03 \times (10 - 3)}{0.075} \times \dfrac{(0.799)^2}{2g} + \dfrac{2}{3} \times \dfrac{0.03 \times 3}{0.075} \times \dfrac{(2.512)^2}{2g} \right]$$

$$= [3.0 + 0.0091 + 0.257]$$

$$= 3.348 \ \text{m}$$

Total pressure $(H_t)_d$ during delivery stroke

$$= \left[H_d + f \dfrac{(l_d - l_{dv})}{d_d} \times \dfrac{U_d^2}{2g} + f \dfrac{l_{dv}}{d_d} \left(\dfrac{A \omega r}{a_d} \right)^2 \right]$$

$$= \left(25 + 0.03 \times \dfrac{(40 - 5)}{0.050} \times \dfrac{(1.798)^2}{2g} + \dfrac{2}{3} \times \dfrac{0.03 \times 5}{0.05} \times \dfrac{(5.65)^2}{2g} \right)$$

$$= (25 + 3.46 + 3.25)$$
$$= 31.71 \text{ m}$$

$$\text{Power required} = \frac{w\,Q\,(H_{ts} + H_{td})}{\eta_0}$$

$$= \frac{9810 \times 0.00353\,(3.348 + 31.71)}{0.84} \text{ watts}$$

$$= 1.445 \text{ kW}$$

16.12 Calculate the work saved in overcoming friction by fitting large air vessels near the suction and delivery valves of a reciprocating pump of the following specifications. Pump is single acting and has single cylinder, speed 60 rpm, diameter of the cylinder = 200 mm, stroke 350. mm; delivery pipe 100 mm diameter and 50 m long; suction pipe 150 mm diameter and 8 m long. Take Darcy's friction coefficient f = 0.04. Water is supplied by this pump.

Solution

Discharge $\quad Q = \dfrac{A\,L\,N}{60}$

$$= \frac{\pi}{4} \times (0.2)^2 \times \frac{0.350 \times 60}{60}$$

$$= 0.011 \text{ m}^3/\text{s}$$

Work done/sec against friction (without air vessel)

$$E_1 = w\,Q\left(\frac{2}{3}\,h_f\right)$$

$$= w\,Q\,\frac{2}{3}\left(\frac{f\,l_s}{2\,g\,d_s}\right)\left(\frac{A}{a_s}\cdot \omega\,r\right)^2$$

Work done/sec against friction (with air vesel)

$$E_2 = w\,Q\,h_{fs}$$

$$= w\,Q \times \frac{f\,l_s}{d_s} \times \frac{U_s^2}{2g}$$

$$= w\,Q \times \left(\frac{f\,l_s}{2\,g\,d_s}\right) \times \left(\frac{A}{a_s}\cdot \frac{\omega\,r}{\pi}\right)^2$$

Work saved/sec on suction side,

$$E_3 = w\,Q\,\frac{f\,l_s}{2\,g\,d_s}\left(\frac{A\,\omega\,r}{a_s}\right)^2\left(\frac{2}{3} - \frac{1}{\pi^2}\right) \qquad (1)$$

Similarly work saved/sec on delivery side

$$E_4 = w\,Q\left(\frac{f\,l_d}{2\,g\,d_d}\right) \times \left(\frac{A\,\omega\,r}{a_d}\right)^2\left(\frac{2}{3} - \frac{1}{\pi^2}\right) \qquad (2)$$

Mean velocity of flow in the suction pipe

$$U_d = \left(\frac{A}{a_s} \times \frac{\omega r}{\pi} \right)$$

$$= \left(\frac{0.20}{0.15} \right)^2 \times \frac{2\pi \times 60}{60} \times \frac{0.350}{2} \times \frac{1}{\pi}$$

$$= 0.622 \, m/s$$

Mean velocity of flow in the delivery pipe

$$U_d = \frac{A}{a_d} \times \left(\frac{\omega r}{\pi} \right)$$

$$U_d = \left(\frac{0.2}{0.1} \right)^2 \times \frac{2\pi \times 60}{60} \times \frac{0.35}{2 \times \pi}$$

$$= 1.4 \, m/s$$

$$\left(\frac{A \omega r}{a_s} \right) = 0.622 \, \pi$$

$$\frac{A \omega r}{a_d} = 1.4 \, \pi$$

From Eq. 1,

$$E_3 = 9810 \times 0.011 \times \frac{0.04 \times 8}{2 \times 9.81 \times 0.15}$$

$$\times \left(0.622 \, \pi \right)^2 \left(\frac{2}{3} - \frac{1}{\pi^2} \right)$$

$$= 25.28 \text{ watts or } 0.02528 \text{ kW}$$

From Eq. 2,

$$E_4 = 9810 \times 0.011 \times \left(\frac{0.04 \times 50}{2 \times 9.81 \times 0.10} \right)$$

$$\times (1.4\pi)^2 \left(\frac{2}{3} - \frac{1}{\pi^2} \right)$$

$$= 1201.553 \text{ watts or } 1.2015 \text{ kW}$$

Total work saved/sec

$$= (25.28 + 1201.553) \text{ watts}$$

$$= 1.226 \text{ kW}.$$

Objective Questions

16.1 The coefficient of discharge of a reciprocating pump is given by

(a) $\dfrac{A \, L \, N}{60 \, Q_a}$

(b) $\left(\dfrac{A \, L \, N}{60} - Q_a \right)$

(c) $\dfrac{60 \, Q_a}{A \, L \, N}$

(d) $\left(\dfrac{A \, L \, N}{60} + Q_a \right)$

(e) none.

16.2 The percentage slip of a reciprocating pump is defined as

(a) $(Q_{th} - Q_a)/Q_{th}$

(b) $(Q_{th} + Q_a)/Q_{th}$

(c) $Q_{th} \times Q_a$

(d) $(Q_a - Q_{th})/Q_a$

(e) none.

16.3 The work done per second by a two cylinder double acting reciprocating pump is

(a) $\dfrac{w\,A\,L\,N}{60}\,(H_s + H_d)$

(b) $\dfrac{2\,w\,A\,L\,N}{60}\,(H_s + H_d)$

(c) $4\,w\,\dfrac{A\,L\,N}{60}\,(H_s + H_d)$

(d) $2\,w\,\dfrac{A\,L\,N}{60}\,(H_s - H_d)$

(e) none.

16.4 The mean velocity of flow in the delivery pipe is expressed as

(a) $\dfrac{A}{a_d}\,\omega\,r$

(b) $\dfrac{A}{a_d}\,\omega\,r^2$

(c) $\dfrac{A}{a_d}\,\dfrac{\omega\,r}{\pi}$

(d) $\dfrac{A\,\omega\,r\,\pi}{a_d}$

(e) none.

16.5 The limiting velocity of a reciprocating pump is governed by

(a) $H_s + H_a = H_v$

(b) $H_{atm} + H_s + H_a = H_v$

(c) $H_{atm} - (H_s + H_a) = H_v$

(d) $H_v + H_a = H_s$

(e) none.

16.6 The work done/second per unit weight against friction of water is given by

(a) $\left(H_s + \dfrac{f\,l_s}{d_s}\,\dfrac{U_s^2}{2g} \right)$

(b) $\left(H_s + \dfrac{2\,f\,l_s}{3}\,\dfrac{U_s^2}{d_s}\,\dfrac{1}{2g} \right)$

(c) $\left[H_s + \dfrac{2\,f\,l_s}{3\,g\,d_s}\left(\dfrac{A\,\omega\,r}{\pi}\right)^2 \right]$

(d) $\left[H_s + \dfrac{2}{3}\left(\dfrac{f\,l_s}{2g\,d_s}\right)\dfrac{(A\,\omega\,r)^2}{\pi} \right]$

(e) none.

16.7 The total work done per second per revolution of the crank of a reciprocating pump is expressed as

(a) $W\,(H_s + H_d + H_{as} + H_{ad} + h_{fs} + h_{fd})$

(b) $W\,(H_s + H_d + h_{fs} + h_{fd})$

(c) $W\left(H_s + H_d + \dfrac{1}{3}\,h_{fs} + \dfrac{1}{3}\,h_{fd} \right)$

(d) $W\left(H_s + H_d + \dfrac{2}{3}\,h_{fs} + \dfrac{2}{3}\,h_{fd} \right)$

(e) none.

16.8 The rate of flow from air vessel into delivery pipe of a double acting reciprocating pump is given by

(a) $A\,\omega\,r\left(\dfrac{2}{\pi} - \sin\theta \right)$

(b) $A\,\omega\,r\left(\dfrac{2}{\pi} + \sin\theta \right)$

(c) $A\,\omega\,r\left(\dfrac{1}{\pi} + \sin\theta \right)$

(d) $A\,\omega\,r\left(\dfrac{1}{\pi} - \sin\theta \right)$

(e) none.

16.9 The acceleration head in the pipe length between the location of air vessel and centre line of the cylinder of reciprocating pump is expressed as

(a) $\dfrac{A}{a_s}\dfrac{l_{sv}}{g}\omega^2 r\cos\theta$

(b) $\dfrac{A}{a_s}\dfrac{l_{sv}}{g}\omega r\cos\theta$

(c) $\dfrac{A}{a_s}\dfrac{l_{sv}}{g}\omega r\sin\theta$

(d) $\dfrac{A}{a_s}\dfrac{l_{sv}}{g}\omega^2 r\sin\theta$

(e) None

16.10 The percentage work saved per second by a double acting reciprocating pump is

(a) 84.8 %   (b) 39.2 %   (c) 50 %

(d) 66.67 %   (e) none.

16.11 The maximum efficiency of reciprocating pump is as high as

(a) 65 %   (b) 75 %   (c) 85 %

(d) 95 %   (e) 100 %

Problem

16.1 Define slip, negative slip and coefficient of discharge of a reciprocating pump.

16.2 Explain with the help of a sketch, the working of a double acting reciprocating pump.

16.3 Derive an expression for acceleration head impressed on flow in the case of a reciprocating pump. Assume that the plunger or piston has simple harmonic motion.

16.4 Derive expressions for the acceleration and friction head impressed on the water in the suction and delivery pipes. Sketch indiator diagram and determine the work done per stroke of the pump.

16.5 What is air vessel. Explain its working briefly. How is the indicator diagram is modified by fitting the air vessel on suction and delivery sides.

16.6 Why is the speed of a reciprocating pump lower than that of a centrifugal pump? On what factors does the speed of the reciprocating pump depend.

16.7 Explain how the separation of flow is caused in reciprocating pumps. What preventive measures are usually taken to reduce the same appreciably ?

16.8 A double acting reciprocating pump running at 40 rpm is discharging 1.0 m³ of water per minute. The pump has a stroke of 400 mm and the diameter of its cylinder is 200 mm. The pump is located 5 m above the pump to supply water 20 m above the centre line of the pump. Compute the slip of pump and the power required to derive the pump.

16.9 A double acting reciprocating pump has a stroke of 250 mm and plunger diameter 125 mm. The centre of the pump is 4 m above the lower pump water level and 30 m below the delivery water. The lengths of suction and delivery pipes are 6 m and 35 m respectively. Both pipes are 60 mm in diameter. If the pump is to run at 30 rpm, find the pressure head on the piston at the beginning, middle and end of the suction stroke. If meachnical efficiecny is 75% and f = 0.04, determine the power required to derive the pump.

16.10 A single acting reciprocating pump has a plunger 75 mm diameter and a stroke of 120 mm. It lifts water from a pump 3 m below the pump through a suction pipe 5 m long and 35 mm diameter. It delivers the water to a tank 15 m above the pump through a delivery pipe 25 mm diameter and 15 m long. Determine the maximum speed at which this pump can be run if it is given that separation occurs at a pressure of 7.8 N/cm². Also sketch the indicator diagram assuming plunger motion as simple harmonic.

16.11 A reciprocating pump is 150 mm diameter and has a stroke of 300 mm. It is running at a speed of 30 r.p.m. and supplying water to a heigh of 12 m. The diameter and length of the delivery pipe are 100 mm and 300 mm respectively. If a large air vessel is fitted in the delivery pipe at a distance of 2 m from the pump centre line, find the maximum pressure head in the cylinder at the beginning and middle of delivery stroke.

16.12 The diameter of a plunger of reciprocating pump is 200 mm and stroke 300 mm. Pump is to be driven with SHM at 60 r.p.m. and it draws water from a pump 4 m below pump centre line. Find the least diameter of the suction pipe which is 5 m long in order to prevent separation at this speed.

16.13 A single reciprocating pump has a piston of diameter 250 mm and stroke 450 mm, the delivery pipe is to be 100 mm diameter and water is lifted to a tank whose level is 15 m above the pump and 30 m horizontally from it. If separation takes place at 2.35 m of water absolute, find the speed of the pump in r.p.m. at which separation would occur in the delivery pipe if no air vessel was fitted for the two cases. (a) If the pipe was vertical from pump and then horizontal up to the tank, (b) If the pipe ran horizantally from the pump and then vertically to the tank. Assume atmospheric pressure as 10.3 m of water and SHM of the plunger.

16.14 A double acting reciprocating pump 190 mm diameter and 380 mm stroke runs at 36 double strokes per minute. The suction head impressed on the pump is 3.6 m and discharge head 30 m. The lengths of suction and delivery pipe are 9 m and 60 m respectively and both pipes are 100 mm in diameter. Large air vessels are fitted 3 m and 6 m away from the pump on suction and delivery side respectively. Neglecting entrance and exit losses for the pipes, determine (a) head in the two ends of the cylinder, (b) load on piston rod. Assume f = 0.032 and simple harmonic motion of the crank.

16.15 A single acting reciprocating pump has a cylinder bore of 200 mm and stroke 300 mm. The crank revolves at 30 r.p.m. (motion is simple harmonic). The delivery pipe of the pump is 150 mm diameter and a large air vessel is fitted on it near the delivery valve. Find the discharge to and from the air vessel when crank makes an angle of 60°, 120° and 180° with inner dead centre. Find the crank angles at which there is no flow from or into the air vessel.

16.16 A single acting reciprocating pump has a plunger 375 mm diameter and stroke 600 mm. The delivery pipe is 90 m long and 150 mm in diameter. The pump runs at 50 r.p.m. Find the head lost due to friction in delivery pipe when a large air vessel is fitted near the pump outlet (b) when no air vessel is fitted (c) power saved by installing the air vessel. Assume f = 0.032.

16.17 A single acting reciprocating pump has a plunger of 200 mm diameter and a stroke of 400 mm. The delivery pipe of 100 mm diameter and 45 m long. Determine the power saved in overcoming friction in the delivery pipe by fitting a large air vessel when the pump runs at a speed of 55 r.p.m. Take $f = 0.04$

Centrifugal Pump

17.1 INTRODUCTION

Centrifugal pump is a type of classes of rotodynamic pump. Centrifugal pump may be defined as a pump which increases the dynamic pressure of the fluid by centrifugal action.

Essentially, the pump consists of an impeller mounted over a shaft and driven by an external source. The impeller rotates the fluid and increases its pressure and absolute velocity. As discussed in chapter 5, the magnitude of the centrifugal head imparted to the rotating fluid (at the point) is directly proportional to the product of the square of the angular velocity and the distance of the point from the centre of rotation. Further, most of the centrifugal pumps are of outward radial flow type. During the flow of liquid through its impeller from inner rim to outer rim, the angular momentum of the fluid changes. This further causes an increase in the pressure of the fluid. The increased velocity energy of fluid is later converted into pressure energy in the pump (as discussed later), Thus, in contrast to a reciprocating pump in which the fluid is pushed upward by the force of the plunger, it is rather the pressure generated by the rotation of the fluid by the impeller which modifies the hydraulic gradient line in a way that makes the flow of the fluid invitable (See Fig. 17.7).

Rotodynamic pumps are classified according to the direction of the flow through their impellers. These are :

(i) Radial flow pumps or centrifugal pumps,

(ii) axial flow or propeller pumps, and

(iii) mixed flow or screw pumps.

(i) *Radial flow pump*: The direction of flow through the impeller remains in the radial direction outwardly, i.e. from the inner rim (at the centre) towards the outer circumference. Ordinarily, all the centrifugal pumps are manufactured as radial flow pumps. In construction, they are analogous to a low specific speed Francis turbine.

(ii) *Axial flow pump* : In such pumps the direction of flow is in the axial direction and hence no centrifugal force, as such is developed. The pressure is developed by the flow of liquid over blades of aerofoil section by the same principle as in 'lift theory'. In construction, axial flow pumps are analogous to a propeller turbine.

(iii) *Mixed flow pump* : The direction of flow through the impellers of these pumps is partly radial and partly axial. Thus the shape of the blades of these impeller resemble that of a propeller of a ship. The mixed flow impellers look like a screw and are know n as screw impellers and such pump are sometimes are known as diagonal pumps.

17.2 COMPARISON OF CENTRIFUGAL PUMPS WITH RECIPROCATING PUMPS

The comparison of centrifugal pumps with reciprocating pumps is given below :

1. The centrifugal pumps provide a continuous rate of flow whereas reciprocating pumps supply at fluctuating rate of flow.

2. The centrifugal pumps are cheaper in their initial cost as well as maintenance cost whereas reciprocating pumps are costly on both these accounts.

3. The efficiency of centrifugal pump (of low head) is high as compared to a reciprocating pump.

4. A centrifugal pump is a high speed pump and can be coupled directly through flanged coupling to electric motor whereas reciprocating pump is a low speed pump and can not be directly connected, otherwise there might be separation of flow and cavitation may start in the pump. This makes the belt drive indispensable for reciprocating pump.

5. The centrifugal pump is lighter in weight and their installation is simpler.

6. The construction of centrifugal pump is simpler as it does not have air vessels, glands, non return valves as used with reciprocating pump.

Reciprocating is more suitable to lift oil from deep oil wells as compared to centrifugal pump. It can build up as high pressure as 7×10^4 kN/m^2 (equivalent of 700 kg/cm^2). Moreover, reciprocating pump give higher efficiency at high head and low discharge rate (nearly 90% or so) as compared to a centrifugal pump.

17.3 CENTRIFUGAL PUMP

17.3.1 Construction

As discussed earlier, the centrifugal pump is a rotodynamic pump which increases the pressure of the fluid within it due to centrifugal action. It essentially consists of the following components:

1. *Impeller* A centrifugal pump consists of a rotor called impeller which is mounted over a shaft. It is enclosed in a casing and is driven by the external source of energy (an electric motor).

It consists of a number of curved vanes. The fluid enters in the central portion of the impeller, called eye, and flows out radially outward and then it is discharged around the entire circumference into a casing. The impellers can be classified as, *closed, semi-open and open type.* (Fig. 17.2)

Ordinarily, the impellers are of 'closed type' and the vanes or blades are covered with shrouds (covers) on both their sides. The cover or shroud on the suction side (or upper plate) is known as crown plate and on the outer side (or lower plate) as base plate. Such impellers are used to handle non viscous fluids. e.g. water, hot oil or chemicals.

'Semi open impellers' are provided with only one shroud at its base, that is base plate and no shroud is provided on the upper side, (no crown plate is provided). Semi-open impellers are used to pump sugar molesses, etc. In order to minimise the likelyhood of clogging, the number of vanes is reduced and their height is increased.

'Open type' impellers are not provided with any shroud and the vanes remain open on both of their sides. Open type impellers are used to pump sewerage, mixture of water, sand and pebbles, etc.

2. *Suction pipe* A suction pipe is fitted to the eye of a centrifugal pump. At the other end of the suction pipe, a foot valve (one way valve or non return valve) and a strainer is fitted. These remain submerged in water (or liquid to be pumped) in such a way that they are a few centimetres above the bottom of the lower pump. The strainer prevents the floting material like wooden pieces, leaves and other rubbish material to enter into the impeller.

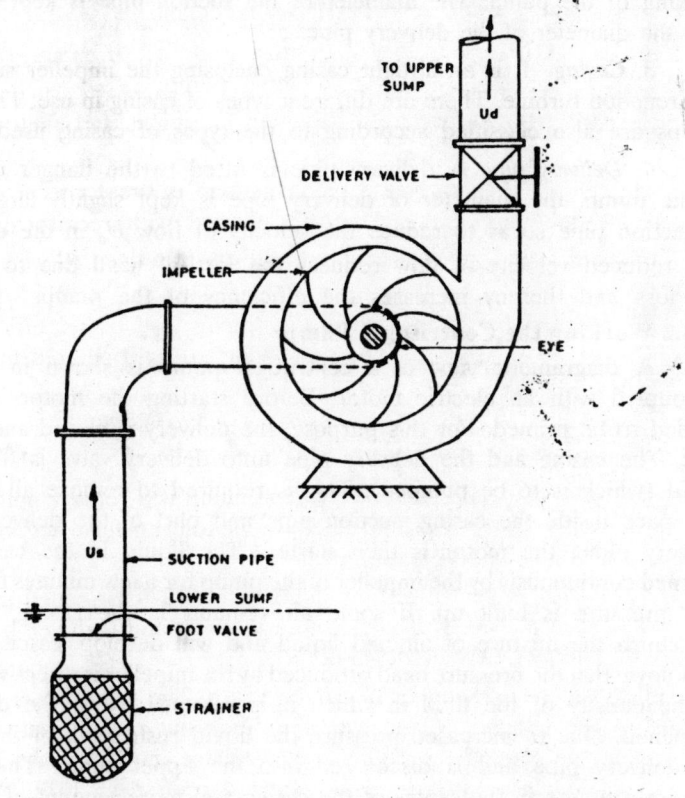

FIG. 17.1. CENTRIFUGAL PUMP—VARIOUS COMPONENTS.

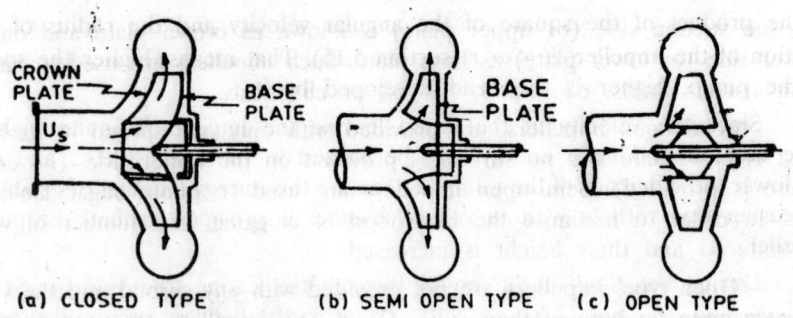

(a) CLOSED TYPE   (b) SEMI OPEN TYPE   (c) OPEN TYPE

FIG. 17.2. DIFFERENT TYPES OF IMPELLERS.

The foot valve is a non-return valve which permits the liquid to flow only in the upward direction. The liquid from the strainer enters the foot valve and then flows upward along the suction pipe. The suction pipe should be so laid that it rises all its way. Any loop in the suction pipe should be avoided otherwise air pockets may be formed in it and will hinder the satisfactory working of the pump. The diameter of the suction pipe is kept slightly less than the diameter of the delivery pipe.

    3. *Casing* It is an airtight casing enclosing the impeller similar to that of a reaction turbine. There are different types of casing in use. The centrifugal pumps are also classified according to the types of casing used. (See 17.4).

    4. *Delivery pipe* A delivery pipe is fitted to the flanger of the casing of the pump, the diameter of delivery pipe is kept slightly larger than that of suction pipe so as to reduce the velocity of flow U_d in the delivery pipe. The reduced velocity of flow reduces the loss of head due to friction and exit loss and thereby increases the efficiency of the pump.

17.3.2 Working the Centrifugal Pump

    A diagrametic view of a centrifugal pump is shown in Fig. 17.1. It is coupled with an electric motor. Before starting the motor, the pump is needed to be primed. For this purpose, the delivery is closed and the suction pipe. The casing and the delivery pipe upto delivery valve is filled with the liquid (which is to be pumped). This is required to remove all the air from the space inside the casing, suction pipe and part of the delivery pipe upto delivery pipe., the motor is then started. The liquid in the casing is being churned continuously by the impeller of the pump for a few minutes till sufficiently high pressure is built up. If some air remains in the casing, the impeller will churn the mixture of air and liquid and will develop lesser head. (Since it is known that the pressure head produced by the impeller is directly proportional to the density of the fluid in which it is rotated). Now, the delivery valve is opened. Due to increased pressure the liquid rushes out of the casing into the delivery pipe and is discharged into the upper sump. This causes the vacuum pressure in the centre of the casing and more amount of water rushes up from the lower sump. Thus a continuous supply of liquid is maintained by the pump. The pressure head developed by the impeller is directly proportional to the product of the square of the angular velocity and the radius of the rotation of the impeller, $h \propto \omega^2 r$ (section 5.15). That means, higher the speed of the pump, higher is the head developed by it.

Since the velocity of the liquid leaving the impeller is quite high, a large amount of kinetic energy may be wasted in the eddies, etc., and this will lower the efficiency of the pump. To recoup this energy a casing of gradually increasing area with or without vortex chamber is provided around the pump impeller.

During the flow of the liquid through the casing, the velocity go on reducing and becomes U_d i.e. velocity of flow in the delivery pipe and thereby the pressure rises continuously. In this way a large amount of kinetic energy of the liquid leaving the impeller is converted into pressure energy. This, in turn, reduces the loss of energy in the casing and the delivery pipe. By these measures, the efficiency of the pump is improved. Further, as the liquid flow around the casing from its narrowest end, more and more liquid is added to it. The casing is usually so designed that the velocity of flow remains uniform. This means, the area of the casing is increased at the same rate at which the liquid is added in the casing.

The total energy line (T.E.L.) and hydraulic gradient line (H.G.L.) are also shown in Fig. 17.7. The total energy line starts from a point 'a' in the suction pipe, falls gradually to account for frictional and other losses in the suction pipe and ends up at 'b'. At the entrance to the pump, the water enters the impeller. It does work on the liquid equal to $(U_{w1}u_1/g)$ and so this amount of energy is added to the flowing liquid. Hence T.E.L. rises suddenly at point 'b' and jumps to point 'c'. From this point, the energy line falls off gradually as the liquid flows along the delivery pipe. It ends up at point 'd' just at the other end of delivery pipe. Point 'd' lies at a distance $U_d^2/2g$ above the liquid level in the upper sump. The hydralic gradient line can now be easily drawn by substracting velocity energy in the respective pipe and is shown plotted in the above figure.

17.4 TYPES OF PUMP

These are mainly two types of casing namely, volute type and diffuser type. These are also the devices which convert a part of the energy ejected by the impeller in the form of velocity energy into useful pressure energy. According to the type of casing, the centrifugal pumps are classified as : (1) Volute pump and (2) Diffuser or turbine pump.

17.4.1 Volute Pump

In this pump, the impeller is surrounded by a spiral casing, the outer boundary of which is in the form of a curve, called volute and hence its name. These may be of constant velocity form or variable velocity form. In the constant velocity form of volute (Fig. 17.3), the cross sectional area of the casing at successive sections is increased in such a way that velocity of fluid 'v' circulating in the casing remains uniform having a value nearly equal to two third of U_{w1}, i.e. whirling velocity of liquid leaving the impeller. The loss of energy due to shock is thus reduced from $U_{w1}^2/2g$ to $(U_{w1} - v)^2/2g$ or even less. As a result of the reduction of velocity in the casing a part of the velocity energy gets converted into pressure energy. In the variable velocity volute the cross sectional area of the casing increases at more rapid rate than in the constant velocity casing. The mean velocity

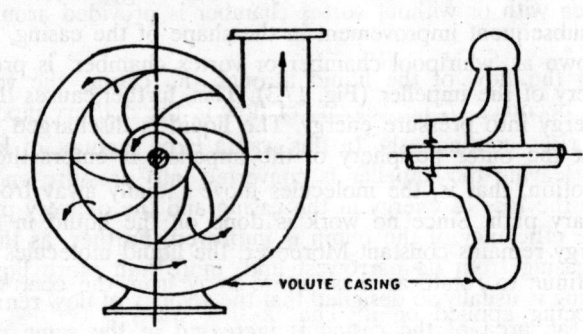

VOLUTE CASING

(a) VOLUTE PUMP

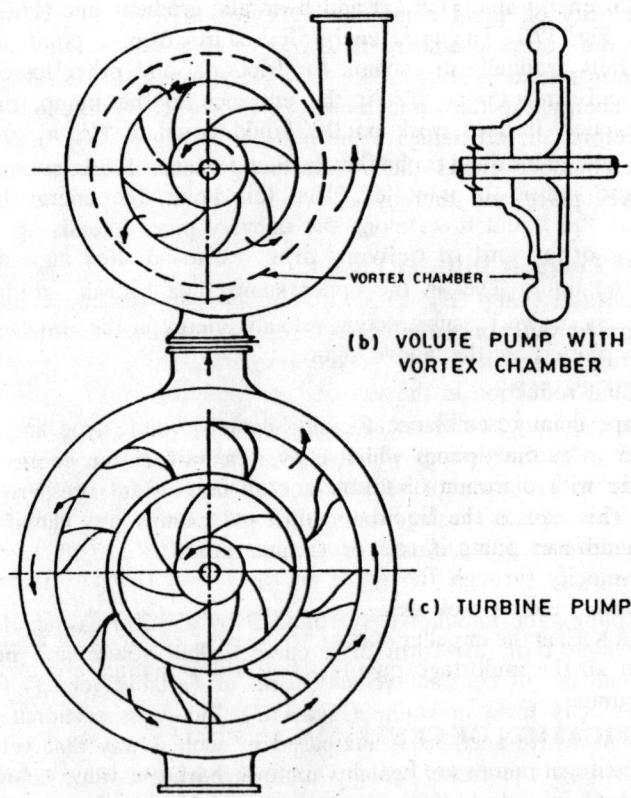

VORTEX CHAMBER

(b) VOLUTE PUMP WITH VORTEX CHAMBER

(c) TURBINE PUMP

FIG. 17.3. VOLUTE PUMP AND DIFFUSER PUMP

of liquid circulating in the casing continuously diminishes from a valve 'v' at the smallest cross section to U_d (velocity in the delivery pipe) at the outlet flange. Thus, the variable velocity casing may be regarded as one long diverging passage wrapped around the entire periphery of the impeller. This slightly increases the efficiency of the pump. In the reduction of velocity from v to U_d, the eddies are formed and thereby some energy is lost in the casing.

As a subsequent improvement in the shape of the casing, an additional chamber, known as 'whirlpool chamber or vortex chamber' is provided at the outer periphery of the impeller (Fig. 17.3). This, further,causes the conversion of kinetic energy into pressure energy. The liquid is discharged with absolute velocity U_1 at the outer periphery of the impeller. It enters the chamber in a whirling motion, that is, the molecules move radially away from the centre following rotary path. Since no work is done on the liquid in the chamber, the total energy remains constant Moreover, the liquid molecules in the vortex chamber continue to rotate as these move away from the centre and without any torque being applied on it. Thus a free votex is formed in it. For a free vortex flow, it is known that the velocity of flow at any point is inversely proportional to the distance of the point from the axis of rotation (i.e., $u \propto 1/r$). Hence, the velocity of liquid continuously decreases as it moves away from the centre in the vortex chamber. This decrees in velocity is accompanied by the increase in pressure. Thus a decrease part of kinetic energy is converted into pressure energy. At the same time, the loss of energy in the casing is reduced. Therefore, the efficiency of the pump is improved. The liquid after leaving vortex chamber enters the volute casing where a further reduction in velocity takes place and thereby a further rise in pressure energy takes piece.

17.4.2 Turbine Pump or Diffuser Pump

In the diffuser pump (Fig. 17.3c), the impeller is surrounded by a series of stationary guide vanes mounted on a diffuser ring. These guide vanes are known as 'diffuse vanes' and they provide gradually enlarging passage. This results in gradual reduction in the velocity and building up of pressure head. Because of superficial resemblance to a reaction turbine, this type of pump is often called a 'turbine pump'. The angle of guide vanes at its entrance should coincide with direction of absolute velocity of liquid at the outlet of the impeller. This causes the liquid to enter over the guide blades without shock. Thus a diffuser pump is considered more efficient because of gradual reduction in velocity through the guide passages and thereby lesser energy loss in the eddies, etc. A well designed diffuser is capable of converting as much as 75% of K.E. at the impeller outlet into pressure energy. This arrangement is employed in all the multistage pumps. The diffuser pumps are more costly than volute pump.

17.5 CLASSIFICATION OF CENTRIFUGAL PUMPS

The centrifugal pumps are further classified according to different criteria as discussed here-in-under:

(1) *Single or double suction* The centrifugal pumps may be classified as single suction pumps or double suction pumps. The latter has the advantage of symmetry and ideally balance the end thrusts or axial thrust on the shaft. They also provide a larger inlet area with lower intake velocities, than would be possible with a single suction pump of the same outside diameter of the impeller.

(2) *Number of stages* The pumps may be classified as single stage pump or multistage pump. In the former there is only one impeller. In the later type of pumps, two or more impellers are arranged in series and are mounted on the same shaft. The quantity of liquid discharged is same as discharged by single impeller alone, but the total head developed is 'n' times the head developed by single impeller (n is the number of impellers used).

(3) *Disposition of shaft* The pumps may be classified on the basis of the disposition of the shaft as horizontal pumps or vertical pumps.

(4) *Working head* Similarly the pumps can be classified on the basis of working head as high head pumps, medium head pumps or low head pumps.

(5) *Specific speed* On the basis of specific speed, the pumps are classified as high specific speed, medium specific speed and low specific speed pumps.

17.6 VELOCITY TRIANGLES APPLIED TO CENTRIFUGAL PUMP

The real flow through an impeller is three dimensional and so quite complex. Let the absolute velocity of flow be U which is a function of three directional coordinates.

$$U = f(r, \theta, Z) \qquad ...(17.1)$$

Thus the velocity varies not only along the radius but also across the blade passage in any plane parallel to impeller rotation, say, from upper side of one blade to the lower side of the adjacent blade, which constitute an abrupt change – a discontinutiy. Also, there is a variation in the velocity in the meridian plane, i.e. in the plane along the axis of the impeller. Thus, it is seen that the velocity distribution is very complex and depends upon the number of blades, their geometric dimensions, (shape, thickness and width) and with radius.

The following assumptions are made to simplify the problem:

(1) The blades are too thin and the pressure difference across them is replaced by an imaginary body force acting on the fluid and producing torque.

(2) The number of blades are infinitely large so that the velocity variation across the blade passage is reduced and tends to zero, i.e. the flow is axisymmetrical. Thus,

$$\frac{\partial U}{\partial \theta} = 0 \qquad ...(17.2)$$

(3) Over that part of the impeller where transfer of energy takes place (blade passages), there is no variation of velocity in the meridian plane, i.e. across the width of the impeller. Thus,

$$\frac{\partial U}{\partial Z} = 0 \qquad \qquad ...(17.3)$$

Thus, Eq. 17.1 reduces to

$$U = f(r) \qquad \qquad ...(17.4)$$

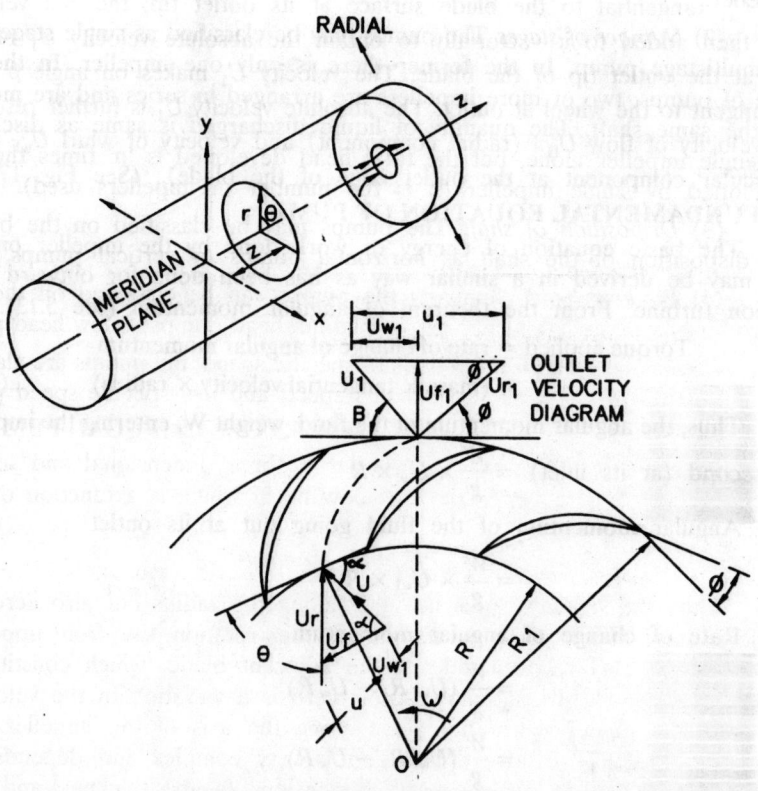

FIG. 17.4. (A) DIRECTIONAL COORDINATES (B) VELOCITY TRIANGLES,

Fig. 17.4 (b) shows diagrammetically the flow through a centrifugal pump impeller. The dotted line shows the fluid streamline through the narrow interblade passage which is congruent with the shape of interblade centre line. The above assumptions simplify the problem. The space between impeller inlet and impeller outlet is treated as 'black box' having an input in the form of inlet velocity triangle and output in the form of outlet velocity triangle.

At inlet, the fluid moving with velocity U enters the impeller through a cylindrical space of radius R and may make an angle α with the tangent at that radius (to the cylindrical surface). At the outlet, the fluid leaves with radius R_1 inclined to the tangent at outlet by angle β.

The inlet velocity triangle is constructed by first drawing the vector representing the absolute velocity U at angle α. The tangential velocity of the impeller u is then substracted from it vectorially in order to obtain

U_r relative velocity of the fluid with respect to impeller blades at radius R. The absolute velocity is then resolved into radial velocity U_f (called velocity of flow) and perpendicular to it, i.e., in the tangenttial direction, U_w (called velocity of whirl).

Similarly, the velocity triangle at outlet consists of relative velocity of fluid U_{r1} tangential to the blade surface at its outlet tip; the rim velocity u_1 is then added to it vectorially to obtain the absolute velocity U_1 of the fluid at the outlet tip of the blade. The velocity U_1 makes on angle β with the tangent to the wheel at outlet. The absolute velocity U_1 is further resolved into velocity of flow U_{f1} (radial component) and velocity of whirl U_{w1} (perpendicular component at the outlet edge of the blade)., (See Fig. 17.4)

17.7 FUNDAMENTAL EQUATION OF PUMP

The basic equation of energy or work done by the impeller on the fluid may be derived in a similar way as has been done for outward flow reaction turbine. From the theorem of angular momentum (see 5.13).

Torque applied = rate of change of angular momentum

$$= \text{(mass} \times \text{tangential velocity} \times \text{radius)} \qquad ...(17.5)$$

Thus, the angular momentum of the fluid, weight W, entering the impeller per second (at its inlet) $= \dfrac{W}{g} \times U_w \times R$

Angular momentum of the fluid going out at its outlet

$$= \frac{W}{g} \times U_{w1} \times R_1$$

Rate of change of angular momentum

$$= \frac{W}{g}(U_{w1}R_1 - U_w R)$$

$$= \frac{W}{g}(U_{w1}R_1 - U_w R)$$

The work done/sec, E = torque × angular velocity

$$= T \times \omega$$

$$= \frac{W}{g}(U_{w1}R_1 - U_w R) . \omega$$

$$= \frac{W}{g}(U_{w1}u_1 - U_w u) \text{ Joules/sec or watts} \quad ...(17.6a)$$

$$\text{(Since } u = \omega R)$$

And, the work done/sec/unit weight of fluid

$$= \frac{E}{W}$$

Work done/sec/unit weight $= \dfrac{(U_{w1}u_1 - U_w u)}{g} \qquad ...(17.6b)$

Eq. 17.6 is known as 'Euler's Equation' for the pump. From its derivation it is seen that Euler's equation applies to pump as well as to a turbine. However, in case of turbine $U_w u > U_{w1} u_1$, so that E would be –ve, indicating reverse direction of energy transfer. It is, therefore, common for a turbine to use the reversed order of terms in the brackets (Eq. 17.6) to yield positive E. Since, the unit of E in Eq. 17.6b is in metre, it is often referred as Euler's head or theoretical (or ideal) head developed by the pump H_{TH}.

The Eq. 17.6b can be modified by re-arrangement of various terms.

From velocity triangles,

$$U_w = U \cos \alpha, \text{ and } U_{w1} = U_1 \cos \beta$$

so that, $\qquad E_t = (U_1 u_1 \cos \beta - U . u \cos \alpha)/g \qquad$ ...(17.6c)

By cosine rule

$$U_r^2 = U^2 + u^2 - 2 U u \cos \alpha$$

so that, $\quad U u \cos \alpha = (U^2 + u^2 - U_r^2)/2$

Similarly, $U_1 u_1 \cos \beta = (U_1^2 + u_1^2 - U_{r1}^2)/2$

Substituting these values in Eq. (17.6c)

$$E_t/\text{unit weight} = \frac{1}{2g} [(U_1^2 + u_1^2 - U_{r1}^2) - (U^2 + u^2 - U_r^2)]$$

$$= \frac{U_1^2 - U^2}{2g} + \frac{u_1^2 - u^2}{2g} + \frac{(U_r^2 - U_{r1}^2)}{2g} \qquad ...(17.7)$$

In this Eq. 17.7, the first term represents the increase in the kinetic energy of the fluid in the impeller, the second term represents the energy used in setting the liquid into a circular motion about the central axis of the impeller (which is also the increase in pressure head due to centrifugal action) and the third term represents the regain of static head due to reduction in relative velocity of fluid passing through the impeller.

A centrifugal pump rarely has any sort of guide vanes at inlet. The liquid, therefore, is assumed to approach the impeller without any appreciable tangential component of velocity. Therefore, in the design of pumps, it is assumed that

(1) absolute velocity of flow U at inlet remains radial,

i.e. $\qquad U = U_f$ and $U_w = 0$

also $\qquad \alpha = 90°$

This means, the initial angular momentum of the fluid is zero.

(2) The blade angle at inlet, i.e. θ is such that liquid enters the blade tangentially. This assumption is known as 'no shock' condition. Similarly, the liquid leaves the blades tangentially.

With these assumptions, it is seen from outlet velocity triangle.

$$\cot \varphi = (u_1 - U_{w1})/U_{f1}$$

or $\qquad U_{w1} = (u_1 - U_{f1} \cot \varphi)$

With this substitution in the Eular's equation

$$\text{Work done/sec/unit weight} = \frac{U_{w1} u_1}{g} \qquad ...(17.6d)$$

$$= \frac{u_1}{g}(u_1 - U_{f1} \cot \varphi) \qquad ...(17.6e)$$

From above Eq. (17.6e), it is found that the work done/sec in independent of u, inlet rim velocity.

As derived for turbines, the rim velocity u_1 and velocity of flow U_{f1} can also be expressed in terms of theoretical velocity of flow $\sqrt{2gH_m}$

Thus, the speed ratio Φ is defined as

$$\Phi = \frac{u_1}{\sqrt{2gH_m}} \qquad ...(17.8a)$$

and the flow ratio ψ is defined as

$$\psi = \frac{U_{f1}}{\sqrt{2gH_m}} \qquad ...(17.8b)$$

where u_1 is the speed of rotation at the output rim and U_{f1} is the velocity of flow at the outlet tip of the blade. The usual range of variation of these coefficients is given below.

	High N_s value	Low N_s value
Φ	0.95	1.25
ψ	0.10	0.25

It is seen from Eq. 17.6 that the energy transferred to the flowing liquid and correspondingly the efficiency of the pump will increase if the outlet blade angle φ is made smaller and smaller. Theoretically, it may be reduced to a very small value, but in practice it is rare to find the value of 'angle φ, less than 20°. The smaller outlet blade angle yields a narrow and long passages, which causes additional energy loss in the blade passage. Thus, it is futile to obtain higher efficiency by the adoption of blade angle φ less than 20°.

17.8 EFFECT OF VARIATION OF BLADE ANGLE

The shape of the blades of centrifugal pump may be either as (a) forward facing, (b) radial or (c) backward facing. Fig. 17.5 (a) shows a forward facing blade ($\theta < 90°$) and it is used for slow moving impellers. Fig. 17.5b shows a radial flow blade, for which $\varphi = 90°$. The liquid leaves such blades (and impeller) in the radial direction. Such blades are suited for medium speed runners. Fig. 17.5(c) depicts a backward facing blade ($\varphi > 90°$) which is used with fast moving impellers. The backward facing blades are so bent that this curvature is in the opposite direction to the direction of rotation of the impeller and these are mostly used in centrifugal pumps.

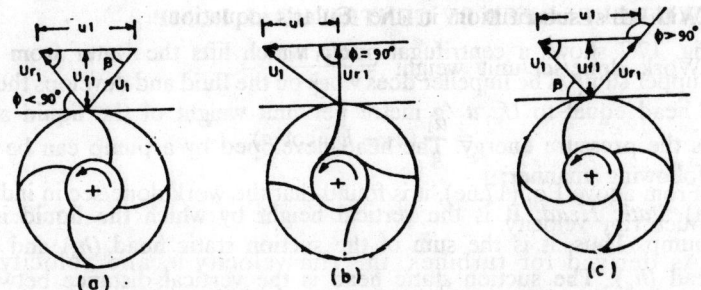

FIG. 17.5. DIFFERENT SHAPE OF BLADES.

The theoretical or ideal head developed by a pump is given by Eq. 17.6d.

$$E_t \text{ (or } H_{th}) = \frac{U_{w1} u_1}{g}$$

$$= \frac{u_1}{g} (u_1 - U_{f1} \cot \varphi)$$

$$= \frac{u_1}{g} \left(u_1 - \frac{Q}{a_{f1}} \cot \varphi \right) \qquad \qquad ...(17.9a)$$

Since $u_1 \, \alpha \, N$, the theoretical head can be expressed as

$$H_{th} = (C N^2 - B N Q)$$

where N is the speed of rotation, A_1 is the area of flow at the outlet section and Q is the discharge supplied by the impeller.

For a constant speed N of the pump, the ideal head developed by the impeller gets plotted with discharge as straight lines for various values of φ (Fig. 17.6). In actual practice, the relationship between H_{th} and Q is parabolic. The disparity between ideal straight line and actual parabolic characteristic can be explained as follows: At low rates of discharge, the head recovered in the guide passages or in the volute chamber has not been considered in the Euler's equation., Eq. 17.6. It causes the actual head to rise above ideal head curve, but later on, especially when the discharge is in excess of that, for which guide passages were designed, the eddy, friction and shock losses in the impeller and in the casing are greater than the regain in the head. This causes the actual curve to fall below ideal one.

Further, the head developed by the impeller is also a function of the outlet blade angle φ. For smaller angle, the curve II falls more sharply as compared to curved I for large value of φ.

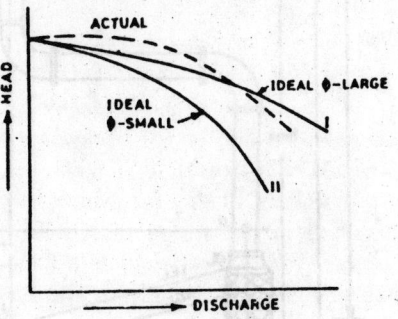

FIG. 17.6. VARIATION OF HEAD WITH ANGLE φ AND DISCHARGE.

17.9 HEAD DEVELOPED BY CENTRIFUGAL PUMP

Fig. 17.7 shows a centrifugal pump which lifts the water from a lower sump to upper sump. The impeller does work on the fluid and develops theoretical or ideal head equal to $U_{w1} u_1/g$ metre per unit weight of the liquid and thus increases the pressure energy. The head developed by a pump can be defined in the following manner:

(a) *Static Head*: It is the vertical height by which the liquid is raised by the pump. Thus, it is the sum of the suction static head (h_s) and delivery static head (h_d). The suction static head is the vertical distance between the liquid level in the lower sump and the centre line of the shaft of the pump. The delivery static head is the vertical height between the centre line of the pump and the liquid level in the upper sump.

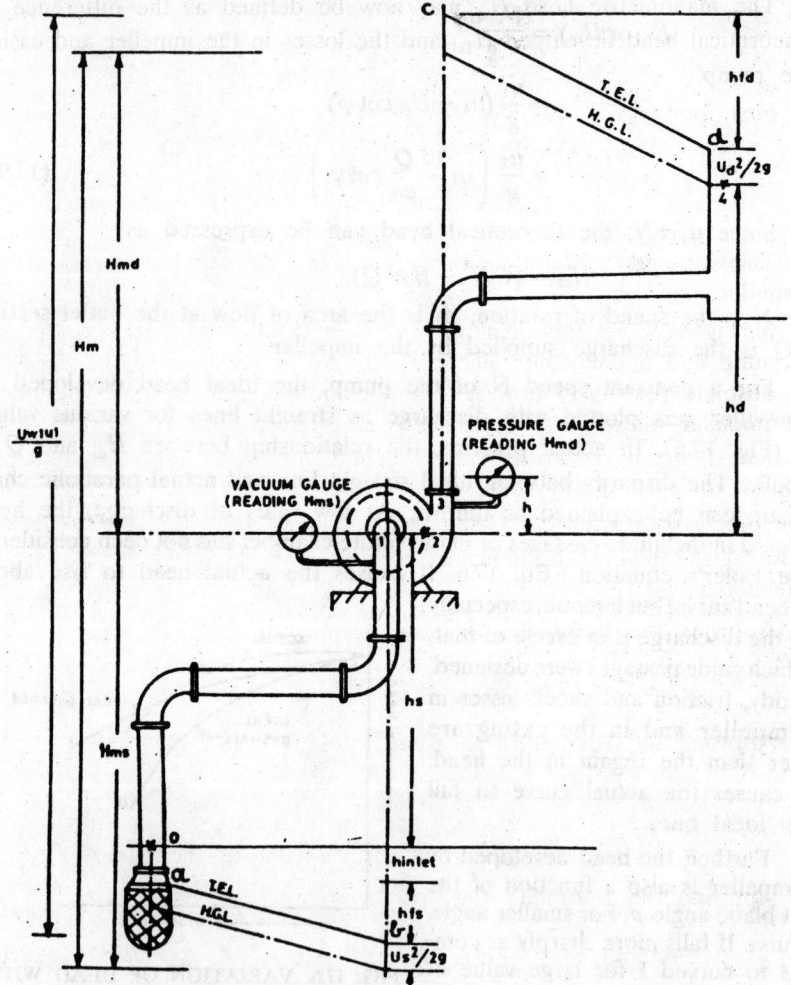

FIG. 17.7. A CENTRIFUGAL PUMP : DEFINITION OF HEAD

$$H_{static} = h_s + h_d \qquad ...(17.10)$$

(b) *Manometric Head* (H_m). It is the amount of total head which a pump must develop to satisfy the external requirements of energy. The impeller of a centrifugal pump (radial flow type) does work on the liquid and generates theoretical head H_{TH} $\left(= \dfrac{U_{w1} u_1}{g} \right)$. Ideally it is the amount of energy which is supposed to be transferred to the liquid. But invariably, the hydraulic losses take place in the various components of the pump (suction pipe, delivery pipe, etc.). Let all the losses occurring in the suction pipe be designated as h_{fs}, in the delivery pipe by h_{fd}. The eddy and friction losses also occur in the impeller and casing of the pump. Let the losses in the former be written as h_{Li} and in the later be written as h_{Lc}.

The manometric head H_m may now be defined as the difference of the theoretical head developed H_{TH} and the losses in the impeller and casing of the pump.

First form.

$$H_m = H_{TH} - h_{Li} - h_{Lc}$$

$$= \frac{U_{w1} u_1}{g} - h_{Li} - h_{Lc} \qquad ...(17.11)$$

The manometric height can be expressed in other ways also as described hereinunder.

In Fig 17.7, let the point '0' and 4 lie at the liquid surface in the lower sump and upper sump. The point 1, lies at the inlet to the impeller, where absolute velocity of flow is U and point 2 lies at the outer periphery of the impeller where absolute of flow is U_1. The point 3 is assumed to be at the outer flange of the casing and at this point a pressure gauge is connected. Let the reading of the pressure gauge be p_d. The velocity of flow in the suction pipe is expressed as U_s and that in the delivery pipe as U_d. Let the pressure at the point 1 as indicated by a vacuum gauge connected to the pump be p_s.

Applying the Bernoulli's theorem between 0 and 1,

$$0 = \frac{p_s}{w} + \frac{U_s^2}{2g} + h_s + h_{fs} \qquad ...(17.12)$$

Applying the Bernoulli's theorem between 1 and 2,

$$\frac{p_s}{w} + \frac{U_s^2}{2g} + \frac{U_{w1} u_1}{g} = \frac{p_2}{w} + \frac{U_1^2}{2g} + h_{Li} \qquad ...(17.13)$$

where h_{Li} is the energy loss in the impeller of the pump

Applying the Bernoull's theorem between 2 and 3.

$$\frac{p_2}{w} + \frac{U_1^2}{2g} = \frac{p_d}{w} + \frac{U_d^2}{2g} + h + h_{Lc} \qquad ...(17.14)$$

where h is the height of pressure gauge above the centre line of the pump and h_{Lc} is the energy loss in the casing. Finally, applying Bernoulli's theorem between 3 and 4,

$$\frac{p_d}{w} + \frac{U_d^2}{3g} = h_d + U_d^2/2g + h_{fd}$$

$$\frac{p_d}{w} = h_d + h_{fd} = H_{md} \qquad (17.15)$$

In the above equation, H_{md}, is known as the delivery manometric head and it is the reading of pressure gauge connected on the delivery side of the pump.

Second form. From Eq. 17.12

$$\frac{p_s}{w} = -h_s - \frac{U_s^2}{2g} - h_{fs} = H_{ms} \qquad ...(17.12)$$

where H_{ms} is the reading of the vacuum gauge connected on the suction side of the pump and is known as suction manomtetric head.

From Eq. 17:13 and 17.14,

$$\frac{p_s}{2} + \frac{U_s^2}{2g} + \frac{U_{w1} u_1}{g} = \left(\frac{p_d}{w} + \frac{U_d^2}{2g} + h + h_{Lc}\right) + h_{Li}$$

$$\frac{U_{w1} u_1}{g} - h_{Li} - h_{Lc} = \frac{(p_d - p_s)}{w} + \frac{U_d^2 - U_s^2}{2g} + h$$

$$H_m = \left(\frac{p_d - p_s}{w}\right) + \frac{U_d^2}{2g} - \frac{U_s^2}{2g} + h \qquad ...(17.16)$$

Eq. 17.16 gives another expression for H_m. Generally, the delivery pipe is slightly larger in diameter than suction pipe and the difference in velocity head in these pipes is of small magnitude. Hence, this difference in velocity head can be neglected.

$$\therefore \qquad H_m = \frac{p_d}{w} - \frac{p_s}{w} + h \qquad ...(17.17)$$

If the pressure gauge is also connected at the centre line of the pump, h is reduced to zero.

$$H_m = \frac{p_d}{w} - \frac{p_s}{w} \qquad ...(17.18)$$

Since, the pressure head in the suction pipe is sub- atmospheric, it means, the manometric head is the arithmatic sum of the readings of the pressure gauge and vacuum gauge.

Third form: Form Eq. 17.13,

$$\frac{U_{w1} u_1}{g} - h_{Li} = \frac{p_2}{w} - \frac{p_s}{w} + \frac{U_1^2}{2g} + \frac{U_s^2}{2g}$$

Substracting h_{Lc} from both sides,

$$\frac{U_{w1}u_1}{g} - h_{Li} - h_{Lc} = \frac{p_2}{w} - \frac{p_s}{w} + \frac{U_1^2}{2g} - \frac{U_s^2}{2g} - h_{Lc}$$

$$H_m = \frac{p_2}{w} - \frac{p_s}{w} + \frac{U_1^2}{2g} + \frac{U_s^2}{2g} - h_{Lc} \qquad ...(17.19)$$

The fluid leaves the impeller with velocity U_1 and comes out at the outlet flange of the casing with velocity U_d – velocity of flow in the delivery pipe. This means, the velocity changes from U_1 to U_d in the casing. The velocity U_1 is quite high and when it is reduced, the pressure recovery takes place in the casing. It is usually expressed as the function of velocity U_1. Therefore, Eq. 17.19 can be written as

$$\frac{U_{w1}u_1}{g} - h_{Li} - h_{Lc} = \left(\frac{p_2}{w} - \frac{p_s}{w}\right) + \left(\frac{U_1^2}{2g} - \frac{U_s^2}{2g}\right) - h_{Lc}$$

Adding the substrating $U_d^2/2g$) on the right hand side,

$$H_m = \left(\frac{p_2}{w} - \frac{p_s}{w}\right) + \left(\frac{U_1^2}{2g} - \frac{U_d^2}{2g}\right) + \left(\frac{U_d^2}{2g} - \frac{U_s^2}{2g}\right) - h_{Lc}$$

The term $(U_1^2/2g - U_d^2/2g)$ represent the recovery of pressure head and is generally written as $k\, U_1^2/2g$.

$$\therefore \qquad H_m = \left(\frac{p_2}{w} - \frac{p_s}{w}\right) + k\frac{U_1^2}{2g} + \left(\frac{U_d^2}{2g} - \frac{U_s^2}{2g}\right) - h_{Lc} \quad ...(17.20)$$

As discussed above, the third bracketed term is of small magnitude,

$$\therefore \qquad H_m = \left(\frac{p_2}{w} - \frac{p_s}{w}\right) + k\frac{U_1^2}{2g} - h_{Lc} \qquad ...(17.21)$$

The manometric head is thus expresses as

(Manometric head) = (Pressure rise in the impeller + Pressure rise

in the casing − Energy loss in the casing)

Fourth Form. Introducing the values of p_s/w and p_d/w in Eq. 17.16 from Eqn. 17.12 and 17.15,

$$H_m = (h_d + h_{rd}) - (-h_s - U_s^2/2g - h_{fs}) + \left(\frac{U_d^2 - U_s^2}{2g}\right) + h$$

$$H_m = (h_s + h_d + h_{fs} + h_{fd} + U_d^2/2g + h) \qquad ...(17.22a)$$

If the pressure gauge is put up at the centre line of the pump

$$H_m = (h_s + h_d + h_{fs} + h_{fd} + U_d^2/2g) \qquad ...(17.22b)$$

= (Static lift + friction losses in the suction and

delivery pipe + velocity energy in the delivery pipe).

17.10 LOSSES AND EFFICIENCIES

A centrifugal pump converts mechanical energy into hydraulic energy and in this process a part of the energy is lost in the various parts of the pump. The distribution of energy loss and the energy available at different stages are shown in Fig. 17.8. Let Q_i be the discharge flowing through the impeller whereas h_{Li} be the loss of head due to friction and eddies in the impeller. The power loss in the impeller is then given by

$$P_i = w Q_i h_{Li} \qquad \qquad ...(17.23)$$

The impeller handles a greater volume than discharged by it, (since some fluid flows back through the inlet clearance between the impeller and the casing. The difference of Q_i and Q is the flow rate of liquid Q_v, that leaks across the impeller. The pump discharges $Q \, m^3/s$. Let H_i be the total head built up across the impeller. The power lost due to leakage can then be expressed as

$$P_v = w Q_v H_i \qquad \qquad ...(17.24)$$

where $\qquad Q_v = Q_i - Q$

As the liquid flows out through the casing, the loss of energy is h_{Lc} through the casing. The power lost in the casing is then given by

$$P_c = w Q h_{Lc} \qquad \qquad ...(17.25)$$

Finally, the energy is also lost in the mechanical friction as in the bearing and sealing glands. It is normal practice to include in it the losses due to disc friction[1] (sometimes referred as windage losses). If P be the power supplied by the shaft, one can write

$$P = P_m + (w Q_v H_i + w Q h_{Lc}) + w Q H_m \qquad ...(17.27)$$

Thus the efficiencies of a centrifugal pump may be defined as

(1) Mechanical efficiency

(2) Manometric efficiency

(3) Volumetric efficiency, and

(4) Overall efficiency.

(1) *Mechanical efficiency* η_{mech}. It is defined as the ratio of the power input to the impeller and the power input to shaft.

$$\eta_{mech} = \left[\frac{P - P_m}{P} \right] \qquad \qquad ...(17.28)$$

It is to be noted that power input to the impeller is also given by $w (Q + Q_v) H_{TH}$, therefore, the mechanical efficiency may also be defined as

$$\eta_{mech} = \frac{w (Q + Q_v) H_{TH}}{P} \qquad \qquad ...(17.29)$$

---

1 This is the power required to spin the impeller at the required speed without any work being done by the impeller on the fluid. This would be only possible if the impeller did not have any blades. Thus, the windage loss accounts for the friction between the outer surfaces of the impeller rotating in the fluids.

(2) *Manometric efficiency* η_{man}. It is defined as the ratio of the power given out of the pump $w\,Q\,H_m$ to the power input to the pump at its impeller, $P - P_m$.

$$\eta_{man} = \left(\frac{w\,Q\,H_m}{P - P_m}\right) \qquad ...(17.30)$$

Since $(P - P_m) = w\,Q_i\,H_{TH} = w\,(Q + Q_v)\dfrac{U_{w1}\,u_1}{g}$

$$\eta_{man} = \frac{w\,Q\,H_m}{w\,(Q + Q_v)\dfrac{U_{w1}\,u_1}{g}} \qquad ...(17.31a)$$

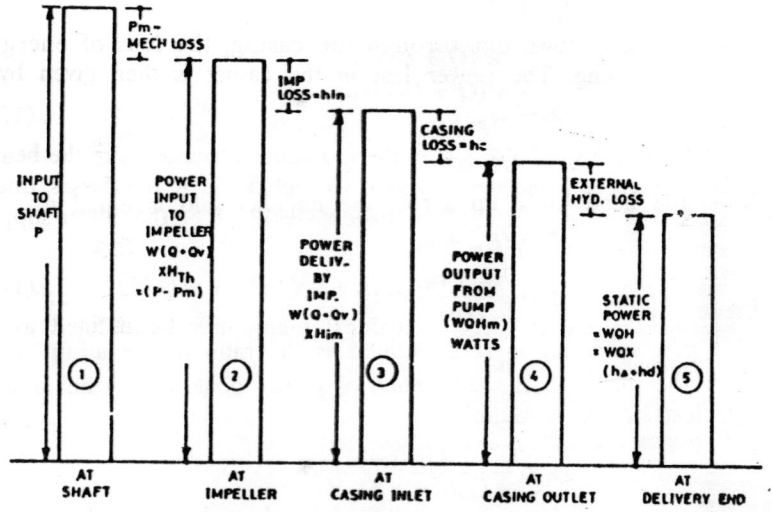

FIG. 17.8.' POWER AVAILABLE AT DIFFERENT STAGES

$$= \left(\frac{Q}{Q + Q_v}\right)\left(\frac{g\,H_m}{U_{w1}\,u_1}\right)$$

If no liquid leaks past the impeller, $Q_v = 0$,

$$\eta_{man} = \frac{g\,H_m}{U_{w1}\,u_1} \qquad ...(17.31b)$$

(3) *Volumetric efficiency* (η_v). It is defined as the ratio of the flow rate supplied by the pump to the flow rate passing through the impeller.

$$\eta_v = \frac{Q}{Q_i}$$

$$= \left(\frac{Q}{Q + Q_v}\right) \qquad ...(17.32)$$

(4) *Overall efficiency* η_0. It is defined as the ratio of power output of the pump to the power input to the pump

$$\eta_0 = \frac{w\,Q\,H_m}{P} \qquad \qquad ...(17.33)$$

The manometric efficiency can also be defined in an alternative form. The hydraulic losses occurring in the pump consists of losses in the impeller, losses in the casing and leakage losses. Therefore, the impeller efficiency and casing efficiency can now be defined separately.

(5) *Impeller efficiency* η_1 It is defined as the ratio of the power developed by the impeller to the power input to the impeller.

$$= \frac{w\,Q_i\,H_i}{P - P_m} \qquad \qquad ...(17.34a)$$

Alternatively,

$$= \frac{w\,(Q + Q_v)\,H_i}{w\,(Q + Q_v)\,H_{TH}}$$

$$= \frac{H_i}{H_{TH}} \qquad \qquad ...(17.34b)$$

where H_i is the head build up across the impeller and is equal to

$$H_i = (H_m + h_{Li})$$

$$\therefore \qquad \eta_i = \frac{H_m + h_{Li}}{H_{TH}} \qquad \qquad ...(17.34c)$$

(6) *Casing efficiency* η_c It is defined as the ratio of the useful power output from the pump to the difference of power built up by the impeller and power lost in the leakage.

$$\eta_c = \frac{w\,Q\,H_m}{w\,Q_i\,H_i - w\,Q_v\,H_i}$$

$$= \frac{w\,Q\,H_m}{w\,Q\,H_i} \qquad \qquad \text{(Since } Q = (Q_i - Q_v))$$

$$= \frac{H_m}{H_i} \qquad \qquad ...(17.35)$$

From Eqs 17.32; 17.34b and 17.35, the manometric efficiency can now be obtained.

$$\eta_{man} = \frac{Q}{(Q + Q_v)} \times \frac{H_i}{H_{TH}} \times \frac{H_m}{H_i}$$

$$= \frac{w\,Q\,H_m}{w\,(Q + Q_v)\,H_{TH}}$$

$$= \frac{w\,Q\,H_m}{w\,(Q + Q_v)\,\dfrac{U_{w1}\,u_1}{g}} \qquad \qquad ...(17.31a)$$

which is same as Eq. 17.31(a) obtained earlier.

Next, it is possible to show that the overall efficiency is equal to the product of all the component efficiencies.

From Eqns, 17.29 to 17.35a,

$$\eta_0 = \eta_{mech} \times (\eta_i \times \eta_c \times \eta_v)$$

$$= \eta_{mech} \times \eta_{man}$$

$$= \frac{w\,(Q + Q_v)\,H_{TH}}{P} \times \frac{w\,Q\,H_m}{w\,(Q + Q_v)\,H_{TH}}$$

$$= \frac{w\,Q\,H_m}{P} \qquad\qquad ..(17.33)$$

which is same expression as given in Eq. 17.33.

17.11 EFFECT OF VARIATION IN THE DISCHARGE

A centrifugal pump attains its maximum efficiency when it runs at the designed speed and supplies designed discharge. At this condition of operation of the pump, the losses are minimum. The liquid enters the impeller tangentially without shock. But if the pump supplies the liquid either at more or at less rate than normal rate of flow, the fluid will not be eentering the impeller tangentially as shown in Fig. 17.9. This causes the energy due to shock at the entry and therefore, the efficiency of the pump is reduced,

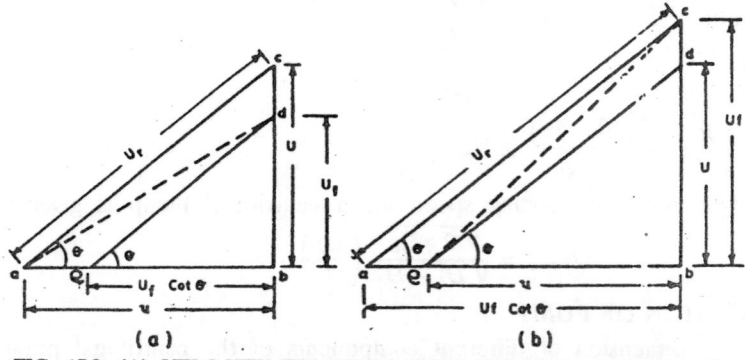

FIG. 17.9. (A) VELOCITY TRIANGLE WITH REDUCED DISCHARGE,
(B) VELOCITY TRIANGLE WITH INCREASED DISCHARGE

Consider first the inlet velocity triangle a b c in Fig. 17.9 (a) when the pump is supplying the normal discharge. If the flow rate is reduced, the velocity of flow U_f is also reduced, and is shown plotted as 'b d', the speed of the pump remains the same. Therefore, the velocity triangle should now modify to abd. But the inlet blade angle remains unaltered hence the inlet velocity triangle is formed by combining the tangential velocity vector $U_f \cot \theta$ (in place of rim speed, u) and reduced velocity of flow U_f, i.e., the new velocity triangle is e b d. This means, that the tangential velocity changes suddenly from u to $U_f \cot \theta$. It results in a shock at entry.

$$\therefore \quad \text{Energy loss at inlet} = \left[\frac{(\text{change in velocity})^2}{2\,g}\right]$$

$$= \frac{(u - U_f \cot \theta)^2}{2\,g} \qquad\qquad ...(17.36)$$

Similarly, when the discharge is increased, the tangential velocity of flow is also increased. The new velocity traingle (Fig. 17.9b) is now formed by combining U_f and $U_f \cot \theta$.

$$\therefore \qquad \text{Energy loss at inlet} = \frac{(U_f \cot \theta - u)^2}{2g} \qquad \qquad ...(17.37)$$

17.12 MINIMUM STARTING SPEED

The pressures at the suction and delivery side of the impeller are found to be $\frac{p_s}{W}$ and $\frac{p_d}{W}$ metre of the liquid which are indicated by the pressure and vacuum gauges connected on the respective sides. The difference of these pressure, Eq. 17.18, is equal to be manometric head H_m. Therefore, the necessary condition for the liquid to be raised to the required height is that the pump must generate at least H_m metre of head. This head is generated as a result of the rotation of the impeller in fluid, (forced vortex flow). The centrifugal head generated should thus be greater or atleast equal to H_m.

$$\therefore \qquad \frac{u_1^2 - u^2}{2g} \geq H_m \qquad \qquad ...(17.38)$$

$$\text{But} \qquad u_1 = \frac{\pi D_1 N}{60} \qquad \qquad ...(16.39a)$$

$$\text{and} \qquad u = \frac{\pi D N}{60} \qquad \qquad ...(17.39b)$$

$$\therefore \qquad \left(\frac{\pi N}{60} \right)^2 \frac{(D_1^2 - D^2)}{2g} \geq H_m$$

The minimum starting speed for a centrifugal pump is given by

$$(N)_{min} = \frac{\sqrt{2 g H_m}}{\sqrt{D_1^2 - D^2}} \left(\frac{60}{\pi} \right) \qquad \qquad ...(17.40)$$

17.13 DESIGN OF PUMP

The dimension of different components of the centrifugal pump can be computed as follows :

17.13.1 Diameter of Impeller

First the outside diameter D_1 of the impeller to generate manometric head H_m is determined. The tangential speed of wheel at its outer rim u_1 is given by Eq. 17.39a.

$$u_1 = \frac{\pi D_1 N}{60} \qquad \qquad ...(17.39a)$$

It can also be expressed in terms of manometric head by Eq. 17.8a.

$$u_1 = \Phi \sqrt{2 g H_m} \qquad \qquad ...(17.30)$$

Equating the two values of u_1

$$\pi D_1 N / 60 = \Phi \sqrt{2 g H_m}$$

$$D_1 = 60 \Phi \sqrt{2 g H_m / \pi N} \qquad \qquad ...(17.41)$$

This equation can also be used to determine the head developed by a pump of given diameter D_1 and running at speed N. Conversely, this expression, Eq. 17.41 can be used to check whether a pump will be able to raise the water to the required height or not.

17.13.2 Inlet diameter of the impeller

The minimum inlet diameter D of the impeller is chosen as 1/3 rd to 2/3rd of the outside diameter of the impeller D_1. The actual value of D/D_1 to be used depends on the head to be built up and the specific speed of the impeller.

17.13.3 Least Outside Diameter of the Impeller

The minimum outside diameter of the impeller D_1 should be such that it generates at least H_m (manometric head). From Eq. 17.40, the least outside diameter of the impeller is given by

$$\left(\frac{\pi N}{60}\right)^2 \left(\frac{D_1^2 - D^2}{2g}\right) \ge H_m$$

$$(D_1^2 - D^2) \ge \frac{2 g H_m (60)^2}{\pi N^2}$$

Putting $\qquad D = 0.5 D_1,$

$$D_1 \ge \frac{\sqrt{9600 g}}{\pi} \times \frac{\sqrt{H_m}}{N}$$

17.13.4 Size of Suction Pipe

If the suction pump is to discharge $Q\,m^3/s$, the diameter of suction pipe d_s, is given by continuity equation.

$$Q = \frac{\pi}{4} d_s^2 U_s$$

or $\qquad d_s = \sqrt{\frac{4Q}{\pi} \times U_s} \qquad \qquad ...(17.42)$

Generally, the velocity of flow U_s in the suction pipe is assumed as 1.5 m/s to 3.0 m/s.

17.13.5 Size of Delivery Pipe

The diameter of the delivery pipe is generally kept slightly larger than suction pipe so as to obtain a lower velocity of flow in the delivery pipe. It is usually taken as 1.5 m/s to 2.5 m/s.

17.14 MULTISTAGE PUMP

A single stage pump consists of a single impeller. It may supply required discharge against a maximum of 150 m or so. If the liquid is to be supplied against a much higher head, one way of doing it is to connect the number of pumps in series. This means, the delivery of one pump is connected to the suction side of the another pump. In this way, a number of pumps are connected to produce the desired pressure head. This arrangement is now obsolete. Moreover, it is not economical to use single stage pump for higher

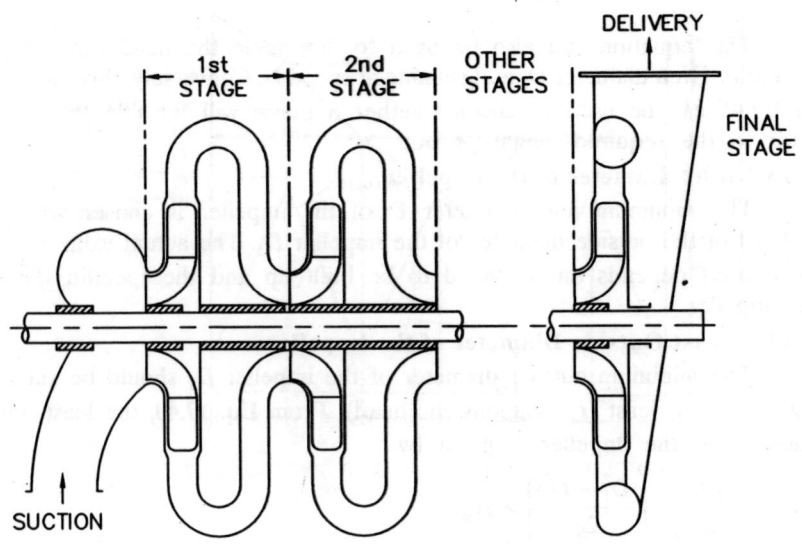

FIG. 17.10. A MULTISTAGE PUMP

heads because the pumps are either to run at higher speed or the diameter of the impeller required is large. In either case, large mechanical and leakage losses result in lower efficiency of the unit.

Instead of the pumps connected in series, nowadays multistage pumps are much in use. In this arragement, two or more impellers are mounted on the same shaft. In this intermediate space between the impellers, stationary return passages are provided. Each return passage includes a set of gradually diverging guide blades. The liquid (with pressure) delivered by one impeller is fed to the succeeding impeller, Fig. 17.10. In this way, the head built by the number of impellers is multiplied. Moreover, additional increase in pressure also takes place in the return passages (where velocity energy is converted into pressure energy), Fig. 17.11.

Thus in each impeller, the absolute velocity of liquid increases and thereafter it decreases in the return passages. In this way, the pressure gain takes place in two stages-first in the impeller and then in the guide or return passage. Both the fixed and rotating elements of the pumps are encased in a combined casing-which is quite often made of forged or welded steel. The total head H_T developed by 'n' number of stages.

$$H_T = n H \qquad \qquad ...(17.43)$$

and $$Q_T = Q_1 = Q_2 \qquad \qquad ...(17.44)$$

The number of stages to be adopted depends on the limitations of the speed of the driving agent, on the head to be developed and on the relationship between head and discharge. In general, not more than 8 to 10 stages are used otherwise the construction of the pump becomes too combersome. The discharge delivered by a multistage pump is same as that of a single

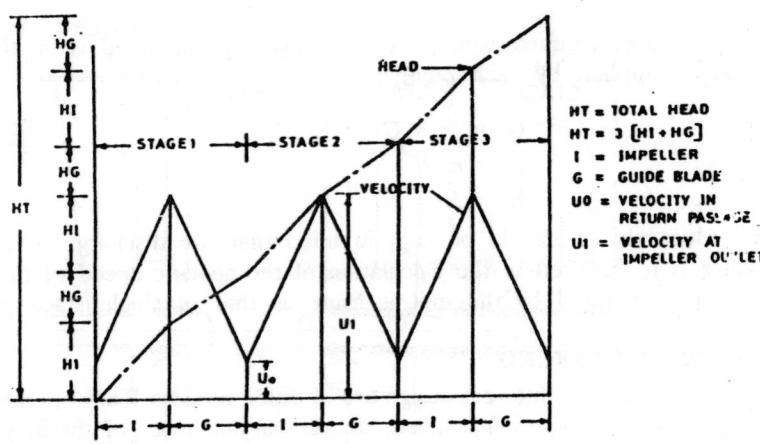

FIG. 17.11. VELOCITY VARIATION AND PRESSURE RISE DURING
VARIOUS STAGES

stage pump. It is to be noted that the specific speed of the multistage pump
is computed as for single stage pump, i.e., using the head developed by
a single impeller $(H = H_T/n)$.

17.15 PUMPS IN PARALLEL

When a single stage pump is not capable of supplying the required
discharge against given head, the pumps are arranged in parallel. In this arrangement, a number of pumps are so connected that each one of them suppllies
liquid to a common delivery pipe (Fig. 17.12). Thus, the total discharge
Q_T supplied by the unit of a number of pumps is equal to the sum of all
the discharges of individual pump. And if all the pumps have same type of

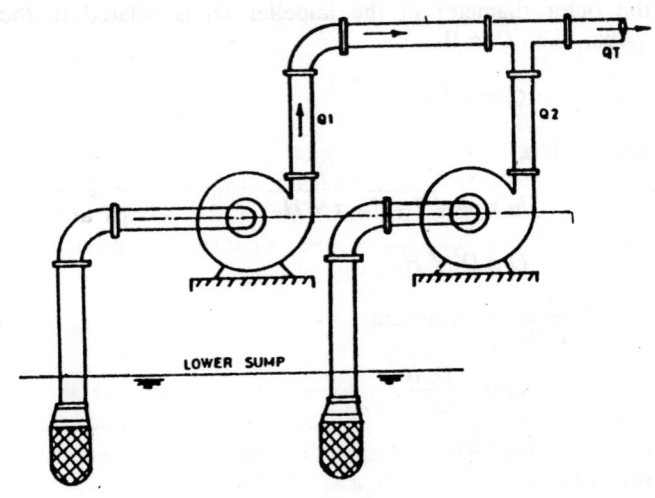

FIG. 17.12. PUMPS CONNECTED IN PARALLEL.

'head discharge characteristics', the total discharge supplied is 'n' times the discharge supplied by each pump

$$Q_T = Q_1 + Q_2 + \ldots Q_n$$

or
$$Q_T = n\, Q$$

and
$$H_T = H_1 = H_2$$

Here also it should be kept in mind that the discharge of only one impeller is to be used in the calculation of the specific speed of the pump. The head generated by the unit is same as that of single stage pump.

17.16 SPECIFIC SPEED

The pumps of different design are of different sizes. They operate within a wide range of operational speed, deliver varying rates of discharge while working against varying heads. This means, a pump of given size and design behaves entirely in different manner to another one. Therefore, two pumps of different design (Fig. 17.13) can be compared by using the criterion of specific speed.

Definition The specific speed of a pump is defined as the speed of a geometrically similar pump of such size that it will deliver a discharge of 1 lit/sec while working against unit head (or 1 metre) under corresponding conditions.

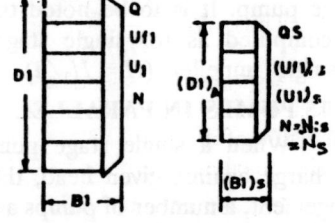

FIG. 17.13 (A) NORMAL RUNNER (B) SPECIFIC RUNNER

From the continuity equation,

$$Q = k\, \pi\, D_1 B_1 U_{f1} \qquad \ldots(17.45)$$
$$Q \propto D_1 B_1 U_{f1}$$

Since the outer diameter of the impeller D_1 is related to the width B_1 of the impeller, i.e. $D_1 \propto B_1$.

$$\therefore \qquad Q \propto D_1^2\, U_{f1}$$

From Eq. 17.8 b,

$$U_{f1} = \psi \sqrt{2g H_m} \, \propto \sqrt{H_m}$$

$$\therefore \qquad Q \propto D_1^2 \sqrt{H_m}$$

$$\frac{Q}{D_1^2 \sqrt{H_m}} = \text{constant} \qquad \ldots(17.46)$$

Also
$$u_1 = \frac{\pi D_1 N}{60}$$

$$u_1 \propto D_1 N$$

From Eq. 17.8 a,

$$\therefore \qquad u_1 = \Phi \sqrt{2g H_m} \, \propto \sqrt{H_m}$$

$\therefore$ $$D_1 N \alpha \sqrt{H_m}$$

or $$D_1 \alpha \sqrt{H_m}/N$$

or $$\frac{D_1 N}{\sqrt{H_m}} = \text{constant} \qquad \qquad ...(17.47)$$

Substituting the value of D_1 from Eq. 17.47 into Eq. 17.46

$$\frac{Q N^2}{H_m \sqrt{H_m}} = \text{constant}$$

$$\frac{N \sqrt{Q}}{(H_m)^{3/4}} = \text{constant} \qquad \qquad ...(17.48)$$

By definition of specific speed, $N = N_s$ when $Q = 1$ lit/sec and $H_m = 1$ m.

$$\frac{N_s \times 1}{1} = \text{constant}$$

Thus, $$N_s = \frac{N \sqrt{Q}}{(H_m)^{3/4}} \qquad \qquad ...(17.49)$$

The specific speed of a pump can be computed by using Eq. 17.49. It is a dimensional quantity and its value is different in S.I. and F.P.S. units. The value of discharge Q and head H_m in Eq. 17.49 must be used corresponding to the maximum efficiency of the pump.

In case of multistage pumps, the head used should correspond to its single stage. Similarly, in case of double suction pump, half the discharge of the pump is to be used in Eq. 17.49. For example if a 4 stage pump develops total head H_T then H_m should be replaced by $H_T/4$ in the expression for specific speed.

17.16 SIMILARITY LAWS

The performance characteristics of a rotodynamic machine depends on the input power P, discharge Q, head H, speed N, diameter of the impeller D_1, including the fluid properties such as mass density ρ, dynamic viscosity μ and bulk modules of elasticity K.

$$P = \varphi\,(\rho, D_1, Q, H, N, \mu, K) \qquad \qquad ...(17.50)$$

By dimensional analysis,

$$\frac{P}{\rho N^3 D_1^5} = \varphi \left[\frac{Q}{N D_1^3}, \frac{gH}{N^2 D_1^2}, \frac{\mu}{\rho N D_1^2}, \frac{K}{\rho N^2 D^2} \right]$$

or $$K_p = \varphi \left[K_Q, K_H, R_e, N_M \right]$$

where $K_p = P/\rho N^3 D_1^5$ is known as power coefficient, $K_Q = Q/N D_1^3$ is discharge coefficient, $g H/N^2 D_1^2$ is head coefficient, and R_e and N_M are Reynolds number and Mach number respectively. The functional relationship could be determined by hydraulic experimentation. Thus, for complete dynamic similarity between model and prototype,

$$\left(K_p \right)_m = \left(K_p \right)_p \qquad \qquad ...(17.52)$$

$$\left(\frac{P}{\rho N^3 D_1^5}\right)_m = \left(\frac{P}{\rho N^3 D_1^5}\right)_p$$

Similarly, $\left(K_Q\right)_m = \left(K_Q\right)_p$

$$\left(\frac{Q}{N D_1^3}\right)_m = \left(\frac{Q}{N D_1^3}\right)_p \qquad \qquad ...(17.53)$$

Also $\left(\dfrac{gH}{N^2 D_1^2}\right)_m = \left(\dfrac{gH}{N^2 D_1^2}\right)_p \qquad \qquad ...(17.54)$

$$\left(R_e\right)_m = \left(R_e\right)_p \qquad \qquad ...(17.55)$$

and $\left(N_M\right)_m = \left(N_M\right)_p \qquad \qquad ...(17.56)$

In case of pumps, K_Q and K_H are two most important parameters and their ratio would indicate the suitability of the pump to the given job (deliver discharge Q against head H_m). If the ratio of $\sqrt{K_Q}$ and $\left(K_H\right)^{3/4}$ is found out, it gives a dimensionless number which is independent of the size of the impeller. It is known as 'type number n_s'.

$$n_s = \sqrt{K_Q}\Big/\left(K_H\right)^{3/4}$$

$$= \frac{\left(\dfrac{Q}{N D_1^3}\right)^{1/2}}{\left(\dfrac{gH}{N^2 D_1^2}\right)^{3/4}}$$

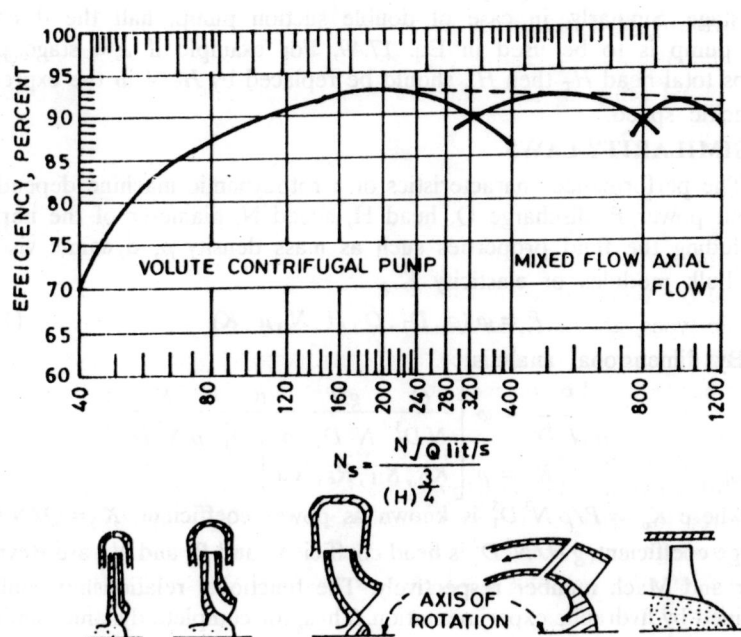

$$N_s = \frac{N\sqrt{Q\ \text{lit/s}}}{(H)^{\frac{3}{4}}}$$

FIG. 17.14. OPTIMUM EFFICIENCY AS A FUNCTION OF SPECIFIC SPEED.

$$= \frac{N\sqrt{Q}}{\left(gH\right)^{3/4}} \qquad\qquad ...(17.57)$$

For practical use, the value of type number n_s, is to be determined at the design point (of the performance curve) which means that it should correspond to maximum efficiency.

Similarly, the ratio of $\left(K_p\right)^{1/2}$ to $\left(K_H\right)^{5/4}$ yields another type number in terms of N, P and H.

$$
\begin{aligned}
n_{s1} &= \left(K_p\right)^{1/2} / \left(K_H\right)^{5/4} \\
&= \left(\frac{P}{\rho N^2 D_3^5}\right)^{1/2} / \left(\frac{gH}{N^2 D_1^2}\right)^{5/4} \\
&= \frac{N\sqrt{P}}{\sqrt{\rho}\left(gH\right)^{5/4}} \qquad\qquad ...(17.58)
\end{aligned}
$$

Eq. 17.57 and 17.58 for type numbers are dimensionless coefficients and as such can be used in any system of units. Pump designers often use another form of these type number. viz. specific speed N_s as given in Eq. 17.49.

$$N_s = \frac{N\sqrt{Q}}{\left(H_m\right)^{3/4}} \qquad\qquad ...(17.49)$$

Obviously N_s differs from n_s by $\left(1/g^{3/4}\right)$. Thus the specific speed N_s is not a dimensionless quantity. Its value $\left(N_s\right)$ differes in different system of units. Usual range of the values of N_s for centrifugal pump lies between 500 to 15,000.

The specific speed is an important characteristic which is widely used for describing the type of the pump. This characteristic is versatile as it is based on three most important parameters of the pump namely, rotational speed N, discharge Q and head H_m. Therefore, the specific speed characterises the type of the pump to a sufficiently large extent. For instance, some pumps differing in types, geometry, and design but having close value of N_s will have many similar features. For instance, low specific speed pumps are always used at higher heads; on the contrary, high specific speed pumps are used at low heads.

Specific speed of a pump largely determines the shape of the impeller (Fig. 17.14). Low specific impellers (300 to 400 r.p.m.) are characterised by the exit area far greater than inlet diameter; its width being relatively small. The flow through such impellers is always radial. As the specific speed increases; so that the impeller becomes a mixed flow type and thereafter it gets changed to axial flow type.

17.18 PERFORMANCE OF PUMPS

The pumps are designed to delivery a constant rate of discharge (design discharge) against a constant head (design head) at maximum efficiency $\left(\eta_0\right)_{max}$ while running at speed N (design speed). but if any of these design conditions are modified, e.g., the discharge Q is increased or it is run at a different speed or it has to work against a different head than design head, the pump will behave differently. The variation in the performance of the pump are usually plotted graphically in the form of various curves and these are known as 'characteristic curves'. Generally, the discharge Q (in lit/sec) is plotted as abscissa and the head, the input power and the efficiency are plotted as ordinates at a constant speed. The various types of characteristic curves can be classified as :

(i) Main and operating characteristic curves.

(ii) Muschel characteristic curves or iso-efficiency curves.

(iii) Constant head and constant discharge characteristic curves.

17.18.1 Main and Operations Characteristic Curves

Main characteristic curves are obtained by performing the tests on a pump at different speeds. In the tests, the discharge Q is varied within a wide range and thereby the head

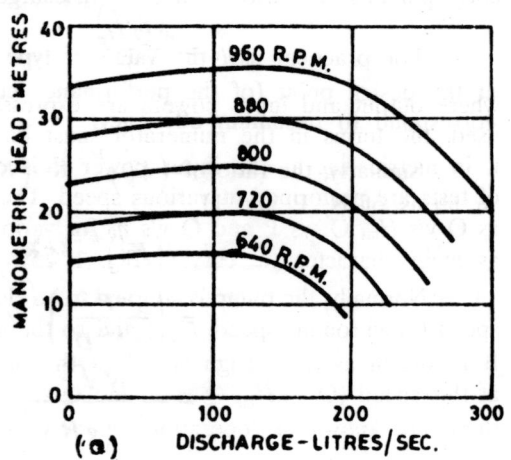

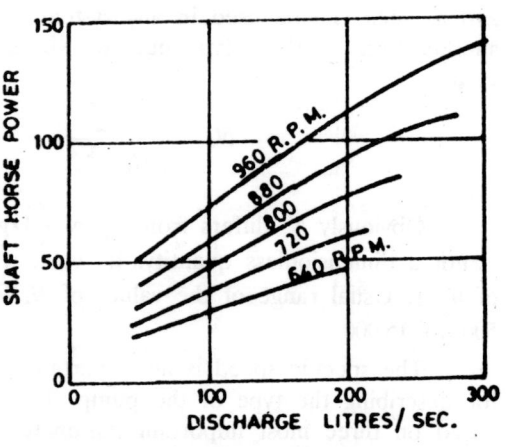

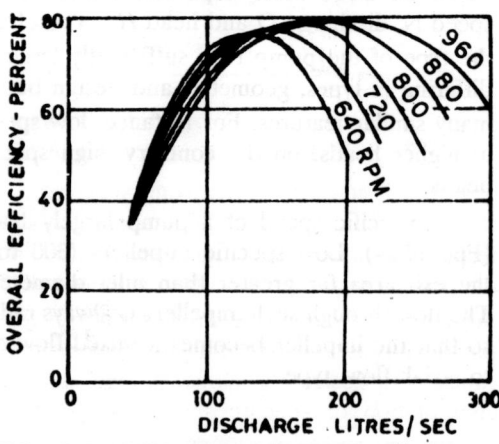

FIG. 17.15. MAIN CHARACTERISTIC CURVES

developed $\left(H_m\right)$, input power (P) also vary. The efficiency of the pump corresponding to various rates of discharge is then computed as

$$\eta_0 = \frac{w \, Q \, H_m}{P}$$

where output and input powers are expressed in watts. (If M.K.S. units are used, the terms in the numerator must be divided by 75 so as to express it in metric h.p. as the input power P is expressed in m.h.p). Similar type of tests are performed at various speed. The results of these tests are plotted as Q v/s H_m, Q v/s P and Q v/s η_0 for various speed. Such curves are known as main characteristic curves (Fig. 17.15).

Normally, the pump is coupled to an electric motor which runs at constant speed (synchronous speed, N_{syn}) and so the pump also runs at constant speed. It is known as the design speed of the pump. Generally, the set of curves at this speed (Q vs H_m, Q vs P and Q vs η_0) are used in practice and hence these are known as 'operating characteristic curves' Fig. 17.16

It is seen from Fig. 17.16, that the head discharge curve is of falling

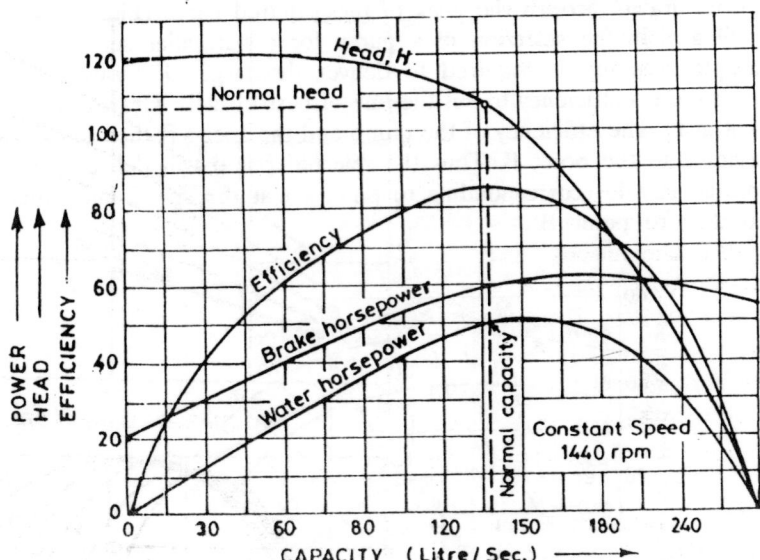

FIG. 17.16. CHARACTERISTICS AT CONSTANT SPEED.

type, i.e., it starts from a certain value rises slightly and then falls continuously with increasing discharge. The input power starts from a minimum value corresponding to zero discharge, rises first and attains a maximum value. Thereafter, the power curve continuously falls down with increase in discharge. Since $P \propto \eta_0$, the efficiency curve is also of similar shape but it starts from the origin. All the quantities corresponding to maximum efficiency are referred as designed values viz. design discharge, design head and design input power. For the computation of specific speed, design head are used in Eq. 17.49.

The input power corresponding to zero discharge is known as shut off power. It is input power which is lost in windage and friction losses.

Usually, these characteristic curves are supplied by the manufacturer alongwith the pump set; otherwise these can be obtained from hydraulic tests. They provide complete information about the performance of the pump.

17.18.2 Iso Efficiency or Muschel Curves

Theses are obtained from efficiency discharge and head- discharge curves. For this purpose the later set of curves is placed below the former. Firstly, the horizontal lines of constant efficiency are drawn at equal interval over η_0 vs Q curve i.e., η_0 corresponding to 10%, 20% an so on. These lines inersect η_0 vs Q curve at different point. Now these points of intersection corresponding to a particular efficiency, say 10%, is transferred on the head-discharge curve corresponding to same running speed N. Similarly, the points of intersection for various efficiencies are transferred over the head discharge curve. Finally, smooth curves corresponding to various efficiencies are drawn on head discharge curve. These are shown as Iso-efficiency for Muschcl cunes Later on, a cuve of best fit is drawn through the peak of these dotted curve (Fig. 17.17). This curve facilitates in the selection of a pump for a particular set of working. For example, a pump is required to deliver discharge Q. Draw a vertical line AB on the iso-efficiency to cut the line of best fit at B. Draw a horizontal line to cut at C. The efficiency of the pump and the speed is then interpolated corresponding to the point B. Thus the selected pump will deliver discharge Q against a head H (corresponding to point C) at the speed and efficiency corresponding to point B.

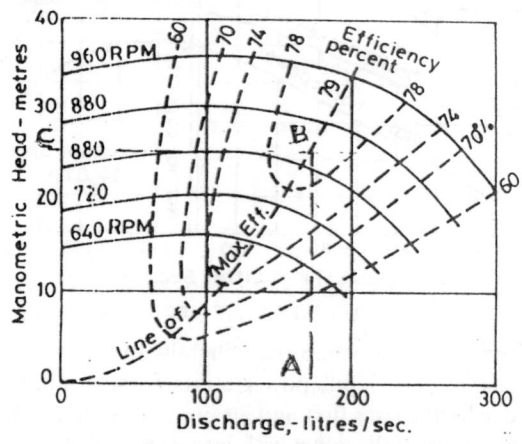

FIG. 17.17. ISO-EFFICIENCY CURVES

17.18.3 Constant Head and Constant Discharge Curve

Pumps are usually designed to run at constant speed. But, in some specified job, they may be required to run at variable speed. At that time, the performance of the pump is determined at variable speed. In such tests, the discharge, head and input power are plotted as ordinates against the speed N as abscissa. As seen from Eq. 17.48, the discharge is directly proportional to speed, hence Q vs N is a straight line. Similarly, H vs N^2, (Eq. 17.47) and P vs N^3, (Eq. 17.52) curves are drawn and are shown in Fig. 17.18.

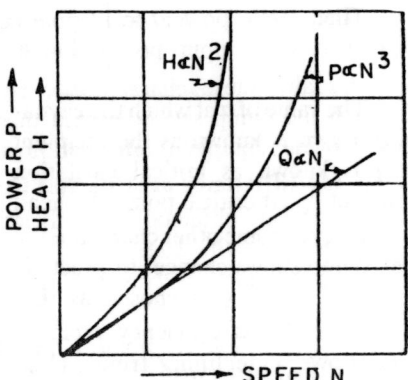

FIG. 17.18 CHARACTERISTIC CUVES AT VARIABLE SPEED

17.19 CAVITATION

Cavitation is the name given to a phenomenon which consists of local vapourisation of a liquid. When the absolute pressure falls to a value equal to or lower than the vapour pressure of the liquid at the given temperature, small bubbles of vapour are formed and boiling occurs. Since normally liquid have air dissolved in them, the lowering of pressure to a value near to the vapour pressure releases this air first. The combination of air released and vapourisation is known as cavitation.

In rotodynamic pumps, the cavitation occurs at pump inlet, where the pressure is lowest. The air bubbles travel along the surface and to the high pressure zone. In this zone, these bubbles get burst and then vanishes along the surface of impeller, casing and other components of the pump, exerting high pressure intensity over small area (pin point zones). In this way, the surfaces of metal (of casing, vanes etc). are repeatedly subjected to such high pressure (which may be as high as a 400 atm), that eventually causes the pitting of surface by actual removal of the solid metal.

The cavitation may cause the operation of the pump noisy, impairment of the hydraulic performance, mechanical vibration or actual material damage. This means, for satisfactory performance of the pump nowhere in the pump the pressure should lower down below vapour pressure of the liquid (at the temperature of the liquid). For cavitation free performance, the most general way is to compute the parameter known as 'Thoma's cavitation coefficient σ'. It is defined as the ratio of suction pressure head H_{sv} (or total head above vapour pressure of liquid) to the total manometric head H_m.

$$\sigma = \frac{H_{sv}}{H_m} \qquad \text{...(17.59)}$$

where
$$H_{sv} = (p_s/w + U_s^2/2g - p_v/w)$$

From Eq 17.12,

$$\frac{p_s}{w} = \left(\frac{p_{atm}}{w} - h_s - h_{fs} - U_s^2/2g \right) \text{ absolute}$$

$$\therefore \qquad H_{sv} = \left(\frac{p_{atm}}{w} - h_s - h_{fs} - \frac{p_v}{w} \right) \qquad \text{...(17.60)}$$

Then
$$\sigma = \left(\frac{p_{atm}}{w} - h_s - h_{fs} - \frac{p_v}{w} \right) / H_m \qquad ...(17.61)$$

The value of σ at which the cavitation starts (it is known as the incipient point) is known as 'critical cavitation coefficient σ_c. At critical point, the head or efficiency or some other characteristic of the pump shows change. In practice, the critical value σ_c is chosen as that point at which the efficiency verses σ curve shows a declining trend. (Fig. 17.19). The value of σ_c is found to depend

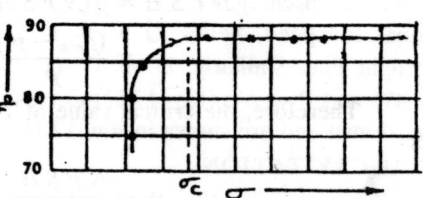

FIG. 17.19. VARIATION OF CAVITATION PARAMETER

on the capacity of the pump and the temperature of the liquid. For safe operation of the pump, it is desirable to run the pump at values of σ above critical value, i.e., $\sigma > \sigma_c$. For any pump installation, the critical value σ_c can be determined by model testing. The value of σ_c is also found to be related to the specific speed of the pump.

$$\sigma_c = 0.103 \, (N_s/1000)^{4/3} \qquad ...(17.62)$$

It is obvious from Eq. 17.61 that σ will increase as the suction static head h_s decreases. Therefore, for cavitation free operation the pump should be installed at proper suction height given by Eq. 17.61.

$$\left(h_s \right) = \left(H_{atm} - H_v \right) - \sigma H_m - h_{fs} \qquad ...(17.61)$$

If the value of h_s as computed by above Eq. 17.61 is –ve, the pump is to be installed below the liquid level in the lower sump. Sir ilarly, when the pumps are to deliver hot liquid (H_v is lower), the pumps may be required to be installed either at the liquid surface in the lower sump or below it as determined from Eq. 17.61.

17.20 NET POSITIVE SUCTION HEAD (OR NPSH)

It is defined as the sum of suction pressure head (in absolute units) above vapour pressure of the liquid and velocity head at the entrance to the impeller. Thus, the NPSH represent the difference between total energy at the inlet flange of the pump and the vapour pressure of the liquid.

Since
$$\frac{p_s}{w} = \left[\frac{p_{atm}}{w} - h_s - h_{fs} - \frac{U_s^2}{2g} \right] \text{ (absolute units) } ...(17.12)$$

$\therefore$
$$NPSH = \left[\frac{p_{atm}}{w} - \frac{p_v}{w} - h_s - h_{fs} \right] \qquad ...(17.63a)$$

It is the minimum pressure which an impeller must built up so that the liquid is raised from lower sump into impeller through suction pipe. If the pressure on the surface of liquid in the lower sump is more than atmospheric the term p_{atm}/w should be replaced by it.

In S.I. units, the NPSH is replaced by net positive suction energy (N.P.S.E) defined as

$$NPSH = g\,(NPSH)$$

$$= \frac{(p_{atm} - p_v)}{\rho} - g\,(h_s + h_{fs}) \qquad ...(17.63b)$$

Therefore, the critical value of Thoma's cavitation coefficiency is defined as

$$\sigma_c = \frac{NPSH}{H_m} \qquad ...(17.64)$$

$$= \frac{NPSH}{gE} \qquad ...(17.65)$$

17.21 SUCTION SPECIFIC SPEED (S)

Since the cavitation is determined by the condition of flow at the entrance to the impeller, another cavitation parameter is commonly used. It is known as suction specific speed S. It is analogous to usual definition of specific speed except that the total head H_m in its expression (Eq. 17.49) is replaced by the suction head above vapour pressure H_{sv}. Thus, it is defined as the speed of a geometrically similar pump which under corresponding similar conditions, would deliver 1 lit/sec against a total suction head of 1 metre (in absolute units).

$$S = \frac{N\sqrt{Q}}{\left(H_{sv}\right)^{3/4}} \qquad ...(17.66)$$

Since the total suction head H_{sv} has been defined as $NPSH$,

$$\therefore \qquad S = \frac{N\sqrt{Q}}{(NPSH)^{3/4}} \qquad ...(17.67)$$

Combining Eqns. 17.49, 17.64 and 17.66 the critical value of Thoma's cavitation coefficient is given by

$$\sigma_c = \left(\frac{N_s}{S}\right)^{4/3} \qquad ...(17.68)$$

For cavitation studies, the dynamic similarity should exist between model and prototype at the corresponding inlet sections. At the same time, the specific speed of the model and prototype should also be same. This is so, since critical cavitation coefficient σ_c depends on the specific speed N_s of the pump. If the second criterion of defining suction specific speed is used, then only a constant value of S for both model and prototype would suffice to satisfy the condition of dynamic similarity between them.

Furthermore for geometrically similar pumps, the similarity laws may be obtained as

$$\frac{(NPSH)_m}{(NPSH)_p} = \frac{(ND)_m}{(ND)_p} \qquad ...(17.69)$$

17.22 PRIMING OF PUMP

Before starting the pump, all the air from the body of the pump, suction pipe and delivery pipe (upto delivery valve) must be removed. It is known that the head built up by the pump impeller is directly proportional to the density of the liquid in which it is rotating. Therefore, if any air remains in the body of the pump, the impeller will churn the air liquid mixture and will generate insufficient head. And the pump will not be able to supply the liquid to the requisite height. Thus, the evacuation of air from pump body and thereby creating a vacuum in it is known as 'priming of the pump'.

There are various priming devices which are discussed hereinunder.

(1) *Pouring liquid* The simplest way of priming the pump is to pour liquid into the pump casing, etc. Fig. 17.20a. Normally the funnel is placed at the top of the casing through which the liquid may be filled into the casing

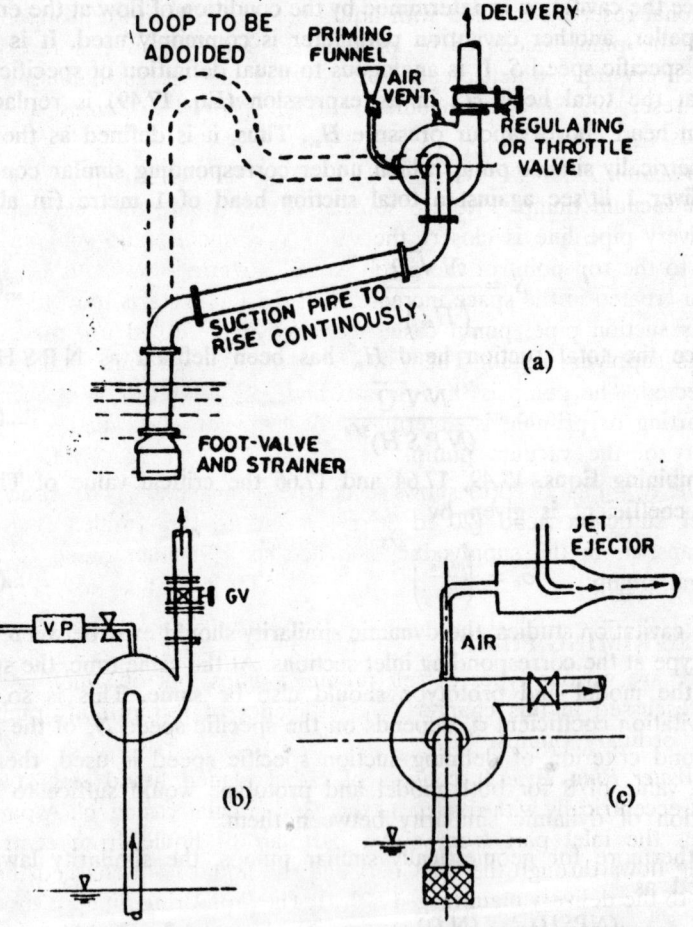

FIG. 17.20. PRIMING DEVICES, (A) POURING OF LIQUID
(B) BY JET (C) BY VACUUM PUMP.

of the pump while the delivery valve is kept closed. The suction pipe and the portion of delivery pipe upto delivery valve is simultaneous filled with liquid. An air vent with a cock is placed at the top of the casing which is kept open while priming the pump. In the beginning, air liquid mixture is ejected out through the air vent. Later on when most of the air has been evacuated, liquid jet issues out of the air vent and then the air vent is closed by means of air cock valve. The pump is now started and allowed to build up sufficient pressure head. Thereafter, the delivery valve is opened and the liquid is delivered at requisite pressure.

(2) *Connection with a City Supply* The pump be connected with city water supply main through a regulation valve. The valve may be operated to prime the pump.

(3) *Additional Reservoir* The centrifugal pumps are sometimes provided with an additional reservoir to which they supply liquid during its running. The additional reservoir is filled with liquid before the pump is stopped. Next time when the pump needs to be primed, the liquid from this reservoir is fed into delivery pipe, which create "piston effect" and sucks that liquid from the lower reservoir. Such arrangement can be used with pumps to handle dirty liquids.

(4) *Vacuum Producing Devices* Fig. 17.20 (b) shows a set up of centrifugal pump with vacuum pump. Prior to starting of the pump. the gate valve GV in the delivery pipe line is closed, the valve V is opened and vacuum pump connected to the top point of the scroll casing is started. As air is evacuated, the vacuum created in the space increases and the liquid starts moving upward. As soon as suction pipe, pump casing and delivery is filled up, the vacuum pump starts supplying liquid. The valve V is now closed and vacume pump is disconnected. The pump is thus primed and gate valve GV is opened. The time of starting or priming is determined by the volume of suction line and the capacity of the vacuum pump.

(5) *Jet type* Fig. 17.20(c) shows a jet type arrangement. The liquid from a jet under sufficient head (20 to 30 m) is fed to the nozzle. The jet of liquid entraps air in the supply duct and acts as a vacuum pump to prime a centrifugal pump.

17.23 SELF PRIMING PUMP

There are various types of self priming pumps; out of which only two types are discussed in this chapter. The efficiency of self priming pumps is lower than ordinary pumps.

(1) *Water Ring Type* It consists of radial bladed liquid ring rotor 'a' which is set eccentrically with respect to the fixed circular casing 'b'. A partition 'c' separates the inlet part from outlet part; air or liquid from centrifugal pump casing flows through the inlet part and the liquid is discharged through outlet part, to the delivery main (Fig. 17.21 a). The liquid ring pump is mounted coaxially in a common casing when the pump is started, the liquid remaining in the liquid ring casing 'a' is compelled by the rotor blades to revolve also

and because of centrifugal force, it is flung against the circumferential wall of the casing 'b'. Each space bounded by the inner surface of this liquid ring, the inner rim of the rotor and by a pair of adjacent rotor blades constitute a compartment of variable speed. As the blades descend, the enclosed volume of the cell increases and as the cell ascend during the remaining half of a revolution, the volume diminishes. Each cell, therefore, draws a definite volume of liquid from inlet part and then discharge it through outlet part.

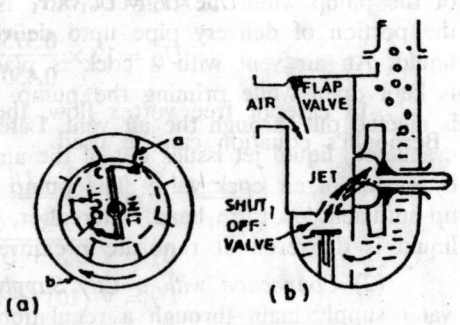

FIG. 17.21. SELF-PRIMING PUMP
(A) WATER RING PUMP
(B) WATER JET PUMPE.

(2) *Water Jet Pump* The machine embodies a water jet as the evaluating element. It is directly projected into the eye of impeller. (Fig. 17.21 b). The casing of the pump is so designed that sufficient liquid remains to keep the impeller submerged. When the pumps is started, the water from the suction chamber is sucked and raised into the delivery chamber which forms the pump casing. The resulting head difference creates flow through the nozzle into the impeller and a continous circulation of liquid is maintained. The jet entrains with it air from the suction side of the casing. The flap valve opens and the air is progressively evaluated from the suction pipe. As the volume increase, so does the pressure difference producing flow through the nozzle, the strength of the jet grows accordingly. The impeller continues to deliver a mixture of air and liquid. The liquid is recirculated and air passes into the delivery pipe. When the pressure difference is sufficiently high, the current approaching the nozzle from below is so powerful that it lifts shut off valve and cut the nozzle out of action. From this movement, the normal flow starts from the pump.

Example 17.1 – 17.18

17.1 A pump impeller is 375 mm diameter and it discharges water with component velocities of 2 m/s and 12 m/s in the radial and tangential directions respectively. The impeller is surrounded by a concentric cylindrical chamber with parallel sides, the outer diameter being 450 mm. If the flow in this chamber is a free vortex, find the component velocities of water on leaving and increase in pressure if there is no loss of energy.

Solution

Since the flow in the volute chamber is free vortex flow (Refer Fig. 17.3 b)

$$U \times r = C = \text{constant}$$

i.e.

$$U_{f1} \times r_1 = U_{f2} \times r_2$$

$$U_{f2} = 2 \times \frac{0.375}{0.450} = 1.667 \text{ m/s}$$

Similarly,

$$U_{w2} \times r_2 = U_{w1} \times r_1$$

$$U_{f2} = 12 \times \frac{0.375}{0.450} = 10 \text{ m/s}$$

In case of free vortex flow, the type of flow is irrotational. Hence, Bernoulli's equation can be used.

$$\left(\frac{p_2 - p_1}{w}\right) = \left(\frac{U_1^2 - U_2^2}{2g}\right)$$

$$U_2 = \sqrt{U_{w2}^2 + U_{f2}^2}$$

$$U_2 = \sqrt{(10)^2 + (1.667)^2}$$

$$U_2 = 10.14 \text{ m/s}$$

$$U_1 = \sqrt{(U_{w1})^2 + (U_{f1}^2)^2}$$

$$= \sqrt{(12)^2 + (2)^2}$$

$$= 12.165 \text{ m/s}$$

$$\frac{\Delta p}{w} = \text{pressure rise} = \frac{(12.165)^2 - (10.14)^2}{2 \times 9.81}$$

$$= \text{pressure rise} = 2.3 \text{ m of water}$$

17.2 A centrifugal pump has an impeller with inner and outer diameters 150 mm and 250 mm respectively. It delivers water at the rate of 50 lit/sec at 1500 r.p.m. The velocity of flow through the impeller is constant at 2.5 m/s. The blades are curved back at an angle of 30° to the tangent at exit. The diameters of suction and delivery pipes are 150 mm and 100 mm respectively. The pressure head at suction end is 4 m below atmospheric and that at delivery end is 18 m above atmospheric pressure. The power required to derive the pump is 18.4 kW. Find (i) the vane angle at inlet, (ii) overall efficiency, and (iii) the manometric efficiency.

Solution

Given Data : $D = 150$ mm, $D_1 = 250$ mm.

$Q = 0.05$ m³/s, $N = 1500$ r.p.m.,

$U_f = 2.5$, $\varphi = 30°$, $d_s = 150$ mm

$d_d = 100$ mm, $h_s = -4$ m (gauge)

$h_d = 18$ m gauge, power $= 18.4$ kW.

(i) $u = \frac{\pi D N}{60}$

$$= \frac{\pi \times 0.150 \times 1500}{60} = 11.78 \text{ m/s}$$

(ii) Refer to inlet velocity triangle, Fig. 17.22.

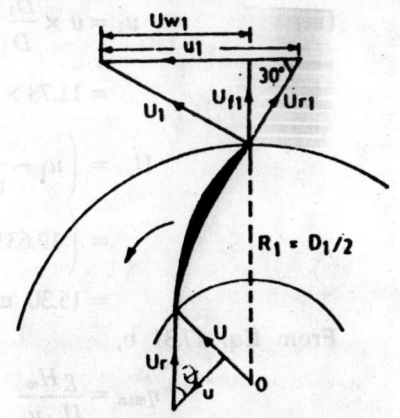

FIG. 17.22. EXAMPLE 17.2

Since the flow is in radial direction at inlet,

$$U = U_f = 2.5 \text{ m/s}$$

$$\tan \theta = \frac{U}{u}$$

$$= \frac{2.5}{11.78} = 0.2122$$

$$\theta = 71°90'$$

$$H_m = \left(\frac{p_d}{w} + \frac{U_d^2}{2g} \right) - \left(\frac{p_s}{w} + \frac{U_s^2}{2g} \right)$$

$$U_s = \frac{Q}{a_s} = \frac{0.050}{\pi/4 \times (0.15)^2} = 2.83 \text{ m/s}$$

$$U_d = \frac{Q}{a_d} = \frac{0.050}{\pi/4 \times (0.10)^2} = 6.36 \text{ m/s}$$

$$H_m = \left(\frac{p_d - p_s}{w} \right) + \left(\frac{U_d^2 - U_s^2}{2g} \right)$$

$$= \left[(18 + 4) + \frac{(6.36)^2 - (2.83)^2}{2 \times 9.81} \right]$$

$$= (22 + 1.653) = 23.653 \text{ m}$$

From Eq. 17.33

$$\eta_0 = \frac{w \, Q \, H_m}{P} \times 100$$

$$= \frac{9810 \times 0.050 \times 23.653}{18.4 \times 1000} \times 100$$

$$= 63 \%$$

(iii)

$$u_1 = u \times \frac{D_1}{D}$$

$$= 11.78 \times \frac{0.250}{0.150} = 19.633 \text{ m/s}$$

$$U_{w1} = \left(u_1 - \frac{U_{f1}}{\tan \varphi} \right) \text{ from outlet velocity triangle}$$

$$= \left(19.633 - \frac{2.5}{\tan 30°} \right)$$

$$= 15.30 \text{ m/s}$$

From Eq. 17.31 b,

$$\eta_{man} = \frac{g \, H_m}{U_{w1} \, u_1}$$

$$\eta_{man} = \frac{9.81 \times 23.653}{15.30 \times 19.633} \times 100 \quad = 77.27 \%$$

17.3 The impeller of a centrifugal pump is 0.3 m diameter and runs at 1450 r.p.m. The pressure gauges on suction and delivery side show the difference of 25 m. If the blades are curved back at an angle of 30° to tangent at outlet tips of the blades and the velocity of flow through the impeller being constant equals to 2.5 m/s, find manometric efficiency. If the frictional losses in the impeller amount to 2 m, find the fraction of total energy which is converted into pressure energy by whirl. Consider zero whirl at entry.

Solution

Given Data $D_1 = 0.3$ m,
$N = 1450$ r.p.m.

$\dfrac{p_d - p_s}{w} = 25$ m, $\varphi = 30°$

$U_f = U_{f1} = 2.5$ m/s, $U_w = 0$

$h_{Li} = 2$ m

$u_1 = \dfrac{\pi D_1 N}{60}$

$= \dfrac{\pi \times 0.3 \times 1450}{60} = 22.78$ m/s

$U_{w1} = (u_1 - U_{f1} \cot \varphi)$

$= (22.78 - 2.5 \cot 30°) = 18.45$ m/s

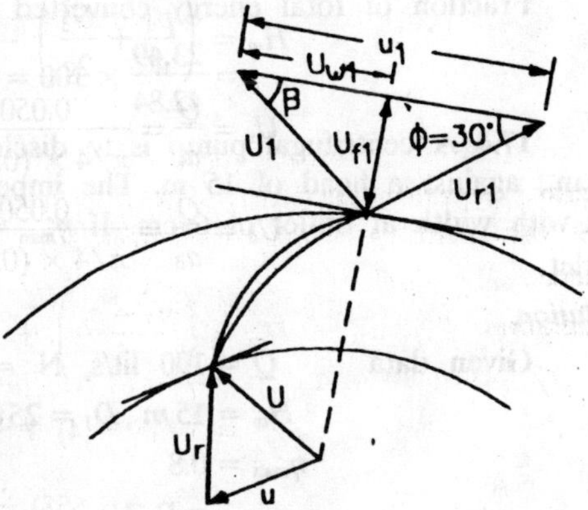

FIG. 17.23. EXAMPLE 17.3

Work done/s $= \dfrac{U_{w1} u_1}{g}$ (Since $U_w = 0$)

Work done/s $= \dfrac{18.45 \times 22.78}{9.81} = 42.84$ m

$\eta_{man} = \dfrac{H_m}{\dfrac{U_{w1} u_1}{g}}$

$= \dfrac{25}{42.84} = 58.35$ %

Now $U_1^2 = (U_{w1}^2 + U_{f1}^2)$

$= (U_{w1}^2 + U_f^2)$ (Since $U_f = U_{f1}$)

$U^2 = (U_w^2 + U_f^2)$

$= U_f^2$ (Since $U_w = 0$)

Hence change in K.E. in the impeller $= \dfrac{(U_1^2 - U_f^2)}{2g}$

$= \dfrac{(U_{w1}^2 + U_f^2 - U_f^2)}{2g} = \dfrac{(U_{w1}^2)}{2g}$

$$= \frac{(18.45)^2}{2 \times 9.81} = 17.35 \text{ m}$$

Energy converted into pressure energy

$$= \left(\frac{U_{w1} u_1}{g} - \frac{U_{w1}^2}{2g} - h_{Li} \right)$$

$$= 42.84 - 17.35 - 2$$

$$= 23.49 \text{ m}$$

Fraction of total energy converted into pressure energy

$$= \frac{23.49}{42.84} \times 100 = 54.83 \text{ \%}$$

17.4 A centrifugal pump is to discharge 100 lit/s at a speed of 1450 r.p.m., against a head of 15 m. The impeller has an outer diameter of 25 cm with width at outlet of 6 cm. If $\eta_{man} = 0.8$, esitmate the blade angle of outlet.

Solution

Given data
$$Q = 100 \text{ lit/s, } N = 1450 \text{ r.p.m.}$$
$$H_m = 15 \, m \, , D_1 = 25 \, cm \, , B_1 = 6 \, cm$$
$$\eta_{man} = 0.8$$
$$u_1 = \frac{\pi D_1 N}{60}$$
$$= \frac{\pi \times 0.25 \times 1450}{60} = 18.97 \text{ m/s}$$

Assuming radial flow at inlet,
$$U_w = 0$$

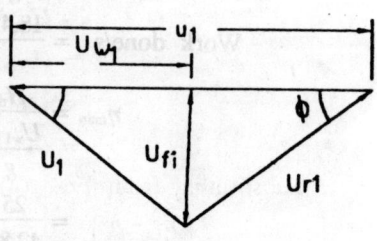

FIG. 17.24 EXAMPLE 17.4

$$\eta_{man} = \frac{g H_m}{U_{w1} u_1}$$

$$0.8 = \frac{9.81 \times 15}{U_{w1} \times 18.97}$$

$$U_{w1} = \frac{9.81 \times 15}{18.97 \times 0.8} = 9.7 \text{ m/s}$$

Discharge
$$Q = \pi D_1 B_1 U_{f1}$$
$$0.100 = \pi \times 0.25 \times 0.06 \times U_{f1}$$

$$U_{f1} = \frac{0.100}{\pi \times 0.25 \times 0.06} = 2.123 \text{ m/s}$$

From outlet velocity triangle
$$\tan \varphi = \frac{U_{f1}}{u_1 - U_{w1}}$$

$$= \frac{2.123}{18.97 - 9.7}$$

$$= 0.2290$$

$$\varphi = 12°53'54''$$

17.5 Show that the pressure rise in the impeller of a centrifugal pump is given by

$$\left(\frac{p_1 - p}{w}\right) = \frac{1}{2g}(U_1^2 + u_1^2 - U_{f1}^2 \, cosec^2 \, \varphi)$$

with usual notations.

Solution

Apply Bernoulli's equation between the inlet and outlet of the impeller. Assumptions are made that both these sections are located at the same elevation and no energy loss takes place in the impeller.

$$\left(\frac{p_1}{w} + \frac{U_1^2}{2g}\right) = \left(\frac{p}{w} + \frac{U^2}{2g} + \frac{U_{w1} u_1}{g}\right)$$

for raidal flow at entry.

or $\quad \left(\frac{p_1 - p}{w}\right) = \left(\frac{U^2}{2g} - \frac{U_1^2}{2g} + \frac{U_{w1} u_1}{g}\right)$ ...(i)

For radial entry (Refer Fig. 17.4)

$$U = U_f \text{ and } U_{w1} = (u_1 - U_{f1} \cot \varphi) \qquad \text{...(ii)}$$

Further,

$$U_1^2 = (U_{f1}^2 + U_{w1}^2)$$

$$= U_{f1}^2 + (u_1 - U_{f1} \cot \varphi)^2$$

$$= (U_{f1}^2 + u_1^2 + U_{f1}^2 \cot^2 \varphi - 2u_1 U_{f1} \cot \varphi)$$

$$= U_{f1}^2 (1 + \cot^2 \varphi) - 2u_1 U_{f1} \cot \varphi + u_1^2$$

$$= U_{f1}^2 \, cosec^2 \, \varphi - 2u_1 U_{f1} \cot \varphi + u_1^2 \qquad \text{...(iii)}$$

Substituting from Eqs. (ii) and (iii) into Eq. (i)

$$\left(\frac{p_1 - p}{w}\right) = \text{pressure rise}$$

$$= \frac{U_f^2}{2g} - \frac{(U_{f1}^2 \, cosec^2 \, \varphi - 2u_1 U_{f1} \cot \varphi + u_1^2)}{2g}$$

$$+ \frac{2u_1 (u_1 - U_{f1} \cot \varphi)}{2g}$$

$$\left(\frac{p_1 - p}{w}\right) = \frac{1}{2g}(U_f^2 + u_1^2 - U_{f1}^2 \, cosec^2 \, \varphi)$$

17.6 Prove that for a centrifugal pump running at N r.p.m. and giving a discharge Q, the manometric head H_m is given by

$$H_m = (AN^2 + BNQ + CQ^2)$$

where A, B and C are constants.

Solution

The manometric head H_m is given by

$$H_m = \left(\frac{U_{a1} u_1}{g} - losses \right)$$

$$= \left(\frac{U_{a1} u_1}{g} - k \frac{U_1^2}{2g} \right) \quad \ldots(i)$$

where $k U_1^2/2g$ is the head loss in the impeller and casing

At the outlet of impeller

$$u_1 = \frac{\pi D_1 N}{60} = k_1 N \quad \ldots(ii)$$

$$U_{f1} = \frac{Q}{a_{f1}} = k_2 Q \quad \ldots(iii)$$

From outlet velocity triangle,

$$U_{w1} = (u_1 - U_{f1} \cot \varphi)$$

$$= (k_1 N - k_2 \cot \varphi) \quad \ldots(iv)$$

$$= (k_1 N - k_3 Q)$$

where k_1, k_2 and k_3 are constants.

Substituting into Eq. (i)

$$H_m = \frac{(k_1 N - k_3 Q) k_1 N}{g} - \frac{k}{2g} [(k_2 Q)^2 + (k_1 N - k_3 Q)^2]$$

where

$$U_1^2 = (U_{w1}^2 + U_{f1}^2)$$

$\therefore$

$$H_m = \frac{1}{2g} [2 k_1^2 N^2 - 2 k_1 k_3 Q N]$$

$$- \frac{k}{2g} [k_2^2 Q^2 + k_1^2 N^2 - 2 k_1 k_3 N Q + k_3^2 Q^2]$$

$$= \frac{1}{2g} [N^2 (2 k_1^2 - k k_1^2) + QN (- 2 k_1 k_3 + 2 k k_1 k_3)$$

$$+ Q^2 (- k k_2^2 - k k_3^2)]$$

Thus

$$H_m = [A N^2 + B N Q + C Q^2]$$

17.7 A centrifugal pump lifts water against a static head of 35 m, of which 4 m is suction. The suction and delivery pipes are both 150 mm diameter; the loss in the suction pipe is 2.25 m and in the delivery pipe 8 m. The impeller is 395 mm diameter and 24.5 mm in width at its outlet. It revolves at 1200 rpm and its effective blade angle at outlet is 35°. If the manometric efficiency of the pump is 82 % and overall efficiency is 70 %, determine the discharge supplied by the pump and power required to derive the pump. Also determine the pressure head at the suction and delivery sides of the pump.

Solution

$$Q = \frac{\pi}{4} (0.150)^2 \times U_d$$

$$= 0.01766 \, U_d \qquad \qquad \text{...(i)}$$

Also

$$Q = \pi D_1 B_1 \times U_{f1}$$

$$= \pi \times 0.395 \times 0.0245 \times U_{f1}$$

$$= 0.0304 \, U_{f1} \qquad \qquad \text{...(ii)}$$

Equating Eqns. (i) and (ii)

$$0.01766 \, U_d = 0.0304 \, U_{f1}$$

$$U_{f1} = \frac{0.01766}{0.0304} \, U_d$$

$$= 0.581 \, U_d$$

Rim velocity at inlet

$$u_1 = \frac{\pi D_1 N}{60}$$

$$= \frac{\pi \times 0.395 \times 1200}{60}$$

$$= 24.81 \text{ m/s}$$

Now

$$H_m = \left(h_s + h_d + h_{fs} + h_{fd} + \frac{U_d^2}{2g} \right)$$

$$= \left(35 + 2.25 + 8 + \frac{U_d^2}{2g} \right)$$

$$\left(45.25 + \frac{U_d^2}{2g} \right) \qquad \qquad \text{...(iv)}$$

But

$$\eta_{man} = \frac{g \, H_m}{U_{w1} \, u_1}$$

$$H_m = \eta_{man} \times \frac{U_{w1} \, u_1}{g}$$

$$= 0.82 \, \frac{(u_1 - U_{f1} \cot \varphi) \, u_1}{g} \quad \text{where } U_{w1} = (u_1 - U_{f1} \cot \varphi)$$

$$= \frac{0.82}{9.81} (24.81 - 0.581 \, U_d \times \cot 35°) \times 24.81$$

$$= 2.073 (24.81 - 0.834 \, U_d) \qquad \qquad \text{...(v)}$$

From Eqns. (iv) and (v)

$$\left(45.25 + \frac{U_d^2}{2g} \right) = 2.073 (24.81 - 0.834 \, U_d)$$

Solving, $\qquad U_d = 3.23$ m/s

From Eq. (i) $\qquad Q = 0.01766 \times 3.23$

$$= 0.057 \text{ m}^3/\text{s}$$

From Eq. (iv) $H_m = [45.25 + (3.23)^2/(2 \times 9.81)] = 45.78$ m

Power required $\qquad = \dfrac{w \, Q \, H_m}{\eta_0}$ watts

$$= \frac{9810 \times 0.057 \times 45.78}{0.70}$$

$$= 25600 \text{ watts or } 25.6 \text{ kW}$$

Pressure on the suction side

$$= \left(h_s + \frac{U_s^2}{2g} + h_s \right)$$

$$= \left(4 + \frac{(3.23)^2}{2 \times 9.81} + 2.25 \right)$$

$$= 6.78 \text{ below atmosphere.}$$

Pressure on the delivery side

$$= (H_m - 6.78)$$

$$= (45.78 - 6.78)$$

$$= 39 \text{ m above atmosphere.}$$

17.8 A multistage centrifugal pump is discharging 45,000 lit/min against a manometric head of 60 m. There are four impellers, keyed to the same shaft which is running at 350 rpm. The vanes are curved back at an angle of 60° to the tangent at the outer periphery. The velocity of flow is 0.27 times the corresponding peripheral velocity and hydraulic losses in the pump are 1/3 the velocity head at exit of the pump. Determine diameter of the impeller and manometric efficiency.

Solution

Since there are four stages, head developed per stage is

H per stage $= \dfrac{60}{4} = 15 \text{ m}$

$$u_1 = \frac{\pi D_1 N}{60}$$

$$= \pi \times D_1 \times \frac{350}{60} = 18.31 D_1 \text{ m/s}$$

$$U_{f1} = 0.27 \times u_1$$

$$= 0.27 \times 18.31 D_1 = 4.9 D_1 \text{ m/s}$$

From outlet velocity triangle (Refer to Fig. 17.4)

$$U_{w1} = (u_1 - U_{f1} \cot 60°) = 15.48 D_1 \text{ m/s}$$

$$U_1 = \sqrt{U_{f1}^2 + U_{w1}^2}$$

$$= \sqrt{(4.9 D_1)^2 + (15.48 D_1)^2} = 16.24 D_1 \text{ m/s}$$

Hydraulic losses $= \dfrac{1}{3} \dfrac{U_1^2}{2g}$

$$= \frac{1}{3} \frac{(16.24 D_1)^2}{2 \times 9.81} = 4.48 D_1^2 \text{ metre}$$

Work done/sec $= \dfrac{U_{w1} u_1}{g}$ for radial inflow

$$= \dfrac{15.48\, D_1 \times 18.31\, D_1}{9.81} = 28.9\, D_1^2 \text{ Nm/s/N (i)}$$

Also work/done/sec/newton $= (H_m + losses)$

$$= (15.0 + 4.48\, D_1^2)$$

Equating Eqns. (i) and (ii)

$$28.9\, D_1^2 = (15 + 4.48\, D_1^2)$$

$$24.42\, D_1^2 = 15$$

$$D_1 = \sqrt{\dfrac{15}{24.42}} = 0.783 \text{ m}$$

Hence $\eta_{man} = \dfrac{g\, H_m}{U_{w1} u_1}$

$$= \dfrac{15 \times 9.81}{(15.48 \times 0.783)\,(18.31 \times 0.783)}$$

$$= 0.845 \text{ or } 84.5 \%$$

17.9 The impellers of a centrifugal pump has an outer diameter of 250 mm and an effective outlet area 150×10^{-4} m^2. The blades are bent back so that the angle at outlet is 148° to the tangent drawn in the direction of impeller rotation. The diameter of suction and delivery openings are 150 mm and 125 mm respectively. At speed of 1500 r.p.m. and discharge 0.025 m^3/s, the pressure heads at delivery and suction sides were found to be 15 m and 5 m above and below atmospheric pressure. Both these pressure points at which pressure were measured were at the same level. The power required

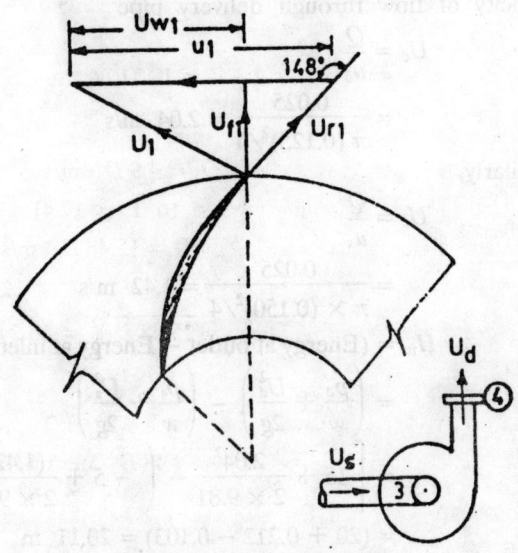

FIG. 17.25. EXAMPLE 17.9

to drive the pump is found to be 9.2 kW. It is found that water enters the pump without shock or whirl. Compute overall and manometric efficiency based on true whirl component. Assuming that true whirl component of velocity is 0.7 times ideal one.

Solution

Given $\qquad D_1 = 250$ mm, $a_{f1} = 150 \times 10^{-4}$ m^2

$$\varphi = (180 - 132) = 48°, d_s = 150 \text{ mm}$$

$$d_d = 125 \text{ mm}, \ N = 1500 \text{ r.p.m.},$$

$$Q = 0.025 \text{ m}^3/\text{s}, \ h_d = 15 \text{ m}, \ h_s = 5 \text{ m},$$

$$P = 9.2 \text{ kW}, \ (U_w)_{\text{true}} = 0.7 \times (U_w)_{\text{ideal}}$$

(i) $\qquad U_{f1} = \dfrac{0.025}{150 \times 10^{-4}} = 1.67$ m/s

(ii) $\qquad u_1 = \dfrac{\pi D_1 N}{60}$

$$= \dfrac{\pi \times 0.025 \times 1500}{60} = 19.63 \text{ m/s}$$

(iii) $\qquad U_{w1} = (u_1 - U_{f1} \cot \varphi)$

$$= (19.63 - 1.67 \cot 32°)$$

$$= (19.62 - 2.67) = 16.96 \text{ m/s}$$

(iv) Actual $\quad U_{w1} = 0.7 \times 16.96 = 11.87$ m/s

(v) Work done/sec $= \dfrac{U_{w1} u_1}{g}$

$$= \dfrac{11.87 \times 19.63}{9.81} = 23.75 \text{ Nm/s/N}$$

(vi) Velocity of flow through delivery pipe

$$U_d = \dfrac{Q}{a_d}$$

$$= \dfrac{0.025}{\pi (0.125)^2/4} = 2.04 \text{ m/s}$$

(vii) Similarly,

$$U_s = \dfrac{Q}{a_s}$$

$$= \dfrac{0.025}{\pi \times (0.150)^2/4} = 1.42 \text{ m/s}$$

(viii) $\qquad H_m = (\text{Energy at outlet} - \text{Energy at inlet})$

$$= \left(\dfrac{p_d}{w} + \dfrac{U_d^2}{2g} \right) - \left(\dfrac{p_s}{w} + \dfrac{U_s^2}{2g} \right)$$

$$= \left[15 + \dfrac{2.04^2}{2 \times 9.81} - \left(-5 + \dfrac{(1.42)^2}{2 \times 9.81} \right) \right]$$

$$= (20 + 0.212 - 0.103) = 20.11 \text{ m}$$

(ix) $\therefore$ $\eta_{man} = \dfrac{g\,H_m}{U_{w1}\,u_1}$

$$= \dfrac{20.11}{23.75} = 0.8460 \text{ or } 84.6 \ \%$$

(x) Also $H_m = \left(h_s + h_{fs} + h_d + h_{fd} + \dfrac{U_d^2}{2g} \right)$

$(h_s + h_d) = \left(H_m - h_{fs} - h_{fd} - \dfrac{U_d^2}{2g} \right)$

$$= \left(20.11 - \dfrac{(2.04)^2}{2 \times 9.81} \right); \text{ neglecting losses}$$

$$= 19.89 \ \text{m}.$$

(xi) $\eta_0 = \dfrac{w\,Q\,H_m}{P}$

$$= \dfrac{9810 \times 0.025 \times 20.11}{9.2 \times 1000} = 0.502 \text{ or } 50.2 \ \%.$$

17.10 The impeller of a centrifugal pump has blades which are bent backwards and make an acute angle β with the tangent at outer periphery. The pump has no diffuser, the velocity of flow is constant and absolute velocity of water at inlet is radial. Assuming the flow through the impeller is frictionless and streamlined, show from first principles that the ratio (rise in pressure head/work done per newton of water through impeller) is

$$\frac{1}{2} \left(1 + \frac{U_{f1}\cot\varphi}{u_1} \right)$$

A similar pump is fitted with a diffuser which converts a certain fraction k of the head due to whirling component of velocity at outlet into pressure head. Show that above would be

$$\frac{1}{2} \left[(1 + k) + (1 - k) \times \frac{U_{f1}\cot\varphi}{u_1} \right]$$

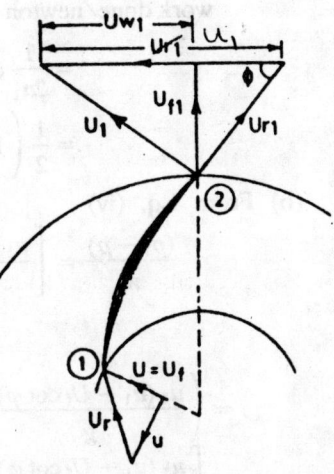

FIG. 17.26. EXAMPLE 17.10

Solution

(a) Since the flow is radial at the inlet

$$U = U_f, U_f = U_{f1} \qquad \qquad \text{...(i)}$$

$\therefore$ $U_{w1} = (u_1 - U_f \cot\varphi)$ ...(ii)

Work done per newton $= \dfrac{U_{w1}\,u_1}{g}$

$$= \frac{u_1}{g}(u_1 - U_f \cot \varphi) \qquad \text{...(iii)}$$

Also, work done per newton $= (H_2 - H_1)$

$$= \left(\frac{p_1}{w} + \frac{U_1^2}{2g} - \frac{p}{w} - \frac{U^2}{2g} \right) \qquad \text{...(iv)}$$

Now, $\quad U_1^2 = \left(U_{f1}^2 + U_{w1}^2 \right)$

$$= \left[U_f^2 + (u_1 - U_f \cot \varphi)^2 \right] \qquad \text{...(v)}$$

$$\therefore \quad \frac{(p_1 - p)}{w} = \text{Work done/newton} - \left(\frac{U_1^2}{2g} - \frac{U^2}{2g} \right)$$

From Eqs. (iii) to (v)

$$\therefore \quad \frac{(p_1 - p)}{w} = \frac{u_1(u_1 - U_f \cot \varphi)}{g} - \frac{U_f^2 + (u_1 - U_f \cot \varphi)^2}{2g} + \frac{U_f^2}{2g}$$

Solving $\quad \dfrac{(p_1 - p)}{w} = \dfrac{(u_1^2 - U_f^2 \cot^2 \varphi)}{2g}$

Hence $\quad \dfrac{(p_1 - p)/w}{\text{work done/newton}} = \dfrac{(u_1^2 - U_f^2 \cot^2 \varphi)}{2g} \times \dfrac{g}{u_1(u_1 - U_f \cot \varphi)}$

$$= \frac{1}{2u_1}(u_1 + U_f \cot \varphi)$$

$$= \frac{1}{2} \left(1 + \frac{U_{f1}}{u_1} \cot \varphi \right)$$

(b) From Eq. (iv)

$$\frac{(p_1 - p)}{w} = \left[\frac{u_1(u_1 - U_f \cot \varphi)}{g} - \frac{U_1^2}{2g} + \frac{U^2}{2g} + k\frac{U_{w1}^2}{2g} \right]$$

$$\left(\text{Since } k\frac{U_{w1}^2}{2g} \text{ is added due to diffuser} \right)$$

$$= \left(\frac{u_1(u_1 - U_f \cot \varphi)}{g} - \frac{(U_{f1}^2 + U_{w1}^2)}{2g} + \frac{U_f^2}{2g} + k\frac{U_{w1}^2}{2g} \right) (\because U_{f1} = U_f)$$

$$= \left[\frac{u_1(u_1 - U_f \cot \varphi)}{g} - \frac{U_{w1}^2}{2g}(1 - k) \right]$$

$$= \left[\frac{u_1(u_1 - U_f \cot \varphi)}{g} - (u_1 - U_f \cot \varphi)^2 \frac{(1 - k)}{2g} \right]$$

$$= \frac{(u_1 - U_f \cot \varphi)}{2g} [2u_1 - (1 - k)(u_1 - U_f \cot \varphi)]$$

$$= \frac{(u_1 - U_r \cot \varphi)}{2g} [(2u_1 - u_1 + U_f \cot \varphi + k u_1 - k U_f \cot \varphi)]$$

$$\therefore \quad \frac{(p_1 - p)/w}{\text{work done/newton}} = \frac{\dfrac{(u_1 - U_f \cot \varphi)}{2g}[u_1(1 + k) + (1 - k)U_f \cot \varphi]}{\dfrac{(u_1 - U_f \cot \varphi) \times u_1}{g}}$$

$$= \frac{1}{2u_1}[u_1(1+k) + (1-k)U_f \cot \varphi]$$

$$= \frac{1}{2}\left[(1+k) + (1-k)\frac{U_f}{u_1} \cot \varphi\right]$$

17.11 A centrifugal pump has inlet diameter of 300 mm and outlet diameter of 600 mm. The velocity of flow is 2 m/s. The vanes are curved backward and make as angle of 45° to the tangent at the outlet tip. Determine minimum starting speed of the pump. Take manometric efficiency as 75%.

Solution

Given $D = 300$ m..n , $D_1 = 600$ mm,

$$U_f = 2 \text{ m/s}, \ \varphi = 45°,$$

$$\eta_{man} = 75\%, U_{f1} = 2 \text{ m/s}.$$

$$u_1 = \frac{\pi D_1 N}{60}$$

$$= \frac{\pi \times 0.6 \times N}{60} = 0.0314 \text{ N}$$

From outlet velocity triangle,

$$U_{w1} = (u_1 - U_{f1} \cot \varphi)$$

$$= (0.0314 N - 2 \cot 45°)$$

$$= (0.0314 N - 2)$$

$$\eta_{man} = \frac{g H_m}{U_{w1} u_1}$$

$$H_m = \frac{U_{w1} u_1 \eta_{man}}{g}$$

For starting the pump, the necessary condition is

$$\frac{u_1^2 - u^2}{2g} = H_m$$

For minimum speed, the limiting condition is

$$\frac{u_1^2 - u^2}{2g} = \frac{U_{w1} u_1 \eta_{man}}{g}$$

or $\frac{1}{2}\left[\left(\frac{\pi D_1 N}{60}\right)^2 - \left(\frac{\pi D N}{60}\right)^2\right] = \eta_{man}\left(U_{w1} \times \frac{\pi D_1 N}{60}\right)$

Dividing by $\left(\frac{\pi N}{60}\right)$ on both sides

$$\frac{\pi N}{120}(D_1^2 - D^2) = \eta_{man} \times U_{w1} \times D_1$$

$$N = \frac{120 \eta_{man} \times U_{w1} \times D_1}{\pi (D_1^2 - D^2)}$$

Substituting the values,

$$N = \frac{120 \times 0.68 \times (0.0314 N - 2) \times 0.6}{\pi (0.6^2 - 0.3^2)}$$

$$= 57.75 (0.0314 N - 2)$$

$$= 1.813 N - 115.49$$

$$N = \frac{115.49}{0.813} = 142.06 \text{ r.p.m.}$$

17.12 A three stage centrifugal pump has impeller 500 mm diameter and 20 mm wide at the outlet. The vanes are curved back at the outlet at 45° and reduces the circuferential area by 10%. The manometric efficiency of the pump is 90% and overall efficiency is 80%. Determine the head developed by the pump when running at 1000 r.p.m., delivering 0.05 m³/s and what is the power required ?

Solution

Given $D_1 = 400$ mm, $B_1 = 20$ mm,

$$\varphi = 45°, k = 0.9, \eta_{man} = 0.90,$$

$$\eta_0 = 0.80, N = 1000 \text{ r.p.m}$$

$$Q = 0.05 \text{ m}^3/\text{s}$$

$$U_{f1} = \frac{Q}{a_{f1}} = \frac{Q}{k \pi D_1 B_1}$$

$$= \frac{0.05}{0.90 \times \pi \times 0.4 \times 0.020} = 2.21 \text{ m/s}$$

$$u_1 = \frac{\pi D_1 N}{60}$$

$$= \frac{\pi \times 0.4 \times 1000}{60} = 20.93 \text{ m/s}$$

From outlet velocity triangle,

$$U_{w1} = (u_1 - U_{f1} \cot \varphi)$$

$$= (20.93 - 2.21 \cot 45°) = 18.72 \text{ m/s}$$

Now $\eta_{man} = \dfrac{g H_m}{U_{w1} u_1}$

$$0.90 = \frac{9.81 \times H_m}{18.72 \times 20.93}$$

$$H_m = \frac{0.9 \times 18.72 \times 20.93}{9.81} = 35.94 \text{ m}$$

Total head generated by the pump $H_T = n H_m$

$$= 3 \times 35.94$$

$$= 107.84 \text{ m}$$

$$\eta_0 = \frac{w Q H_T}{P}$$

$$0.80 = \frac{9810 \times 0.05 \times 107.84}{P}$$

$$P = \frac{9810 \times 0.05 \times 107.84}{0.80}$$

$$= 66119.4 \text{ watts or } 66.12 \text{ kW.}$$

17.13 A single stage centrifugal pump with impeller diameter of 300 mm rotates at 2000 r.p.m and supplies 3 m³/s to a height of 30 m with an efficiency of 75%. Find the number of stages and diameter of each impeller of a similar multistage pump to lift 5 m³/s of water to a height of 200 m when rotating at 1500 r.p.m.

Solution

Given $\qquad D_1 = 300$ mm, $N_1 = 2000$ r.p.m.,

$$Q_1 = 3 \text{ m}^3/\text{s}, \quad H_{m1} = 30 \text{ m},$$

$$\eta_0 = 75 \%, \quad H_T = 200 \text{ m}$$

$$Q_2 = 5 \text{ m}^3/\text{s} \quad N_2 = 1500 \text{ r.p.m.}$$

Since the pumps are of similar design, their specific speed should be same.

$$\frac{N_1 \sqrt{Q_1}}{(H_{m1})^{3/4}} = \frac{N_2 \sqrt{Q_2}}{(H_{m2})^{3/4}}$$

$$(H_{m2})^{3/4} = \frac{N_2}{N_1} \times \frac{\sqrt{Q_2}}{\sqrt{Q_1}} \times (H_{m1})^{3/4}$$

$$= \frac{1500}{2000} \times \sqrt{\frac{5}{3}} \times (30)^{3/4} = 12.411$$

$$H_{m2} = 28.73 \text{ m.}$$

$\therefore \qquad$ Number of stages $= \dfrac{H_T}{H_m}$

$$= \frac{200}{28.73} = 6.97 \approx 7$$

From Eq. 17.47

$$\frac{D_1 N_1}{\sqrt{H_{m1}}} = \frac{D_2 N_2}{\sqrt{H_{m2}}}$$

$$D_2 = D_1 \times \frac{N_1}{N_2} \times \frac{\sqrt{H_{m2}}}{\sqrt{H_{m1}}}$$

$$= 0.30 \times \frac{2000}{1500} \times \frac{\sqrt{28.73}}{\sqrt{30.0}} = 0.3914 \text{ m.}$$

17.14 A centrifugal pump having four stages in parallel delivers 200 lit/sec of liquid against a head of 25 m, the diamter of impeller being 250 mm and its speed 1750 r.p.m.

A pump is to be made up with a number of identical stages in series of similar construction to those in the first pump to run at 1250 r.p.m and to deliver 300 lit/sec against a head of 250 m. Find the diameter and number of stges required.

Solution

Given $(Q_T)_1 = 200$ lit/sec, $(H_m)_1 = 25$ m,

$D_1 = 0.250$ m, $N_1 = 1750$ r.p.m.,

$N_2 = 1250$ r.p.m., $Q_2 = 300$ lit/sec,

$(H_T)_2 = 250$ m

Since the impellers are geometrically similar and will operate under similar conditions of ratios of useful energies to losses of energy, their velocity triangles will also be similar.

Pump 1; $N_s = \dfrac{N_1 \sqrt{Q_1}}{(H_{m1})^{3/4}}$

Since the given pump is four stage in parallel,

Q_1 per stage $= \dfrac{200}{4} = 50$ lit/sec

$N_s = \dfrac{1750 \times \sqrt{50}}{(25)^{3/4}} = 1100$ r.p.m.

Pump 2: Let the number of stages be n for the pumps connected in series

$\therefore$ Head per stage $= \dfrac{250}{n}$

$N_s = \dfrac{1250 \times \sqrt{300}}{\left(\dfrac{250}{n}\right)^{3/4}}$

$\left(\dfrac{250}{n}\right)^{3/4} = \dfrac{1250 \times \sqrt{300}}{1100}$

$= 19.68$

$n = \dfrac{250}{(19.68)^{4/3}}$

$= \dfrac{250}{53.13} = 4.7 \approx 5$

$\therefore$ Head per stage

$= \dfrac{250}{5} = 50$ m

Using Eq. 17.47,

$\dfrac{D_1 N_1}{\sqrt{H_{m1}}} = \dfrac{D_2 N_2}{\sqrt{H_{m2}}}$

$$D_2 = D_1 \times \frac{N_1}{N_2} \times \frac{\sqrt{H_{m2}}}{\sqrt{H_{m1}}}$$

$$= 25 \times \frac{1750}{1250} \times \frac{\sqrt{50}}{\sqrt{25}}$$

$$= 0.495 \text{ m}$$

17.15 The head discharge characteristics of a centrifugal pump is given by the following equation

$$H = (45 + 20 Q - 100 Q^2)$$

where H is in metres and Q is in cubic metre per second. The pump is in an installation where the static head is 15 m and the head lost in the pipe system is given by $h_f = 180 Q^2$, where h_f is in metres and Q in cumec. Find the manometric head at which the pump will operate and the discharge it will deliver.

Solution

Head developed = (static head + losses)

$$H = (15 + 180 Q^2) \qquad\qquad ...(1)$$

Also $\qquad\qquad H = (45 + 20 Q - 100 Q^2) \qquad\qquad ...(2)$

Equating Eqns 1 and 2,

$$15 + 180 Q^2 = 45 + 20 Q - 100 Q^2$$

$$280 Q^2 - 20 Q - 30 = 0$$

Solving, $\qquad\qquad Q = 0.365 \text{ m}^3/\text{s}$

Operating head $H = 15 + 180 Q^2$

$$= 15 + 180 (0.365)^2$$

$$= 38.98 \text{ m.}$$

17.16 Centrifugal pump running at 1500 r.p.m. has the following characteristics

Q (lit/min)	10	15.5	21.5	30.3	36.3	42.5	48
H (m)	35.5	34.5	33.25	30.0	26.75	22.75	18.5
η_0 (%)	60	67.5	72	73.5	71	66	60

Draw the characteristic curves of the pump and find out its specific speed. Also determine the power of the motor required when operating at maximum efficiency.

Solution

The characteristic curves are drawn in Fig. 17.27. The values corresponding to maximum efficiency are

$$(\eta_0)_{man} = 74 \%$$

$$Q = 27.5 \text{ lit/sec}$$

$$H = 31.5 \text{ m}$$

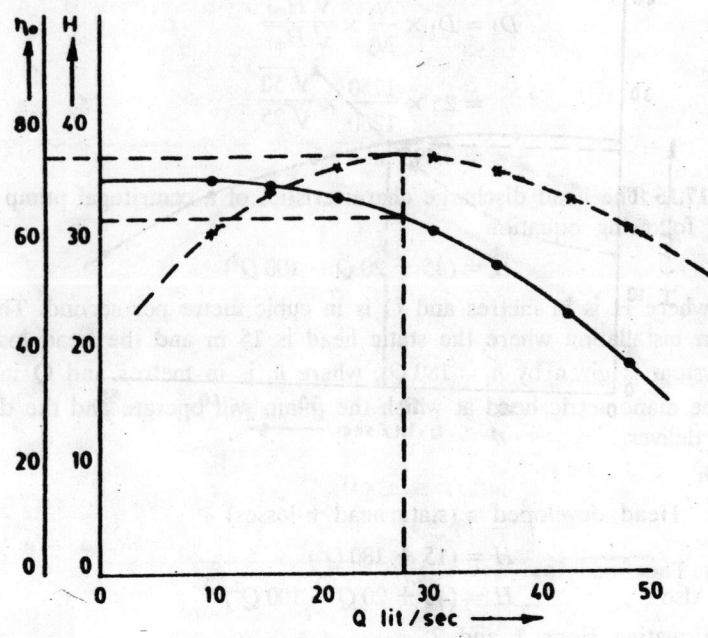

FIG. 17.27. EXAMPLE 17.16

$$N_s = \frac{N\sqrt{Q}}{(H)^{3/4}}$$

$$= \frac{1500\sqrt{27.5}}{(31.5)^{3/4}} = 591.6 \text{ r.p.m.}$$

Power required $= \frac{(w\,Q\,H_m)}{\eta_0}$

$$= \frac{9810 \times 0.0275 \times 31.5}{0.74}$$

$$= 11483.67 \text{ watts or } 11.483 \text{ kW}$$

17.17 The head discharge characteristic of a centrifugal pump is given below

Q (lit/sec)	0	10	20	30	40	50
H (metres)	25.3	25.5	24.5	22.2	18.7	12.0

The pump delivers water through a 500 m long pipe of 140 mm diameter. The static lift is 14 m. Find (a) the discharge of the pump and (b) driving power of the pump. Take f = 0.025 and neglect minor losses. The overall efficiency of the pump may be taken as 70 %.

Solution

Given Data $L = 500$ m, $D = 150$ mm

$$h_s + h_d = 14 \text{ m}, \quad f = 0.025,$$

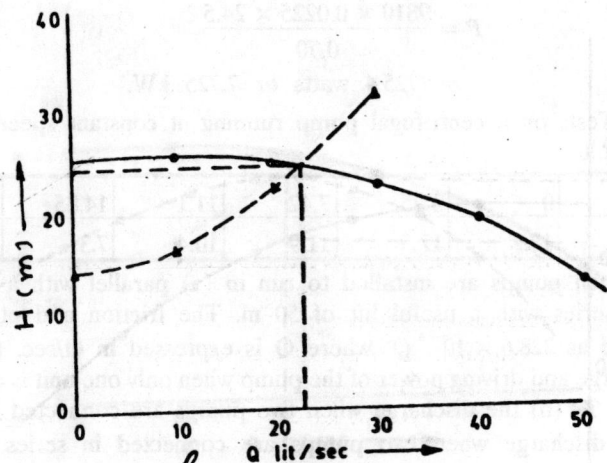

FIG. 17.28. EXAMPLE 17.17

$$\eta_0 = 70 \ \%$$

(i) The head loss due to friction in the pipe

$$h_f = \frac{fL Q^2}{12.1 D^5}$$

$$= \frac{0.025 \times 500 \times Q^2}{12.1 (0.140)^5} = 19208.1 \ Q^2$$

The total head developed by the pump is given by

$$H = (\text{static lift} + \text{losses})$$

$$H = (14 + 19208.1 \ Q^2)$$

Writing Q in lit/sec,

$$H = \left[14 + 19208.1 \left(\frac{Q}{1000} \right)^2 \right] = (14 + 0.0192 \ Q^2)$$

The head computed from above equation is given as

Q lit/sec	0	10	20	30	40	50
H metre	14	15.92	21.68	31.29	44.73	62.02

The data is plotted on the head-discharged graph of the pump as dotted curve. At the point of intersection of these two curves, i.e. the discharge supplied by the pump (Fig. 17.28) and head developed by it are

(a) $\qquad$ $Q = 22.5$ lit/sec

$$H = 24.5 \ m$$

(b) $\qquad$ $P = \dfrac{wQH}{\eta_0}$

$$P = \frac{9810 \times 0.0225 \times 24.5}{0.70}$$

$$= 7725.4 \text{ watts or } 7.725 \text{ kW.}$$

17.18 Tests on a centrifugal pump running at constant speed gave the following results:

Q lit/sec	0	3.75	7.42	11.1	14.85	18.5
H_m metre	12.2	12.5	11.9	10.4	7.3	3.65

Two such pumps are installed to run in (a) parallel with a useful lift of 7 m (b) series with a useful lift of 50 m. The friction and other losses are calculated as $228.6 \times 10^{-4} Q^2$ where Q is expressed in lit/sec. Determine (a) the discharge and driving power of the pump when only one unit is connected. Take $\eta_0 = 75 \%$, (b) the discharge when two pumps are connected in parallel and (c) the discharge when two pumps are connected in series.

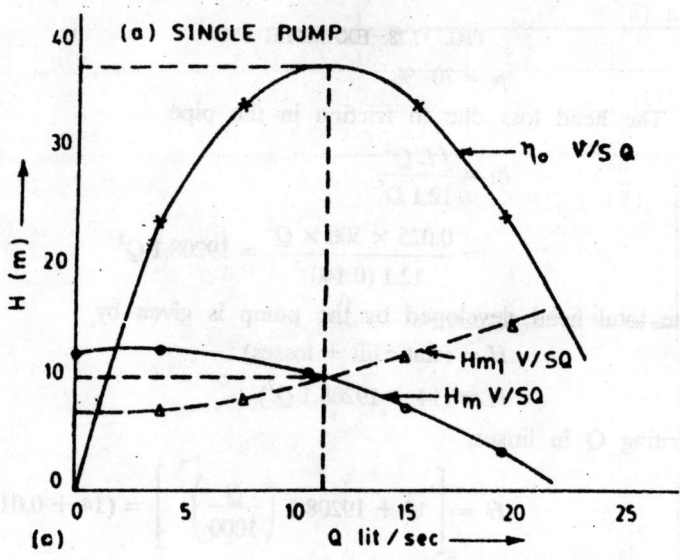

FIG. 17.29. EXAMPLE 17.18

Solution

(a) When only one pump is connected in the pipe line, the pump must generate head H_{m1}.

$$H_{m1} = \text{static lift} + \text{losses}$$

$$= (7 + 228.6 \times 10^{-4} \times Q^2) \qquad \text{...(i)}$$

The values of H_{m1} are computed for various values of Q.

Q lit/sec	0	3.75	7.42	11.1	14.85	18.5
H_m metre	7.0	7.32	8.26	9.82	12.04	14.82

The curves for H_m vs Q and H_{m1} vs Q are plotted in Fig. 17.29. These two curves intersects at point A.

$$Q = 11.25 \text{ lit/sec}; \quad H = 10 \text{ m}, \quad \eta_0 = 75\%$$

$$\therefore \quad P = \frac{wQH_m}{\eta_0}$$

$$= \frac{9810 \times 0.01125 \times 10}{0.75} = 163.5 \text{ watts.}$$

(b) When two pumps are connected in parallel,

The discharge from both the pumps will flow through common suction and delivery pipes.

$$\therefore \quad H_{m2} = (7 + 228.6 \times 10^{-4} \times (2Q)^2)$$

$$= (7 + 914.4 \, Q^2/10^4) \qquad ...(ii)$$

Corresponding to various values of Q, H_{m2} is computed from above equation (ii)

Q	2.5	5.0	7.5	10.0	12.5
Q_T (= 2Q)	5.0	10.0	15.0	20.0	25.0
H_{m2}	7.57	9.29	12.14	16.14	21.28

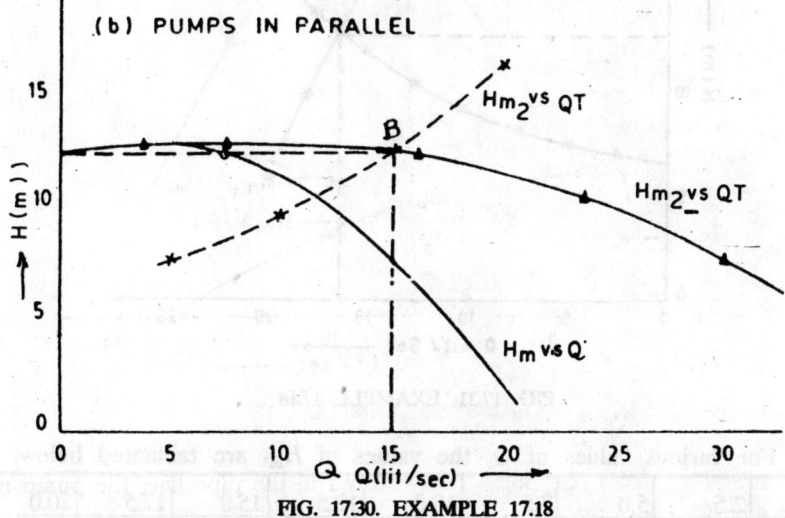

FIG. 17.30. EXAMPLE 17.18

The head discharge characteristic of the pump units connected in parallel is tabulated below. For various values of H_m, Q and hence Q_T (= 2Q) is computed from the given $H_m - Q$ table (or graph).

H_m (m)	2.5	5.0	7.5	10.0	12.0	12.5
Q (lit/sec)	19.0	17.25	14.90	11.75	8.0	3.65
Q_T (lit/sec)	38.0	34.5	29.8	23.5	16.0	7.50

These two curves H_m vs Q_T and H_{m2} vs Q_T are plotted in Fig. 17.30. At the point of intersection B (upper dark curve and dotted curve)

$$Q_T = 15 \text{ lit/sec}$$

$$H_m = 12.25 \text{ m}$$

$$Q = 7.5 \text{ lit/sec from each pump.}$$

(c) When two pumps are connected in series, the head developed by the two units will be added up. The head to be built up by the pump unit is H_{m3}

$$H_{m3} = (\text{Static lift} + \text{losses})$$

$$= (7 + 228.6 \, Q^2/10^4)$$

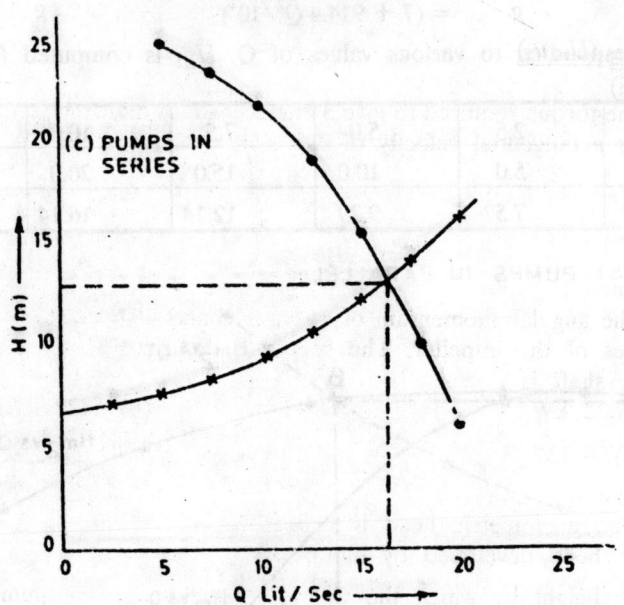

FIG. 17.31. EXAMPLE 17.18

For various values of Q, the values of H_{m3} are tabulated below:

Q	2.5	5.0	7.5	10.0	12.5	15.0	17.5	20.0
H_{m3}	7.14	7.57	8.28	9.29	10.57	12.14	14.0	16.14

The values of H_m vs Q for the pump units connected in series as read from head discharge characteristic curve (given) as

Q	2.5	5.0	7.5	10.0	12.5	15.0	17.5	20.0
H_m	12.6	12.5	11.75	11.0	9.5	7.25	5.0	3.0
$2 H_m$	25.2	25.0	23.5	22.0	19.0	14.5	10.0	6.0

The curves H_{m3} vs Q and $2H_m$ vs Q are drawn in Fig. 17.31. At the point of intersection C.

Discharge $\qquad Q = 16.25$ lit/sec

Total head $\qquad H_{m3} = 13.0$ m.

Objective Question

17.1 The fundamental equation known as Euler's Equation for a centrifugal pump for radial entry is

(a) $H = \dfrac{(U_w u + U_{w1} u_1)}{g}$

(b) $H = \dfrac{(U_{w1} u_1 - U_w u)}{g}$

(c) $H = \dfrac{(U_w u - U_{w1} u_1)}{g}$

(d) $H = \dfrac{(U_w u)}{g}$

(e) $H = \dfrac{(U_{w1} u_1)}{g}$

17.2 The torque required to give 3 cumec water a moment of momentum so that it has a tangential velocity of 3 m/s at a radius of 15 cm from the axis is

(a) 1.35

(b) 0.1376

(c) 1350

(d) 13243.5

(e) none.

17.3 The angular momentum of water is changed by 2800 N-m flowing through blades of the impeller. The speed of the shaft is 400 r.p.m. The power at the shaft is

(a) 117.22 kW

(b) 1120 kW

(c) 7033.6 kW

(d) 7.0 kW

(e) none

17.4 The manometric head is defined as

(a) the head developed by the pump

(b) the height by which the water is lifted above the pump centre line.

(c) the difference in elevations of upper and lower reservoirs or tanks

(d) the difference in the piezometric heads between the points on the delivery and suction side as close to the pump as possible

17.5 The manometric head is given by

(a) $\dfrac{U_{w1} u_1}{g}$

(b) $\dfrac{U_{w1} u_1}{g} + losses$

(c) $\dfrac{U_{w1} u_1}{g} - losses$

(d) $\dfrac{U_w u}{g} + losses$

(e) none.

17.6 The manometric efficiency η_{man} is given as

(a) $\dfrac{w\,Q\,H_m}{P}$

(b) $\dfrac{w\,Q\,H_s}{P}$

(c) $\dfrac{U_{w1}\,u_1}{g\,H_m}$

(d) $\dfrac{g\,H_m}{U_{w1}\,u_1}$

(e) none.

17.7 The minimum starting speed of a centrifugal pump to start the supply of water is given by

(a) $\dfrac{2\,g\,H_m}{(R_1^2 - R^2)}$

(b) $\dfrac{(R_1^2 - R^2)}{2\,g\,H_m}$

(c) $\sqrt{\dfrac{2\,g\,H_m}{(R_1^2 - R^2)}}$

(d) $2\,g\,H_m\,(R_1^2 - R^2)$

(e) none.

17.8 A three stage centrifugal pump supplies water at the rate of 0.16 m³/s while running at 800 rpm. The pump lifts water from 89 m deep well. If it's speed is changed to 1200 rpm. It will supply discharge (m³/s)

(a) 0.24

(b) 0.071

(c) 0.196

(d) 0.106

(e) none.

17.9 A centrifugal pump discharges water at the rate of 0.167 m³/s at 200 r.p.m under a head of 100 m. It consumes 300 kW power. A 1:4 scale model is to run at 1500 r.p.m. The power consumed by model is

(a) 0.1236 kW

(b) 126.56 kW

(c) 75 kW

(d) 25 kW

(e) none.

17.10 The specific speed of a centrifugal pump is given by

(a) $N_u\,\sqrt{Q_u}$

(b) $N\,\sqrt{P}/H_m^{3/4}$

(c) $N\,\sqrt{Q}/H_m^{5/4}$

(d) $\dfrac{H_m^{3/4}\,\sqrt{Q}}{N}$

(e) none.

17.11 For cavitation free operation of the centrifugal pump, the minimum pressure should not fall down below

(a) $[H_a - H_v - U_s^2/2g - h_{fs}]$

(b) $[H_a - H_v - U_s^2/2g + h_{fs}]$

(c) $[H_a - H_v - U_d^2/2g + h_{fd}]$

(d) $\left[H_a - H_v - \dfrac{U_d^2}{2g} - h_{fd}\right]$

(e) none.

17.12 The net positive suction head (NPHS) which represents the suction head at the impeller eye is given by

(a) $\left(\dfrac{p_s}{w} - \dfrac{p_v}{w} + h_s - h_{fs}\right)$

(b) $\left(\dfrac{p_s}{w} - \dfrac{p_v}{w} - h_s - h_{fs}\right)$

(c) $\left(\dfrac{p_a}{w} - \dfrac{p_v}{w} - h_s + h_{fs}\right)$　　　　(d) $\left(\dfrac{p_a}{w} - \dfrac{p_v}{w} + h_s + h_{fs}\right)$

(e) none.

17.13 The net positive suction energy (NPSE) is given by

(a) ρ (NPSH)　　　　　　　　　　(b) g (NPSH)

(c) w (NPSH)　　　　　　　　　　(d) Equal to NPSH

(e) none.

17.14 The suction specific speed S for a centrifugal pump is defined as

(a) $N\sqrt{Q}/H_m^{3/4}$　　　　　　　　(b) $N\sqrt{Q}/(NPSH)^{3/4}$

(c) $N\sqrt{Q}/(NPSE)^{3/4}$　　　　　　(d) $N\sqrt{Q}/H_{su}^{3/4}$

(e) none.

17.15 The hydraulic function of the casing of a centrifugal pump is

(a) to convert hydraulic energy into mechnacial energy

(b) to convert mechanical energy into hydraulic energy

(c) to transform most of the pressure energy into kinetic energy

(d) to transform most of the kinetic energy into pressure energy

(e) no hydraulic function

Problems

17.1 Give a layout of a pumping installation and name the main accessories.

17.2 Explain with neat sketches the working of a single stage centrifugal pump.

17.3 State the difference between a closed, semi open and open impeller.

17.4 Why is the efficiency of a volute casing as an energy conversion device of a centrifugal pump low. How is a whirl pool or vortex chamber superior in performance ?

17.5 What are various methods adopted to increase the efficiency of a centrifugal pump by varying the shape of the casing or chamber surrounding the impeller.

17.6 State various types of losses which may occur in a centrifugal pump.

17.7 Define different types of efficiencies used in reference of a centrifugal pump.

17.8 Explain, why priming is essential before starting a centrifugal pump.

17.9 What is meant by 'Priming' of a centrifugal pump ? What are different arrangements employed for priming of centrifugal pump ?

17.10 Define net positive suction head (NPSH) and net positive suction energy (NPSE).

17.11 Differentitae between specific speed and suction specific speed of a centrifugal pump.

17.12 Why should a centrifugal pump be set within a certain limit ? Or why should its suction lift be within certain limit.

17.13 A centrifugal pump of the radial flow type delivers 5000 lit/min. against a total head of 38 m when coupled to a motor with a speed of 1450 r.p.m. If the outer diameter of the impeller is 30 cm and its width at the outer periphery 1.30 cm, find the blade angle at exit. Assume a manometric efficiency for the pump as 80 %.

17.14 A centrifugal pump has an impeller 29 cm diameter running at 960 r.p.m. with an effective outlet blade angle of 28°. The velocity of flow assumed constant throughout the system is 2 m/s. The static suction lift is 2.8 meters. The energy losses in meters of water are in suction pipe 0.6 m, in impeller 0.40 m, and in volute casing 0.88 m. Determine the reading of the pressure or vacuum gauge fitted (a) at inlet to the impeller (b) at outlet to the impeller (i.e. on the clearance space between the impeller and the volute casing, and (c) at the begining of delivery pipe.

17.15 A centrifugal pump has an impeller 500 mm outler diameter and 250 mm inner diameter when running at 6000 r.p.m., the pump discharge 0.130 m³/s of water against a total head of 12 m. The vane angle of the outlet is 45° to the tangent at the outlet and the area of flow remaining constant from inlet to outlet of the impeller and is equal to 0.061 m². Determine (a) the manometric efficiency of the pump and (b) the loss of head at the inlet to the impeller when the discharge is reduced by 50 %, the speed of rotation being unchanged.

17.16 The axis of a centrifugal pump is 2.5 m above the water level in the sump and the static lit from the pump centre is 33.5 m. The friction losses in the suction and delivery pipes are 1 N-m/N and 8.33 N-m/N respectively. The impeller is 300 mm in diameter and 1.8 mm wide at outlet and its speed is 1700 r.p.m. The water at inlet has radial flow and the blade angle at outlet is 32° to the tangent to the periphery. The suction and delivery pipes are 75 mm diameter. Assuming manometric efficiency of 77 % and overall efficiency of 72 %, calculate (a) the power to be supplied (b) the discharge in lit/sec (c) the reading of the gauges connected to suction and delivery side.

17.17 A centrifugal pump dishcarge 0.226 m³/s of water and develops a head of 23 m when the impeller rotates at 1500 r.p.m. Determine the impeller diameter and the blade at outlet edge of the impeller. Assume that manometric efficiency is 75 %, the loss of head of the pump due to fluid resistance is 0.033 U_1 metres, (where U_1 is the absolute velocity with which the water is discharged from the impeller) and the area of flow at outlet is $1.2 D^2$ sq. m. Assume that the water enters the impeller without whirl.

17.18 The impeller of a centrifugal pump has an outer diameter of 250 mm and an effective outlet area of 170 cm². The blades are bent backward so that the direction of outlet relative velocity makes an angle of 148° with the tangent drawn in the direction of impeller rotation. The diameter of the suction and delivery pipes are 150 mm and 100 mm respectively. The pump delivers 310 lit/sec at 1450 r.p.m. when the gauge show heads of 4.6 m below and 18.0 m above atmosphere respectively. The head losses in the suction and delivery pipes are 2.0 m and 2.9 m respectively. The motor driving the pump supplies 8.71 kW. Find the manometric and overall efficiency of the pump assuming water enters the pump without shock or whirl.

17.19 Two geometrically similar pumps run at the same speed of 100 r.p.m. One pump has impeller diameter of 300 mm and lifts water at the rate of 20 lit/sec against a head of 15 m. Determine the head and diameter of the other pump if it has to supply half the discharge.

17.20 A centrifugal pump has total lift of 15 m from a well to the tank. The pump is located 2 m above the water level in the well. The velocity of delivery is 2 m/s and the radial velocity of flow through the pump is 3 m/s. The outlet blade angle of the pump is 120° and water enters the wheel radially. Find (a) the speed of the pump at its exit (b) the pressure head at the exit from the wheel (c) the velocity head at exit from the wheel and (d) the direction of guide blades. Neglect friction and other losses.

17.21 The unit speed characteristics of a centrifugal pump gave for maximum efficiency of 72 %, the following values, Q/N = 0.0236 lit/s/r.p.m. $H/N^2 = 10^{-5}$ m/r.p.m/r.p.m.. Determine the specific speed of the pump.

17.22 Estimate the number of the impellers required for a multistage pump to lift 60 lit/s against a total head of 150 m at a speed of 750 r.p.m.

17.23 A combination of centrifugal pumps running at 1500 r.p.m. and overall efficiency 75% is required to supply 1 m³/s to a height of 40 m. Determine the number and arrangement of the pump.

17.24 A centrifugal pump running at 1450 r.p.m. has the characteristic indicated in the table below. Draw the characteristic curves of the pump and determine its design values. Also calculate the specific speed of the pump.

Q lit/sec	11.3	16.9	22.6	23.3	34.0	39.6	45.0
H metre	25.8	25.0	24.1	23.2	21.4	18.9	15.8
η_0 %	65	70	73	24.1	23.2	69	62

17.25 Two centrifugal pumps that are available in the market have the head discharge characteristic as folows:

Q (lit/sec)	0	15	30	45	60
H_{m1} (metre)	45.0	43.5	40.0	32.7	23.3
H_{m2} (metre)	40.7	39.0	43.0	27.3	20.7

Both pumps are installed together and are required to pump through a pipe 500 mm diameter (f = 0.032). Determine the heads under which pumps are working and discharge being pumped by them. Both the pumps are connected in parallel. Take static lift of 18 m and lenght of delivery pipe as 15000 m.

Miscellaneous Machines

18.1 INTRODUCTION

A fluid system is a device in which force and power are transmitted through a fluid medium, generally oil or water. There are various types of fluid machines which are employed for storing or magnifying many fold the hydraulic energy. The stored (or magnified) energy is later transmitted to the required machine. Most of these fluid machines work on the principle of either 'fluid statics' or 'fluid kinematics'.

In fluid statics or hydrostatic system, the power or force is transmitted to the required machine by the change in pressure whereas in fluid kinematics or hydro-kinematic system, the effect is obtained primarily by virtue of the change in velocity of flow of the working media, i.e. liquid and changes in pressure are avoided as far as possible. Some of these machines are described hereinunder.

18.2 HYDRAULIC ACCUMULATOR

Hydraulic accumulator is a device which is used for storing or accumulating the water under pressure (hydraulic energy) temporarily and transmitting it either as it is or after magnifying it several times to the machines (hydraulic press, lift, etc.) wherever required. Several hydraulic machines such as hydraulic lift, hydraulic press or hydraulic crane, etc. are required to do a large amount of work during a small interval of time, which is followed by an idle period. The need of these machines is not at uniform rate throughout its stroke whereas the pumps supply water (or liquid) at a uniform rate. For example, a lift or a crane requires the energy to be supplied during its upward motion of the load only. Practically, no energy is used during its downward motion. But the pumps supply water (liquid) under pressure (hydraulic energy) continuously more or less at uniform rate. Hence, this water under pressure (or hydraulic energy) is stored in an accumulator during the idle period of the machine when machine does not need this energy. The energy from the accumulator is being given out at an increased rate during the working period of the machine alongwith the energy supplied by the pump at uniform rate. This means by introducing an accumulator between the pump and machine (lift or crane) the capacity of the pump required need not be as large as required by the machine when doing its maximum rate of work.

(a) *Simple hydraulic accumulator*

(a) An accumulator consists of a vertical cylinder containing a sliding ram Fig. 18.1. The ram is loaded with heavy loads which may consists of slag or dead weights. The accumulator is introduced in between the pump and machine. Initially, the ram is at its lowest position and the water from the pump is delivered into cylinder when not required by the machine.

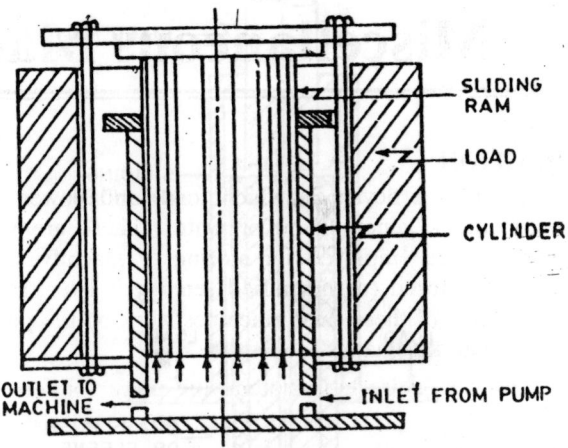

FIG. 18.1 HYDRAULIC ACCUMULATOR

The pressure of water lifts up the heavy ram until the cylinder is full and the accumulator has stored its maximum amount of energy. Later on, when the machine does maximum amount of work, it draws the energy from the accumulator and the ram descends down. This constitutes one cycle of hydraulic accumulator.

The maximum amount of energy, which it can store, is known as the capacity of the accumulator.

Let D be the diameter of the ram and L its lift (or length of the stroke). Let the pump supply the liquid (or water) under pressure p.

Weight of the ram including the dead weight being supported by it,

i.e. $\qquad W = p \times A$ $\qquad$ ...(18.1)

Work done in lifting the ram $= p \times A \times L$ $\qquad$ ...(18.2)

where A is the area of the sliding ram.

The work done in lifting the ram is equal to the energy stored and hence it is the capacity of the accumulator.

Volume of the accumulator $= A \times L$

$\therefore$ Capacity of accumulator $= p \times$ volume

$\qquad\qquad\qquad\qquad = p \times A \times L$ $\qquad$ ...(18.3)

(b) *Differential Hydraulic Accumulator*

Another form of accumulator is known as Twedell's differential accumulator. Its main advantage is that it can store water at a high pressure by comparatively small load on the ram. It consists of a vertical fixed ram, the lower portion of which is made larger than the upper portion by closely fitting a brass bush around it. The fixed ram is surrounded by an inverted cylinder with the collar at the base projecting outward. The loads are being supported over these collars.

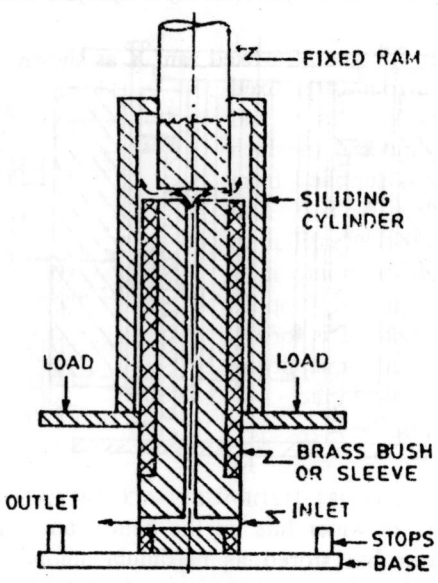

FIG. 18.2 DIFFERENTIAL ACCUMULATOR

The fixed ram is being provided at its centre with a small diameter vertical hole throughout its length. The water under pressure (supplied by the pump) enters the accumulator through this hole. This causes the cylinder to ascend upward and store water under pressure (hydraulic energy). The liquid entering the cylinder exerts pressure on the internal annular area of the cylinder which is equal to the horizontal area of the brass bush. When the machine is working, the liquid under pressure (hydraulic energy) is supplied by the accumulator and the cylinder descends downward.

Let the annular area of the brass bush or sleeve be 'a' and the vertical lift of the cylinder be L. Further let the liquid under pressure p be supplied by the pump which lifts the weight W of the cylinder (including its self weight).

$$W = p \times a$$

or
$$p = \frac{W}{a} \qquad ...(18.4)$$

From Eq. 18.4, it is clear that pressure intensity can be increased with a small load W be making area 'a' small.

Capacity of the accumulator $= (p \times a) \times L$

$$= p \times \text{volume} \qquad ...(18.5)$$

18.3 HYDRAULIC INTESIFIER

The hydraulic intensifier is a device which is used for increasing the pressure intensity of water by means of a large quantity of water at low pressure.

Many times it is necessary to supply water (or liquid) at high pressure which is not available from the direct mains or given pump. In such cases, a hydraulic intensifier can be successfully employed to supply water at high pressure.

An intersifier consists of a fixed ram X as shown in Fig. 18.3. A sliding cylinder or ram Y surrounds the fixed ram X. The cylinder Y slides up and down into a fixed cylinder Z, to which low pressure water is supplied from the main. Four valves A, B, C and D are provided to the intensifier to regulate the flow of water into it or out of it. Valves A and D supplies low pressure water, valve C is for exhaust and valve B is used for supplying high pressure water or liquid.

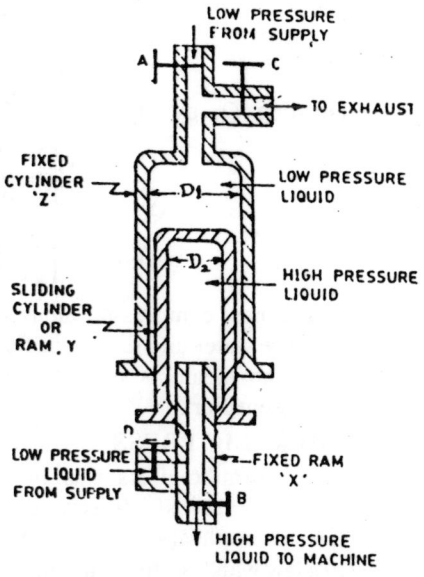

LOW PRESSURE FROM SUPPLY

TO EXHAUST

LOW PRESSURE LIQUID

HIGH PRESSURE LIQUID

FIXED CYLINDER 'Z'

SLIDING CYLINDER OR RAM. Y

LOW PRESSURE LIQUID FROM SUPPLY

FIXED RAM 'X'

HIGH PRESSURE LIQUID TO MACHINE

In the beginning, when the sliding cylinder or ram Y is at its lowest position, the cylinder Z is full of low pressure water. The valves D and C are now opened and low pressure water from the main enters the sliding cylinder Y. The water from the fixed cylinder Z is allowed to flow out through the exhaust valve C. When whole of the water from the cylinder

FIG. 18.3 HYDRAULIC INTENSIFIER

Z flows out, the sliding ram reaches at its topmost position. Now the valves D and C are closed and valves A and B are opened. The low pressure water supply flows into the cylinder Z through valve A. This water exerts pressure on the base of the sliding cylinder and forces the cylinder to move down. This causes the water in the cylinder Y to flow out of the machine (hydraulic press or hydraulic crane, etc.) through the valve B. The same cycle of operation is repeated. The hydraulic intensifier is thus a single acting machine since it supplies high pressure water during downward stroke of the sliding ram. Double acting intensifier are also made which gives a continuous supply of high pressure water. It is possible to raise the pressure of water of 16 kN/cm^2 (16000 tonnes/m^2) by means of an intensifier.

Let the internal diameters of the fixed cylinder Z and sliding ram or cylinder Y be D_1 and D_2 respectively. Let their respective areas of cross section be a_1 and a_2. The pressure of water supplied by the main may be assumed as p_1 which is raised to p_2 by means of the intersifier and supplied to the machines (press, crane, etc.). Then the total upward force on the cylinder Y should be equal to the downward force on it.

∴ $$p_1 A_1 = p_2 A_2$$

or
$$p_2 = \left[\frac{p_1 A_1}{A_2}\right] = p_1 \left[\frac{D_1^2}{D_2^2}\right] \qquad \text{...(18.6)}$$

If Q_1 is the quantity of low pressure water supplied to the cylinder Z and Q_2 is the quantity of high pressure water supplied to the hydraulic machine.

$$Q_1 = A_1 L \qquad \text{...(18.7)}$$

and
$$Q_2 = A_2 L \qquad \text{...(18.8)}$$

Dividing Q_1 by Q_2

$$\frac{Q_1}{Q_2} = \frac{A_1 L}{A_2 L} = \left(\frac{D_1}{D_2}\right)^2$$

$\therefore$
$$Q_2 = Q_1 \left(\frac{D_2}{D_1}\right)^2 \qquad \text{...(18.9)}$$

Sometimes, compressed air is supplied to the larger cylinder Z in place of low pressure water and the intensifier is known as 'Hydropneumatic intensifier'. Similarly if the steam is used in place of low pressure water, it is known as 'steam intensifier'.

18.4 HYDRAULIC PRESS

The hydraulic press was first developed by Ernest Brahma in 1785. Since then it is in use. It is a device which is used to lift large load or weight by the application of a much smaller force. It works on the principle of Pascal's law which states that intensity of pressure in a static fluid is transferred equally in all directions.

Mainly, a hydraulic press consists of two cylinders, one of which is of larger diameter than the other. Both these cylinders are connected by means of a pipe. Two sliding rams are provided in these cylinders as shown in Fig. 18.4. A liquid or water is filled up in the cylinders and pipe to transmit the pressure. When a smaller force F is applied in the downward direction

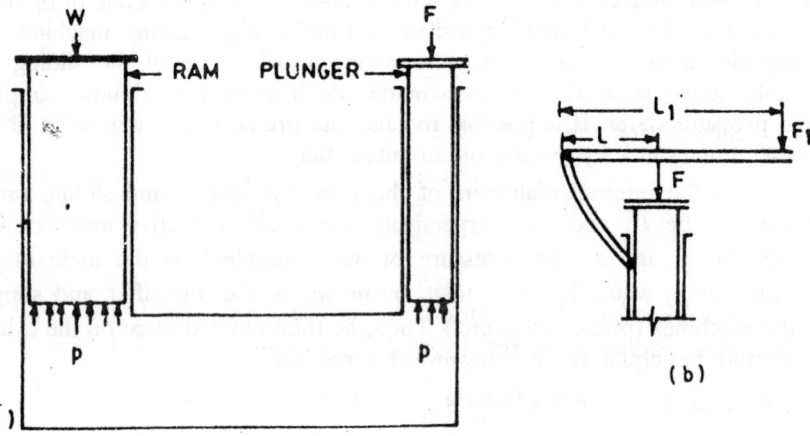

FIG. 18.4 HYDRAULIC PRESS

over the plunger (area 'a'), it creates the pressure intensity in the liquid. This pressure p is distributed throughout the fluid according to Pascal's law. The liquid exerts a pressure intensity p on the larger diameter ram in the upward direction and thus lifts a much heavier load weight. W.

Pressure acting, in the downward direction, on the plunger

$$P = \frac{F}{a}$$

Pressure acting, in the upward direction, on the ram or piston

$$p = \frac{W}{A}$$

According to Pascal's law, the pressure intensity is transmitted equally in all the directions.

$$\therefore \qquad \frac{W}{A} = \frac{F}{a}$$

or
$$W = F \times \frac{A}{a} \qquad \qquad ...(18.10)$$

By making the ratio $\frac{A}{a}$ much larger, a weight (or load) W which is many times heavier than the force applied F may be developed. The ratio of the area of the ram to the area of the plunger is known is the known as the mechanical advantage of the hydraulic press.

$$\text{Mechanical advantage} = \left(\frac{A}{a}\right) \qquad \qquad ...(18.11)$$

The mechanical advantage can further be improved by providing a lever to the plunger. By applying a smaller force F_1 at the end of plunger (which is much smaller than F) it can lift a weight (or force) W as is seen from in Fig. 18.4(b).

Taking moment about hinge O,

$$F_1 \times L_1 = F \times L$$

$$F_1 = F \times \frac{L}{L_1} \qquad \qquad ...(18.12)$$

Substituting the value of F from Eq. 18.10.

$$F_1 = W \times \frac{a}{A} \times \frac{L}{L_1}$$

$$W = F_1 \times \frac{A}{a} \times \frac{L_1}{L}$$

The ratio of L/L_1 is known as the 'leverage of hydraulic press'. The mechanical advantage of the hydraulic press now becomes,

$$\text{Mechanical advantage} = \frac{A}{a} \times \frac{L_1}{L}$$

Hydraulic presses are employed to perform various odd jobs, requiring tremendous pressure. There are various shapes of hydraulic presses depending upon the nature of the work to be performed. Essentially, all the hydraulic presses consist of a ram sliding in a cylinder to which high pressure liquid is forced.

Fig. 18.5 shows one of the actual hydraulic press. It consists of two stationary platens and a movable platen. The latter is carried by a plunger or ram passing through the upper stationary platen and moves in the cylinder. The upper and lower platens are joined by columns.

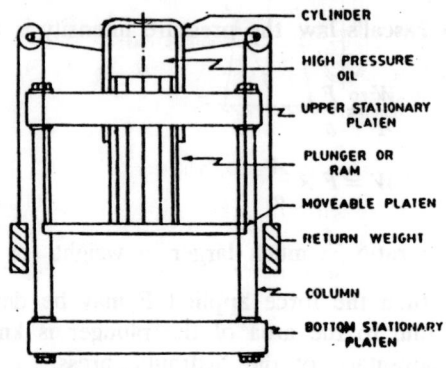

FIG. 18.5 ACTUAL HYDRAULIC PRESS

When the hydraulic press is in operation, the ram under high hydraulic pressure supplied by the pumps , moves down and exerts tremendous pressure upon the job placed between upper (stationary) and lower (moving) platens. Thus the material gets pressed .The force applied on the material equals the product of pressure intensity and the area of the ram. To bring back the ram in the upward position, the liquid from the cylinder is taken out and then by the action of return weights the ram alongwith movable platen moves up.

Usually, a hydraulic accumulator is provided in between the pump and the press. It permits the high pressure liquid to be stored in the accumulator cylinder during the idle period of the hydraulic press during its working period. In this way, the maximum total pressure exerted by the hydraulic press ranges from 5000 tonnes to 10,000 tonnes.

18.5 HYDRAULIC CRANE

A hydraulic crane is a device which is used for raising or transferring the heavy loads. It is widely used in workshops, warehouses, dock sidings etc.

It consists of a (a) mast, (b) tie, (c) jib, (d) guide pulley and (e) a jigger as shown in Fig. 18.6: The jib can be raised or lowered in order to decrese or increase the radius or action of the crane. The mast is supported

over a pedestal and can revolve alongwith the jib and thus the load attached
to the rope can be transferred to any place within the area of the crane's
action.

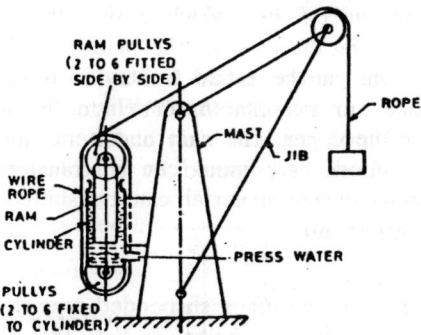

FIG. 18.6 A HYDRAULIC CRANE

The jigger consists of movable ram sliding in a fixed cylinder. On the
upper end of ram, a set of pulleys is attached and its lower end remains
in contact of water or liquid. Another set of fixed pulley block is attached
on the lower end of fixed cylinder. The pulley is attached to the ram moves
up and down alongwith the ram while the pulley block attached to the fixed
cylinder remains stationery.

A wire rope, with one of its end attached to the movable pulley, is
taken round all the pulleys of the two sets of pulley block and finally passes
over the guide pulley attached to the gib. The other end of rope remains
free. Usually a hook is attached to the free end of the rope to suspend the
load.

For lifting the load, high pressure water or liquid is admitted into the
cylinder which forces the ram (of the jigger) to move upward. This causes
upward movement of the upper pulley block thereby increasing the distance
between two sets of pulley block attached to the pulley and hence lifting
of heavy load. While the crane is to be lowered, the outlet valve is opened
out and the high pressure liquid is let out. Thus sliding ram lowered down,
thereby the distance between pulley block reduces. This causes the rope to
be wrapped round the pulleys and free end of the rope to lower down.

The velocity ratio of the hook to the ram of the jigger depends upon
the number of sets of pulleys. Thus, a six sheef pulley block system will have
a velocity ratio of 6 : 1. It means that the load suspended on the hook will
move six times the speed of ram of the jigger. A modern hydraulic crane
can have a lifting speed of nearly 75 m per minute. The hydraulic crane
can lift a load upto 250 tonnes. In the modern times, the electric cranes
are replacing hydraulic cranes.

18.6 HYDRAULIC LIFT

The hydraulic lift is a device which is used for carrying goods or persons
from one floor to another in a multi-storey building. The hydraulic lifts are
to two types, (a) direct acting hydraulic lift and (b) suspended hydraulic lift.

(a) *Direct Acting Hydraulic Lift*

It consists of a ram sliding in a fixed cylinder (Fig. 18.7 a). At the top end of the sliding ram, a platform or a cage is fitted. The liquid under pressure is admitted to the cylinder which pushes the ram in the vertically upward direction, thus lifting the cage or the platform to the required height. The platform or the cage can be made to stay in level with each floor so as to transfer the goods or persons there. When the high pressure liquid from the cylinder is drained out, the ram and hence the cage or platform is lowered. Thus, the goods or persons can be transferred to lower floors. In this way, the persons or the material can be shifted in either direction with the help of hydraulic lift.

(b) *Suspended Type*

Another type of hydraulic lift is suspended type. It is a modified form of direct acting hydraulic lift. As shown in Fig. 18.7 (b), it is fitted with

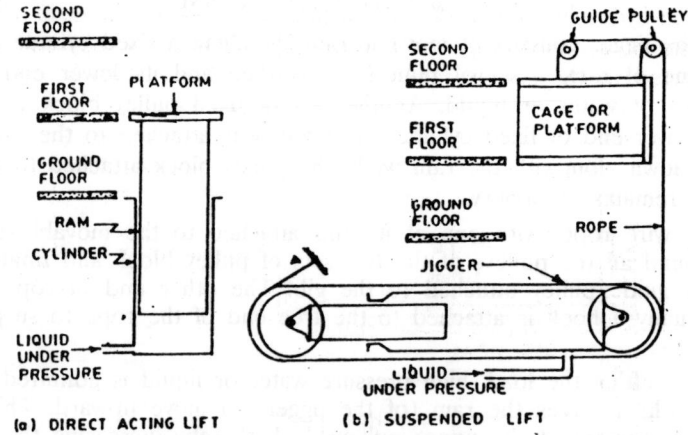

(a) DIRECT ACTING LIFT   (b) SUSPENDED LIFT

FIG. 18.7 (A) AND (B) HYDRAULIC LIFT

a jigger as explained (in section 18.5) with hydraulic crane. A jigger consists of a ram sliding in a fixed horizontal cylinder. On the left side, a movable pulley block is fitted and its right side remains in contact of liquid. Another set of fixed pulley block is fitted to the fixed cylinder. A rope is attached to some point A and is then wrapped round these two pulley blocks. The rope, then passes over the guide pulley and finally supports a cage or plateform. The high pressure liquid is admitted to the cylinder to raise the cage (or plateform).

When the lift is to be raised, the high pressure liquid is admitted to the cylinder at its right side. This forces the sliding ram to be pushed out towards left side. This increases the distance between two sets of pulley blocks and pulls the wire rope. The cage or plateform is thus raised gradually. For its downward journey, the high pressure liquid is taken out and so the ram moves from left to the right side. This decreses the distance between the pulley blocks and increases the length of the rope. The cage is thus lowered down.

The lift cage or plateform runs between guides of hardwood or round steel and is usually suspended by four lifting ropes, each one being of sufficient strength to support the load. Sliding balancing weights are provided to balance the weight of the cage. Modern hydraulic lifts have a lifting speed of 105 to 120 metre per minute. Nowadays, these hydraulic lifts have been replaced by electric lifts which are fast moving and are more convenient.

18.7 HYDRAULIC RAM

The hydraulic ram or hydram is a hydraulically driven pump, in which the energy of a large quantity of water under small head is utilised to lift a small quantity of water to a greater height. Thus, no external energy is utilised to operate this pump. Hydram are chiefly used in country estate and farms at which large quantity of water under low head is available and power is scarce so that all other types of pumps could not be used.

The hydraulic ram works on the principle of water hammer (Fig. 18.8). It consists of a supply pipe or a drive pipe CD, the upper end of which is connected to the supply reservoir A and the lower end is connected to

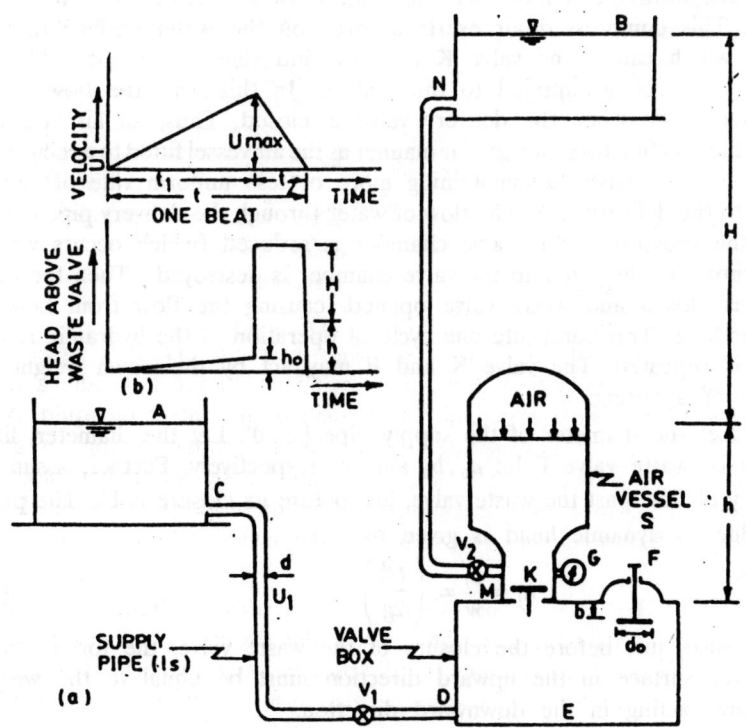

FIG 18.8 (A) HYDRAM OR HYDRAULIC RAM

(B) VARIATION OF VELOCITY AND PRESSURE

a valve box E, The valve box has two automatic 'one way' valves-waste valve or impulsive valve F opening downwards and a delivery valve K opening upwards. Above the delivery valve, an air vessel S is provided. At the foot of air vessel, the delivery pipe alongwith a non return valve V_2 is fitted to it, which leads the water to the supply tank B.

Initially, the valve V_1 in the supply pipe CD is closed and waste valve F is open ; the pressure in the valve box E is zero or atmospheric. When the valve V_1 is opened, the water in the pipe CD begins to move under acceleating head h. It fills the valve box and starts going waste through the waste valve E. As the rate of discharge past the waste valve increases, the pressure in the valve chamber begins to rise. It rapidly reaches a value at which the static thrust together with the dynamic thrust acting on the lower face of the valve becomes greater than downward force on it due to the weight of the valve F. The waste valve F, therefore, closses instantaneously and brings the water in the supply pipe suddenly to rest; causing a further increase in the pressure in the valve chamber. Due to this increase in pressure which is always immediately after the closure of waste valve F is closed, the supply valve K is forced open. The water flows straight from supply tank A into the delivery pipe MN and some portion of it is stored in the air vessel. The air vessel always contains some air, and it is compressed by the incoming water. This compressed air exerts a force on the water surface in the air vessel which causes the valve K to close and valve F to open. The water from air vessel is supplied to the tank B. In this way, the flow of water continues even when the delivery valve is closed. Thus, an air vessel of a hydraulic ram functions in a similar manner as the air vessel fitted to a reciprocating pump, i.e., it assists in maintaining more or less uniform rate of supply of water to the delivery tank. The flow of water through the delivery pipe continues until the pressure in the valve chamber is reduced (which occurs when the momentum of the water in the valve chamber is destroyed). Then the delivery valve is closed and waste valve opened, causing the flow from tank A to recommence. This constitute one cycle of operation of the hydraulic ram. The cycle is repeated. The valve K and F may act by their own weight or by means of a spring.

Let the diameter of the supply pipe be 'd'. Let the diameter, lift and weight of waste valve F be d_0, b_0 and W respectively. Further, assume that velocity of flow past the waste valve, just before its closure is U_0. The pressure rise due to dynamic head is given by

$$h_i = \frac{p_i}{w} = \left(\frac{U_0^2}{2g} \right) \qquad \qquad ...(18.15)$$

Also, just before the closure of the waste valve, the force acting on its lower surface in the upward direction must be equal to the weight of the valve acting in the downward direction.

$$p_i \times \frac{\pi}{4} \times d_0^2 = W$$

$$p_i = \frac{W}{\left(\dfrac{\pi}{4}\right) \times d_0^2}$$

$$\frac{p_i}{w} = \frac{W}{w \times \dfrac{\pi}{4} d_0^2} \qquad \qquad ...(18.16)$$

Now, consider the supply pipe. The maximum velocity of water through the supply pipe is assumed to be U_m. It occurs just before the closure of waste valve. Using continuity equation,

$$\frac{\pi}{4} d^2 \times U_m = \pi \times d_0 \times b_0 \times U_0$$

$$U_m = \frac{4 d_0 b_0 U_0}{d^2} \qquad \qquad ...(18.17)$$

Let the supply tank be located h metre above the valve chamber and the length of supply pipe be l_s. Further, it is assumed that the velocity in the supply pipe varies from 0 to U_m in time t_1. Using Eq. 10.47 b of water hammer,

$$h = \frac{l_s}{g} \times \frac{U_m}{t_1} \qquad \qquad ...(18.18)$$

Similarly, if the delivery tank is located H metre above valve chamber and delivery valve remains open or waste valve remains closed for time t_2, then from Eq. 10.47 b,

$$H = \frac{l_s}{g} \times \frac{U_m}{t_2} \qquad \qquad ...(18.19)$$

The time t taken in one cycle is given by, (Eqs. 18.18 and 18.19),

$$t = (t_1 + t_2)$$

$$= \frac{l_s}{g} \times U_m \left(\frac{1}{h} + \frac{1}{H}\right) \qquad \qquad ...(18.20)$$

The number of beats, N per minute, is given bv:

$$N = \frac{60}{t}$$

$$= \frac{60 \, g}{l_s \, U_m \left(\dfrac{1}{h} + \dfrac{1}{H}\right)} \qquad \qquad ...(18.21)$$

where t is the time taken in one cycle or one beat.

Let q be the discharge actually supplied and Q be the discharge going waste past the waste valve in each cycle. Since the velocity in the supply pipe varies from 0 to U_m, the mean velocity of flow is $\dfrac{U_m}{2}$.

$$\therefore \qquad q = \frac{\pi}{4} d^2 \times \frac{U_m}{2} \times \frac{t_2}{t} \qquad \qquad ...(18.22)$$

and
$$Q = \frac{\pi}{4} d^2 \times \frac{U_m}{2} \times \frac{t_1}{t} \qquad \ldots(18.23)$$

The efficiency of the ram can be expressed in the following two ways.

Rankine Efficiency

In this system the water surface in the supply reservoir is taken as datum. Then,

The energy delivered by the ram $= q \times H$

The energy supplied to the flowing water $= Q \times h$

$\therefore$ Rankine's efficiency $\eta_R = \dfrac{qH}{Qh}$ \qquad \ldots(18.24)

D' Aubuissen's efficiency

In this system. the datum plane is taken as passing through the waste valve.

The energy received by the hydram or input $= (Q + q) \times h$

The energy output of the hydram $= q(H + h)$

$\therefore$ D' Aubuissen's efficiency $\eta_R = \dfrac{q(H+h)}{(Q+q)h}$ \qquad \ldots(18.25)

The valve of η_A is naturally higher than η_R. The chief causes of the energy loss in the hydram are –(i) friction and secondary losses in the supply pipe and in the valves and, (2) the velocity energy carried away by the water leaving the waste valve. Even under the favourable conditions, the efficiency of the hydram is limited to 75 %.

If the head loss due to friction in the supply pipe and delivery pipe are taken into account in Eq. 18.17 and 18.18, these are modified to

$$h - h_{fs} = \frac{l_s}{g} \times \frac{U_m}{t_i} \qquad \ldots(18.26)$$

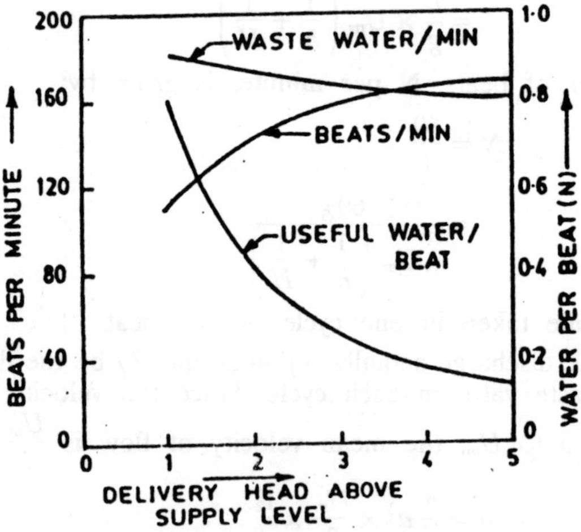

FIG. 18.9 PERFORMANCE CURVE OF HYDRAM

$$H + h_{fd} = \frac{l_s}{g} \times \frac{U_m}{t_2} \qquad\qquad ...(18.27)$$

The characteristic performance of the hydram working under conditions of constant lift of waste valve, constant supply head and varying delivery head is shown in Fig. 18.9. The variation of velocity and pressure during one cycle of operation of hydram is shown in Fig. 18.8 (b).

18.8 HYDRAULIC COUPLING

Hydraulic coupling is a device which is used to transmit power from driving shaft (known as primary) to driven shaft (known as secondary) with the help of a fluid. The fluid used is, generally, a light viscosity oil. Since there is no mechanical connection between two shafts, impulsive shocks and periodic vibrations are prevented by the fluid media.

A hydraulic coupling is shown in Fig. 18.10. It essentially consists of a centrifugal pump impeller (as transmitting element and a turbine runner as receiving element). Both these element together form a casing, completely filled with oil. Each rotating element is shaped as one half of a hollow ring and contains thin, straight, radial blades. Such radial vanes not only are less expensive then curved one, but have the additional advantage of being adopted for rotation in either direction.

In the beginning, both the shafts A and B are stationary. When the shaft A is made to rotate slowly, the forced vortex is generated in the oil. In consequence, the oil starts flowing out from the impeller and strikes turbine runner at its outer periphery. Due to the destruction of the angular momentum corresponding to this velocity of whirl, a tangential force or torque is exerted on the turbine runner blades. Initially, since the turbine runner has not started rotating, there are no centrifugal force to resist and hence the oil flows directly to the runner eye and across to the impeller again, so the circulation of fluid now continues. When the speed of the shaft A is increased further, the torque imposed on the shaft B may rise sufficiently to overcome the resistance of the runner which till now has resisted its motion. Further increase in the speed of the impeller causes further increase in the speed of the runner until at designed full load, the speed of shaft B is slightly less (nearly 2 %) than the speed of the shaft A. In this way for all practical purposes, both the shafts are directly coupled.

Although the forced vortex motion occures in both the elements, i.e. in the impeller and the runner, but for the flow of oil to be maintained, the centrifugal head produced by the impeller must be slightly greater than the centrifugal head of the turbine runner resisting the flow.

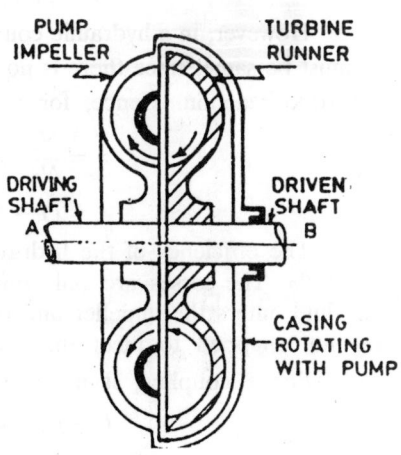

FIG. 18.10 HYDRAULIC COUPLING

This is only possible if the speed of the impeller is greater than the speed of the runner. Thus, for torque transmission there must be a difference in the speed of these two elements giving rise to 'slip'.

Slip

It is defined as the ratio of the difference in the speed of the pump impeller and turbine runner to the speed of the impeller

$$S = \left(\frac{N_1 - N_2}{N_1} \right)$$

$$= \left(1 - \frac{N_2}{N_1} \right) \qquad \text{...(18.28)}$$

where N_1 and N_2 are the speed of the pump impeller and turbine runner respectively. The slip of the hydraulic coupling varies from 2 to 4 %.

Stall

The stall is the condition when the speed of both the shafts are equal. For such condition, the slip is zero and efficiency is unity. At such a condition there is no flow of fluid and hence the coupling does not work. The power input to the pump impeller

$$P_{in} = T_1 \times \frac{2 \pi N_1}{60} = k_0 T_1 N_1$$

The power output to the turbine runner

$$P_{out} = T_2 \times \frac{2 \pi N_2}{60} = k_0 T_2 N_2$$

The efficiency of the hydraulic coupling is defined as

$$\eta = \frac{P_{out}}{P_{in}}$$

$$= \frac{T_2 N_2}{T_1 N_1} \qquad \text{...(18.29)}$$

However, in a hydraulic coupling, the input torque T_1 and output torque T_2 must be same, since there is no other element between two parts to provide a torque reaction. Hence, for a hydraulic coupling

$$\eta = \frac{N_2}{N_1} \qquad \text{...(18.30)}$$

$$= (1 - S) \qquad \text{...(18.31)}$$

The efficiency of the hydraulic coupling is quite high; usually in excess of 94 %. The losses are only due to friction and turbulence created when the fluid enters the impeller and runner blades. This is so because the blades are not shapped to meet the flow without shock or tangentially.

For a coupling, it may be shown by dimensional analysis, that

$$P = f(\rho, D, N_2, N_1, \mu, V)$$

$$\frac{P}{\rho N_1^3 D^5} = f \left[S, \frac{\rho N_1 D^2}{\mu}, \frac{V}{D^3} \right] \qquad \text{...(18.32)}$$

In Eq. 18.32, D is the diameter of the impeller, V is the volume of the fluid, ρ and μ are fluid mass density and dynamic viscosity. Since for a hydraulic coupling, V/D^3 is a constant and the second term is proportional to Reynolds number and the flow is turbulent, these are also not important.

$$\therefore \qquad P \propto N^3 D^5 f(S) \qquad\qquad ...(18.33)$$

The performance characteristic curves for a hydraulic coupling is shown in Fig. 18.11. It is seen that the efficiency increases with increses in slip, becomes maximum (about 98 %) and then reduces suddenly. The reason for high efficiency at low slip is that as the two speeds approach each other, the opposing centrifugal force of the turbine causes the velocity of the circulation to be too low. The dashed line in the above figure shows that the efficiency drops to zero as the slip is reduced to zero. It indicates that the driving torque is no longer adequate and the drived shaft is receiving energy from some other source as in the case of an automobile going downhill.

The fluid coupling are employed in rail road and autombiles to transport power from internal combustion engine to the moving wheel. These are also widely used for power driven excavators. Fluid coupling of capacity 1 to 30,000 kW capacity has been manufactured and are used in practice.

18.9 HYDRAULIC TORQUE CONVERTOR

Hydraulic torque convertor is a device which is used to transmit the increased or decresed torque at the driven shaft. In case of fluid coupling, the torque output is always equal to the torque input. If it is desired to mulitiply or reduce the torque (of the driving shaft) to be transmitted to

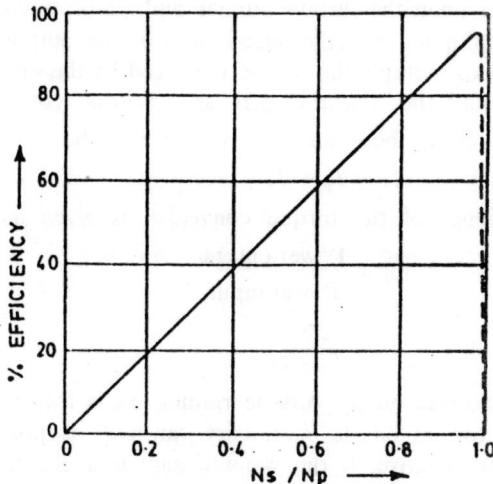

FIG. 18.11 PERFORMANCE CURVE

the driven shaft, then a torque convertor is used.

Fig. 18.12 shows a torque convertor of one stage as it contains only one torque runner. When two or more turbine runners are used, these are correspondingly known as two stage or three stage torque convertors. These are used to have much larger torque multiplication. The main difference between a fluid coupling and a torque convertor is that while the former consists of only one pump impeller and one turbine runner, the latter also has in addition, a set of stationary vanes-known as stator or reactors. These vanes are interposed between two runners. They receive the flow from the turbine and deliver it to the pump. The reactor vanes are so shpaed as to change the direction

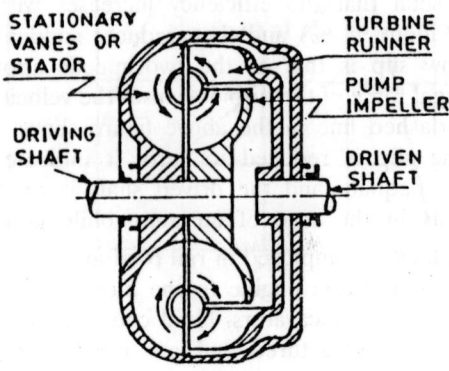

FIG. 18.12 TORQUE CONVERTOR

of flow over it and thus increase the angular momentum. At the same time, the pump impeller also adds angular momentum to the flowing fluid. Thus the flowing fluid through the turbine receives the angular momentum equal to the sum of that from the stator and that in the pump. As a result of the fluid reaction upon the turbine runner and stator vanes, the input torque is increasingly multiplied and the speed ratio of the output falls. In this way, the stationary vanes multiply the torque delivered by the engine (by redirecting the fluid flow) and the assembly acts as a torque convertor.

The relationship between the torques may be written as

$$T_s = T_p + T_v \qquad \qquad ...(18.34)$$

The efficiency of the torque convertor is given as

$$\eta = \frac{\text{Power output}}{\text{Power input}}$$

$$= \frac{T_s \times \omega_s}{T_p \times \omega_p} \qquad \qquad ...(18.35)$$

where T_s is the torque on the turbine runner. T_p is the torque on the pump and T_v is the torque on the stationary vanes. It is possible for T_v to be either positive or negative. If the vanes design is such that they receive the torque from the fluid which is in the opposite direction to that exerted on the driven shaft, T_v is positive. It signifies an increased output torque. It may, in fact, be as much as five times the input torque of the pump impeller. If, on the other hand, the vanes are such that they receive the torque which is in the same direction as that of the driven shaft, T_v is negative and the torque on the turbine runner is reduced.

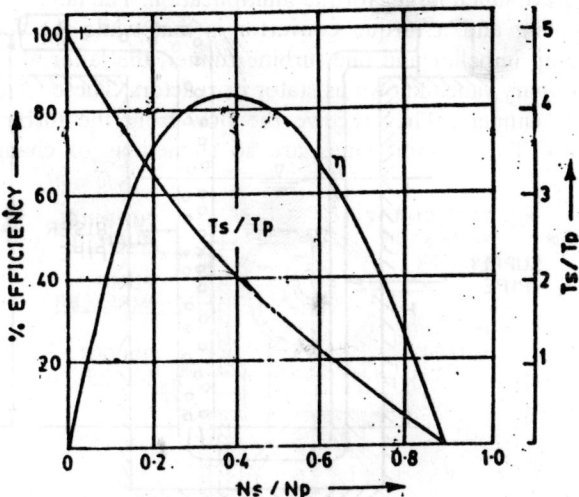

FIG. 18.13 PERFORMANCE CURVE

where ω_s and ω_p are the angular velocities of the turbine and pump respectively. Fig. 18.13 shows the plot of η versus N_s/N_p alongwith the plot of T_s/T_p verses N_s/N_p. It is seen that maximum efficiency may be as high as 87 %. Further, it is found that maximum efficiency of a torque convertor is smaller than that of a fluid coupling due to the additional losses occurring in the reactor or stationary vanes.

Further, it is seen that we $\omega_s \to \omega_p$ ($\omega_s/\omega_p \to 1$), the efficiency of a torque convertor is less while that of a fluid coupling is high. The maximum efficiency of a torque convertor occurs at a much smaller speed ratio.

18.10 AIR LIFT PUMP

An air lift pump is a device which is used to raise the water from a bore hole by utilising the compressed air. It functions on the principle that the density of the mixture of air water column is much less than the density of equal column of water.

An air lift pump is show in Fig. 18.14. It consists of a compressor, a supply pipe with nozzles fitted at the ends and a rising main. One end of the supply pipe is connected to the compressor and other end is kept open. One or more nozzles are fited to open end.

The air from compressor is introduced through one or more nozzles at the bottom of the air supply pipe, into the water at the foot of rising main fixed in a well. As soon as the column in the rising main becomes impregnated with air bubbles the pressure due to water column of length L becomes less than due to the static pressure H. This difference in pressure causes the flow of water to begin through rising main. The flow of air water mixture continues till the supply of air is continued.

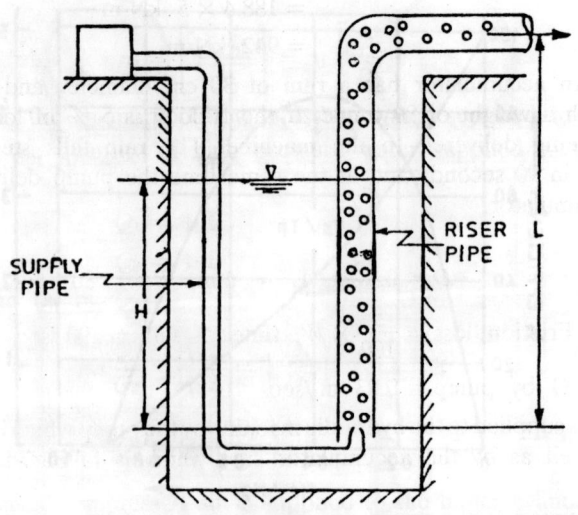

FIG. 18.14 AIR LIFT PUMP

Best results from this pump are obtained if the useful lift (L – H) is less than sugmergence H. The ratio of H/(L – H) varies from 1 to 4 for H varying from 100 to 33 m.

The main advantages of air lift pump are (1) it has no moving parts so that it can not be damaged by solids suspended in the water. This permits the pump to be used to lift sediment ladden water. (2) It can raise more water through a bore hole of given diameter than any other form of pump. (3) It can be used in mines where compressors are already present.

The disadvantage are that (1) its efficiency is too low - 20 to 40 % i.e. only 20 to 40 % of power is available than that used for compressing the air. (2) there is a possibility of leakage of air from supply pipe, rising main, etc.

Example 18-1 to 18.19

18.1 An acculculator has a ram of 20 cm diameter and its lifts is 5 m. If the water is supplied under a pressure of 600 N/cm^2, find the load on the ram and the capacity of the accumulator.

Solution

Given : $D = 0.2$ m, L = 5 m, p = 600 N/cm^2,

(a) Area of the ram $= \frac{\pi}{4}(0.2)^2$

Total weight on the ram $= p \times A$

$$= 600 \times 10^4 \times \frac{\pi}{4} \times (0.2)^2 \text{ N}$$

$$= 188.4 \text{ kN.}$$

(b) Capacity of accumulator $= p \times A \times L$

$$= 188.4 \times 5 \text{ kN-m}$$

$$= 942 \text{ kN-m}$$

18.2 An accumulator has a ram of 30 cm diameter and lift 6 m and is loaded with a weight of 80 tonne. If the friction is 5 % of load, determine the power being delivered to the machine. The ram falls steadily through its full range in 90 seconds and at the same time the pump delivers 30 lit/sec through accumulator.

Solution

Given : $D = 0.3$ m, $L = 6$ m, W $= 80$ tonne,

Friction loss $= \dfrac{5}{100} \times W$, time of fall $= 90$ sec $= 1.5$ min

Q by pump $= 0.03$ m³/sec.

Work is supplied to the hydraulic machine by the pump which is continuously working as well as by the accumulator ram which is falling steadily due to its weight.

(i) Work supplied by the accumulator ram per minute

$$= 80 \,(1 - 0.05) \times 9810 \times \frac{6}{1.5} \text{ N-m/min}$$

$$= 2982.24 \text{ kN m/min}$$

(ii) Intensity of pressure in accumulator

$$p = \frac{W\,(1 - 0.05)}{\pi\, D^2/4}$$

$$= \frac{80 \times 9810 \times 0.95}{\dfrac{\pi}{4} \times (0.3)^2} = 1,05,52,866 \text{ N/m}^2$$

Head H due to this pressure

$$= \frac{10552866}{9810} = 1075.72 \text{ m}$$

Work-supplied by the pump per minute

$$= w\,Q\,H$$

$$= 9810 \times \frac{30}{60 \times 1000} \times 1075.72 \text{ N-m/min}$$

$$= 316.58 \text{ kN-m/min}$$

Total work supplied to the hydraulic machine

$$= (2982.24 + 316.58)$$

$$= 3298.82 \text{ kN-m/min.}$$

18.3 The total weight (including self weight of the ram) placed on the sliding ram of a hydraulic accumulator is 40 tonnes. The diameter of the ram is 50 cm. If the frictional resistance against the movement of the ram is 5 % of the total weight, determine the intensity of pressure of water when

(i) the ram is moving up with uniform velocity, and (ii) the ram is moving down with uniform velocity.

Solution

Given : $W = 40$ tonne, $D = 0.5$ m,

Frictional resistance $= 5$ % of W

(a) *Ram moving up*

Total force on the ram $=$ (total weight $+$ frictional resistance)

$$= W \left(1 + \frac{5}{100} \right) = 1.05 \ W$$

$$p = \frac{\text{total force}}{\text{Area of ram}}$$

$$= \frac{1.05 \times 40 \times 9810}{\frac{\pi}{4} \times (0.5)^2} \ \text{N/m}^2 \ \left(\because 1 \, tonne = 9810 \, N \right)$$

$$= 2099.47 \ \text{kN/m}^2$$

(b) *Ram moving down*

Total force on the ram $=$ (total weight - frictional resistance)

$$= W \left(1 - \frac{5}{100} \right) = 0.95 \ W$$

$\therefore$

$$p = \frac{0.95 \times 40 \times 9810}{\frac{\pi}{4} \times (0.5)^2} \ \text{N/m}^2$$

$$p = 1899.5 \ \text{kN/m}^2$$

18.4 Certain machinery is worked from a weight loaded accumulator through a pipe 700 m long and 10 cm diameter. The accumulator has a ram 27.5 cm diameter and 4 m stroke, loaded with 32 tonnes. It is supplied with water from a three throw pumps running at 42 rpm; the plunger area of 5 cm diameter and a stroke of 25 cm. The slip may be estimated as 4% and the pipe coefficient f as 0.032. If the machinery absorbs 40 kW, calculate the longest period during which it may be operated continuously.

Solution

Given : $l = 700$ m, $d = 0.10$ m, $D = 0.275$ m,

$$L = 4.0 \ \text{m}, \ W = 32 \ \text{tonne}, \ N = 42 \ \text{r.p.m.},$$

Plunger dia $= 0.05$ m, and stroke $= 0.35$ m, slip $= 4$ %.

$$f = 0.032, \ h_f = 40 \ \text{kW}.$$

Pressure intensity supplied by accumulator $= \dfrac{W}{\text{Area of ram}}$

$$p = \frac{32 \times 9810}{\frac{\pi}{4} \times (0.275)^2} \quad \left(\because 1 \, \text{tonne} = 9810 \, N \right)$$

$$p = 5287908.6 \ \text{N/m}^2$$

$$\text{Equivalent head} = \frac{5287908.6}{9810}$$

$$= 539.03 \ \text{m}$$

Friction loss in pipe $h_f = \dfrac{fl\,U^2}{2\,g\,d}$

$$h_f = \frac{0.032 \times 700 \times U^2}{2 \times 9.81 \times 0.10} = 11.417 \ U^2$$

Weight of water supplied per second

$$= \frac{\pi}{4} \times (0.1)^2 \times U \times 9810$$

$$W_1 = 77 \ U \ \text{Newton}$$

Effective head at the machine $= (H - h_f)$

$$= (539.03 - 11.417 \ U^2)$$

Power at machine $= \dfrac{W_1 \times (H - h_f)}{100} \ \text{kW}$

$$= \frac{77 \ U \ (539.03 - 11.417 \ U^2)}{1000}$$

$$= 40 \ \text{(Given)}$$

Solving $\qquad U = 1.19 \ \text{m/s}$

Hence, $\qquad W_1 = 77 \times 1.19$

$$= 91.63 \ \text{N}$$

Corresponding volume per second leaving accumulator

$$Q = \frac{91.63}{9810} = 9.34 \times 10^{-3} \ \text{m}^3/\text{s}$$

Also, the quantity of water entering accumulator

$$= \text{discharge of pump}$$

$$= 3 \frac{ALN}{60} \times (1 - slip)$$

$$= 3 \times \frac{\pi}{4} \times (0.05)^2 \times 0.35 \times \frac{42}{60} \times (1 - 0.04)$$

$$= 1.3847 \times 10^{-3} \ \text{m}^3/\text{s}$$

Hence, net water supplied from accumulator

$$= (9.34 - 1.3875) \times 10^{-3}$$

$$= 7.9553 \times 10^{-3} \ \text{cumec}$$

Therefore, time to empty accumulator = time during which machine may be operated continuously.

$$= \frac{\pi}{4} \times \frac{(0.275)^2 \times 4.0}{7.9553 \times 10^{-3}}$$

$$= 29.85 \text{ seconds.}$$

18.5 Weight of the loaded moving cylinder of a differential accumulator is 50 kN. The diameters of large and smaller ram are 145 mm and 135 mm respectively. Find the pressure of water in the accumulator. Neglect friction.

If the length of stroke of the accumulator is 4m which is executed in 1 minute, determine the power supplied by the accumulator.

Solution

Given : $D_1 = 145$ mm, $D_2 = 135$ mm, W = 50 kN,

$L = 4$ m in 1 minute.

Annular area $A = \frac{\pi}{4} \times (0.145^2 - 0.135^2)$

$$= 2.198 \times 10^{-3} \text{ m}^2$$

$$W = p \times a$$

$$p = \frac{50}{2.198 \times 10^{-3}}$$

$$= 22747.95 \text{ kN/m}^2$$

Power supplied by the accumulator

$$= \frac{W \times L}{time}$$

$$= \frac{50 \times 4}{60}$$

$$= 3.334 \text{ kW}$$

18.6 A hydraulic intensifier supplying water to a hydraulic press gets water at a pressure of 500 N/cm². If the intensity of pressure is increased to 4000 N/cm², find the internal and external diameter of ram. The stroke of the intensifier is 1.2 m and its capacity is 24 litre.

Solution

Given $p_1 = 500 \text{ N/cm}^2$, $p_2 = 4000 \text{ N/cm}^2$,

$L = 1.2$ m, Capacity = 24 litre

Capacity of intensifier = area × stroke

$$\frac{24}{1000} = \frac{\pi}{4} \times D_2^2 \times 1.2$$

$$D_2 = \sqrt{\frac{24 \times 4}{1000 \, \pi \times 1.2}} = 0.1596 \text{ m}$$

∴ Internal diameter of sliding cylinder

$$= 0.1596 \text{ m}$$

Now $p_1 A_1 = p_2 A_2$

$$A_1 = \frac{p_2 A_2}{p_1}$$

$$\frac{\pi}{4} \times D_1^2 = \frac{4000}{500} \times \frac{\pi}{4} \times (0.1596)^2$$

$$D_1 = 0.1596 \sqrt{8}$$

$$= 0.4515 \text{ m}$$

Internal Diameter of fixed cylinder Z

$$= 0.4515 \text{ m}$$

18.7 An intensifier has a ram diameter of 150 mm and a sliding cylinder of 750 mm diameter. Calculate the pressure of water on the low pressure side of the intensifier if the pressure on the high pressure side is 20600 kN/m². The loss of head due to friction at each of the packings of the intensifies is 5% of the total force on each side of the packings.

Solution

Given D_1 = 150 mm , D_2 = 750 mm,

p_1 = 20600 kN/m², Loss = 5 % of force.

Force on the end of the sliding cylinder = $p_1 A_1$ Since 5 % of this force is lost in the friction, therefore, the net force on the sliding cylinder = $0.95 \times p_1 \times A_1 = F$

Again 5 % of this force is lost in the friction in the packing between the sliding cylinder and fixed ram.

Thus net force on the fixed ram = $0.95 \times F$

$$= 0.95 (0.95 \times p_1 \times A_1) \tag{i}$$

The force exerted by the fixed ram of the intensifier is also given by

$$= p_2 A_2$$

From Eqs. (i) and (ii)

$$0.95 \left[0.95 \times p_1 \times \frac{\pi}{4} \times (0.750)^2 \right] = 20600 \times \frac{\pi}{4} \times (0.150)^2$$

$$p_1 = \frac{20600 \times (0.150)^2}{(0.95)^2 \times (0.750)^2} = 913.02 \text{ kN/m}^2$$

18.8 A hydraulic press has a ram of 20 cm diameter and a plunger of 3 cm diameter. It is used for lifting a weight of 3 tonnes. Find (a) the force required at the plunger. (b) If a lever is used for applying force on the plunger, find the force required at the end of the lever if the ratio of l/l_1 is 1 : 10.

Solution

Given D = 0.2 m, d = 0.03 m,

$$W = 3 \times 9810 \text{ N}, \ l/l_1 = 1/10.$$

(a) From Eq. 18.10,

$$W = \frac{F \times A}{a}$$

$$3 \times 9810 = \frac{F \times \frac{\pi}{4} \times (0.2)^2}{\frac{\pi}{4} \times (0.03)^2}$$

$$F = \frac{3 \times 9810 \times (0.03)^2}{(0.2)^2} = 662.18 \text{ N}$$

(b) When a lever is used, Eq. 18.12 b yields,

$$F_1 = W \times \frac{A}{a} \cdot \times \frac{l}{l_1}$$

$$= 3 \times 9810 \times \frac{(0.03)^2}{(0.2)^2} \times \frac{1}{10} = 62.6 \text{ N}$$

18.9 A hydraulic press lifts 3 tonne load to a height of 1 metre in 2 minutes. The diameter of ram and plunger are 150 mm and 25 mm respectively. The stroke of the plunger is twice the diameter of the ram. Find (a) the power of the motor to drive the plunger of the press (b) the number of beats required by the plunger, and (c) the pressure on the plunger and the ram.

Solution

Given $W = 3$ tonne, $H = 1 \text{ m}$ in 2 min, $D = 0.15 \text{ m}$

$$d = 0.025 \text{ m}, \quad L = 2D$$

(a) Work done by the press per second

$$= \frac{\text{Weight lifted} \times \text{distance travelled}}{\text{time}}$$

$$= \frac{3 \times 9810 \times 1}{2 \times 60} \quad (\text{Since 1 tonne} = 1000 \text{ kg} = 9810 \text{ N})$$

$$= 245.25 \text{ N m/s}$$

Power required to drive the plunger

$$= 245.25 \text{ N m/s}$$

$$= 245.25 \text{ watts}$$

(b) Volume of water displaced as the ram is lifted through 1 m

$$= \left[\frac{\pi}{4} \times (0.15)^2 \times 1 \right] \text{ m}^3$$

Volume of water displaced by the plunger during each stroke

$$= \left[\frac{\pi}{4} \times (0.025)^2 \times 2 \times 0.15 \right] \text{ m}^3$$

$$\therefore \text{ Number of beats} = \frac{\frac{\pi}{4} \times (0.15)^2 \times 1}{\frac{\pi}{4} \times (0.025)^2 \times 2 \times 0.15}$$

No. of beats = 120.

(c) Force on the plunge $F = \dfrac{W \times a}{A}$

$$= \dfrac{3 \times 9810 \times \dfrac{\pi}{4} \times (0.025)^2}{\dfrac{\pi}{4} \times (0.15)^2}$$

$$= 817.5 \ N$$

18.10 The ram of a hydraulic press is 200 mm in diameter and is worked from an intensifier. The intensifier gets its low pressure supply of water from a tank whose surface level is 16 m above the level of intensifier, through a pipe 50 mm in diameter and 150 m long. The intensifier ram is 75 mm in diameter and sliding cylinder 900 mm in diameter. The friction of each of three packings may be taken as 3 % of the total pressure on the appropriate ram. The friction coefficient for low pressure pipe is 0.02. Calculate the speed of advance of the press ram in cm/min when exerting a force on 50 tonne. Neglect all other losses.

Solution

Given Press $D = 200$ mm, $W = 50$ tonne,

Intensifier $D_1 = 0.075$ m, $D_2 = 0.9$ m,

            $l = 150$ m, $d = 0.05$ m,

            $H = 16$ m,   Friction $= 3$ % of pressure,

            $f = 0.02$.

Since there is 3 % friction loss in the package of the hydraulic press, the force due to water acting on its ram $= \dfrac{50}{0.97}$ tonne.

Pressure intensity on ram of press

$$= \dfrac{50}{0.97} \times \dfrac{1}{\dfrac{\pi}{4} \times (0.2)^2}$$

$$= 1641 \ \text{tonne/m}^2$$

As there is the same pressure transmitted by the fixed ram of the intensifier, the intensity of pressure on (intensifier) ram

$$= \dfrac{1641}{0.97} \ \text{tonne/m}^2$$

$$= 1691.75 \ \text{tonne/m2}$$

From Eq. 18.6 for the intensifier,

$$p_1 A_1 = p_2 A_2$$

$$p \times \dfrac{\pi}{4} \times (0.9)^2 \times 0.97 = 1691.75 \times \dfrac{\pi}{4} \times (0.075)^2$$

where p is the pressure of water supplied from the water tank and there is 3 % friction loss in the gland packings outside the sliding ram.

Solving,
$$p = \frac{1691.75 \times (0.075)^2}{(0.9)^2 \times 0.97}$$

$$= 12.11 \text{ tonne/m}^2$$

Equivalent head of water $= \dfrac{12.11 \times 9810}{9810}$

$$= 12.11 \text{ m.}$$

The intensifier is supplied water (on its low pressure side) from a water tank 16m high.

The head lost in friction $= (16 - 12.11)$

$$= 3.89 \text{ m}$$

$\therefore$
$$h_f = \frac{f L \, U^2}{2 g d}$$

$$3.89 = \frac{0.02 \times 150 \times U^2}{2 \times 9.81 \times 0.05}$$

$$U = \sqrt{\frac{3.89 \times 2 \times 9.81 \times 0.05}{0.02 \times 150}}$$

$$= 1.128 \text{ m/s}$$

Discharge flowing in the pipe or discharge entering in the low pressure side of intensifier

$$= 1.128 \times \frac{\pi}{4} \times (0.05)^2 = 2.214 \times 10^{-3} \text{ m}^3/\text{s}$$

Discharge flowing into the cylinder of the press from the high pressure side of intensifier is reduced in the ratio of area of intensifier ram A_2 and area A_1 of fixed cylinder.

Discharge of high pressure water into the press cylinder

$$= 2.214 \times 10^{-3} \times \left(\frac{0.075}{0.09}\right)^2 = 1.537 \times 10^{-5} \text{ m}^3/\text{s}$$

Now if U_1 is the speed of the advance of the press ram, then

$$U_1 \times \frac{\pi}{4} \times (0.2)^2 = 1.537 \times 10^{-5}$$

$$U_1 = \frac{1.537 \times 10^{-5} \times 4}{\pi \times (0.2)^2}$$

$$U_1 = 4.89 \times 10^{-4} \text{ m/s} = 2.93 \text{ cm/min.}$$

18.11 A hydraulic crane is used to lift a weight through a height of 10 m. It is supplied water under a pressure of 700 N/cm^2. The diameter of the ram of the crane is 15 cm, the velocity ratio of hook to ram is 5 : 1

and efficiency of the ram is 65 %. Find (a) the volume of water required to lift the weight, and (b) the weight lifted by the crane.

Solution

Given lift $\quad = 10$ m, p $= 700$ N/cm^2, D $= 15$ cm.

velocity ratio $= 5 : 1$. $\quad \eta = 65 \%$.

(a) Let L be the stroke of the ram, then

$$\text{Velocity ratio} = \frac{\text{Distance travelled by hook}}{\text{Distance travelled by ram}}$$

$$5 = \frac{10}{L}$$

$$L = \frac{10}{5} = 2 \text{ m.}$$

Since distance L travelled by crane ram is its stroke, volume of water required $=$ Area $\times$ stroke

$$= \frac{\pi}{4} \times (0.15)^2 \times 2 = 0.03533 \text{ m}^2$$

(b) $\quad$ Efficiency $= \dfrac{\text{Ouput}}{\text{Input}} = \dfrac{\text{Work done in lifting weight}}{\text{work done by ram}}$

$$0.65 = \frac{W \times \text{Distance moved by weight (or hook)}}{F \times \text{Distance moved by ram}}$$

$$= \frac{W}{F} \times 5$$

$$W = \frac{0.65 \times F}{5}$$

The force F acting on the ram $= p \times A$

$$= 700 \times 10^4 \times \frac{\pi}{4} \times (0.15)^2$$

$$\therefore \quad W = \frac{0.65}{5} \times 700 \times 10^4 \times \frac{\pi}{4} \times (0.15)^2$$

$$= 1672.8 \text{ N or } 1.672 \text{ kN}$$

18.12 A hydraulic crane is used to lift a load at a speed of 0.6 m per second. It is supplied water from an accumulator at a pressure of 600 N/cm^2 through a pipe line 50 mm in diameter. The crane is situated at 250m from the accumulator. The diameter of the ram of the crane is 225 mm and the velocity ratio of the hook to the ram is 4 : 1. Assume that a pressure of 27.5 N/cm^2 on the ram pulleys, etc., of the crane is lost in mechanical friction. Assuming friction coefficient of the pipe line is 0.4, calculate the load lifted.

Solution

Given Crane, $\quad p = 600$ N/cm^2, p_1 lost $= 27.5$ N/cm^2,

$$D = 0.225 \text{ m, velocity ratio} = 4 : 1,$$

Speed of lifting = 0.6 m/min,

Pipe, l = 250 m, d = 0.5 m , f = 0.04.

$$\text{Velocity ratio} = \frac{\text{Speed of hook}}{\text{Speed of ram}}$$

$$\text{Speed of ram} = \frac{0.6}{4} = 0.15 \text{ m/s.}$$

Let U be the velocity of flow of water through the pipe line. The quantity of water flowing through the pipe is same as the quantity of water entering the cylinder of the crane.

$$U \times \frac{\pi}{4} \times (0.05)^2 = 0.15 \times \frac{\pi}{4} \times (0.225)^2$$

$$U = 3.0375 \text{ m/s.}$$

Now, head of water in the accumulator $= \dfrac{600 \times 10^4}{9810}$

$$= 611.2 \text{ m.}$$

Head lost in friction in the pipe line, $h_f = \dfrac{f l U^2}{2 g d}$

$$h_f = \frac{0.04 \times 250 \times (3.0375)^2}{2 \times 9.81 \times 0.05} = 94.05 \text{ m}$$

Head lost in mechanical friction in the ram, pulleys etc

$$= \frac{27.5 \times 10^4}{9810} = 28.03$$

Total head lost = (94.05 + 28.03)

$$= 122.08 \text{ m}$$

Net head available on the ram of crane

$$= (611.2 - 122.08)$$

$$= 489.12 \text{ m}$$

∴ Net pressure intensity on the ram = 9810 × 489.12 N/m²

$$= 479.824 \text{ N/cm}^2$$

$$\text{Load on the ram} = \frac{479.824 \times 10^4 \times \frac{\pi}{4} \times (0.225)^2}{9810} \text{ tonne}$$

$$= 19.438 \text{ tonne}$$

Load lifted by crane = load on ram/velocity ratio

$$= 19.438 \times \frac{1}{4}$$

$$= 4.86 \text{ tonne.}$$

18.13 The following particulars refer to a hydraulic crane : Diameter of ram = 300 mm, velocity ratio of crane hook to ram = 5 : 1, length of supply pipe from accumulator = 160 m, diameter of supply pipe = 50 mm, pressure at accumulator $= 600$ N/cm^2, mechanical friction of ram, pulleys, etc., equivalent to 40 N/cm^2, coefficient of friction for pipe $= 0.04$.

Obtain a relationship between the load lifted and speed of lifting

Solution

Given $\qquad D = 0.3$ m, velocity ratio $= 5 : 1$, $l_s = 160$ m,

$\qquad\qquad d_s = 0.05$ m, p $= 600$ N/cm^2, f $= 0.04$,

$\qquad\qquad$ Friction $= 40$ N/cm^2.

Load on the ram $\times$ velocity of ram $=$ Load lifted $\times$ Velocity of lifting

or $\qquad$ load on the ram $= W \times \dfrac{\text{Velocity of lifting}}{\text{Velocity of ram}}$

$$= W \times \frac{1}{1/5} = 5\,W$$

Since there is frictional resistance equivalent of 40 N/cm^2

Pressure intensity acting on the ram of crane

$$= \left[\frac{5\,W}{\frac{\pi}{4} \times (0.3)^2} + 40 \times 10^4 \right]$$

$$= (70.77\,W + 40 \times 10^4)$$

Pressure head on the ram $= \dfrac{(70.77\,W + 40 \times 10^4)}{9810}$ m

$$= (0.00721\,W + 40.77) \qquad\qquad ...\text{(i)}$$

Pressure head on accumulator$= \dfrac{600 \times 10^4}{9810}$

$$= 611.621 \text{ m} \qquad\qquad ...\text{(ii)}$$

Head lost in friction in pipe$= \dfrac{0.04 \times 160 \times U^2}{2 \times 9.81 \times 0.05}$

$$h_f = 6.524\,U^2 \text{ m} \qquad\qquad ...\text{(iii)}$$

Also from Eqs. (i) and (ii)

$$h_f = [611.621 - (0.00721\,W + 40.77)] \qquad\qquad ...\text{(iv)}$$

From Eqs (iii) and (iv)

$$6.524\,U^2 = (611.621 - 0.00721\,W - 44.77)$$

$$U = [87.50 - 1.105 \times 10^{-3}\,W]^{1/2} \qquad\qquad ...\text{(v)}$$

Speed of lifting weight $=$ speed of ram $\times$ velocity ratio

$$U_2 = U_1 \times 5$$

or $\qquad\qquad U_1 = \dfrac{U_2}{5} \qquad\qquad ...\text{(vi)}$

From continuity equation, discharge flowing through pipe is same as the discharge entering the cylinder of the crane, U is velocity in pipe.

$$\therefore \quad \left[\frac{\pi}{4} \times (0.05)^2 \times U \right] = \left[\frac{\pi}{4} \times (0.3)^3 U_1 \right]$$

$$U_1 = \frac{(0.05)^2}{(0.3)^2} \times U \qquad \qquad \text{...(vii)}$$

From Eqs (vi) and (vii)

$$U_2 = 5 U_1 = 5 \times \left(\frac{0.05}{0.3} \right)^2 U$$

$$= \frac{5}{36} U$$

Substituting the valve of U from Eq. (v)

$$U_2 = \frac{5}{36} [87.5 - 1.105 \times 10^{-3} \, W]^{1/2} \qquad \qquad \text{...(viii)}$$

Eq. (viii) is the required relationship.

For load $W = 0$, Speed of lifting $U_2 = 1.3$ m/s

For load $W = 1$ tonne $= 9810$ N, Speed $U_2 = 1.216$ m/s

For load $W = 5$ tonne $= 49050$ N, Speed $U_2 = 0.801$ m/s

18.14 The load on a hydraulic machine is applied by means of a water pressure acting on its ram 355 mm diameter. The machine rises by 600 mm in 20 seconds. The maximum load to be applied on the hydraulic machine is 200 tonne and the frictional resistance of the ram is equivalent to a additional load of 5 tonne. The accumulator has a ram of diameter 112.5 mm and machine remains idle for 0.9 times of the working period of the machine. Determine (a) the load on the accumulator, (b) minimum volumetric capacity of the accumulator and (c). the power continuously supplied by the pump to the accumulator and machine (while it is working).

Solution

Given Machine, $D_1 = 0.375$ m, $L = 0.6$ m in 20 sec, W = 200 tones, Frictional resistance = 5 tonne,

Accumulator, $D = 0.1125$ m,

Machine remains idle $= 0.9 \times 20 = 18$ sec.

(a) The total load to be overcome by hydraulic pressure

$$= (200 + 5) = 205 \text{ tonnes.}$$

The pressure intensity on the ram of hydraulic machine

$$= \frac{205}{\frac{\pi}{4} \times (0.375)^2} = 1857.04 \text{ tonnes/m}^2$$

The load on the accumulator

$$= (1857.04 \times \text{area of ram of accumulator})$$

$$= 1857.04 \times \frac{\pi}{4} \times (0.1125)^2$$

$$= 18.45 \text{ tonne.}$$

(b) Let q be the discharge supplied by the pump continuously and Q be the discharge supplied to the machine during the working period of

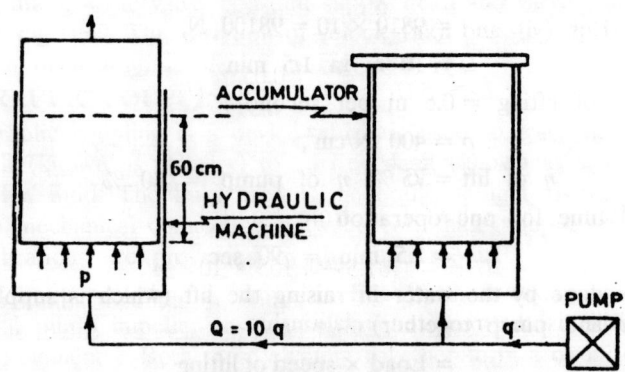

FIG 18.15 EXAMPLE 18.14

the machine. During the idle period, the discharge is stored in the accumulator i.e. 9q is stored in the accumulator. Thus, during the working period of the machine, it receives 9 q from the accumulator and q directly from the pump.

$$\therefore \qquad Q = 10 \ q.$$

Also, quantity of water per second entering the machine

$$= \frac{\text{Volume of the cylinder of the machine}}{\text{Time}}$$

$$Q = \frac{\pi}{4} \times (0.375)^2 \times 0.6 \times \frac{1}{20} = 3.311 \times 10^{-3} \text{ m}^3/\text{s}$$

$$\therefore \qquad q = \frac{Q}{10}$$

$$= 3.311 \times 10^{-4} \text{ m}^3/\text{s}$$

Capacity of accumulator

$$= 9q = 9 \times 3.311 \times 10^{-4}$$

$$= 2.98 \times 10^{-3} \text{ m}^3/\text{s}$$

(c) Power supplied by the pump

$$= q \times p \text{ watts}$$

$$= 3.311 \times 10^{-4} \times 1857.04 \times 9810$$

$$= 603.83 \text{ watts or } 6.032 \text{ kW}$$

18.15 A hydraulic lift raises a load of 10 tonne through a height of 10 m once every 1.5 minute, the speed of lifting being 0.6 m per second. It is worked from an accumulator which is being supplied water by a pump. The pressure of water supplied is 400 N/cm². The efficiency of lift is 75 % and that of pump is 80 %. Find the power required to drive the pump and minimum capacity of the accumulator. Frictional losses in the pipeline may be neglected.

Solution

Given $\quad W = 10$ tonnes

$$= 9810 \times 10 = 98100 \text{ N},$$

$$L = 10 \text{ m in } 1.5 \text{ min},$$

Speed of lifting $= 0.6$ m per second,

$$p = 400 \text{ N/cm}^2,$$

η of lift $= 75\%$, η of pump $= 80\%$

Total time for one operation

$$= 1.5 \text{ min} = 90 \text{ sec} \qquad \qquad ...(i)$$

Work done by the water in raising the lift (which is supplied by the accumulator and pump together)

$$= \text{Load} \times \text{speed of lifting}$$

$$= 98100 \times 0.6 \qquad \left(\because 1 \, tonne = 9810 \, N \right)$$

$$= 58860 \text{ N m/s}$$

Power supplied $= 58860$ watts.

Actual power supplied to the lift together by the pump and accumulator

$$= \frac{58860}{0.75} = 78480 \text{ watts} \qquad \qquad ...(ii)$$

Now let the power supplied by the pump be P_1 and that by the accumulator be P_2

$$P_1 + P_2 = 78480 \qquad \qquad ...(iii)$$

Working period of lift $= \dfrac{\text{lift}}{\text{speed of lifting}}$

$$= \frac{10}{0.6} = 16.67 \text{ sec} \qquad \qquad ...(iv)$$

From Eqns (i) and (iv)

Idle period of the lift

$$= \text{ total time - Working period}$$

$$= (90 - 16.67)$$

$$= 73.33 \text{ sec} \qquad \qquad ...(v)$$

During the idle period of the lift, the energy is stored in the accumulator. The energy is then given by the accumulator to the lift during its working period of 16,67 seconds.

$\therefore$ Energy stored in the accumulator during idle period

$$= \text{output of pump} \times \text{idle period}$$

Energy stored $= P_1 \times 73.33$ N- m $\qquad \qquad ...(vi)$

$$= \frac{P_1 \times 73.33}{16.67} = 4.398 \, P_1 \quad \text{N} \quad \text{m/s}$$

Power supplied by the accumulator

$$P_2 = 4.398 \, P_1 \quad \text{watts} \qquad\qquad ...(vii)$$

From Eqs (iii) and (vii)

$$P_1 + 4.398 \, P_1 = 78480$$

$$P_1 = 14538.72 \quad \text{watts}$$

Input to the pump $= \dfrac{14538.27}{0.80}$

$$= 18173.4 \quad \text{watts or} \quad 18.173 \quad \text{kW}$$

Power required to drive the pump

$$= 18.173 \quad \text{kW}$$

(b) Minimum capacity of the accumulator

= energy stored during idle period of lift.

From Eq. (vi)

Minimum capacity $= \dfrac{14538.72 \times 73.33}{100}$ kN-m

$$= 1066.12 \quad \text{kN-m}$$

18.16 The following observations were obtained from a hydraulic ram.

Supply head = 3m, length of supply pipe = 6 m, diameter of supply pipe = 25 mm, delivery head = 7.5 m, length of delivery pipe = 7.5 m, diameter of delivery pipe = 12.5 mm, time taken to supply 13.5 N of water = 33.8 second, water wasted during this time = 60 N, Assume f = 0.04, determine the efficiency of the ram.

Solution

Given :

$$h = 3 \text{ m}, \ l_s = 6\text{m}, \ d_s = 0.025 \text{ m}, \ H = 7.5 \text{ m}$$

$$l_d = 7.5 \text{ m}, \ d_d = 0.0125 \text{ m}, \ t = 35 \text{ sec},$$

$$wQ = 60 \text{ N}, \ wq = 13.5 \text{ N}, \ f = 0.04.$$

Total quantity of water supplied from supply reservoir in 35 seconds

$$= (w \, Q + w \, q)$$

$$= (60 + 13.5) = 73.5 \text{ N}$$

Total discharge $(Q + q)$

$$= \frac{73.5}{9810 \times 35} = 2.14 \times 10^{-4} \text{ m}^3\text{/s}$$

Velocity of flow in the supply pipe

$$= \frac{Q + q}{a_s}$$

$$= \frac{2.14 \times 10^{-4}}{\frac{\pi}{4} \times (0.025)^2} = 0.436 \text{ m/s}$$

Water actually lifted,

$$q = \frac{13.5}{35 \times 9810} = 3.93 \times 10^{-5} \text{ m}^3/\text{s}$$

Water wasted per second $= \dfrac{60}{35 \times 9810}$

$$= 1.747 \times 10^{-4} \text{ m3/s}$$

Velocity of flow through delivery pipe

$$= \frac{3.93 \times 10^{-5}}{\frac{\pi}{4} \times (0.0125)^2}$$

$$= 0.32 \text{ m/s}$$

Head lost due to friction in the supply pipe,

$$h_{fs} = \frac{0.04 \times 6 \times (0.436)^2}{2 \times 9.81 \times 0.025}$$

$$= 0.093 \text{ m}$$

Head lost due to friction in the delivery pipe,

$$h_{fd} = \frac{0.04 \times 7.5 \times (0.32)^2}{2 \times 9.81 \times 0.0125}$$

$$= 0.125 \text{ m.}$$

Effective supply head $= (h - h_{fs})$

$$= (3 - 0.093) = 2.907\text{m}$$

Effective delivery head $= (7.5 + 0.125) = 7.625$ m developed by the ram.

Rankine's efficiency $= \dfrac{q\,(H + h_{fd})}{Q\,(h - h_{fs})} \times 100$

$$= \frac{3.93 \times 10^{-5} \times 7.625}{1.747 \times 10^{-4} \times 2.907} \times 100$$

$$= 58.98 \text{ \%}$$

18.17 A hydram has a supply head of 1.5 m and delivery head (above the waste valve) of 11 m. The diameter of supply pipe is 75 mm and its length is 10 m. The waste valve, which is 125 mm diameter and weights 15 N, has a travel of 6 mm. Determine (a) the number of beats per minute, and (b) the weight of water lifted per minute.

Solution

Given : $\qquad h = 1.5$ m, $(H + h) = 11$ m, $d_s = 75$ mm,

$\qquad\qquad l_s = 10$ m, $d_0 = 125$ mm,

Weight of waste valve $= 15$ N, $b_0 = 6$ mm.

(a) Upward pressure head required to close the waste valve, from Eq. 18.16

$$h_0 = \frac{W}{w \times \frac{\pi}{4} \times d_0^2}$$

$$= \frac{15}{9810 \times \frac{\pi}{4} \times (0.125)^2} = 0.1246 \text{ m}$$

Maximum velocity past waste valve just before closure, from Eq. 18.15,

$$U_0 = \sqrt{2 g h_0}$$
$$= \sqrt{2 \times 9.81 \times 0.1246}$$
$$= 1.563 \text{ m/s}$$

Let maximum velocity in the supply pipe be U_m just before the closure of the waste valve. From continuity equation,

$$\frac{\pi}{4} \times (0.075)^2 \times U_m = \pi \times 0.125 \times 0.006 \times 1.563$$

$$U_m = 0.832 \text{ m/s}$$

Since the velocity increases gradually from 0 to 0.832 metre per second in the supply pipe, the time t_1 for it is given by Eq. 18.18.

$$h = \frac{l_s}{g} \times \frac{U_m}{t_1}$$

or
$$t_1 = \frac{10}{9.81} \times \frac{0.832}{1.5} = 0.565 \text{ sec.}$$

Let t_2 be the time during one beat for which the waste valve remains closed or delivery valve remains open.

∴
$$H = \frac{l_s}{g} \times \frac{U_m}{t_2}$$

or
$$t_2 = \frac{10}{9.81} \times \frac{0.832}{(11 - 1.5)} = 0.0893 \text{ sec.}$$

∴ Total time for one beat,
$$t = (t_1 + t_2)$$
$$= (0.565 + 0.0893) = 0.6543 \text{ sec.}$$

∴ Number of beats per minute $= \dfrac{60}{0.6543}$

$$N = 91.7 \approx 92.$$

(b) Quantity of water lifted per second

$$= w q \times \frac{t_2}{t}$$

$$= 9810 \times \frac{\pi}{4} \times (0.075)^2 \times \frac{0.832}{2} \times \frac{0.0893}{0.6543}$$

$$= 2.46 \text{ N}$$

Quantity of water lifted per minute= $2.46 \times 60 = 147.56$ N

18.18 The load of 400 tonne in a hydraulic machine is applied by means of four jacks with a ram of 20 cm diameter. The frictional resistance on each ram is equivalent to a load of 2.5 tonne. The jacks are applied with water under pressure from an intensifier. Find the pressure of water applied to the jacks and the ratio of external diameter of fixed ram and external diameter of sliding ram of the intensifier with inlet pressure of 0.1 tonne/cm^2

Solution

Given : Load on four jacks= 400 tonne,

$\qquad$ Frictional resis = 2.5 tonne on each ram,

$$p_1 = 0.1 \text{ tonne/cm}^2$$

Since there are four jacks which support the load of 400 tonne, the load of each ram of the jack.

$$= \left(\frac{400}{4} + 2.5 \right)$$

$$= 102.5 \text{ tonne}$$

Water under pressure of p_2 is needed to be supplied by the intensifier.

$$p_2 = \frac{102.5}{\frac{\pi}{4} \times (0.2)^2} = 3264.3 \text{ tonne/m}^2$$

Now $\qquad p_1 A_1 = p_2 A_2$

$$\frac{A_1}{A_2} = \frac{p_2}{p_1}$$

$$= \frac{3264.3}{0.04 \times 10^4}$$

$$= 8.16$$

18.19 A hydram has got a waste valve, 100 mm in diameter, weighing 16 N. The waste valve has a travel of 6 mm and makes 110 beats per minute. The supply pipe is 10 m long and 75 mm diameter. Determine the discharge supplied to a delivery tank located 6 m above the waste valve. Assume there is no slip.

Solution

Given : $\qquad W = 16$ N, $d_0 = 100$ mm, $b_0 = 6$ mm,

$\qquad N = 110, l_s = 10$ m, $d_s = 75$ mm

$\qquad H = 6$ m.

Upward pressure required to close the waste valve,

$$h_0 = \frac{W}{w \times \frac{\pi}{4} \times d_0}$$

$$= \frac{16}{9810 \times \frac{\pi}{4} \times (0.100)^2}$$

$$= 0.2077 \text{ m}$$

Maximum velocity past waste valve just before closure,

$$U_0 = \sqrt{2 g h_0}$$

$$= \sqrt{2 \times 9.81 \times 0.2077}$$

$$= 2.02 \text{ m/s}$$

The discharge flowing in the supply pipe

= discharge going waste past waste valve.

Maximum velocity in the supply pipe U_m is given by

$$U_m = \frac{U_0 \times \pi \times d_0 \times b_0}{\frac{\pi}{4} \times d^2} = \frac{4\, U_0 \times d_0 \times b_0}{d^2}$$

$$= \frac{4 \times 2.02 \times 0.1 \times 0.006}{(0.075)^2}$$

$$= 0.862 \text{ m/s}$$

Kinetic energy of water in the supply pipe just at the time of closure of waste valve

$$= \frac{1}{2} \text{Mass} \times U_m^2 = \frac{1}{2} \times \frac{w}{g} \times a_s\, l_s \times U_m^2$$

$$= \frac{1}{2} \times \frac{9810}{9.81} \times \frac{\pi}{4} \times (0.075)^2 \times 10 \times (0.862)^2$$

$$= 16.405 \text{ N-m}$$

Neglecting slip, this kinetic energy can lift W_1 newton water against 6 m delivery head in each beat,

$$\therefore \qquad 6\, W_1 = 16.405$$

$$W_1 = \frac{16.405}{6}$$

$$= 2.734 \text{ N per beat}$$

Since the hydram makes 110 betas per minute, the discharge supplied per minute is

$$q = \frac{2.734 \times 110}{9810}$$

$$= 0.0306 \text{ m}^3/\text{minute}$$

$$= 30.658 \text{ lit/min.}$$

Objective Questions

18.1 A hydraulic accumulator is a device which is used

(a) to increase the intensity of pressure of water,

   (b) to store the energy during idle period of machine,

   (c) to supply water from lower tank to higher tank,

   (d) to increase the velocity of flow,

   (e) none.

18.2 The capacity of a hydraulic accumulator, with usual notation, is given by

   (a) w A/L   (b) p AL

   (c) pL/w   (d) w AL

   (e) none.

18.3 A hydraulic intensifier increases the pressure intensity of water given by

   (a) $p_1 A_2/A_1$ (b) $p_1 Q_2/Q_1$

   (c) $p_1 A_1$ (d) $p_1 A_1 L/Q_2$ (e) none.

18.4 A hydraulic press is used to apply a force of 3 tonne on a job with its ram of 200 mm diameter and plunger of 30 mm diameter. The operator applies a force of 60.2 N through a lever (levarage of 1 : 10). The mechanical advantage obtained is

   (a) 488.88   (b) 44.44

   (c) 4.04   (d) 0.248

   (e) none.

18.5 The velocity of a hydraulic crane is defined as the ratio of

   (a) Weight lifted/force applied as the ram

   (b) Speed of ram to the speed of lifting weight

   (c) distance moved by the ram to the distance moved by weight

   (d) none.

18.6 A hydraulic ram is used to lift water from a supply tank, h metre above it and supply it to a tank H metre above the supply tank. The head loss in the supply and delivery pipes are h_{fs} and h_{fd} respectively. The efficiency (Rankine's) of hydram is

   (a) $q (H + h_{fd})/Q (h - h_{fs})$ (b) $q (H - h_{fd})/Q (h + h_{fs})$

   (c) $q (H - h_{fd})/Q (h - h_{fs})$ (d) $q (H + h_{fd})/Q (h + h_{fs})$

   (e) none.

18.7 Mark the correct statements

   (a) A hydram is used to lift large quantity of water against low head

   (b) A hydram is used to lift small quantity of water against large head

   (c) A hydram works on the principle of water hammer

   (d) A hydram is a positive displacement pump.

18.8 The maximum velocity of water in a supply pipe of a hydram is given by one or more of the following statement. Mark the correct one/s.

   (a) $\sqrt{2 g p_i/w}$ (b) $4 b_0 d_0 U_0/d^2$

   (c) $gh\, t_1/l_s$ (d) q/a_s (e) none.

18.9 A hydraulic coupling is used to transfer the torque from driving shaft to driven shaft while transmitting

(a) it increases the torque of driving shaft

(b) it decreases the torque

(c) it does not change the torque

(d) none.

18.10 The term 'stall' of a hydraulic coupling refers to

(a) when the speed of primary shaft is maximum

(b) when the speeds of primary and secondary shafts are same

(c) when the speed of secondary is maximum

(d) when the speed of secondary shaft is zero

(e) none.

18.11 The slip of a hydraulic coupling is necessary

(a) to obtain maximum efficiency

(b) to obtain minimum shock losses

(c) to transmit torque from primary to secondary

(d) it is unnecessary

(e) none.

18.12 The reactor blades of a torque convertor are such that they

(a) change the momentum of flowing fluid

(b) increases the velocity of flowing fluid through it

(c) change the direction of flow of the fluid

(d) change the torque of fluid

(e) none.

PROBLEMS

18.1 Explain the working of a hydraulic accumulator. Deduce an expression for the capacity of the accumulator.

18.2 Describe the working of a hydraulic intensifier and its use. Use neat sketch to explain your answer.

18.3 Draw a neat sketch of a hydram. Describe the working principle of a hydraulic ram.

18.4 Explain with neat sketches the working of the following devices: (a) hydraulic crane, (b) hydraulic lift, (c) hydraulic press, and (d) hydraulic coupling.

18.5 Explain the term - (a) stall, (b) slip, (c) velocity ratio, (d) mechanical advantage, (e) leverage.

18.6 Discuss about the working of a torque convertor. Draw a neat sketch to explain your answer.

18.7 State and draw the characteristics of fluid coupling and torque convertor.

18.8 The ram of a hydraulic accumulator is loaded with 150 tonnes. It supplies water through a 100 mm diameter pipe, 1500 m long. The loss in the pipe is estimated to be 2 % of the power supplied by the accumulator. The diameter of ram, working frictionless is 0.75 m. Determine the maximum power it can supply.

18.9 An intensifier of 100 mm diameter ram and 1 meter diameter piston is connected to a press having a ram of 300 mm diameter. Water is supplied to the intensifier from a tank 15 m above the intensifier through 50 diameter pipe, 200 m long. Take f = 0.032. Calculate the speed of advance of the press ram when exerting a load of 60 tonne.

18.10 A hydraulic press has a ram of 150 mm diameter and a plunger of 20 mm diameter. The stroke of the plunger is 200 mm and the weight lifted is 8 tonne. If the distance moved by the weight is 1 meter in 20 minutes. Determine (a) the number of strokes performed by the plunger, and (b) power required to drive the plunger.

18.11 A hydraulic crane is used to lift a weight of 12 kN through a height of 12 m with a speed of 18 m per minute, once in every 2 minutes. The efficiency of hydraulic crane is 65 % and it is working under a pressure of 500 N/cm² of water. The crane is fed from an accumulator to which water is supplied by a pump. Find (a) the capacity of the accumulator, (b) capacity of the cylinder of the jigger, and (c) the power required to drive the pump.

18.12 In a hydram, a following data are given: Diameter of supply pipe = 75 mm, diameter of waste valve = 100 mm, lift of waste valve = 6 mm, weight of waste valve = 15 N. Calculate the maximum velocity that can occur in the supply pipe.

18.13 Diameter of two parts of the ram of a differential accumulator are 150 mm and 140 mm respectively and the stroke is 1.5 m. If the pressure of water is 9800 kN/m² when the load is at rest at the upper end of stroke, what will be the weight of loaded cylinder and how much energy can be stored in the accumulator?

18.14 A hydraulic lift situated at a distance of 1000 m from the accumulator is supplied water (under a pressure of 800 N/cm²) by means of a pipe 150 mm diameter. The weight of the ram of the lift, inclusive its own weight, is 15 tonne and its diameter is 200 mm. Assuming the friction of the ram to be equivalent to an 6 % of gross load on the ram, determine the speed of ascend of the lift. Take f = 0.032.

18.15 The following particulars relate to a hydram. Drive pipe diameter = 60 mm, drive pipe lengths = 10 m, supply head = 3 m, area past waste valve = 3600 mm², delivery head above waste value = 9 m, head needed to close waste valve = 0.5 m. Compute the quantities of useful and waste water per minute and Rankine efficiency of the hydram.

19

Compressible Flows

19.1 INTRODUCTION

In general all the fluids are compressible, i.e. they can be compressed under the influence of pressure, velocity or temperature. Any change in volume causes also change in the density of fluid. In a flow system, if the density of fluid does not change appreciably, it is treated as incompressible fluid whereas if large variation in the density of fluid takes place, it is treated as compressible fluid. Problems involving large variations in volume and hence large variation in density include flights of aeroplanes and projectiles, flow of gas through orifices and nozzles, problems of flow of gas in machines such as compressors, etc. Thus significant density changes may usually be produced under the following conditions:

(i) when there is a great change in the elevation as in the case of flight of air planes at varying altitudes, and also in the meteorology.

(ii) when gases flow at very high velocities. This occurs when bodies (like projectiles, air planes, etc.) travel in air at very high velocities or when two regions, between which there is pressure difference (comparable with the absolute pressure) are connected by a tube; and

(iii) when large accelerations occur. This occurs in the case of fluids (stationary or moving) when the solid body in contact of it moves with large acceleration. The phenomena of water hammer and accoustical problems are examples of this class.

Since the fluid density is a function of pressure and temperature in the flow, therefore, thermodynamic relations are required to establish definite relationship between these parameters.

19.2 BASIC CONCEPTS OF THERMODYNAMICS

1. Equation of State

A perfect gas (sometimes also called as ideal gas) is the one which satisfies the equation of state given by

$$pv = RT \qquad \qquad ...(19.1\ a)$$

or

$$p = \rho RT \qquad \qquad ...(19.1\ b)$$

in which p is the absolute pressure, T is the absolute temperature ($^\circ K$) and $\rho\ (= 1/v)$ in the mass density of the gas. R is the gas constant and in measured is joule per kilogram per Kelvin (J kg^{-1} K^{-1}).

For air $\qquad R = 287\, J\, kg^{-1} K^{-1}$.

2. Internal Energy

It is the energy possessed by the molecules of a fluid due to molecular activity and is also known as microscopic energy. It is different to that of external energy or macroscopic energy, viz., kinetic energy or potential energy associated with fluid mass. If H unit of total heat energy is transferred to unit fluid mass, a part of it is stored in the gas as internal energy and remaining part is utilized in increasing the volume of the gas. The internal energy (I) is a function of temperature; higher the temperature, higher is the internal energy of the gas and vice versa. The change in internal energy, (I_2-I_1) of unit mass of fluid depends only on the initial and final state of gas or compressible fluid and does not depend on the manner in which these states are attained. In other words, the internal energy is solely a function of temperature, that is

$$(I_2 - I_1) = C_v (T_2 - T_1) \qquad \qquad ...(19.2)$$

where T_1 and T_2 are absolute temperatures.

3. Enthalpy

The enthalpy or total head of a gas is defined as the sum of internal energy of the gas and the work done by the gas due to its increase in the volume. Since work done per unit mass is given by p/ρ, the enthalpy is given by

$$H = (I + p/\rho) \qquad \qquad ...(19.3)$$

The total head or enthalpy H of a gas at given temperature is defined as the amount of heat required to raise the temperature of unit mass of a gas from $0°K$ to the given temperature, when heated at constant pressure. Hence

$$H = C_p (T - 273) \qquad \qquad ...(19.4)$$

where T is the absolute temperature in degrees Kelvin.

4. Specific Heat

Since pressure, temperature and density of a gas are inter-related, the amount of heat energy H required to raise the temperature from T_1 to T_2 will depend upon whether the gas is allowed to expand during the process (so that some of the energy is used in doing the external work) or not. Therefore two different definitions of specific heat are given for a gas corresponding to two extreme conditions of constant volume and constant pressure.

(a) Specific heat at constant volume, c_v :

It is the amount of heat given for a temperature change from T_1 to T_2 at constant volume.

Heat supplied per unit mass

$$H = c_v (T_2 - T_1) \qquad \qquad ...(19.5)$$

Since there is no change in volume no external work is done so that the increase in internal energy per unit mass of gas is given by $c_v (T_2 - T_1)$ heat units.

(b) Specific heat at constant pressure c_p

It is the amount of heat given at constant pressure. If the pressure is kept constant, the gas will expand as the temperatures increases from T_1 to T_2.

∴ Heat supplied per unit mass $= c_p (T_2 - T_1)$ heat units   ...(19.6)

Only part of this energy is used to raise the temperature of gas, the rest of the energy is used to do external work.

For air $c_p = 1.005 \text{ kJ kg}^{-1}\text{K}^{-1}$

and $c_v = 0.718 \text{ kJ kg}^{-1}\text{K}^{-1}$

Further it can be shown that $k\,(= c_p/c_v), R, c_p$ and c_v are related as follows

$$\frac{c_p}{c_v} = k \qquad ...(19.7)$$

$$c_p - c_v = R \qquad ...(19.8)$$

$$c_v = \left(\frac{R}{k-1}\right) \qquad ...(19.9)$$

$$c_p = \left(\frac{k}{k-1}\right) R \qquad ...(19.10)$$

Average values of k and R for some of the gases are given in Table 19.1

TABLE 19.1

Values of index k and gas constant R

Gas	k	R(m/K)
Air	1.4	29.57
Carbon Monoxide	1.4	30.64
Carbon di Oxide	1.3	19.50
Oxygen	1.29	20.80
Hydrogen	1.41	215.00
Helium	1.66	425.00

5. First Law of Thermodynamics

First law of thermodynamics is the law of conservation of energy. It states that the energy can neither be created nor destroyed; of course, its form can be changed.

If a gas is expanded in such a manner that it performs some form of external work, it follows that heat absorbed, work done and change in internal energy must satisfy the principle of conservation of energy (all expresed in heat units), viz.,

$$\begin{pmatrix} Heat\ absorbed \\ by\ unit\ mass \end{pmatrix} = \begin{pmatrix} Work\ done \\ by\ unit\ mass \end{pmatrix} + \begin{pmatrix} Increase\ of \\ internal\ energy \\ of\ unit\ mass \end{pmatrix}$$

$$H = W + (I_2 - I_1) \qquad ...(19.11)$$

where H is heat energy absorbed, W is work done and $(I_2 - I_1)$ is the increase in internal energy. It should be noted that if the gas rejects heat then H is -ve; if external work is being done on the gas in compressing it, then W is -ve; and if the term $(I_2 - I_1)$ is -ve, it represents a decrese in the internal energy.

6. Thermodynamic Processes

A gas can be expanded or compressed under two different thermodynamic processes.

(a) *Isothermal Process*: If a gas is expanded or compressed whilst its temperature is maintained constant, the process is said to be isothermal. The equation of state, Eq. 19.1, becomes

$$p\,v = p_1\,v_1 = \text{constant}$$

$$p = \frac{p_1 v_1}{v} \qquad ...(19.12a)$$

Alternatively since $\rho = 1/v$,

$$\frac{p}{\rho} = \frac{p_1}{\rho_1} = \text{constant}$$

$$p = p_1 \rho / \rho_1 \qquad ...(19.12b)$$

As there is no change of temperature in this process of expansion (or compression), there can not be any change of internal energy of gas. Therefore, Eq. 19.11,

$$H = W \qquad ...(19.11a)$$

In isothermal process, the external work is done by a gas as shown in Fig. 19.1

Work done by unit mass of gas during its expansion

= Area under p-v curve between v_1 and v_2 (shaded)

$$W = \int_{v_2}^{v_1} p\,dv \qquad ...(19.13)$$

Substituting for p from Eq. 19.12a

$$W = \int_{v_2}^{v_1} \frac{p_1 v_1}{v}\,dv$$

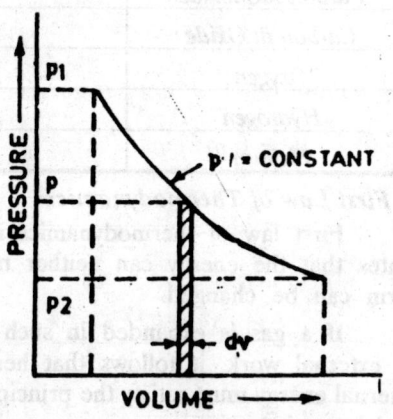

FIG. 19.1 ISOTHERMAL EXPANSION OF GAS

$$W = p_1 v_1 \log_e (v_2/v_1)$$
$$= p_1 v_1 \log_e (p_1/p_2)$$

But $\qquad p_1 v_1 = R_1 T_1$ from Eq. 19.1

$$W = R T_1 \log (p_1/p_2) \qquad \qquad ...(19.14a)$$
$$W = H = R T_1 \log (p_1/p_2) \qquad \qquad ...(19.14b)$$

Eq. 19.14a and Eq. 19.14b represents the work done by a gas which is also equal to the heat energy absorbed during expansion. If the gas is compressed, the work done W by a gas is −ve. This means the work is done on the gas and consequently the heat is rejected.

(b) *Adiabatic Process*: If a gas is expanded or compressed in such a manner that no interchange of heat takes place during the process, this process is known as adiabatic. For such a process

$$p v^k = p_1 v_1^k = p_2 v_2^k = \text{constant} \qquad \qquad ...(19.15a)$$

or $\qquad \dfrac{p}{\rho^k} = \dfrac{p_1}{\rho_1^k} = \dfrac{p_2}{\rho_2^k} = \text{constant} \qquad \qquad ...(19.15b)$

where $k (= c_p/c_v)$ is the ratio of specific heats c_p and c_v.

Applying the law of conservation of energy to this process, Eq. 19.11 and putting H = 0,

$$0 = W + (I_2 - I_1)$$

or $\qquad W = (I_1 - I_2) \qquad \qquad ...(19.16)$

Thus if work is performed by the gas adiabatically, its internal energy decreases. The work done by a gas adiabatically is shown diagrammetically in Fig. 19.2.

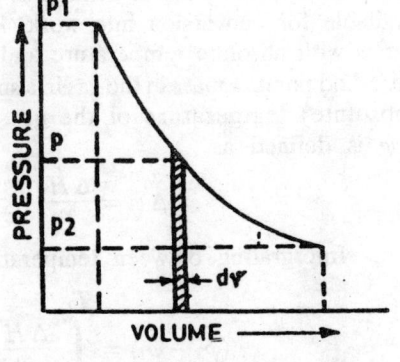

FI.G 19.2 ADIABATIC EXPENSION OF GAS

Work done by unit mass of gas

$$= \int_{v1}^{v2} p \, dv$$

From Eq. 19.15b, $p = p_1 v_1^k/v^k$

$\therefore \qquad W = \int_{v1}^{v2} p_1 \dfrac{v_1^k}{v^k} \, dv$

$$= p_1 v_1^k \dfrac{[v_2^{(1-k)} - v_1^{(1-k)}]}{(1-k)}$$

But $\qquad p_1 v_1^k = p_2 v_2^k$

$\therefore \qquad W = \dfrac{[p_2 v_2^k v_2^{(1-k)} - p_1 v_1^k v_1^{(1-k)}]}{(1-k)}$

$$= \dfrac{(p_2 v_2 - p_1 v_1)}{(1-k)} \qquad \qquad ...(19.17a)$$

But $\qquad p_1 v_1 = R T_1$ and $p_2 v_2 = R T_2$,

$$W = \frac{R(T_2 - T_1)}{(1 - k)} = \frac{R(T_1 - T_2)}{(k - 1)} \qquad ...(19.17b)$$

(c) *Polytropic Process*: In general, the relationship between pressure and density (or specific volume) can be expressed as

$$pv^n = \text{constant}$$

or $\qquad \dfrac{p}{\rho^n} = \text{constant} \qquad\qquad ...(19.18)$

where n is a constant or index for given process.

(i) Thus, for $n = 0$, p = constant, means the process is isobaric.

(ii) for $n = 1$, T = constant, means the process is isothermal.

(iii) for $n = k$, entropy = constant, means the process is isentropic.

7. Reversible and Irreversible Process

When the physical property of a gas is changed, it is said to undergo a process. The process is said to be reversible if the gas and its surroundings could subsequently be completely restored to their initial conditions by adding to (or substracting from) the gas exactly the same amount of heat and work taken from (or added to) it during the process.

A reversible process is an ideal situation which is never achieved in practice. Since it is known that viscous friction dissipate a part of mechanical energy into heat energy and it is not easily possible to convert it back into mechanical energy. In practice, therefore, all processes are irreversible.

8. Entropy

Entropy of a gas is defined as the measure of the maximum heat energy available for conversion into work. It is the physical property of a gas and varies with absolute temperature and the state of the gas. If ΔH is the heat absorbed per unit mass of the gas in a small time interval and if T is thermodynamic (absolute) temperature of the gas at that instant, the change in entropy $\Delta \varphi$ is defined as

$$\Delta \varphi = \frac{\Delta H}{T} \qquad\qquad ...(19.19)$$

Intergrating between temperatures T_1 to T_2,

$$(\varphi_2 - \varphi_1) = \int_{T_1}^{T_2} \frac{\Delta H}{T} \qquad\qquad ...(19.20)$$

If heating of gas takes place isothermally, the temperature of gas remains constant. Therefore,

$$(\varphi_2 - \varphi_1) = \frac{\Delta H}{T} = \frac{p_1 v_1 \log_e (v_2/v_1)}{J T} \qquad\qquad ...(19.21)$$

where J is the conversion factor for work into heat units.

For adiabatic process, since no transfer of heat occurs, i.e. $\Delta H = 0$, hence

$$(\varphi_2 - \varphi_1) = 0$$

or $\qquad\qquad \varphi = \text{constant}$ ...(19.22)

A process in which entropy remains constant is termed as isentropic process. However, the entropy does not change in an adiabatic process only which is frictionless. Thus a frictionless adiabatic process which is also reversible is termed as 'isentropic'.

19.3 FUNDAMENTAL EQUATIONS

The following fundamental equations, in addition to equation of state, are required to solve the problems of compressible fluid. These are (1) continuity equation, (2) momentum equation, and (3) energy equation.

1. Continuity Equation

The continuity equation, in cartesian co-ordiantes, applicable to compressible fluids has been developed in section 4.6. It is expressed as

$$\frac{\partial \rho}{\partial t} + \frac{\partial}{\partial x}(\rho u) + \frac{\partial}{\partial y}(\rho v) + \frac{\partial}{\partial z}(\rho w) = 0 \qquad\qquad ...(19.23)$$

For one dimensional flow of compressible fluid, the continuity equation reduces to

$$\rho A U = \text{constant} \qquad\qquad ...(19.24)$$

where ρ is the mass density of the fluid at any given section, A is the area of cross section and U is the mean velocity of flow at that section.

Differentiating Eq. 19.24

$$A U d\rho + \rho A \, dU + \rho U \, dA = 0$$

Dividing on both sides by $\rho A U$.

$$\frac{d\rho}{\rho} + \frac{dU}{U} + \frac{dA}{A} = 0 \qquad\qquad ...(19.25)$$

Eq. 19.25 is the differential form of continuity equation.

2. Momentum Equation

The momentum equation for incompressible fluids derived in section 5.10 is also applicable to compressible fluids. This is so because the rate of change of momentum is being equated to the net force required to cause this change. And the momentum flux is equal to the product of mass flux $\rho A U$ and the velocity component in the required direction. But the mass flux $\rho A U$ remains constant from section to section (principle of continuity). As such, the momentum equation is independent of compressibility effect.

The momentum equation in X-direction may be expressed as

$$F_x = \rho_1 A_1 U_1 (U_{2x} - U_{1x}) \qquad\qquad ...(19.26a)$$

Similarly, the momentum equation in Y and Z direction is expressed as

$$F_y = \rho_1 A_1 U_1 (U_{2y} - U_{1y}) \qquad\qquad ...(19.26b)$$

$$F_z = \rho_1 A_1 U_1 (U_{2z} - U_{1z}) \qquad \qquad ...(19.26c)$$

3. Energy Equation

The general energy equation for steady flow of compressible fluid has beed discussed in Section 5.5 and 5.6. The energy equation applicable to compressible fluid can be written between two points 1 and 2 along a stream line as

$$d(p/w) + dz + \frac{U\,dU}{g} + dI = de_M + de_H$$

or $\qquad \dfrac{(p_2 - p_1)}{\rho} + g(z_2 - z_1) + \dfrac{(U_2^2 - U_1^2)}{2} + (I_2 - I_1) = e_M + e_H \qquad ...(19.27)$

where p/ρ is the pressure energy per unit maxx, gz is datum energy per unit mass and $U^2/2$ is the kinetic energy per unit mass. I is the internal energy, e_M is mechanical work done and e_H is heat energy added. All the forms of energy are expressed for unit mass of ompressible fluid. Since enthalpy H is given by Eq. 19.3,

$$H = (p/\rho + I)$$

Above Eq. 19.27 may be written as

$$\left(\frac{U_1^2}{2} + gz_1 + H_1 + e_M + e_H \right) = \left(\frac{U_2^2}{2} + gz_2 + H_2 \right) \qquad ...(19.28)$$

In case of isothermal process, since the temperature remains constant, no change in internal energy takes place. Hence $I_1 = I_2$. From Eq. 19.1,

$$\frac{p_1}{\rho_1} = \frac{p_2}{\rho_2}$$

Therefore, $\qquad H_1 = H_2.$

Further, if no energy is lost due to mechanical friction (i.e. the fluid is frictionless), $e_M = 0$. Also, for isothermal process, the heat energy added e_H is equal to the work done given by Eq. 19.14b.

$$e_H = W = R\,T \log\left(p_1/p_2 \right)$$

Therefore, Eq. 19.28 becomes

$$\left[\frac{U_1^2}{2} + gz_1 + R\,T \log_e (p_1/p_2) \right] = \left(\frac{U_2^2}{2} + gz_2 \right)$$

$$[R\,T \log_e (p_1/p_2)] = \left[\left(\frac{U_2^2 - U_1^2}{2} \right) + g(z_2 - z_1) \right]$$

Dividing on both sides by g and writing $p_1 = \rho_1 R\,T$

$$\frac{p_1}{w_1} \log_e (p_1/p_2) = \left[\frac{(U_2^2 - U_1^2)}{2g} + (z_2 - z_1) \right] \qquad ...(19.29)$$

In case of adiabatic process, no heat energy is added to or substracted from the system, hence, $e_H = 0$. For this case, the change in internal energy $(I_1 - I_2)$ is equal to the work done, Eq. 19.17a, viz..

$$W = \frac{(p_1 v_1 - p_2 v_2)}{(k-1)} = (I_1 - I_2) \qquad \ldots(19.17a)$$

The change of entropy between two section 1 and 2 is given by

$$H_1 - H_2 = \left(\frac{p_1}{\rho_1} + I_1\right) - \left(\frac{p_2}{\rho_2} + I_2\right)$$

$$= \left(\frac{p_1}{\rho_1} - \frac{p_2}{\rho_2}\right) + (I_1 - I_2)$$

$$= \frac{k}{(k-1)}\left(\frac{p_1}{\rho_1} - \frac{p_2}{\rho_2}\right) \qquad \ldots(19.30)$$

If no mechanical work is done against friction. $e_M = 0$, that is, the flow is frictionless adiabatic or isentropic. Eq. 19.28 becomes

$$\frac{k}{(k-1)}\left(\frac{p_1}{\rho_1} - \frac{p_2}{\rho_2}\right) = \left(\frac{U_2^2}{2} - \frac{U_1^2}{2}\right) + g(z_2 - z_1)$$

$$\left(\frac{p_1}{\rho_1}\right)\left(\frac{k}{k-1}\right)\left[1 - \frac{p_2}{p_1} \times \frac{\rho_1}{\rho_2}\right] = \left[\left(\frac{U_2^2}{2} - \frac{U_1^2}{2}\right) + g(z_2 - z_1)\right] \quad \ldots(19.31)$$

which is the same as Eq. 5.30b derived earlier. From Eq. 19.15,

$$\frac{p_1}{\rho_1^k} = \frac{p_2}{\rho_2^k}$$

Substituting the value of ρ_1/ρ_2 in Eq. 19.31,

$$\left(\frac{p_1}{\rho_1}\right)\left(\frac{k}{k-1}\right)\left[1 - \left(\frac{p_2}{p_1}\right)^{(k-1)/k}\right]$$

$$= \left[\left(\frac{U_2^2 - U_1^2}{2}\right) + g(z_2 - z_1)\right] \qquad \ldots(19.32)$$

For compressible fluid, the change in potential energy term is quite small, because of low specific mass. Neglecting the last term

$$\left(\frac{k}{k-k}\right)\frac{p_1}{\rho_1}[1 - (p_2/p_1)^{(k-1)/k}] = \left(\frac{U_2^2 - U_1^2}{2}\right) \qquad \ldots(19.33a)$$

$$\left(\frac{k}{k-k}\right)\frac{p_1}{w_1}[1 - (p_2/p_1)^{(k-1)/k}] = \left(\frac{U_2^2 - U_1^2}{2g}\right) \qquad \ldots(19.33b)$$

19.4 PROPAGATION OF ELASTIC WAVE DUE TO COMPRESSION OF FLUID

If there occurs a change in pressure at a point in the fluid, it is transmitted throughout the fluid. The fluid molecules transmit the pressure change to the adjoining fluid molecules and so on. Thus an elastic wave or pressure wave is generated which travels at a certain velocity. If the fluid is incompressible, the transmission of pressure occurs instantaneously, i.e., with infinite velocity. However, all the fluids can be compressed to some extent, hence the velocity of pressure wave is finite. It has been found that the velocity of pressure wave is equal to the velocity of sound in the same fluid media. An expression for velocity of pressure wave or elastic wave can now be derived as follows.

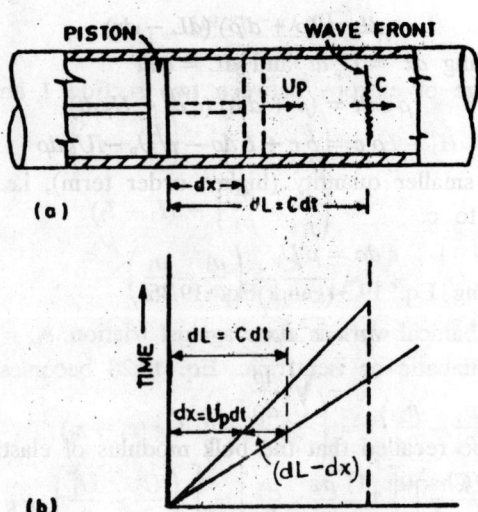

FIG 19.3 PROPAGATION OF A PRESSURE WAVE -

Consider a long rigid tube of uniform cross sectional area A fitted with a piston at one end which is initially at rest as show in Fig. 19.3. The tube is filled with a compressible fluid. If the piston moves instataneously with a velocity U_p, a pressure wave is propagated ahead of the piston at the sonic velocity 'c'. During the time interval dt, the piston has advanced through a distance dx $(= U_p\, dt)$ while the pressure wave travels ahead of the piston through a distance dL $(= c\, dt)$. Between the pressure wave front and the piston, there is a region of compressed fluid which is being increased in length at the rate of $(dL - dx)/dt = (c - U_p)$, as shown in Fig. 19.3b.

Within the region of compressed fluid, the fluid particles have acquired a velocity U_1 which is apparently equal to the velocity of the piston U_p accompanied by an increase in pressure dp due to sudden motion of the piston. Applying the momentum equation for the compressed region during time interval dt,

$$dp \times A = \frac{\rho\, dL\, A}{dt}\, (U_p - 0)$$

which may be simplified as

$$dp = \frac{\rho\, dL}{dt}\, U_p = \rho\, c\, U_p \left(\text{since } \frac{dL}{dt} = c \right) \qquad ...(19.34)$$

Before, the sudden motion of the piston, the fluid within the compressed region, length dL has an initial density ρ and its total mass is $\rho\, A\, dL$. After the piston has moved a distance dx, the fluid density within the compressed region of length $(dL - dx)$ will be increased to $(\rho + d\rho)$ and the total mass of the fluid in the compressed region is $(\rho + d\rho)\, A\, (dL - dx)$. Applying continuity equation,

$$\rho\, A\, dL = (\rho + d\rho)\, A\, (dL - dx)$$

$$\rho \, dL = (\rho + d\rho)(dL - dx)$$

Substituting $dx = U_p \, dt$ and $dL = c \, dt$

$$\rho c \, dt = (\rho + d\rho)(c \, dt - U_p \, dt)$$

$$\rho c = \rho c + c \, d\rho - \rho U_p - U_p \, d\rho$$

Neglect smaller quantity (higher order term), i.e. $U_p \, d\rho$, since U_p is much smaller to c.

$$c \, d\rho = \rho U_p \qquad\qquad \text{...(19.35)}$$

Combining Eq. 19.34 and Eq. 19.35

$$dp = c^2 \, d\rho$$

$$c = \sqrt{\frac{dp}{d\rho}} \qquad\qquad \text{...(19.36)}$$

It may be recalled that the bulk modulus of elasticity of fluid, E_v has been defined (Chapter 1) as

$$E_v = -\frac{dp}{dv/v}$$

where v is the specific volume and dv is the change in specific volume. Writing v as $1/\rho$

$$\rho v = \text{constant}$$

Differentiating,

$$\rho \, dv + v \, d\rho = 0$$

or

$$\frac{dv}{v} = \frac{-d\rho}{\rho}$$

Substituting for dv/v in Eq. 1.18,

$$E_v = \frac{dp}{d\rho/\rho}$$

$$= \frac{\rho \, dp}{d\rho}$$

or

$$\frac{dp}{d\rho} = \frac{E_v}{\rho} \qquad\qquad \text{...(19.37)}$$

Combining Eq. 19.36 and Eq. 19.37

$$c = \sqrt{\frac{E_v}{\rho}} \qquad\qquad \text{...(19.38)}$$

Eq. 19.38 shows that the velocity of elastic wave depends on the ratio of bulk modulus of elastocity E_v and the mass density of the fluid. Since the sound wave is also an elastic wave, the velocity of elastic wave is same as the velocity of sound in the fluid and is given by $\sqrt{E_v/\rho}$

(a) For isothermal process, it has been shown in Section 1.46, that $E_v = p$.

$$\therefore \qquad c = \sqrt{p/\rho}$$

But for perfect gas, $pv = RT$ or $p/\rho = RT$

$$\therefore \quad c = \sqrt{RT} \qquad \qquad ...(19.39)$$

(b) for isentropic process, $E_v = kp$

$$c = \sqrt{\frac{kp}{\rho}} = \sqrt{kRT} \qquad \qquad ...(19.40)$$

19.5 MACH NUMBER AND ITS IMPORTANCE

Mach number is the ratio of the inertia forces to the elastic forces or compressibility forces. It is also defined as the ratio of the velocity of free stream U_0 to the velocity of elastic wave, i.e., velocity of sound

$$N_M = \frac{U}{c}$$

The effects of compressibility is, therefore, studied in terms of Mach number. A brief mention of the effect of compressibility has been made in Chapter 6 on 'Dimensional Analysis and Similitude'. Since very significant changes occur in the flow at Mach number equal to unity, the flows are classified as follows.

(1) *Incompressible flow region*: For such flows, the Mach number is much less than unity ($0 < N_M < 0.4$). In this range, the effects of comressibility are considered to be negligible.

(2) *Subsonic flows* : The Mach number in this region ranges between 0.4 to 1.0.

(3) *Transonic flows* : The Mach number of flow in this region ranges from slightly less than unity to slightly greater than unity ($0.9 < N_M < 1.1$).

(4) *Supersonic flows* : The Mach number in this region is always greater than unity but less than 6.0.

(5) *Hypersonic flows* : The Mach number exceeds an approximate value of 6.0.

When the Mach number is unity, the flow is said to be sonic flows.

In subsonic flow at relatively low velocities, the viscous forces and hence Reynolds number are of predominance. The changes in density are small and Mach number N_M for the flows are small and hence influence is negligible. As the velocity of flow increases, simultaneously Mach number also increases and its influence become more and more pronounced. When Mach number becomes unity, the effects to Re ceases to have any significance and are replaced by the compressibility effects indicated by the value of Mach number.

In supersonic flows, shock waves are generated. They not only effect the boundary layer but also skin friction and the position of separation, which controls the form drag, and hence produces an abrupt change of pressure. This gives rise to additional drag known as 'wave drag'. To reduce the wave drag in supersonic flows, the streamlining the rear part of the body (in contrast to subsonic flows), has little effect. For such flows, the nose of the body should be made sharp and pointed. This confines the shock wave to only a small region.

19.6. PROPAGATION OF ELASTIC WAVE DUE TO DISTURBANCE IN FLUID (SHOCK WAVES)

As has been discussed in Chapter 11 (Forces on Immersed Bodies), if some disturbances are created in compressed fluid, these causes the pressure changes in them. These pressure changes are propagated uniformly throughout the fluid, with the velocity of sound and in the form of spherical waves. Such disturbances may be caused when an object moves in a relatively stationary fluid.

(i) In order to study the pattern of pressure waves, let us consider a tiny object (such as a small projectile) which starts from point S in a stationary fluid at a time t = 0. It causes a periodic pressure disturbance in the fluid and resulting pressure waves travel radially outwards from point S as concentric spheres. If the period of disturbances is Δt, then the distance travelled by a wave between first and second disturbance will be $c \Delta t$. By the time, the second wave covers the distance $c \Delta t$, the first wave being $c \Delta t$ ahead of second wave, would have travelled a distance $2 c \Delta t$ from the source. In this way, all the successive waves are equidistance from each other in all directions; the distance being $c \Delta t$ (See Fig. 19.4a).

(ii) Now consider that the fluid is also moving with a velocity U_0 which is less than the velocity of sound c, i.e. $U_0 < c$. The pressure waves are still concentric spheres but these are swept away by the moving fluid. The lateral distance over which each spherical wave travels during the periodic time t is $U_0 \Delta t$, thus the absolute velocity with which the pressure disturbance is propagated is $(U_0 + c)$ in the direction of motion of the fluid and $(U_0 - c)$ in the opposite direction. But still the source or body remains within the spheres. As is seen from Fig. 19.4 b, the distance between consecutive waves is large downstream of the body S and small upstream of it.

(iii) As the velocity of fluid U_0 increases and approaches to the velocity of sound c, the concentration of spherical waves on the upstream side of the object go on increasing. When $U_0 = c, N_M = 1$, all the spherical waves become tangential to each other at the source of disturbance or the body S (Fig. 19.4 c). In this case, the spherical waves are unable to move upstream against the oncoming fluid and hence the fluid ahead of this pressure wave surface is not influenced by the motion of the body.

(iv) Finally, when the velocity of the fluid U_0 becomes more than the velocity of sound $(U_0 > c)$, the Mach number of flow becomes more than unity $(N_M > 1)$. In this case, the object moves much more faster than the pressure wave itself. The object moves $U_0 \Delta t$ distance in time Δt whereas the pressure wave travels $c \Delta t$ (Fig. 19.4 d). If the tangents are drawn to the consecutive waves generated at Δt time intervals from the initial position of the object S, it forms a conical surface. The pressure disturbances caused

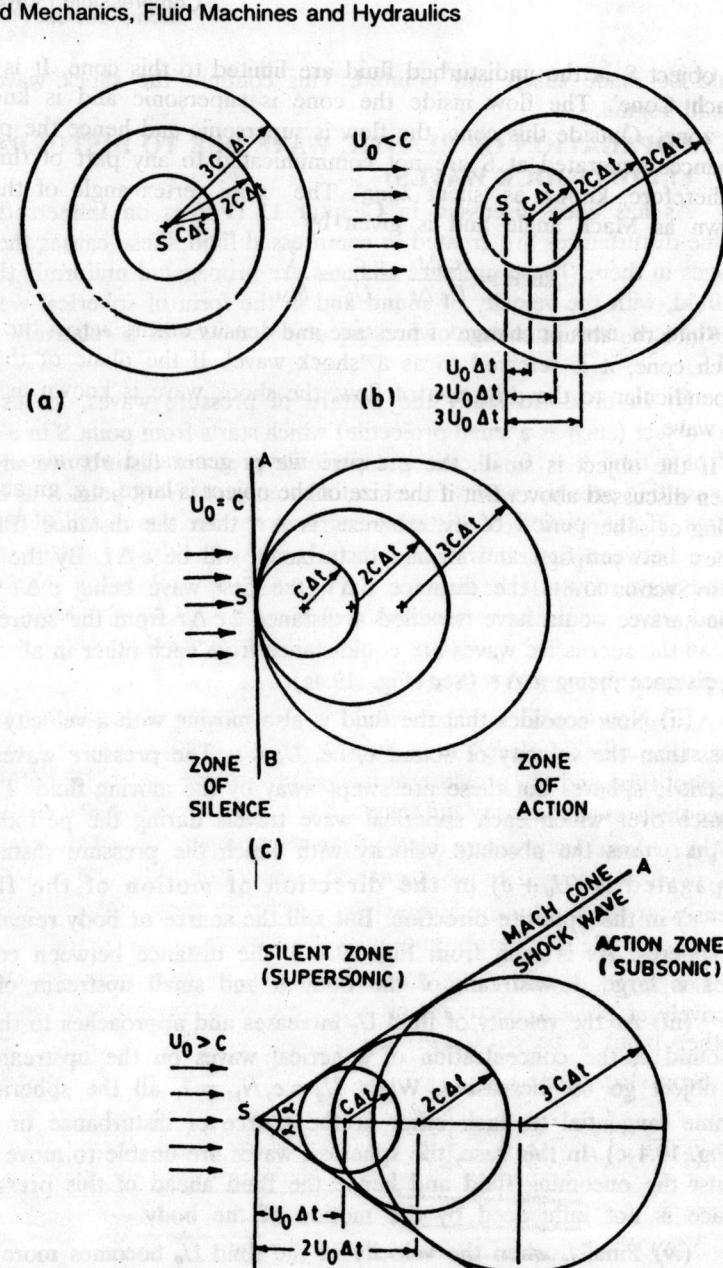

FIG. 19.4 PROPAGATION OF PRESSURE WAVE DUE TO DISTURBANCE

by the object S in the undisturbed fluid are limited to this cone. It is known as 'Mach Cone'. The flow inside the cone is supersonic and is known as 'action zone'. Outside this cone, the flow is supersonic and hence the pressure disturbances generated at S are not communicated to any part of this zone. It is, therefore, known as 'silent zone'. The semi vertex angle of this cone is known as Mach angle and is given by

$$\sin \alpha = \frac{c\,\Delta t}{U_0\,\Delta t} = \frac{c}{U_0} = \frac{1}{N_M}$$

Since the abrupt change of pressure and density occurs across the surface of Mach cone, it is referred to as a 'shock wave'. If the plane of the shock is perpendicular to the direction of flow, the shock wave is known as normal shock wave.

If the object is small, the pressure waves generated are also small as has been discussed above. But if the size of the object is large, e.g. an aeroplane travelling at supersonic velocity, the resulting pressure waves are of large size and these are propagated with a velocity greater than the velocity of sound (see also Section 11.8). If the flow is two dimensional, the surface of discontinuity, i.e., the surface of pressure waves A and B (Fig. 19.4 d) is known as Mach line.

19.7 STAGNATION PRESSURE

A stagnation point is chacterised by the existence of zero velocity. When a pitot static tube is placed in a fluid, the velocity becomes zero at the tip of the pitot tube and the pressure at this point is known as 'stagnation pressure p_{st}. Since the pressure, density and temperature are inter-related in a compressible fluid, the change in pressure also affect the temperature. The temperature at this point is referred to as stagnation temperature T_{st}. At the same time, the density of the fluid also changes appreciable, in contrast to incompressible fluid (constant density fluid) and it is known as stagnation density ρ_{st}.

Let ρ_1, U_1, p_1 and T_1 be the density, velocity, pressure and temperature respectively at point 1 upstream of an object. The corresponding quantity at any other point 2 be ρ_2, U_2, p_2 and T_2 respectively

From Eq. 19.31,

$$\frac{k}{(k-1)}\left(\frac{p_1}{\rho_1} - \frac{p_2}{\rho_2}\right) = \left(\frac{U_2^2}{2} - \frac{U_1^2}{2}\right) + g\,(z_2 - z_1)$$

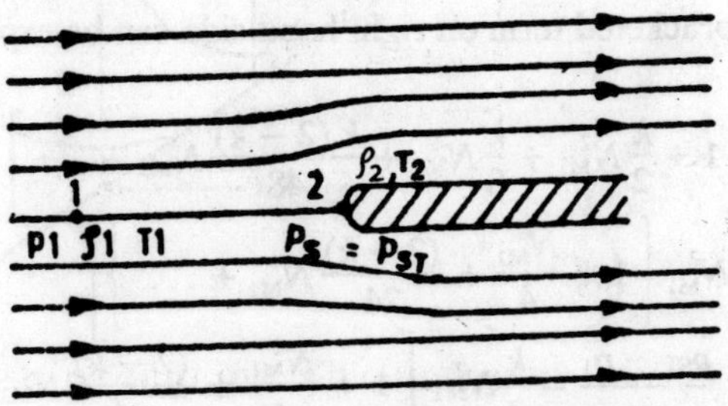

FIG. 19.5. STAGNATION PRESSURE

Since $\quad z_1 = z_2$

$$\left(\frac{U_2^2}{2} - \frac{U_1^2}{2}\right) = \frac{k}{(k-1)}\left(\frac{p_1}{\rho_1} - \frac{p_2}{\rho_2}\right)$$

$$= \frac{k}{(k-1)} \cdot \frac{p_1}{\rho_1}\left(1 - \frac{p_2}{\rho_2} \times \frac{\rho_1}{p_1}\right)$$

But $\quad \dfrac{p_1}{\rho_1^k} = \dfrac{p_2}{\rho_2^k}$, so that $\left(\dfrac{\rho_1}{\rho_2}\right) = \left(\dfrac{p_1}{p_2}\right)^{1/k}$

$$\therefore \quad \left(\frac{U_2^2}{2} - \frac{U_1^2}{2}\right) = \frac{k}{(k-1)} \cdot \frac{p_1}{\rho_1} \cdot \left[1 - \left(\frac{p_2}{p_1}\right)\left(\frac{p_1}{p_2}\right)^{1/k}\right]$$

$$\left(\frac{U_2^2}{2} - \frac{U_1^2}{2}\right) = \frac{k}{(k-1)} \cdot \frac{p_1}{\rho_1} \cdot \left[1 - \left(\frac{p_1}{p_2}\right)^{(1-k)/k}\right]$$

But $\quad c = \sqrt{kp_1/\rho_1}$, so that $c^2 = kp_1/\rho_1$

$$\therefore \quad \left(\frac{U_2^2}{2} - \frac{U_1^2}{2}\right) = \frac{c^2}{(k-1)}\left[1 - \left(\frac{p_1}{p_2}\right)^{(1-k)/k}\right]$$

or $\quad \left(\dfrac{p_2}{p_1}\right)^{(k-1)/k} = \left[1 - \dfrac{(k-1)}{c^2} \cdot \left(\dfrac{U_2^2 - U_1^2}{2}\right)\right]$

or $\quad \left(\dfrac{p_2}{p_1}\right) = \left[1 - \dfrac{(k-1)}{c^2}\left(\dfrac{U_2^2 - U_1^2}{2}\right)\right]^{k/(k-1)}$ ...(19.41)

If the point 2 lies at the point of stagnation, $U_2 = 0$ and $p_2 = p_{sT}$ stagnation pressure.

$$\therefore \quad \frac{p_{sT}}{p_1} = \left[1 + \frac{(k-1)}{c^2}\frac{U_1^2}{2}\right]^{k/(k-1)}$$

Putting $\quad N_{M1}^2 = U_1^2/c^2$,

$$\frac{p_{sT}}{p_1} = \left[1 + \frac{(k-1)}{2}N_{M1}^2\right]^{k/(k-1)} \qquad ...(19.42a)$$

Since $N_{M1} < 1$ for subsonic flows, the term $\dfrac{(k-1)}{2} N_{M1}^2$ is also less than unity. Hence the bracketed term on right hand side can be expanded by binomial theorem.

$$\frac{p_{sT}}{p_1} = \left[1 + \frac{k}{2}N_{M1}^2 + \frac{k}{8}N_{M1}^4 + \frac{k(2-k)}{48}N_{M1}^6 + \dots\right] \qquad ...(19.42b)$$

$$= \left[1 + \frac{k}{2}N_{M1}^2\left\{1 + \frac{N_{M1}^2}{4} + \frac{(2-k)}{24}N_{M1}^4 + \dots\right\}\right]$$

$$\frac{p_{sT} - p_1}{p_1} = \frac{k}{2}N_{M1}^2\left[1 + \frac{N_{M1}^2}{4} + \frac{(2-k)}{24}N_{M1}^4 + \dots\right]$$

Further,

$$p_1 k \frac{N_{M1}^2}{2} = \frac{p_1}{2} \cdot k \cdot \frac{U_1^2}{C^2} = \frac{p_1}{2} \cdot k \cdot \frac{U_1^2}{(k \, p_1/\rho_1)} = \frac{\rho \, U_1^2}{2}$$

$$\therefore \qquad \frac{(p_{sT} - p_1)}{(\rho \, U_1^2/2)} = \left[1 + \frac{N_{M1}^2}{4} + \left(\frac{2-k}{24} \right) N_{M1}^4 + \ldots \right] \qquad \ldots(19.43a)$$

For incompressible fluid $(p_{sT} - p_1)/(\rho \, U_1^2/2)$ must be equal to unity. However, for compressible fluid it has a value greater than unity. The difference between the two values is a function of Mach number, N_{M1}. The ratio of $(p_{sT} - p_1)/0.5 \rho \, U_1^2$ is known as 'compressibility factor', i.e.,

Compressibility correction factor

$$= \left(\frac{p_{sT} - p_1}{\rho \, U_1^2/2} \right)$$

$$= \left(1 + \frac{N_{M1}}{4} + \frac{N_{M1}^4}{24} + \ldots \right) \qquad \ldots(19.43b)$$

The above equation shows that the compressibility correction factor depends upon initial Mach number. For $N_{M1} < 0.2$, the error in assuming the flow to be incompressible is less than 1 %; for $N_{M1} > 0.5$, the error is 6.55 % and if $N_{M1} = 1$, the error introduced is 28 %. Therefore variation of pressure coefficient with Mach number should be taken into account while calibrating the Pitot tube (as discussed in Section 13.10b) as well as in the determination of the velocity of an object moving in compressible fluid.

The measurement of stagnation pressure as well as velocity of compressible fluids are discussed in Chapter 13 on 'Fluid Flow Measurement'

The expression for density ρ_2 can now be determined. From Eq. 19.15b.

$$\left(\frac{\rho_1}{\rho_2} \right) = \left(\frac{p_1}{p_2} \right)^{1/k}$$

$$\rho_2 = \rho_1 \left(\frac{p_2}{p_1} \right)^{1/k}$$

Substituting the value of p_2/p_1 from Eq. 19.42a.

$$\rho_2 = \rho_{sT} = \rho_1 \left[\left\{ 1 + \frac{(k-1)}{2} N_{M1}^2 \right\}^{k/(k-1)} \right]^{1/k}$$

$$\rho_{sT} = \rho_1 \left[1 + \frac{(k-1)}{2} N_{M1}^2 \right]^{1/(k-1)} \qquad \ldots(19.44)$$

The temperature T_{sT} at the stagnation point 2 is determined from Eq. of state, Eq. 19.1

$$\frac{p_{sT}}{\rho_{sT}} = R T_{sT}$$

$$T_{sT} = \frac{1}{R} \cdot \frac{p_{sT}}{\rho_{sT}}$$

Substituting the value of p_{sT} and ρ_{sT} from Eq. 19.42a and Eq. 19.44,

$$T_{sT} = \frac{1}{R} \frac{p_1 \left[1 + \left(\dfrac{k-1}{2} \right) N_{M1}^2 \right]^{k/(k-1)}}{\rho_1 \left[1 + \dfrac{(k-1)}{2} N_{M1}^2 \right]^{1/(k-1)}}$$

$$= \frac{1}{R} \cdot \frac{p_1}{\rho_1} \cdot \left[1 + \frac{(k-1)}{2} N_{M1}^2 \right]$$

Since $\qquad \dfrac{p_1}{\rho_1} = RT_1$

$$T_{sT} = T_1 \left[1 + \frac{(k-1)}{2} N_{M1}^2 \right] \qquad ...(19.45)$$

19.8 FRICTIONLESS ADIABATIC FLOW THROUGH PIPE OF VARYING SECTION

Although isentropic flow is an ideal condition of flow which occurs under adiabatic process and is frictionless. The condition of flow can never be fully realised in practice. even then the assumption of isentropic flow conditions gives a satisfactory approximation for the analysis of flow through short transitions, orifices, venturimeters and nozzles in which friction and heat transfer are minor effects which can be neglected.

For steady flow of incompressible fluid, since the mass density remains constant, the continuity equation is

$$AU = \text{constant}$$

Differentiating, one gets,

$$U\,dA + A\,dU = 0$$

or $\qquad \dfrac{dA}{A} = \dfrac{-dU}{U}$

For compressible fluids, the continuity equation is

$$\rho A U = \text{constant}$$

Differentitating, one gets

$$\rho U\,dA + A\,d(\rho U) = 0$$

$$\rho U\,dA + A\,U d\rho + \rho A\,dU = 0$$

Dividing by $\rho A U$ on both sides

$$\frac{dA}{A} + \frac{d\rho}{\rho} + \frac{dU}{U} = 0$$

or $\qquad \dfrac{dA}{A} = -\left(\dfrac{dU}{U} + \dfrac{d\rho}{\rho} \right) \qquad ...(i)$

Further, the application of momenturm equation to an elementary volume yields

$$dp \times A = \rho A U [0 - dU]$$

or
$$dp = - \rho U dU \qquad \qquad ...(ii)$$

Combining Eqs (i) and (ii)

$$\frac{dA}{A} = \left[\frac{dp}{\rho U^2} - \frac{d\rho}{\rho} \right]$$

$$= \frac{dp}{\rho U^2} \left[1 - \frac{U^2 d\rho}{dp} \right] \qquad \qquad ...(iii)$$

But
$$c^2 = \frac{dp}{d\rho} , N_M^2 = \frac{U^2}{c^2}$$

$$\frac{dA}{A} = \frac{dp}{\rho U^2} [1 - N_M^2] \qquad \qquad ...(iv)$$

From Eq. (ii)

$$\frac{dp}{\rho U^2} = - \frac{\rho U dU}{\rho U^2} = - \frac{dU}{U} \qquad \qquad ...(v)$$

From Eqs (iv) and (v)

$$\frac{dA}{A} = \frac{dU}{U} [N_M^2 - 1] \qquad \qquad ...(19.46)$$

From Eq. 19.46, it is possible to formulate the following conclusions of practical significance

(1) For subsonic flow (i.e. $N_M < 1$)

$$\frac{dU}{U} > 0, \frac{dA}{A} < 0 \qquad \qquad \text{(convergent nozzle)}$$

$$\frac{dU}{U} < 0, \frac{dA}{A} > 0 \qquad \qquad \text{(divergent nozzle)}$$

(2) For supersonic flow (i.e. $N_M > 1$)

$$\frac{dU}{U} > 0, \frac{dA}{A} > 0 \qquad \qquad \text{(divergent nozzle)}$$

$$\frac{dU}{U} < 0, \frac{dA}{A} < 0 \qquad \qquad \text{(convergent nozzle)}$$

(3) For sonic flow (i.e. $N_M = 1$)

$$\frac{dA}{A} = 0 \qquad \qquad \text{(straight flow passage)}$$

This can be written as

$$\frac{dA}{A} = \frac{dA}{dx} \times \frac{dx}{dU} = \left(\frac{dA}{dx} \right) / \left(\frac{dU}{dx} \right)$$

and since $\frac{dU}{dx}$ can not be infinite, the value of $\frac{dA}{dx}$ must be zero, indicating that the cross sectional area must be minimum. It is also seen Eq. 19.46 that the second derivative of A is positive.

Thus the effect of area variation on subsonic flow of compressible fluid is same as that for incompressible fluid, i.e. the area should be reduced to increase the velocity (that is to accelerate the flow) but the effect of area variation on supersonic flow of compressible fluid is seen to be exactly opposite, viz. the area should be increased to increase the velocity of flow (that is to accelerate the flow). This means, the flow passage must have divergence to accelerate a supersonic flow. This divergence is necessary because in supersonic flow of compressible fluid, the decrease in fluid density is greater than increase in flow velocity, and the area of flow passage must increase in order for the mass flow rate $G = (\rho\,UA)$ to remain constant.

When the flow takes place at sonic velocity, $U = c$, $N_M = 1$, Eq. 19.46 yields $dA = 0$. Since the second derivative of A is positive, A must be minimum. It thus shows that if anywhere in the flow the velocity of flow is equal to the velocity of sound, it must do so at a section where area is minimum. However, dA could also be zero when $dU = 0$(Eq. 19.46). As such at a position of minimum cross sectional area, the velocity is either equal to sonic velocity or it is maximum velocity for subsonic flow or it is minimum velocity for supersonic flow.

It is seen from the above discussion that to convert a subsonic flow through a nozzle into supersonic flow, it is necessary to have a convergent section followed by a divergent section. The flow at the throat must be sonic ($N_M = 1$) where the area is minimum. Of course, it will necessitate a relatively high pressure gradient to accelerate the flow in the convergent passage to obtain a sonic velocity at the throat. Otherwise the divergent passage will simply function as a diffuser and the compressible flow is decelerated in the divergent section.

19.9 FLOW OF COMPRESSIBLE FLUID THROUGH A CONVERGENT NOZZLE

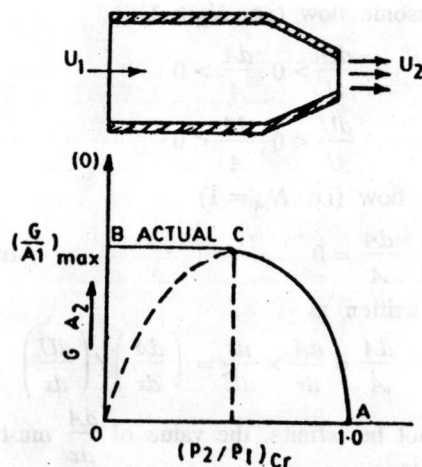

FIG. 19.6 (A) FLOW THROUGH A CONVERGENT NOZZLE
(B) VARIATION OF MASS FLOW RATE WITH PRESSURE RATIO.

The flow of a compressible fluid through a nozzle or an orifice may be regarded as frictionless adiabatic or isentropic process if the pressure drop is appreciable. On the other hand, if the pressure drop is small, the process can be considered to be isothermal.

Let us consider a convergent passage or nozzle through which compressible fluid is flowing out. Let the flow be isentropically. Let the velocity in the approach section be U_1 which is small in comparison with exit velocity U_2 at the throat (Fig. 19.6). The areas of cross section at section 1 and 2 are A_1 and A_2 respectively. Since the approach velocity U_1 is too small, the Mach number N_{M1} of the approaching flow may be assumed to be zero. The flow accelerates subsonically in the convergent nozzle. For a reversible adiabatic process, with approach velocity $U_1 = 0$, the velocity of flow at the throat, section 2, is given be Eq. 19.32.

$$\left(\frac{k}{k-1}\right)\left(\frac{p_1}{\rho_1} - \frac{p_2}{\rho_2}\right) = \left(\frac{U_2^2}{2} - \frac{U_1^2}{2}\right) + g(z_2 - z_1) \qquad ...(19.32)$$

Neglecting the elevation terms, being small in comparison of other terms and $U_1 = 0$,

$$\frac{U_2^2}{2} = \frac{k}{(k-1)}\left(\frac{p_1}{\rho_1} - \frac{p_2}{\rho_2}\right)$$

$$\frac{U_2^2}{2} = \frac{k}{(k-1)}\frac{p_1}{\rho_1}\left(1 - \frac{p_2}{p_1} \cdot \frac{\rho_1}{\rho_2}\right)$$

From Eq. 19.15b, $\left(\frac{\rho_1}{\rho_2}\right) = \left(\frac{p_1}{p_2}\right)^{1/k}$;

$$\therefore \quad \frac{U_2^2}{2} = \frac{k}{(k-1)}\frac{p_1}{\rho_1}\left[1 - \left(\frac{p_2}{p_1}\right)\left(\frac{p_2}{p_1}\right)^{-1/k}\right]$$

$$= \frac{k}{(k-1)}\frac{p_1}{\rho_1}\left[1 - \left(\frac{p_2}{p_1}\right)^{(k-1)/k}\right]$$

$$U_2 = \sqrt{\frac{2k}{(k-1)} \cdot \frac{p_1}{\rho_1} \cdot \left[1 - \left(\frac{p_2}{p_1}\right)^{(k-1)/k}\right]} \qquad ...(19.47)$$

Mass rate of flow at the throat section 2 is given by

$$G = \rho_2 A_2 U_2$$

$$= \rho_1 \left(\frac{p_2}{p_1}\right)^{1/k} A_2 \cdot \sqrt{\frac{2k}{(k-1)} \cdot \frac{p_1}{\rho_1} \cdot \left[1 - \left(\frac{p_2}{p_1}\right)^{(k-1)/k}\right]} \qquad ...(19.48)$$

Putting $(p_2/p_1) = P =$ Pressure ratio

$$G = \rho_1 (P)^{1/k} \cdot A_2 \cdot \sqrt{\frac{2k}{(k-1)} \cdot \frac{p_1}{\rho_1}} \cdot [1 - P^{(k-1)/k}] \qquad ...(19.48b)$$

In practice, the actual discharge will be C_d G where C_d is the coefficient of discharge. The Mach number N_{M2} at the throat section may be determined by putting $c_2 = \sqrt{k p_2/\rho_2}$

$$N_{M2} = \left[\frac{2}{(k-1)} \left(\frac{p_1}{p_2}\right)^{(k-1)/k} - 1 \right]^{1/2} \qquad ...(19.49)$$

The variation of mass rate of flow for given conditions at the approach section 1 is shown in Fig. 19.6b. It is found from Eq. 19.48 that G is a function of pressure ratio P ($= p_2/p_1$). As the throat pressure p_2 is reduced below p_1 (i.e. $p_2/p_1 < 1$), the mass flow increases as shown by curve AC in Fig. 19.6b. The mass flow is maximum at a certain pressure ratio $p_2/p_1 = (p_2/p_1)_{cr}$, called critical pressure ratio. The critical pressure ratio is determined by differentitating Eq. 19.48 and setting the resulting expression equal to zero.

$$\frac{d}{dp} \left[\rho_1 A_2 \sqrt{\frac{2k}{(k-1)}} \sqrt{P^{2/k} \{1 - P^{(k-1)/k}\}} \right] = 0$$

$$\text{or} \qquad \left[\frac{2}{k} P^{2/k-1} - \left(\frac{k+1}{k}\right) P^{\left(\frac{k+1}{k}\right)-1} \right] = 0$$

Solving $\qquad P = (p_2/p_1)_{cr} = \left[\frac{2}{k+1} \right]^{k/(k-1)} \qquad ...(19.50)$

which for air at normal conditions (with k = 1.4), has the value of $(p_2/p_1)_{cr} = 0.528$. With this value of $p_2/p_1 = (p_2/p_1)_{cr}$, the mass rate of flow is given by

$$G_{cr} = A_2 \sqrt{k p_1/\rho_1} \left(\frac{2}{k+1}\right)^{(k+1)/2(k-1)} \qquad ...(19.51)$$

Eq. 19.48 states that with further decrease in the throat pressure p_2 below the critical value [i.e. $(p_2/p_1) < (p_2/p_1)_{cr}$], the mass rate of flow will decrease as shown by dotted line OC in Fig. 19.6b. The decrease is evidently physically unreasonable and indeed the decreasing values of mass rate of flow for pressure ratios lower than critical pressure ratio do not occur in a convergent nozzle. At critical pressure ratio, the corresponding throat Mach number may be determined by substituting the value of $(p_2/p_1)_{cr}$ in Eq. 19.49 from Eq. 19.50. Therefore,

$$N_{M2} = \left[\left(\frac{2}{k-1}\right) \left(\frac{k+1}{2} - 1\right) \right]^{1/2} = 1 \qquad ...(19.52)$$

which indicates that the throat velocity to be sonic at critical pressure ratio. The mass rate of flow increases with decreasing throat pressure until the throat velocity becomes sonic at the critical pressure ratio. For any further reduction in throat pressure (i.e. $p_2/p_1) < (p_2/p_1)_{cr}$) the throat velocity must remain sonic since the velocity of an accelerating compressible fluid is physically limited to the subsonic in a convergent nozzle with a maximum velocity at the throat (Section 19.8). The mass rate of flow must, therefore, remain constant (as indicated by the horizontal line BC in Fig. 19.6b) for all subcritical pressure ratios and mass rate of flow is given by Eq. 19.51. This phenomenon is called "restricted or chocked flow". At subcritical pressure ratios, the actual pressure in the fluid flowing out of throat remains constant at the critical value and is therefore higher than that prevailing in the surroundings.

19.10 FLOW THROUGH CONVERGENT DIVERGENT NOZZLE OR LAVAL NOZZLE

This type of nozzle was first introduced by a Swedish Engineer and is named after its inventor de Laval (1885-1913). It is a convergent divergent nozzle (Fig. 19.7) with subsonic flow occuring in the convergent section, critical or transonic conditions in the throat and supersonic flow in the divergent section. Thus, the main purpose of this type of nozzle is to produce supersonic flow in a nozzle.

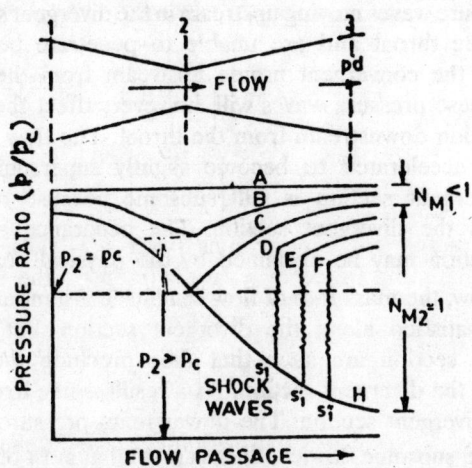

FIG. 19.7 FLOW DEVELOPMENT IN A CONVERGENT DIVERGENT NOZZLE

Fig. 19.7 illustrates the flow phenomenon in a convergent divergent passage. If the pressures at both, inlet section 1 and discharge section 3, are same (i.e. $p_3/p_1 = 1$), there is no flow (as indicated by curve A of Fig. 19.7(b)). Now as the downstream pressure, p_d, is gradually reduced, the pressure disturbances moving upstream within the passage cause the flow to accelerate in the convergent section. There are four possible flow conditions in this type of nozzle depending on the values of downstream pressure p_d prevailing beyond the discharge section.

1. So long as the downstream pressure p_d is of such a value that $(p_2/p_1) > (p_2/p_1)_{cr}$, the flow is subsonic throughout the entire passage. The flow accelerates in the convergent nozzle and decelerates in the subsequent divergent diffuser isentropically as shown by curve B (Fig. 19.7(b)). The discharge pressure p_3 equals p_d and the corresponding mass rate of flow which depends

on the value of pressure ratio (p_3/p_1) is given by Eq. 19.48 with A_2 and p_2 being replaced by A_3 and p_3 respectively. Thus

$$G = A_3 \rho_1 (p_3/p_1)^{1/k} \sqrt{\frac{2k}{(k-1)} (1 - p_3/p_1)^{(k-1)/k}} \qquad \ldots (19.53)$$

2. When p_d is reduced to a value such that the flow just attains a sonic velocity at the throat and immediately reverts to subsonic conditions in the subsequent divergent section, the flow decelerates in the divergent diffuser at subsonic velocity (curve C, Fig. 19.7(b)). In this case, the gas expands isentropically to p_{cr} in the throat and diffuses isentropically along curve C to $(p_d)_c$. The mass rate of flow is then given by Eq. 19.51.

3. If the downstream pressure p_d is further reduced, new flow conditions occur in the divergent flow section, although the throat pressure ratio (p_2/p_1) remains at critical value (as discussed in the section 19.2) and, consequently, the mass rate of flow also remains unchanged (that is, G is still given by Eq. 19.51). The pressure waves moving upstream in the divergent section encounter the sonic flow at the throat and are unable to penetrate beyond the throat so that the flow in the convergent nozzle upstream from the throat remains the same as in 2. These pressure waves will, however, affect the flow conditions in the divergent section downstream from the throat. The flow just downstream from the throat is accelerated to become slightly supersonic, but the flow in most of the divergent section is still subsonic because of the formation of normal shock in the divergent section. The occurance of normal shock in the divergent section may be explained by the physical conditions of flow.

For steady flow, the mass rate of flow remains constant and the continuity equation must be satisfied along the divergent section. but the area ratios along the divergent section are such that they preclude the occurrance of an isentropic flow in the divergent section. As a result, some irreversible process takes place in the divergent section. The downstream pressure, p_d, being more than critical pressure, subsonic flow conditions prevail in most of the downstream portion of the divergent section. However, the flow immediately downstream from the throat section is accelerated to become slightly supersonic and re-adjustment of flow conditions occurs abruptly. This results in the formation of a shock front.

The flow across the shock front is non-isentropic. The velocity changes abruptly from supersonic to subsonic across the shock as shown by curve D. (Fig. 19.7b). There is also a finite pressure difference across the shock. The position of the shock is fixed by the physical conditions, that the momentum difference across the shock is just balanced by the pressure difference between the supersonic flow (on upstream side of shock). With further reduction in the downstream pressure, p_d, new pressure waves moving upstream reduce the pressure difference across the shock so that new dynamic equilibrium position must be established further downstream in the divergent section (as shown by successive curves E and F, Fig. 19.7b). This happens, until pressure wave moves all the wave to the exit of the divergent passage and the pressure at exit is then $p_d = p_3'$ (curve H). The mass rate of flow remains the same and is given by Eq. 19.51, regardless of the position of the shock in the divergent section.

4. A $p_d = p_3'$ the flow accelerates steadily throughout the entire passage. It is subsonic in the convergent section, sonic in the throat and supersonic in the divergent section. The gas expansion is isentropic to a pressure p_{cr} in the throat and continues its isotropic expansion in the divergent section. It is marked as curve H in Fig. 19.7b. There is no shock front in the divergent section and G may be computed either by Eq. 19.48 or Eq. 19.51.

Further lowering of downstream pressure below p_3' does not have any effect on the flow in the nozzle. The flow conditions throughout the entire passage remain exactly the same as in stage 4.

This shows that convergent divergent passage should be properly designed for an isentropic supersonic flow to occur in the divergent section. This means that throat area A_2 and exit area A_3 should be proportioned in accordance with the operating pressure ratio p_3/p_1. To obtain the area ratio A_2/A_3, equate the right hand side of Eq. 19.48 and 19.51.

$$\rho_1 A_3 \, (p_3/p_1)^{1/k} \sqrt{\frac{2k}{(k-1)} (1 - p_3/p_1)^{(k-1)/k}}$$

$$= A_2 \sqrt{k \, p_1 \rho_1} \left(\frac{2}{k+1} \right)^{(k+1)/(2(k-1))}$$

Solving for A_2/A_3

$$\frac{A_2}{A_3} = \frac{\rho_1 \sqrt{\dfrac{2k}{k-1}} \sqrt{[1 - p_3/p_1]^{(k-1/k)} (p_3/p_1)^{4/k}}}{\sqrt{k \, p_1 \rho_1} \left[\dfrac{2}{k+1} \right]^{(k+1)/2(k-1)}}$$

$$= \left(\frac{k+1}{2} \right)^{(k+1)/2(k-1)} \left(\frac{2}{k-1} \right)^{1/2} (p_3/p_1)^{1/k} [1 - (p_3/p_1)^{(k-1)/k}]^{1/2}$$

$$...(19.54)$$

19.11 NORMAL SHOCK WAVES

As discussed in Section 19.10, whenever the flow changes abruptly from supersonic to subsonic it is accompanied by a rise in pressure and density and reduction in velocity of flow. Thus, a shock wave is generated. In case of one dimensional stationary shock wave, the supersonic flow at upstream is converted into subsonic flow in a very short reach. And it is accompanied by a sudden change in pressure. At the same time, the velocity and hence the Mach number of the flow is reduced across a shock wave. The thickness of the shock front across the discontinuity may be of the order of 10^{-3} cm to 10^{-5} cm. The shock wave may occur in the divergent section of a nozzle, in the diffuser throat of a supersonic wind tunnel, in front of blunt bodies as well as in pipes. Although the discussion here is devoted entirely to shock waves in the gas flow; shock waves are frequently encountered in the flow of liquid. Water hammer in pipe flow is a typical example of shock wave. Similarly, the formation of a hydraulic jump in an open channel is another example. It is analogous to shock wave and the flow changes from supercritical to subcritical, accompanied by the increase in depth and decrease in velocity. For shock waves, the critical velocity is the velocity of sound (or sonic velocity).

The shock waves may be either normal or oblique with respect to the direction of flow. However, only normal shock waves have been discussed here. The elements of shock waves can be obtained by the application of continuity equation, momentum equation and energy equation.

Let ρ_1, U_1 and p_1 be the density, velocity and pressure upstream of a shock front respectively. The corresponding values of density, velocity and pressure downstream of shock front are ρ_2, U_2 and p_2 respectively (Fig. 19.8).

For continuity equation, Eq. 19.24

$$G = \rho_1 A_1 U_1 = \rho_2 A_2 U_2$$

$$\frac{G}{A} = \rho_1 U_1 = \rho_2 U_2 ...(19.55)$$

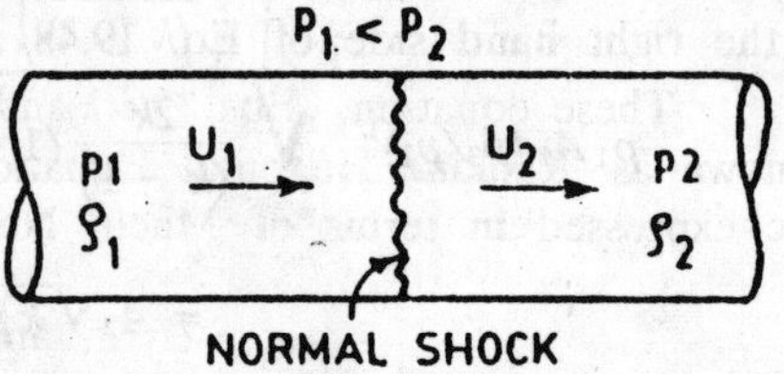

From momentum equation, Eq. 19.26,

$$(p_1 - p_2) A = \rho_1 A U_1 (U_2 - U_1)$$

$$(p_1 - p_2) = (\rho_1 U_1 U_2 - \rho_1 U_1^2)$$

where A is the area of cross section.

NORMAL SHOCK

FIG. 19.8 STATIONARY NORMAL SHOCK FRONT

But from Eq. 19.55, $\rho_1 U_1 = \rho_2 U_2 = G/A$

$$(p_1 - p_2) = \rho_2 U_2^2 - \rho_1 U_1^2$$

$$(p_1 + \rho_1 U_1^2) = (p_2 + \rho_2 U_2^2) \qquad ...(19.56)$$

Now, from energy equation, Eq. 19.31, neglecting elevation term and $e_H = 0$.

$$\left[\frac{U_1^2}{2} + \frac{k}{(k-1)} \frac{p_1}{\rho_1} \right] = \left[\frac{U_2^2}{2} + \frac{k}{(k-1)} \frac{p_2}{\rho_2} \right] \qquad ...(19.57)$$

Combining Eqs. 19.55 and 19.56 yields the Eq. of Rayleigh's line

$$\left[p_1 + \frac{(G/A)^2}{\rho_1} \right] = \left[p_1 + \frac{(G/A)^2}{\rho_2} \right] \qquad ...(19.58)$$

Similarly, combining Eq. 19.53 and 19.57 yields the Eq. of Fanno line.

$$\left[\frac{(G/A)^2}{2\rho_1^2} + \frac{k}{(k-1)} \frac{p_1}{\rho_1} \right] = \left[\frac{(G/A)^2}{2\rho_2^2} + \frac{k}{(k-1)} \frac{p_2}{\rho_2} \right] \qquad ...(19.59)$$

Solving, $\qquad (G/A)^2 = \dfrac{2k}{(k-1)} \dfrac{(p_2/\rho_2 - p_1/\rho_1)}{(1/\rho_1^2 - 1/\rho_2^2)} \qquad ...(i)$

From Eq. 19.58,

$$(G/A)^2 (1/\rho_1 - 1/\rho_2) = (p_2 - p_1) \qquad ...\text{(ii)}$$

From Eqs. (i) and (ii)

$$\frac{(p_2 - p_1)}{(1/\rho_1 - 1/\rho_2)} = \frac{\dfrac{2k}{(k-1)}[p_2/\rho_2 - p_1/\rho_1]}{[1/\rho_1^2 - 1/\rho_2^2]}$$

Solving for p_2/p_1,

$$\left(\frac{p_2}{p_1}\right) = \frac{\dfrac{2k}{(k-1)}(\rho_2/\rho_1 - 1)}{\left[\left(\dfrac{(k+1)}{(k-1)}\right) - \dfrac{\rho_2}{\rho_1}\right]} \qquad ...\text{(19.60)}$$

Similarly,

$$\left(\frac{\rho_2}{\rho_1}\right) = \left(\frac{U_1}{U_2}\right) = \frac{\left[1 + \dfrac{(k+1)}{(k-1)} \cdot \dfrac{p_2}{p_1}\right]}{\left[\left(\dfrac{(k+1)}{(k-1)}\right) + \dfrac{p_2}{p_1}\right]} \qquad ...\text{(19.61)}$$

These equations, Eqs 19.60 and 19.61 were developed in 1870 and are known as 'Rankine Hugoniot Equation'. The above two equations can also be expressed in terms of Mach Number $\left(N_{M1}\right)$, using .

$$N_{M1} = U_1/c_1 \text{ and } c_1 = \sqrt{k R T_1}.$$

$$\left(\frac{p_2}{p_1}\right) = \left[\frac{2 k N_{M1}^2 - (k-1)}{(k+1)}\right] \qquad ...\text{(19.62)}$$

$$\left(\frac{\rho_2}{\rho_1}\right) = \left(\frac{U_1}{U_2}\right) = \frac{(k+1) N_{M1}^2}{(k-1) N_{M1}^2 + 2} \qquad ...\text{(19.63)}$$

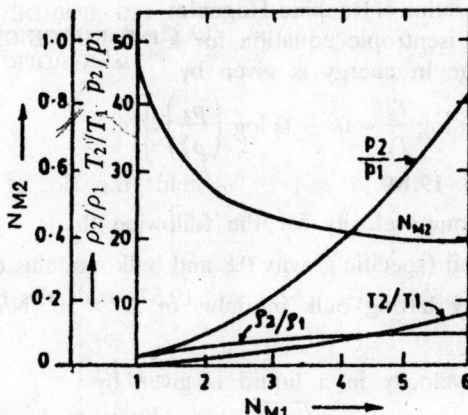

FIG. 19.9 CHANGES OF PARAMETERS ACROSS A SHOCK FRONT

Since $N_{M1} > 1$ and $k = 1.4$, the pressure ratio $p_2/p_1 > 0$, i.e., a pressure rise occurs across a shock front.

The corresponding equation for temperature ratio T_2/T_1 is given by

$$\frac{T_2}{T_1} = \frac{[(k-1)\,N_{M1}^2 + 2]\,[2\,k\,N_{M1}^2 - (k-1)]}{(k+1)^2\,N_{M1}^2} \qquad ...(19.64)$$

Further, Mach number for downstream flow, M_{M2} may be found in terms of upstream flow Mach number, N_{M1} by combinins Eq. 19.56 and Eq. 19.57.

$$N_{M2} = \frac{[(k-1)\,N_{M1}^2 + 2]}{[2\,k\,N_{M1}^2 - (k-1)]} \qquad ...19.65)$$

It is seen that Eqs. 19.62, 19.63 and 19.64 are functions of Mach number N_{M1} and k only and are shown plotted in Fig. 19.9.

The strength of a shock wave is defined as the ratio of the pressure rise across the shock to the upstream pressure. Thus,

Shock strength

$$= \left(\frac{p_2 - p_1}{p_1}\right) = \left(\frac{p_2}{p_1} - 1\right) \qquad ...(19.66a)$$

By substituting the value of p_2/p_1 from 19.60,

Shock strength $= \left(\dfrac{2k}{k+1}\right)(N_{M1}^2 - 1)$

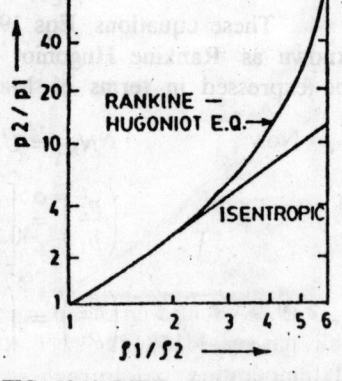

FIG. 19.10 DEVIATION OF RANKING–HUGONIOT RELATION FROM ISENTROPIC FLOW (k = 1.4)

It is to be noted, that although the energy of the flow is conserved as the fluid crosses a shock wave, there is, however, an increase in the entropy of the flow and the flow crossing a shock must be considered as a thermodynamically irreversible process. Fig. 19.10 shows the deviation of Rankine-Hugoniot relation from the isentropic equation for k = 1.4. The change in energy is given by

$$\left(\frac{H_2 - H_1}{C_v}\right) = \left[k \log \frac{T_2}{T_1} - (k-1) \log \left(\frac{p_2}{p_1}\right)\right] \qquad ...(19.67)$$

Examples 19.1 to 19.14

19.1 Find the sonic velocity for the following fluids

(a) Crude oil (specific gravity 0.8 and bulk modulus of 1.56×10^5 N/cm^2

(b) Mercury having bulk modulus of 2.7×10^6 N/cm^2.

Solution

The sonic velocity in a liquid is given by

$$c = \sqrt{\frac{E_v}{\rho}}$$

(a) For crude oil,

$$c = \sqrt{\frac{1.56 \times 10^5 \times 10^4}{0.8 \times 1000}}$$

$$= 1396.4 \text{ m/s}$$

(b) For crude oil,

$$c = \sqrt{\frac{2.7 \times 10^6 \times 10^4}{13.6 \times 1000}} = 1409.4 \text{ m/s}$$

19.2 Find the velocity of bullet fired in standard air if the Mach angle is 30°. Take R = 29.27 m/°K, k = 1.4 and assume temperature of air as 15° C.

Solution

Temperature of air = (273 + 15) = 288 °K.

The velocity of sound in air $c = \sqrt{kRT}$,

where R is to be expressed in J/kg K.

$$\therefore \qquad c = \sqrt{1.4 \times (29.27 \times 9.81) \times 288} = 340.25 \text{ m/s}$$

$$\sin \alpha = \frac{1}{N_M}$$

$$\sin 30° = 1/N_M \,; N_M = 2$$

Now $\qquad N_M = \dfrac{U}{c}$

$$U = c \times N_M$$

$$= 340.25 \times 2$$

$$= 680.5 \text{ m/s}$$

19.3 A schlieven photograph showing the wave formed by a bullet moving in air gave a Mach angle of 40°. Find the speed of bullet if the pressure and temperature of atmosphere are 9 N/cm² and − 2 °C respectively.

Solution

Velocity of sound in air $c = \sqrt{kRT}$

Taking $\qquad R = 29.27 \text{ m/°K} = 29.27 \times 9.81 = 287.1 \text{ J/kg K}$

$$c = \sqrt{1.4 \times 287.1 \times (273 - 2)} = 330 \text{ m/s}$$

Now Mach angle represents the half the vertex angle of Mach cone and is given by

$$\sin \alpha = \frac{c}{U} = \frac{1}{N_M}$$

$$\sin \alpha = \frac{330}{U}$$

$$U = 330/\sin 40° = 513.38 \text{ m/s}.$$

19.4 A supersonic plane is flying at a height of 200 m where the air temperature is 3° C. Calculate the speed of the plane if its sound is heard 4.5 seconds after its passage over the head of the observer.

Solution

Let the plane be at P directly over the head of the observer at time t. After 4.5 seconds it reaches at Q when the observer listens its sound.

Thus OQ is the wave front, making an angle α with the horizontal (half the angle of Mach cone). See Fig. 19.11.

Let the velocity of the supersonic plane is U and velocity of sound wave is c.

$$c = \sqrt{kRT}$$
$$= \sqrt{1.4 \times 290 \times (273 + 3)} = 334.74 \ \text{m/s}$$

Now from Eq. 11.15

$$\sin \alpha = \frac{c}{U} = \frac{334.74}{U} \qquad ...(i)$$

From Fig. 19.11

$$\tan \alpha = \frac{2500}{4.5 \, U} \qquad ...(ii)$$

From Eqs. (i) and (ii)

$$\cos \alpha = 0.6025$$
∴ $$\sin \alpha = 0.7981$$

From Eq. (i)

$$U = \frac{334.74}{0.7981} = 419.42 \ \text{m/s}$$

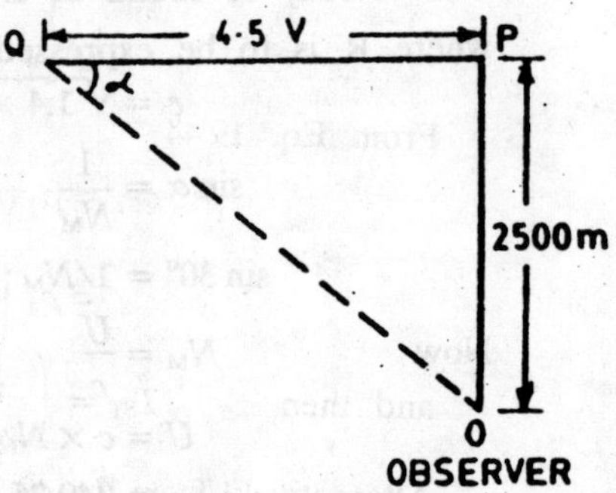

FIG. 19.11 EXAMPLE 19.4

19.5 Find the Mach number when an aeroplane is flying at 1100 km/hr through still air having a pressure of 8.5 N/cm^2 and temperature of $-5\,°C$. Wind may be assumed still and assume R = 287.1 J/kg °K. Calculate the pressure, density and temperature of air at stagnation point on the nose of the plane.

Solution

Velocity of sound in air $c = \sqrt{kRT}$

$$c = \sqrt{1.4 \times 287.1 \times (273 - 5)} = 328.15 \ \text{m/s}$$

Velocity of the aeroplane

$$= \frac{1100 \times 1000}{60 \times 60} = 305.5 \ \text{m/s}$$

∴ $$N_M = \frac{U}{c}$$

$$= \frac{305.5}{328.15} = 0.931$$

The mass density of air in the still air is given by

$$\rho_1 = \frac{p_1}{R\,T_1}$$

$$= \frac{8.5 \times 10^4}{287.1 \times (273 - 5)} = 1.1\ \text{kg/m}^3$$

From Eq. 19.43 a,

$$\frac{(p_{ST} - p_1)}{(\rho_1 U_1^2/2)} = \left[1 + \frac{N_{M1}^2}{4} + \cdots\right]$$

$$= \left[1 + \frac{(0.931)^2}{4} + \cdots\right] = 1.2167$$

$$P_{ST} = \left[p_1 + 1.2167\frac{\rho_1 U_1^2}{2}\right]$$

$$= \left[8.5 \times 10^4 + \frac{1.2167 \times 1.1 \times (305.5)^2}{2}\right]$$

$$= 14.74 \times 10^4\ \text{N/m}^2 \text{ or } 14.74\ \text{N/cm}^2$$

From Eq. 19.44

$$\rho_{ST} = \rho_1\,(p_2/p_1)^{1/k}$$

$$= \rho_1\left[1 + \frac{(k - 1)}{2} N_{M1}^2\right]^{1/(k-1)}$$

and then

$$T_{ST} = \left(\frac{p_{ST}}{\rho_{ST}\,R}\right)$$

Alternatively, from Eq. 19.31, neglecting elevation term and putting $U_2 = 0$ at stagnation point, i.e. $U_2 = U_{ST} = 0$

$$\left(\frac{k}{k-1}\right)\left(\frac{p_1}{\rho_1} - \frac{p_2}{\rho_2}\right) + \frac{U_1^2}{2} = 0$$

$$\left(\frac{k}{k-1}\right)R\,T_1 - \left(\frac{k}{k-1}\right)R\,T_2 + \frac{U_1^2}{2} = 0$$

$$T_2\,(= T_{ST}) = \frac{(k-1)}{k}\frac{1}{R}\left[\frac{U_1^2}{2} + \left(\frac{k}{k-1}\right)R\,T_1\right]$$

$$= \left[\frac{(k-1)}{k} \cdot \frac{1}{R} \cdot \frac{U_1^2}{2} + T_1\right]$$

$$= \left[\frac{(1.4 - 1)}{1.4 \times 287.1} \times \frac{(305.5)^2}{2} + (273 - 5)\right]$$

$$= 314.43°\ K$$

$$= 41.44°\ C$$

Now

$$\rho_{ST} = \frac{p_{ST}}{R\,T_{ST}}$$

$$= \frac{14.74 \times 10^4}{287.1 \times 314.33} = 1.633 \ \text{kg/m}^3$$

19.6 Air mass 3 kg, expands from an initial state $p_1 = 90$ N/cm² (gauge) and $T_1 = 250°\,C$ to a final state $p_2 = 10$ N/cm² gauge. Find the final volume and temperature and the work done on the gas in (a) isothermal, and (b) adiabatic expansion. Take gas constant R = 293 J/kg°K and specific heat ratio k = 1.4.

Solution

Absolute temperature $T_1 = (273 + 250) = 523\,°K$

Absolute pressure $p_1 = (90 \times 10^4 + 10^5) = 10 \times 10^5$ N/m².

$$p_2 = (10 \times 10^4 + 10^5) = 2 \times 10^5 \ \text{N/m}^2$$

From equation of state.

$$\frac{p_1}{\rho_1} = R\,T_1$$

$$\rho_1 = \left(\frac{p_1}{R\,T_1}\right) = \frac{10 \times 10^5}{293 \times 523} = 6.525 \ \text{kg/m}^3$$

Initial volume $v_1 = \dfrac{3}{59.38} = 0.46 \ \text{m}^3$

(a) For isothermal expansion,

$$\frac{p_1}{\rho_1} = \frac{p_2}{\rho_2}$$

$$\rho_2 = \left(\frac{p_2}{p_1} \times \rho_1\right)$$

$$= \left(\frac{10 \times 10^4 + 10^5}{10 \times 10^5}\right) \times 6.525 = 1.305 \ \text{kg/m}^3$$

Final volume $v_2 = \dfrac{3}{1.305} = 2.298 \ \text{m}^3$

Now $T_2 = \dfrac{p_2}{\rho_2\,R}$

where absolute pressure $p_2 = (10 \times 10^4 + 10^5)$ N/cm²

$$= 2 \times 10^5 \ \text{N/cm}^2$$

$$T_2 = \frac{2 \times 10^5}{1.305 \times 293} = 523.06\,°K$$

$$= 250.06\,°C$$

From Eq. 19.14 b,

Work done $= R\,T_1 \log_e (p_1/p_2)$

$$= 293 \times 523 \times \log_e \left(\frac{10 \times 10^5}{2 \times 10^5} \right)$$

$$= 246628.66 \text{ Nm}$$

(b) For adiabatic expansion,

$$\frac{p_1}{\rho_1^k} = \frac{p_2}{\rho_2^k}$$

$$\rho_2 = \rho_1 \, (p_2/p_1)^{1/k}$$

$$= 6.525 \left(\frac{2 \times 10^5}{10 \times 10^5} \right)^{1/1.4} = 2.067 \text{ kg/m}^3$$

Final volume $\quad v_2 = \dfrac{3}{2.067} = 1.451 \text{ m}^3$

Now $\quad T_2 = \dfrac{p_2}{\rho_2 R}$

$$= \frac{2 \times 10^5}{1.451 \times 293} = 470.28°K$$

$$= 197.28°C$$

From Eq. 19.17 b,

Work done $\quad = \dfrac{R \, (T_1 - T_2)}{(k - 1)}$

$$= \frac{293 \, (523 - 470.28)}{(1.4 - 1)}$$

$$= 38617.4 \text{ N-m}$$

19.7 At a certain section of a duct in which air is flowing at a temperature of $40°C$ and pressure of 8.25 N/cm^2 with the velocity of 360 m/s. Assuming isentropic flow, determine the velocity and temperature at a section where the pressure is 12.5 N/cm^2 and Mach number at both sections. Take R $=$ 287 J/kg $°K$ and k $= 1.4$.

Solution

$$p_1 = 8.25 \times 10^4 \text{ N/m}^2$$

$$p_2 = 12.5 \times 10^4 \text{ N/m}^2$$

$$T_1 = (273 + 40) = 313°K$$

$$U_1 = 360 \text{ m/s}$$

$$R_1 = 287 \text{ J/kg}°K$$

From Eq. 19.31, neglecting elevation term

$$\left(\frac{k}{k - 1} \right) \left(\frac{p_1}{\rho_1} - \frac{p_2}{\rho_2} \right) = \left(\frac{U_2^2 - U_1^2}{2} \right)$$

$$\left(\frac{k}{k-1}\right)\left(\frac{p_1}{\rho_1}\right)\left(1 - \frac{p_2 \rho_1}{p_1 \rho_2}\right) = \left(\frac{U_2^2 - U_1^2}{2}\right)$$

But $\qquad \left(\dfrac{p_1}{p_2}\right) = \left(\dfrac{\rho_1}{\rho_2}\right)^k$; so that $\left(\dfrac{\rho_1}{\rho_2}\right) = \left(\dfrac{p_1}{p_2}\right)^{1/k}$

and $\qquad \left(\dfrac{p_1}{\rho_1}\right) = R\,T_1$

$\therefore \quad \left(\dfrac{k}{k-1}\right) R\,T_1 \left[1 - \left(\dfrac{p_2}{p_1}\right)\left(\dfrac{p_1}{p_2}\right)^{1/k}\right] = \left(\dfrac{U_2^2 - U_2^2}{2}\right)$

$\left(\dfrac{k}{k-1}\right) R\,T_1 \left[1 - \left(\dfrac{p_2}{p_1}\right)^{(1-1/k)}\right] = \left(\dfrac{U_2^2 - U_1^2}{2}\right)$

$\dfrac{1.4 \times 2.87}{0.4} \times 2 \times 313 \left[1 - \left(\dfrac{12.5 \times 10^4}{8.25 \times 10}\right)^{(1-1/1.4)}\right] = (U_2^2 - U_1^2)$

Solving, $(U_2^2 - 360^2) = 628817\,(1 - 1.126)$

$\qquad U_2^2 = (-79230.94 + 129600)$

$\qquad U_2 = 224.43 \text{ m/s}$

Now $\qquad p = \rho R T \text{ and } \left(\dfrac{p}{\rho k}\right) = \text{constant}$

Eleminating ρ.

$\left(\dfrac{T_2}{T_1}\right) = \left(\dfrac{p_2}{p_1}\right)^{(k-1)/k}$

$\qquad = \left(\dfrac{12.5 \times 10^4}{8.25 \times 10^4}\right)^{(1.4-1)/1.4}$

$\qquad = 1.126$

$\qquad T_2 = 1.126 \times 313 = 352.42°K$

$\qquad = 79.45\,°C$

The Mach numbers can now be determined.

$N_{M1} = \dfrac{U_1}{c_1} = \dfrac{U_1}{\sqrt{k R T_1}}$

$\qquad = \dfrac{360}{\sqrt{1.4 \times 287 \times 313}} = 1.015$

$N_{M2} = \dfrac{224.43}{\sqrt{1.4 \times 287 \times 352.42}} = 0.596$

19.8 A large tank contains a gas at a temperature of 15 °C and 5 atmospheric pressure. An orifice of 1.0 cm diameter is provided at the side of container through which the gas is supplied. Determine the velocity of jet and its mass rate of flow. Take R = 189 J/kg ° K, k = 1.3 and atmospheric pressure = 10.13 N/cm^2

Solution

The density of gas in the container is given by

$$\rho_1 = \frac{p_1}{R\,T_1}$$

$$= \frac{5 \times 10.13 \times 10^4}{189 \times (273 + 15)} = 9.305 \text{ kg/m}^3$$

Now

$$\left(\frac{p_2}{p_1}\right) = \left[\frac{10.13 \times (10)^4}{5 \times 10.13 \times (10)^4}\right] = 0.20$$

For **chocked flow** of orifice, the critical pressure p_2/p_1, i.e. $(p_2/p_1)_{cr}$ is given by Eq. 19.50

$$\left(\frac{p_2}{p_1}\right)_{cr} = \left[\frac{2}{k+1}\right]^{k/(k-1)}$$

$$= \left(\frac{2}{1.3 + 1}\right)^{1.3/(1.3-1)}$$

$$= 0.545$$

Since $(p_2/p_1) < (p_2/p_1)_{cr}$, the flow at orifice exit is chocked. This means, that the velocity of jet is critical or sonic and temperature is T_c.

$$\frac{p_1}{\rho_1^k} = \frac{p_2}{\rho_2^k}$$

and

$$p_1 = \rho_1\,R\,T_1$$

$$p_2 = \rho_2\,R\,T_2$$

Eliminating (ρ_2/ρ_1)

$$\left(\frac{T_2}{T_1}\right) = \left(\frac{T_2}{T_1}\right)_c = \left(\frac{p_2}{p_1}\right)_c^{(1-k)/k}$$

$$(T_2/T_1)_c = (0.545)^{(1.3-1)/1.3}$$

$$= 0.8693$$

$$(T_2)_c = 0.8693 \times (273 + 15)$$

$$= 250.35 \text{ °K}$$

The velocity of jet $c = \sqrt{k\,R\,T_2}$

$$c = \sqrt{1.3 \times 189 \times 250.35}$$

$$= 248 \text{ m/s}$$

Density of gas at orifice exit

$$\rho_2 = \frac{(p_2)_c}{R\,(T_2)_c} = \frac{(p_2/p_1)_c \times p_1}{R\,(T_2)_c}$$

$$= \frac{0.545 \times 5 \times 10.13 \times 10^4}{189 \times 250.35}$$

$$= 5.834 \text{ kg/m}^3$$

Mass rate of flow $G = \rho_2 A_2 (U_2)_c$

$$= 5.834 \times \frac{\pi}{4} (0.001)^2 \times 248$$

$$= 0.1136 \text{ kg/m}^3$$

19.9 A pitot static tube is inserted into an air stream of velocity U_1 and pressure $1.02 \times 10^5 \text{ N/m}^2$ and temperature of 28°C. It is connected to a mercury differential U-tube manometer. Calculate the difference of mercury in the two limbs of manometer if the velocity U_1 is (a) 50 m s^{-1} (b) 250 m s^{-1}, and (c) 400 m s^{-1}. Take R = 287 J kg^{-1} K^{-1} and k = 1.4.

Solution

(a) velocity of sound $c = \sqrt{kRT}$

$$c = \sqrt{1.4 \times 287 \times (273 + 28)}$$

$$= 347.77 \text{ m/s}$$

Since $N_M = 0.4$, the compressibility effects are not important and the flow may be considered as incompressible.

$$(p_{ST} - p) = \frac{1}{2} \rho U_1^2$$

But $\qquad \dfrac{p}{\rho} = RT$

From which $\qquad \rho = \dfrac{p}{RT}$

$$\rho_{air} = \frac{1.02 \times 10^5}{287 \times (287 + 28)} = 1.18 \text{ kg/m}^3$$

$$(p_{ST} - p) = \frac{1}{2} \times 1.18 \times (50)^2 = 1475 \text{ N/m}^2$$

The deflection of mercury in the two limbs of U-tube is given by h.

$$h = \frac{(p_{ST} - p_1)}{w_{Hg}}$$

$$= \frac{1475}{13.6 \times 9810}$$

$$= 11.06 \times 10^{-3} \text{ m or } 11.06 \text{ mm of mercury}$$

(b) When $\qquad U_1 = 250 \text{ m/s}$,

$$N_{MI} = \frac{250}{374.77} = 0.719 > 0.4$$

Since Mach number is more than 0.4, the compressibility effects must be taken into account. From Eq. 19.42 a.

$$\frac{p_{ST}}{p} = \left[1 + \frac{(k-1)}{2} N_{M1}^2\right]^{k/(k-1)}$$

$$\frac{p_{ST}}{p} = \left[1 + \left(\frac{1.4-1}{2}\right)(0.719)^2\right]^{1.4/(1.4-1)}$$

$$\frac{p_{ST}}{p} = 1.411$$

$$p_{ST} = 1.411 \times 1.02 \times 10^5$$

$$\therefore \quad (p_{ST} - p_1) = (1.411 \times 1.02 \times 10^5 - 1.02 \times 10^5)$$

$$= 0.42 \times 10^5 \text{ N/m}^2$$

$$h = \frac{(h_{ST} - p_1)}{w_{Hg}}$$

$$= \frac{0.42 \times 10^5}{13.6 \times 9810} = 0.3148 \text{ m of mercury}$$

$$= 314.8 \text{ mm of mercury}$$

(c) When $\qquad U_1 = 400$ m/s

$$N_{m1} = \frac{400}{347.77} = 1.208 > 1$$

This means the flow is supersonic and therefore, a shock wave will be formed due to the disturbance created by the pitot-static tube. As the nose of the tube is rounded it is reasonable to assume that the shock will be detched and a section of it just upstream of the pitot static tube will be normal to it. Thus, the pressure downstream of the shock and upstream of the tube will be given by Eq. 19.62.

$$\frac{p_2}{p_1} = \left[\frac{2k N_{M1}^2 - (k-1)}{(k+1)}\right]$$

$$p_2 = 1.02 \times 10^5 \left[\frac{2 \times 1.4 \times (1.208)^2 - (1.4-1)}{(1.4+1)}\right]$$

$$= 1.567 \times 10^5 \text{ N/m}^2$$

In order to determine the stagnation pressure p_{ST}, it is necessary to determine the Mach number in the action zone between the shock wave and pitot static tube.

From Eq. 19.65,

$$N_{M2} = \frac{[(k-1) N_{M1}^2 + 2]}{[2k N_{M1}^2 - (k-1)]}$$

$$= \frac{[(1.4-1)(1.208)^2 + 2]}{[2 \times 1.4 \times (1.208)^2 - (1.4 - 1)]} = 0.7$$

From Eq. 19.42 a,

$$\frac{p_{ST}}{p_2} = \left[1 + \left(\frac{k-1}{2}\right) N_{M1}^2\right]^{k/(k-1)}$$

$$= \left[1 + \frac{(1.4-1)}{2} (0.7)^2\right]^{1.4/(1.4-1)}$$

$$= 1.387$$

$$p_{ST} = 1.387 \times 1.567 \times 10^5 \text{ N/m}^2$$

$$= 2.173 \times 10^5 \text{ N/m}^2$$

Deflection of mercury is then given by

$$\therefore \qquad h = \frac{p_{ST} - p_2}{w_{Hg}}$$

$$= \frac{(2.173 - 1.567) \times 10^5}{13.6 \times 9810}$$

$$= 0.4542 \text{ m or } 454.2 \text{ mm}$$

19.10 A tank contains air at a pressure of 3.5 N/cm² and a temperature of 25°C. The local atmospheric pressure is 1 bar. Air discharges out of the tank and into the atmosphere through a convergent nozzle. The exit opening of the nozzle is 2.54 cm in diameter. Assume isentropic flow and take $C_d = 1.0$, (a) what is the mass rate of flow through the nozzle (b) what will be the mass rate of flow if the pressure in the tank is 35 N/cm². Take R = 287 J kg^{-1} °K and k = 1.4.

Solution

(a) From Eq. 19.50

$$\left(\frac{p_2}{p_1}\right)_{cr} = \left[\frac{2}{k+1}\right]^{k/(k-1)}$$

$$= \left[\frac{2}{1.4+1}\right]^{1.4/(1.4-1)}$$

$$= 0.528$$

The mass density of the air in the tank is determined from the equation of state.

Since absolute pressure = $(p_{atm} + p_1 \text{ gauge})$

$$p_1 = (10^5 + 3.5 \times 10^4)$$

$$= 1.35 \times 10^5 \text{ N/m}^2$$

$$\rho_1 = \frac{p_1}{R T_1}$$

$$= \frac{1.35 \times 10^5}{287 \times (173 + 25)}$$

$$= 1.58 \text{ kg/m}^3$$

Now $\quad \dfrac{p_a}{p_1} = \dfrac{10^5}{1.35 \times 10^5}$

$$= 0.741$$

Since $\left(\dfrac{p_a}{p_1}\right) > \left(\dfrac{p_2}{p_1}\right)_{cr}$, Eq. 19.47 or Eq. 19.48 may be used.

$$U_2 = \sqrt{\dfrac{2k}{(k-1)} + \dfrac{p_1}{p_1} \times [1 - (p_2/p_1)^{(k-1)/k}]}$$

and $\quad G = \rho_2 A_2 U_2$

$$= \rho_1 (p_2/p_1)^{1/k} \times A_2$$

$$\times \sqrt{\left(\dfrac{2k}{k-1}\right)(p_1/\rho_1)[1 - (p_2/p_1)^{(k-1)/k}]}$$

$$= A_2 \sqrt{\left(\dfrac{2k}{k-1}\right)} \sqrt{p_1\rho_1} \left(\dfrac{p_2}{p_1}\right)^{1/k} \sqrt{[1 - (p_2/p_1)^{(k-1)/k}]}$$

$$= \dfrac{\pi}{4} \times (2.54 \times 10^{-2})^2 \sqrt{\dfrac{2 \times 1.4}{1.4-1}} \times 1.35 \times 10^5 \times 1.58$$

$$\times (0.741)^{1/1.4} \times \sqrt{1 - (0.741)^{(1.4-1)/1.4}}$$

$$= (5.06 \times 10^{04}) \times 1221.92 \times 0.807 \times 0.2865$$

$$= 0.1429 \text{ kg/s}$$

(b) The absolute pressure of air in the tank

$$= (10^5 + 35 \times 10^4) \text{ N/m}^2$$

$$= 4.5 \times 10^5$$

The mass density ρ of air in the tank is

$$= \left(\dfrac{p_1}{R T_1}\right)$$

$$= \dfrac{4.5 \times 10^5}{287 \times (273 + 25)}$$

$$= 5.26 \text{ kg/m}^3$$

The ratio of pressure at the exit of nozzle, p_2, which is discharging in atmosphere to the pressure p_1 in the tank is

$$\left(\dfrac{p_2}{p_1}\right) = \dfrac{10^5}{4.5 \times 10^5}$$

$$= 0.222 < (p_2/p_1)_{cr}$$

It is less than critical pressure ratio of $(p_2/p_1)_{cr}$. Therefore, the velocity of air at nozzle exit is critical. The rate of flow is, now, given by Eq. 19.51.

$$G = A_2 \sqrt{k p_1 \rho_1} \left[\frac{2}{(k+1)} \right]^{(k+1)/2(k-1)}$$

$$= \frac{\pi}{4} \times (2.54 \times 10^{-2})^2 \sqrt{1.4 \times (4.5 \times 10^5)(5.26)}$$

$$\times \left(\frac{2}{1.4+1} \right)^{(1.4+1)/2(1.4-1)}$$

$$= (5.064 \times 10^{-4}) \times 1820.38 \times 0.5787$$

$$= 0.5334 \text{ kg/s.}$$

19.11 Air from a reservoir is supplied through a convergent divergent nozzle. The ratio of exit area to throat area is 2.5, the throat being 12.5 cm². The pressure of the air contained in the reservoir is 70 N/cm² whereas its temperature is 24°C. The nozzle discharges into atmosphere where local barometric pressure as 1 bar. Assume the air flow to be isentropic with R = 29.3 m/k and k = 1.4. Calculate (a) the mass rate of flow of air through the nozzle (b) exit pressure, (c) exit temperature, (d) exit Mach number, and (e) exit velocity for the following two conditions

(i) Sonic flow at the throat with supersonic flow in the divergent section,
and

(ii) Sonic flow at the throat with subsonic flow in the diverget section.

Solution

Apply energy equation, Eq.19.33 to throat section 2 and exit section 3.

$$\frac{p_2}{\rho_2} \left(\frac{k}{k-1} \right) [1 - (p_3/p_2)^{(k-1)/k}] = \left[\frac{U_3^2 - U_2^2}{2} \right]$$

To express this equation in term of Mach number, introduce following conversion.

$$p = \rho R T \qquad \qquad ...(19.1b)$$

and
$$c = \sqrt{k R T} = \sqrt{k p/\rho}$$

$$N_M = \frac{U}{c} = \frac{U}{\sqrt{k p/\rho}}$$

so that,
$$U^2 = \frac{kp}{\rho} \cdot N_M^2 \qquad \qquad ...(a)$$

$$\therefore \quad \frac{p_2}{\rho_2} \times \left(\frac{k}{k-1} \right) [1 - (p_3/p_2)^{(k-1)/k}] = \frac{1}{2} \left[k \frac{p_3}{\rho_3} N_{M3}^2 - k \frac{p_2}{\rho_2} N_{M2}^2 \right]$$

Divide by p_2/ρ_2

$$\left(\frac{2}{k-1} \right) \left[1 - \left(\frac{p_3}{p_2} \right)^{(k-1)/k} \right] = \left[\frac{p_3}{\rho_3} \times \frac{\rho_2}{p_2} N_{M3}^2 - N_{M2}^2 \right]$$

But
$$\left(\frac{\rho_2}{\rho_3} \right) = \left(\frac{p_2}{p_3} \right)^{1/k} \quad \text{and put} \quad \frac{p_3}{p_2} = P$$

$$\left(\frac{2}{k-1}\right)\left[1-\left(\frac{p_3}{p_2}\right)^{(k-1)/k}\right] = \left[\left(\frac{p_3}{p_2}\right)\left(\frac{p_2}{p_3}\right)^{1/k} \times N_{M3}^2 - N_{M2}^2\right]$$

$$\left(\frac{2}{k-1}\right)-\left(\frac{2}{k-1}\right)P^{(k-1)/k} = (P)^{(1-1/k)} \times N_{M3}^2 - N_{M2}^2$$

$$(P)^{(k-1)/k}\left[\left(\frac{2}{k-1}\right)+N_{M3}^2\right] = N_{M2}^2 + \left(\frac{2}{k-1}\right)$$

Divided by $\left(\dfrac{2}{k-1}\right)$

$$P^{(k-1)/k}\left[1+\frac{(k-1)}{2}N_{M3}^2\right] = \left[1+\frac{(k-1)}{2}N_{M2}^2\right]$$

$$P = \left(\frac{p_3}{p_2}\right) = \left[\frac{1+\dfrac{(k-1)}{2}N_{M2}^2}{1+\dfrac{(k-1)}{2}N_{M3}^2}\right]^{\left(\frac{k}{k-1}\right)} \qquad ....(b)$$

Now $\qquad p_2 = \rho_2 R\, T_2, p_3 = \rho_3 R\, T_3 \text{ and } (\rho_2/\rho_3) = (p_2/p_3)^{1/k}$

$$\frac{T_2}{T_3} = \left(\frac{p_3}{p_2}\right)\left(\frac{\rho_2}{\rho_3}\right) = \left(\frac{p_3}{p_2}\right)\left(\frac{p_2}{p_3}\right)^{1/k}$$

$$= \left(\frac{p_3}{p_2}\right)^{(k-1)/k}$$

Hence from Eq. (b)

$$\left(\frac{T_3}{T_2}\right) = \left[\frac{1+\dfrac{(k-1)}{2}N_{M3}^2}{1+\dfrac{(k-1)}{2}N_{M2}^2}\right] \qquad ...(c)$$

Now from Eq. (a)

$$U_3^2 = k\left(\frac{p_3}{\rho_3}\right)(N_{M2})^2$$

and $\qquad U_2^2 = k\dfrac{p_2}{\rho_2}(N_{M2})^2$

$$\left(\frac{U_3^2}{U_2^2}\right) = \left(\frac{p_3}{p_2}\right)\left(\frac{\rho_2}{\rho_3}\right)\left(\frac{N_{M3}}{N_{M2}}\right)^2$$

But $\qquad \left(\dfrac{\rho_2}{\rho_2}\right) = \left(\dfrac{p_2}{p_3}\right)^{1/k}$

$$\left(\frac{U_3}{U_2}\right)^2 = \left(\frac{p_3}{p_2}\right)^{k-1/k}\left(\frac{N_{M3}}{N_{M2}}\right)^2$$

$$\left(\frac{U_3}{U_2}\right) = \left(\frac{p_3}{p_2}\right)^{(k-1)/2k} \left(\frac{N_{M3}}{N_{M2}}\right)$$

Substituting the value of p_3/p_2 from Eq. (b)

$$\left(\frac{U_3}{U_2}\right) = \left(\frac{N_{m3}}{N_{M2}}\right) \left[\frac{1 + \dfrac{(k-1)}{2} N_{M2}^2}{1 + \dfrac{(k-1)}{2} N_{M3}^2}\right]^{1/2} \qquad ...(d)$$

Now from continuity Eq

$$\rho_2 A_2 U_2 = \rho_3 A_3 U_3$$

$$\left(\frac{A_2}{A_3}\right) = \left(\frac{\rho_3}{\rho_2}\right)\left(\frac{U_3}{U_2}\right)$$

$$= \left(\frac{U_3}{U_2}\right)\left(\frac{p_3}{p_2}\right)^{1/k}$$

$$= \left(\frac{N_{M3}}{N_{M2}}\right)\left(\frac{p_3}{p_2}\right)^{(k-1)/2k}\left(\frac{p_3}{p_2}\right)^{1/k}$$

$$= \left(\frac{N_{M3}}{N_{M2}}\right)\left(\frac{p_3}{p_2}\right)^{(k+1)/2k}$$

Substituting the value of (p_3/p_2) from Eq. (b)

$$\frac{A_2}{A_3} = \left(\frac{N_{M3}}{N_{M2}}\right)\left[\frac{1 + (k-1)\dfrac{N_{M2}^2}{2}}{1 + \dfrac{(k-1)}{2} N_{M3}^2}\right]^{\frac{(k+1)}{2(k-1)}} \qquad ...(e)$$

Using Eq. (e) with throat area A_2 to, exit area A_3 as 2.5 and $N_{M2} = 1$

$$\frac{1}{2.5} = N_{M3}\left[\frac{1 + \dfrac{(1.4-1)}{2}(1)^2}{1 + \dfrac{(1.4-1)}{2} N_{M3}^2}\right]$$

Solving by trial error,

$$N_{M3} = 2.44 \text{ or } 0.24$$

The former value is for divergent section acting as a nozzle and the later value corresponds to the condition when the divergent section acts as a diffuser.

(a) When sonic velocity occurs at the throat, the mass rate of flow is same for both conditions and is determined by using Eq. 19.51.

$$G_{cr} = A_2 \sqrt{k p_1 \rho_1} \left(\frac{2}{k+1}\right)^{(k+1)/2(k-1)}$$

in which $\quad \rho_1 = \dfrac{p_T}{R T_1} = \dfrac{70 \times 10^4}{(29.3 \times 9.81)(273 + 24)}$

$$= 8.2 \ \text{kg/m}^3$$

$\therefore \qquad G = 12.5 \times 10^{-4}$

$$\times \sqrt{1.4 \times 70 \times 10^4 \times 8.2} \left[\dfrac{2}{1.4 + 1} \right]^{(1.4 + 1)/2(1.4 - 1)}$$

$$= 2.05 \ \text{kg/s}$$

(i) When $\quad N_{M3} = 2.44$

Using Eq. b, with $N_{M1} = 0$ and $p_1 = 70 \times 10^4 \ \text{N/m}^2$, the exit pressure

is

$$\frac{p_3}{70 \times 10^4} = \left[\frac{1}{1 + \dfrac{1.4 - 1}{2} (2.44)^2} \right]^{1.4/(1.4 - 1)}$$

$$p_3 = 44998.5 \ \text{N/m}^2 \quad \text{or} \quad 4.49 \ \text{N/cm}^2$$

The exit temperature T_3 is calculated from Eq. (c) with $N_{M1} = 0$ and temperature in the reservoir $T_1 = (273 + 24) = 297 \,^\circ K$

$$\frac{T_3}{T_1} = \left[\frac{1 + \dfrac{(k - 1)}{2} N_{M1}^2}{1 + \dfrac{(k - 1)}{2} N_{M3}^2} \right]$$

$$= \left[\frac{1}{1 + \dfrac{(1.4 - 1)}{2} (2.44)^2} \right] = 0.4564$$

$$T_3 = 135.57 \,^\circ K \quad \text{or} \quad -137.4 \,^\circ C$$

The exit velocity is given by Eq. (d)

$$U_3 = N_{M3} \sqrt{k R T_3}$$

$$U_3 = (2.44) \sqrt{1.4 \times 29.3 \times 9.81 \times 135.57}$$

$$= 569.9 \ \text{m/s}$$

(ii) When $\quad N_{M3} = 0.24,$

$$p_3 = p_1 \left[\frac{1}{1 + \dfrac{(k - 1)}{2} N_{M3}^2} \right]^{k/(k - 1)}$$

$$= 70 \times 10^4 \left[\frac{1}{1 + \dfrac{(1.4 - 1)}{2} (0.24)^2} \right]^{1.4/(1.4 - 1)}$$

$$= 67.24 \times 10^4 \ \text{N/m}^2 \quad \text{or} \quad 67.24 \ \text{N/cm}^2$$

$$T_3 = T_2 \left[\cfrac{1}{1 + \cfrac{(k-2)}{2} N_{M3}^2} \right]$$

$$= 297 \left[\cfrac{1}{1 + \left(\cfrac{1.4 - 1}{2} \right) (0.24)^2} \right]$$

$$= 293 \, °K$$

$$U_3 = N_{M3} \sqrt{k R T_3}$$

$$= 0.24 \sqrt{1.4 \times 29.3 \times 9.81 \times 293.61}$$

$$= 82.49 \ m/s.$$

19.12 The air is flowing through a duct and a normal shock wave is formed at a cross section at which the Mach number is 2.0. The upstream pressure and temperature are 105 bar and 15 °C respectively. Find Mach number, pressure, and temperature immediately downstream of the shock wave. Take k = 1.4.

Solution

From Eq. 19.65

$$N_{M2}^2 = \left[\frac{(k-1) N_{M1}^2 + 2}{2k N_{M1}^2 - (k-1)} \right]$$

$$= \left[\frac{(1.4-1)(2)^2 \times 2}{2 \times 1.4 \times (2)^2 - (1.4-1)} \right]$$

$$= 0.333$$

$$N_{M2} = 0.577$$

From Eq. 19.62,

$$p_2 = p_1 \left[\frac{2k N_{M1}^2 - (k-1)}{(k+1)} \right]$$

$$= 105 \times 10^5 \left[\frac{2 \times 1.4 \times (2)^2 - (1.4-1)}{(1.4+1)} \right]$$

$$= 105 \times 4.5 \times 10^5 = 472.5 \times 10^5 \ N/m^2$$

From Eq. 19.63

$$\left(\frac{p_2}{\rho_1} \right) = \left(\frac{U_1}{U_2} \right) = \left[\frac{(k+1) N_{M1}^2}{(k-1) N_{M1}^2 + 2} \right]$$

Combining Eqs. 19.62 and 19.63

$$\frac{T_2}{T_1} = \left(\frac{p_2}{p_1} \right) \left(\frac{\rho_1}{\rho_2} \right)$$

$$= \left[\frac{2k N_{M1}^2 - (k-1)}{k+1} \right] \left[\frac{(k-1) N_{M1}^2 + 2}{(k+1) N_{M1}^2} \right]$$

$$= \left[\frac{2 \times 1.4 \times (2)^2 - (1.4 - 1)}{(1.4 + 1)} \right] \left[\frac{(1.4 - 1)(2)^2 + 2}{(1.4 + 1)(2)^2} \right]$$

$$= (4.5)(0.375)$$

$$= 1.6875$$

$$T_2 = 1.6875 \, T_1$$

$$= 1.6875 \times (273 + 16)$$

$$= 487.7 \,°K \ \text{or} \ 214 \,°C$$

19.13 A normal shock wave moves through still air (pressure is 100 kN/m^2 and temperature is 300 K) with constant velocity of 1500 m/s. Calculate the velocity of the air behind the wave, static pressure and temperature. Take $R = 29.27 \ \text{m}/°\text{K}$.

Solution

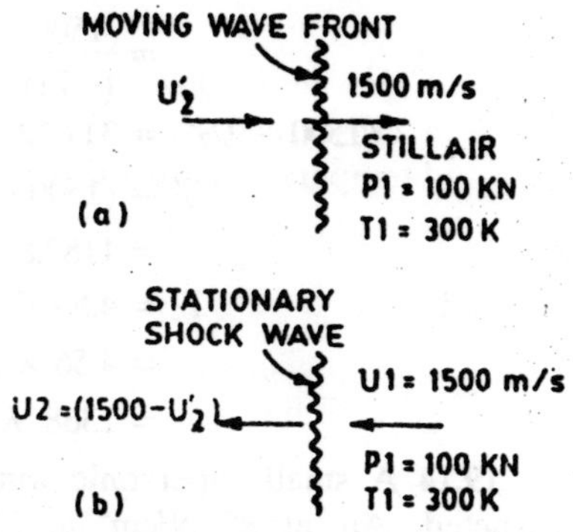

Since the shock wave is moving, it should be made stationary by super-imposing a velocity of 1500 m/s in the opposite direction. Then only the equations of the shock may be applied to this problem.(Fig. 19.12)

The velocity of sound c_1 is given by

FIG. 19.12 EXAMPLE 19.13

$$c_1 = \sqrt{k \, R \, T_1}$$

$$= \sqrt{1.4 \times (29.27 \times 9.81) \times 300}$$

$$= 347.27 \ \text{m/s}$$

$$N_{M1} = \frac{U_1}{c_1}$$

$$= \frac{1500}{347.27} = 4.32$$

From Eq. 19.62,

$$\frac{p_2}{p_1} = \left[\frac{2k \, N_{M1}^2 - (k - 1)}{(k + 1)} \right]$$

$$= \left[\frac{2 \times 1.4 \times (4.32)^2 - (1.4 - 1)}{(1.4 + 1)} \right] = 21.60$$

From Eq. 19.63,

$$\left(\frac{\rho_2}{\rho_1} \right) = \left(\frac{U_1}{U_2} \right) = \left[\frac{(k + 1) \, N_{M1}^2}{(k - 1) \, N_{M1}^2 + 2} \right]$$

$$= \left[\frac{(1.4 + 1)(4.32)^2}{(1.4 - 1)(4.32)^2 + 2} \right] = 4.73$$

From Eq. 19.1b,

$$\frac{T_2}{T_1} = \left(\frac{p_2}{p_1} \times \frac{\rho_2}{\rho_1} \right)$$

$$= \left(21.60 \times \frac{1}{4.73} \right) = 4.56$$

Therefore, $\quad p_2 = 21.60 \, p_1$

$$= 21.60 \times 100 \;\; kN/m^2$$

$$= 2160 \;\; kN/m^2$$

$$U_2 = U_1/4.73$$

$$= \frac{1500}{(4.73)} = 317.12 \;\; m/s$$

$\therefore \qquad (1500 - U_2') = 317.12$

$$U_2' = (1500 - 317.12)$$

$$= 1182.87 \;\; m/s$$

and $\qquad T_2 = 4.56 \, T_1$

$$= 4.56 \times 300$$

$$= 1368 \,^\circ K \;\; or \;\; 1095 \,^\circ C$$

19.14 A small supersonic wind tunnel with Mach number 2.0 is to be constructed. Air at 85 N/cm^2 at 21 °C is available. The throat diameter is 2.5 cm. Determine the diameter of exit as well as the pressure intensity and temperature at exit. Neglect losses.

Solution

Since the flow is to be supersonic in the divergent section 3, i.e. $N_{M3} > 1.0$, the flow at the throat will be critical or sonic. The critical mass rate of flow is given by Eq. 19.51.

$$G_{cr} = A_2 \sqrt{k \, p_1 \rho_1} \times \left(\frac{2}{k+1} \right)^{(k+1)/2(k-1)}$$

$$= \frac{\pi}{4} \times (2.5 \times 10^{-2})^2 \sqrt{1.4 \times 85 \times 10^4 \times \rho_1}$$

$$\times \left(\frac{2}{1.4+1} \right)^{(1.4+1)/2(1.4-1)}$$

Assuming $\qquad C_d = 1.0$

$$\rho_1 = \left(\frac{p_1}{R \, T_1} \right)$$

$$= \frac{85 \times 10^4}{290 \times (273 + 21)} = 9.97 \;\; kg/m^3$$

$\therefore \qquad G = \frac{\pi}{4} (2.5 \times 10^{-2})^2 \sqrt{1.4 \times 85 \times 10^4 \times 9.97} \times (0.578)$

$$= 0.97678 \text{ kg/s}$$

Now
$$c_3 = \sqrt{k R T_3}$$
$$= \sqrt{1.4 \times 290 \times T_3} = 20.15 \sqrt{T_3}$$

Since the Mach number of flow at the exit of divergent section is given as 2.0.

$$N_{M3} = \frac{U_3}{c_3}$$

$$U_3 = 2 \times c_3$$
$$= 2 \times 20.15 \sqrt{T_3} = 40.30 \sqrt{T_3} \qquad \text{...(i)}$$

From the isentropic flow equations,
$$T_3 = T_1 (p_3/p_1)^{(k-1)/k} \qquad \text{...(ii)}$$

From Eqs. (i) and (ii)
$$U_3 = 40.30 \sqrt{T_1} (p_3/p_1)^{(k-1)/2k} \qquad \text{...(iii)}$$

From Eq. 19.31, assuming $U_1 \approx 0$

$$\frac{U_3^2}{2} = \frac{k}{(k-1)} \frac{p_1}{\rho_1} \left[1 - \left(\frac{p_3}{p_1} \right)^{(k-1)/k} \right] \qquad \text{...(iv)}$$

Solve Eqs. (iii) and (iv) for p_3 and U_3

$$\frac{p_3}{p_1} = 0.1278$$

$$p_3 = 0.1278 \times 85 \times 10^4 \text{ N/m}^2$$
$$= 10.86 \times 10^4 \text{ N/m}^2$$

From Eq. (iii),
$$U_3 = 40.30 \sqrt{(273 + 21)} (10.1278)^{(1.4-1)/2 \times 1.4}$$
$$= 515.04 \text{ m/s}$$

Then
$$T_3 = T_1 [p_3/p_1]^{(k-1)/k}$$
$$= (273 + 21) [0.1278]^{(1.4-1)/1.4}$$
$$= 163.33 \text{ °K or } -109.67 \text{ °C}$$

From continuity equation,

$$A_3 = \frac{G}{\rho_3 U_3} = \frac{G}{U_3 (p_3/R T_3)}$$

$$= \frac{G R T_3}{U_3 P_3}$$

$$= \frac{0.9768 \times 290 \times 162.33}{515.04 \times 10.86 \times 10^4}$$

$$= 8.27 \times 10^{-4} \text{ m}^2$$

Diameter d_3 of exit section of the divergent section is

$$d_3 = \sqrt{\frac{4}{\pi} A_3}$$
$$= \sqrt{\frac{4 \times 8.27 \times 10^{-4}}{3.14}}$$
$$= 3.246 \times 10^{-2} \text{m or } 3.25 \text{ cm,}$$

OBJECTIVE QUESTIONS

19.1 The relationship between pressure and density of a compressible fluid is given by p/ρ^n = constant, where n is a index which varies for different types of process. Match the value of n for different process.

(a) Isothermal   (i) $n = k$

(b) isentropic   (ii) $n = 1$

(c) Isobaric   (iii) $n = 0$

19.2 The gas constant R is related to k ($= c_p/c_v$) by the one of following relationship. Mark the correct one.

(a) $c_p (k - 1)$ (b) $(k - 1) c_v/k$

(c) $(c_p + c_v)$ (d) $c_p (k - 1)/k$

(e) none.

19.3 The expressions for work done for two different processes are given below. Mark the correct expression or expressions for isentropic process.

(a) $R T \log (p_1/p_2)$ (b) $p_1 v_1 - p_2 v_2/(k - 1)$

(c) $R (T_1 - T_2)/(k - 1)$ (d) $(I_2 - I_1)$

(e) none.

19.4 An isentropic process is the one in which

(a) temperature remains constant

(b) heat does not change

(c) entropy remains constant

(d) adiabatic and reversible

(e) adiabatic and irreversible

19.5 The continuity equation for a compressible fluid states that

(a) the net mass rate of inflow in any given volume is zero

(b) applied to irrotational flow only

(c) the energy remains constant along a stream line

(d) the product of area and volume remains constant from section to section

(e) none.

19.6 The differential energy equation in an isentropic flow may take the form

(a) $dp + d (\rho U^2) = 0$ (b) $U d U + dp/\rho = 0$

(c) $2U\,dU + dp/\rho = 0$ (d)$dv/v + dp/\rho + dA/A = 0$

(e) none.

19.7 Mark the correct statement for work done when the process is isentropic

(a) $\dfrac{p_1}{w_1}\log{(p_1/p_2)} = \left(\dfrac{U_2^2 - U_1^2}{2g}\right) + (z_2 - z_1)$

(b) $\left(\dfrac{p_1}{w_1} + z_1 + \dfrac{U_1^2}{2g}\right) = \left(\dfrac{p_2}{w_2} + z_2 + \dfrac{U_2^2}{2g}\right)$

(c) $\dfrac{k}{(k-1)}\left(\dfrac{p_1}{\rho_1} - \dfrac{p_2}{\rho_2}\right) = \left(\dfrac{U_2^2 - U_1^2}{2}\right)$

(d) $\dfrac{k}{k-1}\left(\dfrac{p_1}{\rho_1}\right)\left[1 - (p_2/p_1)^{(k-1)/k}\right] = \left(\dfrac{U_2^2 - U_1^2}{2}\right)$

(e) none.

19.8 Select the statement which does not give the speed of sound

(a) $\sqrt{kRT}$ (b) $\sqrt{p/\rho}$

(c) $\sqrt{dp/d\rho}$ (d) $\sqrt{E_v/\rho}$

(e) $\sqrt{kp/\rho}$

19.9 The speed of sound in water (in metre per second) under normal conditions is

(a) 1483 (b) 741.5

(c) 2000 (d) 344.9

(e) none.

19.10 The speed of sound in an ideal gas varies directly as

(a) the density (b) the absolute pressure

(c) the absolute temperature (d) the bulk modulus of elasticity

(e) none.

19.11 An elastic wave is propagated in the fluid due to disturbance and flow is divided into silent zone and action zone. The silent zone is region where the velocity is

(a) zero (b) sonic

(c) subsonic (d) supersonic

(e) none.

19.12 A pitot static tube is used to measure the velocity in an isentropic flow. The stagnation pressure is given in terms of $(p_{ST} - p_1)/0.5\rho\,U_1^2$. It is related to Mach number of upstream flow N_{M1} by one of the following relationship.

(a) $\left[1 + \dfrac{N_{M1}^2}{4} + \dfrac{N_{M1}^4}{16}\right]$

(b) $[1 + N_{M1}^2 + N_{M1}^4]$

(c) $\left[1 + \dfrac{N_{M1}}{4} + \dfrac{(2-k)}{48} N_{M1} \right]$

(d) N_{M1}

(e) none.

19.13 The compressibility correction factor is defined as $(p_{ST} - p_1)/0.5 \rho U_1^2$. It is equal to

(a) 1.0   (b) 1.0655

(c) 1.28   (d) none.

when the Mach number N_{M1} of the flow is 0.5.

19.14 The density of the compressible fluid at stagnation point is

(a) more   (b) less

(c) equal   (d) zero   (e) none.

as compared to its counterpart in the ambient fluid.

19.15 Select the correct statement regarding flow through converging diverging passage

(a) when the Mach number at exit is greater than unity, no shock wave develops in the passage.

(b) when the critical pressure ratio is exceeded, the Mach number at the throat is greater than unity.

(c) For sonic velocity at the throat, one and only one pressure or velocity can occur at a given section downstream

(d) The Mach number at the throat is always unity.

(e) The density increases in the downstream direction throughout the converging portion of the passage.

19.16 The critical pressure ratio for carbon dioxide ($k = 1.3$) flowing through a converging nozzle is

(a) 0.528   (b) 0.545

(c) 6.467   (d) 0.968

(e) none.

19.17 In a normal shock wave in one dimensional flow, the

(a) velocity, pressure and density increases,

(b) pressure, density and temperature increases,

(c) velocity, temperature and density increases,

(d) pressure, density and momentum per unit time increases

(e) mechanical energy remains constant.

19.18 A normal shock wave is analogous to

(a) an elementary wave in still liquid

(b) the hydraulic jump

(c) open channel flow with $N_F > 1$

(d) flow of liquid through an expanding nozzle

(e) none.

19.19 If the Mach number immediately before a normal shock wave in air is 1.5, the Mach number after the shock wave is

(a) 0.44   (b) 0.49

(c) 0.70   (d) 0.82   (e) none.

19.20 A gas flow situation at $N_M = 2.3$ might be analogous to an open channel flow situation at Froude number.

(a) 0.43   (b) 0.77

(c) 1.0   (d) 2.3   (e) 6.9

PROBLEMS

19.1 Show, from first principle, that the velocity of sound in an adiabatic gas flow is given by

$$c = \sqrt{kRT}$$

19.2 Define the following

(a) Enthalpy

(b) Internal energy

(c) Entropy

(d) Reversible and irreversible process.

19.3 Derive the continuity equation and energy equation for compressible fluid.

19.4 Define and state the significane of Mach number in the fluid flow. Upto what limit of Mach number can one neglect the compressibility effects and treat the fluids as incompressible.

19.5 Show by means of a diagram the nature of propagation of disturbance in compressible fluid flow when Mach number is less than unity, equal to unity and more than unity.

19.6 State the area velocity relationship for one dimensional stready, compressible, adiabatic and frictionless flow. Show the effects of variation of area on subsonic, sonic and supersonic flows.

19.7 Drive an expression for Mach number downstream of a normal shock wave in terms of Mach number of upstream flow and k. And show that (for k = 1.4)

$$N_{M2} = \frac{(N_{M1}^2 + 5)}{(7\,N_{M1}^2 - 1)}$$

19.8 A closed container contains 5 kg of helium at 80 kN/m^2 pressure and 30 °C temperature. It is so heated that its pressure rises to 200 kN/m^2. Calculate its final temperature, heat added, changed in internal energy and work done.

19.9 Air flows through the transitional section of a conduit. The pressure, velocity and temperature upstream of the transition are 35 kN/m³, 30 m/s and 150 °C. If at the downstream section, the velocity is measured as 150 m/s, determine the temperature and pressure at this section. Assume the process as isentropic and take k = 1.4 and R = 29.57 m/°K.

19.10 A jet airplane is propelled at a velocity of 1000 km/hr through air in which atmospheric pressure is 9 N/cm². The temperature of air at this section is − 5°C and the wind speed is negligible. Calculate the pressure intensity, density of air and temperature at the stagnation point on the nose of the jet and determine its Mach number. Take R = 290 J kg⁻¹ K⁻¹.

19.11 A supersonic plane is flying at Mach number of 1.80. It is observed flying directly overhead at a high of 12000 m. How far it will be when one hears the sonic boom.

19.12 A tank contains air at a temperature of 30°C. Air flows from the tank into atmosphere through a convergent nozzle. The diameter of the nozzle exit is 2.5 cm. Find the mass rate of flow through the nozzle if the pressure in the tank is (a) 4 N/cm² gauge (b) 35 N/cm² gauge. Assume the process to be adiabatic. Take R = 287 J kg⁻¹ K⁻¹ and k = 1.4. The atmospheric pressure may be taken as 1 bar.

19.13 For an normal shock wave in air, with $N_{M1} = 2.0$, determine the flow conditions before and after the shock wave. The atmospheric pressure and density are respectively 0.26×10^5 N/m² and 0.4 kg/m². Take k for air = 1.4.

19.14 An ideal gas flows through a convergent divergent nozzle and discharge into atmosphere. The pressure and temperature at the nozzle inlet are 42 N/cm² and 27°C respectively. For the complete expansion of air as it leaves the exit, determine, (a) the velocities at the throat, inlet and exit section of the nozzle and (b) the temperature at the throatand exit sections of the nozzle. It is known that barometric pressure is equivalent to 74 cm of mercury. The process be assumed as isentropic, k = 2.0 and R = 225.63 J kg⁻¹ K⁻¹.

Appendix I

Consider a parallelopiped fluid element as shown in Fig. 5.1, having sides dx, dy and dz in the three co- ordinate directioins X, Y and Z respectively. The forces acting on a fluid element are of two types, namely (i) body forces B and (ii) surface forces, P.

The body force, B, has got three components X, Y and Z in the three co-ordinate directions, i.e.,

$$B = iX + jY + kZ \qquad \text{...(A-1)}$$

Referring to Fig. 5.1, let the surface forces acting in the X-direction on two opposite faces ABFE and DCGH be P_{xx}. (Convetionally, the first letter of the subscript denotes the direction of normal to the plane on which the stress vector is acting and the second letter denotes the direction of stress vector). Hence the surface forces acting on the pair of faces ABFE and DCGH are

$$P_{xx} = \left[\left(p_x + \frac{\partial p_x}{\partial x} dx \right) - p_x \right] dy \, dz = \frac{\partial p_x}{\partial x} dx \, dy \, dz \qquad \text{...(A-2a)}$$

where p_x is the surface force acting on a face normal to X axis.

Similarly $\qquad P_{yy} = (\partial p / \partial y) \, dx \, dy \, dz \qquad \text{...(A-2a)}$

and $\qquad P_{zz} = (\partial p / \partial z) \, dx \, dy \, dz \qquad \text{...(A-2b)}$

∴ Resultant surface force/unit volume,

$$P = \left(\frac{\partial p_x}{\partial x} + \frac{\partial p_y}{\partial y} + \frac{\partial p_z}{\partial z} \right) \qquad \text{...(A-3)}$$

Since P_{xx}, P_{yy} and P_{zz} are vectors, these can be resolved in the three co-ordinate directions.

$$P_{xx} = i \, \sigma_x + j \, \tau_{xy} + k \, \tau_{xz} \qquad \text{...(A-4a)}$$

$$P_{yy} = i \, \tau_{yx} + j \, \sigma_y + k \, \tau_{yz} \qquad \text{...(A-4b)}$$

$$P_{zz} = i \, \tau_{zx} + j \, \tau_{zy} + k \, \sigma_z \qquad \text{...(A-4c)}$$

This can be expressed as stress matrix

$$n = \begin{pmatrix} \sigma_x & \tau_{xy} & \tau_{xz} \\ \tau_{yx} & \sigma_y & \tau_{yz} \\ \tau_{zx} & \tau_{zy} & \sigma_z \end{pmatrix} = \begin{pmatrix} \sigma_x & \tau_{xy} & \tau_{zx} \\ \tau_{xy} & \sigma_y & \tau_{yz} \\ \tau_{zx} & \tau_{xz} & \sigma_z \end{pmatrix}$$

Since $\qquad \tau_{xy} = \tau_{xy}$ and so on.

Hence, the surface force P can be written as

$$P = \partial/\partial x \, (i \, \sigma_x + j \, \tau_{xy} + k \, \tau_{xz}) + \partial/\partial y \, (i \, \tau_{yz} + j \, \sigma_y + k \, \tau_{yz})$$
$$+ \partial/\partial_x (i \, \tau_{zx} + j \, \tau_{zy} + k \, \sigma_z)$$

$$P = i \left(\frac{\partial}{\partial x} \sigma x + \frac{\partial}{\partial y} \tau_{xy} + \frac{\partial}{\partial z} \tau_{zx} \right) + j \left(\frac{\partial}{\partial x} \tau_{xy} + \frac{\partial}{\partial y} \sigma_y + \frac{\partial}{\partial x} \tau_{yz} \right)$$

$$+ k \left(\frac{\partial}{\partial x} \tau_{zx} + \frac{\partial}{\partial y} \tau_{yz} + \frac{\partial}{\partial z} \sigma_z \right) \qquad \text{...(A-5)}$$

Now, the n-matrix for an elastic body can be written by Hooke's law.

$$\pi = \begin{pmatrix} \bar{\sigma} & 0 & 0 \\ 0 & \bar{\sigma} & 0 \\ 0 & 0 & \bar{\sigma} \end{pmatrix} + G \begin{pmatrix} \partial\xi/\partial x & \partial\xi/\partial y & \partial\xi/\partial z \\ \partial\eta/\partial x & \partial\eta/\partial y & \partial\eta/\partial z \\ \partial\gamma/\partial x & \partial\gamma/\partial y & \partial\gamma/\partial z \end{pmatrix}$$

$$+ G \begin{pmatrix} \partial\xi/\partial x & \partial\eta/\partial x & \partial\gamma/\partial x \\ \partial\xi/\partial y & \partial\eta/\partial y & \partial\gamma/\partial y \\ \partial\xi/\partial z & \partial\eta/\partial z & \partial\gamma/\partial z \end{pmatrix} - 2/3\ G \begin{pmatrix} \text{div s} & 0 & 0 \\ 0 & \text{div s} & 0 \\ 0 & 0 & \text{div s} \end{pmatrix}$$

where G is the shear modulus of elasticity and s is the shear strain. For a fluid, strain s is replaced by the rate of change of strain and G by dynamic viscosity μ. The arithmetic mean of normal stress σ is replaced by bulk fluid pressure, $-p$. Thus, the Stokes law is obtained as,

$$\pi = \begin{pmatrix} -p & 0 & 0 \\ 0 & -p & 0 \\ 0 & 0 & -p \end{pmatrix} + \mu \begin{pmatrix} \partial u/\partial x & \partial u/\partial y & \partial u/\partial z \\ \partial v/\partial x & \partial v/\partial y & \partial v/\partial z \\ \partial w/\partial x & \partial w/\partial y & \partial w/\partial z \end{pmatrix}$$

$$+ \mu \begin{pmatrix} \partial u/\partial x & \partial v/\partial x & \partial w/\partial x \\ \partial u/\partial y & \partial v/\partial y & \partial w/\partial y \\ \partial u/\partial z & \partial v/\partial z & \partial w/\partial z \end{pmatrix} - 2/3\ \mu \begin{pmatrix} \text{div}\ \overline{U} & 0 & 0 \\ 0 & \text{div}\ \overline{U} & 0 \\ 0 & 0 & \text{div}\ \overline{U} \end{pmatrix}$$

The normal fluid stress σ_x consists of static fluid stress, $-p$ and dynamic pressure σ_x

$$\sigma_x = -p + \sigma_x' \quad \text{and similar other terms.} \qquad \text{...(A-6)}$$

Hence, normal and frictional terms of surface stress can be written as

$$\sigma_x' = \mu\ (2\ \partial u/\partial x - 2/3\ div\ \overline{U});\ \tau xy = \mu\ (\partial u/\partial y + \partial v/\partial x)$$
$$\sigma_y' = \mu\ (2\ \partial v/\partial y - 2/3\ div\ \overline{U});\ \tau_{yz} = \mu\ (\partial v/\partial z + \partial w/\partial y)$$
$$\sigma_z' = \mu\ (2\ \partial w/\partial z - 2/3\ div\ \overline{U});\ \tau zx = \mu\ (\partial w/\partial x + \partial u/\partial z) \quad \text{...(A-7)}$$

Substituting these values from Eq. A-7 in Eq. A-4,

$$P_x = i \left(-\frac{\partial p}{\partial x} + \frac{\partial}{\partial x} \sigma_x' + \frac{\partial}{\partial y} \tau_{yx} + \frac{\partial}{\partial z} \tau_{zx} \right)$$

$$= -\frac{\partial p}{\partial x} + \frac{\partial}{\partial x} \left(2\mu \frac{\partial u}{\partial x} - \frac{2}{3} \mu\ div\ \overline{U} \right) + \mu \frac{\partial}{\partial y} \left(\frac{\partial u}{\partial y} + \frac{\partial v}{\partial x} \right)$$

$$+ \mu \frac{\partial}{\partial z} \left(\frac{\partial w}{\partial x} + \frac{\partial u}{\partial z} \right) \qquad \text{...(A-8)}$$

Similar expressions can be written for Y and Z directions.

Newton's second law of motion is written as

$$\Sigma F_x = M\ a_x$$

or $\qquad \rho\ a_x = \Sigma f_x = $ Body forces + Surface forces ...(A-9)

Substituting the values of body forces and surface forces,

$$\rho \frac{Du}{Dt} = X - \frac{\partial p}{\partial x} + \frac{\partial}{\partial x}\left\{\mu\left(2\frac{\partial u}{\partial x} - \frac{2}{3}\, div\,\overline{U}\right)\right\}$$

$$+ \frac{\partial}{\partial y}\left[\mu\left(\frac{\partial u}{\partial y} + \frac{\partial v}{\partial x}\right)\right] + \frac{\partial}{\partial z}\left\{\mu\left(\frac{\partial w}{\partial x} + \frac{\partial u}{\partial z}\right)\right\}$$

$$\rho \frac{Du}{Dt} = \left[X - \frac{\partial p}{\partial x} + \mu\left\{\frac{\partial^2 u}{\partial x^2} + \frac{\partial^2 u}{\partial y^2} + \frac{\partial^2 u}{\partial z^2}\right\}\right.$$

$$\left. + \mu\left\{\frac{\partial}{\partial x}\left(\frac{\partial u}{\partial x}\right) + \frac{\partial}{\partial x}\left(\frac{\partial v}{\partial y}\right) + \frac{\partial}{\partial x}\left(\frac{\partial w}{\partial z}\right)\right\} - \frac{2}{3}\mu\,\nabla.\overline{U}\right]$$

$$\rho \frac{Du}{Dt} = \left[X - \frac{\partial p}{\partial x} + \mu\,\nabla^2 u + \mu\frac{\partial}{\partial x}\left(\nabla.\overline{U}\right) - \frac{2}{3}\mu\left(\nabla.\overline{U}\right)\right] \quad ...(A\text{-}9a)$$

Similarly, other two equations in Y and Z directions can be written.

Eq. A-9a and similar equation in Y and Z direction are known as Navier Strokes equation for viscous fluid. For incmpressible fluid, the mass density remains constant and the continuity equation is written as

$$\nabla.\overline{U} = 0$$

Hence, Eq. A-9a modifies to

$$\rho\, Du/Dt = X - (\partial p/\partial x) + \mu\,\nabla^2 u \qquad ...(A\text{-}10a)$$

$$\rho\, Dv/Dt = Y - (\partial p/\partial y) + \mu\,\nabla^2 v \qquad ...(A\text{-}10b)$$

$$\rho\, Dw/Dt = Z - (\partial p/\partial z) + \mu\,\nabla^2 w \qquad ...(A\text{-}10c)$$

Eq. A-10a in expanded form is written as

$$\rho\left(\frac{\partial u}{\partial t} + u\frac{\partial u}{\partial x} + v\frac{\partial u}{\partial y} + w\frac{\partial u}{\partial z}\right)$$

$$= X - \frac{\partial p}{\partial x} + \mu\left(\frac{\partial^2 u}{\partial x^2} + \frac{\partial^2 u}{\partial y^2} + \frac{\partial^2 u}{\partial z^2}\right)$$

Eqs. A-10a to A-10c aré solved for viscours flow alongwith equation of continuity and equation of state to determine the unknown quantities.

Appendix II

Some Important conversion Factors

1. *Length*

1 cm = 0.394 in

1 m = 3.28 ft

1 km = 0.621 mile

2. *Area*

1 cm^2 = 0.155 in^2

1 m^2 = 10.764 ft^2

1 hactare = 10^4 m^2 = 2.471 acres

1 acres = 43560 ft^2

3. *Volume*

1 cm^3 = 0.061 in^3

1 cm^3 = 35.315 ft^3

1 litre = 0.0353 ft^3 = 0.220 imp.gall = 0.264 U.S.gal

4. *Mass*

1 msl = 0.672 slug = 9.81 kg(m)

1 kg(m) = 2.205 lb(m) = 0.0685 slug

5. *Force*

1 kg (f) = 2.205 lb (f)

1 N = 0.1020 kg (f) = 10^5 dynes = 0.2248 lb (f)

1 tonne = 1000 kg = 0.984 ton

6. *Mass density*

1 msl/m^3 = 0.019 slug/ft^3

1 gm/cc = 102 msl/m^3 = 1.94 slug/ft^3

1 gm/cc = 62.4 lb (m)/ft^3

1 gm/cc = 1kg (m)/litre = 1000 kg (m)/m^3

1 slug/ft^3 = 0.5154 gm/cc

7. *Weight density*

1 kg (f)/m^3 = 0.0624 lb (f)/ft^3

1 kg (f)/m^3 = 9.81 N/m^3

8. *Viscosity*

1 poise = 0.1 Ns/m^2

Answers to Objective Questions

Chapter 1

1.1 (d)	1.2 (c)	1.3 (b)	1.4 (a), (b), (c), (d)
1.5 (b)	1.6 (a)	1.7 (b)	1.8 (b)
1.9 (d)	1.10 (c)	1.11 (a)	1.12 (c)
1.13 (b)	1.14 (d)	1.15 (a), (b)	1.16 (a)
1.17 (d)	1.18 (c)	1.19 (c)	1.20 (b)

Chpater 2

2.1 (c)	2.2 (b)	2.3 (c)	2.4 (b)
2.5 (b)	2.6 (c)	2.7 (a)	2.8 (d)
2.9 (c)	2.10 (b), (c)	2.11 (c)	2.12 (b)
2.13 (a)	2.14 (a)	2.15 (c)	

Chapter 3

3.1 (b)	3.2 (c)	3.3 (a)	3.4 (c)
3.5 (a), (b)	3.6 Defination	3.7 (c)	3.8 (b)
3.9 (d)			

Chpater 4

4.1 (a)	4.2 (b)	4.3 (a)	4.4 (c)
4.5 (a)	4.6 (a)	4.7 (b)	4.8 (a)
4.9 (d)	4.10 (b)	4.11 (d)	

Chapter 5

5.1 (d)	5.2 (c)	5.3 (a)	5.4 (a)
5.5 (a) (iii), (b) (ii), (c) (i)			5.6 (b)
5.8 (d)	5.9 (b)	5.10 (b)	5.11 (e)
5.12 (b)	5.13 (d)	5.14 (c)	5.15 (e)
5.16 (b)	5.17 (d)	5.18 (b)	5.19 (c)
5.20 (b)	5.21 (b)	5.22 (a) & (b),	5.23 (c)

5.24 (a) free vortex   (b) free vortex
     (c) forced vortex   (d) free vortex
     (e) free vortex   (f) free vortex
     (g) free vortex

Chapter 6

6.1 (f)   6.2 (a) (i), (b) (v), (c) (vi), (d) (iii), (e) (iv), (f) (ii)
6.3 (a) (ii), (b) (iv), (c) (iii), (d) (v),   (e) (vi), (f) (i)
6.4 (a) no; (b) no; (c) no; (d) no; (e) no; (f) no;

6.5 (a) 6.6 (a) 6.7 (a) 6.8 (a) (i), (b) (iii), (c) (ii), (d) (iv)

6.9 (a)   6.10 (a)   6.11 (c)

6.12 (a) (iv), (b) (vi) (c) (v), (d) (ii), (e) (iii),   (f) (i)

6.13 (b) 6.14 (c)

Chapter 7

7.1 (d)   7.2 (d)   7.3 (a)   7.4 (d)

7.5 (d)   7.6 (d)   7.7 (a)   7.8 (c)

7.9 (c)   7.10 (b)   7.11 0.1948 stokes, use $C_1 = 0.0022$ and

$C_2 = -1.8$ 7.12 (b)

Chapter 8

8.1 (c)   8.2 (b)   8.3 (a) (iv), (b) (ii) (c) (i), (d) (iii),

8.4 (b)   8.5 (a)   8.6 (d)   8.7 (a)

8.8 (c), (d) 8.9 (b)   8.10 (c)

Chapter 9

9.1 (b)   9.2 (c)   9.3 (c)   9.4 (b)

9.5 (b)   9.6 (b)   9.7 (c)   9.8 (b)

9.9 (c)   9.10 (b)

Chapter 10

10.1 (d),(e) 10.2 (a)   10.3 (e)   10.4 (b)

10.5 (e)   10.6 (b)   10.7 (a)   10.8 (e)

10.9 (a)   10.10 (c)   10.11 (b)   10.12 (b)

10.13 (a)   10.14 (a)   10.15 (b)   10.16 (b)

10.17 (d)

Chapter 11

11.1 (b)   11.2 (b)   11.3 (b)   11.4 (d)

11.5 (d)   11.6 (d)

11.7 (a) (iii), (b) (i), (c) (iv), (d) (ii), (e) (iv)

11.8 (e)   11.9 (c)   11.10 (c)

11.11 (a) (iii), (b) (ii), (c) (i)   11.12 (d)

11.13 (c)   11.14 (b)

11.15 (a) Operation of parachute, (b) mixing of chemicals.

Chapter 12

12.1 (a)   12.2 (c)   12.3 (b)   12.4 (c)

12.5 (b)   12.6 (b)   12.7 (d)   12.8 (b)

12.9 (c)   12.10 (b)   12.11 (d)   12.12 (c)

12.13 (a)   12.14 (b), (c) 12.15 (a)   12.16 (a)

12.17 (b)   12.18 (b)   12.19 (a) $M_2 . S_2$ (b) M_2 (c) M_1 (d) H_2 (e) S_2

12.20 (c)

Chapter 13

13.1 (b)	13.2 (a)	13.3 (c)	13.4 (a)
13.5 (c)	13.6 (d)	13.7 (d)	13.8 (b)
13.9 (b)	13.10 (d)	13.11 (c)	13.12 (b)
13.13 (b)	13.14 (b)	13.15 (b)	

Chapter 14

14.1 (e)	14.2 (b)	14.3 (a)	14.4 (a)
14.5 (a)	14.6 (c)	14.7 (b)	14.8 (a)
14.9 (d)	14.10 (a)		

Chapter 15

15.1 (d)	15.2 (c)	15.3 (a)	15.4 (c)
15.5 (d)	15.6 (c)	15.7 (d)	15.8 (a)
15.9 (c)	15.10 (b)	15.11 [a] (iii) [b] (iv) [c] (i), [d] (ii)	
15.12 (b)	15.13 (a)	15.14 (a)	15.15 (a)

Chapter 16

16.1 (c)	16.2 (a)	16.3 (c)	16.4 (c)
16.5 (c)	16.6 (d)	16.7 (d)	16.8 (d)
16.9 (a)	16.10 (39.2%)	16.11 (d)	

Chapter 17

17.1 (e)	17.2 (c)	17.3 (a)	17.4 (d)
17.5 (c)	17.6 (d)	17.7 (c)	17.8 (b)
17.9 (a)	17.10 (a)	17.11 (a)	17.12 (b)
17.13 (b)	17.14 (b)	17.15 (c)	

Chapter 18

18.1 (b)	18.2 (b)	18.3 (d)	18.4 (a)
18.5 (a)	18.6 (a)	18.7 (b), (c)	18.8 (b),(c)
18.9 (c)	18.10 (a)	18.11 (c)	18.12 (c),(d)

Chapter 19

19.1 [a] (ii) [b] (i)		19.2 (d)	19.3 (b) [c] (iii)
19.4 (c),(e)	19.5 (a)	19.6 (b)	19.7 (c),(d)
19.8 (b)	19.9 (a)	19.10 (c)	19.11 (b)
19.12 (c)	19.13 (b)	19.14 (a)	19.15 (d)
19.16 (b)	19.17 (b)	19.18 (b)	19.19 (b)
19.20 (d)			

Answers to Problems

Chapter 1

1.1 $16.285 \, \text{N/m}^3$;
$0.602 \times 10^{-3} \, \text{m}^3/\text{kg}$

1.2 $1.27 \times 10^{-3} \, \text{m}^3/\text{kg}$

1.3 1.203 , 14.8×10^{-6} m²/s   1.4 $\partial u/\partial y = 0 , 3.265, 6.53 , 9.80\, s^{-1}$,
                                                    $\tau = 0 , 2.61 , 5.22 , 7.84$ N/m²

1.5 $\partial u/\partial y = \infty$, $6.32, 5.02\, s^{-1}$;   1.6 1 N s/m² and 2 N s/m²
     u in m/s and y in metre

1.7 $x = \left(h/\sqrt{1 + 1/k} \right)$ from   1.8 0.348 N m
     the lower plate

1.9 0.0496 N s/m³   1.10 53.6 N, neglecting buoyant force

1.11 $\left(\omega_1 - \omega_2 \right) = \left[16\, y\, T/\pi\, \mu\, d^4 \right]$ 1.12 $T = \left[\pi\, \mu\, \omega\, H^4/2\, h \cos \alpha \right]$

1.13 1.415 N s/m².   1.14 $\Delta p = 29.4$ N/m²

1.15 15 mm rise, 4.9 mm   1.16 0.225×10^{-3} N/m
      depression

1.17 0.00577 N   1.18 0.0149 mm

1.19 $p = 50$ mm, error   1.20 $p = 400$ mm, error = 0.199%
      $= 1.596$ %

1.21 1483.24 m/s, 343 m/s   1.22 1078.4 kg/m³

Chapter 2

2.9   127.045 kPa   2.10 62. 72 kPa ; 73.32 kPa

2.11 35.3 kN ; 7.36 kN   2.12 1.54 m

2.13 62.7 kPa,   2.14 Difference of pressure (a) 1.47 kPa
                                          (b) 0.29 kPa

2.15 $P = \left[w_0 H^2/2 + k\, H^3/3 \right]$,   2.16 33.74 kN, 45° with the horizontal
      $M = \left[w_0 H^3/3 + k\, H^4/4 \right]$ & normal to the area, 2.32 m

2.17 400.0 kN, 2.0625 m from   2.18 3.678 kN
      the top

2.19 0.72 kN-m   2.20 $l = 15.64$ m $h = 0.642$ m from W.S

2.21 4.86 m   2.22 7.38 m below W.S.

2.23 2.12 m   2.24 92.05 kN at 43°40′ with the vertical

2.25 12.054 kN upwards   2.26 2.12 m

Chapter 3

3.1   46.062°   3.2 58 cm

3.4   0.392 kN   3.5 8.83 m from bottom for 1 m draft,
                                          4.58 m from bottom for 2.5 m draft

3.6   0.0583 kN   3.7 0.707 m

3.8   (a) 0.705 m from bottom   3.9 4.92 N
      (b) 0.738 m from bottom
      (c) 1.078 m

Chapter 4

4.2 C/r^2 4.3 (a) Rotational
                                          (b) Irrotational (c) Rotational
                                          (d) Irrotational

4.4 $w = -xz(6 + 2z) + f(x, y)$ 4.5 $q = t/4$

4.6 $U = (3 - 6x)i + 6yj - 12tk$ 4.7 (a) no (b) yes (c) no

4.8 (a) $\psi = \left(x^2y + xy - y^3/2\right) + c$

$\varphi = -\left(x^3/3 + x^2/2 - xy^2 + y^2/2\right) + c$

(b) $\psi = axy + c$; $\varphi = a/2\left(x^2 - y^2\right) + c$

4.10 (c) $u = 2x, v = -2y$; $U = -4j$; $U = 8.94, \theta = 116°33'$ with X- axis

(e) $\varphi = y^2 - x^2 + c$

Chpater 5

5.1 1.029 m^3/s

5.2 $d = 0.074$ m

5.3 $d = 241$ mm

5.4 0.0105 m^2

5.5 $K = 1.9$

5.6 0.821 m; flow from A to B

5.7 -43.06 kPa, 94.3 kPa
     38.76 m, 6.42 cm

5.8 12.45 m

5.9 (a) 3.471 m^3/s/m width
     (b) 2.6 m (c) 1.8 m at
     the tip of gate

5.10 0.224 m^3/s, 142.75 mm

5.11 (a) 61.4 lit/s (b) 110 kPa

5.13 148.35 kPa

5.14 449.3 kW

5.15 $\alpha = \dfrac{\left\{(n + 1)(2n + 1)\right\}^3}{4n^4(2n + 3)(n + 3)}$

$\beta = \dfrac{(n + 1)(2n + 1)^2}{4n^2(n + 2)}$

5.16 225.3 N, 61.95%

5.17 39.184 kN, 40 kN

5.18 1523 N to the right
     5697.1 N upwards

5.19 9.87 kN, 155.95 kN

5.20 15.87 m/s   0.33 Nm

5.21 7.396 kPa and 12.22 kPa

5.22 $pa = 17.53$ kPa

5.23 Volume spilled $= 0.41$ m^3
     Depth at centre $= 1.076$ m

5.24 146.867 kPa
     176.3 kPa

5.25 184.64 kPa,   104.21 kPa

5.26 446.6 kPa

5.27 25.15 m

Chapter 6

6.12 (a) 2 km/hr,
     Force ratio $\doteq$ 1
     Scale ratio $= 1/100$

6.14 $Qm = 2$ lit/s
     $U_p = 8$ m/s,
     $E_p = 1.17 \times 10^4$ kW

6.15 $L_r = 1/50$

6.16 $N_p = 2828$ rpm
     $P_p = 565$ kW
     $H_p = 60$ m

6.17 $Q_p = 3.26$ m^3/s

6.18 $L_r = 1/600, Dr = 1/60$

$\left(Pressure \right)_p = 50.17$ mm $\qquad T_r = 1/77.52, T_m = 9.6$ m

$\left(Power \right)_p = 0.895$ kW

6.19 $Q_m = 0.064$ m³/s

$\left(h_f \right)_p = 1.44$ m

$\left(f \right)_p = 0.027$

$\mu_p = 98 \times 10^{-5}$ Ns/m²

Chapter 7

7.1 0.321 kN/m²

7.2 0.403 m/s

7.3 1067 N/m²

7.4 1 in 167.5

$\quad$ − 2.67 N/m²; 5.33 N/m²

7.5 (a) 100.6 kN/m²

7.6 $\mu = 3.082 \times 10^{-3}$ N s/m²

$\quad$ (b) 795.19 kN/m²

$\quad$ (c) 594 kN/m² increase

7.8 1.488 kW

7.9 895.35 W

7.10 0.067 Ns/m²

7.11 (a) − 29.54 kN/m²/m length

$\qquad$ (b) 1.113×10^{-3} m³/s (c) 4.326 N

Chapter 8

8.1 (a) $\theta/\delta_* = \dfrac{1}{2}$

8.2 6.35 kN

$\quad$ (b) $\theta/\delta_* = \dfrac{1}{3}$

$\qquad$ 0.854 kN

$\quad$ (c) $\theta/\delta_* = 1/2.655$

8.3 0.055 m, 28.53 kN

8.4 (a) $5.835 x/\sqrt{R_{ex}}$; $\left(0.6854/\sqrt{R_{ex}} \right) \rho\, U_o^2/2$, $1.36/\sqrt{R_{eL}}$

$\quad$ (b) $\left[0.0275\,(n+1)\dfrac{(n+2)}{n} \right]^{4/5} x/\sqrt{R_{ex}^{0.2}}$,

$\quad$ $0.0902 \left[\dfrac{n}{(n+1)\,(n+2)} \right]^{1/5} \times 1/R_{ex}^{0.2}$, $0.11275 \left[\dfrac{n}{(n+1)\,(n+2)} \right]^{1/5}$

8.6 11.377 W

8.7 4.45, 2.41

8.8 24 N

8.9 $\delta = 0.418 x/(R_{ex})^{1/5}$

$$\tau_0 = \frac{0.0547}{(R_{ex})^{1/5}} \frac{\rho\, U_0^2}{2}$$

$$C_f = 0.0684/(R_{eL})^{1/5}$$

8.10 17.967 kN ; 7.032 kN

Chapter 9

9.3 $U_* = 0.3732$ m/s   9.4 $k_s = 3.85 \times 10^{-4}$ m   9.7 $h_f = 31$ m
     $u = 5.1$ m/s $\tau_0 = 0.116$ m/s $\tau_0 = 6.31$ N/m^2
     $f = 0.0428$ $f = 0.0237$ $U_{max} = 1.89$ m/s

9.6 $Q = 44.5 \times 10^{-3}$ m^3/s $\tau_{25} = 4.1$ N/m^2
     $f = 0.053$ 9.10 $f = 0.032$ $u_{25} = 1.672$ m/s
     $k_s = 5.2$ mm $\partial' = 0.0285$ cm

9.9 Smooth,   9.11 (a) Smooth turbulent
     $U_{max} = 2.778$ m/s $f = 0.043$
     $U = 2.403$ m/s   (b) Rough turbulent
     $Q = 42.443$ m^3/s $f = 0.018$

Chapter 10

10.1 7.8×10^{-3} m^3/s   10.2 376 kPa, 87.4 %
      11.8×10^{-3} m^3/s

10.3 58.5×10^{-3} m^3/s,   10.4 51.78×10^{-3} m^3/s

10.5 12 cm φ 10.6 18.35 %

10.7 13.85×10^{-3} m^3/s;   10.8 75.71 m
      7.63×10^{-3} m^3/s;
      18.52×10^{-3} m^3/s

10.10 $Q_B = 0.1087$ m^3/s,   10.12 Upper left corner = 50
      $Q_C = 0.1789$ m^3/s;   Upper right corner = 50
      $Z_C = 20.60$ m   Lower left corner -= 45
                                                  Lower right corner = 30

10.13 43.3×10^3 kPa   10.14 $U_y = 0.3732$ m/s;
      21.65×10^3 kPa $U = 5.1$ m/s; $f = 0.0428$

Chapter 11

11.1 85.07 N, 0.271 kW   11.2 2.67 m
11.3 32.9 km/hr, 46 N   11.4 (a) 19.69 kW (b) 1.97 kW
11.5 0.225 N m   11.6 38 %
11.8 219°32′ and 320°27′   11.9 20.83 m^3/s
      32.73 m/s; − 7.27 m/s   55.85 N/m^2, 40 N/m^2
11.10 5.49 H_z, 64.68 N/m

Chapter 12

12.1 (a) $2.664 y^{8/3}$ (b) $15.29 y^{8/3}$ 12.2 7.70 m^2/s, 7.74 m^3/s,
12.3 6034 m^3/m length, 0.0016
12.5 6.56×10^{-4}, 390 m^3/s   12.6 0.2955 m, 0.2875 m
12.7 6.21 m^3/s   12.8 65.05 km

12.9 3.89 m, 0.217 m, 4.46%   12.10 (a) 1.9 m (b) 3.22 m^3/s/m length
                                                 (c) 0.26 m

12.11 0.11 m, 2.11 m

Chapter 13

13.1 42.4×10^{-3} m^3/s, 0.1584 m   13.2 3.07 m, 0.97
    73.6 kPa   13.4 0.1272 m^2

13.5 876.4 seconds   13.6 1413.4 seconds

13.7 40.24 seconds, 0.18 m^3/s   13.8 0.9810 , 0.0638 , 0.65

13.9 2.7 m, 4.98 m vacuum,   13.10 15.65×10^{-3} m^3/s, 0.54 m,
    12.42 m, 98×10^{-3} m^3/s   71.8 kPa absolute

13.11 78.5×10^{-3} m^3/s   13.13 0.14 m^3/s

13.14 6.2 m/s   13.15 3.26 kPa

13.16 0.74 m^3/s   13.17 0.34 m^3/s

13.18 21.2 m^3/s   13.19 61.4 m

13.20 15.196 h

Chapter 14

14 5 110.36 N , 70.63 N 14.6 (a) 1030 N (b) 1275.3 N
                                       (c) 1638.27 N at 51°12′ with the direct-
                                          ion of jet

14.7 35.31 N , 35°   14.8 15039 N 30° ; 10800 N , 30°;
                                       116.05 kN-m; 60 %

14.9 0.576   14.10 25.8 m/s; 2383.8 m/s at 7.5°;
                                       2364.1 m/s in the direction of motion;
                                       6.7 m/s at 82.5°

14.11 129.3 rpm, 61.7 J/s/N, 59.8 %   14.12 26.3° and 68.9° ; 23.8 J/s/N; 47.0 %

Chapter 15

15.12 9.61 m; 2.22 m; 0.246 m; 5 ; 21.24 rpm

15.13 (a) 786 rpm (b) 94.47 kN   (c) 475.22 kN   (d) 90.5 %

15.14 (a) 7549.8 kW   15.15 B = 0.606 m ; D = 6.06 m;
    (b) 312.15 rpm B_1 = 1.212 m ; D_1 = 3.03 m;
                                 α = 46.18° ; θ = 1.68° ;
                                 φ = 3.27°

15.16 (a) α = 13.20°   15.17 (a) 14.0 m/s; 139.2 mm
    (b) β = 25.20°   (b) 95.8 %
    (c) 69.6 mm;

15.18 (a) 692.4 rpm   15.19 23627.44 kW
    (b) 13.077 kW

15.20 65.5° , 76%   15.22 (a) − 5.323 m; 0.135 m;
                                  0.09 m (b) 779.7 W;
                                  519.8 W ; 259.89 W

15.23 74.68 %

2.61 N/cm^2 vacuum

15.25 (a) 141.4 rpm

(b) 4419.3 (c) 76.9 %

15.24 (a) 1002.4 rpm;

(b) 7937.37 kW (c) 88 %

15.26 77.46 rpm; 2925.24 kW

15.27 76.65 rpm; 7.28 m; 14 %

Chapter 16

16.8 9×10^{-5} m^3/s;

411 kW

16.10 46.75 rpm, 3.82 m,

10.78 m, 42.1 m, 2.5 m

16.12 185 rpm

16.14 3.38 m of water, 48.88 m of water,

12.9 kN

16.9 7.28 m gauge, 4.6 m gauge,

0.72 m gauge, 2.0 kW

16.11 12.75 m; 12.116 m

16.13 13.4 rpm, 18 rpm

16.17 1.24 kW

Chapter 17

17.13. $\varphi = 70.5°$

17.15 55.25 % ; 0.785 m

17.17 25.7 cm; 30°

17.19 9.5 m, 0.283 m

17.21 847 rpm

17.23 3 in parallel

17.14 3.614 m, 6.04 m; 11.12 m

17.16 26.13 kW, 39.6 lit/sec

– 7.24 N/cm^2; 40.22 N/cm^2

17.18 82.89 % , 89.9 %

17.20 11.5 m/s : 8.2 m; 17°

17.22 10.0

17.24 730 rpm 17.25 29 m, 93 lit/sec

Chapter 18

18.8 12.19 kW

18.10 281 , 6.54 W

18.12 0.87 m/s

18.14 3.02 m/s

18.9 1.66 cm/min

18.11 29.5 lit, 44.3 lit, 1.811 kW

18.13 22.54 kN, 338.1 kN- m

18.15 Useful water = 1.1047 kN/min

Waste water = 2.211 kN/min

Chapter 19

19.8 486.74° C , 1684.7 kCal,

1684.7 kCal , no work

19.10 $p_2 = 1.428$ bar ,

$\rho_2 = 1.6$ kg/m^3 ,

$N_{M_0} = 0.84$

19.12 0.146 kg/s ; 0.494 kg/s

19.14 (a) 200° K , 146.7° K

19.9 139.34° C , 32.015 kN/m^2

19.11 17.96 km

19.13 $N_{M_2} = 0.577$,

$p_2 = 1.193$ bar; $\rho_2 = 1.101$ kg/m^3 ;

$T_2 = 373.43°$ K $U_2 = 224.66$ m/s

$U_1 = 599.44$ m/s ; $T_1 = 221.29°$ K

(b) 368 m/s , 300.4 m/s ; 257.3 m/s

Selected Bibliography

Addison, H.,A Treatise on Applied Hydraulics. Chapman and Hall, 1956.

Addision, H., Hydarulic Measurements. Chapman and Hall.

Binder, R. C., Fluid Mechanics. Prentice Hall Inc., 1949.

Chow, V.T., Open Channel Hydraulics Mc Graw, Hill, New York, 1959.

Daugherty, R.L., and Ingersoll, A.C., Fluid Mechanics. Mc. Graw Hill, New York, 1954.

Gill, H.A., Exact solution of gradually varied flow. Jnl. Hyd. Div., Proc ASCE, Sept, 1978.

Handerson, F.M., Open Channel Flow. Mac Millan, New York, 1966

Hamilton, J.B., The suppression of intake losses by various degrees of rounding. Univ. Wash Engg. Expt. Station, Bull. 51, 1929.

Hickox, G.H., Aeration of spillways. Tran. ASCE, vol. 109, p. 517-556, 1944.

Jain, A.K., Accurate Explicit Equation for friction factor. Tech. Note, Proc. ASCE, Jnl of Hyd. Div., May, 1976

Keulegan, G.H., Laws of turbulent flow in open channels, Research paper, RP 1151, Jnl. of Res. U.S. NBS. Vol. 21, p. 707-741, Dec. 1938.

King, H.W., Handbook of Hydraulic. John Wiley.

Lansford, W.M., The use of elbow in a pipeline for determination of the flow in the pipe. Engg. Expt. station, Univ., Ill., Bulletin, 289, 1936.

Malika, J., Flow in non-circular conduiuts. Proc. ASCE, Jnl. Hyd. Div., Nov., 1962.

Pao., R, Fluid Mechanics. John Wiley, 1961.

Prandtl, L and Titjons, Applied hydro and aeromachines, Dover Rajaratnam, N. and Subramanya, K., Profile of the hydraulic jump. Jnl. of Hyd. Div., Proc., ASCE May, 1968.

Ranga Raju, K.G. and Asawa, G.L., Viscosity and surface tension effects on weir flow. Jnl. Hyd. Div. Proc. ASCE, Oct, 1977.

Rouse, H., Elementary Mechanics of Fluids. John Wiley and Sons, 1956.

Rouse, H. Engineering Hydraulics. John Wiley and sons, 1950.

Schlichting, H., Boundary layer theory. Mc Graw Hill, 1955.

Shames, I., Mechanics of Fluid. Mc Graw Hill, 1962.

Streater, V.L., Fluid Mechanics. Mc Graw Hill, 1958.

Streater, V.L., Fluid Dynamics. Mc Graw Hill, 1948.

Venard, J.K., Elementary Fluid Mechanics, John Wiley and Sons, 1962.

Yuan, S Y., Fundamentals of Fluid Mechanics, Prentice Hall of India, Private Ltd., 1969.

Index